The Esophagus

The Esophagus

EDITED BY

Joel E. Richter MD FACP MACG
Professor of Medicine
Hugh F Culverhouse Chair for Esophagology
Director, Division of Digestive Diseases and Nutrition
Director, Joy McCann Culverhouse Center for Swallowing Disorders
University of South Florida
Tampa, FL, USA

Donald O. Castell MD
Professor of Medicine and Director
Esophageal Disorders Program
Division of Gastroenterology
Department of Internal Medicine
Medical University of South Carolina
Charleston, SC, USA

FIFTH EDITION

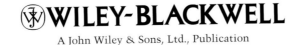

A John Wiley & Sons, Ltd., Publication

This edition first published 2012 © 2012 by Blackwell Publishing Ltd,
Previously published by Lippincott Williams and Wilkins, 2004

Blackwell Publishing was acquired by John Wiley & Sons in February 2007. Blackwell's publishing program has been merged with Wiley's global Scientific, Technical and Medical business to form Wiley-Blackwell.

Registered office: John Wiley & Sons Ltd, The Atrium, Southern Gate, Chichester, West Sussex, PO19 8SQ, UK

Editorial offices: 9600 Garsington Road, Oxford, OX4 2DQ, UK
The Atrium, Southern Gate, Chichester, West Sussex, PO19 8SQ, UK
350 Main Street, Malden, MA 02148-5020, USA

For details of our global editorial offices, for customer services and for information about how to apply for permission to reuse the copyright material in this book please see our website at www.wiley.com/wiley-blackwell

Library of Congress Cataloging-in-Publication Data
The esophagus / editors, Joel E. Richter, Donald O. Castell. – 5th ed.
    p. ; cm.
  Includes bibliographical references and index.
  ISBN-13: 978-1-4051-9864-6 (hardcover : alk. paper)
  ISBN-10: 1-4051-9864-8
  1. Esophagus–Diseases. I. Richter, Joel E. II. Castell, Donald O.
  [DNLM: 1. Esophageal Diseases. WI 250]
  RC815.7.E763 2012
  616.3'2-dc23

                        2011016563

A catalogue record for this book is available from the British Library.

Wiley also publishes its books in a variety of electronic formats. Some content that appears in print may not be available in electronic books.

Set in 9/12 pt Meridien by Toppan Best-set Premedia Limited
Printed and bound in Singapore by Markono Print Media Pte Ltd

1 2012

Contents

Section V Malignant Disease

Section VI Miscellaneous

Companion website

This book is accompanied by a website:

www.wiley.com/go/richter/esophagus

The website features:

- PowerPoints of all figures from the book for downloading

List of Contributors

Sami R. Achem MD FACP FACG AGAF
Professor of Medicine
Gastroenterology Consultant
Mayo College of Medicine
Mayo Clinic
Jacksonville, FL, USA

Edgar Achkar MD
Consultant
The Cleveland Clinic Foundation
Cleveland, OH, USA

Amit Agrawal
Assistant Professor of Gastroenterology and Hepatology
Medical University of South Carolina
Charleston, SC, USA

Stephen J. Antonik MD
Gastroenterology Associates, P.L.L.C.
Leesburg, VA, USA

Albert J. Bredenoord MD
Consultant Gastroenterologist
Department of Gastroenterology and Hepatology
Academic Medical Center
Amsterdam, The Netherlands

Donald Castell MD
Professor of Medicine and Director
Esophageal Disorders Program
Division of Gastroenterology
Department of Internal Medicine
Medical University of South Carolina
Charleston, SC, USA

Kenneth R. DeVault MD
Professor and Chair
Department of Medicine
Mayo Clinic
Jacksonville, FL, USA

Nicholas Diamant MD
Professor of Medicine and Physiology (Emeritus)
University of Toronto
Professor of Medicine
Queen's University
Kingston, Ontario, Canada

Carlo Di Lorenzo MD
Chief, Division of Pediatric Gastroenterology
Nationwide Children's Hospital
Professor of Clinical Pediatrics
The Ohio State University
Columbus, OH, USA

Siva Doma MD
Gastroenterologist
Temple University School of Medicine
Gastroenterology Section
Philadelphia, PA, USA

Christy M. Dunst MD
Director of Research and Education
Division of Gastrointestinal and Minimally Invasive Surgery
The Oregon Clinic
Portland, OR, USA

Gary W. Falk MD MS
Professor of Medicine
Division of Gastroenterology
Hospital of the University of Pennsylvania
Philadelphia, PA, USA

Ronnie Fass MD
Professor of Medicine
University of Arizona
Chief of Gastroenterology and Head Neuroenteric
Clinical Research Group
Southern Arizona VA Health Care System
Tucson, AZ, USA

Robert S. Fisher MD
Lorber Professor of Medicine
Division of Gastroenterology
Temple University School of Medicine
Philadelphia, PA, USA

Janice Freeman RN
Clinical Research Coordinator
Esophageal Function Laboratory
Medical University of South Carolina
Charleston, SC, USA

Frank Friedenberg MD MS
Professor of Medicine
Temple University Hospital
Philadelphia, PA, USA

John R. Goldblum MD
Chairman, Department of Anatomic Pathology
Cleveland Clinic
Professor of Pathology
Cleveland Clinic Lerner College of Medicine
Cleveland, OH, USA

Susana Gonzalez MD
Assistant Professor of Medicine
Division of Gastroenterology
Mount Sinai School of Medicine
New York, NY, USA

Tiberiu Hershcovici MD
Research Fellow
University of Arizona
The Neuroenteric Clinical Research Group
Tucson, AZ, USA

Peter J. Kahrilas MD
Gilbert H. Marquardt Professor in Medicine
Department of Medicine
The Feinberg School of Medicine
Northwestern University
Chicago, IL, USA

Arne Kandulski MD
GI Fellow Department of Gastroenterology, Hepatology
and Infectious Diseases
Otto-von-Guericke University Magdeburg
Magdeburg, Germany

Philip O. Katz MD
Clinical Professor of Medicine
Jefferson Medical College;
Chairman
Division of Gastroenterology
Albert Einstein Medical Center
Philadelphia, PA, USA

David A. Katzka MD
Professor of Medicine
Mayo Clinic, College of Medicine
Rochester, MN, USA

Robert T. Kavitt MD
Gastroenterology Fellow
Division of Gastroenterology,
Hepatology, and Nutrition
Vanderbilt University Medical Center
Nashville, TN, USA

James Walter Kikendall MD
Staff Gastroenterologist
National Naval Medical Center
Uniformed Services University of the Health Sciences
Division of Gastroenterology
Bethesda, MD, USA

Jason M. Lake MD
Major, Medical Corps, U.S. Army
Division of Gastroenterology
Uniformed Services University of the Health Sciences
Walter Reed Army Medical Center
Washington, DC, USA

Marc S. Levine MD
Professor of Radiology and Advisory Dean
University of Pennsylvania School of Medicine;
Chief, Gastrointestinal Radiology Section
Hospital of the University of Pennsylvania
Philadelphia, PA, USA

Harvey Licht MD
Professor of Clinical Medicine
Division of Gastroenterology
Temple University School of Medicine
Philadelphia, PA, USA

Charles J. Lightdale MD
Professor of Clinical Medicine
Division of Digestive and Liver Diseases
Columbia University Medical Center
New York, NY, USA

Xiuli Liu MD PhD
Assistant Professor of Pathology
Cleveland Clinic Lerner College of Medicine
Department of Anatomic Pathology
Cleveland Clinic
Cleveland, OH, USA

Ryan D. Madanick MD
Assistant Professor of Medicine
Center for Esophageal Diseases and Swallowing
Division of Gastroenterology and Hepatology
University of North Carolina School of Medicine
Chapel Hill, NC, USA

Peter Malfertheiner MD
Professor of Medicine and Chairman
Department of Gastroenterology,
Hepatology and Infectious Diseases
Otto-von-Guericke University of Magdeburg
Magdeburg, Germany

Francisco J. Marrero MD
Director
Digestive Health Center
Lake Charles Memorial Hospital
Lake Charles, LA, USA

Ravinder K. Mittal MD
Professor of Medicine
Director Gastrointestinal Function Laboratory
University of California, San Diego;
Gastroenterology Section
San Diego Veterans Health Care Center
La Jolla, CA, USA

Pamela A. Morganroth MD
Medical student
Philadelphia VA Medical Center;
Department of Dermatology
University of Pennsylvania School of Medicine
Philadelphia, PA, USA

Brant K. Oelschlager MD
Byers Endowed Professor in Esophageal Research
Director, Center for Videoendoscopic Surgery
Director, Center for Esophageal and Gastric Surgery
Department of Surgery
University of Washington
Seattle, WA, USA

Roy C. Orlando MD
Mary Kay and Eugene Bozymski and Linda and William
Heizer Distinguished Professor of Gastroenterology
Adjunct Professor of Cell and Molecular Physiology
University of North Carolina School of Medicine
Chapel Hill, NC, USA

John E. Pandolfino MD
Associate Professor
Department of Medicine
Division of Gastroenterology
The Feinberg School of Medicine
Northwestern University
Chicago, IL, USA

Henry P. Parkman MD
Professor of Medicine
Gastrointestinal Section
Temple University School of Medicine
Philadelphia, PA, USA

Carlos A. Pellegrini MD
The Henry Harkins Professor and Chairman
Department of Surgery
University of Washington
Seattle, WA, USA

Roberto Penagini
Associate Professor of Gastroenterology
Università degli Studi of Milan
Division of Gastroenterology
Fondazione IRCCS Cà Granda Ospedale Policlinico
Milan, Italy

David A. Peura MD FACP MACG AGAF
Emeritus Professor
Division of Gastroenterology and Hepatology
University of Virginia
Charlottesville, VA, USA

Daniel Pohl MD
Research and Gastroenterology Fellow
Division of Gastroenterology and Hepatology
University Hospital Zurich
Zurich, Switzerland

Daniel von Renteln MD
Department of Interdisciplinary Endoscopy
University Medical Center Hamburg
Hamburg, Germany

Thomas W. Rice MD
Professor of Surgery at the Cleveland Clinic Lerner College of Medicine
Daniel and Karen Lee Chair of Thoracic Surgery
Head of the Section of General Thoracic Surgery
Heart and Vascular Institute
Department of Thoracic and Cardiovascular Surgery, Cleveland Clinic
Cleveland, OH, USA

Joel E. Richter MD FACP MACG
Professor of Medicine
Hugh F Culverhouse Chair for Esophagology
Director, Division of Digestive Diseases and Nutrition
Director, Joy McCann Culverhouse Center for Swallowing Disorders
University of South Florida
Tampa, FL, USA

Jason Fellow R. Roberts MD
Division of Gastroenterology and Hepatology
Medical University of South Carolina
Charleston, SC, USA

Richard I. Rothstein MD
Professor of Medicine and of Surgery
Dartmouth Medical School;
Chief, Section of Gastroenterology and Hepatology
Dartmouth-Hitchcock Medical Center
Lebanon, NH, USA

Pauline Roumeguère
Resident Gastroenterology Department
Saint André Hospital
Université Bordeaux Segalen
Bordeaux, France

Stephen E. Rubesin
Professor of Radiology
Department of Radiology
University of Pennsylvania School of Medicine
Philadelphia, PA, USA

Nicholas J. Shaheen MD MPH
Professor of Medicine and Epidemiology
Director, Center for Esophageal Diseases and Swallowing
Division of Gastroenterology and Hepatology
University of North Carolina School of Medicine
Chapel Hill, NC, USA

Reza Shaker MD
Joseph E. Geenen Professor and Chief
Division of Gastroenterology and Hepatology
Froedtert Memorial Lutheran Hospital
Medical College of Wisconsin
Milwaukee, WI, USA

Prateek Sharma MD
Professor of Medicine
University of Kansas
School of Medicine and Veterans Affairs Medical Center
Kansas City, MO, USA

Neeraj Sharma MD
Gastroenterology Fellow
Medical University of South Carolina
Charleston, SC, USA

Steven S. Shay MD
Staff Gastroenterologist
Cleveland Clinic Foundation
Cleveland, OH, USA

Daniel Sifrim MD PhD
Professor of Gastrointestinal Physiology
Barts and the London School of Medicine and Dentistry
Queen Mary University of London
Wingate Institute of Neurogastroenterology
London, UK

Michael S. Smith MD MBA
Medical Director, Esophageal Program
Gastroenterology Section
Department of Medicine
Temple University School of Medicine
Philadelphia, PA, USA

André J. P. M. Smout MD
Professor of Gastroenterology and Motility
Department of Gastroenterology and Hepatology
Academic Medical Center
Amsterdam, The Netherlands

Joseph R. Spiegel MD
Associate Professor of Otolaryngology-Head & Neck Surgery
Thomas Jefferson University
Philadelphia, PA, USA

Ellen M. Stein MD
Assistant Professor of Medicine
Division of Gastroenterology & Hepatology
The Johns Hopkins Hospital
Baltimore, MD, USA

Lee Swanstrom MD
Clinical Professor of Surgery
Oregon Health Sciences University
Chief, Gastrointestinal and Minimally Invasive Surgery
The Oregon Clinic
Portland, OR, USA

Roger P. Tatum, MD
Associate Professor of Surgery
VA Puget Sound Health Care System
University of Washington
Seattle, WA, USA

Radu Tutuian MD
Staff Gastroenterologist University Clinic for Visceral Surgery and Medicine
Bern University Hospital
Switzerland

Michael F. Vaezi MD PhD MSc (Epi)
Professor of Medicine and Clinical Director
Division of Gastroenterology, Hepatology and Nutrition
Vanderbilt University Medical Center
Nashville, TN, USA

Babac Vahabzadeh MD
Gastroenterology Fellow
The University of Kansas Medical Center
Kansas City, KS, USA

Yvan Vandenplas MD
Professor of Pediatrics
Universitair Ziekenhuis Brussel
Brussels, Belgium

Melina C. Vassiliou MD MEd FRCS (C)
Assistant Professor of Surgery
Department of Surgery
McGill University
Montreal, Quebec, Canada

Marcelo F. Vela MD MSCR
Associate Professor of Medicine
Director of Gastrointestinal Motility, Gastroenterology Section
Baylor College of Medicine &
Michael E. DeBakey VA Medical Center
Houston, TX, USA

Andrew Y. Wang MD
Assistant Professor of Medicine
Co-Medical Director of Endoscopy
Division of Gastroenterology and Hepatology
University of Virginia Health System
Charlottesville, VA, USA

Victoria P. Werth MD
Professor of Dermatology and Medicine Philadelphia
VA Medical Center;
Department of Dermatology
University of Pennsylvania School of Medicine
Philadelphia, PA, USA

C. Mel Wilcox MD
Professor
Department of Medicine
Division of Gastroenterology and Hepatology
University of Alabama at Birmingham
Birmingham, AL, USA

John M. Wo MD
Professor of Medicine
Division of Gastroenterology, Hepatology and Nutrition
University of Louisville School of Medicine
Louisville, KY, USA

Roy K. H. Wong MD
Chief of Gastroenterology
Walter Reed Army Medical Center
Washington, DC, USA;
Professor of Medicine
Director, Division of Digestive Diseases
Uniformed Services University of the Health Sciences
Bethesda, MD, USA

Patrick E. Young MD
Director of Clinical Research and Assistant Professor of Medicine
Director, Medical Operations, USNS COMFORT (T-AH 20)
National Naval Medical Center
Uniformed Services University of the Health Sciences
Division of Gastroenterology
Bethesda, MD, USA

Frank Zerbib MD PhD
Head of Gastroenterology Department
Saint André Hospital
Université Bordeaux Segalen
Bordeaux, France

Preface

The 5th edition of *The Esophagus* is finally ready! As with previous editions, we have made changes in chapters and authors to achieve our goal of maintaining the highest level of clinical usefulness and new information for our readership. Over half of the chapters have new authors from the United States and internationally. New chapters have been added, including GERD and obesity, eosinophilic esophagitis, and new esophageal testing, especially high resolution manometry.

Since the last edition, we have changed publishers and are delighted to be working with the esteemed group Wiley-Blackwell. They are a dominant publishing company and we are confident they will continue the tradition of helping us disseminate the important information on esophageal function and disease more widely throughout the world.

The preparation of the text material for *The Esophagus* remains a labor of love and a collaboration for the two co-editors that now spans nearly 35 years. All the members of our team have strived to provide information that will be of clinical importance to the internists, gastroenterologists and surgeons who care for patients with esophageal disorders and their sometimes perplexing clinical scenarios. It is our hope that you will find the material in this 5th edition as helpful and exciting as we do.

Joel E. Richter, MD and Donald O. Castell, MD
October 2011

I

Esophageal Symptoms

1 Symptom Overview and Quality of Life

Ryan D. Madanick and Nicholas J. Shaheen

Center for Esophageal Diseases and Swallowing, Division of Gastroenterology & Hepatology, University of North Carolina School of Medicine, Chapel Hill, NC, USA

Introduction

In the first century AD, the Roman scientist Pliny the Elder described the first treatment for heartburn, coral powder, which contains calcium carbonate, a buffer still used in today's antacids. In the second century, the Greek physician Galen defined the problem as *kardialgia*, or heart pain [1]. Although this problem was recognized over 2000 years ago, heartburn and other esophageal disorders remain a major source of distress for patients today. The esophagus is unique in gastrointestinal disease, because it is the only structure of the gastrointestinal tract that resides normally within the thorax. As a result, the symptoms of esophageal disease are distinct from the typical symptoms related to disorders affecting other gastrointestinal organs, but they often overlap with symptoms that result from organs outside of the gastrointestinal tract, as Galen recognized.

This chapter will begin with a discussion of how esophageal symptoms develop. The particular symptoms that relate to the esophagus will then be discussed (Table 1.1). Finally, the impact of esophageal disorders on quality of life (QOL) will conclude the chapter.

Sensory pathways and symptom production

The development of symptoms related to the esophagus is a complex neurophysiologic phenomenon that is incompletely understood. A stimulus at the level of the esophagus acts upon one of several types of afferent neurons (nociceptors) that may be responsible for esophageal sensation. The nociceptors transmit the signal to the central nervous system, where it is processed at a subcortical level. If the signal is of sufficient strength to pass through subcortical suppressive pathways, it is transmitted to the cortical level, to allow the individual to respond to the signal. A patient can respond to the internal signal (sensation) in a variety of ways, depending on their circumstances and background. Each of these steps is briefly considered below.

Several types of chemo-, thermo-, and/or mechano-sensitive nociceptors have been identified within the esophagus. These nociceptors carry various sensors, such as the acid-sensitive transient receptor potential vanilloid receptor 1 (TRPV1), which stimulate an action potential within the nociceptor [2]. These receptors are ion channels that can be activated by various mediators of injury, such as hydrogen ions, histamine, bradykinin or serotonin. The impulses are transmitted by two types of nerve fibers, Aδ-fibers and C-fibers. Aδ-fibers are myelinated fibers that carry pain impulses relatively rapidly, and typically generate a sensation of sharp, localized pain of sudden onset. C-fibers are unmyelinated fibers that transmit their signals more slowly, and lead to a pain sensation that is dull, poorly localized, and of a more gradual onset [3].

Afferent input from the esophagus is transmitted by vagal (parasympathetic) and spinal (sympathetic) nerves. Parasympathetic afferent signals are carried to the vagus nerve via the superior laryngeal nerves, recurrent laryngeal nerves, and vagal branches within the esophageal plexus. The cell bodies of the vagal afferent neurons are located in the jugular and nodose ganglia, with central projections to the nucleus of the solitary tract in the brainstem [3, 4]. Sympathetic afferent signals are carried to the spinal cord via the splanchnic nerves. The cell bodies of the spinal afferent neurons are located in the thoracic and cervical dorsal root ganglia [4]. These first-order neurons synapse with second-order neurons in the dorsal horn of the spinal cord. Pain signals then ascend via the spinoreticular and spinothalamic tracts to synapse with third-order neurons in the reticular nuclei and thalamus, respectively. These signals are

The Esophagus, Fifth Edition. Edited by Joel E. Richter, Donald O. Castell.
© 2012 Blackwell Publishing Ltd. Published 2012 by Blackwell Publishing Ltd.

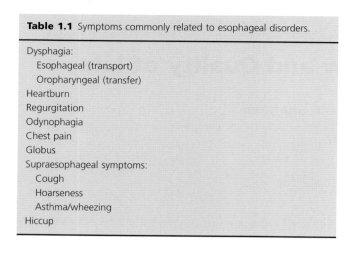

Table 1.1 Symptoms commonly related to esophageal disorders.

Dysphagia:
   Esophageal (transport)
   Oropharyngeal (transfer)
Heartburn
Regurgitation
Odynophagia
Chest pain
Globus
Supraesophageal symptoms:
   Cough
   Hoarseness
   Asthma/wheezing
Hiccup

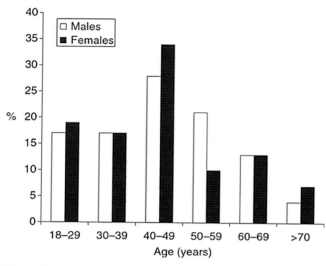

Figure 1.1 Population prevalence rates of dysphagia by age and gender (reproduced from Eslick *et al.* [7], with permission).

subsequently transmitted to higher centers for processing [3]. Vagal afferents also appear to influence spinal nociceptive transmission [5]. Vagal afferent input from other intrathoracic organs, such as the heart, lungs and tracheobronchial tree, converges with input from the esophagus before these afferent signals are transmitted to the higher medullary centers. This overlap in part explains the difficulty in separating visceral symptoms from these organs, such as chest pain.

Central processing of the peripheral signals has two dimensions, sensation and affect [5]. The sensation dimension of the stimulus is responsible for determining the location and intensity of the symptom. The affective dimension relies on a very complex interplay of emotions, words, and personal experiences to modulate the sensation into a particular expression. Four predominant cortical regions have been hypothesized to be involved in central processing: the primary somatosensory cortex, secondary somatosensory cortex, insula, and cingulate cortex. The primary and secondary somatosensory cortices receive nociceptive projections from the ventroposterior lateral nuclei of the thalamus. The primary somatosensory cortex appears to be important in determining the concrete dimensions of the symptom (duration, location, intensity), whereas the secondary somatosensory cortex appears to play a principle role in recognizing the nature of the symptom (mechanical, thermal, chemical) [5]. The insula is thought to be responsible for integrating input from both the secondary somatosensory cortex and the thalamic nuclei, and for transmitting this information to limbic structures for affective processing. The anterior cingulate cortex (ACC) appears to be responsible for the affective-motivational aspects of symptom processing. This area appears to be especially active in symptom generation in functional bowel disorders [6].

Descending pathways are also important in the modulation of pain transmission. Neurons descend from the primary somatosensory cortex, secondary somatosensory cortex, ACC, and insula, and couple with neurons from other regions of the brain, such as the periventricular and periaqueductal gray matter, and brainstem to synapse with neurons in the dorsal horns of the spinal cord to inhibit afferent pain signals [3].

Symptoms

Dysphagia

The word dysphagia, derived from the Greek *phagia* (to eat) and *dys* (with difficulty), is any sensation of ingested material being hindered in its normal passage from the mouth to the stomach. The epidemiology of dysphagia remains incompletely assessed. A recent study from Australia found that the prevalence of dysphagia among adults was 16%, a proportion that is similar to that in other epidemiologic investigations [7]. The majority of individuals with dysphagia only reported having difficulty once a month or less. Interestingly, this study found that the prevalence of dysphagia peaked in the 40–49-year-old age group, with declining prevalence in the older age groups (Figure 1.1).

There are two types of dysphagia: transfer (oropharyngeal) and transport (esophageal). Generally, these two types of dysphagia can be distinguished based on historical features. Certain symptoms, such as drooling, coughing, and gurgling upon eating, are more strongly suggestive of oropharyngeal dysphagia than of esophageal dysphagia. Patients may also complain of nasal regurgitation of food or liquid. The timing of dysphagia can guide the initial evaluation toward oropharyngeal dysphagia. Dysphagia that occurs very soon after the onset of eating, especially if a cervical location of the dysphagia is described, often indicates an oropharyngeal source. The localization of the bolus hold-up in the cervical region usually indicates a pharyngeal source of dysphagia, but patients with esophageal dysphagia can occasionally report sticking in the cervical region [8].

Identification of the specific location at which a patient reports sticking may be helpful to determine the site of the esophageal pathology. Patients with esophageal dysphagia usually complain that food sticks or "hangs up" retrosternally during meals. Dysphagia is not often painful, although some individuals complain of a painful squeezing sensation or fullness in the chest. This type of discomfort should not be confused with painful swallowing or odynophagia (see below), which is more often described as a very sharp localized pain or as a severe pain that seems to move down the chest in tandem with each swallow.

Esophageal dysphagia may be caused by obstruction to luminal flow (mechanical) or by altered esophageal motility (neuromuscular) (Table 1.2). Esophageal obstruction can be caused by rings, webs, strictures, or masses, both intrinsic and extrinsic. Neuromuscular causes include disorders such as achalasia or scleroderma, in which peristalsis has completely failed, and esophageal spasm, in which a hypercontractile region of esophageal musculature induces luminal obstruction. Eosinophilic esophagitis, a disorder that has

been recently recognized to be a cause of dysphagia among children and young adults, typically presents with features more suggestive of an obstructive phenomenon. Occasionally, patients who have undergone antireflux surgery (fundoplication) complain of dysphagia even though there is no motility disorder or physical obstruction. In the case of post-fundoplication dysphagia, altered compliance at the region of the gastroesophageal junction is thought to result in an increase in intrabolus pressure, which subsequently leads to dysphagia [9].

In evaluating a patient with esophageal dysphagia, a good clinical history is paramount, and can suggest an etiology in approximately 80% of patients [10]. In addition to location, three characteristics of the dysphagia are crucial during the initial assessment: (1) the type of bolus eliciting symptoms (liquid or solid); (2) the frequency (intermittent or continual); and (3) the presence or absence of associated heartburn. Other pertinent information to gather during the initial assessment includes the onset (sudden or gradual), duration, and associated features, such as pain, weight loss, and coughing. A drug history is also important, with specific reference to medications such as non-steroidal anti-inflammatory drugs, bisphosphonates, and vitamins. An algorithm of the common causes of esophageal dysphagia based on the clinical history is shown in Figure 1.2.

Patients with dysphagia related to a physical obstruction usually complain of dysphagia to solids only, although if the obstruction becomes severe enough, the patient may complain of dysphagia for both solids and liquids. When the obstruction is fixed (or worsening), the swallowing difficulty is continual and sometimes progressive, unless the patient adapts to the smaller caliber lumen by changing their eating style. On the other hand, patients with a distal esophageal ring usually complain of solid-food dysphagia on a much more intermittent basis. Dysphagia that begins after a long-standing history of heartburn often indicates a peptic stricture. Rapidly progressive dysphagia, especially when accompanied by weight loss, strongly suggests an esophageal malignancy. Patients with dysphagia associated with eosinophilic esophagitis are usually in the younger decades of life [11, 12], and often present with long-standing, often indolent, nonprogressive dysphagia. Many patients only come to the attention of the gastroenterologist following a food impaction, but further history reveals that the patient has adapted to their disease over many years by eating slowly, chewing carefully, and cutting solid food well. They often describe fullness in the chest during meals, instead of the typical sensation of food hanging up. Additionally, a rare but well-known cause of long-standing dysphagia is extrinsic compression by a vascular structure, most commonly an aberrant right subclavian artery, a condition known as dysphagia lusoria [13].

As opposed to patients with obstructive dysphagia, patients with esophageal motility disorders often complain of dysphagia for both solids and liquids that is usually slowly

Table 1.2 Etiologies of esophageal dysphagia.

Structural/mechanical	Neuromuscular
Strictures:	Primary:
Peptic	Achalasia
Radiation	Esophageal spasm
Caustic	Nutcracker esophagus
Pill induced	Hypertensive lower esophageal sphincter
Rings and webs	Ineffective esophageal motility
Eosinophilic esophagitis	Secondary:
Malignant neoplasms:	Systemic sclerosis
Adenocarcinoma	Chagas disease
Squamous cell carcinoma	Polymyositis/dermatomyositis
Benign tumors:	
Leiomyoma	
Fibrovascular polyps	
Diverticula	
Post-fundoplication	
Extrinsic compression:	
Vascular	
Mediastinal tumors	
Cervical osteophytes	
Congenital anomalies:	
Esophageal stenosis	
Duplication cysts	

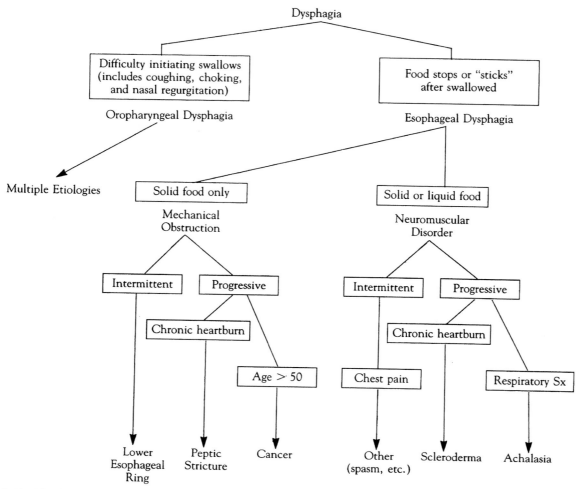

Figure 1.2 Algorithm for dysphagia (reproduced from Johnston BT, Castell DO. Symptom overview and quality of life. In: Castell DO, Richter JE, eds. *The Esophagus*, 4th edn. Philadelphia: Lippincott Williams & Wilkins, 2004:37–46).

progressive. Continual symptoms are indicative of persistent peristaltic dysfunction, as in achalasia and systemic sclerosis, whereas intermittent symptoms indicate either esophageal spasm or a milder peristaltic dysfunction, such as ineffective esophageal motility. When the dysphagia is constant, associated symptoms can help differentiate between achalasia and systemic sclerosis as the etiology. In patients with achalasia, there is often regurgitation of undigested food, especially at night. Patients often describe compensatory techniques that increase intrathoracic pressure to try to help food to pass, such as lifting the arms over the head, jumping up and down, standing up, and performing a modified Valsalva maneuver. Patients with systemic sclerosis often complain of severe, long-standing heartburn, and occasionally develop frank strictures as a result of the unrelenting gastroesophageal reflux.

Physical examination in patients with esophageal dysphagia is usually unremarkable. Careful attention should be paid to the head and neck, particularly in patients whose symptoms suggest oropharyngeal dysphagia. The oral cavity should be examined for the presence of an adequate salivary pool. Cranial nerve examination, especially examination of the tongue, should be performed. The neck should be closely examined for key findings, such as goiter, radiation fibrosis, and lymphadenopathy. Patients should be examined for other manifestations of CREST syndrome (calcinosis, Raynaud's phenomenon, esophageal dysmotility, sclerodactyly, telangiectasia). Tightening of the skin in CREST syndrome may also affect the skin of the face, and lead to a limited ability to open the mouth. The palms of the hands should also be examined for tylosis (palmoplantar keratoderma), as this may be an indicator of the presence of squamous cell carcinoma.

Further evaluation of dysphagia is directed by the history and physical examination. Both barium swallow (esophagram) and upper endoscopy can be used as an initial diagnostic modality. Traditionally, the investigation of dysphagia began with barium swallow, but with the widespread availability of endoscopy, many patients undergo this procedure as a primary examination [14]. The use of a barium tablet (usually 12.5 or 13 mm wide) during the esophagram can help detect subtle esophageal strictures that go unnoticed at upper endoscopy [15]. When a motility disorder is suspected, an esophageal manometry can clarify or confirm the abnormality. Special investigations, such as a modified (video) barium swallow or flexible endoscopic evaluation of swallowing (FEES) test, are usually required for further investigation of oropharyngeal dysphagia [8].

Heartburn

Heartburn (pyrosis) is the classic, cardinal symptom of gastroesophageal reflux disease (GERD). Heartburn is defined as a burning sensation in the retrosternal area (behind the breastbone) [16]. It usually occurs in the post-prandial period, between 30 min and 2 h after meals, especially large meals or meals with refluxogenic contents, such as fat, caffeine, or alcohol. Heartburn can sometimes be accompanied by other symptoms, including an acidic or bitter taste in the mouth, regurgitation of food or liquid contents, or water brash, which is recognized as a sudden rush of salty fluid exuded by the salivary glands into the oral cavity. Heartburn often occurs at night and is a common cause of nocturnal awakenings, particularly if reclining within 2 h after eating a large meal. Most patients with heartburn report that over-the-counter antacids ameliorate the heartburn, but these compounds only last for a short period of time. Some patients obtain relief of symptoms by drinking milk or water, presumably by inducing buffering of the refluxed acid or by washing refluxate down into the stomach. Heartburn and regurgitation can be exacerbated by bending over or by activities that increase strain on the abdomen, including certain types of exercise.

Although heartburn is considered a strong indication of GERD, several other conditions should be considered in the differential diagnosis (Table 1.3). When a patient reports the symptom of heartburn, it is imperative to clarify exactly what the patient means. The term "heartburn" is often used by patients indiscriminately to indicate another symptom, such as abdominal pain, nausea, or bloating. In one study, among patients who endorsed heartburn, the most commonly chosen symptom description was "a pain or discomfort in the stomach" [17]. Coronary artery disease should be considered in the appropriate patient population, particularly if the symptoms routinely occur with exertion. Pill-induced esophagitis can present as the sudden onset of heartburn or chest pain, but may also induce more chronic symptoms. Eosinophilic esophagitis can present with both heartburn and dysphagia. Patients with achalasia often report heartburn or chest pain in addition to dysphagia. The pathophysiology of heartburn in achalasia however, is not well understood. A more recently described entity is functional heartburn, which is defined as a burning retrosternal discomfort or pain in the absence of GERD or a defined motility disorder such as achalasia or esophageal spasm [18].

Regurgitation

Regurgitation is defined as the perception of flow of refluxed gastric contents into the mouth or hypopharynx [16]. In patients who are not taking any antisecretory therapy, it often accompanies heartburn. However, if the patient is using potent antisecretory agents, regurgitation may occur in the absence of heartburn. Although GERD is the most common etiology of regurgitation, especially when associated with heartburn, regurgitation can also occur as a result of intraesophageal stasis, as seen in achalasia. At times, patients may complain of vomiting, when in effect they are actually describing regurgitation. Vomiting is the forceful retrograde evacuation of gastric contents caused by a pressure gradient generated by repetitive contraction of the abdominal musculature [19]. Vomiting is usually, but not always, preceded by nausea. Regurgitation should also be differentiated from rumination, which is repetitive regurgitation of food into the mouth, followed by rechewing and reswallowing or expulsion [20].

Odynophagia

Odynophagia indicates pain upon swallowing. It is strongly suggestive of pathology in the pharynx or esophagus. True odynophagia must be differentiated from the discomfort that often accompanies swallowing in patients with diffuse esophageal spasm. Odynophagia strongly suggests the presence of mucosal injury, and can often be localized quite well. It can occur in any type of disorder that produces a mucosal break, including peptic esophagitis, pill-induced esophagitis or infectious esophagitis. In some patients, the odynophagia is severe enough to produce dysphagia or fear of swallowing.

Chest pain

Retrosternal chest pain can often be caused by esophageal pathology. Because the sensory innervation of the

Table 1.3 Differential diagnosis of heartburn.

Esophageal disorders
Gastroesophageal reflux disease
Achalasia
Esophageal spasm
Eosinophilic esophagitis
Pill-induced esophagitis
Infectious esophagitis

Non-esophageal disorders
Coronary artery disease
Pericarditis
Functional heartburn

intrathoracic organs is intertwined, differentiating esophageal from cardiac chest pain is virtually impossible based on characteristics of the pain alone. Certain features such as pain upon exertion are more strongly suggestive of a cardiac etiology, whereas pain during meals is more suggestive of an esophageal etiology. However, these features lack the accuracy to make a diagnosis based on symptoms alone. Once a cardiac cause has been excluded, esophageal diseases account for the majority of chest pain [21]. Among esophageal causes, GERD is the most common source of pain. Other causes of chest pain, such as musculoskeletal disorders (e.g. costochondritis), pulmonary disorders (e.g. pleuritis), and psychiatric disorders (e.g. anxiety), should be considered in addition to esophageal diseases. Evaluation and management of chest pain as it pertains to the esophagus are discussed in detail in Chapter 2.

Globus

Globus is defined as a frequent or continual non-painful sensation of a lump or fullness in the throat, usually located in the region of the sternal notch [18]. Many patients with a globus sensation often complain about trouble swallowing, which often leads to the patient being labeled as having dysphagia. However, globus is a more constant, continual symptom that does not interfere with the normal swallowing process, and may actually decrease during meals. The sensation of globus has often been ascribed to patients with anxiety or other psychiatric conditions. Historically, the symptom was believed to occur predominantly in women and was called "globus hystericus," indicating a relationship of the symptom to the uterus. This term has been abandoned in most of the recent literature. Several studies have identified a relationship between globus and GERD, but this relationship is not strong [22–25]. The role of esophageal motility disorders in globus remains uncertain [22, 26, 27]. Recent data indicate that hyperdynamic changes in upper esophageal sphincter pressure occur as a response to respiration in some patients with globus [28]. Psychologic factors have been extensively studied in patients with globus sensation. Globus has been associated with several psychopathologic states, including depression, anxiety, and somatization [29–31]. The presence of a gastric inlet patch has also been associated with globus, and endoscopic ablation of the patch may ameliorate symptoms [32].

Respiratory and supraesophageal symptoms

Over the last two decades, the recognition of the relationship of GERD with several pulmonary and otolaryngologic problems, such as cough, hoarseness, and asthma, has brought many patients to seek consultation with gastroenterologists and esophageal specialists. These problems are often grouped together and called "supraesophageal" or "extraesophageal" manifestations of GERD. In some spheres, this association has led to an overdiagnosis of GERD as the sole cause of a

patient's complaints. More recent research indicates that the association may be weaker than has been noted previously, and many recent publications have questioned the true relationship between GERD and many extraesophageal symptoms [33–35].

Hiccup (singultus)

A hiccup is an involuntary spastic contraction of the diaphragm and intercostal muscles associated with an abrupt closure of the glottis, which leads to the characteristic sound. Virtually everyone experiences hiccups at some point or another, but a very small number of patients present with hiccups as a persistent problem. Reports in the literature have defined persistent hiccups as bouts lasting 48h or longer, with intractable hiccups lasting at least 1 month [36]. The Guinness World Record for the longest bout of hiccups is held by Charles Osborne, who had one continuous attack that lasted 68 years [37]. Unlike some other noxious recurrent symptoms like cough or vomiting, hiccups are not known to serve any beneficial function [38]. Most self-limited bouts of hiccups are caused by gastric distention, but can also be associated with sudden changes in the ambient or gastrointestinal temperature, or with sudden emotional changes [38]. In rare instances, medical complications have been seen with hiccups, such as malnutrition, exhaustion, depression, even death [38, 39]. The esophagus is often implicated in the pathophysiology of persistent or intractable hiccups, usually in association with GERD [40–42]. In normal volunteers, rapid stretch of the proximal esophagus with a barostat was able to induce hiccups by stimulating local mechanoreceptors [43]. However, the association between GERD and hiccups may be coincidental, and failure of antisecretory therapy to control intractable hiccups should not be construed as an indication for surgery [44]. Nonesophageal pathology should also be considered when patients present with persistent or intractable hiccups. Any irritation of the diaphragm or phrenic nerve, including mass lesions, can lead to hiccups. Pathology in the central nervous system, most notably within the brainstem, should also be considered in the differential diagnosis.

Quality of life

In 1993, the World Health Organization defined "quality of life" as "an individual's perception of their position in life in the context of the culture and value systems in which they live and in relation to their goals, expectations, standards, and concerns" [45]. When QOL specifically refers to patient-reported outcomes, it is often referred to interchangeably as health-related quality of life (HRQOL). Any symptom, illness, or disease can reduce QOL. In chronic conditions, it becomes important to measure the effect of the disorder on QOL [46]. Symptom frequency and severity often correlate

Table 1.4 Examples of instruments available for the assessment of quality of life in esophageal disorders.

Generic:
Short Form 36 (SF-36) [48]
Psychological General Well-Being Index (PWGBI) [103]

Gastrointestinal specific:
Gastrointestinal Quality of Life Index (GIQLI) [49]

Region specific:
Patient Assessment of Upper Gastrointestinal Disorders-Quality of Life (PAGI-QOL)[50]

Symptom specific:
SWAL-QOL [51]
M.D. Anderson Dysphagia Inventory [81]

Disease/syndrome specific:
Quality of Life in Reflux and Dyspepsia (QOLRAD) [52]
GERD-Health Related Quality of Life Scale (GERD-HRQL) [62, 104]
Quality of Life scale for Achalasia [91]
European Organization for Research and Treatment of Cancer Quality of Life Questionnaire-Esophageal Cancer Module (EORTC QLQ-OES24) [84]

with the impairment in QOL, so symptom scores have traditionally been used as a surrogate marker, especially in the absence of a validated QOL instrument. However, using a symptom-based assessment to quantify QOL does not take many of the non–symptom-based dimensions of QOL into account, such as the anxiety associated with the symptoms or the limitations in life activities. Formal assessment of QOL should quantify the impact of symptoms on at least three core dimensions, including physical, social, and psychologic functioning [47].

An individual's HRQOL can be assessed in a variety of manners (Table 1.4). A general QOL questionnaire, such as the SF-36 [48], can quantify QOL irrespective of the condition, and permits the comparison of QOL across illnesses. However, a generic QOL measure may lack detail to assess the impact of symptoms specific to the disease state. For instance, the SF-36 may not accurately demonstrate the decrement in QOL associated with dysphagia in achalasia. A system-specific questionnaire, such as the Gastrointestinal Quality of Life Index (GIQLI) [49], or a region-specific questionnaire, such as the Patient Assessment of Upper Gastrointestinal Disorders–Quality of Life (PAGI-QOL) [50], can quantify how dysfunction in the gastrointestinal system (or upper digestive tract in the case of the PAGI-QOL) is affecting QOL. Symptom-based instruments, such as the SWAL-QOL instrument, a questionnaire on swallowing problems [51], can quantify the impact of one particular symptom on an individual's QOL. Finally, disease- or syndrome-specific instruments, such as the Quality of Life in Reflux and Dyspepsia (QOLRAD) [52], take into account certain key features of a particular condition that are not

assessed on more general scales (e.g. the impact of GERD on sleep). As the instruments become more specific, more accurate comparisons can be made between patients with similar conditions, at the expense of the ability to compare patients with different illnesses.

Gastroesophageal reflux disease

HRQOL has been extensively investigated in GERD. Patients with GERD score lower in every dimension measured on the SF-36 than the general population [53]. GERD has a greater negative impact on QOL than heart failure and angina pectoris [54]. Erosive and non-erosive reflux diseases seem to have similar decrements in QOL [55], but patients with Barrett's esophagus have better QOL than either of these groups [56] Nocturnal reflux also has a significant impact on QOL. In 2000, the American Gastroenterological Association sponsored a Gallup telephone survey of 1000 adults who admitted to having heartburn at least once per week [57]. Nocturnal heartburn was reported by 79% of respondents, 70% of whom reported moderate (28%) or severe (42%) night-time discomfort. About half of these respondents indicated that their nocturnal symptoms had a greater negative impact on their lives than daytime symptoms [58]. According to the 2005 NIDDK-sponsored investigation, Burden of Digestive Diseases in the United States, GERD accounts for a greater proportion of encounters in the ambulatory setting and has more direct costs (US$12 billion in 2005) than any other gastrointestinal disorder [59].

Numerous generic and disease-specific instruments are available to measure HRQOL in GERD, but none has been clearly shown to be the gold standard for use as a primary endpoint in clinical trials [58, 60, 61]. An ideal instrument would be both sensitive and specific for measuring GERD symptoms, would cover both typical and atypical symptoms, and would be easy for a patient to use on a daily basis [60]. The Gastroesophageal Reflux Disease Health-Related Quality of Life Scale (GERD-HRQL) is one example of a disease-specific instrument that can be used to quantify QOL in GERD [62]. Each QOL instrument has its own benefits and limitations. Some instruments that can monitor changes in symptom severity over time have less utility in monitoring daily changes in symptoms. Instruments such as the Gastrointestinal Symptom Rating Scale (GSRS) [63] and the QOLRAD are frequently used in clinical trials for GERD, but have less specificity for GERD than other disease-specific instruments, such as the GERD-HRQL.

Because QOL has been recognized as an important outcome of therapy, the effects of both acid-suppressive medications and antireflux surgery on QOL have been the subject of numerous recent publications [64–77]. Proton-pump inhibitors (PPIs) have been shown to improve HRQOL in GERD, during both the acute and maintenance phases of treatment. Treatment can restore HRQOL to levels similar to those in the normal population [77]. Therapy with histamine-2-receptor antagonists has been found to improve HRQOL in GERD as well, but PPIs appear to have a more beneficial effect on HRQOL in both erosive and non-erosive reflux disease [67, 69, 78, 79]. Antireflux surgery also improves HRQOL in GERD in most patients, although a small proportion of patients do experience long-term side effects. Short-term studies comparing medical and surgical therapy for GERD often show greater improvements in HRQOL with surgical therapy, but with long-term follow-up, the difference disappears [80].

Dysphagia

Very limited data exist that quantify QOL in patients with esophageal dysphagia. Most of the QOL-based research in dysphagia surrounds oropharyngeal dysphagia, esophageal carcinoma, and achalasia to a limited degree, with virtually no studies that discuss QOL in other esophageal motor disorders. Compared to individuals without dysphagia, people who report dysphagia have been found to have impaired QOL overall and on many of the individual subscales of the SF-36 instrument (e.g. role-physical, general health perception). Furthermore, increasing frequency of dysphagia was independently associated with impaired general health (OR 0.95; 95% CI 0.90–0.99) [7]. Only a few instruments are available that specifically address the impact of dysphagia on QOL. Both the SWAL-QOL instrument [51] and the M.D. Anderson Dysphagia Inventory [81] measure QOL in patients with oropharyngeal dysphagia. To date, no instrument has been developed to assess QOL in patients specifically with esophageal (transport) dysphagia. The Mayo Dysphagia Questionnaire [82] is available for measuring the impact and severity of dysphagia; however, this instrument has not been validated to assess QOL *per se*.

In patients with esophageal cancer, QOL is highly associated with the degree of dysphagia [83]. The European Organization for Research and Treatment of Cancer (EORTC) has developed a specific QOL module for esophageal cancer that encompasses a variety of issues related to esophageal cancer in addition to dysphagia [84]. Many options are available to manage patients with malignant esophageal dysphagia, including stents, chemotherapy, radiotherapy, and intraluminal ablation, and optimal management of these patients should ideally take QOL and personal preferences into account. Palliative care for dysphagia usually, but not always, improves QOL in patients with inoperable esophageal cancer, although QOL may continue to deteriorate as a result of progressive disease [85–88]. In patients who have undergone surgical management of head and neck malignancies, the presence of dysphagia is associated with a higher decrement in QOL [89, 90], and this impairment in QOL is most common in patients who have undergone adjuvant therapy with radiotherapy or chemoradiotherapy [89].

Untreated achalasia is also associated with an impaired QOL. Increasingly, recent studies of achalasia have begun to incorporate measures of QOL as secondary, or even primary, outcomes. The vast majority of these investigations report on the effects of surgical management. Recently, an instrument has been developed to specifically measure QOL in achalasia [91], which has facilitated a structured assessment, but few published studies have yet incorporated this instrument. As is the case with esophageal cancer, the dysphagia associated with achalasia appears to be the major contributor to the decrement in QOL, but other symptoms such as chest pain may also play a role in this impairment as well [92, 93]. Both cardiomyotomy (Heller myotomy) and pneumatic dilation have been found to improve QOL in several small studies [92, 94–102]. Although cardiomyotomy has recently been shown to have more durable effects than pneumatic dilation on the improvement in swallowing, a similar benefit on QOL has not been seen in studies comparing these two therapies [100, 102].

Conclusion

Symptoms related to esophageal diseases are highly prevalent and significantly affect patients' QOL. Symptoms develop through complex interactions between the esophagus and the nervous system, and can be modulated by a patient's emotional and psychologic status. The evaluation of a patient's esophageal symptom should also include an assessment of the patient's QOL. These concepts underscore the importance of open communication and a strong physician–patient relationship in esophageal disease, whether the patient is faced with a life-threatening diagnosis such as advanced stage esophageal cancer, or a more indolent chronic condition.

References

1. Available at: http://www.heartburnalliance.org/press_ages.php [Accessed February 7, 2010].
2. Knowles CH, Aziz Q. Visceral hypersensitivity in non-erosive reflux disease. *Gut* 2008;57:674–83.
3. Orlando RC. Esophageal perception and noncardiac chest pain. *Gastroenterol Clin North Am* 2004;33:25–33.
4. Sengupta JN. An overview of esophageal sensory receptors. *Am J Med* 2000;108 (Suppl 4a):87S–89S.
5. Hobson AR, Aziz Q. Brain processing of esophageal sensation in health and disease. *Gastroenterol Clin North Am* 2004;33: 69–91.
6. Drossman DA. Brain imaging and its implications for studying centrally targeted treatments in irritable bowel syndrome: a primer for gastroenterologists. *Gut* 2005;54:569–573.
7. Eslick GD, Talley NJ. Dysphagia: epidemiology, risk factors and impact on quality of life—a population-based study. *Aliment Pharmacol Ther* 2008;27:971–979.
8. Cook IJ, Kahrilas PJ. AGA technical review on management of oropharyngeal dysphagia. *Gastroenterology* 1999;116:455–478.

9. Scheffer RC, Samsom M, Haverkamp A, *et al*. Impaired bolus transit across the esophagogastric junction in postfundoplication dysphagia. *Am J Gastroenterol* 2005;100:1677–1684.

10. Ingelfinger FJ, Kramer P, Soutter L, Schatzki R. Panel discussion on diseases of the esophagus. *Am J Gastroenterol* 1959;31: 117–131.

11. Pasha SF, DiBaise JK, Kim HJ, *et al*. Patient characteristics, clinical, endoscopic, and histologic findings in adult eosinophilic esophagitis: a case series and systematic review of the medical literature. *Dis Esophagus* 2007;20:311–319.

12. Dellon ES, Gibbs WB, Fritchie KJ, *et al*. Clinical, endoscopic, and histologic findings distinguish eosinophilic esophagitis from gastroesophageal reflux disease. *Clin Gastroenterol Hepatol* 2009;7:1305–1313.

13. Levitt B, Richter JE. Dysphagia lusoria: a comprehensive review. *Dis Esophagus* 2007;20:455–460.

14. Spechler SJ. AGA technical review on treatment of patients with dysphagia caused by benign disorders of the distal esophagus. *Gastroenterology* 1999;117:233–254.

15. Gallo SH, McClave SA, Makk LJ, Looney SW. Standardization of clinical criteria required for use of the 12.5 millimeter barium tablet in evaluating esophageal lumenal patency. *Gastrointest Endosc* 1996;44:181–184.

16. Vakil N, van Zanten SV, Kahrilas P, *et al*. The Montreal definition and classification of gastroesophageal reflux disease: a global evidence-based consensus. *Am J Gastroenterol* 2006;101: 1900–1920.

17. Carlsson R, Dent J, Bolling-Sternevald E, *et al*. The usefulness of a structured questionnaire in the assessment of symptomatic gastroesophageal reflux disease. *Scand J Gastroenterol* 1998;33:1023–1029.

18. Galmiche JP, Clouse RE, Balint A, *et al*. Functional esophageal disorders. *Gastroenterology* 2006;130:1459–1465.

19. Quigley EMM, Hasler WL, Parkman HP. AGA technical review on nausea and vomiting. *Gastroenterology* 2001;120:263–286.

20. Tack J, Talley NJ, Camilleri M, *et al*. Functional gastroduodenal disorders. *Gastroenterology* 2006;130:1466–1479.

21. Eslick GD, Fass R. Noncardiac chest pain: evaluation and treatment. *Gastroenterol Clin North Am* 2003;32:531–552.

22. Hill J, Stuart RC, Fung HK, *et al*. Gastroesophageal reflux, motility disorders, and psychological profiles in the etiology of globus pharyngis. *Laryngoscope* 1997;107:1373–1377.

23. Anandasabapathy S, Jaffin BW. Multichannel intraluminal impedance in the evaluation of patients with persistent globus on proton pump inhibitor therapy. *Ann Otol Rhinol Laryngol* 2006;115:563–570.

24. Chevalier JM, Brossard E, Monnier P. Globus sensation and gastroesophageal reflux. *Eur Arch Otorhinolaryngol* 2003;260: 273–276.

25. Wilson JA, Heading RC, Maran AG, *et al*. Globus sensation is not due to gastro-oesophageal reflux. *Clin Otolaryngol Allied Sci* 1987;12:271–275.

26. Wilson JA, Pryde A, Piris J, *et al*. Pharyngoesophageal dysmotility in globus sensation. *Arch Otolaryngol Head Neck Surg* 1989;115:1086–1090.

27. Watson WC, Sullivan SN. Hypertonicity of the cricopharyngeal sphincter: a cause of globus sensation. *Lancet* 1974;2: 1417–1419.

28. Kwiatek MA, Mirza F, Kahrilas PJ, Pandolfino JE. Hyperdynamic upper esophageal sphincter pressure: a manometric observation in patients reporting globus sensation. *Am J Gastroenterol* 2009;104:289–298.

29. Moser G, Wenzel-Abatzi TA, Stelzeneder M, *et al*. Globus sensation: pharyngoesophageal function, psychometric and psychiatric findings, and follow-up in 88 patients. *Arch Intern Med* 1998;158:1365–1373.

30. Wilson JA, Deary IJ, Maran AG. Is globus hystericus? *Br J Psychiatry* 1988;153:335–339.

31. Gale CR, Wilson JA, Deary IJ. Globus sensation and psychopathology in men: the Vietnam experience study. *Psychosom Med* 2009;71:1026–1031.

32. Bajbouj M, Becker V, Eckel F, *et al*. Argon plasma coagulation of cervical heterotopic gastric mucosa as an alternative treatment for globus sensations. *Gastroenterology* 2009;137: 440–444.

33. American Lung Association Asthma Clinical Research Centers, Mastronarde JG, Anthonisen NR, *et al*. Efficacy of esomeprazole for treatment of poorly controlled asthma. *N Engl J Med* 2009;360:1487–1499.

34. Vaezi MF, Richter JE, Stasney CR, *et al*. Treatment of chronic posterior laryngitis with esomeprazole. *Laryngoscope* 2006;116: 254–260.

35. Vavricka SR, Storck CA, Wildi SM, *et al*. Limited diagnostic value of laryngopharyngeal lesions in patients with gastroesophageal reflux during routine upper gastrointestinal endoscopy. *Am J Gastroenterol* 2007;102:716–722.

36. Kolodzik PW, Eilers MA. Hiccups (singultus): review and approach to management. *Ann Emerg Med* 1991;20:565–573.

37. Available at: http://en.wikipedia.org/wiki/Hiccup [Accessed February 28, 2010].

38. Rousseau P. Hiccups. *South Med J* 1995;88:175–181.

39. Lewis, J.H. Hiccups: causes and cures. *J Clin Gastroenterol* 1985;7:539–552.

40. Schreiber LR, Bowen MR, Mino FA, Craig TJ. Hiccups due to gastroesophageal reflux. *South Med J* 1995;88:217–219.

41. Mattox HE, 3rd, Richter JE. Prolonged ambulatory esophageal pH monitoring in the evaluation of gastroesophageal reflux disease. *Am J Med* 1990;89:345–356.

42. Shay SS, Myers RL, Johnson LF. Hiccups associated with reflux esophagitis. *Gastroenterology* 1984;87:204–207.

43. Fass R, Higa L, Kodner A, Mayer EA. Stimulus and site specific induction of hiccups in the oesophagus of normal subjects. *Gut* 1997;41:590–593.

44. Fisher MJ, Mittal RK. Hiccups and gastroesophageal reflux: cause and effect? *Dig Dis Sci* 1989;34:1277–1280.

45. Study protocol for the World Health Organization project to develop a Quality of Life assessment instrument (WHOQOL). *Qual Life Res* 1993;2:153–159.

46. Guyatt GH, Feeny DH, Patrick DL. Measuring health-related quality of life. *Ann Intern Med* 1993;118:622–629.

47. Wiklund I. Quality of life in patients with gastroesophageal reflux disease. *Am J Gastroenterol* 2001;96:S46–53.

48. McHorney CA, Ware JE, Jr, Raczek AE. The MOS 36-Item Short-Form Health Survey (SF-36): II. Psychometric and clinical tests of validity in measuring physical and mental health constructs. *Med Care* 1993;31:247–263.

49. Eypasch E, Williams JI, Wood-Dauphinee S, *et al.* Gastrointestinal Quality of Life Index: development, validation and application of a new instrument. *Br J Surg* 1995;82:216–222.

50. de la Loge C, Trudeau E, Marquis P, *et al.* Cross-cultural development and validation of a patient self-administered questionnaire to assess quality of life in upper gastrointestinal disorders: the PAGI-QOL. *Qual Life Res* 2004;13:1751–1762.

51. McHorney CA, Robbins J, Lomax K, *et al.* The SWAL-QOL and SWAL-CARE outcomes tool for oropharyngeal dysphagia in adults: III. Documentation of reliability and validity. *Dysphagia* 2002;17:97–114.

52. Wiklund IK, Junghard O, Grace E, *et al.* Quality of Life in Reflux and Dyspepsia patients: psychometric documentation of a new disease-specific questionnaire (QOLRAD). *Eur J Surg Suppl* 1998;583:41–49.

53. Revicki DA, Wood M, Maton PN, Sorensen S. The impact of gastroesophageal reflux disease on health-related quality of life. *Am J Med* 1998;104:252–258.

54. Dimenas E. Methodological aspects of evaluation of quality of life in upper gastrointestinal diseases. *Scand J Gastroenterol* 1993;28:18–21.

55. Kovacs Z, Kerekgyarto O. Psychological factors, quality of life, and gastrointestinal symptoms in patients with erosive and non-erosive reflux disorder. *Int J Psychiatry Med* 2007;37:139–150.

56. Lippmann QK, Crockett SD, Dellon ES, Shaheen NJ. Quality of life in GERD and Barrett's esophagus is related to gender and manifestation of disease. *Am J Gastroenterol* 2009;104: 2695–2703.

57. Shaker R, Castell DO, Schoenfeld PS, Spechler SJ. Nighttime heartburn is an under-appreciated clinical problem that impacts sleep and daytime function: the results of a Gallup survey conducted on behalf of the American Gastroenterological Association. *Am J Gastroenterol* 2003;98:1487–1493.

58. Shaker R, Brunton S, Elfant A, *et al.* Review article: impact of night-time reflux on lifestyle—unrecognized issues in reflux disease. *Aliment Pharmacol Ther* 2004;20 (Suppl 9):3–13.

59. Everhart JE, Ruhl CE. Burden of digestive diseases in the United States part I: overall and upper gastrointestinal diseases. *Gastroenterology* 2009;136:376–386.

60. Fass R. Symptom assessment tools for gastroesophageal reflux disease (GERD) treatment. *J Clin Gastroenterol* 2007;41: 437–444.

61. Talley NJ, Wiklund I. Patient reported outcomes in gastroesophageal reflux disease: an overview of available measures. *Qual Life Res* 2005;14:21–33.

62. Velanovich V, Vallance SR, Gusz JR, *et al.* Quality of life scale for gastroesophageal reflux disease. *J Am Coll Surg* 1996;183: 217–224.

63. Revicki DA, Wood M, Wiklund I, Crawley J. Reliability and validity of the Gastrointestinal Symptom Rating Scale in patients with gastroesophageal reflux disease. *Qual Life Res* 1998;7:75–83.

64. Amato G, Limongelli P, Pascariello A, *et al.* Association between persistent symptoms and long-term quality of life after laparoscopic total fundoplication. *Am J Surg* 2008;196:582–586.

65. Slim K, Bousquet J, Kwiatkowski F, *et al.* Quality of life before and after laparoscopic fundoplication. *Am J Surg* 2000;180: 41–45.

66. Pidoto RR, Fama F, Giacobbe G, *et al.* Quality of life and predictors of long-term outcome in patients undergoing open Nissen fundoplication for chronic gastroesophageal reflux. *Am J Surg* 2006;191:470–478.

67. Mathias SD, Colwell HH, Miller DP, *et al.* Health-related quality-of-life and quality-days incrementally gained in symptomatic nonerosive GERD patients treated with lansoprazole or ranitidine. *Dig Dis Sci* 2001;46:2416–2423.

68. Johanson JF, Siddique R, Damiano AM, *et al.* Rabeprazole improves health-related quality of life in patients with erosive gastroesophageal reflux disease. *Dig Dis Sci* 2002;47: 2574–2578.

69. Kovacs TO, Freston JW, Haber MM, *et al.* Long-term quality of life improvement in subjects with healed erosive esophagitis: treatment with lansoprazole. *Dig Dis Sci* 2010;55:1325–1336.

70. de Souza Cury M, Ferrari AP, Ciconelli R, *et al.* Evaluation of health-related quality of life in gastroesophageal reflux disease patients before and after treatment with pantoprazole. *Dis Esophagus* 2006;19:289–293.

71. Pace F, Negrini C, Wiklund I, *et al.* Quality of life in acute and maintenance treatment of non-erosive and mild erosive gastro-oesophageal reflux disease. *Aliment Pharmacol Ther* 2005;22:349–356.

72. Bjornsson E, Abrahamsson H, Simren M, *et al.* Discontinuation of proton pump inhibitors in patients on long-term therapy: a double-blind, placebo-controlled trial. *Aliment Pharmacol Ther* 2006;24:945–954.

73. Aanen MC, Weusten BL, Numans ME, *et al.* Effect of proton-pump inhibitor treatment on symptoms and quality of life in GERD patients depends on the symptom-reflux association. *J Clin Gastroenterol* 2008;42:441–447.

74. Ciovica R, Gadenstatter M, Klingler A, *et al.* Quality of life in GERD patients: medical treatment versus antireflux surgery. *J Gastrointest Surg* 2006;10:934–939.

75. Fernando HC, Schauer PR, Rosenblatt M, et al. Quality of life after antireflux surgery compared with nonoperative management for severe gastroesophageal reflux disease. *J Am Coll Surg* 2002;194:23–27.

76. Lundell L, Miettinen P, Myrvold HE, *et al.* Continued (5-year) followup of a randomized clinical study comparing antireflux surgery and omeprazole in gastroesophageal reflux disease. *J Am Coll Surg* 2001;192:172–179.

77. Havelund T, Lind T, Wiklund I, *et al.* Quality of life in patients with heartburn but without esophagitis: effects of treatment with omeprazole. *Am J Gastroenterol* 1999;94:1782–1789.

78. Pare P, Armstrong D, Pericak D, Pyzyk M. Pantoprazole rapidly improves health-related quality of life in patients with heartburn: a prospective, randomized, double blind comparative study with nizatidine. *J Clin Gastroenterol* 2003;37:132–138.

79. Revicki DA, Sorensen S, Maton PN, Orlando RC. Health-related quality of life outcomes of omeprazole versus ranitidine in poorly responsive symptomatic gastroesophageal reflux disease. *Dig Dis* 1998;16:284–291.

80. Lundell L, Attwood S, Ell C, *et al.* Comparing laparoscopic antireflux surgery with esomeprazole in the management of patients with chronic gastro-oesophageal reflux disease: a 3-year interim analysis of the LOTUS trial. *Gut* 2008;57: 1207–1213.

81. Chen AY, Frankowski R, Bishop-Leone J, *et al.* The development and validation of a dysphagia-specific quality-of-life questionnaire for patients with head and neck cancer: the MD Anderson dysphagia inventory. *Arch Otolaryngol Head Neck Surg* 2001;127:870–876.

82. Grudell AB, Alexander JA, Enders FB, *et al.* Validation of the Mayo Dysphagia Questionnaire. *Dis Esophagus* 2007;20:202–205.

83. Wildi SM, Cox MH, Clark LL, *et al.* Assessment of health state utilities and quality of life in patients with malignant esophageal dysphagia. *Am J Gastroenterol* 2004;99:1044–1049.

84. Blazeby JM, Alderson D, Winstone K, *et al.* Development of an EORTC questionnaire module to be used in quality of life assessment for patients with oesophageal cancer. *Eur J Cancer* 1996;32:1912–1917.

85. Dallal HJ, Smith GD, Grieve DC, *et al.* A randomized trial of thermal ablative therapy versus expandable metal stents in the palliative treatment of patients with esophageal carcinoma. *Gastrointest Endosc* 2001;54:549–557.

86. Barr H, Krasner N. Prospective quality-of-life analysis after palliative photoablation for the treatment of malignant dysphagia. *Cancer* 1991;68:1660–1664.

87. Loizou LA, Rampton D, Atkinson M, *et al.* A prospective assessment of quality of life after endoscopic intubation and laser therapy for malignant dysphagia. *Cancer* 1992;70:386–391.

88. Maroju NK, Anbalagan P, Kate V, Ananthakrishnan N. Improvement in dysphagia and quality of life with self-expanding metallic stents in malignant esophageal strictures. *Indian J Gastroenterol* 2006;25:62–65.

89. García-Peris P, Parón L, Velasco C, *et al.* Long-term prevalence of oropharyngeal dysphagia in head and neck cancer patients: impact on quality of life. *Clin Nutr* 2007;26:710–717.

90. Nguyen NP, Frank C, Moltz CC, *et al.* Impact of dysphagia on quality of life after treatment of head-and-neck cancer. *Int J Radiat Oncol Biol Phys* 2005;61:772–778.

91. Urbach DR, Tomlinson GA, Harnish JL, *et al.* A measure of disease-specific health-related quality of life for achalasia. *Am J Gastroenterol* 2005;100:1668–1676.

92. Youssef Y, Richards WO, Sharp K, *et al.* Relief of dysphagia after laparoscopic Heller myotomy improves long-term quality of life. *J Gastrointest Surg* 2007;11:309–313.

93. Frankhuisen R, van Herwaarden MA, Heijkoop R, *et al.* Persisting symptoms and decreased health-related quality-of-life in a cross-sectional study of treated achalasia patients. *Aliment Pharmacol Ther* 2007;26:899–904.

94. Mineo TC, Ambrogi V. Long-term results and quality of life after surgery for oesophageal achalasia: one surgeon's experience. *Eur J Cardiothorac Surg* 2004;25:1089–1096.

95. Ben-Meir A, Urbach DR, Khajanchee YS, *et al.* Quality of life before and after laparoscopic Heller myotomy for achalasia. *Am J Surg* 2001;181:471–474.

96. Dan D, Seetahal S, Mohammed S. Quality of life before and after laparoscopic Heller procedures—a Caribbean perspective. *J Natl Med Assoc* 2009;101:174–178.

97. Luketich JD, Fernando HC, Christie NA, *et al.* Outcomes after minimally invasive esophagomyotomy. *Ann Thorac Surg* 2001;72:1909–1912.

98. Dang Y, Mercer D. Treatment of esophageal achalasia with Heller myotomy: retrospective evaluation of patient satisfaction and disease-specific quality of life. *Can J Surg* 2006;49:267–271.

99. Decker G, Borie F, Bouamrirene D, *et al.* Gastrointestinal quality of life before and after laparoscopic Heller myotomy with partial posterior fundoplication. *Ann Surg* 2002;236:750–758.

100. Meshkinpour H, Haghighat P, Meshkinpour A. Quality of life among patients treated for achalasia. *Dig Dis Sci* 1996;41:352–356.

101. Kostic S, Kjellin A, Ruth M, *et al.* Pneumatic dilatation or laparoscopic cardiomyotomy in the management of newly diagnosed idiopathic achalasia: results of a randomized controlled trial. *World J Surg* 2007;31:470–478.

102. Kostic S, Johnsson E, Kjellin A, *et al.* Health economic evaluation of therapeutic strategies in patients with idiopathic achalasia: results of a randomized trial comparing pneumatic dilatation with laparoscopic cardiomyotomy. *Surg Endosc* 2007;21:1184–1189.

103. Dupuy HJ. The psychological general well-being (PGWB) index. In: Wenger NK, Mattson ME, Furberg CF, Elinson J (eds). *Assessment of Quality of Life in Clinical Trials of Cardiovascular Therapies*. New York: Le Jacq Publishing, 1984, pp. 170–183.

104. Velanovich V. The development of the GERD-HRQL symptom severity instrument. *Dis Esophagus* 2007;20:130–134.

2 Non-Cardiac Chest Pain

Ronnie Fass[1] and Tiberiu Herschcovici[2]
[1]University of Arizona, Southern Arizona VA Health Care System, Tucson, AZ, USA
[2]University of Arizona, The Neuroenteric Clinical Research Group, Tucson, AZ, USA

Introduction

Non-cardiac chest pain (NCCP) is defined as recurring, angina-like, retrosternal chest pain of non-cardiac origin. A patient's history and characteristics do not reliably distinguish between cardiac and esophageal causes of chest pain [1, 2]. When it comes to chest pain, the cardiologist's first priority is to exclude any acute life-threatening cardiovascular condition[3]. These include acute coronary syndrome, aortic dissection, pulmonary thromboembolism, and pericardial tamponade. If these acute conditions have been excluded, evaluation for chronic ischemic heart disease or pericardial disease must be pursued. Various tests can help determine the presence and severity of ischemia, left ventricular function, appearance of the coronary arteries, and functional capacity. They include exercise test electrocardiography (EKG), echocardiography or nuclear single photon emission computed tomography (SPECT), and if patients are unable to exercise, pharmacologic echocardiography, nuclear SPECT, or cardiac magnetic resonance imaging (MRI). The decision about what tests to pursue should be left to the discretion of the treating cardiologist [4]. The heightened awareness about the potentially devastating ramifications of chest pain may drive patients to seek further medical attention despite a negative cardiac work-up [5].

Compared to patients with cardiac angina, those with NCCP are usually younger, less likely to have typical symptoms, and more likely to have a normal resting EKG [6]. Additionally, levels of anxiety of NCCP patients seen in a rapid access chest pain clinic significantly exceeded those of patients with cardiac angina and remained above community norms for at least 2 months after the clinic visit [7]. NCCP patients view their condition as significantly less controllable and less understandable than those whose pain is of cardiac origin [8].

NCCP may be the manifestation of gastrointestinal or non–gastrointestinal-related disorders (Figure 2.1). An important step toward understanding the underlying mechanisms of NCCP was the recognition that gastroesophageal reflux disease (GERD) is the most common contributing factor for chest pain. While chest pain has been considered an atypical manifestation of GERD, it is an integral part of the limited repertoire of esophageal symptoms. In patients with non–GERD-related NCCP, esophageal motility disorders and functional chest pain of presumed esophageal origin are the main underlying mechanism for symptoms. The Rome III Committee does not specifically address NCCP, but rather a subset of patients with NCCP termed "functional chest pain of presumed esophageal origin" to describe recurrent episodes of substernal chest pain of visceral quality with no apparent explanation (Table 2.1). As with all other functional esophageal disorders, GERD and esophageal dysmotility should also be ruled out before the diagnosis is established [9]. However, up to 20% of patients with functional chest pain exhibit other functional disorders, primarily irritable bowel syndrome (IBS) (27%) and abdominal bloating (22%) [10].

Epidemiology

Information about the epidemiology of NCCP in the United States and around the world is relatively limited. Presently, chest pain is the second most common presentation to hospital emergency departments; however, only 25% of the individuals who experience chest pain actually present to a hospital [11].

The mean annual prevalence of NCCP in six population-based studies was approximately 25%. However, these studies differ in many aspects, such as NCCP definition, geography, sample size, sampling order, and ethnicity [12].

The Esophagus, Fifth Edition. Edited by Joel E. Richter, Donald O. Castell.
© 2012 Blackwell Publishing Ltd. Published 2012 by Blackwell Publishing Ltd.

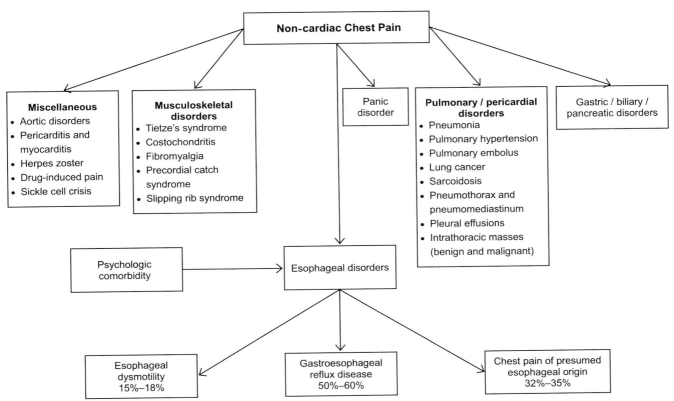

Figure 2.1 Underlying mechanisms of non-cardiac chest pain. LES, lower esophageal sphincter (modified from Fass and Navarro-Rodriquez [2], with permission).

Table 2.1 Rome III Diagnostic Criteria for Functional Chest Pain of Presumed Esophageal Origin [9].

Must include all of the following:
- Midline chest pain or discomfort that is not of burning quality
- Absence of evidence that gastroesophageal reflux is the cause of the symptom
- Absence of histopathology-based esophageal motility disorders
Criteria fulfilled for the last 3 months with symptom onset at least 6 months prior to diagnosis.

A population-based survey in the United States assessed the prevalence of GERD in Olmsted County, Minnesota [13] and reported an overall NCCP prevalence of 23%. Gender distribution among NCCP patients was similar (24% among males and 22% among females). Eslick *et al.* have evaluated the prevalence of NCCP in Australia by mailing a validated Chest Pain Questionnaire (CPQ) to 1000 randomly selected individuals. The study demonstrated a prevalence rate of 33% with almost equal gender distribution (32% in males vs 33% in females). This study also showed that the population prevalence of NCCP decreases with increasing age [14, 15].

Although females with NCCP tend to consult healthcare providers more often than men, the disorder affects both genders equally [13]. Additionally, females are more likely to present to hospital emergency departments with NCCP than males. However, there are no gender differences regarding chest pain intensity, although women tend to use terms like "burning" and "frightening" more often than men [16].

Epidemiologic studies report a decrease in the prevalence of NCCP with increasing age. Women under 25 years of age and those between 45 and 55 years of age have the highest prevalence rates [15]. Patients with NCCP are younger, consume greater amounts of alcohol, smoke more, and are more likely to suffer from anxiety than their counterparts with ischemic heart disease. Patients with NCCP continue to seek treatment on a regular basis after the diagnosis is established for both chest pain and other unrelated symptoms [17].

A recent US-based survey revealed that cardiologists managed about half of the patients who were diagnosed with NCCP [18]. Of those NCCP patients who were referred, 45.9% were sent back to the primary care physician (PCP), and only 29.3% to a gastroenterologist. In a survey of PCPs, Wong *et al.* demonstrated that most NCCP patients were diagnosed and treated by PCPs (79.5%), without being referred to a gastroenterologist [19]. The most preferred subspecialty for the initial diagnostic evaluation of a patient presenting with chest pain was cardiology (62%), followed by gastroenterology (17%). However, the mean percentage of such referrals was only 22%. The most preferred subspecialty for the further management of NCCP was gastroenterology (76%), followed by cardiology (7.8%).

A study by Eslick *et al.* reported that 78% of patients who presented to a hospital emergency department with acute chest pain had seen a healthcare provider in the last 12 months [20]. The most common healthcare provider seen was a general practitioner (85%), followed by a cardiologist (74%), gastroenterologist (30%), pulmonologist (14%), alternative therapist (8%), and psychologist (10%) [20]. Additionally, work absenteeism rates because of NCCP were high (29%), as were interruptions to daily activities (63%) [20].

Natural history

The long-term prognosis of NCCP patients is excellent, and very few eventually succumb to coronary artery disease (CAD) or other cardiovascular-related disorders. In a study following 46 NCCP patients over a period of 11 years, only 4.3% died from a cardiovascular-related event [21]. However, most of the NCCP patients continued to report episodes of long-term chest pain: 75% of the surviving patients reported chest pain 11 years later, with 34% reporting chest pain weekly.

In a survey study, 119 NCCP patients, of whom 63 were diagnosed as having pain that originated from the esophagus, were followed for 21.8 months [22]. Patients with esophageal-related chest pain usually continued to have recurrent pain. Importantly, a specific diagnosis did not significantly increase the likelihood of pain resolution. However, patients who understood that the esophagus was the source of their pain were significantly less likely to feel disabled by their pain and require continued physician evaluation.

A study by Eslick *et al.* followed for 4 years 126 patients with NCCP and 71 with CAD who presented in the emergency room [23]. The majority of the NCCP (71%) and CAD patients (81%) continued to have symptoms 4 years later. The authors found no difference in the mortality rate between the two groups (CAD 11% vs NCCP 5.5%, *P* = .16).

A recent study compared the characteristics, natural history, and long-term survival of NCCP and GERD patients using data collected between 1984 and 1996 from the Veterans Affairs Decentralized Hospital Computer Program (VA DHCP) storage system [24]. During the 12-year enrollment period, 1218 GERD and 161 NCCP patients were referred for endoscopy [all of them in the pre-proton pump inhibitor (PPI) era]. The mean follow-up period was 9.8

years. NCCP patients had a significantly lower prevalence of GERD-related findings, such as erosive esophagitis, Barrett's esophagus, esophageal adenocarcinoma, and hiatal hernia. In the NCCP group, there was a significantly higher prevalence of cardiac factors, such as CAD, and there was a trend toward greater cardiac clinic enrollment and cardiac medication usage. The level and duration of antireflux therapy consumption, such as histamine-2 receptor antagonists (H_2RAs) and PPIs, were significantly less in the NCCP group as compared to the GERD group. Interestingly, the diagnosis of NCCP disappeared from the electronic hospital record in 96% of patients within 2 years of follow-up. There was no significant difference in long-term survival between the NCCP and the GERD groups. The study supported previous findings that patients with NCCP have an excellent long-term prognosis, similar to that for patients with GERD.

In one study, health-related quality of life (HRQOL) was assessed in 167 NCCP patients and compared with general population norms utilizing the SF-36 [25]. NCCP patients reported a significantly more impaired HRQOL as compared to controls. Gender, age, marital status, years of education, sum of chronic illnesses, neuroticism, and presence of panic disorder and depression symptoms accounted for 17–67% of the variance in SF-36 scales.

Overall, the aforementioned data support the conclusion that increased mortality is uncommon in NCCP patients. However, patients with NCCP demonstrate poor QOL, primarily due to the continuation of symptoms many years after diagnosis. Furthermore, studies have demonstrated that many NCCP patients have long-term impaired functional status and utilize healthcare resources because of their chest pain [14]. In one study, the rates of work absenteeism and interruption to daily activities were 29% and 63%, respectively, over a 1-year period [20].

Pathophysiology

Gastroesophageal reflux disease

Many studies have shown an association between GERD and NCCP. However, association does not confer causality. Resolution or improvement of chest pain symptoms in response to treatment with antireflux medications provides the missing causal link. Locke *et al.* have found that NCCP is more commonly reported by patients who experience heartburn symptoms at least weekly (37%), as compared with those who have infrequent heartburn (less than once a week) (30.7%) and those without any symptoms of GERD (7.9%) [13]. In this study, 5% of the individuals with NCCP reported severe or very severe heartburn symptoms. In another community-based study, 53% of all patients with NCCP experienced heartburn and 58% acid regurgitation [15].

Table 2.2 Value of endoscopy in non-cardiac chest pain patients from a large multicenter consortium study [34].

Findings	Chest pain group (n = 3688)	Reflux group (n = 32 981)	P value
Barrett's esophagus	163 (4.4%)	3016 (9.1%)	<.0001
Esophageal inflammation	715 (19.4%)	9153 (27.8%)	<.0001
Hiatal hernia	1053 (28.6%)	14775 (44.8%)	<.0001
Normal	1627 (44.1%)	12801 (38.8%)	<.0001
Stricture/stenosis	132 (3.6%)	1223 (3.7%)	.69

Ambulatory 24-h esophageal pH testing studies have demonstrated that about half of NCCP patients have an abnormal esophageal acid exposure [26–29]. In three different studies evaluating the role of the PPI test, the authors found an abnormal pH test in 37.5–67% of the NCCP patients [30–32]. In a study from Asia, 34.3% of the NCCP patients had at least one abnormal pH parameter [33].

In the studies evaluating the role of the PPI test in patients with NCCP, GERD-related endoscopic findings (most frequent abnormality: low-grade erosive esophagitis) were reported in 44–75% of the NCCP patients [30–32]. A recent study by Dickman et al. using a large multicenter consortium, evaluated upper gastrointestinal findings in patients with NCCP as compared to those with GERD-related symptoms only[34]. Of the NCCP group, 28.6% had hiatal hernia, 19.6% erosive esophagitis, 4.4% Barrett's esophagus, and 3.6% esophageal stricture/stenosis (Table 2.2). The prevalence of these findings was significantly lower in the NCCP group when compared with the GERD group. From this study, it appears that GERD-related mucosal abnormalities are not uncommon in the esophagus of NCCP patients. However, the prevalence of these anatomic findings is lower than that observed in GERD patients.

The presence of an abnormal acid exposure and/or esophageal mucosal inflammation in patients with NCCP suggests an association with GERD. Studies have shown that approximately 80% of NCCP patients with an abnormal pH test and/or endoscopy report marked improvement in their chest pain when PPIs are administered [35, 36]. In contrast, response to PPI treatment in non–GERD-related NCCP patients ranges from 10% to 14% [30–32]. These data suggest a causal relationship between GERD and chest pain symptoms.

Linked angina

The esophagus and the heart share similar sensory innervation and several studies have demonstrated that acidification of the distal esophagus may influence the flow of the coronary circulation [37–39]. Chauhan et al. have shown a reduction in coronary artery blood flow in response to acid perfusion into the distal esophagus in patients with syndrome X. Syndrome X is defined as typical chest pain and electrocardiographic changes suggestive of myocardial ischemia on stress test, but patent coronary arteries on angiogram [40]. The reduction in coronary blood flow was also associated with typical anginal pain, suggesting the presence of an esophagocardiac inhibitory reflex. These findings were later confirmed by Rosztoczy et al. who showed a decrease in coronary artery blood flow in 19 of 42 (45%) patients undergoing acid perfusion of the esophagus [41].

Esophageal dysmotility

The role of esophageal dysmotility in NCCP is likely very limited, even though it is often entertained as an etiology for NCCP in the absence of GERD. More than 70% of patients with non–GERD-related NCCP have normal esophageal motility [42, 43]. Esophageal dysmotility when documented by esophageal manometry is rarely associated with reports of chest pain [44]. Furthermore, in NCCP patients who underwent simultaneous esophageal manometry and pH testing, chest pain was more commonly associated with acid reflux events than motility abnormalities [45, 46]. Studies have repeatedly shown that chest pain will often improve without any normalization of the esophageal motor abnormalities. Unlike in patients with GERD, in whom PPIs are highly effective in alleviating symptoms, we are still devoid of pharmacologic agents that can effectively treat esophageal dysmotility. The latter further complicates our ability to determine any relationship between chest pain and manometric findings. That said, esophageal motility disorders still can be demonstrated in 30% of patients with non–GERD-related NCCP. Dekel et al. demonstrated, via the Clinical Outcomes Research Initiative Database, that hypotensive lower esophageal sphincter (LES) was the most common (61%) esophageal motor disorder found in patients with NCCP [43]. It has been suggested that this is due to an increased rate of GERD in these patients. Spastic esophageal motility disorders were shown to be the second most common cause, with nutcracker esophagus affecting 10%, hypertensive LES 10%, and diffuse esophageal spasm (DES) 2% of the NCCP cases with esophageal dysmotility. However, in another study of non–GERD-related NCCP, Katz et al. reported that nutcracker esophagus was the most common motor disorder documented during esophageal manometry,

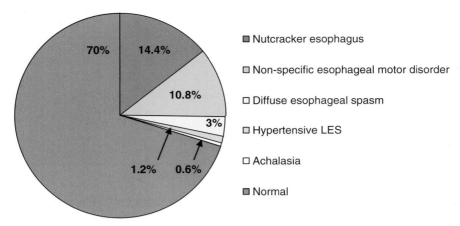

Figure 2.2 Distribution of esophageal motility abnormalities in non-cardiac chest pain patients without gastroesophageal reflux disease (n = 910). LES, lower esophageal sphincter (modified from Katz *et al.* [42], with permission).

followed by non-specific esophageal motility disorders, DES, hypertensive LES, and achalasia [42] (Figure 2.2).

High-resolution manometry (HRM) has shown that patients with a clear link between esophageal motor abnormalities and chest pain usually have high-pressure amplitude waves, and prolonged, repetitive contractions in the distal esophagus [47, 48]. Occasionally, as reported by ultrasonographic studies (*vide infra*), esophageal shortening due to longitudinal muscle spasm is detected by HRM during episodes of chest pain [49].

The aforementioned studies led some investigators to speculate that the motility abnormalities documented in NCCP patients in fact represent an epiphenomenon rather than the direct cause of pain. One possibility is that the abnormal motor response originates from activation of esophageal sensory afferents that trigger a secondary motor contraction in response to the sensory input. Another theory speculates that chest pain may arise from esophageal intramural ischemia that is induced by increased esophageal motor activity [50]. However, studies evaluating the blood supply of the esophagus suggested that the presence of vast arterial perfusion for this organ argues against such a theory [51]. Recent studies have suggested that esophageal pain may originate from other muscle layers of the esophagus that escape detection by conventional esophageal manometry. Investigators have proposed that sustained esophageal longitudinal muscle contractions detected by high-frequency ultrasound may serve as a marker for esophageal-induced chest pain [52].

Sustained esophageal contractions

High-frequency intraluminal ultrasonography, a technique useful for the evaluation of smooth muscle contractions, has been employed to assess the esophageal motor corollary of chest pain in NCCP patients [53]. Using this method, Balaban *et al.* have shown a close correlation between longitudinal

muscle contractions and reports of chest pain [52]. In the 10 subjects, esophageal longitudinal muscle contractions preceded 18 of 24 spontaneous chest pain events. These muscle contractions could not be detected by conventional esophageal pressure recordings that solely evaluate the esophageal circular muscle. It was also demonstrated that edrophonium-induced chest pain was preceded by sustained esophageal muscle contractions. The authors further demonstrated that swallow-associated contractions of the longitudinal muscle on average lasted 6.4 s, whereas contractions associated with chest pain on average lasted 68.0 s. Pehlivanov *et al.* demonstrated that the duration of the sustained esophageal muscle contractions correlated with the type of symptom perceived by patients. Shorter durations of these contractions were more commonly associated with heartburn, while longer durations were linked more with chest pain [49]. Furthermore, sustained esophageal muscle contractions were observed in patients who reported heartburn that was unrelated to an acid reflux event, giving further credence to the hypothesis that sustained esophageal contractions are responsible for the generation of esophageal-related symptoms, such as chest pain.

High-frequency intraluminal ultrasonography is highly operator dependent and consequently may not always be an objective evaluative tool. Whilst sustained esophageal muscle contractions appear to be predictive of chest pain, it is still unclear if they represent the underlying cause or just an epiphenomenon.

Esophageal hypersensitivity

Numerous studies have consistently documented alteration in pain perception regardless of whether esophageal dysmotility is present or absent.

Visceral hypersensitivity is a phenomenon in which the conscious perception of visceral stimulus is enhanced independent of the intensity of the stimulus [54, 55]. Peripheral and central mechanisms have been proposed to be responsible for visceral hypersensitivity in patients with NCCP. It has been hypothesized that peripheral sensitization of esophageal sensory afferents leads to subsequently heightened responses to physiologic or pathologic stimuli of the esophageal mucosa. Additionally, central sensitization at the brain level or the dorsal horn of the spinal cord may modulate afferent neural function and thus enhance perception of intraesophageal stimuli [56]. What causes peripheral or central sensitization remains to be determined. Studies have shown that acute tissue irritation results in subsequent peripheral and central sensitization, which is manifested as increased background activity of sensory neurons, lowering of nociceptive thresholds, changes in stimulus–response curves, and enlargements of receptive fields [57]. Peripheral sensitization involves a reduction in esophageal pain threshold and an increase in the transduction processes of primary afferent neurons. Esophageal tissue injury, inflammation, spasm, or repetitive mechanical stimuli can all sensitize peripheral afferent nerves. The presence of esophageal hypersensitivity can be subsequently demonstrated long after the original stimulus is no longer present and the esophageal mucosa has healed.

Several studies have demonstrated that patients with non–GERD-related NCCP have lower perception thresholds for pain. Barish et al. evaluated 50 patients with NCCP and 30 healthy volunteers using a graded balloon distention protocol [58]. Of the patients with NCCP, 56% experienced their "typical" chest pain during balloon distention as compared to 20% of the normal controls. Of those with NCCP who experienced pain, 86% reported pain at volumes less than 8 mL. There was no difference in esophageal tone between the two groups.

Rao et al. used impedance planimetry to evaluate 24 patients with NCCP and 12 healthy controls, and demonstrated that during balloon distention those with NCCP had lower perception thresholds for first sensation, moderate discomfort, and pain in comparison to healthy controls [59]. Rao et al. also performed graded balloon distentions of the esophagus using impedance planimetry in 16 consecutive patients with NCCP (normal esophageal evaluation) and 13 healthy controls [60]. Patients who experienced chest pain during the balloon distention were subsequently restudied after receiving intravenous atropine. Balloon distentions reproduced chest pain at lower sensory thresholds than controls in most NCCP subjects. Similar findings were documented after atropine administration despite a relaxed and more deformable esophageal wall. Thus, the investigators concluded that hyperalgesia, rather than motor dysfunction, is the predominant mechanism for functional chest pain.

Sarkar et al. recruited 19 healthy volunteers and seven patients with NCCP. Hydrochloric acid was infused into the distal esophagus over a period of 30 min [61]. Sensory responses to electrical stimulation were monitored within the acid-exposed distal esophagus and the non-exposed proximal esophagus both before and after infusion. In the healthy subjects, acid infusion into the distal esophagus lowered the pain threshold in the upper esophagus. Patients with NCCP already had a lower resting esophageal pain threshold than healthy subjects. After acid perfusion, their pain threshold in the proximal esophagus fell even further and for a longer duration than was the case for the healthy subjects (Figure 2.3). Additionally, there was a decrease in the pain threshold of the anterior chest wall after acid infusion. This study demonstrated the development of secondary allodynia (visceral hypersensitivity to an innocuous stimulus

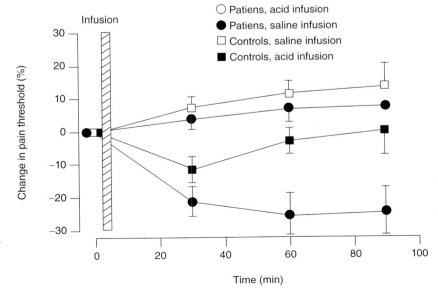

Figure 2.3 Mean change in pain threshold of the upper esophagus after 5-min infusion of acid or saline into the lower esophagus (non-cardiac chest pain vs control). (modified from Sarkar et al. [61], with permission).

in normal tissue that is in proximity to the site of tissue injury) in the proximal esophagus by repeated acid exposure of the distal esophagus. The concurrent visceral and somatic pain hypersensitivity is, most likely, caused by central sensitization (increase in excitability of spinal cord neurons induced by activation of nociceptive C-fibers in the area of the tissue injury). The patients with NCCP demonstrated both visceral hypersensitivity and amplified secondary allodynia in the esophagus.

In another study, perceptual responses to intraluminal esophageal balloon distention (using electronic barostat) were recorded in subjects who underwent either 0.1 N HCl or normal saline perfusion of the distal esophagus [62]. Acid perfusion was associated with reduced sensation thresholds (perception of an innocuous stimulus) and tended to reduce pain thresholds (perception of an aversive stimulus). The study demonstrated short-term sensitization of mechanosensitive afferent pathways by transient exposure to acid. It was suggested that in patients with NCCP, acid reflux induces sensitization of the esophagus and this may subsequently alter the way in which otherwise normal esophageal distentions are perceived.

Sarkar *et al.* evaluated the response of visceral hypersensitivity to acid suppression [63]. Fourteen patients with GERD-related NCCP and eight healthy controls were studied. All subjects underwent an esophageal electrical stimulation protocol in the proximal esophagus and those with NCCP demonstrated lower perception thresholds for pain than normal controls. After a 6-week course of high-dose PPI (omeprazole 20 mg twice daily), there was an increase in the perception thresholds for pain during electrical stimulation in the group of patients with NCCP (Figure 2.4). This study demonstrated that patients with NCCP and evidence of GERD have a component of esophageal hypersensitivity that is responsive to high-dose PPI therapy.

Abnormal cerebral processing of visceral stimulation

During the early 1990s, investigators suggested that NCCP patients demonstrate altered central processing of intraesophageal stimuli [64]. Investigators have used cerebral-evoked potentials as an objective measurement to assess the subjective sensation of pain by NCCP patients. In response to esophageal balloon distention, evoked potential quality scores and amplitude of the major peaks increased significantly with increased sensation, both in NCCP patients and healthy controls. However, in NCCP patients, quality score and amplitude of all four peaks of the evoked potentials were lower, and latencies of two of the four peaks were longer than in the controls. The volumes of air required to produce the various sensations were lower in the NCCP patients. The investigators concluded that increased perception of esophageal stimulation in NCCP patients is caused by altered cortical processing of intraesophageal stimuli. Kamath *et al.* studied the effect of esophageal electrical stimulation on cortical evoked potentials in patients with NCCP. The authors demonstrated that in patients with NCCP, the evoked potentials were of greater amplitude and the peak latencies were slightly longer than in controls [65]. They concluded that increased perception of esophageal stimulation in NCCP reflects an altered cortical processing of visceral sensation.

Hollerbach *et al.*, who studied 20 subjects (eight with NCCP and 12 healthy controls), demonstrated an abnormal cerebral processing of esophageal stimuli in patients with NCCP. Cortical-evoked responses were lower in intensity during electrical esophageal stimulation in patients with NCCP in comparison to the healthy controls. Because of the smaller cortical-evoked potentials, it was hypothesized that the increased perception of esophageal stimuli might in fact be the result of enhanced cerebral processing of visceral sensory input rather than hyperalgesic responses of visceral afferent pathways [55].

Positron emission tomography (PET) and functional magnetic resonance imaging (fMRI) have been increasingly used to evaluate the brain–gut relationship in patients with functional bowel disorders. However, thus far there are no studies using any of these techniques in patients with NCCP.

Altered autonomic activity

Tougas *et al.* have performed several studies exploring autonomic nervous system function and its role in the pathogenesis of NCCP. In one study, autonomic activity was assessed using spectral analysis of heart rate variability, before and during distal esophageal acidification of patients with NCCP and matched healthy controls [66]. Of those with NCCP,

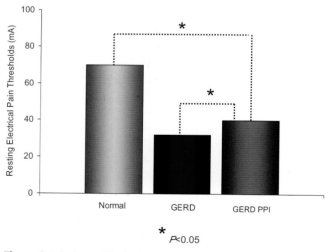

Figure 2.4 Patients with chest pain and occult gastroesophageal reflux (GERD) demonstrate visceral pain hypersensitivity that may be partially responsive to acid suppression with a proton pump inhibitor (PPI) (modified from Sarkar *et al.* [63], with permission).

68% developed angina-like symptoms during the esophageal acidification. These patients had a higher baseline heart rate and a lower baseline vagal activity than patients without acid sensitivity. During acid infusion, vagal cardiac outflow increased in acid-sensitive patients as compared to patients without acid sensitivity. Additionally, Tougas *et al.* have documented increased vagal activity in patients with NCCP during other intraesophageal stimuli, both mechanical and electrical. These studies indicate that autonomic dysregulation may be present in at least a subset of patients with NCCP [67]. The authors further hypothesized that increased perception of esophageal stimulation may also reflect an exaggerated brainstem response. However, it was further hypothesized that in most cases in which both central and autonomic factors are involved, central factors will likely lead to autonomic dysregulation.

Psychologic comorbidity

Between 17% and 43% of patients with NCCP are estimated to suffer from some type of psychologic abnormality [68]. Psychologic comorbidity can modulate esophageal perception and cause subjects to perceive low-intensity esophageal stimuli as being painful [69–72]. Anxiety, depression, neuroticism, and hypochondriac behavior have all been described in NCCP patients [73–76]. However, these findings have been inconsistent when NCCP patients were compared to subjects with CAD, with some authors reporting increased anxiety and depression in NCCP patients and others reporting no significant difference between the two disorders. In a large population-based study in Australia, a random sample of 1000 residents in the Sydney area were surveyed [15]. Among those with NCCP, the prevalence of anxiety was 23% and of depression 7%. In a telephone survey from Hong Kong that included 2209 subjects, it was demonstrated that depression and anxiety were significantly more common in NCCP patients than in those without NCCP [77].

Among all esophageal symptoms, chest pain was shown to closely correlate with psychometric abnormalities. In some patients, chest pain is part of a host of symptoms that characterize panic attack [11]. Panic attack is a common cause for emergency room visits due to chest pain. In a large study that encompassed 441 consecutive ambulatory patients presenting with chest pain to the emergency department of a heart center, 25% were diagnosed as suffering from a panic disorder [78]. Whilst the reason for the observed association between NCCP and panic disorder remains to be fully understood, hyperventilation was demonstrated to precipitate chest pain in 15% of the patients with NCCP [79]. Additionally, it was demonstrated that hyperventilation could provoke reversible esophageal manometric abnormalities, such as esophageal spasm (4%) and a non-specific esophageal motor disorder (22%) [80]. It was also shown that HRQOL scores in NCCP patients with panic disorder were significantly lower than those in NCCP patients without panic disorder [25]. All SF-36 domains were affected and the values were similar to those of panic disorder patients seeking treatment in psychiatric care [25].

NCCP patients with psychologic disorders show diminished QOL, more frequent chest pain, and less treatment satisfaction than NCCP patients without psychologic comorbidity [81]. One study suggested that NCCP patients with more than one psychologic disorder are more difficult to treat than those with a single psychologic disorder [82].

Diagnosis

GERD should be excluded first in all NCCP patients who are referred to a gastroenterologist. GERD as a cause of NCCP appears to be common knowledge that traverses specialties and subspecialties [18–20]. Consequently, empiric therapy directed towards GERD is common in clinical practice as the initial management strategy. Presently, there is no gold standard for diagnosing GERD-related NCCP. The currently available diagnostic tests to detect GERD in patients with NCCP include barium swallow, upper endoscopy, acid perfusion test, pH testing, esophageal impedance + pH sensor, and the PPI test.

Barium esophagram

The barium esophagram has very little use in the diagnosis of GERD. It has a low sensitivity (20%) for diagnosing GERD in general due to lack of anatomic and mucosal abnormalities in most GERD patients. Furthermore, the significance of barium reflux during the procedure as a diagnostic for GERD is questionable. Johnston *et al.* found that the proportion of patients with an abnormal 24-h esophageal pH study was similar to the proportion of patients with a normal study and who had spontaneous barium reflux during the test [83]. Additionally, spontaneous barium reflux has been demonstrated in up to 20% of healthy subjects [84].

The role of the barium esophagram is unclear in patients with GERD-related NCCP, primarily due to the rare presence of esophageal mucosal abnormalities. However, performing a barium esophagram may be considered as the initial diagnostic test in patients who report dysphagia in addition to chest pain.

Upper endoscopy

Once a patient is referred to a gastroenterologist for evaluation of NCCP, if any alarm symptoms (decreased appetite, weight loss, dysphagia, odynophagia, hematemesis, and anemia) are present, an upper endoscopy is warranted to rule out mucosal abnormalities, such as benign or malignant tumors, esophageal ulceration or peptic stricture.

In the 1990s, the routine use of endoscopy in the evaluation of NCCP was recommended by the American

Gastroenterological Association guidelines for chest pain of esophageal origin [85]. Since then, several studies have reported a variable rate of diagnostic yield in NCCP. In one of the earlier endoscopic studies, Hsia *et al.* evaluated 100 consecutive patients with NCCP and demonstrated that 38% of the patients had a normal test, 24% had erosive esophagitis (grades II–IV), 18% had gastritis and/or duodenitis, 14% had a sliding hiatal hernia without evidence of erosive esophagitis, and 6% had gastric or duodenal ulcers [86].

In the largest study thus far addressing the role of upper endoscopy in NCCP, Dickman *et al.* reported mucosal findings from 3688 consecutive patients undergoing endoscopic evaluation for NCCP [34]. Patients were seen in 76 community, university, and Veteran Administration Centers. Of the NCCP patients, 44% had a normal endoscopy. In those with an abnormal endoscopy, 28.6% had hiatal hernia, 19.4% erosive esophagitis, 4.4% Barrett's esophagus, 3.6% esophageal stricture or stenosis, and 2% peptic ulcer. The authors concluded that most of the mucosal findings in NCCP patients were GERD related. A significant finding of this study was that 4.4% of the patients with NCCP were also found to have Barrett's esophagus. This was significantly lower than the Barrett's esophagus rate (9.1%) found in GERD patients in the same study. Two other small studies have also reported the presence of Barrett's esophagus in 5.2–6.7% of NCCP patients undergoing upper endoscopy [87, 88].

In conclusion, the value of upper endoscopy in NCCP is limited, because the anatomic findings are primarily related to GERD (Table 2.3). Potentially, the test may be indicated as a screening tool for Barrett's esophagus in GERD-related NCCP.

Ambulatory 24-h esophageal pH monitoring

Ambulatory 24-h esophageal pH monitoring with symptom correlation is still commonly used to evaluate patients with NCCP [89]. Approximately 50–60% of the NCCP patients have abnormal esophageal acid exposure or a positive symptom index alone. However, the presence of abnormal distal esophageal acid exposure during pH testing does not necessarily imply that the patient's chest pain is GERD related. Richter *et al.* examined 100 consecutive patients

with NCCP and detected abnormal acid exposure in 48% [89]. Of the 83 patients who had spontaneous chest pain during the study, 37 (46%) had abnormal reflux parameters, and 50 (60%) had a normal study but a positive symptom index (calculated as the percentage of symptoms that were associated with acid reflux events). The authors concluded that 24-h esophageal pH testing with symptom index is the single best test for evaluating patients with NCCP. In contrast, Dekel *et al.* demonstrated that a positive symptom index is a relatively uncommon phenomenon in NCCP patients because most do not experience chest pain during the pH study [35].

Overall, the pH test is invasive, inconvenient to patients, costly, and not readily available to many physicians. Additionally, the yield of the test in NCCP has not been rigorously assessed. This is compounded by the rarity of chest pain symptoms during the test in many patients, making it difficult to determine the relationship between patients' symptoms and acid reflux events [90].

pH testing appears to be of value in patients with NCCP in whom objective evidence of abnormal esophageal acid exposure is required (off therapy), e.g. in patients with NCCP who are candidates for antireflux surgery. Otherwise, the role of pH testing in NCCP is relatively limited. In NCCP patients who have failed PPI twice daily for at least 2 months, the pH test is likely to be normal [91].

While impedance + pH sensor have been proposed to be more sensitive in evaluating patients with typical or atypical manifestations of GERD who have failed at least twice-daily PPI, studies addressing NCCP patients specifically are still lacking [92, 93]. This is compounded by the fact that the role of non-acidic reflux in causing NCCP remains to be elucidated.

Wireless pH system

The wireless Bravo (Medtronic, Shoreview, MN, USA) pH monitoring system is a "catheterless" pH system. It involves the attachment of a radiotelemetry pH capsule to the wall of the esophagus. It simultaneously measures pH and transmits data to a pager-sized receiver clipped onto the patient's belt, thereby circumventing the need for a nasally placed pH catheter, which is uncomfortable for many patients. Unlike

Table 2.3 Endoscopic mucosal findings in patients with noncardiac chest pain.

Study	n	Normal (%)	Erosive esophagitis (%)	Barrett's esophagus (%)	Hiatal hernia (%)	Other (%)
Hsia *et al.* [86]	100	38	24	0	14	Peptic ulcer: 6
						Gastritis/duodenitis: 18
Frobert *et al.* [258]	49	N/A	31	N/A	N/A	6
Wong *et al.* [259]	78	90	2.6	0	N/A	Peptic ulcer: 7
Battaglia *et al.* [260]	61	N/A	10	N/A	N/A	N/A
Dickman *et al.* [34]	3688	44	19.4	4.4	28.6	Stricture/stenosis: 3.6

the traditional pH catheter system, the wireless pH system can collect data for 48 h or even longer. The system is well tolerated, reliable, and provides reproducible results [94].

Prakash *et al.* found that by extending the recording time to 48 h, using the wireless pH system, the number of subjects recording symptoms during the test increased by 6.8% and the number of symptoms available for association with an acid reflux event was doubled [95]. The study also demonstrated that patients with NCCP benefited the most from extending the duration of the pH test. In the only study available addressing the impact of extended pH testing (48 h) in patients with NCCP, the same authors demonstrated that the wireless pH system increased the detection of patients with an abnormal pH test and/or positive reflux–symptom association probability. Overall, extending pH testing to 48 h provided meaningful information in 19.4% of the NCCP patients [96].

In conclusion, extended wireless pH testing provides a modest but meaningful advantage in the evaluation of patients with NCCP that is suspected to be GERD related. It increases the window of opportunity for detecting more symptoms associated with gastroesophageal reflux events.

Proton pump inhibitor test

The PPI test (or short therapeutic trial) is defined as a short course of high-dose PPI for diagnosing GERD. This is a simple and non-invasive diagnostic tool for GERD. It is readily available and at the disposal of every PCP. Additionally, it increases the role of PCPs in evaluating and treating patients with different manifestations of GERD. It also offers significant cost savings when compared to the other diagnostic tests for GERD [32, 97].

The doses used in the PPI test have ranged from 40 to 80 mg/day for omeprazole; 30 to 60 mg/day for lansoprazole; and 40 mg.day for rabeprazole, over a duration of treatment of 1–28 days, in patients with symptoms suggestive of GERD or NCCP [28, 30, 31, 33, 98–105]. By far the most commonly used PPI in most of the PPI test trials is omeprazole, which has led to the term the "omeprazole test" [28, 32, 97–104]. However, studies using other PPIs have demonstrated that they are equally efficacious in short therapeutic trials [30, 31, 33].

An important factor in determining the sensitivity of a PPI test is the definition of a positive test. In most studies, a symptom score cut-off was used: if the symptom assessment scores for heartburn, chest pain, or other symptoms improved by more than 50–75% (depending on the study) relative to baseline, the test was considered positive. As with any diagnostic test, the optimal cut-off is critical in defining test accuracy [105]. The symptom score cut-off values that were used among studies that evaluated PPI tests for GERD were chosen arbitrarily. Rarely, studies calculated the receiver operator curve (ROC) by varying the percentage reduction in the symptom tested to ascertain the optimal value for detecting patients with GERD [32, 97, 105]. This cut-off point provides the greatest sensitivity, specificity, positive predictive value, and accuracy of the short therapeutic trial tested.

The diagnostic accuracy of the PPI test is limited by the lack of a gold standard for the diagnosis of GERD. In the absence of a gold standard, studies evaluating the PPI test have used a combination of upper endoscopy and ambulatory 24-h esophageal pH monitoring as the closest approximation to a gold standard. Factors that may determine the sensitivity of the PPI test include type of antireflux medication used, dosage, treatment duration, definition of a positive test (symptom score cut-off, change in symptom grading, ROC analysis), and the GERD-related symptom evaluated. Only one study attempted to compare the accuracy of the PPI test to 24-h esophageal pH monitoring in diagnosing GERD [106]. The study used the presence of erosive esophagitis as indicative of GERD in patients who were not on Aspirin or non-steroidal anti-inflammatory drugs. Thirty-five patients were included, and they underwent both pH testing and the PPI test (omeprazole 40 mg before breakfast and 20 mg before dinner). The PPI test was significantly more sensitive than total acid contact time during pH testing (83% vs 60%, $P < .03$). The sensitivity of the pH test increased to 80% only after adding patients with a positive symptom index, and patients with abnormal acid contact time, in the supine and/or erect positions despite normal total acid contact time. The authors concluded that the PPI test was at least as sensitive as ambulatory 24-h esophageal pH monitoring in diagnosing GERD in patients with documented erosive esophagitis.

In different studies, the sensitivity of the PPI test for GERD-related NCCP ranged from 69% to –95% and the specificity from 67% to 86% [28, 32, 33, 103, 104, 107]. The dosages of PPIs used ranged from 60 to 80 mg/day for omeprazole [28, 32, 103, 104]; 30 to 90 mg for lansoprazole [33]; and 40 mg for rabeprazole [108]. The trial durations ranged from 1 to 28 days.

In a double-blind, placebo-controlled trial, 37 patients with NCCP were randomized to either placebo or high-dose omeprazole (40 mg before breakfast and 20 mg before dinner) for 7 days [32]. After a wash-out period and repeated baseline symptom assessment, patients crossed over to the opposite arm. The PPI test was considered positive if the chest pain improved by at least 50% after treatment. The presence of GERD-related anatomic changes during upper endoscopy and/or abnormal 24-h esophageal pH monitoring was used as the gold standard for diagnosing NCCP. Sixty-two percent (23 of 37) of the patients had evidence by both or one of the diagnostic tools as having GERD. Of the GERD-positive group, 78.3% had a positive PPI test, and 22.7% had a positive placebo response. In contrast, of the GERD-negative group, 14.2% had a positive PPI test and 7.1% had a positive placebo response. Thus, the calculated sensitivity was 78.3%, specificity 85.7%, and the positive predictive value was 90%. When different percentages in chest pain symptom reduction were evaluated, as previously mentioned, the greatest accuracy of predicting GERD-related NCCP was obtained with 65% symptom reduction, producing a sensitivity of 85.7% and specificity of 90.9%. Using a similar design, other investigators confirmed the usefulness of the PPI test for diagnosing GERD-related NCCP [28, 33]. Furthermore, subsequent studies demonstrated that short therapeutic trials with PPIs other than omeprazole achieved similar efficacy for the diagnosis of GERD-related NCCP [30, 31, 33].

The PPI test in NCCP has been scrutinized in two meta-analyses. In the first, the pooled risk ratio for continued chest pain after PPI therapy was 0.54 (95% CI 0.41–0.71) [109]. The overall number needed to treat was 3 (95% CI 2–4). The pooled sensitivity, specificity, and diagnostic odds ratio for the PPI test versus 24-h esophageal pH monitoring and upper endoscopy were 80%, 73%, and 13.83 (95% CI 5.48–34.91), respectively. The authors concluded that PPI therapy reduces symptoms in NCCP and may be useful as a diagnostic test in identifying abnormal esophageal acid reflux. Wang *et al.* have also performed a meta-analysis of the PPI test in patients with NCCP [110]. The overall sensitivity and specificity of a PPI test were 80% (95% CI 71%–87%) and 74% (95% CI 64%–83%), respectively, compared with 19% (95% CI 12%–29%) and 77% (95% CI 62%–87%), respectively, in the placebo group. The PPI test showed significantly higher discriminative power, with a summary diagnostic odds ratio of 19.35 (95% CI 8.54–43.84) compared to 0.61 (95% CI 0.20–1.86) in the placebo group. Thus, the authors concluded that the use of PPI treatment as a diagnostic test for detecting GERD in patients with NCCP has an acceptable sensitivity and specificity, and could be used as an initial approach by PCPs to detect GERD in selected patients with NCCP.

There is evidence that when using the PPI test, there is a significant correlation between the extent of esophageal acid exposure in the distal esophagus as determined by ambulatory 24-h esophageal pH monitoring and the change in symptom intensity score after treatment, suggesting that the higher the esophageal acid exposure, the greater the response to the PPI test in patients with GERD-related NCCP [36].

Economic analysis also showed that the PPI test for GERD-related NCCP is a cost-saving approach, primarily due to significant reduction in the usage of various costly, invasive diagnostic tests [32]. In patients with NCCP, the PPI test was evaluated using a cost minimization analysis. The PPI test was found to save US$573 per average patient with NCCP undergoing diagnostic evaluation. The test was associated with an 81% reduction in the number of upper endoscopies and 79% reduction in the number of ambulatory 24-h esophageal pH tests. This significant reduction is due to the high positive predictive value of the PPI test for patients with GERD-related NCCP.

When a decision-analytic model utilizing Bayesian analysis was developed to compare the costs and outcomes of alternative diagnostic strategies for NCCP, non-invasive strategies utilizing the PPI test as the initial step resulted in significant cost savings as compared to invasive strategies [111]. These cost savings were the direct result of a significant reduction in the utilization of invasive diagnostic tests that are of unproven utility in the diagnosis and subsequent management of patients with NCCP.

Esophageal manometry

Esophageal manometry is one of the best tools to detect motor disorders of the esophagus. The test provides an assessment of the amplitude of the esophageal contraction wave, its configuration and propagation, as well as the function of the upper and lower esophageal sphincters [112].

In approximately a third of patients with non–GERD-related NCCP, various esophageal motility abnormalities have been described [42, 43]. Thus, in NCCP, esophageal manometry is commonly performed if GERD has been initially excluded as the underlying cause [10].

The relationship between motility abnormalities diagnosed in NCCP patients and chest pain remains controversial. In a large retrospective study of patients with NCCP, only 28% were found to have esophageal dysmotility during esophageal manometry [42]. Nutcracker esophagus was the most common motility disorder (48%), followed by non-specific esophageal motility disorder (36%), DES (10%), hypertensive LES (4%), and achalasia (2%).

In NCCP patients with esophageal dysmotility, some have stipulated that esophageal spasm, for example, may be the cause of chest pain either by distending the proximal segment of the esophagus (activation of mechanoreceptors) or by producing myoischemia (activation of chemoreceptors). However, in patients with NCCP, documented esophageal manometry abnormalities are rarely associated with symptoms.

The role of esophageal manometry in NCCP has evolved over the last few years, primarily due to lack of effective treatment for the various esophageal motility abnormalities. This was compounded by clinical evidence that patients with non–GERD-related NCCP, who were treated with pain modulators, reported symptom improvement regardless of whether or not esophageal dysmotility was present (except for achalasia) [113]. Consequently, the role of esophageal manometry in non–GERD-related NCCP appears to be limited to identifying the small number of patients with achalasia who present with chest pain only [44].

Pharmacologically-induced provocative tests

Edrophonium (Tensilon) test

Edrophonium is an anticholinesterase that increases cholinergic activity at muscarinic receptors [114]. The aim of the edrophonium test is to induce greater esophageal body amplitude contractions in the hope of provoking the patient's typical chest pain [115]. The sensitivity of the edrophonium test is relatively low and has varied from as high as 55% to as low as 0% [46, 116–118]. Presently, the test is rarely used in clinical practice.

Bethanechol test

The bethanechol test is presently rarely performed in clinical practice because of its questionable diagnostic value and frequent side effects. Bethanechol chloride, a cholinergic agonist, is a synthetic ester that is structurally and pharmacologically related to acetylcholine and induces chest pain in 12–33% of NCCP patients [119–121]. Side effects reported after the bethanechol test included symptomatic bradycardia requiring atropine treatment, hypotension, headache, increased salivation, sweating, and nervousness, among others [115].

Ergonovine test

The intravenous ergonovine stimulation test has been demonstrated to induce augmentation of esophageal contractions and chest pain in many NCCP patients [122]. Ergonovine is a sympathomimetic agent of the ergoalkaloid group. Because side effects are common and serious cardiac effects and even death have been reported, the test should not be used for standard esophageal testing [123].

Pentagastrin stimulation test

Pentagastrin directly stimulates esophageal smooth muscle, especially in patients with primary esophageal dysmotility. Its sensitivity to inducing pain in patients with NCCP is low, and the drug is no longer used for NCCP provocative testing.

High-frequency intraluminal ultrasonography

High-frequency intraluminal ultrasonography has been recently introduced as a novel modality to study the relationship between esophageal motor events and symptoms. The technique has been a useful tool for evaluating smooth muscle contractions [53]. Esophageal ultrasonography can be performed continuously using a catheter-based probe, which allows direct visualization of changes in smooth muscle conformation [52]. The capability of intraluminal ultrasonography to evaluate changes in the thickness of the longitudinal muscle of the esophagus has been used to determine the relationship between esophageal symptoms and motor changes of the esophageal wall. Although the technique is yet to be standardized, investigators have used an esophageal catheter assembly that included a 12.5-MHz ultrasound transducer, solid-state pressure catheter, and monocrystant antimony pH catheter [52]. The ultrasound transducer was placed 5 cm above the LES. The 24-h recordings were analyzed every 2 s for a period of 2 min before and 30 s after the onset of the studied symptom. Rules for image analysis remain at the discretion of the investigator. Because of the limited number of centers that are proficient with this technique, image analysis is primarily operator dependent, and interobserver and intraobserver agreements have yet to be determined.

Even though high-frequency intraluminal ultrasonography has been a valuable research tool to assess the biomechanics of the human esophagus, its exact role in evaluating esophageal-related symptoms has not been fully elucidated [124]. Sustained contractions of the esophageal longitudinal muscle may represent an epiphenomenon that occurs with symptoms, rather than being the trigger for symptoms.

Acid perfusion test (Bernstein test)

Bernstein and Baker introduced the acid perfusion test as an objective method to identify esophageal chemosensitivity to acid [125]. A nasogastric tube was passed through the nares of a fasting, sitting subject and into the stomach [125, 126]. After the gastric content was aspirated, the tube was withdrawn until it measured 30 cm from the nares to the tip [126]. This maneuver assumed that the solution would be delivered at a level near the junction of the upper and middle thirds of the esophagus. The tube was connected to an intravenous bottle. A control administration of 0.9% NaCl was perfused for 10–15 min at a rate of 6–7.5 mL/min. This was followed by administration of 0.1 N HCl acid, at a similar rate, for 30 min or until discomfort was induced [126]. If symptoms appeared, the test was discontinued and saline solution was given.

The acid perfusion test was originally devised to distinguish between chest pain of cardiac and esophageal origin. However, since the initial description, many modifications have been made to the original Bernstein test. Although the basic principal of the test remained similar, many investigators have tried different acid perfusion rates, concentrations, and durations in the hope of increasing the sensitivity of the test [89, 127–133]. Furthermore, some have even suggested the addition of bile salts to the acid solution [134]. Others required that, for a result to be positive, the acid-induced symptoms should quickly disappear with the reinfusion of saline or bicarbonate [119].

Many attempts were made to change the test from a qualitative to a quantitative tool. Time to onset of symptoms during acid perfusion was used to compare the extent of chemosensitivity to acid between GERD and Barrett's patients [135]. Fass *et al.* placed a manometry catheter 10 cm above the upper border of the LES to ensure sufficient exposure of the esophageal mucosa to acid [56]. Saline was infused initially for 2 min, and then without the patient's knowledge 0.1 N HCl acid was infused for 10 min at a rate of 10 mL/min. Patients were instructed to report whenever their typical symptoms were reproduced. Esophageal chemosensitivity was assessed by both the duration until typical symptom perception was induced (expressed in seconds) and the total sensory intensity rating reported by the subject at the end of acid perfusion by using a verbal descriptor scale. The scale consisted of a 20-cm vertical bar flanked by descriptors of increasing intensity (no sensation, faint, very weak, weak, very mild, mild, moderate, barely strong, slightly intense, strong, intense, very intense, and extremely intense). Placement of words along each scale was determined from their relative log intensity rating in a normative study [136]. The validity of these scales for assessing the perceived intensity of visceral sensations has been confirmed [137].

An acid perfusion test intensity score (cm x s) was then calculated as follows:

$$I \times T/100$$

where I is the total intensity rating at the end of acid perfusion and T is the duration of report of typical symptom perception during the test. For convenience, the score was divided by 100.

Although the test appears to be highly specific, its sensitivity is relatively low, with figures ranging from 6% to almost 60% [46, 116–118, 138]. A negative test result has little clinical value and does not exclude an esophageal origin of the chest pain. Patients with Barrett's esophagus have been reported to demonstrate a decrease in esophageal chemosensitivity to acid, resulting in even more false-negative results [135]. However, this alteration in pain perception disappeared after esophageal ablation resulted in complete Barrett's reversal [139].

Presently, the acid perfusion test is rarely performed in clinical practice due to its limited diagnostic value in NCCP and other esophageal disorders. The modified version of the test is still used as a research tool to assess esophageal chemosensitivity to acid.

Electrical stimulation

Electrical stimulation of the esophagus has been used by very few research groups to study esophageal sensitivity and cortical responses to different intensities of intraesophageal stimuli. The technique has yet to be standardized and published protocols are difficult to compare. The technique is currently used only as a research tool.

Electrical stimulation of the esophageal mucosa is performed using a stainless steel electrode attached to a standard manometric catheter assembly [140, 141]. Electrical stimuli are applied repeatedly in a series of 24 stimuli (duration 200 μs at 0.2 Hz). A reference electrode is placed on the abdominal wall. Electrical stimulation of the upper and lower esophagus can be achieved with two pairs of electrodes located at 5 and 20 cm proximal to the tip of the catheter [61]. The ascending stimulus paradigm includes stimuli that are delivered at a frequency of 0.2 Hz at intensi-

ties between 0 and 100 mA [61]. Severity and qualitative perceptual responses are usually assessed by a verbal descriptor [142]. The sensory threshold is the intensity (measured in mA) at which the participant reports faint sensation, and the pain threshold is the intensity at which the participant reports an intense sensation [61]. Different stimulus paradigms have been used in various studies [55].

Balloon distention

Balloon distention has been used primarily for research purposes to determine perception thresholds for pain. This modality has been used extensively in studies of various functional bowel disorders, most notably IBS, functional dyspepsia, and NCCP [143–145].

More than 40 years ago, intraesophageal balloon distention in humans was reported to produce pain referred to the chest [146]. Early data indicated that, in patients with documented ischemic heart disease, balloon distention of the esophagus produced pain indistinguishable from anginal pain, but without electrocardiographic changes [147]. This may be explained by convergence of sensory pathways at the level of the spinal cord or in the midbrain. Despite this similarity in pain, it seems that esophageal balloon distention by itself has no effect on coronary function or blood flow [148].

Several painful clinical syndromes are associated with esophageal distention. These include esophageal dilation and aperistalsis induced by the ingestion of cold liquids [149], acute food impaction, the drinking of carbonated beverages [150], and dysfunction of the belch reflex [151]. It has also been suggested that esophageal pain is, at times, due to esophageal dilation secondary to a lack of coordination between the esophageal body and the LES [152].

The introduction of the electronic barostat, a computer-driven volume-displacement device, has helped to ensure proper location of the balloon, regardless of the inflation paradigm that was used [153]. The basic principle of the barostat is to maintain a constant pressure within the balloon/bag in the lumen despite muscular contractions and relaxations [153, 154]. To maintain a constant pressure, the barostat aspirates air with contractions and injects air with relaxations. Presently, many prefer the use of a polyethylene bag to that of a latex balloon. Bags are infinitely compliant and show no increase in intrabag pressure until about 90% of the maximum bag volume has been achieved [153, 155]. In contrast, latex balloons resist inflation and thus show a rapid increase in intraballoon pressure with small volumes of distention [153, 156]. When the pressure increases above the elastance threshold, the balloon becomes plastic and accommodates large volumes of air with very little change in pressure [125, 126]. For tubular organs in the gastrointestinal tract, such as the esophagus, experts recommend the use of a cylindrical (rather than a spherical) bag with a fixed length [56, 153].

Barostat has been used extensively in studies evaluating rectosigmoid and gastric perception thresholds for pain. However, this technique has been rarely used to assess esophageal mechanosensitivity in humans. Unlike the rectum and the stomach, the esophagus does not serve as a storage organ, but rather as a conduit. Consequently, intraesophageal distentions do not mimic a normal, physiologic stimulus, and thus perceptual responses to such a stimulus may have no scientific merit. This factor, in addition to the patient's difficulties in tolerating balloon distention, which commonly results in poor recruitment rates as well as the potential for esophageal perforation, have made esophageal balloon distentions by a barostat a less attractive research tool.

Various distention protocols have been used in different studies. Like any other technique that assesses esophageal sensation, balloon distention has yet to be standardized. Slow ramp distention is an ascending method that involves slow (rate varies from one study to another) increase in volume or pressure of the balloon usually until the desired perceptual response has been reported by the subject [56, 62, 157]. In contrast, phasic distentions are rapid inflations of the balloon that can be delivered in random sequence or double random staircase [56, 62]. The latter includes two series of distention stimuli (staircases), and the computer alternates between the two staircases on a random basis. With the tracking method, the barostat is programmed to deliver a series of intermittent phasic stimuli separated by an interpulse rest period within an interactive stimulus tracking procedure [158, 159]. If the subject indicates a sensation below the tracked intensity, then the following stimulus will increase in pressure. If the subject reports the desired sensation, then the following pressure step is randomized to stay the same or decrease. The random element is placed to mask the relationship between ratings and subsequent stimulus change, and therefore, decrease potential scaling bias.

Quantification of perceptual responses depends on the characteristics of the mechanoreceptors in a specific region of the gastrointestinal tract. Volume or pressure distention can be considered the most physiologic stimuli [145, 160]. The most reliable reports of sensory thresholds are obtained during volume distention. Although the overall pressure–volume curve is linear, the pressure at any given volume may vary because of the presence or absence of a superimposed esophageal phasic contractions [56]. Despite this physiologic phenomenon, other investigators rely primarily on pressure when performing balloon studies in the esophagus.

Commonly, qualitative and quantitative perceptual responses are evaluated during balloon distention studies. Qualitative perceptual responses include symptom reports in response to balloon distention, such as chest pain, heartburn, bloating, and fullness, among others [49, 56].

Heartburn is a common sensation that occurs during balloon distention and may mimic the patient's typical heartburn symptom [49]. Quantitative perceptual responses are commonly obtained during slow-ramp distention and include the minimal distention volume or pressure at which the individual first reports moderate sensation (innocuous sensation), discomfort, and pain (aversive sensation). Discomfort threshold is commonly defined as the first unpleasant esophageal sensation, and the pain threshold is defined as the first sensation of pain [56].

Pitfalls that may modify perceptual responses to balloon distention are presented in Table 2.4 [161]. An increased rate of balloon distention results in reported perception at lower volumes or pressures [162]. Longer durations of balloon distention are more likely to elicit sensation than shorter durations [162]. Elderly subjects demonstrate diminished visceral pain perception and female patients seem to have lower perception thresholds for pain compared with male patients [163–165]. The proximal esophagus has been suggested to be more sensitive to chemical and mechanical stimuli than the distal esophagus [56, 166]. Additionally, reduced sensitivity to intraluminal stimuli has been

Table 2.4 Factors that modulate esophageal sensation [161].

Factors	Effect on sensory response
Rate of balloon inflation	
Increase	Reduced perception threshold for pain
Decrease	Increased perception threshold for pain
Duration of balloon distention	
Longer	Increased sensation
Shorter	Reduced sensation
Gender	
Female	Reduced perception threshold for pain
Male	Increased perception threshold for pain
Age	
Elderly	Increased perception threshold for pain
Younger	Reduced perception threshold for pain
Esophageal region	
Proximal	Reduced perception threshold for pain
	Secondary allodynia in distal portion
Distal	Increased perception threshold for pain
	Secondary allodynia in proximal portion
Patient population	
Barrett's esophagus	Increased perception threshold for pain
Peptic stricture	Increased perception threshold for pain
Functional heartburn	Decreased perception threshold for pain
Anxiety	Decreased perception threshold for pain
Stress	Decreased perception threshold for pain

demonstrated in specific patient populations, such as those with Barrett's mucosa or esophageal stricture [167, 168]. The development of secondary allodynia (visceral hypersensitivity to innocuous stimulus in normal tissue that is in proximity to the site of tissue injury) in the adjacent portion of the esophagus that was not sensitized by a chemical stimulus (acid) was also demonstrated [61].

Balloon distention has been commonly used also to assess the effect of various drugs on esophageal sensory perception. Imipramine [169, 170], octreotide [171], and nifedipine [172, 173] have all been shown to increase perception thresholds for pain in normal controls or patients with NCCP.

Central assessment of esophageal sensation

Esophageal evoked potentials

Cerebral evoked potentials reflect electrical activity of the brain in response to visual, auditory, somatosensory, and visceral stimuli. There is a clear relationship between stimulus frequency, using esophageal electrical stimulation, and amplitude of cerebral evoked potentials [174]. Studies have demonstrated that a significant and progressive decrease of evoked potential amplitudes was documented with increasing stimulus frequency. This suggests a rapid attenuation of the cerebral autonomic responses with increased frequency of electrical stimulation [174]. Furthermore, a dose–response relationship has been shown in brain response to increasing stimulus intensity, which is probably explained by increased recruitment of afferent fibers [174, 175].

Balloon distention and electrical stimulation protocols have been used in studies assessing cerebral evoked potentials in response to esophageal stimulation. It is unclear if one of the sensory tests better than the other.

Esophageal balloon distention triggers a characteristic triphasic evoked potential [176]. Two negative peaks (N1 and N2) and one positive peak (P1) can be demonstrated. Latency is the time in milliseconds from the stimulus to the peak. There is considerable intersubject variability but almost no intrasubject variability when recording cerebral evoked potentials. Studies in normal subjects have shown significantly shorter latencies during balloon distention in the proximal esophagus as compared with the distal esophagus [177].

Assessment of patients with NCCP, using an esophageal balloon distention paradigm, revealed that amplitude and quality of cerebral evoked potentials increased with increasing sensation, while the latencies remained stable [176]. Additionally, the amplitude and quality of evoked potentials were lower in NCCP patients as compared with controls. Similar levels of sensation were produced by lower balloon volumes in NCCP patients [174].

Esophageal stimulation and cerebral evoked potentials may provide clues to the pathway and type of neurons involved in nociception [178]. Additionally, cerebral evoked potentials were used to identify brain areas that are responsible for esophageal pain sensation [179, 180].

Brain imaging

In addition to cortical evoked potentials, other techniques have been increasingly used to evaluate the brain–gut relationship in patients with esophageal disorders. These techniques include PET and fMRI. The gastrointestinal tract is intricately connected to the central nervous system by pathways that are continuously sampling and modulating gut function [152].

PET scanning is an established method to study the functional neuroanatomy of the human brain [153, 154]. Radiolabeled compounds allow the study of biochemical and physiologic processes involved in cerebral metabolism [152]. Tomographic images represent spatial distribution of radioisotopes in the brain. Regional cerebral blood flow is studied with labeled water ($H_2^{15}O$) and glucose metabolism with ^{18}F-labeled fluorodeoxyglucose. Unlike PET, fMRI does not require radioisotopes and hence is considered a safer imaging technique. fMRI detects increases in oxygen concentration in areas of heightened neuronal activity [147, 153, 155]. This imaging technique is best suited for locating the site but not the sequence or duration of neuronal activity. Overall, fMRI provides both anatomic and functional information.

Thus far, only a few studies have attempted to assess the cortical process of esophageal sensation in humans [181, 182]. Studies assessing cerebral activation in patients with NCCP are still unavailable. Furthermore, it would have been of great interest to determine whether there are differences in central processing of intraesophageal stimuli among patients with NCCP, non-erosive reflux disease, or functional heartburn. It is also important to begin to examine the role of psychophysiologic states, such as stress, anxiety, and depression, and their effects on central nuclei involved with perception of esophageal stimuli in patients with NCCP.

Treatment

Treatment for NCCP should be targeted toward the specific underlying mechanism responsible for a patient's symptoms. Since GERD is by far the most common condition observed in patients with NCCP, treatment of GERD is indicated in all patients presenting with NCCP unless a specific alternative diagnosis is present. Table 2.5 provides a general treatment plan and Figure 2.5 provides a proposed management algorithm for NCCP.

Gastroesophageal reflux disease-related non-cardiac chest pain

Lifestyle modifications include elevation of the head of the bed, weight loss, smoking cessation, avoidance of alcohol, coffee, fresh citrus juice, carbonated beverages, and other food products, as well as medications that can exacerbate reflux, such as narcotics, benzodiazepines, and calcium-channel blockers. Whilst these lifestyle modifications are commonly advocated as first-line treatment in GERD patients, there is no evidence to support their efficacy in

GERD-related NCCP. Regardless, enthusiasm about lifestyle modifications is very high among physicians, and thus it is highly likely that GERD-related NCCP subjects will be instructed to follow them [183, 184].

The beneficial effect of acid suppression in NCCP was first suggested by DeMeester *et al.* [29]. The authors reported in an uncontrolled study of 50 patients with GERD-related chest pain that 10 (91%) of 11 surgically treated patients became chest pain free as compared with five (42%) of 12 medically treated patients.

The efficacy of H$_2$RAs in controlling symptoms in patients with GERD-related NCCP has been shown to range from 42% to 52% [185]. In one study, cimetidine (unknown dose) and antacids were shown to be effective in only 42% of the patients with GERD-related NCCP who were followed for a period of 2–3 years [186]. Stepping down GERD therapy from a PPI to an H$_2$RAs has proved to be a disappointing therapeutic strategy in GERD-related NCCP patients.

Very few studies have assessed the value of a full course of PPIs in patients with NCCP. Omeprazole 20 mg twice daily

Table 2.5 Treatment plan for non-cardiac chest pain (NCCP).

GERD-related NCCP	PPIs, double dose for at least 2 months
Dysmotility-related NCCP	• Achalasia: medical, endoscopic, and surgical therapy
	• Nutcracker esophagus: treat for GERD first. If no response, pain modulators
	• Spastic motility disorders: muscle relaxants and pain modulators
Chest pain of presumed esophageal origin	Pain modulators, nonmood altering low dose, and at bed time (long term)

GERD, gastroesophageal reflux disorder, PPI, proton pump inhibitor.

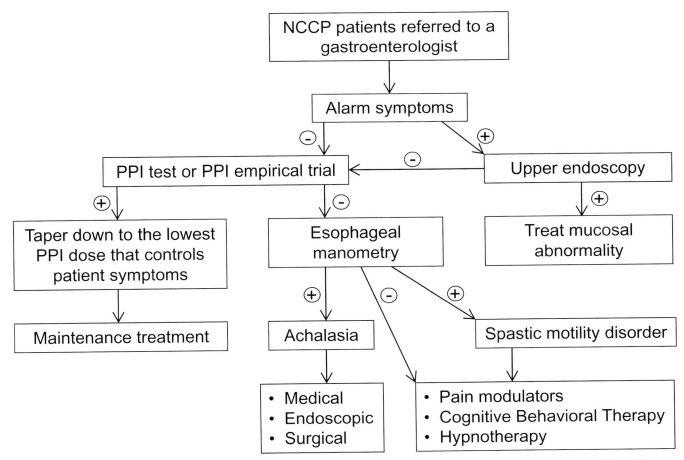

Figure 2.5 Management algorithm for non-cardiac chest pain (NCCP). PPI, proton pump inhibitor (modified from Fass and Navarro-Rodriquez [2], with permission).

or placebo was administered over a period of 8 weeks to GERD-related NCCP patients in the only double-blind, placebo-controlled trial that has been performed thus far [187]. Patients who received omeprazole had a significant reduction in both the number of days with chest pain and in their chest pain severity scores compared to patients who received placebo. Thus far, most of the studies assessing the efficacy of PPIs in NCCP primarily utilized omeprazole. However, it is likely that all other PPIs would demonstrate similar efficacy. In fact, an open-label study using esomeprazole 40 mg/day over a period of 1 month, demonstrated complete resolution of symptoms in 57.1% of patients with either NCCP or laryngeal manifestations of GERD [188]. In another open-label study, 85% of NCCP patients reported symptom relief or improvement after receiving PPI twice daily (different brands) for a period of 3 months [189].

The duration of treatment for GERD-related chest pain has not been critically determined. Three studies have shown successful response to acid inhibition for up to 8 weeks [26, 187, 190] and in one additional study for 6 weeks [191]. Patients with GERD-related NCCP should be treated with at least double the standard dose of PPI until symptoms remit, followed by dose tapering to determine the lowest PPI dose that can control patients' symptoms. As with other extraesophageal manifestations of GERD, NCCP patients may require more than 2 months of therapy for optimal symptom control.

The value of antireflux surgery in GERD-related NCCP is unclear. Several studies have demonstrated a significant improvement in symptoms following laparoscopic fundoplication in patients with GERD-related NCCP. For instance, Patti *et al.* reported improvement in chest pain symptoms following laparoscopic fundoplication in 85% of patients with GERD-related NCCP [192]. Farrell *et al.* reported that 90% of NCCP patients who underwent antireflux surgery experienced improvement in chest pain and 50% reported complete symptom resolution [193]. Rakita *et al.* reported the results of Nissen fundoplication in palliating GERD-associated extraesophageal symptoms including chest pain. Chest pain was noted to be greatly improved or resolved in 81% of the patients [194]. In contrast, So *et al.* reported that after laparoscopic fundoplication, relief of atypical GERD symptoms (e.g. chest pain) was less satisfactory than relief of typical GERD symptoms (e.g. heartburn) [195]. The authors evaluated symptom improvement with a questionnaire given 3 months and 12 months after antireflux surgery. Overall, heartburn was relieved in 93% of patients, whereas only 48% of patients reported relief of chest pain symptoms. Unfortunately, these studies were performed in order to evaluate the effect of surgery on all the GERD-associated extraesophageal symptoms and not specifically for NCCP. None of the surgical studies was a randomized, sham-controlled trial. Also, all available studies originate from tertiary referral centers specializing in the management of esophageal disorders. Further studies are still needed to better determine the role of antireflux surgery in GERD-related NCCP.

Non–gastroesophageal-related non-cardiac chest pain

The treatment of non–GERD-related NCCP is primarily based on esophageal pain modulation. Muscle relaxants appear to have a limited therapeutic value, but are associated with many side effects and thus should be used judiciously. An important development in this field was the recognition that NCCP patients with spastic esophageal motor disorders are more likely to respond to pain modulators than to muscle relaxants. Unfortunately, no large, well-designed studies to assess pain modulators in patients with non–GERD-related NCCP have been performed.

Several recent studies have shown that most NCCP patients are managed by cardiologists and PCPs who appear to know little about the role and treatment of esophageal hypersensitivity in NCCP [18, 19, 196]. Even gastroenterologists appeared somewhat uninformed about the role of visceral hypersensitivity in NCCP [197].

Muscle relaxants

Nitroglycerin and long-acting nitrates cause relaxation of gastrointestinal smooth muscles by stimulating cyclic guanosine monophosphate (cGMP)-dependent pathways. Several open-label studies have reported that nitrates improve symptoms and esophageal motility patterns in patients with chest pain and esophageal dysmotility. Several investigators reported symptomatic improvement in patients with DES, accompanied by normalization of esophageal motility during treatment with nitrates [198, 199]. In a small study, five patients with DES experienced a 4-year clinical and manometric remission when placed on long-term management with long-acting nitrates [200]. However, other studies have failed to demonstrate similar efficacy [201, 202].

Overall, studies that have evaluated the value of nitrates in NCCP have been limited by small numbers of patients and inconsistent results in regard to drug efficacy. However, side effects such as headaches and hypotension have limited their use. It is also possible that patients may become refractory to therapy following long-term use. A placebo-controlled trial that excludes patients with GERD has yet to be performed.

Since calcium plays an important role in esophageal muscle contraction, the role of calcium-channel blocking agents in patients with NCCP and esophageal spastic motility disorders has been the focus of research. Nifedipine (10–30 mg PO tid) decreased the amplitude and duration of esophageal contractions in patients with nutcracker esophagus after only 2 weeks [203]. However, the effect of the drug disappeared after 6 weeks of treatment with the complete recurrence of symptoms. Davies *et al.* used a placebo-controlled trial to assess the efficacy of nifedipine in the prevention of symptomatic episodes of esophageal spasm in eight NCCP patients over a 6-week period [204]. The authors were unable to find statistically significant differences in symptom improvement between the two therapeutic arms. In contrast, symptom improvement was noted in 20 NCCP patients with various esophageal motility disorders, including hypertensive LES, nutcracker esophagus, DES, and vigorous achalasia, treated with nifedipine (10 mg PO tid) [205]. Nifedipine was also found to significantly decrease LES resting pressure, with a direct correlation with the plasma levels of the drug [206].

Diltiazem (60–90 mg PO qid) for 8 weeks significantly improved mean chest pain scores and esophageal motility studies in patients with nutcracker esophagus when compared to placebo [207, 208]. However, in a study evaluating eight patients with DES, the effect of diltiazem in relieving chest pain was no different from that of placebo, possibly due to the small number of patients who participated in the study [209].

Other calcium-channel blockers have been evaluated in patients with primary esophageal motor disorders, including verapamil, fendiline, nimodipine, and nisoldipine, with various effects on LES resting pressure and esophageal amplitude contractions. Regardless, calcium-channel blockers appear to have a transient esophageal motor effect that translates to a short-lived improvement in symptoms, compounded by a variety of side effects such as hypotension, bradycardia, and pedal edema.

Sildenafil (Viagra, Pfizer, New York, NY, USA) is a potent selective inhibitor of cGMP-specific PDE-5 (phosphodiesterase-5), which inactivates the nitric oxide-stimulated GMP. Intracellular accumulation of the latter induces smooth muscle relaxation. In one study sildenafil improved the manometric pattern in nine of 11 patients with various esophageal motility disorders (four with nutcracker esophagus, one with DES, three with hypertensive LES, and three with achalasia). Only four of these patients reported symptomatic improvement, but two discontinued drug therapy due to side effects [210]. Acute administration of sildenafil 50 mg significantly reduced basal pressure in seven patients with symptomatic hypertensive LES as compared to baseline and the placebo period [211]. In a case report of a patient with NCCP whose manometry showed simultaneous features of nutcracker esophagus and DES, symptoms and motility pattern improved with the use of all three commercially available PDE-5 inhibitors [212]. However, thus far, there have been no studies specifically addressing NCCP patients. Consequently, the value of this compound in NCCP remains unknown. Additionally, the usage of this compound in NCCP will likely be limited by its cost and side effects.

The antispasmodic cimetropium bromide has been shown to be efficacious in eight NCCP patients with nutcracker esophagus when taken intravenously, but clinical data regarding the efficacy of an oral formulation are still lacking [213].

Hydralazine, an antihypertensive compound that directly dilates peripheral vessels, was shown to improve chest pain and dysphagia by decreasing the amplitude and duration of esophageal contractions in a small study of only five patients [202].

Pain modulators

Esophageal hypersensitivity is proposed to be the primary underlying mechanism for symptoms of patients with non–GERD-related NCCP, regardless of the presence or absence of esophageal motor disorder. Consequently, drugs that can alter esophageal pain perception have become the mainstay of therapy in these patients. Several drugs have been shown to have a pain modulatory or a visceral analgesic effect, thus alleviating chest pain symptoms.

Tryciclic antidepressants

Several studies have demonstrated that antidepressants have a visceral analgesic effect [214], but they also appear to inhibit calcium channels and thus may have an additional muscle relaxant-like effect [215].

Tryciclic antidepressants (TCAs) have both central neuromodulatory and peripheral visceral analgesic effects. Several clinical trials have found favorable TCA-related effects on esophageal pain perception in both healthy subjects [170] and patients with NCCP. Imipramine, administered at a dose of 75 mg/day, significantly increases the pain threshold of healthy men during intraesophageal balloon distention as compared to baseline [216]. In another study, 60 patients with NCCP and normal coronary angiography were randomized to receive clonidine (0.2 mg/day), imipramine (50 mg before bed time), or placebo for a period of 3 weeks. Patients who received imipramine had a significant (52%) reduction in the frequency of chest pain episodes, independent of cardiac, esophageal, or psychiatric test results, suggesting that imipramine relieves chest pain through visceral analgesic effect [169]. In contrast, amitriptyline failed to show an effect on both perception and esophageal compliance in subjects undergoing a balloon distention protocol [217]. In a retrospective analysis of 21 patients, Prakash *et al.* reported the long-term effects of a variety of TCAs in NCCP after incomplete response to antireflux treatment [218]. The authors found that 75% of the patients with NCCP continued to experience symptomatic relief during long-term use of the medications for up to 3 years. The use of a low-dose TCA in these trials suggests that the benefit of this class of drugs is mediated through their visceral rather than antidepressant properties.

Because of their anticholinergic side effects, TCAs are commonly administered at bed time. Based on our experience, it is recommended that TCA doses are slowly titrated to a maximum of 50–75 mg/day. The incremental increase in dosing should be based on symptom improvement and the development of side effects.

Trazodone is a tetracyclic antidepressant that has been evaluated for the treatment of NCCP. As with TCAs, the visceral analgesic and non–mood-altering effect of the drug has been evaluated in these patients. Trazodone (100–150 mg PO qid) for 6 weeks significantly improved the symptoms of patients with NCCP and esophageal dysmotility as compared to placebo [219]. However, esophageal motility abnormalities remained unchanged. A small, open-label study reported symptom control and improved esophageal motility in patients with NCCP and DES following treatment with both trazodone and clomipramine [220].

Selective serotonin reuptake inhibitors

Serotonin has been shown to play an important role in mediating visceral pain. A recent study demonstrated that citalopram, 20 mg given intravenously in a single dose, reduced chemical and mechanical esophageal hypersensitivity without altering esophageal motility [221].

During a single-blinded, placebo-controlled trial, 30 subjects with NCCP were randomized to receive sertraline or placebo for 8 weeks (starting at 50 mg and adjusted to a maximum of 200 mg). Patients with major depression and panic disorder were excluded. By using intention-to-treat analysis, the investigators have found that sertraline induced a significant reduction in pain scores as compared with placebo. Side effects occurred in 27% of the patient and included delayed ejaculation, decreased libido, and restlessness [222].

Paroxetine has also been evaluated in NCCP. In a double-blind, placebo-controlled trial, patients were randomized to paroxetine versus placebo (27 and 23 patients, respectively) for 8 weeks. Paroxetine-treated patients showed a greater improvement on a physician-rated scale but not on self-rated pain scores [223].

The selective serotonin reuptake inhibitor (SSRI) studies are relatively small but suggest a visceral analgesic effect in NCCP patients that is somewhat limited by their side effects profile.

Adenosine-agonists

Adenosine has been identified as mediator of visceral pain, including esophageal pain [224]. In healthy volunteers, adenosine-induced angina-like pain shortly after infusion. Recent information indicated that adenosine can induce esophageal hypersensitivity and decrease esophageal distensibility in humans [225].

Theophylline, a xanthine derivative, has been shown to inhibit adenosine-induced angina-like chest pain and adenosine-induced pain in other regions of the body [226]. A study using an esophageal balloon distention protocol and impedance demonstrated that intravenous theophylline increased thresholds for sensation and pain in 75% of patients with functional chest pain [227]. Similar results were documented in functional chest pain patients receiving oral theophylline for a period of 3 months. In another study, the same authors showed that oral doses of theophylline 200 mg twice daily were more effective than placebo in preventing chest pain in 19 patients with functional chest pain [228].

The aforementioned studies suggest that research involving adenosine-receptor antagonists may offer new opportunities for the treatment of functional chest pain [229]. The use of theophylline to treat patients with NCCP should be weighed against potential toxicity and side effects.

Anxiolytics

Several anxiolytics have been evaluated for the treatment of NCCP. Benzodiazepines amplify gamma-aminobutyric acid (GABA) throughout the central nervous system.

Alprazolam has been shown in a study to ameliorate chest pain at a mean dose of 4.3 mg/day in patients with NCCP and panic disorder [230]. In this study, 15 of 20 patients reported at least a 50% reduction in panic attack episodes and a corresponding decline in the frequency of chest pain episodes. Clonazepam, given at 1–4 mg/day, was also shown to be effective in the treatment of patients with NCCP and panic disorder [231].

The treatment of a functional disorder such as NCCP with benzodiazepines has been greatly discouraged, primarily due to concerns for long-term addiction to this class of drugs.

Serotonin receptor inhibitors

Serotonin (5-hydroxytryptamine, 5-HT) is a neurotransmitter present in the central nervous system, enteric neurons, and extrinsic afferents of the gut. It is involved in visceral perception and motor activity processes in the gastrointestinal tract [232].

Ondansetron, a 5-HT3 antagonist that is used as an antiemetic, has been shown to increase esophageal perception thresholds for pain in patients with NCCP [232].

The selective 5-HT4 receptor agonist tegaserod (Zelnorm, Novartis, Basel, Switzerland) has been demonstrated to reduce both chemoreceptor sensitivity to acid and mechanoreceptor sensitivity to balloon distention in patients with functional heartburn [233]. Thus far, there are no studies assessing the value of tegaserod in patients with non–GERD-related NCCP.

Octreotide

Octreotide, a synthetic analog of somatostatin, has been shown to increase rectal and sigmoid perception thresholds for pain in IBS patients and healthy subjects [234, 235]. It has been postulated that the effect of octreotide is mediated through the activation of somatostatin receptors at the spinal cord and/or the supraspinal level.

Octreotide, administered at 100 mg subcutaneously, was found to significantly increase perception thresholds for pain as compared to placebo in healthy subjects undergoing intraesophageal balloon distention [171]. Unfortunately, due to cost and the lack of an oral formulation, octreotide is rarely utilized for NCCP in clinical practice.

Endoscopic treatment for noncardiac chest pain

Botulinum toxin (Botox, Allergan, Irvine, CA, USA) interacts selectively with cholinergic neurons to inhibit the release of acetylcholine at the presynaptic terminals. Botulinum toxin injection into the LES has been used in several uncontrolled trials that included patients with NCCP and documented esophageal spastic motor disorder. Cassidy *et al.* in a preliminary communication showed that injection of botulinum toxin (80 U) at the LES produced symptomatic improvement in 80% of patients. At 1-year follow-up, however, only 36% of the patients remained symptom free [236]. Nebendahl *et al.* studied three patients with DES and injected 100 U into four quadrants at five levels of the esophagus and demonstrated symptom improvement in all three subjects [237]. Nebendahl *et al.* used higher doses (260 U) of botulinum toxin in nine patients. The botulinum toxin was injected at five different levels of the esophagus into four quadrants, and symptoms improved in all patients. Persistent improvement of symptoms over a period of 6 months was noted in seven of the patients [238]. Storr *et al.* treated nine DES patients with 100 U of botulinum toxin (100 U at multiple sites in the distal esophagus at 1–1.5-cm intervals). After 6 months, eight patients continued to report symptom improvement, and four required repeat injection to maintain remission [239]. Injecting botulinum toxin into the LES in a small, uncontrolled study resulted in 50% reduction of chest pain episodes in 72% of the subjects with different esophageal motility disorders for a mean duration of 7.3 months [240]. A small case series of nine patients published in abstract form [241] and two additional case reports have also suggested beneficial effects of botulinum toxin injection in patients with hypertensive LES [242, 243]. Recently, a small trial involving 11 patients with DES }compared the effects of botulinum toxin (100 U) to saline injection. This is the only available double-blind placebo-controlled, randomized cross-over trial. As compared with placebo, botulinum toxin significantly improved dysphagia but had no effect on chest pain or GERD-related symptoms [244].

In summary, botulinum toxin appears to have a beneficial effect in the treatment of NCCP patients with spastic motility disorders. However, studies have included only a small number of patients. They were primarily not placebo controlled, and long-term follow-up is still needed.

Psychologic treatment

Psychologic comorbidity, mainly depression and anxiety, is common in patients with NCCP. Psychotherapy may be helpful in the treatment of patients with NCCP, particularly those who also have hypochondriasis, anxiety, or panic disorder.

Reassurance has been proposed as a therapeutic strategy for NCCP. A typical approach has been to offer patients education about the "benign nature" of NCCP and good prognosis in comparison to the prognosis of patients with chest pain due to coronary artery disease. However, despite a favorable medical prognosis [245], patients with NCCP continue to experience chest pain symptoms (50–70%), occupational (19–51%) and functional impairment (46–100%), and high levels of healthcare utilization, including hospitalizations and inappropriate consumption of cardiac medications (27–29%) [246–249].

A number of psychologic techniques have been used in the treatment of NCCP. Cognitive behavioral therapy (CBT) is based on the model of attribution approach. The goal of treatment is to correct the misattributions regarding physical symptoms (e.g. chest pain) as being harmful. Patients must adopt the belief that psychologic factors cause chest pain and attribute the chest pain to panic attacks, anxiety, and/or other psychologic factors. CBT has been reported to be effective in the treatment of NCCP. In one study, CBT was compared to "usual care." Patients receiving CBT reported significant improvement in frequency and intensity of chest pain. Fifteen (48%) of the 31 patients in the treatment group were pain free at 12-month follow-up as compared with four (13%) of the 33 patients in the control group (P = .002) [250]. In another trial, 31 patients with NCCP were randomized to either immediate CBT or to assessment only (control group). The treatment group demonstrated significant reductions in chest pain, limitations and disruption of daily life, autonomic symptoms, distress and psychologic morbidity as compared with the control group. The assessment-only group were subsequently treated with CBT and showed comparable improvements. The improvements were sustained by both treated groups at 4–6-month follow-up [251]. CBT has also been successfully used for the treatment of NCCP patients without an existing panic disorder [252].

Biofeedback was assessed in a study that compared it to primary care visits only in patients with NCCP [253]. Patients in the biofeedback group demonstrated a significantly lower symptom frequency and severity. However, a large group of patients assigned to the biofeedback arm (52%) did not complete the study.

A Cochrane analysis of psychologic intervention in NCCP evaluated eight studies involving 403 randomized participants. The authors found significant reduction in chest pain in the first 3 months following the intervention (relative risk 0.68, 95% CI 0.57–0.81). This was maintained for a period of 3–9 months post intervention (relative risk 0.58, 95% CI 0.45–0.76). There was also a significant increase in the number of days without chest pain up to 3 months following the intervention (standardized mean difference 0.85, 95% CI 0.38–1.31) [254].

Hypnotherapy has been recently evaluated in the treatment of NCCP patients. Jones *et al.* reported an 80% improvement in symptoms, with a significant reduction in pain intensity, among patients who were receiving 12 sessions of hypnotherapy, compared to only 23% symptom improvement in the control group [255]. Hypnotherapy also resulted in a significantly greater improvement in overall wellbeing in addition to a reduction in medication usage. The study concluded that hypnotherapy appears to have a role in treating NCCP and that further studies are needed.

Future therapy

Future research in NCCP therapy will continue to focus on mechanisms for pain and will attempt to identify new therapeutic modalities aimed to reduce or reverse esophageal hypersensitivity. Research will likely concentrate primarily on the role of central and peripheral sensitization in enhancing perception of intraesophageal stimuli. Furthermore, currently available treatments for other functional gastrointestinal disorders, such as IBS and nonulcer dyspepsia, may be tested in NCCP as well.

The serotonin-related drugs, such as 5-HT type 3 antagonist and 5-HT type 4 agonist, appear to have a pain-modulatory effect, probably by altering the initiation, transmission, or processing of extrinsic sensory information from the gastrointestinal tract.

Phosphorylation of N-methyl-D-aspartate (NMDA) receptors expressed by dorsal horn neurons leads to central sensitization via an increase in their excitability and receptive field size [61]. Potentially, this central sensitization may be prevented or even reversed by antagonism of NMDA receptors within the spinal cord.

Potential targets that are currently under consideration include vanilloid receptor ion channels, acid-sensing ion channels, sensory neuron-specific Na^+ channels, P2X purinoceptors, cholecystokinin (CCK) receptors, bradykinin and prostaglandin receptors, glutamate receptors, tachykinin, and calcitonin gene-related peptide receptors [256]. The peripheral opioid receptor agonists are of high interest because they may offer visceral analgesic effect without crossing the blood–brain barrier and thus affecting the central nervous system.

Spinal afferents, which may play a role in visceral nociception, express tachykinins that include substance P, neurokinins A and B, and neuropeptide K. Tachykinin antagonists may confer a visceral analgesic effect that can be used in NCCP patients. Neurokinin (NK)-1, NK-2, and NK-3 receptor antagonists were only evaluated in preclinical trials.

Cholecystokinin receptor antagonists may alter visceral pain perception [257].

Another important area that is likely to attract future attention when treating patients with NCCP is complementary and alternative therapeutic modalities that can interfere with the mind and body axis.

References

1. Jerlock M, Welin C, Rosengren A, Gaston-Johannson F. Pain characteristics in patients with unexplained chest pain and patients with ischemic heart disease. *Eur J Cardiovasc Nurs* 2007;6:130–136.
2. Fass R, Navarro-Rodriguez T. Noncardiac chest pain. *J Clin Gastroenterol* 2008;42:636–646.
3. Fenster PE. Evaluation of chest pain: a cardiology perspective for gastroenterologists. *Gastroenterol Clin N Am* 2004;33:35–40.
4. Fenster PE, Sorrell VL. Evaluation of chest pain—A cardiology perspective for the gastroenterologist. In: Fraeg D, ed. *Noncardiac Chest Pain—A Growing Medical Problem.* San Diego: Plural Publishing, 2007.
5. Ockene IS, Shay MJ, Alpert JS, Weiner BH, Dalen JE. Unexplained chest pain in patients with normal arteriograms. *N Engl J Med* 1980;30:1249–1252.
6. Dumville JC, MacPherson H, Griffith K, Miles JNV, Lewin RJ. Non-cardiac chest pain: a retrospective cohort study of patients who attended a Rapid Access Chest Pain Clinic. *Fam Pract* 2007;24:152–157.
7. Sekhri N, Feder GS, Junghans C, Hemingway H, Timmis AD. How effective are rapid access chest pain clinics? Prognosis of incident angina and non-cardiac chest pain in 8762 consecutive patients. *Heart* 2007;93:458–463.
8. Robertson N, Javed N, Samani NJ, Khunti K. Psychological morbidity and illness appraisals of patients with cardiac and non-cardiac chest pain attending a rapid access chest pain clinic: a longitudinal cohort study. *Heart* 2008;93:e12.
9. Rome III Committee. *The Functional Gastrointestinal Disorders,* 3rd edn. Mc Lean, VA: Degnon Associates Inc, 2006.
10. Mudipalli RS, Remes-Troche JM, Andersen L, Rao SSC. Functional Chest Pain—Esophageal or Overlapping Functional Disorder. *J Clin Gastroenterol* 2007;41:264–269.
11. Potokar JP, Nutt DJ. Chest pain: panic attack or heart attack? *Int J Clin Pract* 2000;54:110–114.
12. Katerndahl DA, Trammell C. Prevalence and recognition of panic states in STARNET patients presenting with chest pain. *J Fam Pract* 1997;45:54–63.
13. Locke GR, 3rd , Talley NJ, Fett SL, Zinsmeister AR, Melton LJ, 3rd. Prevalence and clinical spectrum of gastroesophageal reflux: a population-based study in Olmstead County, Minnesota. *Gastroenterology* 1997;112:1448–1456.
14. Eslick GD. Noncardiac chest pain: epidemiology, natural history, health care seeking, and quality of life. *Gastroenterol Clin North Am* 2004;33:1–23.
15. Eslick GD, Jones MP, Talley NJ. Non-cardiac chest pain: prevalence, risk factors, impact and consulting–a population-based study. *Aliment Pharmacol Ther* 2003;17:1115–1124.

16. Mousavi S, Tosi J, Eskandarian R, Zahmatkesh M. Role of clinical presentation in diagnosing reflux-related non-cardiac chest pain. *J Gastroenterol Hepatol* 2007;22:218–221.

17. Tew R, Guthrie E, Creed F, *et al*. A long-term follow-up study of patients with ischemic heart disease versus patients with nonspecific chest pain. *J Psychosom Res* 1995;39:977–985.

18. Wong WM, Risner-Adler S, Beeler J, *et al*. Noncardiac chest pain: the role of the cardiologist—a national survey. *J Clin Gastroenterol* 2005;39:858–862.

19. Wong WM, Beeler J, Risner-Adler S, Habib S, Bautista J, Fass R. Attitudes and referral patterns of primary care physicians when evaluating subjects with noncardiac chest pain—a national survey. *Dig Dis Sci* 2005;50:656–661.

20. Eslick GD, Talley NJ. Non-cardiac chest pain: predictors of health care seeking, the types of health care professional consulted, work absenteeism and interruption of daily activities. *Aliment Pharmacol Ther* 2004;20:909–915.

21. Potts S, Bass C. Psychological morbidity in patients with chest pain and normal or near-normal coronary arteries: a long-term follow-up study. *Psychol Med* 1995;25:339–347.

22. Ward BW, Wu WC, Richter JE, Hackshaw BT, Castell DO. Long-term follow-up of symptomatic status of patients with noncardiac chest pain: is diagnosis of esophageal etiology helpful? *Am J Gastroenterol* 1987;82:215–218.

23. Eslick GD, Talley NJ. Natural history and predictors of outcome for non-cardiac chest pain: a prospective 4-year cohort study. *Neurogastroenterol Motil* 2008;20:989–997.

24. Williams JF, Sontag SJ, Schnell T, Leya J. Non-cardiac chest pain: the long-term natural history and comparison with gastroesophageal reflux disease. *Am J Gastroenterol* 2009; 104:2145–2152.

25. Dammen T, Ekeberg O, Arnesen H, Friis S. Health-related quality of life in non-cardiac chest pain patients with and without panic disorder. *Int J Psychiatry Med* 2008;38:271–286.

26. Stahl WG, Beton RR, Johnson CS, Brown CL, Waring JP. Diagnosis and treatment of patients with gastroesophageal reflux and noncardiac chest pain. *South Med J* 1994;87: 739–742.

27. Beedassy A, Katz PO, Gruber A, Peghini PL, Castell DO. Prior sensitization of esophageal mucosa by acid reflux predisposes to a reflux-induced chest pain. *J Clin Gastroenterol* 2000;31: 121–124.

28. Pandak WM, Arezo S, Everett S, *et al*. Short course of omeprazole: a better first diagnostic approach to noncardiac chest pain than endoscopy, manometry, or 24-hour esophageal pH monitoring. *J Clin Gastroenterol* 2002;35:307–314.

29. DeMeester TR, O'Sullivan GC, Bermudez G, Midell A, Cimochowski GE, O'Drobinak J. Esophageal function in patients with angina-type chest pain and normal coronary angiograms. *Ann Surg* 1982;196:488–498.

30. Bautista J, Fullerton H, Briseno M, Cui H, Fass R. The effect of an empirical trial of high-dose lansoprazole on symptom resonse of patients with non-cardiac chest pain–a randomized, double-blind, placebo-controlled, crossover trial. *Alimentary Pharmacol Ther* 2004;19:1123–1130.

31. Dickman R, Emmons S, Cui H, *et al*. The effect of a therapeutic trial of high-dose rabeprazole on symptom response of patients with non-cardiac chest pain: a randomized, double-blind,

placebo-controlled, crossover trial. *Aliment Pharmacol Ther* 2005;22:547–555.

32. Fass R, Fennerty MB, Ofman JJ, *et al*. The clinical and economic value of a short course of omeprazole in patients with noncardiac chest pain. *Gastroenterology* 1998;115:42–49.

33. Xia HH, Lai KC, Lam SK, *et al*. Symptomatic response to lansoprazole predicts abnormal acid reflux in endoscopy-negative patients with non-cardiac chest pain. *Aliment Pharmacol Ther* 2003;17:369–377.

34. Dickman R, Mattek N, Holub J, Peters D, Fass R. Prevalence of upper gastrointestinal tract findings in patients with non-cardiac chest pain versus those with gastroesophageal reflux disease (GERD)-related symptoms: results from a national endoscopic database. *Am J Gastroenterol* 2007;102:1173–1179.

35. Dekel R, Martinez-Hawthorne SD, Guillen RJ, Fass R. Evaluation of symptom index in identifying gastroesophageal reflux disease-related noncardiac chest pain. *J Clin Gastroenterol* 2004;38:24–29.

36. Fass R, Fennerty MB, Johnson C, Camargo L, Sampliner RE. Correlation of ambulatory 24-hour esophageal pH monitoring results with symptom improvement in patients with noncardiac chest pain due to gastroesophageal reflux disease. *J Clin Gastroenterol* 1999;28:36–39.

37. Kaski JC. Cardiac syndrome X and microvascular angina. In: Kaski JC, ed. *Chest Pain with Normal Coronary Angiograms: Pathogenesis, Diagnosis and Management*. London: Kluwer Academic Publishers, 1999, pp. 1–12.

38. Kaski JC, Rosano GM, Collins P, Nihoyannopoulos P, Maseri A, Poole-Wilson PA. Cardiac syndrome X: clinical characteristics and left ventricular function. Long-term follow-up study. *J Am Coll Cardiol* 1995;25:807–814.

39. Kaski JC. Pathophysiology and management of patients with chest pain and normal coronary arteriograms (cardiac syndrome X). *Circulation* 2004;109:568–572.

40. Chauhan A, Petch MC, Schofield PM. Cardio-oesophageal reflex in humans as a mechanisms for "linked angina". *Eur Heart J* 1996;17:407–413.

41. Rosztoczy AI, Vass A, Wittmann T, *et al*. Esophageal acid stimulation combined with transesophageal echocardiography shows high clinical impact in the establishment of esophago-cardiac reflex [abstract]. *Gastroenterology* 2003;1244 (Suppl): A534, #T1618.

42. Katz PO, Dalton CB, Richter JE, Wu WC, Castell DO. Esophageal testing of patients with noncardiac chest pain or dysphagia. Results of three years' experience with 1161 patients. *Ann Intern Med* 1987;106:593–597.

43. Dekel R, Pearson T, Wendel C, DeGarmo P, Fennerty MB, Fass R. Assessment of oesophageal motor function in patients with dyspepsia or chest pain—the Clinical outcomes research initiative experience. *Aliment Pharmacol Ther* 2003;18:1083–1089.

44. Fass R, Winters GF. Evaluation of the patient with noncardiac chest pain: is gastroesophageal reflux disease or an esophageal motility disorder the cause? *Medscape Gastroenterol* 2001;36: 1–10.

45. Lam HG, Dekker W, Kan G, Breedijk M, Smout AJ. Acute noncardiac chest pain in a coronary care unit. Evaluation by 24-hour pressure and pH recording of the esophagus. *Gastroenterology* 1992;102:453–460.

46. Peters L, Maas L, Petty D, *et al*. Spontaneous noncardiac chest pain. Evaluation by 24-hour ambulatory esophageal motility and pH monitoring. *Gastroenterology* 1988;94:878–886.

47. Clouse RE, Staiano A, Alrakawi A. Topographic analysis of esophageal double-peaked waves. *Gastroenterology* 2000;118: 469–476.

48. Pandolfino JE, Ghosh SK, Rice J, Clarke JO, Kwiatek MA, Kahrilas PJ. Classifying esophageal motility by pressure topography characteristics: a study of 400 patients and 75 controls. *Am J Gastroenterol* 2008;103:27–37.

49. Pehlivanov N, Liu J, Mittal RK. Sustained esophageal contraction: a motor correlate of heartburn symptom. *Am J Physiol Gastrointest Liver Physiol* 2001;28:G743–751.

50. MacKenzie J, Belch J, Land D, Park R, McKillop J. Oesophageal ischaemia in motility disorders associated with chest pain. *Lancet* 1988;286:592–595.

51. Liebermann-Meffert DM, Luescher U, Neff U, Rüedi TP, Allgöwer M. Esophagectomy without thoracotomy: is there a risk of intramediastinal bleeding? A study on blood supply of the esophagus. *Ann Surg* 1987;206:184–192.

52. Balaban DH, Yamamoto Y, Liu J, *et al*. Sustained esophageal contraction: a marker of esophageal chest pain identified by intraluminal ultrasonography. *Gastroenterology* 1999;116: 29–37.

53. Holloway RH. Esophageal ultrasonography: A new view on esophageal motility. *Am J Gastroenterol* 2007;102:146–148.

54. Lembo AJ. Visceral hypersensitivity in noncardiac chest pain. *Gastroenterol Clin North Am* 2004;33:55–60.

55. Hollerbach S, Bulat R, May A, *et al*. Abnormal cerebral processing of oesophageal stimuli in patients with noncardiac chest pain (NCCP). *Neurogastroenterol Motil* 2000;12:555–565.

56. Fass R, Naliboff B, Higa L, *et al*. Differential effect of long-term esophageal acid exposure on mechanosensitivity and chemosensitivity in humans. *Gastroenterology* 1998;115:1363–1373.

57. Handwerker HO, Reeh PW. Nociceptors: chemosensitivity and sensitization by chemical agents. In: Willis WD, Jr, ed. *Hyperalgesia and Allodynia*. New York: Raven Press, 1992, p. 107.

58. Barish CF, Castell DO, Richter JE. Graded esophageal balloon distention. A new provocative test for noncardiac chest pain. *Dig Dis Sci* 1986;31:1292–1298.

59. Rao S, Gregersen H, Hayek B, Summers RW, Christensen J. Unexplained chest pain: the hypersensitive, hyperreactive, and poorly compliant esophagus. *Ann Intern Med* 1996;124: 950–958.

60. Rao S, Hayek B, Summers RW. Functional chest pain of esophageal origin: hyperalgesia or motor dysfunction. *Am J Gastroenterol* 2001;96:2584–2589.

61. Sarkar S, Aziz Q, Woolf CJ, Hobson AR, Thompson DG. Contribution of central sensitisation to the development of non-cardiac chest pain. *Lancet* 2000;356:1154–1159.

62. Hu WH, Martin CJ, Talley NJ. Intraesophageal acid perfusion sensitizes the esophagus to mechanical distension: a Barostat study. *Am J Gastroenterol* 2000;95:2189–2194.

63. Sarkar S, Thompson DG, Woolf CJ, Hobson AR, Millane T, Aziz Q. Patients with chest pain and occult gastroesophageal reflux demonstrate visceral pain hypersensitivity which may be partially responsive to acid suppression. *Am J Gastroenterol* 2004;99:1998–2006.

64. DeVault KR, Castell DO. Esophageal balloon distention and cerebral evoked potential recording in the evaluation of unexplained chest pain. *Am J Med* 1992;925A:20S–6S.

65. Kamath MV, May A, Hollerbach S, *et al*. Effects of esophageal stimulation in patients with functional disorders of the gastrointestinal tract. *Crit Rev Biomed Eng* 2000;28:87–93.

66. Tougas G, Spaziani R, Hollerbach S, *et al*. Cardiac autonomic function and oesophageal acid sensitivity in patients with non-cardiac chest pain. *Gut* 2001;49:706–712.

67. Tougas G. The autonomic nervous system in functional bowel disorders. *Gut* 2000;47 (Suppl 4):iv78–80.

68. Aziz Q. Acid sensors in the gut: the taste of things to come. *Eur J Gastroenterol Hepatol* 2001;13:885–888.

69. Bass C, Wade C. Chest pain with normal coronary arteries: a comparative study of psychiatric and social morbidity. *Psychol Med* 1984;141:51–61.

70. Channer KS, Papouchado M, James MA, Rees JR. Anxiety and depression in patients with chest pain referred for exercise testing. *Lancet* 1985;284:820–823.

71. Costa PT, Jr. Influence of the normal personality dimension of neuroticism on chest pain symptoms and coronary artery disease. *Am J Cardiol* 1987;60:20J–26J.

72. McCroskery JH, Schell RE, Sprafkin RP, Lantinga LJ, Warner RA, Hill N. Differentiating anginal patients with coronary artery disease from those with normal coronary arteries using psychological measures. *Am J Cardiol* 1991;67:645–646.

73. Flugelman MY, Weisstub E, Galun E, *et al*. Clinical, psychological and thallium stress studies in patients with chest pain and normal coronary arteries. *Int J Cardiol* 1991;33:401–408.

74. Mayou R, Bryant B, Forfar C, Clark D. Non-cardiac chest pain and benign palpitations in the cardiac clinic. *Br Heart J* 1994;72:548–553.

75. Chignon JM, Lepine JP, Ades J. Panic disorder in cardiac outpatients. *Am J Psychiatry* 1993;150:780–785.

76. Tennant C, Mihailidou A, Scott A, *et al*. Psychological symptom profiles in patients with chest pain. *J Psychosom Res* 1994;38: 365–371.

77. Wong WM, Lam KF, Cheng C, *et al*. Population based study of noncardiac chest pain in southern Chinese: prevalence, psychosocial factors and health care utilization. *World J Gastroenterol* 2004;105:702–712.

78. Fleet RP, Dupuis G, Marchand A, Burelle D, Arsenault A, Beitman BD. Panic disorder in emergency department chest pain patients: prevalence, comorbidity, suicidal ideation, and physician recognition. *Am J Med* 1996;101:371–380.

79. Stollman NH, Bierman PS, Ribeiro A, Rogers AI. CO2 provocation of panic: symptomatic and manometric evaluation in patients with noncardiac chest pain. *Am J Gastroenterol* 1997;92:839–842.

80. Cooke RA, Anggiansah A, Wang J, Chambers JB, Owen W. Hyperventilation and esophageal dysmotility in patients with noncardiac chest pain. *Am J Gastroenterol*. 1996;91:480–484.

81. Demiryoguran NS, Karcioglu O, Topacoglu H, *et al*. Anxiety disorder in patients with non-specific chest pain in the emergency setting. *Emerg Med J* 2006;232:99–102.

82. Beitman BD, Basha I, Flaker G, *et al*. Atypical or nonanginal chest pain. Panic disorder or coronary artery disease? *Arch Intern Med* 1987;147:1548–1552.

83. Peghini PL, Johnston BT, Leite LP, Castell DO. Mucosal acid exposure sensitizes a subset of normal subjects to intra-oesophageal balloon distension. *Eur J Gastroenterol Hepatol* 1996;8:979–983.

84. Eslick GD, Fass R. Diagnosis of noncardiac chest pain. In: Fass R, Eslick GD, eds. *Noncardiac Chest Pain—A Growing Medical Problem*. San Diego: Plural Publishing, 2007, pp. 83–101.

85. Browning TH. Diagnosis of chest pain of esophageal origin. A guideline of the Patient Care Committee of the American Gastroenterological Association. *Dig Dis Sci* 1990;35:289–293.

86. Hsia PC, Maher KA, Lewis JH, Cattau EL, Jr., Fleischer DE, Benjamin SB. Utility of upper endoscopy in the evaluation of noncardiac chest pain. *Gastrointest Endosc* 1991;37:22–26.

87. García-Compeán D, González MV, Galindo G, *et al.* Prevalence of gastroesophageal reflux disease in patients with extraesophageal symptoms referred from otolaryngology, allergy, and cardiology practices: a prospective study. *Dig Dis Sci* 2000;18:178–182.

88. Canavan JB, Grainger RJ, Murray FE, Patchett SE. The diagnostic value of endoscopy in evaluating non-cardiac chest pain. *Gastrointest Endosc* 2005;61:AB128, #S1147.

89. Richter JE, Hewson EG, Sinclair JW, Dalton CB. Acid perfusion test and 24-hour esophageal pH monitoring with symptom index. Comparison of tests for esophageal acid sensitivity. *Dig Dis Sci* 1991;36:565–571.

90. Paterson WG. Canadian Association of Gastroenterology Practice Guidelines: management of noncardiac chest pain. *Can J Gastroenterol* 1998;12:401–407.

91. Charbel S, Khandwala F, Vaezi MF. The role of esophageal pH monitoring in symptomatic patients on PPI therapy. *Am J Gastroenterol* 2005;100:283–289.

92. Zerbib F, Roman S, Ropert A, *et al.* Esophageal pH-impedance monitoring and symptom analysis in GERD: a study in patients off and on therapy. *Am J Gastroenterol* 2006;101:1956–1963.

93. Fass R, Sifrim D. Management of heartburn not responding to proton pump inhibitors. *Gut* 2009;58:295–309.

94. Pandolfino JE, Richter JE, Ourts T, Guardino JM, Chapman J, Karhrilas PJ. Ambulatory esophageal pH monitoring using a wireless system. *Am J Gastroenterol* 2003;98:740–749.

95. Prakash C, Clouse RE. Value of extended recording time with wireless pH monitoring in evaluating gastroesophageal reflux disease. *Clin Gastroenterol Hepatol* 2005;34:329–334.

96. Prakash C, Clouse RE. Wireless pH monitoring in patients with non-cardiac chest pain. *Am J Gastroenterol* 2006;101:446–452.

97. Fass R, Ofman JJ, Gralnek IM, *et al.* Clinical and economic assessment of the omeprazole test in patients with symptoms suggestive of gastroesophageal reflux disease. *Arch Intern Med* 1999;150:2161–2168.

98. Schenk B, Kuipers E, Klinkenberg-Knol E, *et al.* Omeprazole as a diagnostic tool in gastroesophageal reflux disease. *Am J Gastroenterol* 1997;92:1997–2000.

99. Schindlbeck NE, Klauser AG, Voderholzer WA, Muller-Lissner SA. Empiric therapy for gastroesophageal reflux disease. *Arch Intern Med* 1995;155:1808–1812.

100. Johnsson F, Weywadt L, Solhaug J, Hernqvist H, Bengtsson L. One-week omeprazole treatment in the diagnosis of gastro-oesophageal reflux disease. *Scand J Gastroenterol* 1998;33:15–20.

101. Bate C, Riley S, Chapman R, Durnin A, Taylor M. Evaluation of omeprazole as a cost-effective diagnostic test for gastro-oesophageal reflux disease. *Aliment Pharmacol Ther* 1999;13:59–66.

102. Juul-Hansen P, Rydning A, Jacobsen C, Hansen T. High-dose proton-pump inhibitors as a diagnostic test of gastro-esophageal reflux disease in endoscopic-negative patients. *Scand J Gastroenterol* 2001;36:806–810.

103. Squillace SJ, Young MF, Sanowski RA. Abstract: Single dose omeprazole as a test for noncardiac chest pain. *Gastroenterology* 1993;107:A197.

104. Young MF, Sanowski RA, Talbert GA, *et al.* Omeprazole administration as a test for gastroesophageal reflux (Abstract). *Gastroenterology* 1992;102:192.

105. Fass R. Empirical trials in treatment of gastroesophageal reflux disease. *Dig Dis* 2000;18:20–26.

106. Fass R, Ofman JJ, Sampliner RE, Camargo L, Wendel C, Fennerty MB. The omeprazole test is as sensitive as 24-h oesophageal pH monitoring in diagnosing gastro-oesophageal reflux disease in symptomatic patients with erosive oesophagitis. *Aliment Pharmacol Ther* 2000;14:389–396.

107. Maev IV, Iurenev GL, Burkov SG, V'iuchnova ES. Rabeprazole test and comparison of the effectiveness of course treatment with rabeprazole in patients with gastroeseophageal reflux disease and non-coronary chest pain. *Klin Med (Mosk)* 2007;85:45–51.

108. Fass R, Pulliam G, Hayden CW. Patients with noncardiac chest pain (NCCP) receiving an empirical trial of high dose rabeprazole, demonstrate early symptom response—a double blind, placebo-controlled trial [abstract]. *Gastroenterology* 2001;116;129A-221.

109. Cremonini F, Wise J, Moayyedi P, Talley NJ. Diagnostic and therapeutic use of proton pump inhibitors in noncardiac chest pain: a meta-analysis. *Am J Gastroenterol* 2005;100:1226–1232.

110. Wang W, Huang J, Zheng G, *et al.* Is proton pump inhibitor testing an effective approach to diagnose gastroesophageal reflux disease in patients with noncardiac chest pain? *Arch Intern Med* 2005;165:1222–1228.

111. Ofman JJ, Gralnek IM, Udani J, Fennerty MB, Fass R. The cost-effectiveness of the omeprazole test in patients with non-cardiac chest pain. *Am J Med* 1999;107:219–227.

112. Knippig C, Fass R, Malfertheiner P. Tests for the evaluation of functional gastrointestinal disorders. *Dig Dis* 2001;19:232–239.

113. Clouse RE, Lustman PJ, Eckert TC, Ferney DM, Griffith LS. Low-dose trazodone for symptomatic patients with esophageal contraction abnormalities. A double-blind, placebo-controlled trial. *Gastroenterology* 1987;92:1027–1036.

114. London RL, Ouyang A, Snape WJJ, *et al.* Provocation of esophageal pain by ergonovine or edrophonium. *Gastroenterology* 1981;81:10–14.

115. Nostrant TT. Provocation testing in noncardiac chest pain. *Am J Med* 1992;925A:56S–64S.

116. Ghillebert G, Janssens J, Vantrappen G, Nevens F, Piessens J. Ambulatory 24 hour intraesophageal pH and pressure recordings v provocation tests in the diagnosis of chest pain of oesophageal origin. *Gut* 1990;31:738–744.

117. Nevens F, Janssens J, Piessens J, Ghillebert G, De Geest H, Vantrappen G. Prospective study on prevalence of esophageal chest pain in patients referred on an elective basis to a cardiac unit for suspected myocardial ischemia. *Dig Dis Sci* 1991; 36:229–235.

118. Soffer EE, Scalabrini P, Wingate DL. Spontaneous noncardiac chest pain: value of ambulatory esophageal pH and motility monitoring. *Dig Dis Sci* 1989;34:1651–1655.

119. Benjamin SB, Richter JE, Cordova CM, Knuff TE, Castell DO. Prospective manometric evaluation with pharmacologic provocation of patients with suspected esophageal motility dysfunction. *Gastroenterology* 1983;84:893–901.

120. Mellow M. Symptomatic diffuse esophageal spasm. Manometric follow-up and response to cholinergic stimulation and cholinesterase inhibition. *Gastroenterology* 1977;73: 237–240.

121. Nostrant TT, Sams J, Huber T. Bethanechol increases the diagnostic yield in patients with esophageal chest pain. *Gastroenterology* 1986;91:1141–1146.

122. Richter JE, Bradley LA, Castell DO. Esophageal chest pain: current controversies in pathogenesis, diagnosis, and therapy. *Ann Intern Med* 1989;110:66–78.

123. Buxton A, Goldberg S, Hirshfeld JW, *et al*. Refractory ergonovine-induced coronary vasospasm: importance of intracoronary nitroglycerin. *Am J Cardiol* 1980;46:329–334.

124. Takeda T, Kssab G, Liu J, *et al*. A novel ultrasound technique to study the biomechanics of the human esophagus in vivo. *Am J Physiol Gastrointest Liver Physiol* 2002;28:G785–793.

125. Bernstein LM, Baker LA. A clinical test for esophagitis. *Gastroenterology* 1958;34:760–781.

126. Bernot R, Norton RA. The esophageal acid perfusion test. *Lahey Clinic Foundation Bull* 1965;142:58–63.

127. Price SF, Smithson KW, Castell DO. Food sensitivity in reflux esophagitis. *Gastroenterology* 1978;75:240–243.

128. Kaul B, Petersen H, Grette K, Myrvold HE, Halvorsen T. The acid perfusion test in gastroesophageal reflux disease. *Scand J Gastroenterol* 1986;21:93-6.

129. Howard PJ, Maher L, Pryde A, Heading RC. Symptomatic gastro-oesophageal reflux, abnormal oesophageal acid exposure, and mucosal acid sensitivity are three separate, though related, aspects of gastro-oesophageal reflux disease. *Gut* 1991;32:128–132.

130. Battle WS, Nyhus LM, Bombeck CT. Gastroesophageal reflux: diagnosis and treatment. *Ann Surg* 1973;177:560–565.

131. Behar J, Biancani P, Sheahan DG. Evaluation of esophageal tests in the diagnosis of reflux esophagitis. *Gastroenterology* 1976;71:9–15.

132. Breen KJ, Whelan G. The diagnosis of reflux oesophagitis: an evaluation of five investigative procedures. *Aust NZ J Surg* 1978;48:156–161.

133. Fisher RS, Cohen S. Gastroesophageal reflux. *Med Clin North Am* 1978;62:3–20.

134. Bachir GS, Leigh-Collis J, Wilson P, Pollak EW. Diagnosis of incipient reflux esophagitis: a new test. *South Med J* 1981;74:1072–1074.

135. Johnson DA, Winters C, Spurling TJ, Chobanian SJ, Cattau EL, Jr. Esophageal acid sensitivity in Barrett's esophagus. *J Clin Gastroenterol* 1987;91:23–27.

136. Gracely RH, McGrath F, Dubner R. Ratio scales of sensory and affective verbal pain descriptors. *Pain* 1978;51:5–18.

137. Silverman DH, Munakata JA, Ennes H, Mandelkern MA, Hoh CK, Mayer EA. Regional cerebral activity in normal and pathological perception of visceral pain. *Gastroenterology* 1997; 112:64–72.

138. De Caestecker JS, Pryde A, Heading RC. Comparison of intravenous edrophonium and oesophageal acid perfusion during oesophageal manometry in patients with non-cardiac chest pain. *Gut* 1988;29:1029–1034.

139. Fass R, Yalam JM, Camargo L, Johnson C, Garewal HS, Sampliner RE. Increased esophageal chemoreceptor sensitivity to acid in patients after successful reversal of Barrett's esophagus. *Dig Dis Sci* 1997;42:1853–1858.

140. Hollerbach S, Kamath MV, Fitzpatrick D, *et al*. The cerebral response to electrical stimuli in the oesophagus is altered by increasing stimulus frequencies. *Neurogastroenterol Motil* 1997;92:129–139.

141. Tougas G, Hudoba P, Fitzpatrick D, et al. Cerebral-invoked potential responses following direct vagal and esophageal electrical stimulation in humans. *Am J Physiol* 1993;294: G486–491.

142. Heft MW, Parker SR. An experimental basis for revising the graphic rating scale for pain. *Pain* 1984;19:153–161.

143. Richter JE, Barish CF, Castell DO. Abnormal sensory perception in patients with esophageal chest pain. *Gastroenterology* 1986;91:845–852.

144. Ritchie J. Pain from distention of the pelvic colon by inflating a balloon in the irritable colon syndrome. *Gut* 1973;14: 125–132.

145. Mertz H, Walsh JH, Sytnik B, Mayer EA. The effect of octreotide on human gastric compliance and sensory perception. *Neurogastroenterol Motil* 1995;7:175–185.

146. Kramer P, Hollander W. Comparison of experimental esophageal pain with clinical pain of angina pectoris and esophageal disease. *Gastroenterology* 1955;29:719.

147. Lipkin M, Sleisenger MH. Studies of visceral pain: measurements of stimulus intensity and duration associated with the onset of pain in esophagus, ileum and colon. *J Clin Invest* 1958;37:28.

148. Yakshe PN, *et al*. Does provocative esophageal testing influence coronary blood flow or coronary flow reserve? Preliminary results of concurrent esophageal and cardiac testing (abstract). *Gastroenterology* 1993;104:A227.

149. Meyer GW, Castell DO. Human esophageal response during chest pain induced by swallowing cold liquids. *JAMA* 1981;246:2057–2059.

150. Kaye MD, Kilby AE, Harper PC. Changes in distal esophageal function in response to cooling. *Dig Dis Sci* 1987;32:22–27.

151. Kahrilas PJ, Dodds WJ, Hogan WJ. Dysfunction of the belch reflex. A cause of incapacitating chest pain. *Gastroenterology* 1987;93:818–822.

152. Kaye MD. Anomalies of peristalsis in idiopathic diffuse oesophageal spasm. *Gut* 1981;22:217–222.

153. Whitehead WE, Delvaux M, Team TW. Standardization of barostat procedures for testing smooth muscle tone and sensory thresholds in the gastrointestinal tract. *Dig Dis Sci* 1997;42:223–241.

154. Azpiroz F, Malagelada JR. Physiological variations in canine gastric tone measured by electronic barostat. *Am J Physiol* 1985;248:G229–237.

155. Toma TD, Zighelboim J, Phillips SF, *et al.* Methods for studying intestinal sensitivity and compliance: in vitro studies of balloons and a barostat. *Neurogastroenterol Motil* 1996;8:19–28.

156. Khan MI, Feinle C, Read DW. Investigating gastric and sensory response to distention: comparative studies using flaccid bags and latex balloons. *2nd United European Gastroenterology Meeting* 1992;13:175.

157. Sun WM, Read NW, Prior A, *et al.* Sensory and motor responses to rectal distention vary according to rate and pattern of balloon inflation. *Gastroenterology* 1990;99:1008–1015.

158. Munakata J, Naliboff B, Harraf F, *et al.* Repetitive sigmoid stimulation induces rectal hyperalgesia in patients with irritable bowel syndrome. *Gastroenterology* 1997;112:55–63.

159. Whitehead WE, Crowell MD, Shone D, *et al.* Sensitivity to rectal distention: validation of a measurement system (abstract). *Gastroenterology* 1993;104:A600.

160. Lembo T, Niazi M, Mayer EA. Do mucosal mechanoreceptors contribute to rectal hyperalgesia in IBS patients? (abstract). *Gastroenterology* 1993;104:A540.

161. Fass R. Sensory testing of the esophagus. *J Clin Gastroenterol* 2004;38:628–641.

162. Nguyen P, Castell DO. Stimulation of esophageal mechanoreceptors is dependent on rate and duration of distention. *Am J Physiol* 1994;267:G115–118.

163. Lasch H, Castell DO, Castell JA. Evidence of diminished visceral pain with aging: studies using graded intraesophageal balloon distention. *Am J Physiol* 1997;272:G1–G3.

164. Fass R, Pulliam G, Johnson C, Garewal HS, Sampliner RE. Symptom severity and oesophageal chemosensitivity to acid in older and young patients with gastro-oesophageal reflux. *Age Aging* 2000;29:125–130.

165. Nguyen P, Lee SD, Castell DO. Evidence of gender differences in esophageal pain threshold. *Am J Gastroenterol* 1995;90:901–905.

166. Niemantsverdriet EC, Timmer R, Breumelhof R, *et al.* Regional differences in esophageal acid sensitivity studied with pH-controlled segmental acid perfusion (abstract). *Gastroenterology* 1997;112:A237.

167. Grade A, Pulliam G, Johnson C, Garewal HS, Sampliner RE, Fass R. Reduced chemoreceptor sensitivity in patients with Barrett's esophagus may be related to age and not to the presence of Barrett's epithelium. *Am J Gastroenterol* 1997;92:2040–2043.

168. Winwood PJ, Mavrogiannis CC, Smith CL. Reduced sensitivity to intra-oesophageal acid in patients with reflux-induced strictures. *Scand J Gastroenterol* 1993;28:109–112.

169. Cannon 3rd RO, Quyyumi AA, Mincemoyer R, *et al.* Imipramine in patients with chest pain despite normal coronary angiograms. *N Engl J Med* 1994;330:1411–1417.

170. Peghini PL, Katz PO, Castell DO. Imipramine decreases oesophageal pain perception in human male volunteers. *Gut* 1998;42:807–813.

171. Johnston B, Shils J, Leite L, *et al.* Effects of octreotide on esophageal visceral perception and cerebral evoked potentials induced by balloon distension. *Am J Gastroenterol* 1994;94:65–70.

172. DeVault KR. Nifedipine does not alter barostat determined esophageal smooth muscle tone (abstract). *Gastroenterology* 1995;108:A591.

173. Smout AJ, DeVore MS, Dalton CB, Castell DO. Effects of nifedipine on esophageal tone and perception of esophageal distension. *Dig Dis Sci* 1992;37:598–602.

174. DeVault KR. Provocative tests for pain of esophageal origin. In: Castell DO, Richter JE, eds. *The Esophagus*, 3rd edn. Philadelphia: Lippincott Williams & Wilkins, 1999, pp. 135–143.

175. Hollerbach S, Kamath MV, Fitzpatrick D, *et al.* The cerebral response to electrical stimuli in the oesophagus is altered by increasing stimulus frequencies. *Neurogastroenterol Motil* 1997;92:129–139.

176. Smout AJ, DeVore MS, Castell DO. Cerebral potentials evoked by esophageal distension in human. *Am J Physiol* 1990;259:G955–959.

177. Frieling T, Enck P, Wienbeck M. Cerebral responses evoked by electrical stimulation of the esophagus in normal subjects. *Gastroenterology* 1989;97:475–478.

178. DeVault KR, Beacham S, Castell DO, Streletz LJ, Ditunno JF. Esophageal sensation in spinal cord-injured patients: balloon distension and cerebral evoked potential recording. *Am J Physiol* 1996;271:G937–941.

179. Franssen H, Weusten BL, Wieneke GH, Smout AJ. Source modeling of esophageal evoked potentials. *Electroencephalogr Clin Neurophysiol* 1996;100:85–95.

180. Aziz Q, Furlong PL, Barlow J, *et al.* Topographic mapping of cortical potentials evoked by distension of the human proximal and distal oesophagus. *Electroencephalogr Clin Neurophysiol* 1995;96:219–228.

181. Kern MK, Birn RM, Jaradeh S, *et al.* Identification and characterization of cerebral cortical response to esophageal mucosal acid exposure and distention. *Gastroenterology* 1998;115:1353–1362.

182. Aziz Q, Andersson JL, Valind S, et al. Identification of human brain loci processing esophageal sensation using positron emission tomography. *Gastroenterology* 1997;113:50–59.

183. Fass R, Bautista J, Janarthanan S. Treatment of gastroesophageal reflux disease. *Clin Cornerstone* 2003;5:18–29.

184. Kitchin L, Castell D. Rationale and efficacy of conservative therapy for gastroesophageal reflux disease. *Arch Intern Med*. 1991;151:448–454.

185. Fang J, Bjorkman D. A critical approach to noncardiac chest pain: pathophysiology, diagnosis, and treatment. *Am J Gastroenterol* 2001;96:958–968.

186. DeMeester T, O'Sullivan G, Bermudez G, *et al.* Esophageal function in patients with angina-type chest pain and normal coronary angiograms. *Ann Surg* 1982;196:488–498.

187. Achem SR, Kolts BE, MacMath T, *et al.* Effects of omeprazole versus placebo in treatment of noncardiac chest pain and gastroesophageal reflux. *Dig Dis Sci* 1997;42:2138–2145.

188. Louis E, Jorissen L, Bastens B, *et al.* Atypical symptoms of GORD in Belgium: epidemiological features, current management and open label treatment with 40 mg esomeprazole for one month. *Acta Gastroenterol Belg* 2006;69:203–208.

189. Dore MP, Pedroni A, Pes GM, *et al.* Effect of antisecretory therapy on atypical symptoms in gastroesophageal reflux disease. *Dig Dis Sci* 2007;52:463–468.

190. Achem SR, Kolts BE, Wears R, Burton L, Richter JE. Chest pain associated with nutcracker esophagus: a preliminary study of the role of gastroesophageal reflux. *Am J Gastroenterol* 1993;88:187–192.

191. Chambers J, Cooke R, Anggiansah A, Owen W. Effect of omeprazole in patients with chest pain and normal coronary anatomy: initial experience. *Int J Cardiol* 1998;65:51–55.

192. Patti M, Molena D, Fisichella P,*et al*. Gastroesophageal reflux disease (GERD) and chest pain. Results of laparoscopic antireflux surgery. *Surg Endosc* 2002;16:563–566.

193. Farrell T, Richardson W, Trus T,*et al*. Response of atypical symptoms of gastro-oesophageal reflux to antireflux surgery. *Br J Surg* 2001;88:1649–1652.

194. Rakita S, Villadolid D, Thomas A, *et al*. Laparoscopic Nissen fundoplication offers high patient satisfaction with relief of extraesophageal symptoms of gastroesophageal reflux disease. *Am Surg* 2006;72:207–212.

195. So J, Zeitels S, Rattner D. Outcomes of atypical symptoms attributed to gastroesophageal reflux treated by laparoscopic fundoplication. *Surgery* 1998;124:28–32.

196. Cheung TK, Lim PWY, Wong BC. Noncardiac chest pain—An Asia-Pacific Survey on the Views of Primary Care Physicians. *Dig Dis Sci* 2007;52:3043–3048.

197. Cheung TK, Lim PWY, Wong BCY. The view of gastroenterologists on non-cardiac chest pain in Asia. *Aliment Pharmacol Ther* 2007;26:597–603.

198. Orlando R, Bozymski E. Clinical and manometric effects of nitroglycerin in diffuse esophageal spasm. *N Engl J Med* 1989;289:23–25.

199. Millaire A, Ducloux G, Marquand A, Vaksmann G. [Nitroglycerin and angina with angiographically normal coronary vessels. Clinical effects and effects on esophageal motility]. *Arch Mal Coeur Vaiss* 1989;82:63–68.

200. Swamy N. Esophageal spasm: clinical and manometric response to nitroglycerine and long acting nitrites. *Gastroenterology* 1977;72:23–27.

201. Kikendall J, Mellow M. Effect of sublingual nitroglycerin and long-acting nitrate preparations on esophageal motility. *Gastroenterology* 1980;79:703–706.

202. Mellow M. Effect of isosorbide and hydralazine in painful primary esophageal motility disorders. *Gastroenterology* 1982;83:364–370.

203. Richter J, Dalton C, Buice R,*et al*. Nifedipine: a potent inhibitor of contractions in the body of the human esophagus. Studies in healthy volunteers and patients with the nutcracker esophagus. *Gastroenterology* 1985;89:549–554.

204. Davies H, Lewis M, Rhodes J,*et al*. Trial of nifedipine for prevention of oesophageal spasm. *Digestion* 1987;36:831–832.

205. Nasrallah S, Tommaso C, Singleton R,*et al*. Primary esophageal motor disorders: clinical response to nifedipine. *South Med J* 1985;78:312–315.

206. Konrad-Danhoff I, Baunack A, Ramsch K,*et al*. Effect of the calcium antagonists nifedipine, nirendipine, nimodipine, and nisoldipine on esophageal motility in man. *Eur J Pharmacol* 1991;41:313–316.

207. Richter J, Spurling T, Cordova C,*et al*. Effects of oral calcium blocker diltiazem, on esophageal contractions. Studies in volunteers and patients with nutcracker esophagus. *Dig Dis Sci* 1984;29:649–656.

208. Cattau Jr. E, Castell D, Johnson D,*et al*. Diltiazem therapy for symptoms associated with nutcracker esophagus. *Am J Gastroenterol* 1991;86:272–276.

209. Drenth J, Bos L, Engels L. Efficacy of diltiazem in the treatment of diffuse oesophageal spasm. *Aliment Pharmacol Ther* 1990;4:411–416.

210. Eherer AJ, Schwetz I, Hammer HF, *et al*. Effect of sildenafil on oesophageal motor function in healthy subjects and patients with oesophageal motor disorders. *Gut* 2002;50:758-64.

211. Bortolotti M, Pandolfo N, Giovannini M, Mari C, Miglioli M. Effect of Sildenafil on hypertensive lower oesophageal sphincter. *Eur J Clin Invest* 2002;32:682–685.

212. Agrawal A, Tutuian R, Hila A, Castell DO. Successful use of phosphodiesterase type 5 inhibitors to control symptomatic esophageal hypercontractility: a case report. *Dig Dis Sci* 2005;50:2059–2062.

213. Bassoti G, Gaburri M, Imbimbo B, *et al*. Manometric evaluation of cimetropium bromide activity in patients with the nutcracker oesophagus. *Scand J Gastroenterol* 1988;23: 1079–1084.

214. Egbunike I, Chaffee B. Antidepressants in the management of chronic pain syndromes. *Pharmacotherapy* 1990;10:262–270.

215. Becker B, Morel N, Vanbellinghen A,*et al*. Blockade of calcium entry in smooth muscle cells by the antidepressant imipramine. *Biochem Pharmacol* 2004;68:833–842.

216. Peghini P, Katz P, Castell D. Imipramine decreases oesophageal pain perception in human male volunteers. *Gut* 1998;42: 807–813.

217. Gorelick A, Koshy S, Hooper F,*et al*. Differential effects of amitriptyline on perception of somatic and visceral stimulation in healthy humans. *Am J Physiol* 1998;275:G460–466.

218. Prakash C, Clouse RE. Long-term outcome from tricyclic antidepressant treatment of functional chest pain. *Dig Dis Sci* 1999;44:2373–2379.

219. Clouse RE, Lustman PJ, Eckert TC, *et al*. Low-dose trazodone for symptomatic patients with esophageal contraction abnormalities. A double-blind, placebo-controlled trial. *Gastroenterology* 1987;92:1027–1036.

220. Handa M, MIne K, Yamamoto H,*et al*. Antidepressant treatment of patients with diffuse esophageal spasm: a psychosomatic approach. *J Clin Gastroenterol* 1999;28:228–232.

221. Broekaert D, Fischler B, Sifrim D, *et al*.. Influence of citalopram, a selective serotonin, reuptake inhibitor, on oesophageal hypersensitivity: a double-blind, placebo-controlled study *Aliment Pharmacol Ther* 2006;23:365–370.

222. Varia I, Logue E, O'Connor C, *et al*.. Randomized trial of sertaline in patients with unexplained chest pain of noncardiac origin. *Am Heart J* 2000;140:367–372.

223. Doraiswamy PM, Varia I, Hellegers C, *et al*. A randomized controlled trial of paroxetine for noncardiac chest pain. *Psychopharmacol Bull* 2006;39:15–24.

224. Bueno L, Fioramonti J, Delvaux M, Frexinos J. Mediators and pharmacology of visceral sensitivity: from basic to clinical investigations. *Gastroenterology* 1997;112:1714–1743.

225. Remes-Troche JM, Chahal P, Mudipalli R, Rao SS. Adenosine modulates oesophageal sensorimotor function in humans. *Gut* 2009;58:1049–1055.

226. Crea F, Pupita G, Galassi A, *et al*.. Role of adenosine in pathogenesis of anginal pain. *Circulation* 1990;81:164–172.

227. Rao SS, Mudipalli RS, Mujica VR, *et al.* An open-label trial of theophylline for functional chest pain. *Dig Dis Sci* 2002;47: 2763–2768.

228. Rao SS, Mudipalli RS, Remes-Troche JM, *et al.* Theophylline improves esophageal chest pain–a randomized, placebo-controlled study. *Am J Gastroenterol* 2007;102:930–938.

229. Achem SR. New frontiers for the treatment of noncardiac chest pain: the adenosine receptors. *Am J Gastroenterol* 2007;102:939–941.

230. Beitman B, Basha I, Trombka L,*et al.* Pharmacotherapeutic treatment of panic disorder in patients presenting with chest pain. *J Fam Pract* 1989;28:177–180.

231. Wulsin L, Maddock R, Beitman B, *et al.* Clonazepam treatment of panic disorder in patients with recurrent chest pain and normal coronary arteries. *Int J Psychiatry Med* 1999;29: 97–105.

232. Tack J, Sarnelli G. Serotonergic modulation of visceral sensation: upper gastrointestinal tract. *Gut* 2002;51 (Suppl 1): i77–i80.

233. Rodriguez-Stanley S, Zubaidi S, Proskin H, *et al.*. Effect of tegaserod on esophageal pain threshold, regurgitation, and symptom relief in patients with functional heartburn and mechanical sensitivity. *Clin Gastroenterol Hepatol* 2006;4: 442–450.

234. Bradette M, Delvaux M, Staumont G, *et al.* Octreotide increases thresholds of colonic visceral perception in IBS patients without modifying muscle tone. *Dig Dis Sci* 1994;39: 1171–1178.

235. Schwetz I, Naliboff B, Munakata J, *et al.* Anti-hyperalgesic effect of octreotide in patients with irritable bowel syndrome. *Aliment Pharmacol Ther* 2004;19:123–131.

236. Cassidy MJ, Schiano TD, Adrain AL, *et al.* Botulinum toxin injection for the treatment of diffuse esophageal spasm (abstract). *Am J Gastroenterol* 1996;91:1884.

237. Nebendahl JC, Brand B, von Schrenck T, *et al.* Effective treatment of diffuse esophageal spasm by endoscopic injection of botulinum toxin (abstract). *Gastroenterology* 1998;114:A240.

238. Nebendahl JC, Brand B, von Schrenck T, *et al.* Treatment of diffuse esophageal spasm with botulinum toxin: a prospective study with 6 month follow up (abstract). *Gastroenterology* 1999;116:A802.

239. Storr M, Allescher HD, Rosch T, Born P, Weigert N, Classen M. Treatment of symptomatic diffuse esophageal spasm by endoscopic injections of botulinum toxin: a prospective study with long-term follow-up. *Gastrointest Endosc* 2001;54:754–759.

240. Miller L, Pullela S, Parkman H, *et al.* Treatment of chest pain in patients with noncardiac, nonreflux, nonachalasia spastic esophageal motor disorders using botulinum toxin injection into the gastroesophageal junction. *Am J Gastroenterol* 2002;97:1640–1646.

241. Mathews S, Cohen H, Kline M. Botulinum toxin injection improves symptomatic hypertensive lower esophageal sphincter. *Gastroenterology* 1998;114 (Suppl 1):A800.

242. Jones MP. Botulinum toxin in hypertensive lower esophageal sphincter. *Am J Gastroenterol* 1996;91:1283–1284.

243. Lacy BE, Zayat EN, Crowell MD. Case report: botulinum toxin in hypertensive lower esophageal sphincter: a manometric case study. *Dysphagia* 2002;17:75–80.

244. Vanuytsel T, Bisschops R, Mimidis K, *et al.* A sham-controlled study of injection of botulinum toxin in diffuse esophageal spasm. *Gastroenterology* 2008;134 (Suppl 1):A-14.

245. Ockene IS, Shay MJ, Alpert JS, Weiner BH, Dalen JE. Unexplained chest pain in patients with normal coronary arteriograms: a follow-up study of functional status. *N Engl J Med* 1980;303:1249–52.

246. Papanicolaou MN, Califf RM, Hlatky MA, *et al.* Prognostic implications of angiographically normal and insignificantly narrowed coronary arteries. *Am J Cardiol* 1986;58:1181–1187.

247. Beitman BD, Kushner MG, Basha I, Lamberti J, Mukerji V, Bartels K. Follow-up status of patients with angiographically normal coronary arteries and panic disorder. *JAMA* 1991;265:1545–1549.

248. Channer KS, James MA, Papouchado M, Rees JR. Failure of a negative exercise test to reassure patients with chest pain. *Q J Med* 1987;63:315–322.

249. Kemp HG, Kronmal RA, Vlietstra RE, Frye RL. Seven year survival of patients with normal or near normal coronary arteriograms: a CASS registry study. *J Am Coll Cardiol* 1986;73: 479–483.

250. van Peski-Oosterbaan AS, Spinhoven P, van Rood Y, van der Does JW, Bruschke AV, Rooijmans HG. Cognitive-behavioral therapy for noncardiac chest pain: a randomized trial. *Am J Med* 1999;106:424–429.

251. Klimes I, Mayou RA, Pearce MJ, Coles L, Fagg JR. Psychological treatment for atypical non-cardiac chest pain: a controlled evaluation. *Psychol Med* 1990;203:605–611.

252. van Peski-Oosterbaan A, Spinhoven P, van Rood Y, Smith. Cognitive-behavioral therapy for noncardiac chest pain: a randomized trial. *Am J Med* 1999;106:424–429.

253. Ryan M, Gervirtz R. Biofeedback-based psychophysiological treatment in a primary care setting: an initial feasibility study. *Appl Psychophysiol Biofeedback* 2004;29:79–93.

254. Kisely S, Campbell LA, Skerritt P. Psychological interventions for symptomatic management of non-specific chest pain in patients with normal coronary anatomy. *Cochrane Database Syst Rev* 2005;(1):CD004101.

255. Jones H, Cooper P, Miller V, *et al.*. Treatment of non cardiac chest pain: a controlled trial of hypnotherapy. *Gut* 2006;55: 1403–1408.

256. Holzer P. Gastrointestinal afferents as targets of novel drugs for the treatment of functional bowel disorders and visceral pain. *Eur J Pharmacol* 2001;429:177–193.

257. Scarpignato C, Pelosini I. Management of irritable bowel syndrome: novel approaches to the pharmacology of gut motility. *Can J Gastroenterol* 1999;13(Suppl A):50A–65A.

258. Frobert O, Funch-Jensen P, Jacobsen NO, Kruse A, Bagger JP. Upper endoscopy in patients with angina and normal coronary angiograms. *Endoscopy* 1995;275:365–370.

259. Wong WM, Lai KC, Lau CP, *et al.* Upper gastrointestinal evaluation of Chinese patients with non-cardiac chest pain. *Aliment Pharmacol Ther* 2002;163:465–471.

260. Battaglia E, Bassotti G, Buonafede G, *et al.* Noncardiac chest pain of esophageal origin in patients with and without coronary artery disease. *Hepatogastroenterology* 2005;52:792–795.

3

Disorders Causing Oropharyngeal Dysphagia

Stephen J. Antonik[1] and Reza Shaker[2]
[1]Gastroenterology Associates, P.L.L.C., Leesburg, VA, USA
[2]Division of Gastroenterology and Hepatology, Froedtert Memorial Lutheran Hospital, Medical College of Wisconsin, Milwaukee, WI, USA

Introduction

Swallowing requires the voluntary and involuntary coordination of a large number of structures of the oral cavity, pharynx, larynx, and esophagus. The major function of swallowing is successful bolus transit to the esophagus while preventing aspiration. The term oropharyngeal dysphagia (OPD) refers to difficulty in swallowing because of abnormalities in either the delivery of oral contents to the proximal esophagus or misdirection of the bolus to the airway or nasopharynx.

OPD is not rare and has a significant morbidity and mortality, including decreased rehabilitation potential, decreased quality of life, increased hospital length of stay, and increased healthcare cost. The prevalence in a population survey is 6.9%, 30% in acute care, post traumatic and single hemispheric cardiovascular accident (CVA), and 59–66% in a chronic care setting. In one study in an acute and community mental health setting, the prevalence of OPD of 32% [1]. OPD is seen in 50% of patients after surgery and chemotherapy for head and neck cancer [2], 6.6–29.8% after anterior cervical decompression and fusion [3], and 7% of patients with inflammatory myopathies [4]. There is a growing population of patients with OPD who have had Parkinson's disease (50%) or Alzheimer's disease (28%). As high as 80% of patients with multiple sclerosis experience OPD [5]. Bulbar palsy, amyothrophic lateral sclerosis, and progressive muscular atrophy have a prevalence of 89%, 29%, and 45%, respectively.

Despite the myriad causes of OPD, the pathophysiologic end result falls into one of two interrelated categories: (1) abnormalities of bolus transfer and (2) abnormalities of airway protection. Abnormalities of bolus transfer can be further grouped into those caused by (1) oropharyngeal pump failure; (2) oral/pharyngeal and pharyngo-upper esophageal sphincter (UES) discoordination; or (3) pharyngeal outflow obstruction. Abnormalities of airway protection may manifest themselves as pre-, intra-, and post-deglutitive aspiration. Whereas intradeglutitive aspiration is usually caused by a defective deglutitive laryngeal closure mechanism, the predeglutitive aspiration is mainly caused by disorders affecting oral pharyngeal transit and its coordination with deglutitive airway closure. Post-deglutitive aspiration for the most part results from pharyngeal outflow compromise and incomplete clearance. These distinctions carry with them important therapeutic implications. For instance, in a patient diagnosed with post-deglutitive aspiration, therapy will be directed to enhance UES deglutitive opening and improve pharyngeal clearance. In a patient diagnosed with intradeglutitive aspiration, however, therapy will be directed at repairing/improving the closure mechanism of the larynx. In a patient with predeglutitive aspiration, postural techniques, bolus modification, and swallow maneuvers will need to be instituted.

In light of the wide array of clinical presentations and a large number of patients with swallow-induced silent aspiration, the diagnosis of OPD requires a high index of suspicion. Some patients may be completely asymptomatic and present with pneumonia, whereas others may complain of difficulty swallowing, or demonstrate frequent throat clearing, repetitive swallowing, and hoarseness (Table 3.1). The investigating physician should seek out a history of recurrent pneumonia, weight loss, and regurgitation, as well as a garbled voice after meals, nasal regurgitation with meals, hoarseness, nasal speech, swallow-related coughing, and avoidance of social dining.

OPD develops as a result of a large number of local and system causes leading to abnormal oropharyngeal bolus transit, compromise of airway protection, and compromise

The Esophagus, Fifth Edition. Edited by Joel E. Richter, Donald O. Castell.
© 2012 Blackwell Publishing Ltd. Published 2012 by Blackwell Publishing Ltd.

Table 3.1 Symptoms of oropharyngeal dysphagia.

Inability to keep the bolus in the oral cavity
Difficulty gathering the bolus at the back of the tongue
Hesitation or inability to initiate the swallow
Food sticking in the throat
Nasal regurgitation
Inability to propel the food bolus caudad into the pharynx
Difficulty swallowing solids
Frequent repetitive swallowing
Frequent throat clearing
Gargly voice after meal
Hoarse voice
Nasal speech and dysarthria
Swallow-related cough: before, during, or after swallowing
Avoidance of social dining
Weight loss
Recurrent pneumonia

of-volition and cognition. OPD must be distinguished from globus and esophageal dysphagia as the causes of orpharyngeal pathology are often much different from those of esophageal dysphagia. OPD frequently requires a multidisciplinary approach as the etiology is often diverse and requires multiple expertise for management (Table 3.2). Therefore, it is imperative that the physiology be properly defined in order to address all modifiable aspects of the swallow to improve quality of life. Potential key participants in the care of the patient include gastroenterologists, radiologists, speech pathologists, neurologists, dietitians, otolaryngologists, geriatricians, palliative care physicians, and home caregivers who provide assistance with meals and medications. A managing physician needs to coordinate the care of dysphagic patients.

Table 3.2 Causes of oropharyngeal dysphagia (modified from Cook I. Disorders causing oropharyngeal dysphagia. In: *The Esophagus*, 4th edn, Lippincott, Williams & Wilkins, and *Edelman, Sleisenger & Fordtran's Gastrointestinal and Liver Disease*, 8th edn, Saunders, 2006.

Structural	Posterior pharyngeal diverticulum (Zenker's)
	Lateral pharyngeal diverticulum
	Cricophryngeal bar
	Cervical or esophageal web
	Oropharyngeal tumors benign and malignant
	Thyroid enlargement or tumor
	Esophageal tumors benign and malignant
	Postsurgical
	Cervical stenosis
	Vertebral spur or osteophytes
	Esophageal stricture
	Inflammatory disease (pharyngitis, tonsillar abscess)
	Foreign body
	Cervical lymphadenopathy
	Vascular anomalies
	Diffuse idiopathic skeletal hyperstosis
Central nervous system	Stroke
	Parkinson's disease
	Huntington's chorea
	Wilson's disease
	Brainstem tumor
	Amyotrophic lateral sclerosis
	Multiple sclerosis
	Cerebral palsy
	Spinal cord injury
	Tabes dorsalis
	Spinocerebellar degeneration
	Stringobulbia
	Progressive bulbar paralysis
	Alzheimer's
	Other congenital or degenerative disorders or motor neuron diseases

(continued)

Table 3.2 (continued)

Peripheral nervous system	Spinal muscular atrophy
	Guillain-Barré syndrome
	Polimyelitis, post polio syndrome
	Diabetes
	Recurrent laryngeal nerve palsy (mediastinal tumor, post surgery)
	Transection or injury
	Diphtheria
	Rabies
	Lead poisoning
	Other neurotoxins
Myogenic	Myasthenia gravis, botulism
	Inflammatory myopathies
	Polymyositis/dermatomyositis
	Scleroderma
	Mixed connective tissue disease
	Inclusion body myositis
	Muscular dystrophies (oculopharyngeal muscular dystrophy, myotonia dystrophica)
	Sarcoidosis
	Hyperthyroidism
	Myxedema
	Stiff-man syndrome
	Cricopharyngeal dysfunction
	Paraneoplastic syndromes
	Mitochondriopathies
Miscellaneous	Chronic obstructive pulmonary disease
	Xerostomia
	Botulinum toxin
	Procainamide
	Cytotoxins, phenothiazines
	Benzodiazepines
	Amiodarone
	Alcohol
	Cholesterol-lowering drugs

Swallowing

Mechanisms

Swallowing occurs under three distinct conditions: volitional, subconscious, and reflexive pharyngeal. Volitional is mostly for nutritional purposes and is so effortless that it is often taken for granted. Subconscious occurs at a rate of one per minute on average. This is considered airway housekeeping and reflux clearing. Reflexive pharyngeal is an airway protective mechanism against aspiration of food inadvertently falling into the pharynx during chewing or materials refluxed into the pharynx from the stomach.

From a functional perspective there are four phases of swallowing: preparatory, oral, pharyngeal, and esophageal. Preparatory and oral are volitional and require cognition. However, the pharyngeal phase is essentially reflexive.

Preparatory, oral, and pharyngeal are all responsible for bolus transit while protecting the airway. The esophageal phase is involved in bolus transit and is discussed in Chapter 5.

During the preparatory phase, the bolus essentially remains in the oral cavity, is altered physically by being subjected to mastication, and altered chemically by mixing with saliva, all resulting in a bolus with suitable characteristics for safe transit through the aerodigestive tract. It is during this phase that the bolus is sized, shaped, and positioned on the dorsum of the tongue for initiation of the upcoming oral phase of swallowing.

During the oral phase, a sequential contraction of the tongue against the hard and soft palates, a peristaltic pressure wave, is generated that propels the bolus from the oral cavity into the pharynx [6, 7] It is in the pharyngeal phase that the pharynx, UES, and larynx [8] are all elevated, and three of the four routes for exit from the pharynx (namely the nasal cavity, oral cavity, and larynx) become sealed off, while the fourth route, the UES, opens. Contraction of the superior pharyngeal constrictor and elevation of the soft palate and its contact with the posterior pharyngeal wall (velopharyngeal closure) close off the nasopharynx. The oral cavity is closed by elevation of the tongue base and its contact with the hard and soft palates [6]. The bolus is then transported into the esophagus by rapid forceful posterior tongue movements that persist from the oral phase, as well as the peristaltic contraction of the pharyngeal constrictors against the soft palate, base of the tongue, and larynx.

It is during the oropharyngeal swallow that important biomechanical events involving the intrinsic glottis, as well as supra- and infra-hyoid muscles, take place that result in the closure of the airway, [9–11] as well as in the opening of the UES [12–14]. These events include (1) adduction of the true vocal cords and arytenoids (first tier of airway closure), followed by vertical approximation of the adducted arytenoids to the base of the epiglottis (second tier of closure) (Figure 3.1); (2) descent of the epiglottis covering the closed

glottis, thereby closing the laryngeal vestibule third tier of closure); and (3) the entire larynx is pulled upward and forward by the contraction of the suprahyoid muscle group at the time of vocal cord closure or shortly thereafter. This displacement results in the positioning of the closed larynx under the tongue base, away from the path of the bolus, thereby providing additional protection against aspiration [15, 16] (Figure 3.2).

During oropharyngeal swallowing, the UES transiently relaxes and is subsequently pulled upward/forward by the contraction of the same suprahyoid muscles that displace the larynx. This traction results in active opening of the UES, which is also modified by the bolus size [17–19]. The temporal relationship of the events that take place during the oropharyngeal phase of swallowing is shown in Figure 3.3. Under normal conditions, oropharyngeal swallowing begins with the closure of the vocal cords, marking the initiation of airway protection [11], and ends when the cords return to their resting positions. During this time, respiration is reflexively inhibited and the protective mechanisms of swallowing are fully activated. Finally, the esophageal phase of

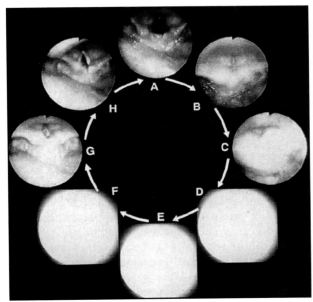
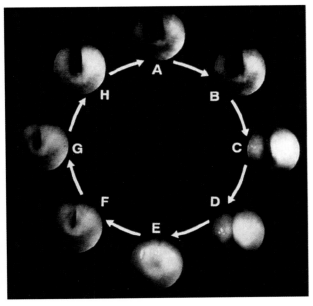

A

B

Figure 3.1 Still frames of deglutitive vocal cord closure seen by (A) transnasal videoendoscopy in a normal volunteer and (B) transtrachael videoendoscopy in a patient with tracheostomy. (A) A, Glottis immediately before initiation of swallow. Vocal cords are open at their resting position. B, Complete deglutitive vocal cord and arytenoid adduction. C, Adducted arytenoids have approximated the base of the epiglottis. D–F, Obscured view because of pharyngeal contraction and laryngeal elevation. G, Vocal cords can be seen still adducted following the descent of the larynx and opening of the pharynx after passage of the bolus. H, Vocal cords are beginning to open at the completion of swallow. (B) A, Inferior view of the glottis at rest. The introitus to the trachea is wide open immediately before the initiation of swallow. B and

C, Vocal cords are in the process of adduction narrowing the introitus. D, Cords are in contact with each other in the anterior part. However, the posterior gap is still open. E, Posterior gap is now closed, resulting in complete closure of the introitus to the trachea. F, Posterior gap is partially reopened while the anterior parts of the cords are still in contact. G and H, Cords are further opened returning to resting position. Note that contrary to the transnasal view, in the transtracheal view, the introitus to the trachea remained visible during the entire period of swallowing (reproduced from Shaker R, Milbrath M, Ren J, *et al.* Deglutitive aspiration in patients with tracheostomy: effect of tracheostomy on the duration of vocal cord closure. *Gastroenterology* 1995;108:1357–1360, with permission).

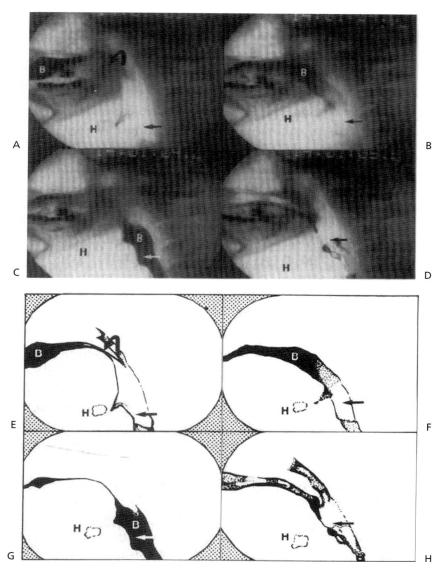

Figure 3.2 Sequence of events during primary swallows. (A–D) The primary swallow resulted in bolus transport form the mouth into the pharynx and esophagus. Straight arrows indicate pharyngeal lumen. (A, E) Bolus of 5 mL of barium is held in the oral cavity immediately before the onset of swallowing. Tongue base and soft palate are in contact (curved arrow), segregating the oral bolus from the pharyngeal cavity. (B, F) Tongue base is depressed and soft palate has elevated and is in contact with the posterior pharyngeal wall. This resulted in closing off the nasopharynx and allowing the bolus to enter the pharynx (C, G). Bolus transferring the pharynx while the nasopharynx and oral cavity are sealed off by approximation of the soft palate and posterior pharyngeal wall, and apposition of the tongue base and soft palate, respectively. The hyoid bone has moved upward and forward (D, H). The barium bolus has cleared the pharynx; the oral cavity and nasopharynx are open; and the larynx and hyoid bone have returned to the resting position. B, barium bolus; H, hyoid bone (reproduced from Shaker et al. [32], with permission).

swallowing transports the bolus further into the esophagus and stomach.

As stated earlier, the elaborate mechanism of oropharyngeal swallowing ensures two important functions: (1) transit of the bolus and (2) protection of the airway. Normal oropharyngeal swallowing is therefore defined as complete transit of the ingested material from the mouth into the esophagus, without compromising the airway. OPD may result when the efficacy and/or coordination of either the transport or protective aspect of oropharyngeal swallowing are compromised.

Control

The cerebral cortical swallowing network is comprised of the sensory motor cortex, insular cingulate gyrus, and prefrontal cortex. In this network neural control of swallowing consists

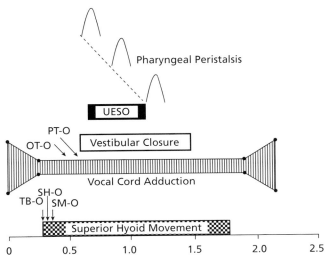

Figure 3.3 Relationship of deglutitive vocal cord kinetics to other events of the oropharyngeal phase of swallowing during 5-mL barium swallows. Bolus transit through the pharynx and across the upper esophageal sphincter (UES) begins and ends with the vocal cords at maximal adduction. TB-O, onset of tongue base movement; SH-O, onset of superior hyoid movement; SM-O, onset of submental myoelectrical activity; UESO, UES opening; OT-O, onset of bolus movement from the mouth; PT-O, arrival of bolus into pharynx.

of three major components: (1) sensory afferent fibers contained in the cranial nerves, (2) central organizing centers, and (3) efferent motor fibers contained in the cranial nerves and ansa cervicalis.

Sensory afferent signals

Sensory afferent signals originating from the oropharyngeal cavity are carried by the branches of the glossopharyngeal (IX) and vagus nerves (X) to the nucleus tractus solitarius (NTS) in the medulla. These afferent sensory fibers also carry sensory information from the pulmonary stretch receptors, as well as chemoreceptors located in the carotid and aortic bodies. They also play a role in the control of the respiratory system.

Central organizing center

The medulla oblongata houses paired swallowing centers responsible for processing afferent sensory signals and programming the motor swallowing sequences [20–22]. These centers are poorly defined areas and are comprised of the NTS, ventromedian reticular formation (VMRF), and nucleus ambiguous (NA). There is increasing evidence that cortical structures have a significant influence on the brainstem swallowing centers [23]. Cortical areas in the preorbital gyrus and lateral precentral gyrus have been implicated in modulation of deglutition. Cortical projections have been found connecting the cortical and medullary swallowing centers. Although poorly understood, experimental evi-

dence suggests the presence of a close functional, structural, and physiologic interaction between deglutitive and respiratory centers and their afferent and efferent inputs.

Motor efferent signals

Motor output to the muscular apparatus of the oropharynx for swallowing is transmitted by axons, whose cell bodies are located in the brainstem swallowing centers. These include motor nuclei of the trigeminal (V), facial (VII), and hypoglossal (XII) nerves. It also includes the NA, which not only consists of the premotor commanding neuron, but also houses large motor neurons that are distributed to striated muscles innervated by the glossopharyngeal (IX) and vagus (X) nerves.

Musculature

The muscular apparatus of oropharyngeal swallowing consists of a total of 30 paired striated muscles. Cranial nerve XII and the ansa cervicalis (C1–C2) control the tongue, while the vagus nerve exerts predominant control over the muscles of the palate, pharynx, and larynx, as well as the cricopharyngeus muscle. Deglutitive orad movement of the hyoid bone, larynx, and UES, and active opening of the UES following its relaxation, are induced by the supra- and infra-hyoid muscles that are innervated by the ansa cervicalis (C1–C2), cranial nerve V3, and cranial nerve VII.

Presentation

Most patients with OPD seek help because of symptoms, although a subset are silent aspirators who may present with recurrent pneumonia. Dysphagia symptoms reflect a breakdown in the transport or protective functions of oropharyngeal swallowing (Table 3.1). These symptoms are highly specific and should not be simply dismissed as functional or psychogenic. Every effort should be exerted to arrive at a specific diagnosis, although subtle abnormalities often escape detection.

A sensation of "food sticking in my throat" is often reported and reflects inadequate clearance of the bolus from the pharynx. Although this sensation may be caused by the presence of a large amount of residue in the pyriform sinus or valleculae, an obstructive lesion of the proximal or distal esophagus may lead to the very same complaint. Thus, patients with complaints of cervical dysphagia should undergo a thorough evaluation of the esophagus. Of course, careful direct visualization of the hypopharyngeal area must also rule out inflammation, abrasion, or tumors in this area.

Misdirection of the bolus into the airway leading to swallow-related coughing or choking is another common complaint. Invasion of the upper airway by the bolus may occur before initiation of, during, or after completion of oropharyngeal swallowing, and results in a coughing or choking sensation [24]. Aspiration into the airway may also occur prior to deglutition, because of the premature loss of the bolus into the hypopharynx from the mouth while the path to the airway is still open—a condition commonly encountered in post-stroke dysphagic patients. An inability to segregate the oral bolus from the pharynx by apposition of the tongue base and soft palate results in this premature spillage, called predeglutitive aspiration. If pharyngeal sensation is deranged, and swallowing is not initiated by entry of the prematurely passed bolus into the pharynx, predeglutitive aspiration and its concomitant complications follow. Deglutitive aspiration occurs either because of an incompetent glottis or one that does not close properly during the swallowing sequence, which leads to invasion of the airway by the bolus while it is being transported through the hypopharynx. Finally, post-deglutitive aspiration develops when the bolus transport is incomplete and a large residue remains in the pyriform sinus or valleculae—a condition encountered in parkinsonism, post stroke, myasthenia gravis, and multiple sclerosis. When the glottis opens and respiration is resumed, the large residue is either inhaled or overflows into the trachea.

The history is helpful to distinguish OPD from globus. Globus is a sensation of a lump or tightness in the throat. Globus is purely sensory and occurs between meals without impairment in bolus transfer [25–28]. It should not be diagnosed in the presence of dysphagia. Patients occasionally have associated psychiatric disorders, such as anxiety, depression, panic disorder, etc. Evaluation often involves otolaryngology.

Similar to esophageal dysphagia, the history can be helpful in narrowing the differential diagnosis in OPD. Solid food dysphagia is often indicative of a structural abnormality. Progressive symptoms associated with weight loss raise the concern for malignancy. Sudden onset of symptoms associated with other neurologic deficit suggests stroke. Foul breath and delayed regurgitation may be indicative of a Zenker's diverticulum. Myopathies often present as slowly progressive dysphagia. Other systemic symptoms such as features of Parkinson's or memory loss may be helpful in determining a diagnosis.

A history of aspiration pneumonia is an important clue to oropharyngeal pneumonia. Langmore *et al.* found that dysphagia is an important risk factor in elderly patients, but is generally insufficient to cause pneumonia unless other risk factors are present. Risk factors include feeding and oral care dependence, decayed teeth, tube feeding, medications, and smoking [29].

In the preparatory phase of swallowing, several protective reflexes are present, including the reflexive pharyngeal swallow, pharyngoglottal reflex, and the laryngeal adductor reflex. All of these protective reflexes are impaired with aging, and the reflexive pharyngeal swallow and pharyngoglottal reflex are impaired with smoking and alcohol [30–33]. These deficits can predispose to aspiration.

Older adults demonstrate slower swallowing process, decreased isometric lingual pressure, unchanged deglutitive lingual pressure, decreased UES opening, and decreased functional reserve [34]. As the population ages, the prevalence for swallow difficulties grows, which is evidenced by the 93% increase of Medicare beneficiaries for aspiration pneumonia from 1991 to 1998 [35]. Abnormal UES opening or pharyngeal outflow obstruction may be caused by primary mechanisms, i.e. myogenic or neurogenic, or secondary, such as inadequate suprahyoid muscle traction, aging deconditioning, and stroke. The evaluation and treatment of abnormal UES opening is discussed below.

Evaluation

Physical examination

The evaluation of OPD begins when the patient enters the room with appearance and gait. A thorough neuromuscular examination is essential as many causes of OPD will have systemic findings. The oropharynx should be inspected for dentition, symmetry, as well as the presence of saliva. Xerostomia is a common cause of OPD in the elderly. This finding should be followed by eye evaluation, joint examination, and a careful history regarding anticholinergic medications and a history of head and neck surgery or radiation. Change in voice such as hoarseness or nasal speech may be observed with nerve dysfunction and soft palate dysfunction, respectively. The neck should be palpated for masses. Before proceeding to a radiologic test or swallow study, it is helpful to ask the patient to perform a dry swallow in the office for visual inspection of movement and symmetry, and with gentle pressure on the thyroid and hyoid cartilage. Normal movement is elliptical anterosuperior motion. Abnormal ascent is seen in neurologic disorders.

Laboratory tests

Although no specific laboratory tests are required in the evaluation of OPD, many clinicians obtain a thyroid stimulating hormone (TSH) measurement to evaluate for hyperthyroid [36]. Systemic symptoms may direct the clinician to order other laboratory tests for the evaluation of a myopathy, connecting tissue diseases, or drug toxicity or poisoning, etc.

Dynamic studies

The approach to the OPD patient is evolving. Until recently, barium studies were the only modality available for evaluation of OPD patients. During the past decade, several other modalities, such as manometry, endoscopy, ultrasonography, and scintigraphy have been introduced into this field. Ongoing intensive research by various disciplines is making the approach to the OPD patient a dynamic and improving phenomenon. Quantitative normalcy data are now available, and study recordings and test substances are more standardized, allowing for interstudy comparison. With the advent of digitalization technology, endoscopic and fluoroscopic images are digitized and analyzed using the slow motion and frame-by-frame movement capability. This technology permits synchronization of several modalities and accurate timing of the events. This synchronization allows determination of the temporal relationship of various events, such as bolus movement and airway closure during oropharyngeal swallowing. Since all the structures of the oropharynx are not adequately seen during swallowing with one single modality, this multisystem recording is essential for studying the coordination of oropharyngeal swallowing events.

Modified barium swallow

Currently, videofluoroscopic recording of a modified barium swallow is the diagnostic modality of choice for initial investigation of the patient with OPD. During this study, recordings of a variety of boluses with different consistencies and volumes are made for subsequent analysis. These recordings may be used subsequently for future comparisons to evaluate progress. This technique not only provides adequate information about the movement of the barium bolus through the aerodigestive tract and documents misdirection of the bolus into the airway, but also vital information about the anatomy and function of the individual anatomic components of the aerodigestive tract involved in swallowing [37, 38]. Additionally, this modality is used to evaluate the effect of various postural and breathing techniques on the efficiency, as well as safety, of swallowing [13, 39]. Normal and abnormal videofluoroscopic findings of swallowing have been published extensively [13, 17, 40]. On videofluoroscopy, abnormalities of the oral phase of swallowing may manifest themselves as inadequate clearance of the barium bolus from the mouth (leaving a barium residue behind), piece-meal swallowing due to inadequate tongue function, or difficulty initiating the swallowing sequence due to impaired cognitive or neural function [13]. Patients with difficulty controlling the labial or facial muscles will not be able to hold the barium bolus in their anterior mouth, and will end up drooling during swallow. Premature spilling of the oral contents into the pharynx before the pharyngeal phase is activated will catch the airway off guard, and may result in predeglutitive aspiration. This abnormality commonly occurs with impaired palatal and/or lingual control.

Abnormalities of the pharyngeal phase of swallowing documented by videofluoroscopy include concomitant absent or diminished upward/forward movement of the larynx and hyoid bone, indicating inadequate suprahyoid muscle contraction. This abnormality may be accompanied by entry of barium into the airway beyond the level of the true vocal cords (aspiration). An incompetent velopharyngeal closure mechanism, due to inadequate elevation and/or weak posterior movement of the palate and uvula, may result in regurgitation of the barium into the nasopharynx.

This abnormality could develop after CVA in the setting of other neurogenic processes, inflammatory disorders of striated muscles, or following surgical excisions. Abnormalities of the oral phase of swallowing may or may not be accompanied by abnormalities of the pharyngeal phase of swallowing.

Abnormalities in transport function during oropharyngeal swallowing result in hypopharyngeal residue. Abnormal lingual, pharyngeal, or UES function, singularly or in combination, may be responsible. Unilateral involvement of the pharynx results in ipsilateral post-deglutitive bulging of the pharyngeal wall and residue on the same side [17, 10].

Misdirection of the barium into the airway may be due to intrinsic abnormalities of the glottal adductor muscles, resulting in an ineffective glottal sphincteric mechanism or lack of coordination between glottal closure and transport function of the oropharynx, which is commonly seen in neurologically impaired patients.

Abnormal opening of the UES during swallowing, seen by videofluoroscopy, may be due to lack of or impairment of its relaxation, decreased UES compliance, or inadequate traction by the suprahyoid muscles. Correct diagnosis requires manometric evaluation of the UES for its resting pressure and its swallow-induced relaxation. Diagnosis of cricopharyngeal achalasia cannot be made solely from its radiographic appearance.

Videoendoscopy

The chronic nature of OPD requires assessment of therapeutic results and progress with repeat videofluoroscopic study. Because of the radiation exposure and also difficulty in moving some patients to the radiology suite, a videoendoscopic approach to the evaluation of OPD has been developed [41–44]. This technique also allows outpatient/clinic evaluation of dysphagic patients. In this technique, a small diameter endoscope, such as a laryngoscope or bronchoscope, is inserted through the nose and positioned at the level of the posterior nares. In this position, the patient is asked to swallow. During this swallow, normal features of pharyngeal seal, namely the adduction of the superior constrictor and postero/orad elevation of the palate seen as a bulging in the nasopharynx, is examined, and then the scope is advanced to the level of the free margin of the epiglottis. At this position the glottis is clearly seen and its adduction function is examined by having the patient produce different vowels. Following this, a 5–10 mL water bolus colored with blue food dye is given through the mouth, and the patient is instructed to hold the bolus in the mouth for 20 s. During this time, the back of the tongue is observed videoendocopically for presence or absence of unilateral or bilateral spill or entry of colored water into the airway (predegultive aspiration). The presence of spill is seen in patients with abnormalities of the tongue and/or palate control. Following this stage, the scope is withdrawn to the level of the posterior nares and the patient is asked to swallow once. The scope is immediately advanced to the level of the epiglottis. On the way toward the epiglottis, attention is given to the presence or absence of blue staining of the retropalatal pharynx, indicative of nasal regurgitation due to abnormalities of the velopharyngeal closure mechanism. This abnormality may be caused by inadequate elevation and posterior movement of the soft palate and uvula. Then, the inner aspect of the epiglottis, aryepiglottic fold, posterior commissure, and true vocal cords are examined for the presence or absence of staining. In a study of normal volunteers in our laboratory, only the outer edges of the epiglottis and aryepiglottic fold were stained with blue dye. Endotracheal coloring with blue dye is easily seen, proving aspiration. The patients are then asked to cough once and, since during cough the laryngeal vestibule remains open, expulsion of blue material from the trachea can be seen and is indicative of aspiration. Following this phase, the presence or absence of residue in the pyriform sinus and valleculae is determined, and overflow of residue into the trachea through the posterior commissure is sought.

Manometry

Although the use of intraluminal strain gauges for pharyngeal manometry has resulted in a significant increase in our knowledge about the pharyngeal pressure phenomena, this modality still remains mainly a research tool, and its clinical application is limited to the evaluation of dysphagic patients with primary muscle diseases. An example of these disorders is Kearns–Sayre syndrome, where significant diminution of the pharyngeal peristaltic pressure wave amplitude is the prominent finding. Because the pharynx is radially, as well as axially, an asymmetric cavity, orientation of the pressure transducers needs to be ascertained and preferably similar in all studies in order to obtain meaningful data. However, with the recent availability of high-resolution catheters with circumferential pressure sensors, this limitation has been remedied. Concurrent pharyngeal and UES manometry helps detect discoordination between the UES relaxation and the arrival of pharyngeal peristalsis in the hypopharynx. Use of manometry to evaluate the oral phase in dysphagic patients has generally been unsuccessful, and this modality continues to be used for research purposes only.

As discussed previously, normal UES opening basically requires the existence of normal cricopharyngeal relaxation and distensibility, as well as normal contractile force of the suprahyoid muscles. Traditionally, UES resting tone and deglutitive relaxation have been studied by intraluminal manometry. Because of the orad displacement of the UES during swallowing and its to-and-fro movement during breathing, the use of a sleeve sensor, such as the currently available e-sleeve of the high-resolution manometric catheter, has been advocated for this purpose. This sensor provides continuous measurement of the UES pressure [45] and records maximal squeeze pressure regardless of the axial sphincter movement along the length of the device. Shorter pressure sensors, either strain gauges or pneumohydraulic side holes, may remain within the sphincter at rest. However, during swallowing, they will drop into the cervical esophagus, due to the upward movement of the sphincter, and record intraesophageal pressure, which may be misinterpreted as UES relaxation.

Differentiating between deglutitive relaxation and opening of the cricopharyngeal muscle by intraluminal manometry is impossible. The sudden intraluminal UES pressure decline during swallowing, commonly referred to as UES relaxation, reflects the effect of (1) cricopharyngeal relaxation and (2) UES opening of various degrees. Concurrent manometry and fluoroscopy also provide information that is the summation of the two effects of relaxation and opening. For this reason, concurrent manometry, electromyography, and videofluoroscopy are essential to differentiate the effects of these phenomena.

A relatively common change in UES morphology, observed during pharyngoesophageal barium studies, is a prominent posterior indentation at the level of the UES; cricopharyngeal bar. Although rarely associated with dysphagia, its observation has been reported in 5% of patients older than 40 years who did not have symptoms [46]. Despite the common notion of spasm or failed relaxation, the pathogenesis of cricopharyngeal bar is not fully known. A study by Dantas *et al.* has shown a normal resting pressure, as well as normal deglutitive relaxation, in individuals with cricopharyngeal bar [47]. However, the upstream (intrabolus) pressure was found to be higher than that of normal controls. Reduced dimension of UES during passage of barium was also found, suggestive of reduced compliance of the cricopharyngeal muscle.

Ultrasonography

Ultrasound has been successfully used for evaluation of the oral phase of swallowing. Since this modality is non-invasive and does not disturb the physiology of the oral phase of swallowing, it can be used in addition to videofluoroscopy to evaluate the dysphagic patient. Using this modality, Sonies *et al.* have described subtle, subclinical changes of the oral phase of swallowing in the elderly [48].

Management

Although only a minority of patients with OPD are amenable to medical/surgical therapy, the majority do require retraining and use of various swallowing maneuvers and techniques in order to achieve an adequate and safe swallow.

Endoscopic and surgical management

Cricopharyngeal dilatation and myotomy has been performed for a variety of neurogenic and myogenic causes of

OPD, with variable results. However, controlled clinical trials and outcome studies are lacking. In general, myotomy yields good results in cricopharyngeal achalasia due to primary cricopharyngeal muscle involvement. The results are less predictable for primary neurogenic causes if other parts of the swallowing apparatus are also involved. The role of myotomy in secondary cricopharyngeal achalasia is controversial, since deglutitive relaxation is present in this group. The rationale for the cricopharyngeal myotomy, which usually is extended to the lower part of the inferior pharyngeal constrictor and upper part of the cervical esophagus, is to eliminate the resistance of the UES against the flow of the swallowed bolus. Under normal conditions, this resistance is eliminated by timely relaxation, followed by opening and timely closure of the UES. However, in a variety of conditions, because of discoordination of the UES and pharynx or ineffective pharyngeal function, the UES acts as a relative resistor to the bolus flow. It is in these conditions that cricopharyngeal myotomy may improve pharyngeal bolus transit and reduce aspiration. In recent years, endoscopic transmucosal botulinum toxin injection into the cricopharyngeal muscle has been tried in patients with cricopharyngeal achalasia. However, close proximity of the injection area and the vocal cords raises special concern about possible respiratory complications. On the other hand, because of the temporary effect of the botulinum toxin, this new technique could potentially be used to select patients who will benefit from cricopharyngeal myotomy.

Vencovsky *et al.* reported successful resolution of dysphagia after cricopharyngeal myotomy in a patient with acute cricopharyngeal obstruction due to dermatomyositis [49]. Gagic reported excellent results of cricopharyngeal myotomy in patients with Zenker's diverticulum and idiopathic hypertrophy of the cricopharyngeal muscle, and marked improvement in patients with vagal injuries, amyotrophic lateral sclerosis, and post CVA; however, no improvement was achieved in patient with myotonia dystrophica [50]. Two patients developed aspiration pneumonia and respiratory arrest. Logemann has reported that the results of cricopharyngeal myotomy are superior when pathology is mainly in the UES, there are pharyngeal propulsive forces present, and patients are able to close the airway voluntarily [51]. Since the major barrier against pharyngeal regurgitations of gastric acid, namely the UES, is ablated by myotomy, pulmonary complications of gastroesophageal reflux postoperatively should remain a major concern in patients who undergo cricopharyngeal myotomy. In a recent report of 253 patients who underwent cricopharyngeal myotomy, one of 15 patients with neurogenic dysphagia developed persistent aspiration requiring a tracheostomy, four of 139 patients with muscular dystrophy died of respiratory distress syndrome and two required a tracheostomy, while none of the 90 patients with Zenker's diverticulum developed any major respiratory complications [52]. These results suggest the significant role of factors other than myotomy *per se*, such as abnormal esophageal motility, proximal or pharyngeal reflux in the development of post-cricopharyngeal myotomy respiratory complications. Documentation of the absence of proximal esophageal and pharyngeal reflux and normal esophageal motility before surgery may help in the decision-making process.

In patients with an inadequate deglutitive glottal closure mechanism, such as seen in patients with Parkinson's disease or amyotrophic lateral sclerosis, the deglutitive airway closure could be augmented by injection of a non-absorbable material such as Teflon [13, 53, 54] into the lateral thyroarytenoid muscle. These injections will result in bulk formation at the injection site and displace the true cord in a fixed position toward the midline, facilitating glottal closure during swallowing, since the adduction of the functioning cord will result in contact of the two cords and closure of the introitus of the trachea. Teflon injection into the cords has also been successfully used to prevent aspiration in patients with various types of vocal cord paralysis, due to dysfunction of the recurrent laryngeal and/or superior laryngeal nerve as a result of various central nervous system, surgical or inflammatory disorders [55, 56].

Swallowing and postural techniques

Swallowing maneuvers and exercises
The majority of OPD patients require specialized rehabilitation of their swallowing functions. Swallow therapy is performed with the aid of videofluoroscopy and more recently, with unsedated transnasal videoendoscopy. The therapy requires a cooperative patient with intact cognition. Swallow therapies (Table 3.3) are time-consuming, and must be tailored to each individual patient and their specific oropharyngeal abnormalities. At times, attempts at various techniques and maneuvers are required until an efficient and safe swallow is achieved. Swallowing maneuvers are used to improve bolus transfer and airway safety. In our practice, we find that they are more effective than postural techniques.

Multiple swallows
The target population is patients with post-deglutitive residue, poor pharyngeal peristalsis, and posterior tongue thrust. The patient follows the swallow of each bite with two or three additional dry swallows. The desired effect is the enhancement of pharyngeal closure and elimination of post-deglutitive pharyngeal residue.

Supraglottic swallow
The target population is patients with intradeglutitive aspiration. When ready to swallow, the patient takes a deep breath, holds it, then swallows while bearing down, followed by a cough [57]. The desired effect is to close the

airway completely by adducting the vocal cords and aryte-noids, and approximating the adducted arytenoids to the base of the epiglottis in order to prevent aspiration. The subsequent cough expels any contents that potentially may have penetrated the airway.

Postural techniques

Postural changes employ altered angles and/or gravitational forces to allow safe passage of the bolus and therefore reduce or eliminate aspiration. Chin tuck, chin up, head rotation to the affected side, and tilting of the head to the stronger side are examples of postural techniques (see Table 3.3) Abnormalities of oropharyngeal transit are often overlap-ping, and rehabilitation of the swallowing mechanism often requires use of a number of the swallowing maneuvers and postural techniques. Abnormalities of UES opening, which usually present with increased pharyngeal residue and post-deglutitive aspiration, respond to maneuvers that improve transphincteric transit, and a single approach, e.g. Mendelsohn's maneuver, Shaker exercise, may suffice.

Table 3.3 Postural techniques and swallowing maneuvers and exercises.

	Desired effect
Postural changes	
Chin tuck	Position bolus anteriorly and narrow airway entrance
Tilting head to stronger side	Gravitational forces direct bolus to stronger side
Head rotation to affected side	Takes advantage of stronger muscles on unaffected side to improve pharyngeal transfer
Chin up	Improve posterior movement of the bolus
Swallowing maneuvers	
Multiple swallows	Residue is cleared with repeated effort
Supraglottic swallow	Close the true vocal cords and arytenoids and approximate the adducted arytenoids to the base of the epiglottis in order to prevent aspiration. The subsequent cough expels any contents which potentially may have penetrated the airway
Effort-full swallow	Increases posterior tongue thrust
Mendelsohn's maneuver	Prolongs upper esophageal sphincter (UES) opening and laryngeal elevation, thus improving pharyngeal clearance
Shaker exercise	Increases cross-sectional area of UES opening Improves pharyngeal clearance and reduces/eliminates post-deglutitive aspiration

Mendelsohn's maneuver

The target population is patients with abnormal pharyngeal transit and post-deglutitive aspiration. The patient is instructed to generate a sustained laryngeal and hyoid bone elevation following the swallow [58]. The desired effect is to prolong UES opening and thus enhance pharyngeal emptying.

Shaker exercise

The target population is patients with abnormal UES func-tion who present with post-swallow pharyngeal residue and aspiration. An isotonic and isometric head-raising exercise regimen in the supine position is performed three times a day for a 6-week period [59, 60]. The desired effect is an increase in the cross-sectional area of the UES opening by strengthening the traction forces of the suprahyoid muscles responsible for UES opening, and thus improving pharyn-geal clearance and eliminating aspiration.

Cost-effectiveness

There are data to support the use of swallowing measures [61]. Large, randomized, controlled trials are needed to establish the cost-effectiveness of these interventions and their method of delivery [62]. For example, a randomized controlled trial found that limited patient and family instruc-tion regarding the use of diet modification and swallowing techniques was just as effective in decreasing the incidence of complications, as was intervention by a therapist to control diet consistency and provide daily rehearsal of com-pensatory swallowing techniques [63]. For this reason, the frequency of scheduled therapy sessions with healthcare professionals should be re-evaluated, and increased family participation should be encouraged.

Pharmacologic treatment

While as yet no specific pharmacologic treatment is available for enhancement of general oropharyngeal swallowing function, withdrawal of certain pharmacologic agents, such as antihistamines, anticholinergics, and particularly phenothiazines, may resolve medication-induced OPD. Pharmacologic therapy directed at a specific reversible etiology of OPD, such as thyroid hormone replacement in patients with thyroid-induced myopathy resulting in OPD, may result in resolution or amelioration of OPD.

Diet and lifestyle

The patient's diet is dictated by the nature of their OPD. While some patients can tolerate a regular diet, others require soft or pureed foods, because they cannot form a cohesive bolus, or they have a defective preparatory phase of swallowing. A simple intervention consists of manipula-tion of bolus size and consistency. However, dietary modifi-cation should not compromise the patient's pleasure in eating. Patients' families should be advised to make every effort to ensure desirability and palatability of meals by paying particular attention to taste, temperature, and texture, as well as being tolerant about the extra time required for some patients to eat properly. The overall goals of dietary intervention are to afford adequate nutrition while minimizing the sometimes dramatic personal and social ramifications of OPD, and thus allow patients to comfortably function within their social milieu.

Conclusions

In conclusion, OPD results from dysfunction of one or more of the highly coordinated events of the oropharyngeal phase of swallowing, leading to abnormal transport and/or airway protection. Whether due to one of a variety of muscular, peripheral, and central nervous system disorders, malignancies of oropharyngeal cavity, or surgical and radiation therapy for these malignancies, the symptoms of OPD are highly specific and should not be dismissed as psychogenic. Physical examination should focus on detection of neurologic deficits. Although a number of useful diagnostic modalities are available, the videofluroroscopic recording of a modified barium swallow is the diagnostic modality of choice for initial investigation of the patient with OPD. Diagnosis and optimal management of OPD require a systematic approach by a well-trained multidisciplinary team, under the guidance of a single managing physician.

References

1. Regan J, Sowman R, Walsh I. Prevalence of dysphagia in acute and community mental health settings. *Dysphagia* 2006;21: 95–101.
2. Garcia-Peris P, Paron L, Velasco C, *et al*. Long-term prevalence of oropharyngeal dysphagia in head and neck cancer patients: Impact on quality of life. *Clin Nutr* 2007;26:710–717.
3. Riley LH 3rd, Skolasky RL, Albert TJ, Vaccaro AR, Heller JG. Dysphagia after anterior cervical decompression and fusion: prevalence and risk factors from a longitudinal cohort study. *Spine* 2005;30:2564–2569.
4. Oh TH, Brumfield KA, Hoskin TL, Stolp KA, Murray JA, Bassford JR. Dysphagia in inflammatory myopathy: clinical characteristics, treatment strategies, and outcome in 62 patients. *Mayo Clin Proc* 2007;82:441–447.
5. Terre-Boliart R, Orient-Lopez F, Guevara-Espinosa D, Ramon-Rona S, Bernabeu-Guitart M, Clave-Civit P. Oropharyngeal dysphagia in patients with multiple sclerosis. *Rev Neurol* 2004;39:707–710.
6. Ardan GM, Kemp FH. A radiographic study of movements of the tongue in swallowing. *Dent Pract* 1955:5:252–261.
7. Shaker R, Cook IJ, Dodds WJ, Hogan WJ. Pressure-flow dynamics of the oral phase of swallowing. *Dysphagia* 1988:3:79–84.
8. Barclay AE. The normal mechanism of swallowing. *Laryngoscope* 1927;3735–3262.
9. Ardan GM, Kemp FH. The protection of the laryngeal airway during swallowing. *Br J Radiol* 1952;25:406–416.
10. Curtis DJ, Cruess DF, Crain M, *et al*. Lateral pharyngeal outpouchings: comparison of dysphagic and asymptomatic patients. *Dysphagia* 1988;2:156–161.
11. Shaker R, Dodds WJ, Dantas RO, *et al*. Coordination of deglutitive glottis closure with Oropharyngeal swallowing. *Gastro enterology* 1990;98:1478–1484.
12. Ramsey GH, Watson Js, Gramiak R, *et al*. Cinefluorographic analysis of the mechanism of swallowing. *Radiology* 1955;64: 498–518.
13. Logemann JA. *Manual for the Videofluorographic Study of Swallowing*. San Diego: College Hill Press, 1986, pp. 12–14.
14. Kahrilas PJ, Dodd. WJ, Dent J, *et al*. Upper esophageal sphincter function during deglutition. *Gastroenterology* 1988:92: 52–62
15. Curtis DJ, Cruess DF, Dachman AH, *et al*. Timing in the normal pharyngeal swallow. *Invest Radiol* 1984:19:523–529.
16. Logemann JA. Factors affecting ability to resume oral nutrition in the oropharyngeal dysphagic individual. *Dysphagia* 1990:4: 202–208.
17. Dodds WJ, Logemann JA, Stewart ET, Radiologic assessment of abnormal oral and pharyngeal phases of swallowing. *AJR Am J Roentgenol* 1990;154:965–974.
18. Donner MW, Silbiger ML. Cinefluorographic analysis of pharyngeal swallowing in neuromuscular disorders. *Am J Med Sci* 1966;251:600–616.
19. Duranceau A, Lafontaine ER, Taillefer R, *et al*. Oropharyngeal dysphagia and operations on the upper esophageal sphincter. *Surg Annu* 1987;19:317–362.
20. Doty RW. Influence of stimulus pattern on reflex deglutition. *Am J Physiol* 1951;166:142–158.
21. Doty R, Bosma JF. An electrophysiological analysis of reflex deglutition. *J Neurophysiol* 1956:19:44–60.
22. Doty R, Richmond W, Storey A. Effect of medullary lesions on coordination of deglutition. *Exp Neurol* 1967;17:91–106.
23. Kern MK, Jaradeh S, Arndorfer, RC, Shaker R. Cerebral cortical representation of reflexive and volitional swallowing in humans. *Am J Physiol Gastrointest Liver Physiol* 2001;280: G354–360.
24. Bevan K, Griffiths MV, Chronic aspiration and laryngeal competence. *Laryngol Otol* 1989;103:196–199.
25. Thompson W, Heaton K. Heartburn and globus on apparently healthy people. *Can Med Assoc J* 1982;126:46–48.
26. Moser G, Wenzel-Abatzi TA, Stelzeneder M, *et al*. Globus sensation: Pharyngoesophageal function, psychometric and psychiatric findings, and follow-up in 88 patients. *Arch Intern Med* 1998;158:1365.
27. Cook IJ, Dent J, Collins SM. Upper esophageal sphincter tone and reactivity to stress in patients with a history of globus sensation. *Dig Dis Sci* 1989;34:672–676.
28. Cook IJ, Shaker R, Doods WJ, *et al*. Role of mechanical and chemical stimulation of the esophagus in globus sensation. *Gastroenterology* 1989;96:A99.
29. Langmore SE, Terpenning MS, Schork A, *et al*. Predictors of aspiration pneumonia: how important is dysphagia? *Dysphagia* 1998;13:69–81.
30. Jadcherla SR, Gupta A, Stoner E, Coley BD, Wiet GJ, Shaker R. Correlation of glottal closure using concurrent ultrasonography

and nasolaryngoscopy in children: a novel approach to evaluate glottal status. *Dysphagia* 2006;21:75–81.

31. Dua K, Bardan E, Ren J, Sui Z, Shaker R. Effect of chronic and acute cigarette smoking on the pharyngo-upper oesophageal sphincter contractile reflex and reflexive pharyngeal swallow. *Gut* 1998;43:537–541.

32. Shaker R, Ren J, Zamir Z, Sarna A, Liu J, Sui Z. Effect of aging, position, and temperature on the threshold volume triggering pharyngeal swallows. *Gastroenterology* 1994;107:396–402.

33. Dua KS, Surapaneni SN, Santharam R, Knuff D, Hofmann C, Shaker R. Effect of systemic alcohol and nicotine on airway protective relfexes. *Am J Gastroenterol* 2009;104:2431–2438.

34. Robbins J, Levine R, Wood J, Roecker EB, Luschei E. Age effects on lingual pressure generation as a risk factor for dysphagia. *J Gerontol* 1995;50:M257–M262.

35. Baine WB, Yu W, Summe JP. Epidemiologic trends in the hospitalization of elderly Medicare patients for pneumonia, 1991-1998. *Am J Public Health* 2001;91:1121–1123.

36. Chiu WY, Yang CC, Huang IC, Huang TS. Dysphagia as a manifestation of thyrotoxicosis: Report of three cases and literature review. *Dysphagia* 2004;19:120.

37. Dodds WJ, Stewart ET, Logemann JA. Physiology and radiology of the normal oral and pharyngeal phases of swallowing. *AJR Am J Roentgenol* 1990;154:953–963.

38. Logemann JA. *Evaluation and Treatment of Swallowing Disorders.* Boston: College-Hill Press, 1983, pp. 58–133.

39. Jones B, Donner MW. How I do it: examination of the patient with dysphagia. *Dysphagia* 1989;4:162–172.

40. Ekberg O. Epiglottic dysfunction during deglutition in patients with dysphagia. *Arch Otolaryngol* 1983;109:376–380.

41. Splaingard ML, Hurchins B, Sulton LD, Chaudhuri G. Aspiration in rehabilitation patients: video fluoroscopy vs bedside clinical assessment. *Arch Phys Med Rehabil* 1988;69:637–640.

42. Langmore SE, Schatz K, Olsen N. Fiberoptic endoscopic examination of swallowing safety; a new procedure. *Dysphagia* 1988:2:216–219.

43. Bastian RW. Videoendoscopic evaluation of patients with dysphagia: an adjunct to the modified barium swallow. *Otolaryngol Head Neck Surg* 1991;104:339–350.

44. Shaker R, Massey BT. Oral pharyngeal and upper esophageal sphincter motility disorders. GI Motility Online. Available at: http://www.nature.com/gimo/index.html

45. Ghosh SK, Pandolfino JE, Zhang Q, Jarosz, Kahrilas PJ. Deglutitive upper esophageal sphincter relaxation: a study of 75 volunteer subjects using solid-state high-resolution manometry. *Am J Physiol Gastrointest Liver Physiol* 2006;291:G525–531.

46. Seaman WB. Cineroentgenographic observations of the cricopharyngeus. *AJR Am J Roentgenol* 1966;96:922–931.

47. Dantas RO, Cook IJ, Dodds WJ, *et al.* Biomechanics of cricopharyngeal bars. *Gastroenterology* 1990;99:1269–1274.

48. Shawker TH, Sonies BC, Stone M, Baum RJ. Real-time ultrasound visualization of tongue movement during swallowing. *J Clin Ultrasound* 1983;11:485–490.

49. Vencovský J, Rehak F, Pafko P, *et al.* Acute cricopharyngeal obstruction in dermatomyositis. *J Rheumatol* 1988;15:1016–1018.

50. Gagic NM. Cricopharyngeal myotomy. *Can J Surg* 1983:26:47–49.

51. Logemann JA. Swallowing physiology and pathophysiology. *Otolaryngol Clin North Am* 1988;21:613–623.

52. Brigand C, Ferraro P, Martin J, Duranceau A. Risk factors in patients undergoing cricopharyngeal myotomy. *Br J Surg* 2007;94:978–983.

53. Arnold G. Vocal rehabilitation of paralytic dysphonia: IX technique of intracordal injection. *Arch Otolaryngol* 1962;76:358–368.

54. Sessions D, Zill R, Schwartz SL. Deglutition after conservation surgery for cancer of the larynx and hypopharynx. *Otolaryngol Head Neck Surg* 1979;87:779–796.

55. Koufman JA, Isaacson G. Laryngoplastic phonosurgery. *Otolaryngol Clin North Am* 1991;24:1151–1177.

56. Rontal E, Rontal M. Vocal cord injection techniques. *Otolaryngol Clin North Am* 1991;24:1141–1149.

57. Martin BJW, Logemann JA, Shaker R, *et al.* Normal laryngeal valving patterns during three breath hold maneuvers: A pilot investigation. *Dysphagia* 1993, 8:11–20.

58. Bartolome G, Neuman DS: Swallowing therapy in patients with neurological disorders causing cricopharyngeal dysfunction. *Dysphagia* 1993, 8:146–149.

59. Shaker, R, Kern M, Bardan E, *et al.* Augmentation of deglutitive upper esophageal sphincter opening in the elderly by exercise. *Am J Physiol* 1997;272:G1518–G1522.

60. Shaker R, Easterling C, Kern M, *et al.* Rehabilitation of swallowing by exercise in tube fed patients with pharyngeal dysphagia secondary to abnormal UES opening. *Gastroenterology* 2002;122:1314–1321.

61. Odderson IR, Keaton JC, McKenna BS: Swallow management in patients on an acute stroke pathway: quality is cost-effective. *Arch Phys Med Rehabil* 1995;76:1130–1133.

62. Cook IJ, Kahrilas PJ. AGA technical review on management of oropharyngeal dysphagia. *Gastroenterology* 1999;116:455–478.

63. DePippo KL, Holas A, Reding MJ, *et al.* Dysphagia therapy following stroke: A controlled trial. *Neurology* 1994;44:1655–1660.

4 Regurgitation and Rumination

Francisco J. Marrero[1] and Steven S. Shay[2]
[1]Digestive Health Center, Lake Charles, LA, USA
[2]Cleveland Clinic Foundation, Cleveland, OH, USA

Introduction

Physicians commonly evaluate patients with recurrent episodes of regurgitation. Since many disorders present in this manner, a systematic approach is advisable to diagnose the origin of regurgitation in the individual patient with an organic lesion. However, even extensive evaluation may fail to define an underlying disorder. In this situation, consideration of a functional etiology, such as rumination, is warranted. Finally, eating disorders such as bulimia should be considered in the appropriate patient population.

Chronic regurgitation

Regurgitation is the sudden, effortless return of small volumes of gastric or esophageal contents into the pharynx, and implies cricopharyngeal relaxation or insufficiency. Regurgitation is best differentiated from vomiting by its small volume and by the lack of forceful abdominal contractions. Regurgitation is a predominantly recumbent occurrence. It is further characterized by the absence of preceding nausea, retching, or autonomic symptoms.

Differential diagnosis

Chronic regurgitation may result from several primary esophageal disorders or gastroesophageal reflux disease (GERD) (Table 4.1). Structural lesions may obstruct the esophageal lumen and thus cause regurgitation. Furthermore, food particles and secretions may accumulate in diverticula (see Chapter 17) at any level of the esophagus, thus resulting in regurgitation when the contents are discharged into the esophageal lumen. An esophageal motility disorder such as achalasia, hypertensive lower esophageal sphincter (LES), or diffuse esophageal spasm may also be responsible for regurgitation.

Pseudoregurgitation, solid or liquid accumulations in the pharynx not resulting from the upper esophageal sphincter (UES) relaxation, occurs in several circumstances and may be confused with regurgitation. Structural lesions, such as Zenker's diverticula, accumulate food and secretions, and may be the source of perceived regurgitation from below the UES. Additionally, inflammation of the nasal passages (sinuses, pharynx, or hypopharynx) may present with pseudoregurgitation when secretions are mistaken for regurgitant by the patient or physician.

Regurgitation can be difficult to distinguish from vomiting, and both symptoms may occur in the same patient. Chronic vomiting is usually of intra-abdominal origin, as in disorders of the pancreas or the hepatobiliary, genitourinary, or gastrointestinal tract; a broad differential encompassing several different organ systems must be considered (Table 4.2).

Complications

Aspiration is the most feared complication of chronic regurgitation or pseudoregurgitation. Nocturnal coughing, wheezing, a pillow stained with gastric contents, recurrent pneumonia, and interstitial lung disease are suggestive of regurgitation. Referred otic pain, globus sensation [1], dental findings [2], and a variety of otolaryngeal lesions [3] have been reported in patients with regurgitation caused by gastroesophageal reflux.

Diagnostic evaluation

Obtaining a detailed medical history that includes associated symptoms is valuable in discerning the etiology of "regurgitation." Most disorders of esophageal origin can present with dysphagia and, occasionally, odynophagia. Pyrosis suggests GERD, either primary or as a result of gastric retention. Chest pain suggests an esophageal motility disorder or GERD. Regurgitation or vomiting of material eaten many hours previously suggests gastric retention but may also

The Esophagus, Fifth Edition. Edited by Joel E. Richter, Donald O. Castell.
© 2012 Blackwell Publishing Ltd. Published 2012 by Blackwell Publishing Ltd.

Table 4.1 Disorders associated with chronic regurgitation and their initial evaluation (modified from Shay *et al.* [41]).

Disorder	Evaluation
Esophageal origin	
Structural esophageal lesion:	Barium esophagram, esophagoscopy
Tumor	
Stricture	
Diverticulum	
Esophageal motility disorder	Videoesophagram, esophageal manometry
Gastroesophageal reflux	
LES dysfunction:	Esophagoscopy, esophageal manometry, 24-h pH monitoring, 48-h pH monitoring (Bravo)
Primary	
Scleroderma	
Gastric retention:	Gastroscopy, UGI series, scintigraphic solid-food gastric emptying study
Obstruction	
Gastric atony	
Pseudoregurgitation	
Zenker's diverticulum	Videoesophagram, modified barium swallow
Nasopharyngeal structural lesion	Nasopharyngoscopy
Sinus disease	Sinus X-ray, CT scan

LES, lower esophageal sphincter; UGI, upper gastrointestinal; CT, computed tomography.

Table 4.2 Disorder categories in patients with chronic vomiting.

Cerebromedullary
Intra-abdominal:
Intraluminal
Visceral
Toxins
Drugs
Metabolic disturbances
Vestibular abnormalities
Pregnancy
Psychogenic

represent material expelled from a diverticulum (esophageal or pharyngeal) or achalasia. Expectoration of small volumes of mucoid or purulent material suggests a nasopharyngeal origin.

The past history is also valuable. Chronic rhinorrhea and coryza, especially seasonal, suggests nasopharyngeal disease. Other important features to note include a history of peptic ulcer disease (which should lead to suspicion of gastric retention), scleroderma, and Raynaud's disease.

The present and past history should lead to suspicion of an esophageal or gastroesophageal source for chronic regurgitation or to suspicion of pseudoregurgitation. The diagnostic tests available for the evaluation of these disorders are listed in Table 4.1. Occasionally, when the history does not clearly discriminate between the symptoms of regurgitation and vomiting or when they coexist, disorders associated with vomiting must be considered and excluded by appropriate studies. Finally, the patient may have primary rumination or an eating disorder.

The treatment of chronic regurgitation resulting from a primary disorder of the esophagus is detailed in Chapter 25.

Rumination syndrome

The rumination syndrome has many different presentations. Voluntary rumination may occur in the those with learning disabilities. In adults with normal intelligence, presentations can be extremely variable. At one extreme are patients with voluntary rumination performed for a pleasurable or profitable reason. At the other extreme are patients whose rumination is confused with organic disease because the rumination is involuntary and accompanied by other symptoms that mask its diagnosis, such as abdominal pain, weight loss, nausea without vomiting, constipation, and heartburn [4, 5]. This discussion addresses these divergent adult presentations after a review of rumination in animals and in the infant rumination syndrome.

Animal rumination

Animals such as sheep and cows are well-known ruminators that regurgitate, remasticate, and reswallow their food. They have compartmentalized stomachs (*rumens*) that aid in this process.

Rumination in cows was first studied by manometry in 19th-century experiments. These and later studies employing fluid-filled, non-perfused catheters identified two steps in the process [6, 7]. First, a negative intrathoracic pressure (−40 mmHg) occurred during rumen contractions, resulting in gastric contents being delivered to the esophagus. Then, antiperistalsis at a very fast rate (>100 mm/s) was observed, delivering contents from the esophagus to the mouth. In the cow, this occurs in regular 1-min cycles. A complex reflex mediated by the brainstem has been proposed since vagal sectioning prevents rumination in cows [8].

Rumination is also reported in 79% of captive gorillas. Since they do not have rumens, the mechanism is unknown, although regurgitation typically follows a series of other voluntary motor movements, as in infants and individuals with learning disabilities (see later in this chapter). Interestingly, as in some adults and infants, rumination in gorillas may respond to behavior modification. That is, rumination decreases if time spent eating increases, suggesting that rumination by gorillas in the zoo environment is voluntary and a result of artificially short feeding times in comparison to eating in the wild [9].

Infant rumination

The typical features of human infant rumination syndrome begin at 3–8 months of age. Infant rumination occurs when the baby is awake, quiet, and self-absorbed, rather than while asleep or actively interested in objects or surroundings. The act of rumination is typically a stereotyped series of maneuvers. It begins with rhythmic movements of the pharynx, tongue, and abdominal muscles. It culminates in regurgitation to the mouth (and usually spilling of regurgitant outside the oral cavity). Then, the regurgitant is masticated and reswallowed. There may be associated self-stimulatory behavior, such as head rolling, hand sucking, etc. The infant often fails to thrive, does not improve with conservative antireflux therapy, formula changes, etc., and, occasionally, exhibits progressive wasting until death [10]. Table 4.3 shows the Rome III diagnostic criteria for the infant rumination syndrome.

The infant rumination syndrome is thought to be the result of the infant's reaction to an emotionally distant caregiver who is unable to sense the baby's needs. Thus, rumination is self-stimulating and satisfies needs ordinarily supplied by the caregiver [10]. Infants residing in an environment that inhibits or prevents normal handling, such as a neonatal intensive care unit, may suffer sufficient sensory and emotional deprivation as to lead to the infant rumination syndrome [11]. Others consider the etiology is behavioral, and rumination persists as a result of the increased attention gained from the caregiver [12].

Table 4.3 Rome III diagnostic criteria for rumination syndrome in Infants [42].

Must include *all* of the following for at least 3 months:
1. Repetitive contractions of the abdominal muscles, diaphragm, and tongue
2. Regurgitation of gastric content into the mouth, which is either expectorated or rechewed and reswallowed
3. Three or more of the following:
   a. Onset between 3 and 8 months
   b. Does not respond to management for gastroesophageal reflux disease or to anticholinergic drugs, hand restraints, formula changes, and gavage or gastrostomy feedings
   c. Unaccompanied by signs of nausea or distress
   d. Does not occur during sleep and when the infant is interacting with individuals in the environment

The key to diagnosing the infant rumination syndrome is direct observation of the ruminating activity, since rumination can be easily confused with other functional vomiting disorders of infancy, such as nervous or innocent vomiting [10]. In addition, gastroesophageal diseases, such as pyloric stenosis, esophageal obstruction, and especially GERD [13] need to be excluded.

Therapy is behavioral if possible. Increasing social interaction between infant and mother or mother-substitute may stop rumination, especially increased holding during and immediately following meals [14, 15]. If this fails, aversive therapy, such as isolation or placing lemon juice on the tongue after rumination, has been effective [14, 16].

Rumination in adults with learning disabilities

Rumination syndrome has been reported to occur in as many as 10% of retarded adult patients with learning disabilities residing in institutions. It appears to be a voluntary behavior as it is typically repetitive and associated with oropharyngeal movements, such as sucking, belching noises, tongue movements, etc. Identifying those stereotyped maneuvers is the key to the correct diagnosis [17]. However, other causes of chronic regurgitation such as GERD [18] and vomiting need to be considered and excluded in the appropriate clinical situation.

Treatment is often necessary due to concern by caregivers about frequent cleaning of the patient and changes of clothing, bedding, etc. A combination of dietary manipulation, such as prescribing peanut butter [19], and behavioral interventions, such as withdrawal of social reinforcement during and after eating [20], should be tried first. If unsuccessful, individuals with learning disabilities have been treated successfully with a food-satiation approach [17] or aversive therapy, such as applying Tabasco sauce or lemon juice to the tongue [21, 22].

Voluntary rumination syndrome in adults

Some adults willfully ruminate as a pleasurable experience and may be selective in the food type regurgitated [23, 24]. In this situation, the patient may present out of concern for self-injury or the presence of an underlying disease, or if heartburn develops, or be presented by a relative who may observe mastication long after meal completion.

Taking advantage economically of their ability to regurgitate on command, some astonishing acts of controlled regurgitation have been described in circus performers. Among the most remarkable was Hadji Ali, an actor, who swallowed a pint of water and a half-pint of kerosene, then stood about 6 feet from a candle burning in a box open at the front. The kerosene, being of lower specific gravity, was brought up first in small jets which dramatically burst into flame as they approached the candle. When the kerosene was exhausted, the water was regurgitated in a spraying fashion from his mouth and the flames extinguished [25].

The pathophysiology of this kind of voluntary rumination is largely unknown. However, it is likely to be similar to that in those with involuntary rumination (described later), since observation of professional ruminators describe Valsalva- and Müller-like maneuvers preceding or associated with rumination [23, 25]. In addition, upper gastrointestinal (UGI) series in four patients during induced rumination observed Müller maneuvers and abdominal contractions simultaneous with rumination [26].

Despite the voluntary nature of rumination in these patients, cessation of rumination behavior should be recommended because of the potential for oropharyngeal, especially dental, complications.

Involuntary rumination syndrome in adults

Rumination in some patients is involuntary and not accompanied by other symptoms. This has been termed *simple rumination*, and men predominate in most series [24]. However, in some patients, rumination is accompanied by other symptoms, which may dominate the presentation. For example, *dyspeptic rumination* has been described, where epigastric discomfort, bloating, belching, and regurgitation were present [23, 27]. In a report of 16 patients (of whom, unusually, 10 were women), pain (n = 6), nausea (n = 5), constipation (n = 5), and heartburn (n = 1) were present [5]. Weight loss was common. Moreover, four of 16 had been on either total parenteral nutrition (TPN) or a feeding jejunostomy tube.

Diagnostic criteria

Rumination is a diagnosis of exclusion based mainly on signs and symptoms when there is no organic esophageal or gastric disease. Diagnostic criteria have been proposed for the rumination syndrome [28, 29]. There must be regurgita-

Table 4.4 Rome III diagnostic criteria for rumination syndrome in adults [43].

Must include *both* of the following for the last 3 months with symptom onset at least 6 months before diagnosis:
1. Persistent or recurrent regurgitation of recently ingested food into the mouth with subsequent spitting or remastication and swallowing
2. Regurgitation is not preceded by retching

Supportive criteria:
1. Regurgitation events are usually not preceded by nausea
2. Cessation of the process when the regurgitated material becomes acidic
3. Regurgitant contains recognizable food with a pleasant taste

tion of recently eaten food back into the mouth with either spitting or reswallowing. Regurgitation must also not be preceded by retching. Other suggestive features are the lack of nausea, lack of perception of acidity to the regurgitant, and the fact that the regurgitant is recognizable food with a potentially pleasant taste. The Rome III diagnostic criteria for the rumination syndrome are listed in Table 4.4 [29]. Regurgitation, remastication, and swallowing may occur as frequently as 20 times after a meal. Finally, rumination syndrome usually occurs with most meals.

Pathophysiology

Whether the varied presentations of rumination described above have the same pathophysiology and natural history is unknown. Early studies compared human and animal rumination, and separate gastric pouches and antiperistalsis were sought. These were not found. In fact, UGI series in patients not actively ruminating were normal in most cases.

Manometry of the UGI tract described simultaneous pressure spikes at all monitored sites concomitant with regurgitation and reswallowing (termed an *R wave*) in several reports. Furthermore, simultaneous pH changes have also been described [4, 5, 21]. This manometric finding is characteristic of rumination.

Shay *et al.* recorded simultaneous esophageal, gastric, UES, and rectal pressures with esophageal and pharyngeal pH in a 31-year-old patient with rumination and dyspeptic complaints for 20 years [30]. Twenty-five episodes were recorded in the first post-prandial hour and revealed the same pathophysiologic sequence (Figure 4.1). First, a spontaneous increase in intraesophageal pressure occurred, with respiratory excursion being the same as intragastric, i.e., a common cavity due to gaseous reflux [31]. A Valsalva maneuver (*R wave*), documented by sudden increases in intrathoracic and intra-abdominal pressures, occurred within 1–5 s of the common cavity and was simultaneous with the esophageal pH change. Relaxation of the UES at

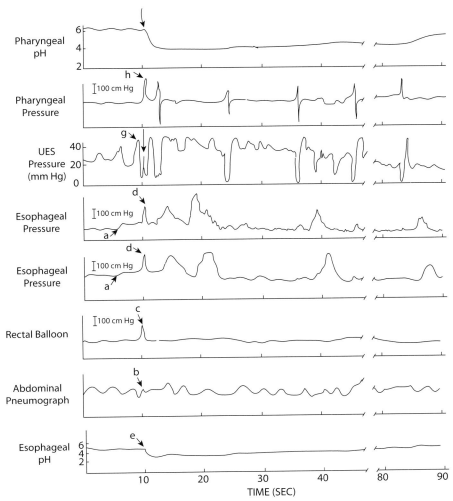

Figure 4.1 Simultaneous hypopharyngeal and esophageal pH monitoring and manometry during a rumination event. a, A spontaneous increase in intraesophageal pressure occurred with a respiratory excursion that coincided with that of the intragastric environment, i.e. the common cavity phenomenon. b, 5 s after the onset of the common cavity, a Valsalva maneuver (R wave) occurred, documented by splinting of respiration. c, Sudden increase in intra-abdominal pressure and d, spikes in intraesophageal pressure. This sequence was the rumination event, simultaneously documented by e, the decrease in esophageal pH and f, pharyngeal pH. g, Simultaneous relaxation of the upper esophageal sphincter (UES) pressure at the time of the Valsalva maneuver (R wave) appeared to facilitate esophagopharyngeal regurgitation.. The velocity of esophagopharyngeal regurgitation was 100 cm/s over the 20-cm distance between the pH probes. Acid reflux was then cleared from both the esophagus and the pharynx by primary peristalsis.

the time of the Valsalva maneuver resulted in near simultaneous pH changes in the pharynx and esophagus. In fact, the calculated velocity of the esophagopharyngeal regurgitation was 100 cm/s over the 20-cm distance between the two pH probes. Acid reflux was then cleared from the esophagus and pharynx by primary swallows [30].

In the patient above, rumination was a learned response to the common cavity phenomenon [30], which is gaseous gastroesophageal reflux. A review also postulates that rumination is a learned adaptation of the belch reflex [32]. Another etiology proposed for rumination is voluntary induction of transient LES relaxation after abdominal contractions [33].

Diagnosis

The rumination syndrome is underdiagnosed and often difficult to diagnose. In one study, patients saw a mean of five physicians and had symptoms for a mean of 2.8 years before diagnosis [4].

As already mentioned, rumination syndrome is a diagnosis of exclusion. Since any cause of regurgitation can potentially meet the definition of rumination syndrome if the patient chooses (or prefers for social reasons) to reingest the regurgitant, the disorders listed in Table 4.1 need to be excluded by the studies suggested. Once excluded, if the characteristic history is present, therapy as described below should be prescribed.

If primary GERD is suspected, the pattern of reflux and symptoms recorded during 24-h pH monitoring can be helpful. That is, predominantly upright post-prandial reflux, especially when accompanied by symptoms during the reflux events, is characteristic. Finally, if the diagnosis is in question because of the accompanying dyspeptic complaints or if abdominal pain is present, gastroduodenal manometry can identify the characteristic R waves from abdominal and thoracic contractions and exclude other disorders.

Tutuian *et al.* demonstrated a case of a 26-year-old man with suspected rumination where the diagnosis was made with combined multichannel intraluminal impedance–esophageal manometry (MII–EM) [34]. This method of diagnosis is the method we favor when the diagnosis needs to be confirmed (Figure 4.2).

Therapy

A number of aversive therapies have been attempted in adults, such as alkalis, acids, bitter potions, and gastric lavage [35]. However, no generally accepted and reliable aversive treatment has been reported. We are also unaware of any

reports showing prokinetic or antisecretory drugs to be effective in rumination. Nissen fundoplication has been shown to be effective in the treatment of the rumination syndrome in a case series of five patients [36]; however, there was no long-term follow-up or report of complications related to these cases.

Non-aversive behavioral therapy employs explanations of the mechanism of rumination and/or behavioral therapy, such as biofeedback, by a behavioral therapist. An eating habit regulation program (six of seven patients), biofeedback and Jacksonian relaxation (two of two patients), and psychotherapy (one of one patient) were associated with improvement or complete cessation of rumination in nine of 10 patients in one study [37]. Shay *et al.* found that biofeedback directed against the abdominal and thoracic contractions stopped rumination, and documented a decrease in acid exposure and reflux event frequency by 24-h pH monitoring [30]. Several other authors have demonstrated the effectiveness of diaphragmatic breathing techniques in the rumination syndrome [38, 39]. Chitkara *et al.* provides an excellent summary of how to teach breathing techniques

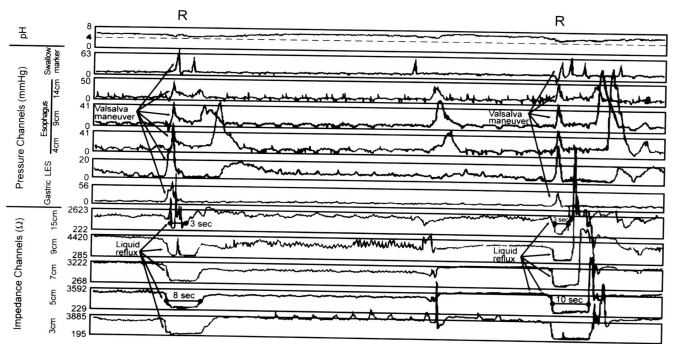

Figure 4.2 Combined multiluminal intraluminal impedance–esophageal manometry (MII–EM) tracings demonstrating simultaneous measurements of esophageal impedance (MII), intra-abdominal (gastric) and intrathoracic (esophageal) manometry along with pH measurement. There are two episodes of non-acid regurgitation (note pH > 4) where regurgitation (R) is identified by impedance as rapid liquid bolus transits to ≥17 cm above the lower esophageal sphincter (LES) almost instantaneously. Manometry shows that this is caused by a Valsalva maneuver recognized by the pressure spike at all gastric and esophageal pressure sites.

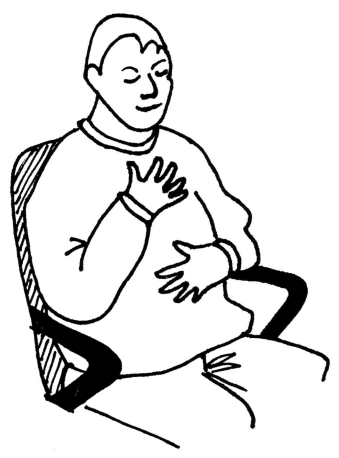

Figure 4.3 Position assumed by patients to employ breathing techniques for treating rumination. Alternatively, the patient may lie down. The patient is instructed to place one hand on their chest and the other on their abdomen. The patient is taught to breathe in such a manner that the hand on the abdomen rises with each breath while the hand on the chest remains relatively motionless. This usually takes observed practice until the patient can get it right.

to patients during a regular clinic visit [40]. Figure 4.3 displays how this is done.

Thus, non-aversive behavioral therapy is the modality of choice for rumination in adults of normal intelligence and it may be possible to employ some techniques in the physician's office.

References

1. Wilson JA, Pryde A, Piris J, *et al.* Pharyngoesophageal dysmotility in globus sensation. *Arch Otol Laryngol Head Neck Surg* 1989;115:1086–1090.
2. Schroeder PL, Filler SJ, Ramirez B, Lazarchik DA, Vaezi MF, Richter JE. Dental erosion and acid reflux disease. *Ann Intern Med* 1995;122:809–815.
3. Koufman JA. The otolaryngeal manifestations of gastroesophageal reflux disease. *Laryngoscope* 1991;101 (Suppl 53):1.
4. O'Brien MD, Bruce BK, Camilleri M. The rumination syndrome: clinical features rather than manometric diagnosis. *Gastroenterology* 1995;108:1024–1029.
5. Soykan I, Chen J, Kendall BJ, McCallum RW. The rumination syndrome: clinical and manometric profile, therapy, and long-term outcome. *Dig Dis Sci* 1997;42:1866–1872.
6. Doughterty RW. Physiology of eructation in ruminants. In: *Handbook of Physiology*, Vol 5. Baltimore: Williams & Wilkins, 1968, p. 2695.
7. Stevens CE, Sellers AF. Rumination. In: *Handbook of Physiology*, Vol 5. Baltimore: Williams & Wilkins, 1968, p. 2699.
8. Clark C. The nerve control for rumination and reticuloruminal motility. *Am J Vet Res* 1953;14:376.
9. Gould E, Bres M, Regurgitation and reingestion in captive gorillas: description and intervention. *Zoo Biol* 1986;5:241.
10. Fleisher DR. Functional vomiting disorders in infancy: innocent vomiting, nervous vomiting, and infant rumination syndrome. *J Pediatr* 1994;125 (Suppl):84.
11. Heymen PE, Milla PJ, Benninga MA, Davidson GP, Fleisher DF, Taminiau J. Childhood functional gastrointestinal disorders: neonate/toddler. *Gastroenterology* 2006;130;1519–1526.
12. Wolf MM, Birnbrauer J, Lawler J, Williams T. The operant extinction, reinstatement and re-extinction of vomiting behavior in a retarded child. In: Ulrich R, Statnik T, Mabry J, eds. *Control of Human Behavior*, Vol 2. Glenview, IL: Scott, Foresman, 1970, p. 146.
13. Taminiau JA. Gastro-esophageal reflux in children. *Scand J Gastroenterol* 1997;32 (Suppl 223):18.
14. Murray ME, Keele DK, McCarver JW. Behavioral treatment of rumination. *Clin Pediatr* 1976;15:591–593.
15. Whitehead WE, Drescher VM, Morrill-Corbin E, Cataldo MF. Rumination syndrome in children treated by increased holding. *J Pediatr Gastroenterol Nutr* 1985;4:550–556.
16. Sajwaj T, Libet J, Agras S. Lemon juice therapy: the control of life-threatening rumination in a six-month-old infant. *J Appl Behav Anal* 1974;7:557–563.
17. Fox RM, Snyder MS, Schroeder F. A food satiation and oral hygiene punishment program to suppress chronic rumination by retarded persons. *J Autism Dev Disorder* 1979;9:399–412.
18. Byrne WJ, Euler AR, Achcraft E, Nash D, Seibert J, Golladay ES. Gastroesophageal reflux in the severely retarded who vomit: criteria for and results of surgical intervention in twenty-two patients. *Surgery* 1982;91:95–98.
19. Greene KS, Johnson JM, Rossi M, Rawal A, Winston M, Barron S. Effects of peanut butter on ruminating. *Am J Mental Retard* 1991;95:631–645.
20. Luiselli JK, Haley S, Smith A. Evaluation of a behavioral medicine consultative treatment for chronic, ruminative vomiting. *J Behav Ther Exp Psychiatry* 1993;24:27–35.
21. Bright PJ, George GC, Smart DE. Suppression of regurgitation and rumination with aversive events. *Mich Mental Health Res Bull* 1968;11:17.
22. White JD, Taylor D. Noxious conditioning as a treatment for rumination. *Mental Retard* 1967;5:30.
23. Brockbank EM. Mercyism or rumination in man. *Br Med J* 1907;1:421.

24. Parry-Jones B. Mercyism or rumination disorder: a historical investigation and current assessment. *Br J Psychiatry* 1994;165: 303.

25. Long C. Rumination in man. *Am J Med Sci* 1929;178:814.

26. Van Trappen G, Hellemans J. *Diseases of the Esophagus*. New York: Springer-Berlag, 1974:418.

27. Geffen N. Rumination in man. *Am J Dig Dis* 1966;11:963.

28. Richter JE. Functional esophageal disorders. In: Drossman DA, ed. *Functional Gastrointestinal Disorders, Diagnosis, Pathophysiology and Treatment—A Multinational Consensus*. Boston: Little, Brown and Company, 1994, p. 35.

29. Tack J, Talley NJ, Camilleri M, Holtmann G, Hu P, Malagelada J, Stanghellini V. Functional gastroduodenal disorders. *Gastroenterology* 2006;130:1466–1479.

30. Shay SS, Johnson LF, Wong RK, *et al.* Rumination, heartburn, and daytime gastroesophageal refulx: a case study with mechanisms defined and successfully treated with biofeedback therapy. *J Clin Gastroenterol* 1986;8:115–126.

31. Butterfield DG, Struthers JE, Showalter BS. A test of gastroesophageal sphincter competence: the common cavity test. *Dig Dis Sci* 1972;17:415–421.

32. Malcolm A, Thumshirn MB, Camilleri M, Williams DE. Rumination syndrome. *Mayo Clin Proc* 1997;72:646–652.

33. Smout AJ, Breumelhof R. Voluntary induction of transient lower esophageal sphincter relaxations in an adult patient with the rumination syndrome. *Am J Gastroenterol* 1990;85:1621.

34. Tutuian R, Castell DO. Rumination documented by using combined multichannel intraluminal impedance and manometry. *Clin Gastroenterol Hepatol* 2004;2:340.

35. Kanner L. Historical notes on rumination in man. *Med Life* 1936;43:27.

36. Oelschlager BK, Chan MM, Eubanks TR, Pope CE, Pellegrini CA. Effective treatment of rumination with Nissen fundoplication. *J Gastrointest Surg* 2002;6:638–644.

37. Amarnath RP, Abell TL, Malagelada J. The rumination syndrome in adults. *Ann Intern Med* 1986;105:513–518.

38. Chial HJ, Camilleri M, Williams DE, Litzinger K, Perrault J. Rumination syndrome in children and adolescents: diagnosis, treatment and prognosis. *Pediatrics* 2003:111:158–162.

39. Wagaman JR, Williams DE, Camilleri M. Behavioral intervention for the treatment of rumination. *J Pediatr Gastroenterol Nutr* 1998;27:596–598.

40. Chitkara DK, Van Tilburg MV, Whitehead WE, Talley NJ. Teaching diaphragmatic breathing for rumination syndrome. *Am J Gastroenterol* 2006;101:2449–2452.

41. Shay SS, Johnson LF. Regurgitation, rumination, and disorders of eating. In: Castel DO, ed. *Esophageal Function in Health and Disease*. New York: Elsevier Science, 1983, p. 140.

42. Hyman P, Milla P, Benninga M, Davidson G, Fleisher D, Taminau J. Childhood functional gastrointestinal disorders: neonate/ toddler. *Gastroenterology* 2006;130:1519–1526.

43. Tack J, Talley NJ, Camilleri M, Holtman G, Hu P, Malagelada JR, Stanghellini V. Functinal gastrointestinal disorders. *Gastroenterology* 2006;130:1466–1479.

II Esophageal Physiology and Testing

5 Functional Anatomy and Physiology of Swallowing and Esophageal Motility

Nicholas E. Diamant

Queen's University, Kingston, Ontario, Canada

Introduction

As part of the swallowing process, esophageal function is dependent on a variety of interacting control mechanisms that intimately link it to the oral and pharyngeal stages of swallowing, gastric function, and other thoracic organs. Connections with the central nervous system (CNS) provide elements of motor control, and sensory pathways that impact on normal motor activity as well as contribute to clinical motility disorders and esophageal pain syndromes.

Anatomically and physiologically the esophagus is an unusual organ. The swallowing process combines voluntarily-induced central control mechanisms for the oral and proximal pharyngeal stages with involuntary/reflex controls, both central and peripheral, as the process proceeds through the distal pharynx and the esophagus. The human esophagus is composed of both striated and smooth muscles, each with different control mechanisms that must integrate effectively. The esophagus passes through and/or connects cavities of different pressures, from atmospheric pressure at the mouth, to negative intrathoracic pressure, to positive intra-abdominal pressure. Valves (sphincters) at each end of the esophagus serve to separate the pressures and organ contents in each location, preventing reflux of gastric contents into the esophagus and esophageal contents into the pharynx. The sphincters must also open temporarily when needed to allow the passage of food aborally, and air and gastric contents orally with belching and vomiting.

The majority of information on the central and peripheral control mechanisms for swallowing, and particularly esophageal function, derive from animal experimentation. Species differ in many aspects and some care is required in imparting animal findings to the human situation. Studies of the central mechanisms are mainly in animals with a totally striated muscle esophageal body (such as the sheep, rat, mouse, ferret, and dog), and this information has relevance to human physiology in terms of the oropharynx and upper striated muscle esophageal body, and to the lower esophageal sphincter (LES). The LES is composed of smooth muscle in all species. Studies in species with a significant portion of the esophageal body composed of smooth muscle, such as the opossum, cat, and to a lesser extent the non-human primate and humans, have provided a large amount of information about the peripheral control mechanisms in the smooth muscle esophageal body and LES, but only limited insight into the central mechanisms.

Swallowing

Swallowing occurs about 600 times a day, mainly while awake and during eating, but a small number, 50 swallows, occur while asleep [1]. Central control of the swallowing process is required for orderly contraction of muscles in the mouth and pharynx (oropharynx), upper esophageal sphincter (UES), and upper esophagus. These regions are striated muscle and need guiding motor input for their contraction. The more distal smooth muscle esophagus, including the LES, has a number of intrinsic control mechanisms for orderly contractile function that must interact and cooperate with the central control. Sensory information from the mouth and pharynx, and peripheral sensory–motor control mechanisms in the esophagus integrate and coordinate with the central control. This combination is a remarkable example of the brain–gut axis at work. It combines the central and peripheral sensory–motor control of an essential human and gut function with the social and pleasurable aspects of eating. Although clinical disorders of the esophagus, especially the smooth muscle portion, are usually considered from the view of the peripheral neuromuscular dysfunction, a central contribution to these disorders must also be considered.

The Esophagus, Fifth Edition. Edited by Joel E. Richter, Donald O. Castell.
© 2012 Blackwell Publishing Ltd. Published 2012 by Blackwell Publishing Ltd.

Swallowing pattern generator

Groups of neurons in the brainstem make up a "swallowing center" composed of a network of swallowing-related neurons that form a central pattern generator (CPG). This CPG programs sequential motor output to the muscles along the entire swallowing pathway, including to the esophagus, and is called the swallowing program generator (SPG). The SPG can be activated in total by cortical input for the voluntary initiation of the swallow, or in part by peripheral sensory input from peripheral locations for reflex initiation of activity such as the "pharyngeal swallow", and secondary peristalsis at one or other level in the esophagus. Once the oral stage is initiated voluntarily, or reflex activity is initiated beyond this stage by sensory input, the process proceeds sequentially through the remaining program under control of the SPG.

The SPG is not a single unit. Food is first masticated, and formed into a bolus that is placed on the tongue and moved posteriorly in the mouth in a preswallow phase. Swallowing is then voluntarily initiated and is composed of three functional stages—oral, pharyngeal and esophageal—that always occur in sequence to move the bolus out of the mouth and through the pharynx and esophagus into the stomach. Each functional stage of the process has its own CPG, and these are hooked in series to form the SPG, each stage activating the subsequent stage. This interactive connectivity serves a number of functions: (1) efficient propulsion of the bolus distally through the entire pathway; (2) protection of the airway; (3) initiation of the process in the pharynx or at different levels in the esophagus independent of voluntary swallowing; (4) contraction and relaxation of the UES and LES; (5) a mechanism for deglutitive and distal inhibition; and (6) involvement with various reflexes that connect the pharynx and esophagus to a number of organ systems, such as the respiratory system and airways, the cardiovascular system including the heart, and the more distal gut for such actions as belching and vomiting.

The SPG is in the medulla portion of the brainstem, and is bilaterally represented. The two sides are connected but able to function independently if necessary, thus providing a protective redundancy. The SPG has complex connections to higher regions in the midbrain and the cerebral cortex, and to the motor nuclei of cranial nerves serving over 50 different muscles along the swallowing pathway. Peripheral sensory input from the mouth, pharynx, and esophagus feed into the SPG and modulate its functions and behavior in response to the nature of the bolus ingested.

A number of features characterize the complexity of the central program and its functional behavior, and these will be summarized in this chapter. Detailed descriptions are given in more recent [2–7] and earlier reviews [8–13].

Organizational structure and function

Each stage of the SPG has a similar overall structure that includes sensory input into a programming circuitry of neurons, and a group of appropriate motor neurons [4]. The programming circuitry has two components: a dorsal group of neurons and interneurons (DSG) in the nucleus of the solitary tract (NTS) and adjacent reticular formation that are triggered and generate the timing and sequencing of events; and a ventral group (VSG) in the ventrolateral medulla that serves as a switching station for signals to the motor neurons of the cranial nerves innervating the muscles. Bilateral connectivity occurs at the level of the NTS. The DSG and VSG are connected either directly or through internerons. Sensory feedback from the periphery modulates the activity of the programming circuitry. Input from higher centers such as the cortex feed into each stage of the SPG.

Figure 5.1 summarizes these aspects for the combined oropharyngeal stages and the esophageal stage of the SPG.

Sensory

Sensory feedback to the oropharyngeal stages is via cranial nerves: trigeminal (V), facial (VII), glossopharyngeal (IX) and vagus (X) [10]. Input from the superior laryngeal nerve (SLN) of the vagus nerve is the primary pathway for sensory initiation of the pharyngeal stage [6, 14]. The maxillary branch of V and sensory input from IX can also initiate swallowing [14–17]. The pharynx is highly sensitive and in humans as little as 0.5 mL of fluid injected quickly into the pharynx can initiate swallowing [18–20]. Esophageal feedback occurs via the vagus nerve with its cell bodies in the nodose ganglion. Afferent information enters into the NTS, where different subdivisions of the NTS can initiate deglutition and program the swallowing sequence, modify ongoing motor activity, or activate reflexes involving the esophagus and its sphincters or reflexes involving supraesophageal structures such as the larynx [6, 21]. There is viscerotopic organization of the afferent input to the NTS [7, 22]. Esophageal afferents may also have a role in modifying cognitive sensation such as pain, acting through higher centers [23]. Although sensory information from the esophagus also passes centrally via sympathetics entering the spinal cord segments C1 to L3 [24, 25], any role of this information in modulating SPG activity is unknown.

Oropharyngeal afferents enter primarily into two subnuclei of the NTS, the interstitial (NTS_{is}) and the intermediate (NTS_{im}), and esophageal afferents enter into the subnucleus centralis (NTS_{ce}) [5–7, 26–29]. In these components of the DSG, programming activity apparently occurs. Other NTS subnuclei are also active and presumably function in the relay to the VSG and to motor neurons, and in the pathways to affected activities such as respiration.

Motor

Motor function of muscles involved with the oropharyngeal stages is mediated by cranial nerves V, VII, and XII (hypoglossal), and the nucleus ambiguous (NA) portion of X [5].

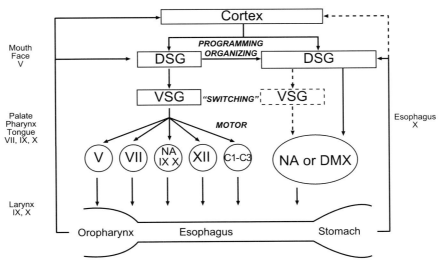

Figure 5.1 Central control of the oropharynx and esophagus. The oropharyngeal circuitry is shown on the left and the esophageal on the right. Both have a dorsal swallowing group (DSG) in the solitary tract nucleus for programming and organizing the sequential events in their respective locations. The oropharyngeal DSG leads the esophageal DSG. The oropharyngeal mechanism has a ventral swallowing group (VSG) in the ventral lateral medulla where "switching" of the DSG signaling distributes excitation to the appropriate cranial nerves for the mouth, pharynx, and larynx. The esophageal circuit likely has a VSG but may be simpler, with a direct connection from the DSG to the motor nuclei. Both circuits can receive inputs from the periphery, the cerebral cortex, and various supramedullary structures. DMX, dorsal motor nucleus of the vagus; NA, nucleus ambiguous (modified from Jean and, Dallaporta [4], with permission).

Innervation of neck muscles through C1–C3 can be considered "facilitative." The striated muscle esophagus receives its innervation from the NA portion of X. A small number of fibers may arise in the dorsal motor nucleus of the vagus (DMNV) in species with a smooth muscle esophagus, perhaps to inhibit the esophageal motor neurons. The smooth muscle receives its motor input from the DMNV, although a small number of fibers may arise in the NA [30]. There is rostral–caudal myotopic organization within the NA for output to the different striated muscles along the swallowing pathway [31–35]. Within the DMNV there are different locations for motor output to the esophageal body and LES, and for function of the LES, with excitation to the LES being distal and inhibition more rostrally positioned [30, 36, 37].

Organization

Once the process is initiated at any stage, sequential activation of the neurons in the remaining program occurs [2, 4, 7]. For example, initiation at the oral stage causes activation of neurons in the pharyngeal and esophageal stages; initiation of the pharyngeal swallow by pharyngeal stimulation activates the esophageal phase; initiation of secondary peristalsis by distention in the mid esophagus activates more distal esophageal programming. Although sequential activation of neurons along the program is the basis for the eventual pattern of motor events in each peripheral location, inhibitory messaging is also present along the entire program circuitry. Two features are evident that affect the esophagus

particularly: excitation decreases along the program pathway, while inhibition increases along it. Figure 5.2 illustrates these features and the place of sensory feedback.

From a functional point of view, the decreasing excitation along the program places added impact on the role of sensory feedback to shape the activity of the central program depending on the bolus requirements, and in the case of the esophagus, sensory feedback may also be necessary to further excite the esophageal stage of the program for muscle contraction and peristalsis to occur [38–43]. These aspects are discussed later. Inhibition within and along the SPG serves at least two purposes. First, inhibition is an essential part of the program timing of events by progressively delaying excitation along the circuitry. Excitation of neurons at any stage in the esophageal program circuitry shuts down activity in all neurons destined for more distal esophageal sites. Excitation at any peripheral level increases excitation at the corresponding level in the SPG, while increasing inhibition below that SPG level. Second, inhibition is also important in the "distal inhibition" of motor events that occur with repetitive swallowing, for example, or distal to a point of distention in the esophagus. Deglutitive inhibition is discussed later.

The oral stage–pharyngeal stage connection and the DSG–VSG–motor neuron activation pathway are well established for the oropharyngeal stages of swallowing, and appear fairly consistent among different species, regardless of the esophageal muscle type. The connection of the pharyngeal stage to the esophageal circuitry is via the subnucleus

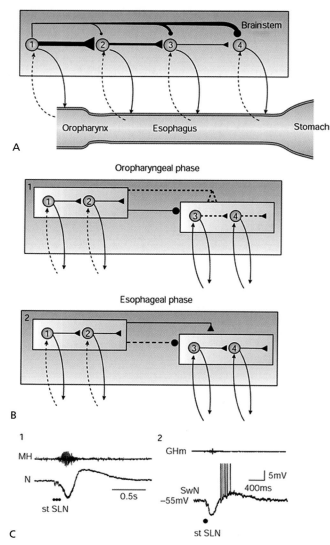

Figure 5.2 Excitation and inhibition in the swallowing network. (A) The swallowing network can be seen as a chain of neurons with excitatory (triangles) and inhibitory (dots) connections, and sensory feedback (broken lines). The power of excitatory inputs decreases along the chain; that of inhibitory inputs increases and can lead to long periods of inhibition of neurons controlling more distal parts of the tract. (B) The central pattern generator can be divided into an oropharyngeal network and an esophageal network. The esophageal network is first inhibited (dot), and then excited (triangle) to provide for successive activation of esophageal neurons. (C) Inhibitory–excitatory sequence recorded in an esophageal motor neuron in the sheep. (1) A single swallow was induced by stimulation of the superior laryngeal nerve (SLN). A biphasic inhibitory hyperpolarization was followed by a depolarization. (2) When spiking occurs on the after-depolarization, a contraction occurs following the inhibitory delay (reproduced from Jean and Dallaporta [4], with permission).

centralis and has its own specific features. The pathway, whether direct or via a VSG, from the DSG program in the NTS_{ce} to the motor neurons for the esophagus is still not fully established [2, 4]. It is also not clear whether the NTS_{ce} organizing program in species with both types of muscles has separate program modules for the striated and smooth muscle portions, and for the two or three segments of the smooth muscle portion including the LES.

There are numerous transmitter mechanisms within the SPG [2]. However, a smaller number provide the major actions. Excitation is largely mediated by excitatory amino acids such as glutamine, while inhibition is largely through the action of gamma-butyric acid (GABA) acting at the $GABA_A$ receptor. Cholinergic excitation also plays a significant role. Nicotinic action is important for activation of premotor neurons in the programming–organizing portions of the SPG, while muscarinic action appears to couple the oropharyngeal with the esophageal stages of the SPG and activate motor neurons. At the level of the NTS_{ce}, two other transmitters are important in activation of the esophageal and LES neurons; nitric oxide (NO) and somatostatin. NO is involved with regulating esophageal contraction amplitude, and LES tone and contraction [44, 45].

Other transmitters such as serotonin, norepinepherine, oxytocin, and vasopressin have modulatory roles, and are likely also connected to other interrelated functions such as hunger, thirst, nausea, and sleep.

Cortical and supramedullary influences

A number of reviews deal with these aspects [10, 12, 46–49].

Voluntary initiation of the entire swallowing process, beginning with the oral preparatory stage or the voluntary component of the oropharyngeal stage, resides in the cerebral cortex. The location involves the frontal cortex; in primates primarily the dorsolateral and anterolateral regions and involving the sensory–motor cortex [50]. The sites are bilaterally represented. There are connections to the SPG in the brainstem and more direct pathways as well to the motor neurons. Transcranial magnetic stimulation (TMS) of these cortical regions in humans has demonstrated a somatotopic organization serving different pharyngeal musculature and the upper striated muscle esophagus [51]. TMS directed at the cortex can also stimulate swallowing in animals but not in humans [52]. This technique has also demonstrated the bilateral representation in humans, with one side, usually the left, being dominant. Cortical stroke on the dominant side results in dysphagia, and recovery from the dysphagia is associated with enhancement of the cortical representation on the non-dominant side [53].

Imaging studies in humans and neurophysiologic studies in animals have demonstrated that many other areas in the cortex and other supramedullary areas are active with swallowing. Generally, these areas are involved in associated events such as feeding behavior, mastication, and respiration, or are connected to peripheral afferent sensory signals that can modify the swallowing process at one or more central levels [54–57]. The other supramedullary areas can include the cerebellum, nuclei in the pons, hypothalamus, and basal ganglia. It is therefore not surprising that strokes in many areas and disorders such as parkinsonism can impact on the swallowing process at many peripheral levels, including the esophagus [46, 58]. Therapeutic interventions directed at one or more of the central areas, such as TMS activation of the sensory feedback pathways, are now practical [59].

Oropharyngeal stage motor activity

A number of reviews detail the anatomy, physiology and investigation of the oropharynx [60–64].

The upper portion of the pharynx is composed of the oropharynx between the soft palate and the tongue, and extending to the valleculae and tip of the epiglottis; and the nasopharynx at the exit of the nasal cavity. The remainder of the pharynx, the hypopharynx, extends from the valleculae to the bottom of the cricoid cartilage. The pharynx is an irregular tube with its walls containing or supported by cartilages, including the cricoid and epiglottis, as well as the superior, middle, and inferior constrictor muscles. The pyriform sinuses situated laterally between the insertion of the inferior constrictor and the lateral wall of the thyroid cartilage end at the cricopharyngeus muscle and add to the axial and radial asymmetry. The hyoid bone pays a critical role as the attachment location for a number of muscles that raise and lower the larynx. The upper esophageal sphincter, formed primarily by the cricopharyngeus muscle, operates closely with the pharynx.

Masticating, forming the food bolus, and positioning it on the tongue for the swallow involves the lips, teeth, hard and soft palates, floor of the mouth, mandible and tongue, and the associated muscles. During mastication the posterior tongue is elevated and the soft palate pulled down against the tongue to prevent spillage into the pharynx, although some leaking of oral content does occur [65]. Once the swallow is initiated, the bolus is rapidly thrust into the pharynx by the tongue, and then the involuntary oral, pharyngeal, and esophageal stages of the SPG-controlled program are initiated. A series of rapid and highly coordinated events occurs through the action of muscles of the soft palate, tongue, and pharynx, including the UES. These events include: closing of the nasopharynx; elevation of the entire soft pharynx and the UES, producing a more tubular structure while protecting the airway; UES opening; and a propulsive contraction to clear the pharynx of content. Respiration is temporarily halted [57, 66] and therefore the swallowing process is considered a temporary switch of the pharynx from a respiratory to an alimentary configuration.

The entire series of events occurs in less than a second and it is not surprising that dysphagia and/or aspiration can occur if any portion of the process fails or becomes abnormal, such as with neurologic or muscle disorders [67–69].

Figure 5.3 shows the multitude of muscles involved in different functions of the pharyngeal swallow. Figures 5.4 and 5.5 illustrate the timing of some of the events and the typical X-ray pattern seen as they occur. Videofluoroscopic examination of the pharyngeal swallow is the most common method of assessing it [62]. Computed imaging techniques have been used for the tongue but these are not practical clinical tools [70, 71]. Recent improvements in manometric recording techniques have added a more precise perspective of pharyngeal bolus pressures, the timing and strength of pharyngeal contractions, and the timing and contractile function of the UES (Figure 5.6). The clinical value of these measurements is yet to be firmly established.

Propulsion of the bolus

With thrust of the tongue and gravity, a liquid bolus moves quickly along the pharynx before the slower moving peristaltic contraction of the three pharyngeal constrictor muscles starts [61, 72]. This peristalsis starts within less than 0.5 s, and then completes its course, with the pressures showing radial and axial asymmetry [73, 74]. The larger the bolus, the quicker it moves [75]. Tongue force and shape change to accommodate bolus size. A more solid bolus depends mainly on the peristaltic contraction for its passage and clearance. The 1-s timing of the process to clearance of either liquid or solid is altered little regardless of bolus consistency or size [75–77], and the pharyngeal peristaltic velocity remains constant.

Protection of the nasal cavity

As the bolus enters the pharynx, the soft palate moves upward and backward to meet the contraction of the upper constrictor muscle that produces a ridge in the posterior pharyngeal wall, called Passavant's ridge [70, 78]. These actions close the nasopharynx. As the contraction of the posterior wall then proceeds distally through the pharynx, the palate remains elevated until the larynx descends [75].

Protection of the airway

The major motor event is elevation and anterior movement of the larynx and tongue, also causing shortening of the pharynx [79]. This occurs through the action of many muscles on the hyoid bone, thyroid cartilage, and tongue (see Figure 5.3). In concert with this movement and the new position of the pharynx, the epiglottis is pulled downwards and the arytenoid cartilages are tilted forward to close entry to the laryngeal vestibule, and the false and true vocal chords are approximated, closing entry to the trachea. The normal repositioning of the larynx and opening of the laryngeal vestibule do not occur until closure of the UES with its

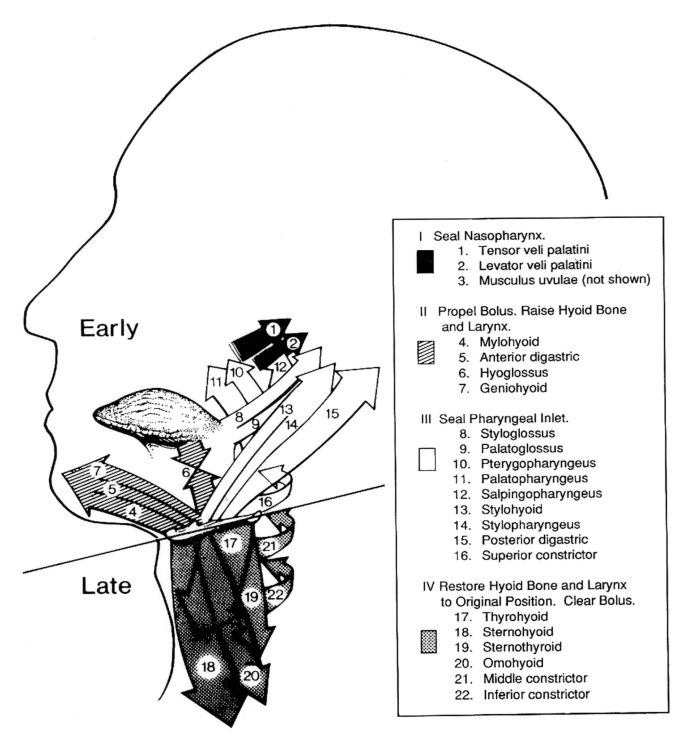

Figure 5.3 Muscular activity during the pharyngeal stage. A schematic view of the muscles and their actions during the early and late parts of the pharyngeal stage of the swallow (reproduced from Jones and Donner [61], with permission).

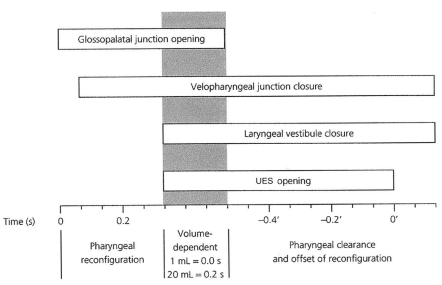

Figure 5.4 Timing of events during the pharyngeal swallow. The volume-induced (1 and 20 mL) modification of timing of events during the pharyngeal swallow. Each horizontal bar depicts the time each one of the oropharyngeal "valves" is moved into position to facilitate bolus passage and protect the airway. Events at the onset and offset of these moves bear a fixed time relationship to each other regardless of bolus volume. This fixed relationship is shown by referencing onset events from time 0, counting forward, and offset events from time 0, counting forward or backward. The middle portion of the events (shaded bar) defines the volume effect. Regardless of bolus size the entire series of events occurs in about a second or less (reproduced from Kahrilas *et al.* [77], with permission).

contraction that follows the laryngeal contraction. A larger bolus is associated with a longer time period of laryngeal elevation.

Respiration is also temporarily halted with a swallow [57, 66]. The apnea commences prior to the swallow, lasts usually 1–1.5 s, and occurs most frequently in expiration.

Upper esophageal sphincter function

The UES "relaxes" with cessation of tonic vagal excitation and opens shortly thereafter, pulled open by the hyoid bone as it moves upward and forward. The sphincter opening ends when the pharyngeal contraction reaches the UES and closes it with a sphincter contraction [63]. The UES is discussed in detail in the next section of the chapter.

Esophageal stage motor activity

Upper esohageal sphincter

There are a number of review articles on this subject [60, 63, 64, 80–82].

Anatomy and innervation

The UES is measured as a 2–4-cm zone of high pressure at the distal end of the pharynx, and at the entry to the esophagus. Its intimate association with the musculature, innervations, and SPG-programmed events of the oropharyngeal stage of swallowing, including its upward movement with

the larynx, makes the UES the inferior pharyngeal sphincter as well. Because of its anatomy, the sphincter has a very asymmetrical shape with pressures higher anteriorly and posteriorly (Figure 5.7). The cricoid cartilage forms the anterior wall. The lateral and posterior walls are formed by the lower portion of the cricopharyngeus muscle that inserts anteriorly into the inferolateral margins of the cricoid lamina and then loops around the esophageal inlet (Figure 5.8). This 1-cm wide portion is situated at approximately the location of maximum pressure [83, 84]. The lower pressures at either end of the high-pressure zone likely make a contribution proximally from the lower end of the inferior constrictor muscle, where a small portion arises from the cricoid cartilage as part of the cricopharyngues muscle, and from circular esophageal muscle distally. A triangular space exists between the cricopharyngeus muscle and the lower border of the inferior constrictor muscle (Killian triangle), the location of a Zenker's diverticulum when it occurs [64].

The UES is striated muscle mainly of the slow twitch type, and has abundant connective and elastic tissue [63, 81, 85, 86]. These aspects potentially contribute to its ability to maintain a small amount of resting tone when excitatory neural input is removed. Of the three UES muscular elements, the inferior constrictor receives its innervation from the pharyngeal branches of the vagus, the cricopharyngeus from both the pharyngeal and recurrent laryngeal (RLN) branches, and the upper striated muscle esophagus from the RLN [87]. These serve both motor and sensory functions.

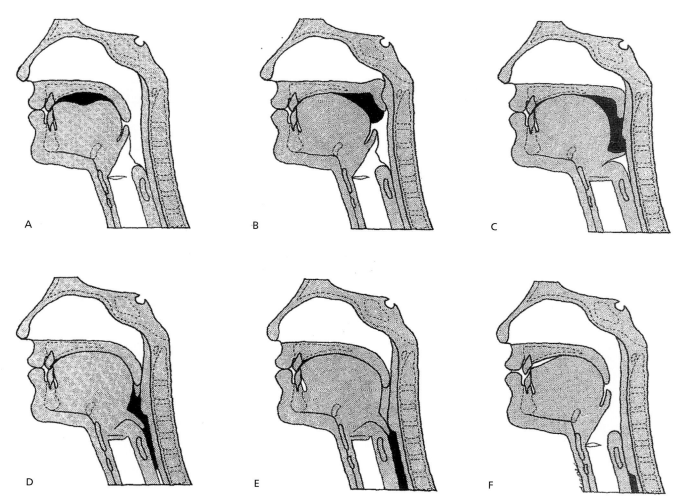

Figure 5.5 Normal oropharyngeal swallow. (A) At rest the bolus is held in the mouth. (B) Bolus is conveyed into the oropharynx. The airway and surrounding larynx have been elevated. (C) Bolus is descending in advance of the descending peristaltic wave. The epiglottis is now horizontal, the larynx is maximally elevated, and the bolus passes into the hypopharynx. (D) Bolus continues to descend, and begins to pass through the open upper esophageal sphincter (UES) into the esophagus, with the peristaltic wave descending behind it. The nasopharynx begins to open and opening progresses in a descending sequence. (E) The pharyngeal contraction moves into the hypopharynx as the bolus continues through the open UES. The nasopharynx continues to open from the top. (F) Bolus is completely in the esophagus. The nasopharynx, pharynx, and entry to the airway have opened, although the larynx has not completely descended to its original position (reproduced from Donner *et al.* [60], with permission).

Motor fibers terminate as motor endplates and release acetylcholine acting on nicotinic receptors for muscle contraction [88]. The motor nuclei for all three muscles are in the nucleus ambiguous with a somatotopic organization there [89]. Sympathetic neural supply is also present, but its role in motor events is unclear [64].

Functional motor activity

The UES is normally closed and has a resting pressure that separates the atmospheric pressure above from the negative intrathoracic pressure, and prevents esophagopharyngeal reflux. The sphincter relaxes with a swallow to allow passage of the bolus into the esophagus, and also relaxes to permit orad movement of content with belching and vomiting. A "pharyngeal swallow" can be initiated by pharyngeal stimulation and involves only the pharynx and UES before proceeding into the esophageal body [18].

Basal pressures

Significant resting pressure is present in the closed UES due to tonic vagal excitation, which if removed leaves a small residual pressure, presumably due to the intrinsic muscle tone [90]. However, resting pressures of the UES are inconsistent and reported to be between 35 and 200 mmHg

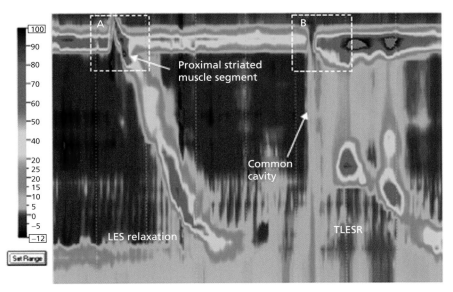
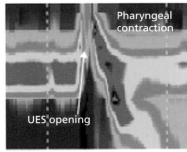
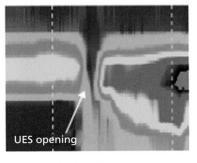

Figure 5.6 Upper esophageal function by high-resolution manometry. The left side of the figure shows the high resolution picture of the timing and pressures of a swallow event, with upper esophageal (UES) and lower esophageal sphincter (LES) relaxation. (A) Typical UES relaxation and opening with a swallow, and its closure with the arrival of the pharyngeal contraction that then propagates through the striated portion of the upper esophagus. (B) UES opening during belching. During a transient LES relaxation (TLESR) a common gastroesophageal cavity develops that leads to UES opening and gas venting. A pharyngeal contraction is absent (reproduced from Kahrilas PJ and Pandolfino JE. Esophageal motor function. In: Yamada T, ed. *Textbook of Gastroenterology*, 5th edn. Hoboken, NJ: Wiley-Blackwell, 2008).

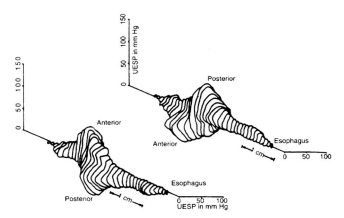

Figure 5.7 Three-dimensional pressure profile of the upper esophageal sphincter (UES). The pressures are higher in the anterior and posterior positions, and lower on the sides. UESP, UES pressure (reproduced from Welsh RW, Gray JE. Influence of respiration on recordings of lower esophageal sphincter pressure in humans. *Gastroenterology* 1982;83:590–594, with permission).

[84, 91–93]: the pressure varies within the UES due to its odd shape (see Figure 5.7); reliable pressure is hard to measure as the UES moves 2–3 cm with a swallow [84, 94] and the recording device may itself increase pressure [90, 95, 96], with larger devices recording higher pressures [97,

98]; pressure falls during sleep [99, 100]; sedation such as anesthesia [101] reduces pressure in humans to about 8 mmHg; pressure varies with respiration [95, 100, 102–104], increasing with each inspiration and coughing [105]; pressure increases with stress [106, 107]; and a number of reflex responses alter pressure, acting, for example, to prevent reflux into the pharynx [108]. Newer techniques such as high-resolution manometry have improved the ability to monitor the pressures, as well as sphincter behavior with swallowing and other events such as belching (see Figure 5.6).

Swallowing

The UES "relaxes" with SPG-controlled cessation of tonic vagal excitation, and a decrease in pressure occurs within 0.2 s of the initiation of the swallow [109]. However, the UES opens about 0.1 s later as a result of traction as the hyoid bone is pulled upward and forward [94, 110]. The degree of opening is enhanced with a larger bolus and the resulting greater bolus pressure developed by more tongue thrust and strength of the descending pharyngeal contraction [70, 76, 79, 109]. Augmentation of the opening can also occur with the Mendelsohn maneuver, forceful voluntary prolongation of the laryngeal excursion [111]. Pharyngeal peristaltic velocity remains unchanged. The UES opening is synchronous with the laryngeal vestibule closure, both occurring earlier

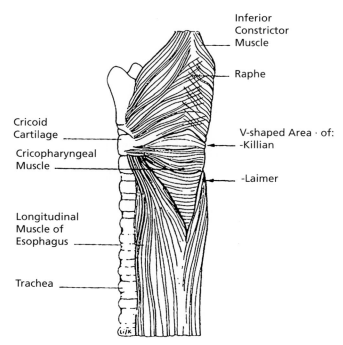

Figure 5.8 Muscular architecture of the pharynx and upper esophagus from the laterodorsal aspect. The cricopharyngeus muscle has an upper portion that is continuous with the inferior constrictor muscle, and a lower portion that encircles the region at the approximate location of the highest upper esophageal sphincter pressure. Between the two portions is a small space, Killian triangle, where a Zenker's diverticulum will occur. The lower border of the cricopharyngeus and the origins of the longitudinal layer of the upper esophageal striated muscle form another triangle, Laimer's triangle (reproduced from Liebermann-Meffert [64], with permission).

with a larger bolus. With arrival of the descending pharyngeal contraction and the following UES contraction, the UES closes just prior to the laryngeal vestibule opening [75, 112].

The remarkable coordination of events during the short 1-s duration of the oropharyngeal stage includes only about a 0.5-s period of UES opening [77]. Therefore, disorders of the UES resulting in dysphagia can readily occur if the sphincter fails to open satisfactorily on swallowing. The UES can become hypertrophic and/or fibrotic, producing a prominent "cricopharyngeal bar" [110], or paralysis or weakness of oropharyngeal musculature, such as with a stroke or parkinsonism, can compromise bolus propulsion by the pharyngeal contraction [113–116], and/or prevent hyoid movement that opens the sphincter.

Esophagopharyngeal reflexes

The UES is highly responsive to a number of events that may occur in the esophagus or pharynx and that either increase UES pressure or result in relaxation. In general, the reflexes act to protect the airway from esophageal content, or allow release of esophageal content such as with belching or vom-

iting. All of the reflexes are mediated by vagal afferent signaling [21, 49, 108, 117].

Esophageal distention with air, liquid or a balloon can either increase or decrease UES pressure, depending on the volume and rapidity of distention [105, 117]. Slow distention causes an increase in pressure [117, 118], which could be seen as protective, the pressure increasing as more air is introduced or balloon volume increases [83, 119]. The effect of distention or infusion of fluid or air increases progressively on approaching the UES [117, 120]. Rapid distention and large volumes are associated with UES relaxation, and in the case of air, an esophageal belch may occur [121]. The more air introduced, the longer the UES relaxation. The belch is also associated with glottic closure [122]. UES relaxation also occurs with vomiting, a gastric belch, and rumination.

Increases in intrathoracic pressure, such as with gagging and a Valsalva maneuver, increase UES pressure.

Acid in the esophagus causes an increase in UES pressure in the dog, and like the response to distention, the response increases with acid closer to the UES and is most vigorous with acid at the location of the UES. Earlier studies indicated a similar response to acid in the human esophagus [117, 119, 123], but the reflex may be less prominent in humans, especially in those who develop esophagitis. Infusion of acid 5 cm below the UES in normal subjects [124] and acid reflux into the distal esophagus of normal subjects and of patients with esophagitis did not increase UES pressure [125].

Pharyngeal stimulation with small volumes of water, 0.1–1.5 cm, will induce the orpharyngeal stage of swallowing with UES relaxation. However, prior to initiation of the swallow, UES pressure increases [18].

Esophageal body

Anatomy, structure, and innervation

The esophagus is 20–22 cm long, the upper 5%, including the UES, being striated muscle. The distal 50–60% is entirely smooth muscle, with the transition from striated to smooth muscle occurring progressively in the middle 35–40% [126]. Measured manometrically, the total length can vary between 17 and 30 cm with a mean of 23 cm [127].The transition occurs more proximally in the circular muscle layer, the longitudinal layer extending further distally. The outer longitudinal muscle originates anteriorly from the cricoid cartilage along with some fibers from the cricopharyngeus muscle, and as it passes distally and posteriorly there is a triangle at the top end that is free of this layer, called Laimer's triangle (see Figure 5.8). The circular muscle can be seen in the triangle and this layer is present through the remainder of the esophageal body to the level of the LES, changing from striated to smooth muscle. There is no serosal cover on the esophagus, only a thin layer of connective tissue, allowing the esophagus to move more freely within the mediastinum.

There is a myenteric plexus of ganglion cells and nerve fibers in both smooth and striated muscle sections, more prominent in the smooth muscle section. The submucosal plexus is sparse [128]. In the smooth muscle portion, these ganglion cells receive the efferent vagal motor fibers from the DMNV and these are the cells that provide excitatory and inhibitory innervation to the muscle layers. Through their connectivity within an enteric nervous system, they provide a local neural mechanism for peristalsis and distal inhibition. From a motor point of view, the sympathetic input is directed primarily to the myenteric plexus [129].

Vagal sensory information is carried centrally by nerves with their cell bodies in the nodose ganglia in the neck, and is responsible for the sensory–motor regulation of the SPG for peristalsis and for the esophageal-initiated reflexes [130]. Sensory receptors include intraganglionic laminar endings (IGLE) [131], and potentially interstitial cells of Cajal (ICC) [132] and intramuscular arrays [133, 134]. Esophageal sensory information also passes to the spinal cord and centrally via the sympathetics through the dorsal root ganglia C1 to L2 [27], and clinically serves cognitive sensation and nociception rather than motor function [24].

Striated muscle

Motor innervation to the striated muscle esophagus originates in motor neurons of the nucleus ambiguous and is carried to the esophagus largely by the recurrent laryngeal nerve. The nerve fibers terminate in motor endplates in both circular and longitudinal layers [135] and release acetylcholine to contract the muscle through nicotinic muscarinic receptors [136]. The ganglion cells in the myenteric plexus send fibers to the motor endplates and contain NO, vasoactive intestinal peptide (VIP), galanin, and neuropeptide Y [137–141]. It is proposed that this coinnervation provides inhibitory modulation of striated muscle contraction and peristalsis through local and/or central reflexes [140, 141]. It is unclear whether vagal fibers from the SPG impact these neurons. IGLE, considered to be sensory receptors, are present. ICC are also present, but their role is unclear, although they may also function as sensory receptors [132, 142]. Sympathetic sensory information is passed from this region through segments C1–T8. The region also receives sympathetic innervation [129].

Smooth muscle

The structure of the smooth muscle layers is of importance in understanding the functional aspects of this region. In this region there is significant redundancy of control mechanisms for peristalsis that must interact effectively.

Vagal fibers enter the esophagus at different levels and travel various distances within the esophagus to reach the neurons within the intramural plexuses. Sympathetic supply arises from spinal segments T1–10 with post-ganglionic fibers passing to the esophagus from paraspinal sympathetic

ganglia [129]. These fibers also go mainly to the intramural plexuses, to modulate neuronal activity. Few sympathetic fibers go directly to the smooth muscle cells. The role of the sympathetics appears to be limited [143, 144], although activation of beta-receptors causes membrane hyperpolarization and muscle relaxation [144, 145], and catecholamines may release other inhibitory peptides from nerves [146]. As in the striated muscle portion, the myenteric ganglion cells have many different peptides [138, 147, 148]. Some of these peptides may have a modulatory role. However, for practical purposes, functionally there are only two types of motor neurons: excitatory cholinergic neurons that also contain substance P; and inhibitory nitrergic (NO) neurons that also contain VIP.

The longitudinal muscle forms a continuous layer of smooth muscle cells that do not make gap junction contact with each other. ICC are present in this layer in the human [149] and cat [132], but not the dog or opossum [150–152]. Nerve fibers enter this layer from the myenteric plexus.

The circular layer is not a continuous sheet of muscle cells, but is separated into lamellae or muscle bundles by connective tissue septa that are in intimate contact with the myenteric plexus region [132, 153]. Smooth muscle cells make gap junction contacts between themselves and the ICCs, but not with nerves. The ICCs are found within the muscle bundles and in the connective tissue septa. There are few ICCs in the myenteric plexus region. It is proposed that many of these ICCs can function as sensory receptors, since the presence and structural integrity of some ICCs are dependent on the presence of intact afferent vagal innervation [132, 154]. IGLE are present that can also function in a sensory mode.

There are other ICCs that likely operate in sensory–motor activity as part of any myogenic control system for peristalsis, as elsewhere in the gut. In such a capacity in the esophagus, the ICCs have the potential to act as transducers for nerve-to-muscle signaling, as pacemakers for the smooth muscles themselves, and as conduction pathways for muscle-to-muscle communication within muscle bundles or between bundles and muscle layers. Independent of the ICCs, there are free nerve endings close to the smooth muscle cells for release of neurotransmitters directly on the cells.

Functional motor activity

Primary peristalsis

The normal swallow-induced contraction of the esophagus is called primary peristalsis. On entry of the bolus into the esophagus and following closure of the UES with a contraction, a progressive circumferential contraction begins in the upper esophagus and passes distally along the esophageal body to reach the relaxed LES. The LES then contracts in sequence. Velocity of the wave varies between 2.5 and 5 cm/s along the esophagus in a bimodal fashion [155–157]

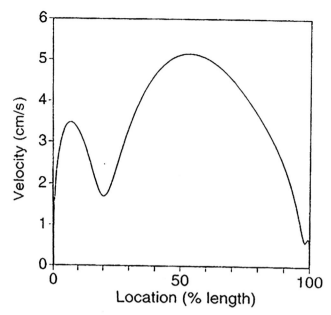

Figure 5.9 Velocity of the peristaltic wave front along the esophagus. The bimodal velocity was apparent using axial reconstructions of pressure data. The two modes represent propagation through the proximal striated muscle and distal smooth muscle regions, with deceleration near the lower esophageal sphincter. There is no break in velocity in the smooth muscle region (reproduced from Clouse RA, Diamant NE. Motor function of the esophagus. In: Johnson LR, ed. *Physiology of the Gastrointestinal Tract*, 4th edn, 2006, with permission).

(Figure 5.9). The duration of normal contractions is usually less than 7 s and contraction amplitudes rarely exceed 200 mmHg [158]. Figure 5.10 shows these events as recorded both by conventional and the more recent high-resolution manometry.

Esophageal shortening of 2–2.5 cm also occurs, longitudinal muscle contraction proceeding distally at 2–4 cm/s and onsetting slightly in advance of the circular muscle contraction [159–161] or very close to it [161–163]. This contraction augments circular muscle contraction and reduces stress on the esophageal wall [164]. Coordination of the longitudinal and circular muscle layers is in part dependent on cholinergic innervation and can be abnormal in some motor disorders such as nutcracker esophagus [165, 166].

Of interest, the amplitude of the circular muscle contraction shows a consistent decrease in a short segment at 4–6 cm below the UES, attributed to the region where striated and smooth muscle have interspersed and/or innervation changes from the RLN proximally to the more distal vagal branches. Within the smooth muscle section there is one other region of decreased contraction amplitude about in its middle, and another near the end of the esophageal body and just above the LES [155, 157, 167]. It is not known if these findings are due to separate neuromuscular units governed by output from subunits in the SPG, or by periph-

eral intramural mechanisms within regional differences in muscle or nerve (see later). If central, it raises the possibility that SPG control of the esophagus may be grouped into three or four functional subunits: UES and upper striated muscle esophagus; proximal and distal smooth muscle esophageal body; and very distal smooth muscle body and LES or LES alone.

The contraction amplitude determines the efficacy of bolus propulsion and esophageal emptying, with this efficacy decreasing as amplitude decreases [168]. At a threshold of 30 mmHg, incomplete bolus transit is identified with a sensitivity of 85% and specificity of 66% [169]. Sensory feedback from the esophagus has an effect on the contractions and peristalsis. Larger boluses and increased viscosity increase contraction amplitude and duration, and slow peristaltic velocity [170–172]. Increased intra-abdominal pressure and esophageal obstruction also increase amplitude and slow velocity. Gravity facilitates transport, especially of liquids, and distal contraction amplitude can decrease in the more upright position [173].

Secondary peristalsis
Secondary peristalsis originates in the esophagus in response to local sensory stimulation, such as from retained food not cleared by the primary wave or from refluxed acid. This peristaltic wave is similar to that of primary peristalsis but begins in the esophagus at or above the level of the stimulus. However, distention high in the esophagus is reported to at times initiate the process at the pharyngeal stage [174].

Tertiary peristalsis
If connections to the central control of the SPG are absent, a local intramural mechanism can produce peristalsis in the smooth muscle segment of the intact animal [175–177]. This contraction is called tertiary peristalsis and is different from the "tertiary" uncoordinated or simultaneous contractions that can occur with central connections intact [178].

Afferent sensory stimulation
Two related questions have arisen. Can the SPG on its own initiate a peristaltic contraction in the esophagus without afferent stimulation from the bolus in the esophagus? Is the bolus-dependent secondary peristalsis a centrally- or peripherally-mediated reflex?

With swallowing the esophageal stage of the SPG is normally activated [4]. This activation is less prominent in the esophageal phase and is enhanced to a maximum with sufficient pharyngeal and esophageal sensory feedback to the SPG. Failed esophageal peristalsis in all or part of the esophagus is common in humans, particularly with "dry" swallows. The presence of a bolus increases the frequency of the peristaltic wave and its completion [170, 171]. Animal studies have been conflicting in determining the necessity for bolus stimulation of the esophagus for primary peristalsis to occur.

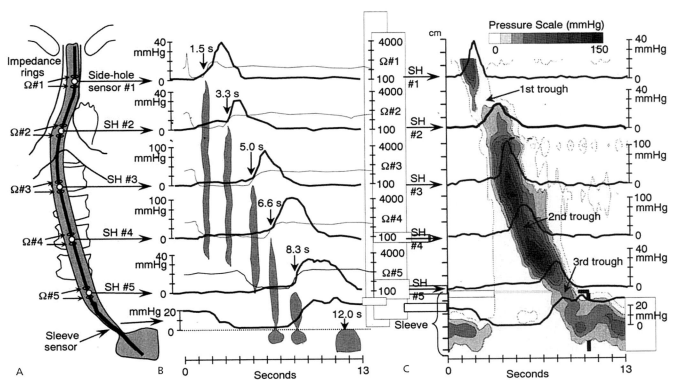

Figure 5.10 Esophageal peristalsis: relationship between videofluoroscopic, manometric, impedance, and topographic representations. (A) Depiction of intraluminal manometry/impedance measurement with five sensors at 4-cm intervals, and a sleeve sensor in the lower esophageal sphincter (LES). (B) Representation by overlaying manometry and impedance measurements with videofluoroscopic appearance of a 5-mL swallowed barium bolus. The pressure scale for the dark thick line is on the left and the impedance scale for the light thin line is on the right. The arrows point to the distribution of the bolus at the times indicated. As the bolus enters the esophagus, there is a slight increase in pressure at most sites, the "bolus pressure." As the contraction reaches each site, the pressure increases and the impedance decreases. As the lumen closes and the upstroke of the pressure wave occurs, the tail of the barium bolus is evident. (C) Comparison of conventional manometric pressure tracing at five sites and the LES, as positioned in A, with the pressure profile obtained with high-fidelity (high-resolution) manometry and displayed topographically as an isocontour plot. The overlay places the two representations at similar locations. In the isocontour plot, deepening shades of gray indicate higher pressures. There are three pressure troughs: at the junction of the striated and smooth muscle esophagus; in the mid portion of the smooth muscle portion; and at the end of the peristaltic segment just before the LES. The troughs separate four different pressure segments, the last fronting the contraction closing the LES. The end of the LES relaxation measured with conventional manometry coincides with arrival of the contraction at the start of the fourth pressure segment and the LES. (reproduced from Pandolfino and Kahrilas [93], with permission).

In dogs that have a totally striated muscle esophagus, and with diversion of the bolus in the cervical esophagus, primary peristalsis is absent in the distal esophagus [179, 180]. In the absence of cortical input (decerebrate) in the cat that has a distal smooth muscle esophagus, the bolus must be present in the cervical esophagus for peristalsis to proceed [108]. In primates that also have a distal smooth muscle esophagus, the bolus is not always necessary [181]. Cortical stimulation with TCMS in the anesthetized cat [52] or awake dog [182] can itself initiate swallowing, and in the dog produces contraction of the upper esophagus without a bolus. TCMS has not initiated swallowing in the human, although muscles in the pharynx and upper and lower esophagus can be induced to contract [183–185]. It is clear that the esophageal stage of the SPG must be adequately activated for primary peristalsis to occur in the esophagus. Therefore, one or more of the three inputs to the SPG— cortical, pharyngeal or esophageal—must be sufficient for activation, and each can facilitate the other [186]. Normally all three inputs are present. However, involvement of all three may not be necessary, depending on species' differences and experimental conditions. Regardless, the swallowed bolus is obviously an important component under normal circumstances, and amplitude, duration, and velocity of the peristaltic wave are subject to the nature and size of the bolus.

Under normal circumstances, secondary peristalsis has been considered as dependent on sensory activation of a central reflex, mediated by activation within the esophageal stage of the SPG [174, 187]. This is always true of the striated muscle esophagus because of its dependence on central control that once initiated, also activates neurons for the smooth muscle segment as well. With secondary peristalsis induced in the striated muscle segment, the contraction wave progressing distally through the smooth muscle segment behaves identically to the primary wave [174, 188]. The SPG program for the esophageal segments involved is as similarly active as those same neurons during primary peristalsis. As long as central connections to the SPG are intact, there is no convincing indication that intramural neural or myogenic mechanisms stimulated locally in the smooth muscle segment could independently produce secondary peristalsis in this segment. In the cat, vagal blockade in the neck abolishes secondary peristalsis [151]. However, local mechanisms in this segment can alter the response to the central control that is initiated by afferent signaling to the SPG, influenced by factors such as the location of the peripheral stimulus and whether the stimulus is a stationary distending balloon, collapsible barostat balloon or a movable bolus. When initiated by a moveable bolus or the barostat balloon, secondary peristalsis proceeds relatively unaltered. A fixed distending balloon, not a physiologic stimulus, induces contractions proximal to the balloon and can significantly alter the distal contraction [41, 189–195]. As with primary peristalsis, the local and central mechanisms must integrate effectively. This integration is discussed later.

Muscle tone

Both the striated and smooth muscle esophagus exhibit some degree of resting tone as measured by a barostat [190, 192]. The tone in the smooth muscle portion has a component due to cholinergic excitation that is largely vagal dependent, and is modulated by nitrergic inhibition. The tone is subject to afferent information, can be enhanced by intraluminal distention, and is inhibited by a swallow [196].

Striated muscle esophageal body: motor activity

Contraction of the striated muscle for both primary and secondary peristalsis is under central control of the SPG esophageal stage [2, 4, 6], with sequential excitation through vagal fibers [40, 41, 197]. As noted above, this activity is sensitive to sensory feedback, and may be modulated by local and/or central reflexes [140, 141, 198].

Smooth muscle esophageal body: motor activity

This segment of the esophageal body is the usual location of the common clinical conditions involving the esophagus, including the esophageal motor disorders, and in association with the LES, gastroesophageal reflux disease (GERD). As with structure, control mechanisms for peristalsis in the smooth muscle layers are of importance in understanding the functional aspects of this region. In this region there are

three potential control mechanisms for peristalsis that must interact and integrate effectively:

1. The central SPG [2–4, 6] sends sequential efferent signals to the esophagus via the vagus nerves [40, 199, 200]. This mechanism and its modulation by sensory feedback have been discussed in previous sections of this chapter.
2. An intramural neural mechanism that can result in peristalsis near the onset of vagal stimulation or intraluminal balloon distention ("on contraction" or "A wave") or after the stimulus or distention are terminated ("off contraction" or "B wave") [201–204].
3. A myogenic mechanism [205–207].

Regardless of the mechanism(s) operating under normal circumstances, the swallow-induced peristaltic contraction is highly atropine sensitive in the human, monkey, and especially the cat [188, 193, 208–210]. That is, final contraction of the smooth muscle is predominantly due to stimulation by intramural cholinergic neurons.

Central control mechanisms

The esophagus receives vagal input providing sequential activation to both the striated and smooth muscle segments during both primary and secondary peristalsis. Figure 5.11 illustrates this vagal activity in the baboon and opossum [40, 200]. The findings in the opossum indicate two different timings of vagal firing patterns, an early rapid-sequence group that would fit with early activation of inhibitory neurons, and a later slower-sequence group that mirrors the timing and velocity of the peristaltic contraction. It is not known if two firing patterns are present in other species. If initial inhibition and subsequent excitation is the function of these two groups, it has been assumed that the early group excites the inhibitory neurons and the later group the excitatory neurons along the smooth muscle esophagus. It is not established if the vagal fibers go directly to these neurons or are routed through interneuronal circuitry. However, this input must integrate effectively with the intramural mechanisms, including this circuitry and the muscle itself.

Intramural neural control mechanisms

In 1970, Christensen demonstrated neurally mediated peristaltic contraction in the isolated opossum smooth muscle esophagus *in vitro* that followed intraluminal balloon distention or electrical stimulation to the external surface [211, 212]. These observations established the presence of a local mechanism capable of producing peristalsis. Thereafter, two main approaches have explored the neural mechanisms involved: studies of the intact animal with or without vagotomy, and studies of smooth muscle strips *in vitro*. The studies have elucidated much of the underlying physiology that can operate, but have not clarified how the central and peripheral neural mechanisms interact under normal circumstances.

Dodds *et al.* stimulated the cut end of the vagus, stimulating all efferent and afferent fibers at once, and found two

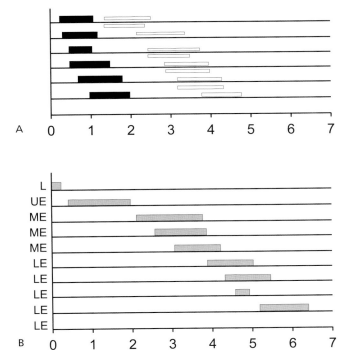

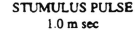

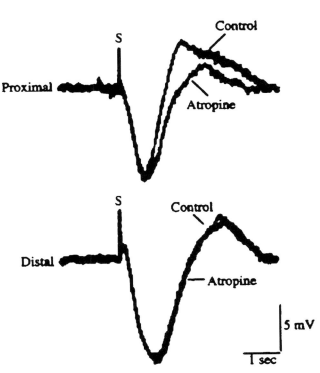

Figure 5.11 Vagus nerve firing patterns with esophageal peristalsis. The firing patterns of the vagus nerve during a swallow in the opossum (A) and the baboon (B). In the opossum there is an early and a late sequential firing pattern, the later pattern corresponding to the timing and velocity of the esophageal peristaltic wave. In the baboon only a sequential firing pattern timed with the presence of the esophageal contraction along the esophagus was recorded. UE, upper esophagus; ME, mid esophagus; LE, lower esophagus (A, reproduced from Gidda JS and Goyal RK [200], with permission; B, reproduced from Roman C and Tieffenbach L [40, with permission).

Figure 5.12 Difference in the duration of the inhibitory junction potential along the opossum esophagus and the effect of atropine. Transmural stimulation produced an inhibitory junction potential (IJP) that was of longer duration at the distal site. Atropine prolonged the duration of the IJP at the proximal site with no effect on the duration at the distal site. The cholinergic effect at only the proximal site is compatible with a gradient of cholinergic activity along the esophagus. (reproduced from Goyal RK, Madhu P, Chang HY. Functional anatomy and physiology of swallowing and esophageal motility. In: Castell DO, Richter JE, eds. *The Esophagus*, 4th edn, 2004, with permission).

peripheral neural mechanisms for peristalsis, an on contraction (A wave) and an off contraction (B wave) [201, 202, 204]. The on contraction was induced by low-frequency stimulation, was atropine sensitive, and had slow propagation velocity similar to normal peristalsis. The off contraction occurred at higher stimulating frequencies, was not atropine sensitive, and had a much more rapid propagation velocity. Varying other stimulus parameters as well can influence the delays to the onset of the A and B waves [213]. The *in vivo* findings correlated well with the *in vitro* muscle strip findings, a cholinergic on contraction and a non-cholinergic off contraction [203, 214]. The cholinergic effect is mediated predominantly via a muscarinic M_3 receptor [215], although the M_2 receptor may also be involved [188, 216]. *In vitro*, the off contraction is associated with a membrane depolarization and spiking activity that follows hyperpolarization of the muscle [217–220], later shown to be due to the action of the inhibitory neurotransmitter NO or similar nitroso compound [221]. Very similar membrane events were observed with the peristaltic contraction *in vivo*

[222–225]. Paired vagal stimulation demonstrated the functional inhibitory effect of one stimulus on the contraction of the other, depending on stimulus frequency and duration [226].

Further studies of muscle strips from along the smooth muscle esophagus have demonstrated regional differences in the smooth muscle responses to electrical stimulation and to pharmacologic agents [203, 227, 228]: (1) with electrical stimulation, the duration of the inhibitory hyperpolarization is shorter in the proximal esophagus and longer distally, and therefore the following muscle depolarization and muscle contraction occur later distally; and (2) atropine decreases the duration of the hyperpolarization and latency to the contraction in the proximal esophagus but not in the distal esophagus (Figure 5.12). This cholinergic effect to shorten

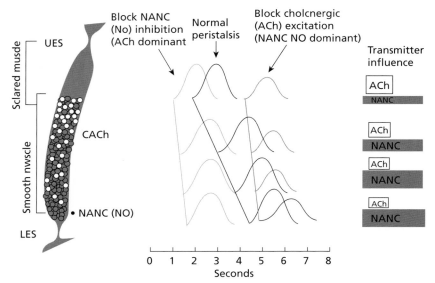

Figure 5.13 Interplay of cholinergic (ACh) and non-cholinergic (NANC) influences along the smooth muscle esophagus in the production of peristalsis. The cholinergic influence is most prominent proximally and decreases distally; the reverse is true for the NANC influence. Proximally the contraction occurs earlier, but is atropine sensitive, cholinergic blockade, delaying its appearance. Distally the contraction normally appears later, but NANC blockade, such as with block of nitric oxide (NO) release, shortens the time to onset of the contraction. In either case of blockade peristaltic velocity can significantly increase. LES, lower esophageal sphincter; UES, upper esophageal sphincter (reproduced from Clouse RE, Diamant NE. Esophageal motor and sensory function and motor disorders of the esophagus. In: Feldman M, Freidman LS, Sleisenger MH, eds. *Sleisenger and Fordtran's Gastrointestinal and Liver Disease*, 8th edn, 2006, with permission).

the latency decreases progressively along the esophagus. These findings are mirrored *in vivo*. Atropine delays the onset of the peristaltic contractions and decreases amplitude in the proximal smooth muscle esophagus, the effect decreasing distally [193, 204, 208, 229]. On the other hand, block of NO release and its inhibitory effect, shortens the delay to the peristaltic contractions at each level and can decrease amplitude, the effect most pronounced distally [230–235]. That is, the intramural neural mechanism combines a balance between a more prominent cholinergic excitatory effect proximally and a more prominent inhibitory nitrergic effect distally. This combination appears to play a major role in ensuring the distal propagation of the peristaltic wave (Figure 5.13). The two mechanisms also have clinical implications. Increased cholinergic effects have been implicated in spastic esophageal motor disorders, such as those with high amplitude contractions [236, 237]. Decreased or absent nitregic innervation is a feature of LES dysfunction in achalasia [238]. The rapid or non-peristaltic wave of achalasia is also in part attributed to absent or decreased nitrergic innervation, while accentuation of the inhibitory NO influence may contribute to slowed propagation velocity and decrease amplitude in the presence of esophagitis and endotoxemia [239, 240]. How the early and late sequential vagal discharges to the smooth muscle esophagus integrate with or exert some control over this local neural or over myogenic mechanisms is not known (see later).

Intramural myogenic (muscle) control mechanisms

Elsewhere in the gut, the myogenic control system has two fundamental characteristics: (1) electrical oscillations of the smooth muscle cells, usually called "slow waves"; and (2) communication among smooth muscle cells allowing the tissue to operate as a functional unit [241, 242]. Both of these features are present in the esophageal smooth muscle and with adequate excitation, for example cholinergic stimulation, can become manifest [205, 207, 243–246]. A significant component of a myogenic system is contributed by the ICCs, as noted above, and appropriately positioned ICCs are present in the esophagus [132, 153]. It is not surprising therefore, that with the esophagus isolated *in vitro* and with nerves blocked, a myogenic peristaltic contraction can be readily demonstrated in the smooth muscle segment [205–207, 246].

It has been assumed that the regional gradients in the cholinergic and nitrergic innervation along the esophagus, discussed above, are sufficient for local control of peristalsis in the smooth muscle section. However, there are also regional differences in the circular smooth muscle along the esophagus that likely contribute significantly to the peristaltic contraction and the delays along the esophagus, including the responses to cholinergic and nitrergic innervation. These differences include a resting membrane potential gradient [217, 247], potassium and calcium ion channel diversity [247–249], and differences in muscle length–tension relationships and responses to cholinergic stimulation [250]. There are also differences in muscle proteins [251], and in intracellular signaling in response to cholinergic stimulation between esophageal body and LES muscles [252, 253], although regional differences in the esophageal body have not been sought.

The longitudinal muscle is not an innocent bystander in the peristaltic process. As noted previously this layer contracts sequentially in close association with the circular muscle contraction during peristalsis and is also involved with reflex activities [254–256]. Cholinergic nerves normally cause this muscle to contract and substance P can also do so [257]. As opposed to the inhibition of circular muscle, NO primarily contracts the longitudinal muscle layer [258, 259]. Heightened sensitivity to stimulation has provided a potential mechanism for esophageal shortening and hiatus hernia production in association with esophagitis [260, 261]. It is not known how the sequencing of longitudinal muscle by cholinergic excitation occurs during peristalsis in the absence of an inhibitory NO mechanism. Stimulation of the cut vagus results in simultaneous contraction [213]. Since the central vagal fibers connect to neurons in the enteric nervous system, excitation must finally result from an intramural mechanism, either primarily directed by the sequential vagal firing or from a coordinating intramural network.

Integration of central and peripheral mechanisms

Clearly all three levels of control, a central mechanism and peripheral neural and myogenic mechanisms, have the potential to direct peristalsis in the smooth muscle segment, and must integrate effectively. Which mechanism is dominant under normal circumstances is not established. The esophagus ordinarily is both mechanically and electrically silent, and for a contraction to occur some form of stimulus is required. With a swallow, the central mechanism controls and initiates contractions in the striated muscles of the oropharygeal stage and in the upper striated muscle portion of the esophagus. For initiation of a contraction in the smooth muscle portion, the excitatory cholinergic neuron must be adequately stimulated by central and/or peripheral neural input. The threshold for muscle contraction, its timing in the peristaltic sequence, and contraction amplitude are determined by the balance between excitatory and inhibitory influences at the muscle level.

The swallow or pharyngeal stimulation initiates the SPG esophageal stage of control and its vagal output to the smooth muscle. Sensory input from a bolus in the esophagus is not necessary for primary peristalsis in this segment, but can alter the intensity and timing of the vagal output that corresponds to the timing and amplitude of the contraction. Finally, secondary peristalsis and its SPG behavior are normally similar to primary peristalsis. Therefore, it could be argued that under normal circumstances the central control runs the show. Vagal inputs would impact directly or indirectly on both excitatory cholinergic and inhibitory nitrergic myenteric neurons, and function as the primary control of the peripheral neural network and the network's excitatory and inhibitory outputs to the muscle [209]. Because of its properties, it is likely that the myogenic control mechanism participates in the final contraction pattern, but how this control mechanism might operate or be controlled is not known. When esophageal sensory input is large and has major impact on the local neural mechanism, such as with a large stationary bolus, this neural mechanism itself can have a significant influence on the final contraction pattern. Final resolution of how the different control mechanisms operate together is yet to be determined. Thankfully, the presence of more than one control mechanism provides for peristalsis to occur if central control is absent or abnormal. Central disorders such as stroke and parkinsonism can affect motility of both striated and smooth muscle segments of the esophagus [114, 262, 263].

Deglutitive inhibition

Deglutitive inhibition is primarily mediated centrally by the SPG. Activation of the SPG at any level is associated with inhibition of neurons and motor neurons distal to this level, with the inhibition increasing more distally (see Figure 5.2). When a first swallow has reached the upper esophagus, a second swallow will inhibit progression of the first swallow after a short period of time, with a delay until the second swallow appears [191, 264, 265]. Centrally, the second swallow shuts down the firing of the motor neurons to the esophagus, with these neurons again active later for the second swallow. The inhibitory neurons in the esophagus may also be activated by separate vagal inputs from the SPG that could normally occur with the second swallow. An experiment suggesting this activation of local inhibitory neurons first produced a zone of high pressure with mild intraluminal balloon distention, likely in large part due to reflex vagovagal activation of the SPG and excitatory output to the esophagus [196]. A second swallow caused a decrease in pressure in the artificial high pressure zone, but would also inhibit the central activation as well. When a sequence of many rapid repetitive swallows occurs, the "chug-a'lug," not only is the first swallow wave inhibited and not present, but all subsequent swallow waves are prevented until after the last swallow, which is then followed by a peristaltic contraction [266].

Secondary peristalsis is also inhibited by a swallow [191, 194]. However, secondary peristalsis initiated in the smooth muscle esophagus may not consistently or effectively inhibit a primary swallow when the stimulus is arriving later in the SPG program.

A previous swallow or the presence of a swallow-induced contraction in the esophagus can alter the nature of a subsequent swallow that occurs within 20–30 s. Amplitude can decrease, and velocity can decrease or increase, even to the point of the wave being non-peristaltic [264, 266]. Therefore, routine clinical studies should space swallows by at least this interval.

Lower Esophageal Sphincter

At the distal end of the esophagus there is a closed 3–4-cm long high-pressure zone that functions as an antireflux barrier and separates negative intrathoracic pressure in the esophagus from positive intra-abdominal pressure in the stomach. This high-pressure zone is considered to normally have two "sphincter" components; an intrinsic smooth muscle sphincter known as the LES, and the surrounding diaphragm that functions as an external sphincter [267]. When normally positioned, the LES is therefore part of a more complex structural arrangement called the "gastro-esophageal junction" that includes the phrenoesophageal membrane and the hiatal portion of the diaphragm.

Anatomy and innervation

Phrenoesophageal membrane

The phrenoesophageal membrane or "ligament" has a thin lower leaf that runs caudally and attaches to the adventitia of the esophageal wall just above the angle of His. A thicker upper leaf arising from the endothoracic fascia of the dia-phragm runs cranially to attach firmly to the esophagus with collagenous extensions that penetrate to the submucosa, at about the level of the squamocolumnar junction [268–270]. This tough ligament serves to limit displacement of the esophagus into the thorax and to draw it back into position while minimizing circumferential traction on the LES. Attenuation of the ligament with age would facilitate the development of hiatus hernia [271].

Diaphragm

The diaphragm, commonly the right crus, surrounds the LES at approximately the mid level of the sphincter [272]. This crus arises from a lumbar vertebra and inclining forward encircles the distal esophagus in a scissor-like fashion to form a 2-cm long hiatal canal (Figure 5.14). The diaphragm receives its motor innervation from second-order neurons in the phrenic motor nucleus of the spinal cord [273]. However, afferent signaling from both the crural diaphragm and the phrenoesophageal ligament pass via the vagus nerve to the SPG and, through efferent vagal pathways from the DMNV, takes part in inhibition of both the LES and crural diaphragm [274, 275]. This inhibition is present with swallow-induced relaxation and with the spontaneous tran-sient LES relaxations (TLESR).

Intrinsic lower esophageal sphincter

In the human the LES is composed of at least two main smooth muscle elements: the circular muscle usually forms only a partial ring (or semicircular "clasp") but can form a complete ring; and the gastric sling muscle runs on the left

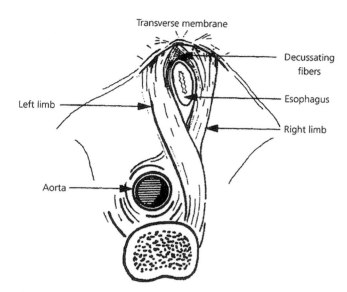

Figure 5.14 Anatomy of the diaphragmatic hiatus: the right crus encircling the distal esophagus. The right crus arises from the anterior longitudinal ligament overlying the lumbar vertebrae. Two muscular elements cross each other in a scissor-like fashion, form the walls of the hiatus, and decussate with each other anteriorly as they encircle the distal esophagus (reproduced from Kahrilas PJ and Pandolfino JE. Esophageal motor function. In: Yamada T, ed. *Textbook of Gastroenterology*, 5th edn. Hoboken, NJ: Wiley-Blackwell, 2008).

lateral aspect to interdigitate with the circular muscle and structurally complete this portion of the sphincter (Figure 5.15) [276–278]. A more recent manometric and ultrasound study has suggested the presence of another smooth muscle component [279, 280], but this finding is yet to be con-firmed [281] as different from either the sling or clasp muscles. It is not clear if the very distal circular smooth muscle of the esophageal body contributes to the proximal end of the LES. In many other species such as the cat, dog, and guinea pig, the LES circular muscle forms a complete ring, but with the sling similarly positioned as in the human [282–287].

The sling contraction and the normal position of the stomach, with its fundus projecting upward under the left diaphragm, act to form an acute angle where the left lateral wall of the esophagus meets the medial aspect of the dome of the stomach, the angle of His. The LES portion of the distal esophagus tends to angle obliquely and to the left to meet the stomach wall. Viewed from the gastric lumen, this region can be seen as a fold or ridge, that has been considered as a flap valve if compressed against the LES opening [288]. As one contributing factor, if the angle of His is less acute, such as with a hiatus hernia or after distal gastrectomy, gastroesopha-geal reflux is more likely to occur [289–292]. A longitudinal smooth muscle layer covers the sphincter region.

As in the esophageal body, LES circular muscle is formed into bundles separated by connective tissue. The LES cells

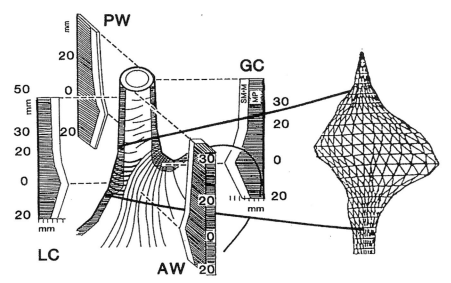

Figure 5.15 Lower esophageal sphincter (LES) radial muscle thickness and three-dimensional (3D) manometric pressure image. Radial thickness shown in millimeters is on the left, and the 3D pressure image in mmHg is plotted on the right around an axis representing atmospheric pressure. The thickest portion of the LES and highest pressure is seen on the left lateral side. GC, greater curve; LC, lesser curve; PW, posterior wall; AW, anterior wall (reproduced from Stein *et al.* [324], with permission).

are somewhat larger and the connective tissue lamina more numerous than in the esophageal body [293]. ICCs are present in both circular and longitudinal muscle layers [152, 154, 294, 295]. Their role as either mechanical receptors and/or transducers of neural input to the smooth muscle cells remains uncertain [294, 296, 297].

The LES receives preganglionic vagal fibers from the DMNV in the brainstem SPG. These fibers enter the esophagus up to 9 cm or more proximal to the LES [298, 299] and synapse on excitatory and inhibitory neurons [300, 301]. Central SPG preganglionic fibers to the LES are also linked to sensory information from the fundus [301]. As in the esophageal body, the neurons have a number of peptides and potential neurotransmitters [302]. However, normally muscle excitation is primarily cholinergic, and inhibition is nitrergic, although the neurons also contain VIP. A VIP or other peptide-mediated component of inhibition may be present under certain circumstances [294, 296, 303–307]. Nitrergic innervation and its effect are greatest in the circular clasp muscle [308, 309]. The inhibitory neurons receive input from the vagus, esophageal body, and gastric fundus, and the clasp and sling are separately innervated [301, 310]. Sympathetic innervation to the LES arrives from the stellate ganglion and from the sympathetic chain via the splanchnic nerve after passing through the celiac ganglion. This innervation excites the muscle directly and through stimulation of acetylcholine release from cholinergic postganglionic nerves, while inhibiting the inhibitory innervation, all by alpha-receptor activation [145, 311, 312]. There is some beta-receptor–mediated inhibition of the muscle, with its effect species dependent and of uncertain importance [144, 311, 313].

Activation of the myenteric plexus excitatory and inhibitory neurons is primarily through cholinergic nicotinic receptors, and the inhibitory neuron to a lesser extent by a muscarinic M_1 receptor. Both may be activated directly or indirectly by other neurotransmitters and these activations can have clinical implications. The inhibitory neuron can be activated directly by serotonin [314], but the importance of this is uncertain, and by cholecystokinin (CCK) [315–317]. CCK excitation of the excitatory neuron can occur by stimulation of preganglionic nerve structures [317].

There appear to be two vagal pathways to the LES, one that is tonically active and likely excitatory to help maintain resting tone. This activity stops with a swallow. The other pathway is normally quiet and activates with a swallow, presumably to stimulate inhibitory neurons for LES relaxation [318, 319]. The inhibitory pathway within the esophageal body to the LES is paucisynaptic and can extend over long sections of the esophageal body [320].

Functional motor activity

To serve its protective function against gastroesophageal reflux, the LES is tonically closed at rest and maintains a basal resting pressure. The sphincter must relax and open to allow the esophageal bolus to pass into the stomach, and to permit retrograde passage with belching and vomiting. LES relaxation occurs with virtually all swallows, even when peristalsis fails to occur. Similarly, distention in the esophagus and secondary peristalsis are associated with LES relaxation. The interactive central and peripheral mechanisms producing the relaxation are related to the mechanisms involved with the production of primary and secondary peristalsis [321, 322], and were discussed previously.

To appreciate the functional behavior at the gastroesophageal junction, it is necessary to consider the functional characteristics of the circular and smooth muscle components of the smooth muscle sphincter and of the diaphragm.

Resting or basal pressure

The resting pressure varies with the measurement method and the respiratory cycle, and maintains an average pressure of about 20 mmHg relative to gastric pressure [93]. With a swallow the LES relaxes and pressure decreases within 1–2.5 s, and remains low until the arrival of the esophageal peristaltic contraction when a sequential LES contraction then occurs and pressure again increases. The decrease in pressure lasts for the duration of the peristaltic esophageal wave in the smooth muscle esophagus that may take 5 s or more. However, esophageal opening depends on a combination of factors. These factors include intrabolus pressure due to peristaltic force and gravity, the abdominothoracic pressure gradient, and the residual LES pressure due to its smooth muscle, the diaphragm, and intra-abdominal pressure surrounding the sphincter. Pressures are higher at the level of the diaphragm and increase with inspiration [269, 323]. Intrinsic sphincter pressure reflected at end inspiration is greater than 5 mmHg. Both radial and axial asymmetry can be demonstrated by high-definition manometric reconstructions (Figure 5.15) [269, 324].

The circular/clasp and sling muscles are functionally different in many ways that impact on resting tone, the responses to neural input and potentially to drugs. The circular muscle has significant spontaneous tone, whereas the sling muscle has little tone and compared to the circular muscle is much more responsive to cholinergic stimulation. The higher pressure in the left lateral position of the sling is reduced by atropine, compatible with the sling contributing to this higher pressure along with the diaphragm. The pressure in the remainder of the LES circumference is unchanged or little changed by cholinergic blockade. These two muscles demonstrate differences in resting membrane potential and voltage-gated K^+ channel densities [325], and in the L-type Ca^{2+} channel and calcium handling [326, 327]. For example, although influx of extracellular calcium is central to the maintenance of myogenic tone and acetylcholine-induced contractility in both LES muscles, this influx occurs through an L-type Ca^{2+} channel in LES circular muscle, and a nifedipine-insensitive, non–L-type Ca^{2+} channel in sling muscle. Therefore, an L-type Ca^{2+} channel blocker such as nifedipine would affect only the circular muscle. The cellular pathways and mechanisms determining contraction in the circular muscle of the esophageal body and LES have been well established and vary depending on the calcium source

[252, 328, 329]. These mechanisms are altered by esophagitis, and these changes carry potential therapeutic implications [330–332].

Regional differences in the LES dictate that the mechanisms maintaining resting LES tone will be different for the LES smooth muscles, cholinergic excitation for the sling and intrinsic myogenic tone for the circular clasp muscle, and set the basal conditions for the mechanisms necessary for LES relaxation. Both muscles have the capacity for repetitive contractile activity [333]. The circular muscle develops membrane electrical slow waves and/or spiking activity, with the intensity of the spiking related to tone development and to changes in pressure with the migrating motor complex (MMC) [334–338]. Potassium- and calcium-activated chloride channels have important opposing roles in the control of the spiking activity and the genesis of LES tone [338]. The circular clasp muscle with its high resting intrinsic tone is relaxed predominantly by release of NO. There is little effect of NO on the sling muscle [308], and relaxation of the sling muscle is likely due predominantly to turning off its cholinergic excitation. That is, the dominant innervation of the circular clasp muscle is nitrergic and inhibitory, whereas that of the sling is cholinergic and excitatory. Therefore, a balance between excitatory and inhibitory innervation to the two muscles sets the level of resting tone at any time. The ability to pharmacologically manipulate this balance has clinical and therapeutic implications. Increasing LES pressure could be advantageous for patients with gastroesophageal reflux. The sling would lend itself to extracholinergic excitation and support the use of cholinergic agonists to raise pressure in these patients [339]. Decreasing tone in disorders where the sphincter is hypertensive or fails to relax, e.g. achalasia, could be directed at the circular muscle with L-type calcium blockers [340] or phosphodiesterase inhibitors such as sildenafil that prevent the degradation of NO [341, 342]. Botulinum toxin injection to lower pressure by decreasing acetylcholine release would involve primarily the sling muscle [343]. The same reasoning can be applied to surgical interventions. Perhaps cutting the circular muscle in patients with achalasia is all that is necessary, while leaving the cholinergic sling activity intact to protect against reflux [344].

A number of influences affect the resting tone and pressure. There is an increase in LES pressure with a rise in intra-abdominal pressure that is mediated by the vagus in the cat [345], but whether the rise is a passive response or a vagally-mediated response in the human is controversial [346–349]. The LES pressure increases in the recumbent position [350, 351]. Fasting pressures are higher during phase III of the MMC and lowest during phase I. Feeding is often associated with a drop in LES pressure, resulting in large part from the secretion of hormones such as secretin and CCK with fat intake [352, 353], or from the nature of the food itself or its contents, such as with chocolate [354],

Table 5.1 Effects of hormones and putative neurotransmitters on the lower esophageal sphincter.

Agent	Effect	Site of Action			Comments
		Circular Smooth Muscle	Inhibitory Neurons	Excitatory Neurons	
Bombesin	Contraction	√	—	√	Releases norepinephrine from adrenergic neurons
Calcitonin gene-related peptide	Relaxation	√	√	—	
Cholecystokinin	Biphasic	√	√	—	Inhibition overrides excitation, causes paradoxical excitation in achalasia patients
Dopamine	Relaxation (D$_2$)	√	—	—	
	Contraction (D$_1$)	√	—	—	
Galanin	Contraction	√	—	—	
Gastric inhibitory polypeptide	Relaxation	?	?	?	
Gastrin	Contraction	√	—	—	
Glucagon	Relaxation	√	—	—	Releases catecholamines from adrenal medulla
Histamine	Contraction	√ (H$_1$)	—	—	
Motilin	Contraction	√	—	√	
Neurotensin	Contraction	√	—	—	
Nitric oxide	Relaxation	√	—	—	
Pancreatic polypeptide	Contraction	√	—	√	
PGF$_{2\alpha}$	Contraction	√	—	—	
PGF$_{1,2}$	Relaxation	√	—	—	
Progesterone	Relaxation	√	—	—	
Secretin	Relaxation	√	—	—	
Serotonin	Contraction	√	—	—	
Somatostatin	Contraction	?	?	?	
Substance P	Contraction	√	—	√	
VIP	Relaxation	√	—	—	

PGE, prostaglandin E; PGF, prostaglandin F; VIP, vasoactive intestinal peptide.

alcohol [355], and caffeine [356]. Even colonic fermentation can lower LES pressure, the mechanism being unclear [357]. Smoking decreases LES pressure [358], as does pregnancy, the latter due in part to the hormone progesterone [359]. Sleep has little or no effect on LES pressure [360, 361]. Psychologic stress can lower the pressure. Many other hormones, neurotransmitters, and ingested medications can alter LES pressure (Table 5.1), such as anticholinergic drugs, nitrates, calcium-channel blockers, and certain prostaglandins, and can potentially predispose to gastroesophageal reflux. Other substances and drugs have therapeutic potential because of their effects [362].

Transient lower esophageal sphincter relaxations
Independent of swallowing, the LES relaxes spontaneously (TLESR), and with belching, retching, and vomiting. In both patients and normal subjects, the TLESR in the face of a normal LES pressure is the most common mechanism of gastroesophageal reflux [363, 364]. Transient LES relaxation occurs largely in the post-prandial period, attributed to a vagal reflex initiated by gastric distention [365, 366]. Belching occurs with a TLESR in response to gastric distention [367]. TLSERs are accompanied by crural diaphragm inhibition except when initiated by laryngeal or pharyngeal stimulation [368–370], and last longer, greater than 10 s, than swallow-related relaxations [366]. The TLESR is mediated centrally in the brainstem SPG in response to afferent input from the stomach, esophagus, pharynx or larynx, and crural diaphragm. The efferent signal is then carried in the vagus to produce relaxation of the LES and via the phrenic nerve to the crural diaphragm [275]. The reflex pathways, neurotransmitters, and chemical mediators involved are shown in Figure 5.16. NO may also be released at the diaphragm as a mediator of inhibition. Knowledge of these pathways had led to the potential for therapies directed at reducing the TLESRs in GERD [371] by inhibiting

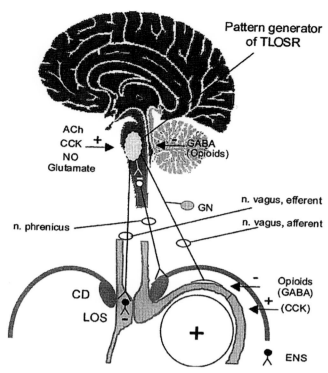

Figure 5.16 Reflex arc underlying transient lower esophageal sphincter relaxations (TLOSRs), and potential sites of actions of different agents. CCK, cholecystokinin; ACh, acetylcholine; GABA, gamma butyric acid; NO, nitric oxide; CD, crural diaphragm; ENS, enteric nervous system; GN, nodose ganglion. NO may also act at the level of the crural diaphragm (reproduced from Hirsch *et al.* [371], with permission).

cholinergic (M_1 receptor), and CCK-A receptor effects, and enhancing GABA-B receptor effects [372–374].

Diaphragm (the "external sphincter")

The contribution of the diaphragm to the LES pressure has been discussed previously, and the contribution of the diaphragm as an antireflux barrier is well described [267, 375]. The relaxation of the crural diaphragm in coordination with the LES relaxations on swallowing and with the TLESR has also been noted previously [371, 376]. A hiatus hernia removes the external sphincter effect at the gastoesophageal junction, the hernia acting as one contributing factor to the occurrence of gastroesophageal reflux.

References

1. Lear CS, Flanagan JB Jr, Moorrees CF. The frequency of deglutition in man. *Arch Oral Biol* 1965;10:83–100.
2. Bieger D, Neuhuber W. Neural circuits and mediators regulating swallowing in the brainstem. GI Motility online. 2006; PART 1 Oral cavity, pharynx and esophagus. http://www.nature.com/gimo/index.html
3. Jean A. Brain stem control of swallowing: neuronal network and cellular mechanisms. *Physiol Rev* 2001;81:929–969.
4. Jean A, Dallaporta M. Electrophysiologic characterization of the swallowing pattern generator in the brainstem. GI Motility online. 2006; PART 1 Oral cavity, pharynx and esophagus. http://www.nature.com/gimo/index.html
5. Lang IM, Dean C, Medda BK, Aslam M, Shaker R. Differential activation of medullary vagal nuclei during different phases of swallowing in the cat. *Brain Res* 2004;1014:145–163.
6. Lang IM. Brain stem control of the phases of swallowing. *Dysphagia* 2009;24:333–348.
7. Broussard DL, Altschuler SM. Brainstem viscerotopic organization of afferents and efferents involved in the control of swallowing. *Am J Med* 2000;108 (Suppl 4a):79S–86S.
8. Jean A. Brainstem control of swallowing: localization and organization of the central pattern generator for swallowing. In: Taylor A, ed. *Neurophysiology of the Jaws and Teeth*. New York: Macmillan Press, 1990, pp. 294–321.
9. Cunningham ET Jr, Sawchenko PE. Central neural control of esophageal motility: a review. *Dysphagia* 1990;5:35–51.
10. Doty RW. Neural organization of deglutition. Code CF, ed. *Handbook of Physiology, Section 6: Alimentary Canal*. Washington, DC: American Physiological Society, 1968.
11. Sumi T. Role of the pontine reticular formation in the neural organization of deglutition. *Jpn J Physiol* 1972;22:295–314.
12. Miller AJ. Deglutition. *Physiol Rev* 1982;62:129–184.
13. Miller AJ. Neurophysiological basis of swallowing. *Dysphagia* 1986;1:91–100.
14. Yoshida Y, Tanaka Y, Hirano M, Nakashima T. Sensory innervation of the pharynx and larynx. *Am J Med* 2000;108 (Suppl 4a):51S–61S.
15. Beyak MJ, Collman PI, Valdez DT, Xue S, Diamant NE. Superior laryngeal nerve stimulation in the cat: effect on oropharyngeal swallowing, oesophageal motility and lower oesophageal sphincter activity. *Neurogastroenterol Motil* 1997;9:117–127.
16. Ciampini G, Jean A. Role of glossopharyngeal and trigeminal afferents in the initiation and propagation of swallowing. II—Trigeminal afferents (author's translation) [in French]. *J Physiologie* 1980;76:61–66.
17. Ciampini G, Jean A. Role of glossopharyngeal and trigeminal afferents in the initiation and propagation of swallowing. I—Glossopharyngeal afferents (author's translation) [in French]. *J Physiologie* 1980;76:49–60.
18. Shaker R, Ren J, Zamir Z, Sarna A, Liu J, Sui Z. Effect of aging, position, and temperature on the threshold volume triggering pharyngeal swallows. *Gastroenterology* 1994;107:396–402.
19. Lang IM, Medda BK, Ren J, Shaker R. Characterization and mechanisms of the pharyngoesophageal inhibitory reflex. *Am J Physiol* 1998;275:G1127–1136.
20. Mansson I, Sandberg N. Oro-pharyngeal sensitivity and elicitation of swallowing in man. *Acta Otolaryngol* 1975;79:140–145.
21. Shaker R. Reflex interaction of pharynx, esophagus, and airways. GI Motility online. 2006; Part 1 Oral cavity, pharynx and esophagus. http://www.nature.com/gimo/index.html
22. Chiang CY, Hu JW, Dostrovsky JO, Sessle BJ. Changes in mechanoreceptive field properties of trigeminal somatosensory brainstem neurons induced by stimulation of nucleus raphe magnus in cats. *Brain Res* 1989;485:371–381.

23. Randich A, Gebhart GF. Vagal afferent modulation of nociception. *Brain Res Brain Res Rev* 1992;17:77–99.

24. Sengupta JN, Saha JK, Goyal RK. Stimulus-response function studies of esophageal mechanosensitive nociceptors in sympathetic afferents of opossum. *J Neurophysiol* 1990;64:796–812.

25. Collman PI, Tremblay L, Diamant NE. The distribution of spinal and vagal sensory neurons that innervate the esophagus of the cat. *Gastroenterology* 1992;103:817–822.

26. Jean A. [The nucleus tractus solitarius: neuroanatomic, neurochemical and functional aspects] [in French]. *Arch Internationales Physiologie Biochimie Biophysique* 1991;99:A3–A52.

27. Amirali A, Tsai G, Schrader N, Weisz D, Sanders I. Mapping of brain stem neuronal circuitry active during swallowing. *Ann Otol Rhinol Laryngol* 2001;110:502–513.

28. Altschuler SM, Bao X, Miselis RR. Dendritic architecture of hypoglossal motoneurons projecting to extrinsic tongue musculature in the rat. *J Comp Neurol* 1994;342:538–550.

29. Barrett RT, Bao X, Miselis RR, Altschuler SM. Brain stem localization of rodent esophageal premotor neurons revealed by transneuronal passage of pseudorabies virus. *Gastroenterology* 1994;107:728–737.

30. Collman PI, Tremblay L, Diamant NE. The central vagal efferent supply to the esophagus and lower esophageal sphincter of the cat. *Gastroenterology* 1993;104:1430–1438.

31. Altschuler SM, Bao XM, Miselis RR. Dendritic architecture of nucleus ambiguus motoneurons projecting to the upper alimentary tract in the rat. *J Comp Neurol* 1991;309:402–414.

32. Bieger D, Hopkins DA. Viscerotopic representation of the upper alimentary tract in the medulla oblongata in the rat: the nucleus ambiguus. *J Comp Neurol* 1987;262:546–562.

33. Lawn AM. The nucleus ambiguus of the rabbit. *J Comp Neurol* 1966;127:307–320.

34. Hyland NP, Abrahams TP, Fuchs K, Burmeister MA, Hornby PJ. Organization and neurochemistry of vagal preganglionic neurons innervating the lower esophageal sphincter in ferrets. *J Comp Neurol* 2001;430:222–234.

35. Kalia M, Mesulam MM. Brain stem projections of sensory and motor components of the vagus complex in the cat: II. Laryngeal, tracheobronchial, pulmonary, cardiac, and gastrointestinal branches. *J Comp Neurol* 1980;193:467–508.

36. Hornby PJ, Abrahams TP. Central control of lower esophageal sphincter relaxation. *Am J Med* 2000;108 (Suppl 4a):90S–98S.

37. Rossiter CD, Norman WP, Jain M, Hornby PJ, Benjamin S, Gillis RA. Control of lower esophageal sphincter pressure by two sites in dorsal motor nucleus of the vagus. *Am J Physiol* 1990;259:G899–906.

38. Umezaki T, Matsuse T, Shin T. Medullary swallowing-related neurons in the anesthetized cat. *Neuroreport* 1998;9:1793–1798.

39. Kalia M. Cerebral pathways in reflex muscular inhibition from type J pulmonary receptors. *J Physiol (Lond)* 1969;204:92–93.

40. Roman C, Tieffenbach L. Recording the unit activity of vagal motor fibers innervating the baboon esophagus [in French]. *J Physiologie* 1972;64:479–506.

41. Roman C. Nervous control of esophageal peristalsis. [French]. *J Physiologie* 1966;58:79–108.

42. Jean A. Localization and activity of medullary swallowing neurones [in French]. *J Physiologie* 1972;64:227–268.

43. Zoungrana OR, Amri MA-C, A., Roman C. Intracellular activity of motoneurons of the rostral nucleus ambiguus during swallowing in sheep. *J Neurophysiol* 1997;77:909–922.

44. Beyak MJ, Collman PI, Xue S, Valdez DT, Diamant NE. Release of nitric oxide in the central nervous system mediates tonic and phasic contraction of the cat lower oesophageal sphincter. *N Engl J Med* 2003;349:801–803.

45. Beyak MJ, Xue S, Collman PI, Valdez DT, Diamant NE. Central nervous system nitric oxide induces oropharyngeal swallowing and esophageal peristalsis in the cat. *Gastroenterology* 2000;119:377–385.

46. Hamdy S. Role of cerebral cortex in the control of swallowing. GI Motility online. 2006; PART 1 Oral cavity, pharynx, and esophagus. http://www.nature.com/gimo/index.html

47. Hockman CH, Bieger D, Weerasuriya A. Supranuclear pathways of swallowing. *Prog Neurobiol* 1979;12:15–32.

48. Martin RE, Sessle BJ. The role of the cerebral cortex in swallowing. *Dysphagia* 1993;8:195–202.

49. Broussard DL, Altschuler SM. Central integration of swallow and airway-protective reflexes. *Am J Med* 2000;108 (Suppl 4a):62S–67S.

50. Martin RE, Kemppainen P, Masuda Y, Yao D, Murray GM, Sessle BJ. Features of cortically evoked swallowing in the awake primate (Macaca fascicularis). *J Neurophysiol* 1999;82:1529–1541.

51. Hamdy S, Aziz Q, Rothwell JC, *et al*. The cortical topography of human swallowing musculature in health and disease. *Nature* 1996;2:1217–1224.

52. Hamdy S, Xue S, Valdez D, Diamant NE. Induction of cortical swallowing activity by transcranial magnetic stimulation in the anaesthetized cat. *Neurogastroenterol Mot* 2001;13:65–72.

53. Hamdy S, Aziz Q, Rothwell JC, *et al*. Recovery of swallowing after dysphagic storke relates to functional reorganization in the intact motor complex. *Gastroenterology* 1998;115:1104–1112.

54. Martin RE, MacIntosh BJ, Smith RC, *et al*. Cerebral areas processing swallowing and tongue movement are overlapping but distinct: a functional magnetic resonance imaging study. *J Neurophysiol* 2004;92:2428–2443.

55. Sumi T. The activity of brainstem respiratory neurons and spinal respiratory motorneurons during swallowing. *J Neurophysiol* 1963;26:466–477.

56. Gestreau C, Milano S, Bianchi AL, Grelot L. Activity of dorsal respiratory group inspiratory neurons during laryngeal-induced fictive coughing and swallowing in decerebrate cats. *Exp Brain Res* 1996;108:247–256.

57. Martin-Harris B. Coordination of respiration and swallowing. GI Motility online. 2006; PART 1 Oral cavity, pharynx and esophagus. http://www.nature.com/gimo/index.html

58. Silva AC, Fabio SR, Dantas RO. A scintigraphic study of oral, pharyngeal, and esophageal transit in patients with stroke. *Dysphagia* 2008;23:165–171.

59. Hamdy S, Rothwell JC, Aziz O, Singh KD, Thompson DG. Long-term reorganization of human motor cortex driven by short-term sensory stimulation. *Nat Neurosci* 1998;1:64–68.

60. Donner MW, Bosma JF, Robertson DL. Anatomy and physiology of the pharynx. *Gastrointest Radiol* 1985;10:196–212.

61. Jones B, Donner MW, eds. *Normal and Abnormal Swallowing. Imaging in Diagnosis and Therapy.* New York: Springer-Verlag, 1990.

62. Jones B. Radiographic evaluation of motility of mouth and pharynx. GI Motility online. 2006; PAET 1 Oral cavity, pharynx and esophagus. http://www.nature.com/gimo/index.html

63. Pouderoux P, Kahrilas PJ. The pharyngoesophageal segment: Normal structure and function. *Dis Esophagus* 1985;8:233–241.

64. Liebermann-Meffert D. The pharyngoesophageal segment: Anatomy and innervation. *Dis Esophagus* 1985;8:242–251.

65. Saitoh E, Shibata S, Matsuo K, Baba M, Fujii W, Palmer JB. Chewing and food consistency: effects on bolus transport and swallow initiation. *Dysphagia* 2007;22:100–107.

66. Preiksaitis HG, Mayrand S, Robins K, Diamant NE. Coordination of respiration and swallowing: effect of bolus volume in normal adults. *Am J Physiol* 1992;263:R624–630.

67. Alberts MJ, Horner J, Gray L, Brazer SR. Aspiration after stroke: lesion analysis by brain MRI. *Dysphagia* 1992;7:170–173.

68. Daniels SK. Neurological disorders affecting oral, pharyngeal swallowing. GI Motility online. 2006; PART 1 Oral cavity, pharynx and esophagus. http://www.nature.com/gimo/index.html

69. Jaradeh S. Muscle disorders affecting oral and pharyngel swallowing. GI Motility online. 2006; PART 1 Oral vavity, pharynx and esophagus. http://www.nature.com/gimo/index.html

70. Ergun GA, Kahrilas PJ, Lin S, Logemann JA, Harig JM. Shape, volume, and content of the deglutitive pharyngeal chamber imaged by ultrafast computerized tomography. *Gastroenterology* 1993;105:1396–1403.

71. Gaige TA, Benner T, Wang R, Wedeen VJ, Gilbert RJ. Three dimensional myoarchitecture of the human tongue determined in vivo by diffusion tensor imaging with tractography. *J Magn Reson Imaging* 2007;26:654–661.

72. Wein B, Bockler R, Klajman S. Temporal reconstruction of sonographic imaging of disturbed tongue movements. *Dysphagia* 1991;6:135–139.

73. Castell JA, Dalton CB, Castell DO. Effects of body position and bolus consistency on the manometric parameters and coordination of the upper esophageal sphincter and pharynx. *Dysphagia* 1990;5:179–186.

74. Sears VW, Jr., Castell JA, Castell DO. Radial and longitudinal asymmetry of human pharyngeal pressures during swallowing. *Gastroenterology* 1991;101:1559–1563.

75. Kahrilas PJ, Logemann JAA-L, S., Ergun GA. Pharyngeal clearance during swallowing: A combined manometric and videofluroscopic study. *Gastroenterology* 1992;103:128–136.

76. Kahrilas PJ, Lin S, Logemann JA, Ergun GA, Facchini F. Deglutitive tongue action: Volume accommodation and bolus propulsion. *Gastroenterology* 1993;104:152–162.

77. Kahrilas PJ, Lin S, Chen J, Logemann JA. Oropharyngeal accommodation to swallow volume. *Gastroenterology* 1996;111:297–306.

78. Dua KS, Ren J, Bardan E, Xie P, Shaker R. Coordination of deglutitive glottal function and pharyngeal bolus transit during normal eating. *Gastroenterology* 1997;112:73–83.

79. Jacob P, Kahrilas PJ, Logemann JA, Shah V, Ha T. Upper esophageal sphincter opening and modulation during swallowing. *Gastroenterology* 1989;97:1469–1478.

80. Lang IM. Upper esophageal sphincter. GI Motility online. 2006; PART 1 Oral cavity, pharynx, and esophagus. http://www.nature.com/gimo/index.html

81. Lang IM, Shaker R. Anatomy and physiology of the upper esophageal sphincter. *Am J Med* 1997;103:50S–55S.

82. Cook IJ, Kahrilas PJ. AGA technical review on management of oropharyngeal dysphagia. *Gastroenterology* 1999;116:455–478.

83. Kahrilas PJ, Dodds WJ, Dent J, Wyman JB, Hogan WJ, Arndorfer RC. Upper esophageal sphincter function during belching. *Gastroenterology* 1986;91:133–140.

84. Welch RW, Luckmann K, Ricks PM, Drake ST, Gates GA. Manometry of the normal upper esophageal sphincter and its alterations in laryngectomy. *J Clin Invest* 1979;63:1036–1041.

85. Bonington A, Mahon M, Whitmore I. A histological and histochemical study of the cricopharyngeus muscle in man. *J Anat* 1988;156:27–37.

86. Kristmundsdottir F, Mahon M, Froes MM, Cumming WJ. Histomorphometric and histopathological study of the human cricopharyngeus muscle: in health and in motor neuron disease. *Neuropathol Appl Neurobiol* 1990;16:461–475.

87. Mu L, Sanders I. The innervation of the human upper esophageal sphincter. *Dysphagia* 1996;11:234–238.

88. Sundman E, Yost CS, Margolin G, Kuylenstierna R, Ekberg O, Eriksson LI. Acetylcholine receptor density in human cricopharyngeal muscle and pharyngeal constrictor muscle. *Acta Anaesthesiol Scand* 2002;46:999–1002.

89. Bao X, Wiedner EB, Altschuler SM. Transsynaptic localization of pharyngeal premotor neurons in rat. *Brain Res* 1995;696:246–249.

90. Asoh R, Goyal RK. Manometry and electromyography of the upper esophageal sphincter in the opossum. *Gastroenterology* 1978;74:514–520.

91. Castell JA, Castell DO, Schultz AR, Georgeson S. Effect of head position on the dynamics of the upper esophageal sphincter and pharynx. *Dysphagia* 1993;8:1–6.

92. Wilson JA, Pryde A, Cecilia A, Macintyre CC, Heading RC. Normal pharyngoesophageal motility. A study of 50 healthy subjects. *Dig Dis Sci* 1989;34:1590–1599.

93. Pandolfino JE, Kahrilas PJ. AGA technical review on the clinical use of esophageal manometry. *Gastroenterology* 2005;128:209–224.

94. Kahrilas PJ, Dodds WJ, Dent J, Logemann JA, Shaker R. Upper esophageal sphincter function during deglutition. *Gastroenterology* 1988;95:52–62.

95. Jacob P, Kahrilas PJ, Herzon G, McLaughlin B. Determinants of upper esophageal sphincter pressure in dogs. *Am J Physiol* 1990;259:G245–251.

96. Isberg A, Nilsson ME, Schiratzki H. Movement of the upper esophageal sphincter and a manometric device during deglutition. A cineradiographic investigation. *Acta Radiol Diagn (Stockh)* 1985;26:381–388.

97. Lydon SB, Dodds WJ, Hogan WJ, Arndorfer RC. The effect of manometric assembly diameter on intraluminal esophageal pressure recording. *Am J Dig Dis* 1975;20:968–970.

98. Cardoso PFG, Miller L, Diamant NE. The effect of catheter diameter on upper esophageal sphincter pressure measurement in normal subjects. *Gullet* 1992;2:145–148.

99. Kahrilas PJ, Dodds WJ, Dent, JD, Haeberle B. Effect of sleep, spontaneous gastroesophageal reflux, and a meal on upper esophageal sphincter pressure in normal human volunteers. *Gastroenterology* 1987;92:466–471.

100. Kahrilas PJ, Dodds WJ, Dent J, Haeberle B, Hogan WJ, Arndorfer RC. Effect of sleep, spontaneous gastroesophageal reflux, and a meal on upper esophageal sphincter pressure in normal human volunteers. *Gastroenterology* 1987;92:466–471.

101. Vanner RG, Pryle BJ, O'Dwyer JP, Reynolds F. Upper oesophageal sphincter pressure and the intravenous induction of anaesthesia. *Anaesthesia* 1992;47:371–375.

102. Vanner RG, Pryle BJ, O'Dwyer JP, Reynolds F. Upper oesophageal sphincter pressure during inhalational anaesthesia. *Anaesthesia* 1992;47:950–954.

103. Goyal RK, Sangree MH, Hersh T, Spiro HM. Pressure inversion point at the upper high pressure zone and its genesis. *Gastroenterology* 1970;59:754–759.

104. Lang IM, Dantas RO, Cook IJ, Dodds WJ. Videoradiographic, manometric, and electromyographic analysis of canine upper esophageal sphincter. *Am J Physiol* 1991;260:G911–919.

105. Preiksaitis HG, Diamant NE. The physiology of swallowing: Pharyngeal and cricopharyngeal mechanisms. In: Pearson FG, Deslauriers J, Ginsberg RJ, Hiebert CA, McKneally MF, Urschel HC, eds. *Esophageal Surgery*. New York: Churchill Livingstone, 1995.

106. Cook IJ, Dent J, Shannon S, Collins SM. Measurement of upper esophageal sphincter pressure. Effect of acute emotional stress. *Gastroenterology* 1987;93:526–32.

107. Cook IJ, Dent J, Collins SM. Upper esophageal sphincter tone and reactivity to stress in patients with a history of globus sensation. *Dig Dis Sci* 1989;34:672–676.

108. Lang IM, Medda BK, Shaker R. Mechanisms of reflexes induced by esophageal distension. *Am J Physiol Gastrointest Liver Physiol* 2001;281:G1246–1263.

109. Ghosh SK, Pandolfino JE, Zhang Q, Jarosz A, Kahrilas PJ. Deglutitive upper esophageal sphincter relaxation: a study of 75 volunteer subjects using solid-state high-resolution manometry. *Am J Physiol Gastrointest Liver Physiol* 2006;291: G525–531.

110. Cook IJ, Dodds WJ, Dantas RO, *et al*. Opening mechanisms of the human upper esophageal sphincter. *Am J Physiol* 1989; 257:G748–759.

111. Kahrilas PJ, Logemann JA, Krugler C, Flanagan E. Volitional augmentation of upper esophageal sphincter opening during swallowing. *Am J Physiol* 1991;260:G450–456.

112. Kahrilas PJ, Logemann JA. Volume accommodation during swallowing. *Dysphagia* 1993;8:259–265.

113. Goyal RK, Martin SB, Shapiro J, Spechler SJ. The role of cricopharyngeus muscle in pharyngoesophageal disorders. *Dysphagia* 1993;8:252–258.

114. Martino R, Terrault N, Ezerzer F, Mikulis D, Diamant NE. Dysphagia in a patient with lateral medullary syndrome: Insight into the central control of swallowing. *Gastroenterology* 2001;121:420–426.

115. Sacco RL, Freddo L, Bello JA, Odel JG, Onesti ST, Mohr JP. Wallenberg's lateral medullary syndrome. Clinical-magnetic resonance imaging correlations. *Arch Neurol* 1993;50:609–614.

116. Kahrilas PJ, Lin S, Rademaker AW, Logemann JA. Impaired deglutitive airway protection: A videofluoroscopic analysis of severity and mechanism. *Gastroenterology* 1997;113:1457–1464.

117. Freiman JM, El-Sharkawy TY, Diamant NE. Effect of bilateral vagosympathetic nerve blockade on response of the dog upper esophageal sphincter (UES) to intraesophageal distention and acid. *Gastroenterology* 1981;81:78–84.

118. Kahrilas PJ, Dodds WJ, Hogan WJ. Dysfunction of the belch reflex. A cause of incapacitating chest pain. *Gastroenterology* 1987;93:818–822.

119. Gerhardt DC, Shuck TJ, Bordeaux RA, Winship DH. Human upper esophageal sphincter. Response to volume, osmotic, and acid stimuli. *Gastroenterology* 1978;75:268–274.

120. Barbara L, Lazzari R, Roda A, *et al*. Serum bile acids in newborns and children. *Pediatr Res* 1980;14:1222–1225.

121. Shaker R, Ren J, Kern M, Dodds WJ, Hogan WJ, Li Q. Mechanisms of airway protection and upper esophageal sphincter opening during belching. *Am J Physiol* 1992;262: G621–628.

122. Shaker R, Dodds WJ, Ren J, Hogan WJ, Arndorfer RC. Esophagoglottal closure reflex: a mechanism of airway protection. *Gastroenterology* 1992;102:857–861.

123. Wallin L, Boesby S, Madsen T. The effect of HCl infusion in the lower part of the oesophagus on the pharyngo-oesophageal sphincter pressure in normal subjects. *Scand J Gastroenterol* 1978;13:821–826.

124. Thompson DG, Andreollo NA, McIntyre AS, Earlam RJ. Studies of the oesophageal clearance responses to intraluminal acid. *Gut* 1988;29:881–885.

125. Vakil NB, Kahrilas PJ, Dodds WJ, Vanagunas A. Absence of an upper esophageal sphincter response to acid reflux. *Am J Gastroenterol* 1989;84:606–610.

126. Meyer GW, Austin MC, Brady CE, Castell DO. Muscle anatomy of the human esophagus. *J Clin Gastroenterol* 1986;8: 131–134.

127. Li Q, Castell JA, Castell DO. Manometric determination of esophageal length. *Am J Gastroenterol* 1994;89:722–725.

128. Christensen J. The oesophagus. In: Christensen J, Wingate DL, eds. *A Guide to Gastrointestinal Motility*. London: Wright PSG, 1983, pp. 75–100.

129. Baumgarten HG, Lange W. Adrenergic innervation of the oesophagus in the cat (Felis domestica) and Rhesus monkey (Macacus rhesus). *Z Zellforsch Mikrosk Anat* 1969;95:529–545.

130. Sengupta JN, Kauvar D, Goyal RK. Characteristics of vagal esophageal tension-sensitive afferent fibers in the opossum. *J Neurophysiol* 1989;61:1001–1010.

131. Rodrigo J, Hernandez CJ, Vidal MA, Pedrosa JA. Vegetative innervation of the esophagus. II. Intraganglionic laminar endings. *Acta Anatomica* 1975;92:79–100.

132. Huizinga JD, Reed DE, Berezin I, *et al*. Survival dependency of intramuscular ICC on vagal afferent nerves in the cat esophagus. *Am J Physiol Regul Integr Comp Physiol* 2008;294: R302–310.

133. Phillips RJ, Powley TL. Tension and stretch receptors in gastrointestinal smooth muscle: re-evaluating vagal mechanoreceptor electrophysiology. *Brain Res Brain Res Rev* 2000; 34:1–26.

134. Powley TL, Wang X-Y, Fox EA, Phillips RJ, Liu LWC, Huizinga JD. Ultrastructural evidence for communication between intramuscular vagal mechanoreceptors and interstitial cells of Cajal in the rat fundus. *Neurogastroenterol Motil* 2008;20:69–79.

135. Zhou DS, Desaki J, Komuro T. Neuro-muscular junctions of longitudinal and circular muscle fibers of the guinea-pig

esophagus and their relation to myenteric plexus. *J Autonom Nerv System* 1996;58:63–68.

136. Toyama T, Yokoyama I, Nishi K. Effects of hexamethonium and other ganglionic blocking agents on electrical activity of the esophagus induced by vagal stimulation in the dog. *Eur J Pharmacol* 1975;31:63–71.

137. Neuhuber WL, Worl J, Berthoud HR, Conte B. NADPH-diaphorase-positive nerve fibers associated with motor end-plates in the rat esophagus: new evidence for co-innervation of striated muscle by enteric neurons. *Cell Tissue Res* 1994; 276:23–30.

138. Singaram C, Sengupta A, Sweet MA, Sugarbaker DJ, Goyal RK. Nitrinergic and peptidergic innervation of the human oesophagus. *Gut* 1994;35:1690–1696.

139. Sang Q, Young HM. Development of nicotinic receptor clusters and innervation accompanying the change in muscle pheno-type in the mouse esophagus. *J Comp Neurol* 1997;386: 119–136.

140. Boudaka A, Worl J, Shiina T, Shimizu Y, Takewaki T, Neuhuber WL. Galanin modulates vagally induced contractions in the mouse oesophagus. *Neurogastroenterol Motil* 2009;21:180–188.

141. Kallmunzer B, Sorensen B, Neuhuber WL, Worl J. Enteric co-innervation of striated muscle fibres in human oesophagus. *Neurogastroenterol Motil* 2008;20:597–610.

142. Baldi F, Ferrarini F, Longanesi A, Ragazzini M, Barbara L. Acid gastroesophageal reflux and symptom occurrence. Analysis of some factors influencing their association. *Dig Dis Sci* 1989;34:1890–1893.

143. Soffer EE, Schneiderman J, Schwartz I, *et al.* Effects of upper dorsal sympathectomy on esophageal motility in humans. *Dig Dis Sci* 1988;33:157–160.

144. Zfass AM, Prince R, Allen FN, Farrar JT. Inhibitory beta adrenergic receptors in the human distal esophagus. *Dig Dis Sci* 1970;15:303–310.

145. Gonella J, Niel JP, Roman C. Mechanism of the noradrenergic motor control on the lower oesophageal sphincter in the cat. *J Physiol (Lond)* 1980;306:251–260.

146. Daniel EE, Jager LP, Jury J. Catecholamines release mediators in the opossum oesophageal circular smooth muscle. *J Physiol (Lond)* 1987;382:489–508.

147. Smid SD, Blackshaw LA. Vagal neurotransmission to the ferret lower oesophageal sphincter: inhibition via GABA(B) receptors. *Br J Pharmacol* 2000;131:624–630.

148. Seelig LL, Jr., Doody P, Brainard L, Gidda JS, Goyal RK. Acetylcholinesterase and choline acetyltransferase staining of neurons in the opossum esophagus. *Anat Rec* 1984;209: 125–130.

149. Faussone-Pellegrini MS, Cortesini C. Ultrastructure of striated muscle fibers in the middle third of the human esophagus. *Histol Histopath* 1986;1:119–128.

150. Christensen J, Rick GA, Soll DJ. Intramural nerves and interstitial cells revealed by the Champy-Maillet stain in the opossum esophagus. *J Autonom Nerv System* 1987;19:137–151.

151. Gabella G. Fine structure of the myenteric plexus in the guinea-pig ileum. *J Anat* 1972;111:69–97.

152. Berezin I, Daniel EE, Huizinga JD. Ultrastructure of interstitial cells of Cajal in the canine distal esophagus. *Can J Physiol Pharmacol* 1994;72:1049–1059.

153. Faussone-Pellegrini MS, Cortesini C. Ultrastructural features and localization of the interstitial cells of Cajal in the smooth muscle coat of human esophagus. *J Submicrosc Cytol* 1985;17: 187–197.

154. Wong WC, Tan SH, Yick TY, Ling EA. Ultrastructure of interstitial cells of Cajal at the gastro-oesophageal junction of the monkey (Macaca fascicularis). *Acta Anatom* 1990;138:318–326.

155. Clouse RE, Alrakawi A, Staiano A. Intersubject and interswallow variability in topography of esophageal motility. *Dig Dis Sci* 1998;43:1978–1985.

156. Clouse RE, Staiano A, Bickston SJ, Cohn SM. Characteristics of the propagating pressure wave in the esophagus. *Dig Dis Sci* 1996;41:2369–2376.

157. Clouse RE, Staiano A. Topography of normal and high-amplitude esophageal peristalsis. *Am J Physiol* 1993;265:G1098–1107.

158. Richter JE, Wu WC, Johns DN, *et al.* Esophageal manometry in 95 healthy adult volunteers. Variability of pressures with age and frequency of "abnormal" contractions. *Dig Dis Sci* 1987;32:583–592.

159. Roman C, Orengo M, Tieffenbach L. Electromyographic study of esophageal smooth muscle in cats [in French]. *J Physiologie* 1969;61 (Suppl 2):390.

160. Edmundowicz SA, Clouse RE. Shortening of the esophagus in response to swallowing. *Am J Physiol* 1991;260:G512–516.

161. Nicosia MA, Brasseur JG, Liu J, Miller LS. Local longitudinal muscle shortening of the human esophagus from high-frequency ultrasonography. *Am J Physiol Gastrointest Liver Physiol* 2001;281:G1022–1033.

162. Jung HY, Puckett JL, Bhalla V, *et al.* Asynchrony between the circular and the longitudinal muscle contraction in patients with nutcracker esophagus. *Gastroenterology* 2005;128:1179–1186.

163. Mittal RK, Padda B, Bhalla V, Bhargava V, Liu J. Synchrony between circular and longitudinal muscle contractions during peristalsis in normal subjects. *Am J Physiol Gastrointest Liver Physiol* 2006;290:G431–438.

164. Pal A, Brasseur JG. The mechanical advantage of local longitudinal shortening on peristaltic transport. *J Biomech Eng* 2002;124:94–100.

165. Korsapati H, Babaei A, Bhargava V, Mittal RK. Cholinergic stimulation induces asynchrony between the circular and longitudinal muscle contraction during esophageal peristalsis. *Am J Physiol Gastrointest Liver Physiol* 2008;294:G694–698.

166. Korsapati H, Bhargava V, Mittal RK. Reversal of asynchrony between circular and longitudinal muscle contraction in nutcracker esophagus by atropine. *Gastroenterology* 2008;135: 796–802.

167. Clouse RE, Staiano A. Topography of the esophageal peristaltic pressure wave. *Am J Physiol* 1991;261:G677–684.

168. Kahrilas PJ, Dodds WJ, Hogan WJ. Effect of peristaltic dysfunction on esophageal volume clearance. *Gastroenterology* 1988;94:73–80.

169. Tutuian R, Castell DO. Clarification of the esophageal function defect in patients with manometric ineffective esophageal motility: studies using combined impedance-manometry. *Clin Gastroenterol Hepatol* 2004;2:230–236.

170. Hollis JB, Castell DO. Effect of dry swallows and wet swallows of different volumes on esophageal peristalsis. *J Appl Physiol (Wash)* 1975;38:1161–1164.

171. Dodds WJ, Hogan WJ, Reid DP, Stewart ET, Arndorfer RC. A comparison between primary esophageal peristalsis following wet and dry swallows. *J Appl Physiol (Wash)* 1973;35:851–857.

172. Dooley CP, Schlossmacher B, Valenzuela JE. Effects of alterations in bolus viscosity on esophageal peristalsis in humans. *Am J Physiol* 1988;254:G8–11.

173. Tutuian R, Elton JP, Castell DO, Gideon RM, Castell JA, Katz PO. Effects of position on oesophageal function: studies using combined manometry and multichannel intraluminal impedance. *Neurogastroenterol Motil* 2003;15:63–67.

174. Siegel CI, Hendrix TR. Evidence for the central mediation of secondary peristals in the esophagus. *Bull Johns Hopkins* 1961;108:297–307.

175. Cannon WB. Oesophageal peristalsis after bilateral vagotomy. *Am J Physiol* 1907;19:436–444.

176. Jurica EJ. Studies on the motility of the denervated mammalian esophagus. *Am J Physiol* 1926;77:371–384.

177. Roman C, Tieffenbach L. Esophageal smooth muscle motility after bivagotomy. Electromyographic study [in French]. *J Physiologie* 1971;63:733–762.

178. Stacher G, Schmierer G, Landgraf M. Tertiary esophageal contractions evoked by acoustical stimuli. *Gastroenterology* 1979;77:49–54.

179. Janssens J, Valembois P, Hellemans J, Vantrappen G, Pelemans W. Studies on the necessity of a bolus for the progression of secondary peristalsis in the canine esophagus. *Gastroenterology* 1974;67:245–251.

180. Longhi EH, Jordan PHJ. Necessity of a bolus for propagation of primary peristalsis in the canine esophagus. *Am J Physiol* 1971;220:698–612.

181. Janssens J, De Wever I, Vantrappen G, Hellemans J. Peristalsis in smooth muscle esophagus after transection and bolus deviation. *Gastroenterology* 1976;71:1004–1009.

182. Valdez DT, Salapatek AM, Niznik G, Linden RD, Diamant NE. Swallowing and upper esophageal sphincter contraction with transcranial magnetic-induced electrical stimulation. *Am J Physiol* 1993;264:G213–219.

183. Aziz Q, Rothwell JC, Hamdy S, Barlow J, Thompson DG. The topographic representation of esophageal motor function on the human cerebral cortex. *Gastroenterology* 1996;111:855–862.

184. Aziz Q, Rothwell JC, Barlow JA-H, A., Alani S, Bancewicz J, Thompson DG. Esophageal myoelectric responses to magnetic stimulation of the human cortex and the extracranial vagus nerve. *Am J Physiol* 1994;267:G827–835.

185. Aziz Q, Rothwell JC, Barlow J, Thompson DG. Modulation of esophageal responses to magnetic stimulation of the human brain by swallowing and by vagal stimulation. *Gastroenterology* 1995;109:1437–1445.

186. Jordan PHJ, Longhi EH. Relationship between size of bolus and the act of swallowing on esophageal peristalis in dogs. *Proc Soc Exp Biol Med* 1971;137:868–871.

187. Meltzer SJ. Secondary peristalsis of the esophagus—a demostration on a dog with a permanent esophageal fistula. *Proc Soc Exp Biol Med* 1906;4:35–42.

188. Blank EL, Greenwood B, Dodds WJ. Cholinergic control of smooth muscle peristalsis in the cat esophagus. *Am J Physiol* 1989;257:G517–523.

189. Winship DH, Zboralske FF. The esophageal propulsive force: esophageal response to acute obstruction. *J Clin Invest* 1967;46:1391–1401.

190. Zhang X, Tack J, Janssens J, Sifrim DA. Neural regulation of tone in the oesophageal body: in vivo barostat assessment of volume-pressure relationships in the feline oesophagus. *Neurogastroenterol Motil* 2004;16:13–21.

191. Pandolfino JE, Shi G, Zhang Q, Kahrilas PJ. Absence of a deglutitive inhibition equivalent with secondary peristalsis. *Am J Physiol Gastrointest Liver Physiol* 2005;288:G671–676.

192. Mayrand S, Diamant NE. Measurement of human esophageal tone in vivo. *Gastroenterology* 1993;105:1411–1420.

193. Paterson WG, Hynna-Liepert TT, Selucky M. Comparison of primary and secondary esophageal peristalsis in humans: effect of atropine. *Am J Physiol* 1991;260:G52–57.

194. Bardan E, Xie P, Aslam M, Kern M, Shaker R. Disruption of primary and secondary esophageal peristalsis by afferent stimulation. *Am J Physiol Gastrointest Liver Physiol* 2000;279:G255–261.

195. Schoeman MN, Holoway RH. Stimulation and characteristics of secondary oesophageal peristalsis in normal subjects. *Gut* 1994;35:152–158.

196. Sifrim D, Janssens J, Vantrappen G. A wave of inhibition precedes primary peristaltic contractions in the human esophagus. *Gastroenterology* 1992;103:876–882.

197. Roman C, Gonella J. Extrinsic control of digestive tract motility. In: Johnson LR, ed. *Physiology of the Gastrointestinal Tract.* New York: Raven Press, 1981, pp. 289–333.

198. Shiina T, Shima T, Worl J, Neuhuber WL, Shimizu Y. The neural regulation of the mammalian esophageal motility and its implication for esophageal diseases. *Pathophysiology* 2010;17:129–133.

199. Tieffenbach L, Roman C. The role of extrinsic vagal innervation in the motility of the smooth-muscled portion of the esophagus: electromyographic study in the cat and the baboon [in French]. *J Physiologie* 1972;64:193–226.

200. Gidda JS, Goyal RK. Swallow-evoked action potentials in vagal preganglionic efferents. *J Neurophysiol* 1984;52:1169–1180.

201. Dodds WJ, Stef JJ, Stewart ET, Hogan WJ, Arndorfer RC, Cohen EB. Responses of feline esophagus to cervical vagal stimulation. *Am J Physiol* 1978;235:E63–73.

202. Dodds WJ, Christensen J, Dent J, Wood JD, Arndorfer RC. Esophageal contractions induced by vagal stimulation in the opossum. *Am J Physiol* 1978;235:E392–401.

203. Crist J, Gidda JS, Goyal RK. Intramural mechanism of esophageal peristalsis: roles of cholinergic and noncholinergic nerves. *Proc Natl Acad Sci USA* 1984;81:3595–3599.

204. Gilbert RJ, Dodds WJ. Effect of selective muscarinic antagonists on peristaltic contractions in opossum smooth muscle. *Am J Physiol* 1986;250:G50–59.

205. Sarna SK, Daniel EE, Waterfall WE. Myogenic and neural control systems for esophageal motility. *Gastroenterology* 1977;73:1345–1352.

206. Helm JF, Bro SL, Dodds WJ, Sarna SK, Hoffmann RG. Myogenic mechanism for peristalsis in opossum smooth muscle esophagus. *Am J Physiol* 1992;263:G953–959.

207. Preiksaitis HG, Diamant NE. Myogenic mechanism for peristalsis in the cat esophagus. *Am J Physiol* 1999;277:G306–313.

208. Dodds WJ, Dent J, Hogan WJ, Arndorfer RC. Effect of atropine on esophageal motor function in humans. *Am J Physiol* 1981; 240:G290–296.

209. Hollis JB, Castell DO. Effects of cholinergic stimulation on human esophageal peristalsis. *J Appl Physiol (Wash)* 1976; 40:40–43.

210. Humphries TJ, Castell DO. Effect of oral bethanechol on parameters of esophageal peristalsis. *Dig Dis Sci* 1981; 26:129–132.

211. Christensen J. Patterns and origin of some esophageal responses to stretch and electrical stimulation. *Gastroenterology* 1970;59:909–916.

212. Christensen J, Lund GF. Esophageal responses to distension and electrical stimulation. *J Clin Invest* 1969;48:408–419.

213. Gidda JS, Cobb BW, Goyal RK. Modulation of esophageal peristalsis by vagal efferent stimulation in opossum. *J Clin Invest* 1981;68:1411–1419.

214. Crist J, Gidda JS, Goyal RK. Characteristics of "on" and "off" contractions in esophageal circular muscle in vitro. *Am J Physiol* 1984;246:G137–144.

215. Preiksaitis HG, Laurier LG, Inculet R. Characterization of muscarinic receptors in human esophageal smooth muscle (abstr). *Gastroenterology* 1996;110:A1108.

216. Daniel EE, Jury J, Bowker P. Muscarinic receptors on nerves and muscles in opossum esophagus muscularis mucosa. *Can J Physiol Pharmacol* 1987;65:1903–1907.

217. Decktor DL, Ryan JP. Transmembrane voltage of opossum esophageal smooth muscle and its response to electrical stimulation of intrinsic nerves. *Gastroenterology* 1982;82:301–308.

218. Diamant NE, Chan WWL. The electrical off-response of cat circular esophageal smooth muscle: The effect of stimulus frequency on its timing. In: Vantrappen G, ed. *Proceedings of the Fifth International Symposium on Gastrointestinal Motility*. Herentals: Typoff-Press, 1975, pp. 158-63.

219. Serio R, Daniel EE. Electrophysiological analysis of responses to intrinsic nerves in circular muscle of opossum esophageal muscle. *Am J Physiol* 1988;254:G107–116.

220. Crist J, Surprenant A, Goyal RK. Intracellular studies of electrical membrane properties of opossum esophageal circular smooth muscle. *Gastroenterology* 1987;92:987–992.

221. Preiksaitis HG, Tremblay L, Diamant NE. Nitric Oxide mediates inhibitory nerve effects in human esophagus and lower esophageal sphincter. *Dig Dis Sci* 1994;39:770–775.

222. Paterson WG. Electrical correlates of peristaltic and nonperistaltic contractions in the opossum smooth muscle esophagus. *Gastroenterology* 1989;97:665–675.

223. Diamant NE. Electrical activity of the cat smooth muscle esophagus: A study of hyperpolarizing responses. In: Daniel EE, ed. *Proceedings of the Fourth International Symposium on Gastrointestinal Motility*. Mitchell Press: Vancouver, 1973, pp. 593–605.

224. Sugarbaker DJ, Rattan S, Goyal RK. Mechanical and electrical activity of esophageal smooth muscle during peristalsis. *Am J Physiol* 1984;246:G145–150.

225. Rattan S, Gidda JS, Goyal RK. Membrane potential and mechanical responses of the opossum esophagus to vagal stimulation and swallowing. *Gastroenterology* 1983;85:922–928.

226. Gidda JS, Goyal RK. Influence of successive vagal stimulations on contractions in esophageal smooth muscle of opossum. *J Clin Invest* 1983;71:1095–1103.

227. Weisbrodt NW, Christensen J. Gradients of contractions in the opossum esophagus. *Gastroenterology* 1972;62:1159–1166.

228. Crist J, Kauvar D, Goyal RK. Gradient of cholinergic innervation in opossum esophageal circular smooth muscle. *Gullet* 1991;1:92–98.

229. Gidda JS, Buyinski JP. Swallow evoked peristalsis in the opossum esophagus: role of cholinergic mechanisms. *Am J Physiol* 1986;251:G779–785.

230. Yamato S, Spechler SJ, Goyal RK. Role of nitric oxide in esophageal peristalsis in the opossum. *Gastroenterology* 1992; 103:197–204.

231. Dodds WJ, Dent J, Hogan WJ, Patel GK, Toouli J, Arndorfer RC. Paradoxical lower esophageal sphincter contraction induced by cholecystokinin-octapeptide in patients with achalasia. *Gastroenterology* 1981;80:327–333.

232. Knudsen MA, Frobert O, Tottrup A. The role of the L-arginine-nitric oxide pathway for peristalsis in the opossum oesophageal body. *Scand J Gastroenterol* 1994;29:1083–1987.

233. Chakder S, Rosenthal GJ, Rattan S. In vivo and in vitro influence of human recombinant hemoglobin on esophageal function. *Am J Physiol* 1995;268:G443–450.

234. Murray JA, Ledlow A, Launspach J, Evans D, Loveday M, Conklin JL. The effects of recombinant human hemoglobin on esophageal motor function in humans. *Gastroenterology* 1995; 109:1241-8.

235. Xue S, Valdez DT, Collman PI, Diamant NE. Effects of nitric oxide synthase blockade on esophageal peristalsis and the lower esophageal sphincter in the cat. *Can J Physiol Pharmacol* 1996;74:1249–1257.

236. Behar J, Biancani P. Pathogenesis of simultaneous esophageal contractions in patients with motility disorders. *Gastroenterology* 1993;105:111–118.

237. Sifrim D, Janssens J, Vantrappen G. Failing deglutitive inhibition in primary esophageal motility disorders. *Gastroenterology* 1994;106:875–882.

238. Mearin F, Mourelle M, Guarner F, *et al.* Patients with achalasia lack nitric oxide synthase in the gastro-oesophageal junction. *Eur J Clin Invest* 1993;23:724–728.

239. Kassim SK, El Touny M, El Guinaidy M, El Moghni MA, El Mohsen AA. Serum nitrates and vasoactive intestinal peptide in patients with gastroesophageal reflux disease. *Clin Biochem* 2002;35:641–646.

240. Park H, Calrk E, Cullen JJ, Conklin JL. Effect of endotoxin on opossum oesophageal motor function. *Neurogastroenterol Motil* 2000;12:215–221.

241. Daniel EE, Bardakjian BL, Huizinga JD, Diamant NE. Relaxation oscillators and core conductor models are needed for understanding of GI electrical activities. *Am J Physiol* 1994;266:G339–349.

242. Bardakjian BL, Diamant NE. Electronic models of oscillator-to-oscillator communications. In: Sperelakis N, Cole W, eds. *Cell Interactions and Gap Junctions*. CRC Press: Florida, 1989, pp. 211–224.

243. Kannan MS, Jager LP, Daniel EE. Electrical properties of smooth muscle cell membrane of opossum esophagus. *Am J Physiol* 1985;248:G342–346.

244. Crist J, Surprenant A, Goyal RK. Intracellular studies of electrical membrane properties of opossum esophageal circular smooth muscle. *Gastroenterology* 1987;92:987–992.

245. Nelson DO, Mangel AW. Acetylcholine induced slow-waves in cat esophageal smooth muscle. *Gen Pharmacol* 1979;10:19–20.

246. Helm JF, Bro SL, Dodds WJ, Sarna SK, Hoffmann RG, Arndorfer RC. Myogenic oscillatory mechanism for opossum esophageal smooth muscle contractions. *Am J Physiol* 1991; 261:G377–383.

247. Salapatek AF, Ji J, Diamant NE. Ion-channel diversity in the feline smooth muscle esophagus. *Am J Physiol Gastrointest Liver Physiol* 2002;282:G288–299.

248. Schulze K, Conklin JL, Christensen J. A potassium gradient in smooth muscle segment of the opossum esophagus. *Am J Physiol* 1977;232:E270–273.

249. Muinuddin A, Ji J, Sheu L, Kang Y, Gaisano HY, Diamant NE. L-type Ca(2+) channel expression along feline smooth muscle oesophagus. *Neurogastroenterol Motil* 2004;16:325–334.

250. Muinuddin A, Xue S, Diamant NE. Regional differences in the response of feline esophageal smooth muscle to stretch and cholinergic stimulation. *Am J Physiol Gastrointest Liver Physiol* 2001;281:G1460–1467.

251. Szymanski PT, Chacko TK, Rovner AS, Goyal RK. Differences in contractile protein content and isoforms in phasic and tonic smooth muscle. *Am J Physiol* 1998;275:C684–692.

252. Biancani P, Sohn UD, Rich HG, Harnett KM, Behar J. Signal transduction pathways in esophageal and lower esophageal sphincter circular muscle. *Am J Med* 1997;24:23S–28S.

253. Cao W, Sohn UD, Bitar KN, Behar J, Biancani P, Harnett KM. MAPK mediates PKC-dependent contraction of cat esophageal and lower esophageal sphincter circular smooth muscle. *Am J Physiol Gastrointest Liver Physiol* 2003;285:G86–95.

254. Liu J, Puckett JL, Takeda T, Jung H-Y, Mittal RK. Crural diaphragm inhibition during esophageal distension correlates with contraction of the esophageal longitudinal muscle in cats. *Am J Physiol Gastrointest Liver Physiol* 2005;288:927–932.

255. Yamamoto Y, Liu J, Smith TK, Mittal RK. Distension-related responses in circular and longitudinal muscle of the human esophagus: an ultrasonographic study. *Am J Physiol* 1998; 275:G805–811.

256. Kahrilas PJ, Wu S, Lin S, Pouderoux P. Attenuation of esophageal shortening during peristalsis with hiatus hernia. *Gastroenterology* 1995;109:1818–1825.

257. Crist J, Gidda J, Goyal RK. Role of substance P nerves in longitudinal smooth muscle contractions of the esophagus. *Am J Physiol* 1986;250:G336–343.

258. Zhang Y, Paterson WG. Nitric oxide contracts longitudinal smooth muscle of opossum esophagus via excitation-contraction coupling. *J Physiol* 2001;536:133–140.

259. Saha JK, Hirano I, Goyal RK. Biphasic effect of SNP on opossum esophageal longitudinal muscle: involvement of cGMP and eicosanoids. *Am J Physiol* 1993;265:G403–407.

260. Paterson WG, Kolyn DM. Esophageal shortening induced by short-term intraluminal acid perfusion in opossum: A cause for hiatus hernia? *Gastroenterology* 1994;107:1736–1740.

261. White RJ, Zhang Y, Morris GP, Paterson WG. Esophagitis-related esophageal shortening in opossum is associated with longitudinal muscle hyperresponsiveness. *Am J Physiol Gastrointest Liver Physiol* 2001;280:G463–469.

262. Weber J, Roman C, Hannequin D, *et al.* Esophageal manometry in patients with unilateral hemispheric cerebrovascular accidents or idiopathic parkinsonism. *J Gastrointest Motil* 1991;3:98–106.

263. Aithal GP, Nylander D, Dwarakanath AD, Tanner AR. Subclinical esophageal peristaltic dysfunction during the early phase following a stroke. *Dig Dis Sci* 1999;44: 274–278.

264. Vanek AW, Diamant NE. Responses of the human esophagus to paired swallows. *Gastroenterology* 1987;92:643–650.

265. Hellemans J, Vantrappen G, Janssens J. Electromyography of the esophagus. 4. The deglutitive inhibition. In: Vantrappen G, Hellemans J, eds. *Diseases of the Esophagus*. New York: Springer-Verlag, 1974, pp. 280–284.

266. Ask P, Tibbling L. Effect of time interval between swallows on esophageal peristalsis. *Am J Physiol* 1980;238:G485–490.

267. Mittal RK, Balaban DH. The esophagogastric junction. *N Engl J Med* 1997;336:924–932.

268. Kwok H, Marriz Y, Al-Ali S, Windsor JA. Phrenoesophageal ligament re-visited. *Clin Anat* 1999;12:164–170.

269. Kahrilas PJ, Lin S, Chen J, Manka M. The effect of hiatus hernia on gastro-oesophageal junction pressure. *Gut* 1999; 44:476–482.

270. Apaydin N, Uz A, Evirgen O, Loukas M, Tubbs RS, Elhan A. The phrenico-esophageal ligament: an anatomical study. *Surg Radiol Anat* 2008;30:29–36.

271. Tierney BJ, Iqbal A, Awad Z, Penka W, Filipi CJ, Mittal SK. Sub-diaphragmatic fascia: role in the recurrence of hiatal hernias. *Dis Esophagus* 2006;19:111–113.

272. Marchand P. The anatomy of esophageal hiatus of the diaphragm and the pathogenesis of hiatus herniation. *J Thorac Surg* 1959;37:81–92.

273. Dobbins EG, Feldman JL. Brainstem network controlling descending drive to phrenic motoneurons in rat. *J Comp Neurol* 1994;347:64–86.

274. Niedringhaus M, Jackson PG, Pearson R, *et al.* Brainstem sites controlling the lower esophageal sphincter and crural diaphragm in the ferret: a neuroanatomical study. *Autonom Neurosci* 2008;144:50–60.

275. Young RL, Page AJ, Cooper NJ, Frisby CL, Blackshaw LA. Sensory and motor innervation of the crural diaphragm by the vagus nerves. *Gastroenterology* 2010;138:1091–1101.

276. Jackson AJ. The spiral constrictor of the gastroesophageal junction. *Am J Anat* 1978;151:265–275.

277. Liebermann-Meffert D, Allgower M, Schmid P, Blum AL. Muscular equivalent of the lower esophageal sphincter. *Gastroenterology* 1979;76:31–38.

278. Apaydin N, Uz A, Elhan A, Loukas M, Tubbs RS. Does an anatomical sphincter exist in the distal esophagus? *Surg Radiol Anat* 2008;30:11–16.

279. Brasseur JG, Ulerich R, Dai Q, Patel DK, Soliman AM, Miller LS. Pharmacological dissection of the human gastro-oesophageal segment into three sphincteric components. *J Physiol* 2007;580:961–975.

280. Miller L, Dai Q, Vegesna A, *et al.* A missing sphincteric component of the gastro-oesophageal junction in patients with GORD. *Neurogastroenterol Motil* 2009;21:813–e52.

281. McCray WH, Jr., Chung C, Parkman HP, Miller LS. Use of simultaneous high-resolution endoluminal sonography (HRES) and manometry to characterize high pressure zone of distal esophagus. *Dig Dis Sci* 2000;45:1660–1666.

282. Wheeler CB, Kohatsu S. Canine gastric sling fibers: contractile properties. *Am J Surg* 1980;139:175–182.

283. Beck CS, Osa T. Membrane activity in guinea pig gastric sling muscle: a nerve dependent phenomenon. *Am J Physiol* 1971; 220:1397–403.

284. Preiksaitis HG, Diamant NE. Regional differences in the cholinergic activity of muscle fibers from the human gastroesophageal junction. *Am J Physiol* 1997;272:G1321–1327.

285. Friedland GW, Kohatsu S, Lewin K. Comparative anatomy of feline and canine gastric sling fibers. Analogy to human anatomy. *Dig Dis* 1971;16:495–507.

286. Lendrum FC. Anatomic features of the cardiac orifice of the stomach (with special reference to cardiospasm). *Arch Intern Med* 1937;59:474–511.

287. Gahagan T. The function of the musculature of the esophagus and stomach inthe esophagogastric sphincter mechanism. *Surg Gynecol Obstet* 1962;114:293–303.

288. Hill LD, Kozarek RA, Kraemer SJ, Aye RW, Mercer CD, Low DE, *et al.* The gastroesophageal flap valve: in vitro and in vivo observations. *Gastrointest Endosc* 1996;44:541–547.

289. Korn O, Csendes A, Burdiles P, Braghetto I, Stein HJ. Anatomic dilatation of the cardia and competence of the lower esophageal sphincter: a clinical and experimental study. *J Gastrointest Surg* 2000;4:398–406.

290. Gordon C, Kang JY, Neild PJ, Maxwell JD. The role of the hiatus hernia in gastro-oesophageal reflux disease. *Aliment Pharmacol Ther* 2004;20:719–732.

291. Fugiwara Y, Nakagawa K, Kusunoki M, Tanaka T, Yamamura T, Utsunomiya J. Gastroesophageal reflux after distal gastrectomy: possiblr significance of the angle of His. *Am J Gastroenterol* 1998;93:3–4.

292. Ismail T, Bancewicz J, Barlow J. Yield pressure, anatomy of the cardia and gastro-oesophageal reflux. *Br J Surg* 1995;82: 943–947.

293. Seelig LL Jr, Goyal RK. Morphological evaluation of opossum lower esophageal sphincter. *Gastroenterology* 1978;75:51–58.

294. Farre R, Wang XY, Vidal E, *et al.* Interstitial cells of Cajal and neuromuscular transmission in the rat lower oesophageal sphincter. *Neurogastroenterol Motil* 2007;19:484–496.

295. Morris G, Reese L, Wang X-Y, Sanders KM. Interstitial cells of Cajal mediate enteric inhibitory neurotransmission in the lower esophageal and pyloric sphincters. *Gastroenterology* 1998; 115:314–329.

296. Zhang Y, Carmichael SA, Wang XY, Huizinga JD, Paterson WG. Neurotransmission in lower esophageal sphincter of W/Wv mutant mice. *Am J Physiol Gastrointest Liver Physiol* 2010; 298:G14–24.

297. Sarna SK. Are interstitial cells of Cajal plurifunction cells in the gut? *Am J Physiol Gastrointest Liver Physiol* 2008;294:G372–390.

298. Higgs RH, Castell DO. The effect of truncal vagotomy on lower esophageal sphincter pressure and response to cholinergic stimulation. *Proc Soc Exp Biol Med* 1976;153:379–382.

299. Temple JG, Goodall RJ, Hay DJ, Miller D. Effect of highly selective vagotomy upon the lower oesophageal sphincter. *Gut* 1981;22:368–370.

300. Collman PI, Tremblay L, Diamant NE. The central vagal efferent supply to the esophagus and lower sphincter of the cat. *J Gastrointest Motil* 1993;104:1430–1438.

301. Hyland NP, Abrahmas TP, Fuchs K, Burmeister MA, Hornby PJ. Organization and Neurochemistry of Vagal Preganglionic Neurons Innervating the Lower Esophageal Sphincter in Ferrets. *J Comp Neurol* 2001;430:222–234.

302. Ny L, Alm P, Ekstrom P, Hannibal J, Larsson B, Andersson K-E. Nitric oxide synthase-containing, peptide-containing, and acetylcholinesterase-positive nerves in the cat lower oesophagus. *Histochem J* 1994;26:721–33.

303. Szewczak SM, Behar J, Billett G, Hillemeier C, Rhim BY, Biancani P. VIP-induced alterations in cAMP and inositol phosphates in the lower esophageal sphincter. *Am J Physiol* 1990;259:G239–244.

304. Imaeda K, Joh T, Yamamoto Y, Itoh M, Suzuki H. Properties of inhibitory junctional transmission in smooth muscle of the guinea pig lower esophageal sphincter. *Jpn J Physiol* 1998;48: 457–465.

305. Imaeda K, Cunnane TC. Electrophysiological properties of inhibitory junction potential in murine lower oesophageal sphincter. *J Smooth Muscle Res* 2003;39:119–133.

306. Biancani P, Beinfeld MC, Hillemeier C, Behar J. Role of peptide histidine isoleucine in relaxation of cat lower esophageal sphincter. *Gastroenterology* 1989;97:1083–1089.

307. Rattan S, Gonnella P, Goyal RK. Inhibitory effect of calcitonin gene-related peptide and calcitonin on opossum esophageal smooth muscle. *Gastroenterology* 1988;94:284–293.

308. L'Heureux MC, Muinuddin A, Gaisano HY, Diamant NE. Feline lower esophageal sphincter sling and circular muscles have different functional inhibitory neuronal responses. *Am J Physiol Gastrointest Liver Physiol* 2006;290:G23–29.

309. Yuan S, Costa M, Brookes SJH. Neuronal pathways and transmission to the lower esophageal sphincter of the guinea pig. *Gastroenterology* 1998;115:661–671.

310. Yuan S, Brookes JH. Neuronal control of the gastric sling muscle of the guinea pig. *J Comp Neurol* 1999;412:669–680.

311. Gonella J, Niel JP, Roman C. Sympathetic control of lower oesophageal sphincter motility in the cat. *J Physiol (Lond)* 1979;287:177–190.

312. Tian ZQ, Liu JF, Wang GY, *et al.* Responses of human clasp and sling fibers to neuromimetics. *J Gastroenterol Hepatol* 2004;19: 440–447.

313. Oriowo MA. Neural inhibition in the rat lower esophageal sphincter: role of beta 3-adrenoceptor activation. *Gen Pharmacol* 1998;30:37–41.

314. Goyal RK, Rattan S. Nature of the vagal inhibitory innervation to the lower esophageal sphincter. *J Clin Invest* 1975;55:1119–1126.

315. Behar J, Biancani P. Effect of cholecystokinin-octapeptide on lower esophageal sphincter. *Gastroenterology* 1977;73:57–61.

316. Rattan S, Goyal RK. Structure-activity relationship of subtypes of cholecystokinin receptors in the cat lower esophageal sphincter. *Gastroenterology* 1986;90:94–102.

317. Salapatek AMF, Hynna-Liepert T, Diamant NE. Mechanism of action of cholecystokinin octapeptide on cat lower esophageal sphincter. *Am J Physiol* 1992;263:G419–425.

318. Miolan JP, Roman C. Activity of vagal efferent fibres innervating the smooth muscle of the dog's cardia [in French]. *J Physiologie* 1978;74:709–723.

319. Miolan JP, Roman C. Discharge of vagal efferent fibers innervating the cardia in dogs [in French]. *J Physiologie* 1973;66: 171–198.

320. Muinuddin A, Paterson WG. Initiation of distension-induced descending peristaltic reflex in opossum esophagus: role of muscle contractility. *Am J Physiol Gastrointest Liver Physiol* 2001;280:G431–438.

321. Paterson WG, Rattan S, Goyal RK. Esophageal responses to transient and sustained esophageal distension. *Am J Physiol* 1988;255:G587–595.

322. Reynolds RPE, El-Sharkawy TY, Diamant NE. Lower esophageal sphincter function in the cat: role of central innervation assessed by transient vagal blockade. *Am J Physiol* 1984;246:G666–674.

323. Mittal RK, Rochester DF, McCallum RW. Electrical and mechanical activity in the human lower esophageal sphincter during diaphragmatic contraction. *J Clin Invest* 1988;81:1182–1189.

324. Stein HJ, Liebermann-Meffert D, DeMeester TR, Siewert JR. Three-dimensional pressure image and muscular structure of the human lower esophageal sphincter. *Surgery* 1995;117:692–698.

325. Salapatek AM, Ji J, Muinuddin A, Diamant NE. Potassium channel diversity within the muscular components of the feline lower esophageal sphincter. *Can J Physiol Pharmacol* 2004;82:1006–1017.

326. Muinuddin A, Kang Y, Gaisano HY, Diamant NE. Regional differences in L-type Ca^{2+} channel expression in feline lower esophageal sphincter. *Am J Physiol Gastrointest Liver Physiol* 2004;287:G772–781.

327. Muinuddin A, Neshatian L, Gaisano HY, Diamant NE. Calcium source diversity in feline lower esophageal sphincter circular and sling muscle. *Am J Physiol Gastrointest Liver Physiol* 2004;286:G271–277.

328. Harnett KM, Cao W, Biancani P. Signal-Transduction Pathways that Regulate Smooth Muscle Function I. Signal transduction in phasic (esophageal) and tonic (gastroesophageal sphincter) smooth muscles. *Am J Physiol Gastrointest Liver Physiol* 2005;288:G407–416.

329. Cao WB, Harnett KM, Chen Q, Jain MK, Behar J, Biancani P. Group I secreted PLA2 and arachidonic acid metabolites in the maintenance of cat LES tone. *Am J Physiol* 1999;277:G585–598.

330. Sohn UD, Harnett KM, Cao W, *et al*. Acute experimental esophagitis activates a second signal transduction pathway in cat smooth muscle from the lower esophageal sphincter. *J Pharmacol Exp Ther* 1997;283:1293–1304.

331. Rich H, Dong Song U, Behar J, Kim N, Biancani P. Experimental esophagitis affects intracellular calcium stores in the cat lower esophageal sphincter. *Am J Physiol* 1997;272:G1523–1529.

332. Cheng L, Cao W, Behar J, Biancani P, Harnett KM. Inflammation induced changes in arachidonic acid metabolism in cat LES circular muscle. *Am J Physiol Gastrointest Liver Physiol* 2005;288:G787–797.

333. Preiksaitis HG, Diamant NE. Phasic contractions of the muscular components of human esophagus and gastroesophageal junction in vitro. *Can J Physiol Pharmacol* 1995;73:356–363.

334. Asoh R, Goyal RK. Electrical activity of the opossum lower esophageal sphincter in vivo. Its role in the basal sphincter pressure. *Gastroenterology* 1978;74:835–840.

335. Holloway RH, Blank EL, Takahashi I, Dodds WJ, Dent J, Sarna SK. Electrical control activity of the lower esophageal sphincter in unanesthetized opossums. *Am J Physiol* 1987;252:G511–521.

336. Walton PD, Huizinga JD. Stimulus-dependent pacemaker activity in the distal canine lower esophageal sphincter. *Can J Physiol Pharmacol* 1989;67:1331–1335.

337. Huizinga JD, Walton PD. Pacemaker activity in the proximal lower oesophageal sphincter of the dog. *J Physiol (Lond)* 1989;408:19–30.

338. Zhang Y, Miller DV, Paterson WG. Opposing roles of K(+) and Cl(–) channels in maintenance of opossum lower esophageal sphincter tone. *Am J Physiol Gastrointest Liver Physiol* 2000;279:G1226–1234.

339. Farrell RL, Roling GT, Castell DO. Cholinergic therapy of chronic heartburn. A controlled trial. *Ann Intern Med* 1974;80:573–576.

340. Bortolotti M, Labo G. Clinical and manometric effects of nifedipine in patients with esophageal achalasia. *Gastroenterology* 1981;80:39–44.

341. Eherer AJ, Schwetz I, Hammer HF, *et al*. Effect of sildenafil on oesophageal motor function in healthy subjects and patients with oesophageal motor disorders. *Gut* 2002;50:758–764.

342. Bortolotti M, Pandolfo N, Giovannini M, Mari C, Miglioli M. Effect of Sildenafil on hypertensive lower oesophageal sphincter. *Eur J Clin Invest* 2002;32:682–685.

343. Birgisson S, Richter JE. Long-term outcome of botulinum toxin in the treatment of achalasia. *Gastroenterology* 1996;111:1162.

344. Korn O, Braghetto I, Burdiles P, Csendes A. Cardiomyotomy in achalasia: which fibers do we cut? *Dis Esophagus* 2000;13:104–107; discussion 108–109.

345. Boyle JT, Altschuler SM, Nixon TE, Pack AI, Cohen S. Responses of feline gastroesophageal junction to changes in abdominal pressure. *Am J Physiol* 1987;253:G315–322.

346. Mittal RK, Fisher M, McCallum RW, Rochester DF, Dent J, Sluss J. Human lower esophageal sphincter pressure response to increased intra-abdominal pressure. *Am J Physiol* 1990;258:G624–630.

347. Crispin JS, McIver DK, Lind JF. Manometric study of the effect of vagotomy on the gastroesophageal sphincter. *Can J Surg* 1967;10:299–307.

348. Dodds WJ, Hogan WJ, Miller WN, Stef JJ, Arndorfer RC, Lydon SB. Effect of increased intraabdominal pressure on lower esophageal sphincter pressure. *Am J Dig Dis* 1975;20:298–308.

349. DiLorenzo C, Dooley CP, Valenzuela JE. Response of lower esophageal sphincter to alterations of intraabdominal pressure. *Dig Dis Sci* 1989;34:1606–1610.

350. Babka JC, Hager GW, Castell DO. The effect of body position on lower esophageal sphincter pressure. *Am J Dig Dis* 1973;18:441–442.

351. Sears VW Jr, Castell JA, Castell DO. Comparison of effects of upright versus supine body position and liquid versus solid bolus on esophageal pressures in normal humans. *Dig Dis Sci* 1990;35:857–864.

352. Nebel OT, Castell DO. Lower esophageal sphincter pressure changes after food ingestion. *Gastroenterology* 1972;63:778–783.

353. Nebel OT, Castell DO. Inhibition of the lower oesophageal sphincter by fat–a mechanism for fatty food intolerance. *Gut* 1973;14:270–274.

354. Wright LE, Castell DO. The adverse effect of chocolate on lower esophageal sphincter pressure. *Am J Dig Dis* 1975;20:703–707.

355. Hogan WJ, DeAndrade SRV, Winship DH. Ethanol-induced acute esophageal motor dysfunction. *J Appl Physiol* 1972;32:755–760.

356. Dennish GW, Castell DO. Caffeine and the lower esophageal sphincter. *Am J Dig Dis* 1972;17:993–996.

357. Piche T, Zerbib F, Varannes SB, *et al.* Modulation by colonic fermentation of LES function in humans. *Am J Physiol Gastrointest Liver Physiol* 2000;278:G578–584.

358. Dennish GW, Castell DO. Inhibitory effect of smoking on the lower esophageal sphincter. *N Engl J Med* 1971;284:1136–1137.

359. Baron TH, Richter JE. Gastroesophageal reflux disease in pregnancy. *Gastroenterol Clin North Am* 1992;21:777–791.

360. Orr WC, Heading R, Johnson LF, Kryger M. Review article: sleep and its relationship to gastro-oesophageal reflux. *Aliment Pharmacol Ther* 2004;20 (Suppl 9):39–46.

361. Pasricha PJ. Effect of sleep on gastroesophageal physiology and airway protective mechanisms. *Am J Med* 2003;115 (Suppl 3A):144S–118S.

362. Farre R, Sifrim D. Regulation of basal tone, relaxation and contraction of the lower oesophageal sphincter. Relevance to drug discovery for oesophageal disorders. *Br J Pharmacol* 2008;153:858–869.

363. Dodds WJ, Dent J, Hogan WJ, *et al.* Mechanisms of gastroesophageal reflux in patients with reflux esophagitis. *N Engl J Med* 1982;307:1547–1552.

364. Mittal RK, McCallum RW. Characteristics and frequency of transient relaxations of the lower esophageal sphincter in patients with reflux esophagitis. *Gastroenterology* 1988;95:593–599.

365. Dent J, Dodds WJ, Friedman RH, *et al.* Mechanism of gastroesophageal reflux in recumbent asymptomatic human subjects. *J Clin Invest* 1980;65:256–267.

366. Mittal RK, Holloway RH, Penagini R, Blackshaw LA, Dent J. Transient lower esophageal sphincter relaxation. *Gastroenterology* 1995;109:601–610.

367. McNally EF, Kelly EJ, Ingelfinger FJ. Mechanism of belching: Effects of gastrin distension with air. *Gastroenterology* 1964;46:254–259.

368. Mittal RK, Fisher MJ. Electrical and mechanical inhibition of the crural diaphragm during transient relaxation of the lower esophageal sphincter. *Gastroenterology* 1990;99:1265–1268.

369. Noordzij JP, Mittal RK, Arora T, *et al.* The effect of mechanoreceptor stimulation of the laryngopharynx on the oesophagogastric junction. *Neurogastroenterol Motil* 2000;12:353–359.

370. Pouderoux P, Verdier E, Kahrilas PJ. Patterns of esophageal inhibition during swallowing, pharyngeal stimulation, and transient LES relaxation. Lower esophageal sphincter. *Am J Physiol Gastrointest Liver Physiol* 2003;284:G242–247.

371. Hirsch DP, Tytgat GN, Boeckxstaens GE. Transient lower oesophageal sphincter relaxations—a pharmacological target for gastro-oesophageal reflux disease? *Aliment Pharmacol Ther* 2002;16:17–26.

372. Lidums I, Checklin H, Mittal RK, Holloway RH. Effect of atropine on gastro-oesophageal reflux and transient lower oesophageal sphincter relaxations in patients with gastro-oesophageal reflux disease. *Gut* 1998;43:12–16.

373. Boulant J, Mathieu S, D'Amato M, Abergel A, Dapoigny M, Bommelaer G. Cholecystokinin in transient lower oesophageal sphincter relaxation due to gastric distension in humans. *Gut* 1997;40:575–581.

374. Lidums I, Lehmann A, Checklin H, Dent J, Holloway RH. Control of transient lower esophageal sphincter relaxations and reflux by the GABA(B) agonist baclofen in normal subjects. *Gastroenterology* 2000;118:7–13.

375. Heine KJ, Mittal RK. Crural diaphragm and lower esophageal sphincter as antireflux barriers. *Viewpoints Dig Dis* 1991;23:1–6.

376. Altschuler SM, Boyle JT, Nixon TE, Pack AI, Cohen S. Simultaneous reflex inhibition of lower esophageal sphincter and crural diaphragm in cats. *Am J Physiol* 1985;249:G586–591.

6 Radiology of the Pharynx and Esophagus

Marc S. Levine and Stephen E. Rubesin

Department of Radiology, Hospital of the University of Pennsylvania, Philadelphia, PA, USA

Introduction

As the population continues to age, pharyngeal disorders have become an increasingly common problem in modern medical practice. Many patients have swallowing dysfunction caused by neurologic conditions such as dementia or strokes, whereas others have morphologic lesions such as pharyngeal carcinoma or Zenker's diverticulum. The videofluoroscopic examination is a valuable technique for demonstrating a wide range of functional and structural lesions of the pharynx in these individuals. Esophagography (primarily double-contrast esophagography) is an equally valuable tool for detecting clinically significant disease of the esophagus in patients with gastroesophageal reflux disease (GERD), infectious esophagitis, esophageal carcinoma, or other structural lesions of the esophagus. Videofluoroscopic evaluation of the esophagus is also a useful technique for assessing esophageal motility and for detecting motility disorders such as achalasia and diffuse esophageal spasm. Thus, pharyngoesophagography has a major role in the evaluation of patients with pharyngeal or esophageal disease. This chapter reviews the various pathologic conditions involving the pharynx and esophagus and their associated findings on barium studies.

Pharynx

Normal pharyngeal anatomy

The pharynx is a tube composed of skeletal muscle lined by squamous epithelium [1] (Figure 6.1). The oropharynx (mesopharynx) is the portion of the pharynx associated with the oral cavity. The oropharynx extends craniocaudally from the soft palate to the pharyngoepiglottic fold. The base of the tongue forms the anterior wall of the oropharynx; the posterior wall of the oropharynx abuts the upper cervical spine. The laryngopharynx (hypopharynx) is the portion of the

pharynx associated with the larynx. The hypopharynx extends craniocaudally from the pharyngoepiglottic fold to the pharyngoesophageal segment [1]. The nasopharynx is the part of the pharynx associated with the nasal cavity. It participates primarily in breathing and is not considered in this chapter. The anatomy and physiology of the oral and pharyngeal cavity are complex. Refer to references 1–12 for a detailed discussion of pharyngeal anatomy and physiology.

The anterior wall of the hypopharynx is shaped by the larynx; its epiglottic and arytenoid cartilages contribute to the anterior wall of the hypopharynx [2] (Figures 6.2 and 6.3). The remainder of the anterior pharyngeal wall is formed by the piriform sinuses and surrounding thyroid cartilage. The posterior wall of the hypopharynx is bordered by the lower cervical spine. The junction of the pharynx and esophagus, the pharyngoesophageal segment, is lined by squamous epithelium and formed by the cricopharyngeus muscle. The pharyngoesophageal segment lies posterior to the cricoid cartilage.

The oropharynx and hypopharynx have four openings: superiorly, the velopharyngeal portal to the nasopharynx; anteriorly, the palatoglossal isthmus to the oral cavity; anteriorly, the laryngeal aditus to the larynx; and inferiorly, the pharyngoesophageal segment to the esophagus [1]. Thus, the pharynx is the crossroads of speech, respiration, and swallowing.

The palatine fossae are bounded by the anterior and posterior tonsillar pillars, also known as the paired palatoglossal and palatopharyngeal folds. The vertical surface of the tongue is nodular because of the underlying circumvallate papillae and lingual tonsil [2]. The valleculae are potential spaces created by a fold of tissue that extends posteriorly to the epiglottis (the median glossoepiglottic fold). The valleculae disappear when the epiglottis inverts during swallowing.

The piriform sinuses form the anterior portion of the lower hypopharynx. The piriform sinuses are pear-shaped spaces created by protrusion of the larynx into the pharynx (Figure 6.4). These spaces are open posteriorly to the

The Esophagus, Fifth Edition. Edited by Joel E. Richter, Donald O. Castell.

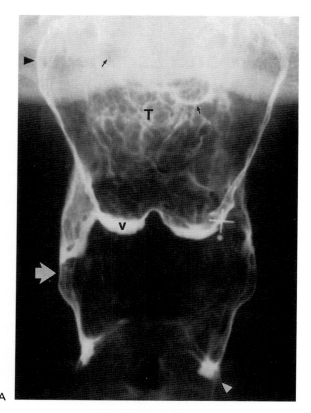

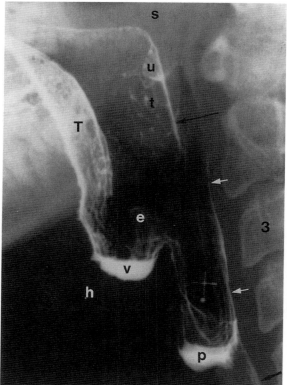

Figure 6.1 Normal pharynx. (A) Frontal view of the pharynx. The surface of the tongue (T) has a reticular appearance due to underlying lingual tonsil. The right tonsillar fossa (black arrowhead), right vallecula (V), tip of the left piriform sinus (white arrowhead), and several of the circumvallate papillae (black arrows) are all identified. The right lateral wall of the hypopharynx is identified with a thick arrow. (B) Lateral view of the pharynx during phonation. The soft palate (s) elevates to appose the posterior pharyngeal wall. The uvula (u) of the soft palate bows anteriorly. The palatopharyngeal fold (posterior tonsillar pillar) (long black arrow) overlies the palatopharyngeal muscle. The palatine tonsils (t) have barium trapped within their interstices. The vertical surface (base) of the tongue (T), epiglottic tip (e), valleculae (v), and tips of the piriform sinuses (p) are identified. The hyoid bone (h) is barely visible. The pharyngoesophageal segment (short black arrow) is closed (reproduced from Rubesin SE, Jones B, Donner MW. Contrast pharyngography: the importance of phonation. *Am J Roentgenol* 1987;148:269–272, with permission).

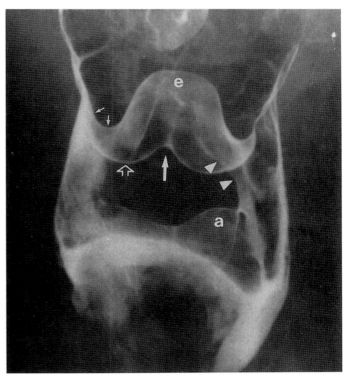

A

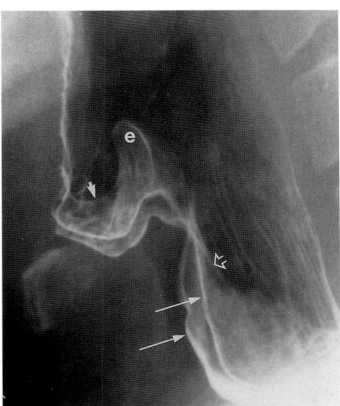

B

Figure 6.2 Folds of the epiglottis in a patient with radiation change. (A) Frontal view of the pharynx. The median glossoepiglottic fold (large arrow) divides the space between the base of the tongue and tip of the epiglottis (e) into two halves. The pharyngoepiglottic folds overlying the paired stylopharyngeal muscles course from the lateral pharyngeal wall to the lateral edge of the epiglottis (right pharyngoepiglottic fold identified with small arrows, forming the posterior wall of the valleculae. The lateral wall of each vallecula is formed by the lateral glossoepiglottic fold. The lowest portion of the right vallecula is identified by an open arrow. The aryepiglottic folds course from the lateral edge of the epiglottis to the mucosa overlying the muscular processes of the arytenoid cartilages (left aryepiglottic fold identified by arrowheads; mucosa overlying left arytenoid cartilage identified by a). (B) Lateral view of the pharynx demonstrates the median glossoepiglottic fold (short arrow), tip of epiglottis (e), aryepiglottic folds (open arrow), and anterior walls of the piriform sinuses (long arrows).

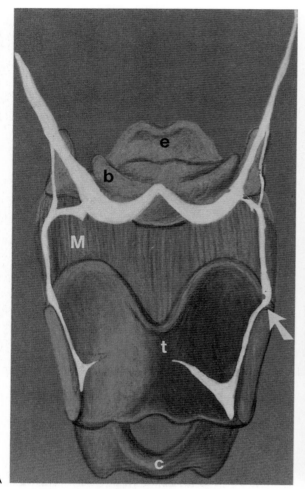

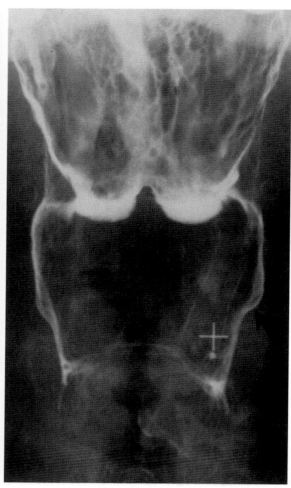

Figure 6.3 Relationship of the laryngeal cartilages to the pharynx. (A) Line drawing in the frontal view demonstrates the tip of the epiglottic cartilage (e) above the level of the hyoid bone (b). The thyrohyoid membrane (M) connects the hyoid bone to the thyroid cartilage (t). The cricoid cartilage (c) is seen inferiorly. The white area represents the barium-coated pharynx posterior to the larynx. (B) Frontal view of the pharynx shows a notch in the lateral hypopharyngeal wall (arrow in both A and B) where the thyrohyoid membrane joins the thyroid cartilage. Inferiorly, the hypopharynx is confined anteriorly by the thyroid cartilage (reproduced from Rubesin *et al.* [2], with permission).

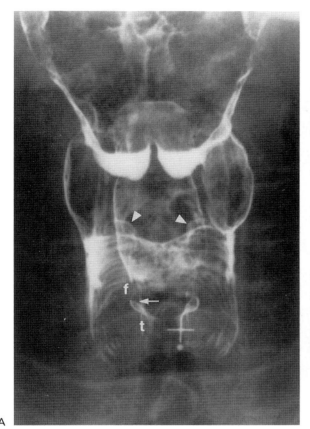

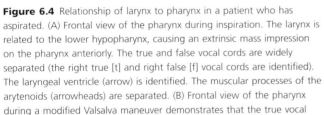

A

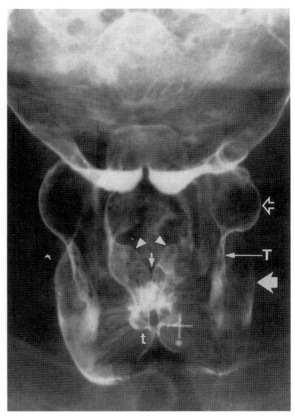

B

Figure 6.4 Relationship of larynx to pharynx in a patient who has aspirated. (A) Frontal view of the pharynx during inspiration. The larynx is related to the lower hypopharynx, causing an extrinsic mass impression on the pharynx anteriorly. The true and false vocal cords are widely separated (the right true [t] and right false [f] vocal cords are identified). The laryngeal ventricle (arrow) is identified. The muscular processes of the arytenoids (arrowheads) are separated. (B) Frontal view of the pharynx during a modified Valsalva maneuver demonstrates that the true vocal cords (right cord—t) are now apposed. The muscular processes of the arytenoids (arrowheads) are close together. The space between them is the interarytenoid notch (small arrow). The pharynx is markedly distended in its posterior portion (large arrow), ballooning posterior to the confines of the thyroid cartilage (arrow—T). The pharynx also bulges at the thyrohyoid membrane (open arrow) (reproduced from Rubesin and Glick [23], with permission).

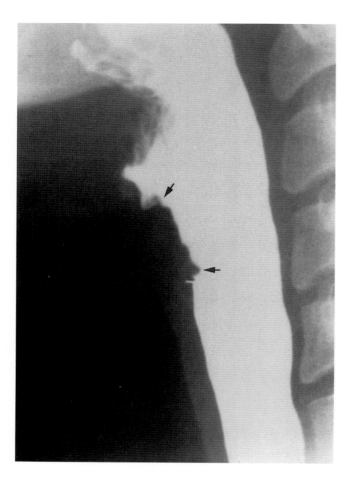

Figure 6.5 Postcricoid squamous mucosa. Just posterior to the cricoid cartilage, the anterior wall of the pharyngoesophageal segment has redundant mucosa that changes size and shape during swallowing. Note how the mucosa has a wavy appearance (arrows). When identified, this mucosa identifies the level of the cricoid cartilage and the level of the cricopharyngeus during pharyngography (reproduced from Rubesin SE. Pharynx: normal anatomy and examination techniques. In: Gore RM, Levine MS, eds. *Textbook of Gastrointestinal Radiology*, 2nd edn. Philadelphia: WB Saunders, 2000, pp. 190–211, with permission).

remainder of the hypopharynx. The aryepiglottic folds and mucosa overlying the muscular process of the arytenoid cartilages form the medial boundaries of the piriform sinuses.

The anterior wall of the pharyngoesophageal segment abuts the cricoid cartilage (Figure 6.5). The mucosa in this region is redundant, and there is abundant submucosal fat [2].

Normal oral and pharyngeal motility

Swallowing is arbitrarily divided into four phases: (1) ingestion and bolus preparation; (2) the oral phase; (3) the pharyngeal phase; and (4) the esophageal phase. In reality, swallowing is a programmed sequence of skeletal then smooth muscle contraction, altered by sensory input [13]. There are no distinct phases of swallowing.

A bolus is selected and brought to the lips by volitional activity. A liquid is sucked or poured into the mouth. A solid is placed on top of the tongue. Liquids do not require much oral manipulation and are therefore easily transferred to the oropharynx. Solids must be chewed and mixed with saliva to achieve a satisfactory consistency for swallowing. During bolus preparation, the bolus is contained in the oral cavity in young adults. Older "normal" adults frequently spill the bolus prematurely into the oropharynx before swallowing [12].

Once the bolus is prepared, the tongue collects and sizes the bolus and transfers it into the oropharynx. The tongue tip rises to appose the hard palate, and the mid tongue forms an inclined plane directing the bolus into the oropharynx [10] (Figure 6.6). The velopharyngeal portal is closed as the soft palate rises to appose the posterior pharyngeal wall and the superior constrictor muscle contracts to appose the soft palate [9].

The pharynx and larynx are elevated by the suprahyoid muscles and intrinsic elevators of the pharynx. Pharyngeal–laryngeal elevation participates in closure of the laryngeal aditus and laryngeal vestibule, epiglottic tilt, and opening of the pharyngoesophageal segment [8].

Epiglottic tilt is accomplished by contraction of the suprahyoid muscles, the thyrohyoid muscle, and the intrinsic epiglottic muscles. Elevation of the hyoid bone by the suprahyoid muscle group pulls on the hyoepiglottic ligament attached to the petiole (lower portion) of the epiglottic cartilage. Hyoid elevation pulls the petiole superiorly, tilting the upper epiglottis towards the horizontal in a fulcrum-like

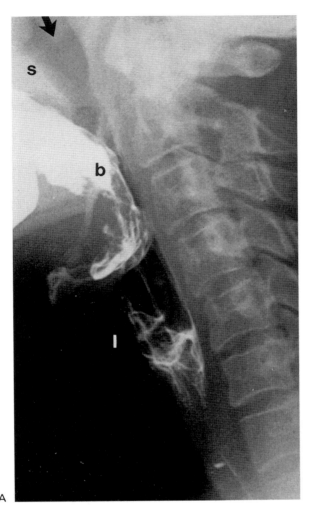
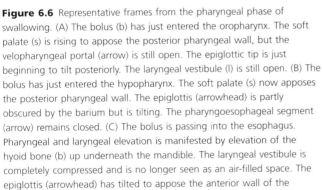

A

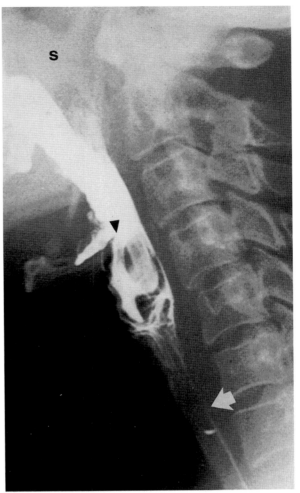

B

Figure 6.6 Representative frames from the pharyngeal phase of swallowing. (A) The bolus (b) has just entered the oropharynx. The soft palate (s) is rising to appose the posterior pharyngeal wall, but the velopharyngeal portal (arrow) is still open. The epiglottic tip is just beginning to tilt posteriorly. The laryngeal vestibule (l) is still open. (B) The bolus has just entered the hypopharynx. The soft palate (s) now apposes the posterior pharyngeal wall. The epiglottis (arrowhead) is partly obscured by the barium but is tilting. The pharyngoesophageal segment (arrow) remains closed. (C) The bolus is passing into the esophagus. Pharyngeal and laryngeal elevation is manifested by elevation of the hyoid bone (b) up underneath the mandible. The laryngeal vestibule is completely compressed and is no longer seen as an air-filled space. The epiglottis (arrowhead) has tilted to appose the anterior wall of the hypopharynx. The posterior pharyngeal contraction wave (long arrow) is in the thyropharyngeal muscle. The pharyngoesophageal segment (short arrow, identified by redundant post-cricoid mucosa on the opposite wall) is open. The C5 vertebral body is labelled 5 to allow a direct comparison to D. (D) The bolus has just passed through the pharynx. The pharynx and larynx have returned to their "resting" position. Compare the levels of the hyoid bone (b) and the pharyngoesophageal segment (thick arrow) on image C during swallowing and image D after swallowing. The epiglottic tip (arrowhead) has returned to its upright position. The soft palate now apposes the tongue and the laryngeal vestibule is open. A small Killian–Jamieson diverticulum (thin arrow) is present. The C5 vertebral body is labelled 5.

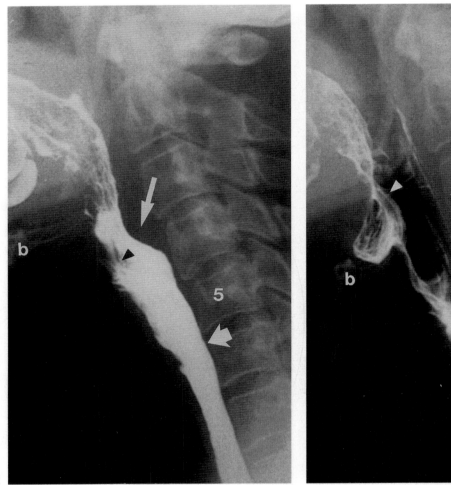

Figure 6.6 (*continued*)

motion. Contraction of the aryepiglottic and oblique arytenoid muscles and the thyroepiglottic muscles then inverts
the epiglottis.

The epiglottis acts as a stream diverter, directing the bolus
into the lateral swallowing channels. The tilting epiglottis
also helps cover the laryngeal vestibule. The larynx closes
in a retrograde fashion. The true vocal cords close at the
beginning of the swallow, followed by the false vocal cords
and the remainder of the laryngeal vestibule. If a portion
of the bolus has penetrated the laryngeal vestibule, it is
pushed back into the hypopharynx by retrograde laryngeal
closure. The bolus flows through the pharynx by a combination of gravity, elevation of the pharynx over the bolus,
tongue push, and sequential contraction of the constrictor
muscles. Although the upper esophageal sphincter relaxes
at the beginning of a swallow, the pharyngoesophageal
segment does not open until the bolus reaches the lower
hypopharynx. Elevation of the larynx and pharynx pulls

the anterior wall of the pharyngoesophageal segment anteriorly. Tongue base retraction, constrictor contraction, and
gravity increase bolus pressure to open the pharyngoesophageal segment.

Neuromuscular disorders

Most patients with swallowing dysfunction have neural or
muscular disorders that alter timing of events or muscular
contraction rather than causing oral or pharyngeal structural
damage. Some diseases affect a patient's ability to self-feed
despite normal swallowing. Other diseases affect both the
ability to feed and to swallow. For example, patients with
Parkinson's disease often have difficulty sitting and manipulating food as well as having abnormal bolus transfer [14].

About one-fourth of cerebrovascular accidents cause dysphagia [14, 15]. In general, left-sided strokes alter the oral
phase of swallowing, whereas right-sided strokes alter the
pharyngeal phase [15, 16]. The corticobulbar pathways in

the internal capsule can be damaged by large hemispheric strokes or small-vessel disease. Acute strokes or small-vessel disease resulting from hypertension, diabetes, or other causes can also affect the swallowing center in the pons and medulla [17].

Diseases that directly damage motor neurons in the swallowing center or cranial nerves in the skull base may result in bulbar palsy with oral and pharyngeal swallowing difficulties [18–22]. Lower motor neural destruction occurs in amyotrophic lateral sclerosis and 10–15% of patients with acute poliomyelitis [19, 20]. Some patients with a history of poliomyelitis have progressive disintegration of axon terminals in surviving but overworked residual motor neurons, resulting in pharyngeal muscle weakness caused by "post-polio muscular atrophy" [21]. Meningeal carcinomatosis may also result in dysphagia. Unilateral pharyngeal paresis is often caused by destruction of motor nerves at the skull base or in the neck as a result of tumor, trauma, or surgery [10]. Abnormal transmission at the myoneural junction in

myasthenia gravis may result in dysphagia that is initiated or exacerbated by prolonged swallowing.

Dysphagia resulting from inflammatory or endocrine-related myopathies is potentially treatable [14]. Dermatomyositis and polymyositis directly damage the intrinsic or extrinsic muscles of the pharynx. Pharyngeal muscle myopathy may be caused by a variety of endocrine disorders, including hyperthyroidism, hypothyroidism, and Cushing's syndrome [22].

The end result of these various neuromuscular disorders is poor timing of oral and pharyngeal events, or abnormal movement of oral and pharyngeal structures. A bolus may be directed in a normal fashion, but because of poor timing, the bolus may enter the laryngeal vestibule or nasopharynx. Laryngeal penetration is defined as passage of the bolus into the laryngeal vestibule either just before the swallow or during swallowing [23, 24]. Abnormal tongue motion, pharyngeal contraction, or epiglottic tilt may also lead to laryngeal penetration (Figures 6.7 and 6.8). Abnormal oral or

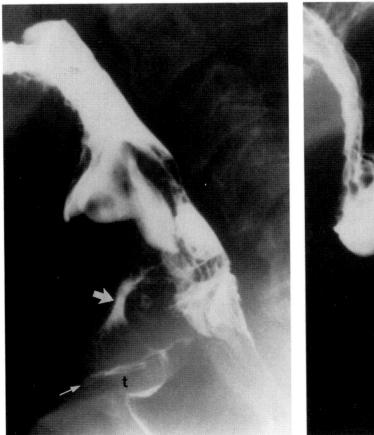 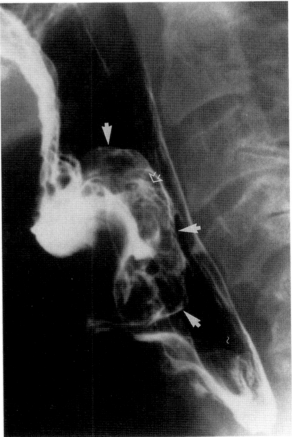

Figure 6.7 Laryngeal penetration. (A) During drinking, barium enters the laryngeal vestibule (thick arrow). The anterior commissure (thin arrow) and true vocal cords (t) are identified. (B) Spot radiograph during phonation shows a huge epiglottic mass (arrows) with nodular mucosa (open arrow) as the cause of the laryngeal penetration (reproduced from Rubesin [10], with permission).

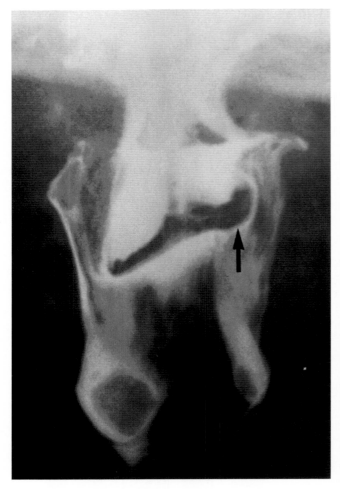

Figure 6.8 Asymmetric epiglottic tilt. There is diminished epiglottic tilt on the left side (arrow).

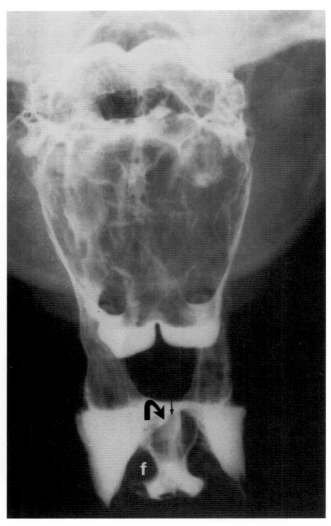

Figure 6.9 Overflow aspiration. This man had global pharyngeal weakness due to polymyositis and poor clearance of barium from the pharynx during swallowing with resultant stasis of barium in the piriform sinuses. Note that the barium level lies above the interarytenoid notch (straight arrow). After the swallow has passed, barium pours over and down into the larynx (curved arrow), outlining the false vocal cords (right cord—f) and laryngeal ventricle.

pharyngeal movement may result from a structural abnormality or neuromuscular disorder. Abnormal epiglottic tilt or pharyngeal muscular contraction may also lead to stasis in either the valleculae or piriform sinuses, respectively. Marked stasis in the piriform sinuses may cause the bolus to overflow into the larynx through the interarytenoid notch when the patient breathes or subsequently swallows for a second time. Thus, overflow aspiration is defined as barium entering the laryngeal vestibule while the patient is breathing normally [23, 24] (Figure 6.9), or as barium entering the laryngeal vestibule as a result of poor timing when the patient swallows for a second time, and there is moderate stasis in the valleculae and piriform sinuses. Aspiration may also result from regurgitation of esophageal contents into the pharynx.

Unilateral pharyngeal paresis should suggest vagal injury from the level of the pons to the recurrent laryngeal nerve, whereas abnormal epiglottic tilt as an isolated finding should suggest recurrent laryngeal nerve damage or intralaryngeal muscle problems. In general, however, the degree and types of swallowing dysfunction on barium swallows do not enable the radiologist to predict the underlying neuromuscular diseases causing this dysfunction.

Pouches and diverticula

Zenker's diverticula
Zenker's diverticulum is an acquired mucosal herniation through an area of congenital muscle weakness in the

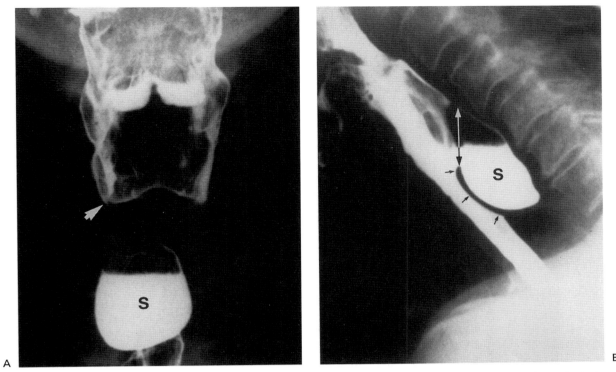

Figure 6.10 Zenker's diverticulum. (A) Frontal view of the pharynx demonstrates a 3- × 2-cm sac (S) with an air–barium level. The sac lies in the midline below the tips of the piriform sinuses (right piriform sinus tip identified by arrow). (B) Lateral view of the pharynx during drinking. The sac has a broad opening (double arrow). The sac (S) lies posterior to the pharyngoesophageal segment and proximal cervical esophagus (small arrows). (Laryngeal penetration resulted from abnormal timing between the oral and pharyngeal phases) (B, reproduced from Rubesin [10], with permission).

cricopharyngeal muscle, known as Killian's dehiscence. This opening is found in about one-third of people at autopsy, and has been described as occurring between the thyropharyngeus and cricopharyngeus or between the oblique and horizontal fibers of the cricopharyngeus itself [25, 26]. The pathogenesis of Zenker's diverticulum is unknown. Manometric studies have produced conflicting findings [27, 28]. Some of these studies have shown a normal tonic pressure in the upper esophageal sphincter (UES) and normal coordination between pharyngeal contraction and relaxation of the UES, whereas others have shown elevated UES pressure or abnormal relaxation of the UES. It also is unknown whether chronic gastroesophageal reflux predisposes patients with Killian's dehiscence to the development of a Zenker's diverticulum. Nevertheless, most patients with Zenker's diverticulum have a hiatal hernia and gastroesophageal reflex [29, 30].

When detected on barium studies, Zenker's diverticulum appears on frontal views as a persistent, barium-filled sac in the midline below the tips of the piriform sinuses (Figure 6.10). On lateral views during swallowing, the opening of the Zenker's diverticulum above the incompletely opened

pharyngoesophageal segment is often surprisingly broad [10, 31]. The sac then courses behind the pharyngoesophageal segment and proximal cervical esophagus. Barium within the diverticulum can be regurgitated back into the lower hypopharynx during breathing or additional swallowing (Figure 6.11), but overflow aspiration is uncommon. Contour deformities in a Zenker's diverticulum may be caused by adherent debris, inflammation, or, rarely, carcinoma [32, 33].

Barium trapped above a prematurely or incompletely opened cricopharyngeus may resemble a small Zenker's diverticulum, and has been termed a *pseudo-Zenker's diverticulum* [24] (Figure 6.12). In such patients, no diverticulum is seen during swallowing. The sac-like structure appears only when the cricopharyngeus closes early or when barium is trapped between the pharyngeal contraction wave and the incompletely opened cricopharyngeus. After a few moments, this barium enters the cervical esophagus, and the sac disappears. It is not known whether a pseudo-Zenker's diverticulum can progress to a true Zenker's diverticulum. Early closure and incomplete opening of the cricopharyngeus have also been associated with GERD [34] (Figures 6.13 and 6.14).

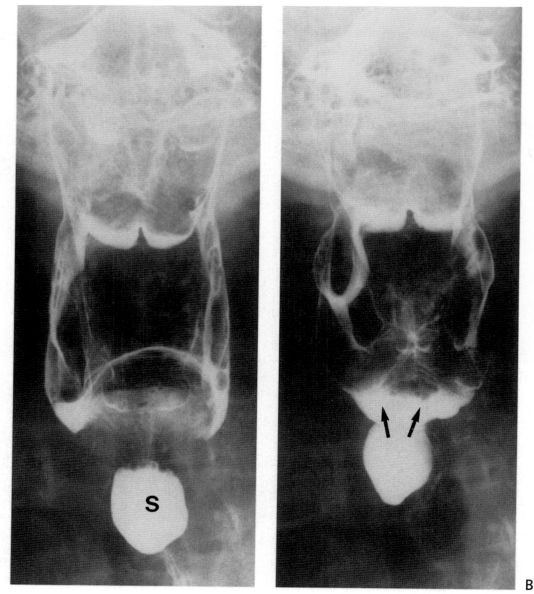

Figure 6.11 Pharyngeal regurgitation from Zenker's diverticulum. (A) Frontal view of the pharynx shows a 2-cm sac (S) in the midline below the tips of the piriform sinuses. (B) Frontal view of the pharynx as the patient begins a second swallow. Barium (arrows) has been regurgitated from the Zenker's diverticulum back into the lower hypopharynx.

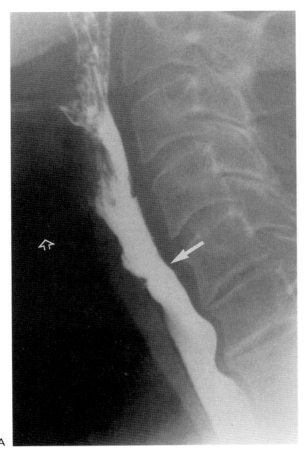

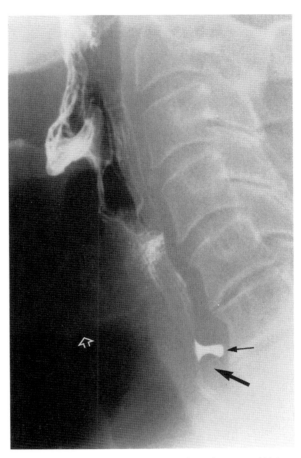

A

B

Figure 6.12 Pseudo-Zenker's diverticulum. (A) Lateral view of the pharynx during drinking shows an open pharyngoesophageal segment (arrow) identified by redundant postcricoid mucosa. (B) Lateral view of the pharynx just after the bolus passes shows how the pharynx is descending to its "resting" position. Barium is trapped (thin arrow) between the early closing pharyngoesophageal segment (thick arrow) and the posterior pharyngeal contraction wave that has just passed. The transiently trapped barium entered the esophagus moments later. Note the difference in height of the pharyngoesophageal segment and the bottom of the vocal cords (open arrows) during and after swallowing.

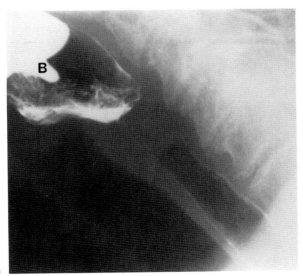

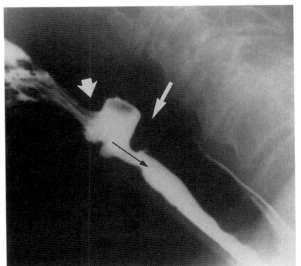

A

B

Figure 6.13 Incomplete opening of the cricopharyngeus. (A) Lateral view of the pharynx obtained just as the bolus (e) is entering the hypopharynx. (B) Lateral view of the pharynx at the end of bolus passage. The cricopharyngeus (long white arrow) is closing before the bolus has cleared the hypopharynx. The posterior pharyngeal contraction wave is identified (thick white arrow). A jet of barium (black arrow) spurts through the anterior wall of the cervical esophagus.

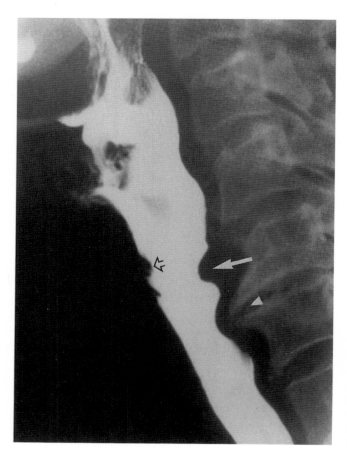

Figure 6.14 Extrinsic impressions during passage of bolus through the pharyngoesophageal segment. A smooth-surface hemispheric impression represents incomplete opening of the cricopharyngeus (white arrow). Osteophytes impress the proximal cervical esophagus (arrowhead). Also note redundant post-cricoid mucosa (open arrow) opposite the cricopharyngeal bar (reproduced from Rubesin SE. Oral and pharyngeal dysphagia. *Gastroenterol Clin North Am* 1995;24:331–352, with permission).

Killian–Jamieson diverticula and pouches

The Killian–Jamieson space is a triangular area of weakness in the upper anterolateral cervical esophagus, not to be confused with Killian's dehiscence. The Killian–Jamieson space is bounded superiorly by the inferior border of the cricopharyngeus, anteriorly by the cricoid cartilage, and inferomedially by the suspensory ligament of the esophagus [35. Transient protrusions through the Killian–Jamieson space are called *lateral proximal cervical esophageal pouches*, whereas persistent protrusions are called *lateral proximal cervical esophageal diverticula*. These structures are also known as Killian–Jamieson pouches and diverticula, respectively [36].

Killian–Jamieson diverticula, which are about one-third as common as Zenker's diverticula, have a characteristic radiographic appearance [36]. They are either unilateral, usually on the left, or bilateral [6]. The diverticula appear on barium studies as persistent 3–20-mm outpouchings with distinct necks (Figure 6.15). The diverticula extend lateral to the cervical esophagus on frontal views and overlap the cervical esophagus on lateral views. In contrast, a Zenker's

diverticulum is in the midline on frontal views and posterior to the cervical esophagus on lateral views (Figure 6.16). When barium is regurgitated from Killian–Jamieson diverticula, it enters the cervical esophagus because the diverticula are below the cricopharyngeal muscle. Thus, there is lower risk of aspiration from Killian–Jamieson diverticula than from Zenker's diverticula. Killian–Jamieson pouches appear as small, transient outpouchings just below the closing cricopharyngeus muscle and are usually detected near the end of swallowing or after the bolus has passed through the cervical esophagus.

Lateral pharyngeal pouches and diverticula

Lateral pharyngeal pouches are transient outpouchings of the proximal anterolateral hypopharyngeal wall, whereas lateral pharyngeal diverticula are persistent sacs through the same area of weakness in the pharyngeal wall [37]. Lateral pharyngeal pouches protrude through an area bounded superiorly by the hyoid bone, anteriorly by the thyrohyoid muscle, inferiorly by the ala of the thyroid cartilage, and

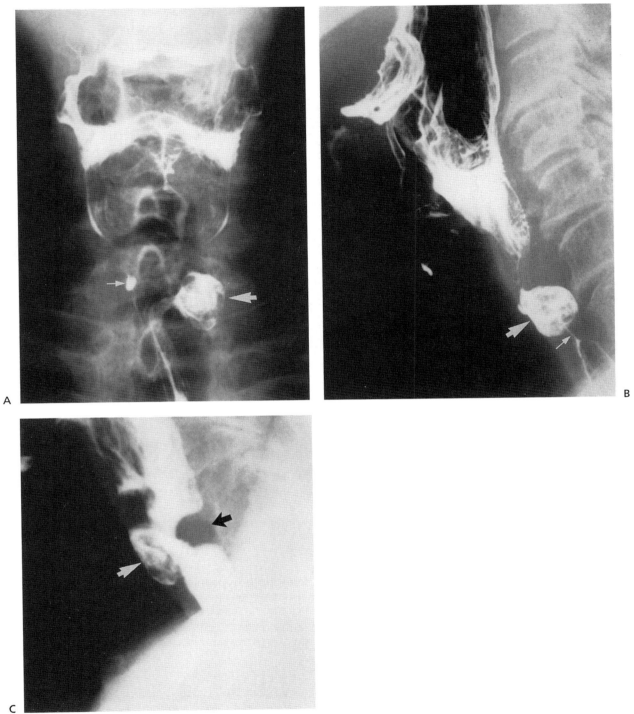

Figure 6.15 Killian–Jamieson diverticula. (A) Frontal view of the pharynx demonstrates a 1.5-cm sac (thick arrow) just below the level of the cricopharyngeus. A tiny sac is also seen on the right (thin arrow). (B) Lateral view of the pharynx shows that the 1.5-cm sac (thick arrow) extends anterior to the expected course of the cervical esophagus (thin arrow). (C) Lateral view of the pharynx during bolus passage demonstrates that the Killian–Jamieson diverticulum (white arrow) lies below the level of an incompletely opening cricopharyngeus (black arrow). The sac arises from the anterolateral wall of the most proximal cervical esophagus (reproduced from Rubesin and Levine [36], with permission).

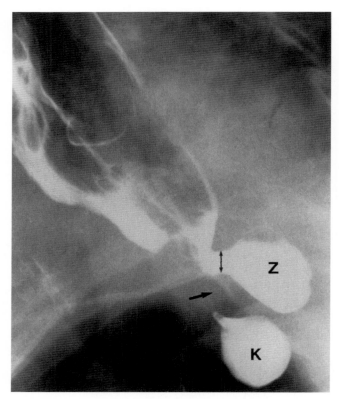

Figure 6.16 Synchronous Zenker's and Killian–Jamieson diverticula. Oblique view of the pharynx shows a 2.5-cm Zenker's diverticulum (Z) with its opening [double black arrow] above the cricopharyngeal bar [thick black arrow]). The Killian–Jamieson diverticulum (K) arises below the cricopharyngeal bar and a portion of the diverticulum extends anterior to the cervical esophagus (reproduced from Rubesin [31], with permission).

posteriorly by the superior cornu of the thyroid cartilage [37] (Figure 6.17A).

Lateral pharyngeal pouches appear on barium studies as smooth-surfaced hemispheric outpouchings of the upper anterolateral hypopharyngeal wall just below the level of the hyoid bone (Figure 6.17B and C). Barium enters the pouches and then spills into the ipsilateral piriform sinus, either late in the swallow or just after swallowing. Overflow aspiration is uncommon. In contrast, barium is retained in lateral pharyngeal diverticula long after the swallow has been completed (Figure 6.18). Lateral pharyngeal pouches are usually bilateral, whereas lateral pharyngeal diverticula are usually unilateral (Figure 6.18).

Lateral pharyngeal pouches are common, and their incidence increases with age. Lateral pharyngeal diverticula are much less common, usually occurring in patients with elevated intrapharyngeal pressures. Most of these patients are asymptomatic, but about 5% with lateral pharyngeal pouches complain of a feeling of incomplete swallowing [38, 39]. Patients with lateral pharyngeal diverticula may also complain of dysphagia, choking, regurgitation of undigested food, or a painless neck mass.

Branchial pouch sinuses and branchial cleft fistulae

In the 4-week embryo, paired grooves of ectodermal origin—the branchial clefts—appear on the sides of the neck. Four outpouchings of endodermal origin—the branchial pouches—grow to meet the branchial clefts [40]. The second branchial cleft forms the middle ear, eustachian tube, and floor of the tonsillar fossa. The third and fourth branchial pouches form the piriform sinuses. Persistence of branchial clefts or pouches may lead to the development of sinus tracks (that end blindly beneath the skin), fistulae (that extend to the skin), or cysts. Branchial pouch sinus tracks arise from the tonsillar fossa (second pouch) (Figure 6.19), the upper anterolateral piriform fossa (third pouch), or the lower anterolateral piriform sinus (fourth pouch).

Inflammatory conditions

Although barium studies are of limited value in immunocompetent patients with an acute sore throat, they may be of value for demonstrating acute inflammatory lesions in the pharynx in immunocompromised patients with suspected *Candida* (Figure 6.20) or herpes esophagitis. In patients with chronic sore throats, barium studies are primarily of value for assessing the presence and severity of gastroesophageal reflux.

Acute ulceration and chronic scarring of the pharynx may be caused by a variety of uncommon diseases, including Behçet's syndrome, bullous pemphigoid, benign mucous membrane pemphigoid, epidermolysis bullosa, erythema multiforme major (Stevens–Johnson syndrome), Reiter's syndrome, and Crohn's disease [41]. Lye ingestion may cause marked ulceration with amputation of the epiglottis and severe scarring (Figure 6.21).

Lymphoid hyperplasia

Lymphoid hyperplasia is a non-specific response to aging, allergies, and repeated infections, involving the palatine tonsils (Figure 6.22) or base of the tongue [42]. Lymphoid hyperplasia of the lingual tonsil may also occur as a compensatory response to prior tonsillectomy. Lymphoid hyperplasia may extend into the valleculae, vallecular surface of the epiglottis, or even the proximal hypopharynx. There are no radiographic criteria for differentiating lymphoid hyperplasia of the tongue base from the normal lingual tonsil. Lymphoid hyperplasia is characterized on barium studies by numerous 3–7-mm smooth-surfaced, ovoid nodules symmetrically distributed over the vertical surface of the tongue [42, 43] (Figure 6.23). These nodules may protrude posteriorly into the oropharynx and valleculae. When lingual tonsil lymphoid hyperplasia is focal or mass-like, it can mimic the appearance of tumor at the base of the tongue

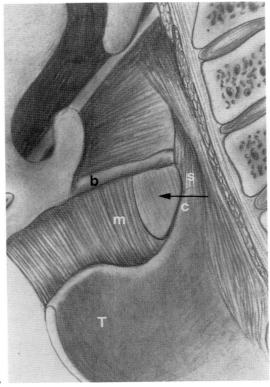

A

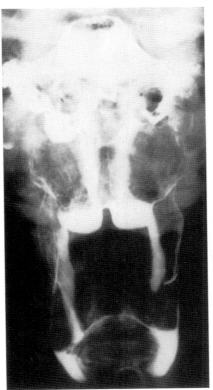

B

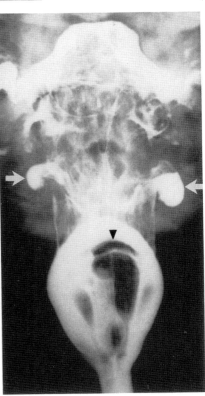

C

Figure 6.17 Lateral pharyngeal pouches.
(A) Line drawing of the pharynx in lateral view shows the area of weakness (arrow) that a lateral pharyngeal pouch protrudes through, bounded by the hyoid bone (b) superiorly, the posterior border of the thyrohyoid muscle (m) anteriorly, the superior cornu of the thyroid cartilage (c), and the insertion of the stylopharyngeal muscle (s) posteriorly. The ala of the thyroid cartilage (T) is identified (reproduced from Rubesin *et al.* [2], with permission).
(B) Frontal view of the pharynx just as the bolus reaches the valleculae shows no evidence of lateral pharyngeal pouches.
(C) Frontal view of the pharynx as the bolus passes through the pharyngoesophageal segment shows 1.5-cm and 1-cm barium-filled sacs (arrows) on the left and right pharyngeal walls, respectively. The tilting epiglottis is identified (arrowhead).

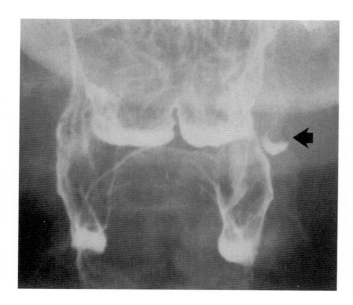

Figure 6.18 Lateral pharyngeal diverticulum. A 0.8-cm barium-filled sac (arrow) persists outside the left lateral wall of the pharynx after the bolus has passed.

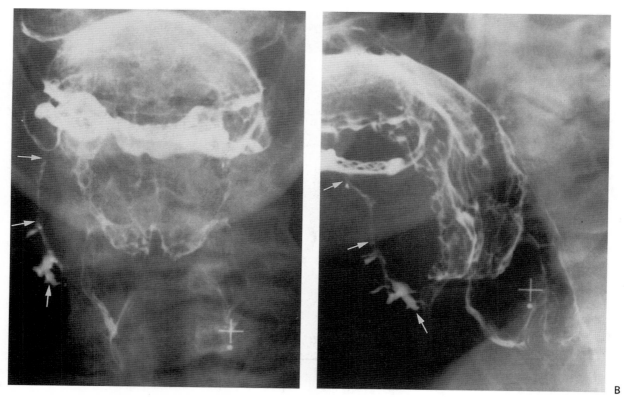

A   B

Figure 6.19 Branchial pouch sinus. (A) Frontal view of the pharynx shows an 8-cm long track (arrows) that courses inferiorly from the floor of the mouth. (B) Steep right posterior oblique view of the pharynx demonstrates the track (arrows) arising from the retromolar trigone/anterior portion of the tonsillar fossa. Dentures are in place (reproduced from Rubesin and Glick [23], with permission).

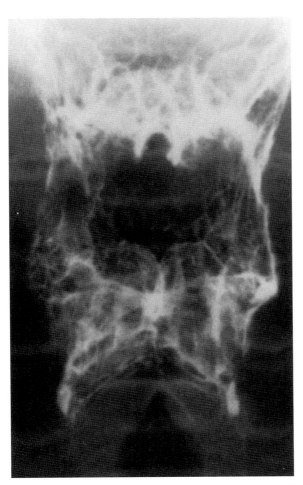

Figure 6.20 *Candida* pharyngitis. Innumerable nodules and plaque-like elevations have disrupted the normally smooth surface of the pharynx.

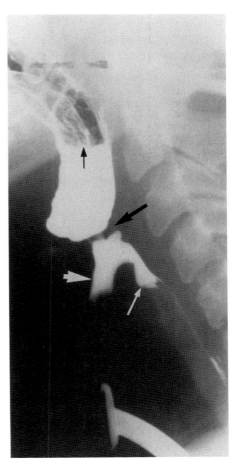

Figure 6.21 Scarring from corrosive ingestion. Lateral view of the pharynx shows a thick radiolucent band of soft tissue (thick black arrow) crossing the hypopharynx. Obstruction is implied by a large standing column of barium (thin black arrow) in the oropharynx. The hypopharynx is small and contracted (thin white arrow). Barium pours into the open laryngeal vestibule (thick white arrow) (reproduced from Rubesin SE. The pharynx: structural disorders. *Radiol Clin North Am* 1994;32:1083–1101, with permission).

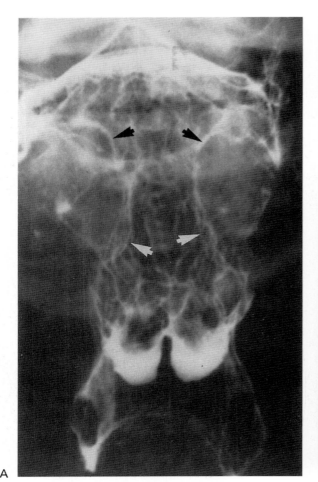

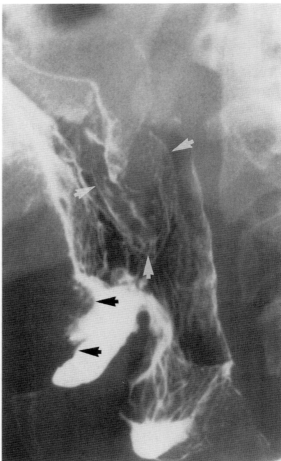

A

B

Figure 6.22 (above) Lymphoid hyperplasia of the palatine tonsils and tongue base. (A) Frontal view of the pharynx demonstrates that the left and right palatine tonsils (arrows) protrude deeply into the oropharynx. Ovoid nodules carpet the base of the tongue. (B) Lateral view of the pharynx during phonation reveals a mass in the tonsillar fossae (white arrows) and nodules at the tongue base (black arrows) (reproduced from Rubesin [31], with permission).

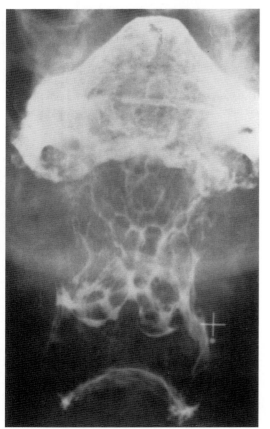

Figure 6.23 Lymphoid hyperplasia of the tongue base. Barium fills the grooves between smooth ovoid nodules symmetrically distributed on the vertical surface of the tongue.

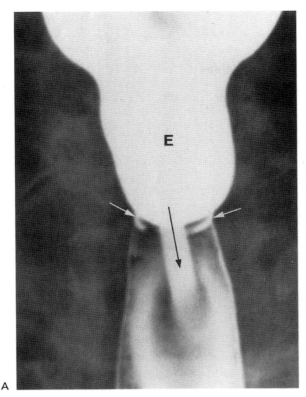

A

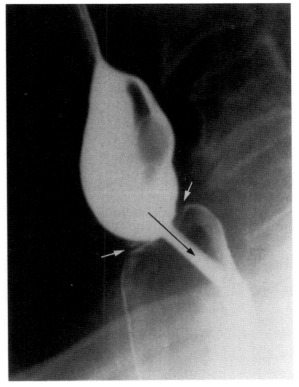

B

Figure 6.24 Cervical esophageal web. (A) Frontal and (B) lateral views demonstrate a thin radiolucent band (white arrows) encircling the cervical esophagus. A jet of barium (black arrow) spurting through the opening in the web indicates that there is partial obstruction. Dilatation of the cervical esophagus (E) proximal to the web is also indicative of obstruction (reproduced from Rubesin SE. Pharynx. In: Levine MS, Rubesin SE, Laufer I, eds. *Double Contrast Gastrointestinal Radiology*, 3d edn. Philadelphia: WB Saunders, 2000, pp. 61–89, with permission).

[42]. Patients with asymmetric nodularity or mass lesions at the tongue base therefore should undergo further investigation to differentiate lymphoid hyperplasia of the lingual tonsil from malignant tumor.

Pharyngeal and cervical esophageal webs

Webs are thin folds composed of mucosa and submucosa arising predominantly from the anterior wall of the pharyngoesophageal segment and proximal cervical esophagus. Cervical esophageal webs are common findings, occurring in 3–8% of patients who undergo upper gastrointestinal barium studies and in 16% of patients at autopsy [44–47]. The pathogenesis of these webs is uncertain. Some webs in the valleculae have been described as normal variants [48]. Other webs result from diseases that cause chronic scarring. Many patients with cervical esophageal webs also have GERD [31, 49].

Webs are thin (1–2 mm in thickness) folds arising from the anterior wall of the pharyngoesophageal segment or proximal cervical esophagus. A web appears on barium studies as a radiolucent bar in the barium pool or as a thin structure etched in white by barium. Some webs extend circumferentially, with a deeper shelf on their anterior surface. Patients with dysphagia usually have circumferential cervical esophageal webs occluding greater than 50% of the luminal diameter (Figure 6.24). Obstruction is implied by dilatation of the cervical esophagus proximal to the web or by a spurt of barium through the web (the so-called jet phenomenon) [50, 51].

Tumors

Benign tumors and cysts

The most common benign lesions of the base of the tongue are retention cysts [43]. Granular cell tumors as well as ectopic thyroid tissue and thyroglossal duct cysts also occur at the tongue base. The most common benign tumor-like lesions of the aryepiglottic folds are retention cysts and saccular cysts [43]. Retention cysts are lined by squamous epithelium and are filled with desquamated debris. Saccular cysts are filled with mucus from glands of the appendix of the laryngeal ventricle [40] and are the mucus-filled variant of internal laryngoceles. True soft tissue tumors are uncommon and include lipomas, neurofibromas, hamartomas, and oncocytomas, usually arising from the aryepiglottic folds or the mucosa overlying the muscular process of the

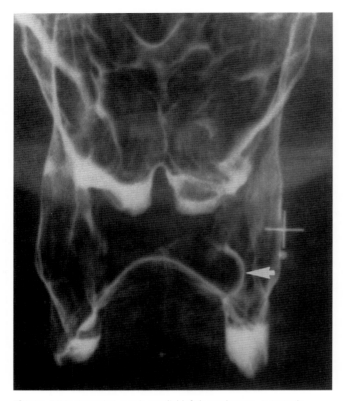

Figure 6.25 Retention cyst in medial left hypopharynx. A smooth-surfaced hemispheric line (arrow) protrudes into the left piriform sinus (reproduced from Rubesin and Glick [23], with permission).

arytenoid cartilages [40]. Benign tumors arising from the mucoserous minor salivary glands are usually found in the soft palate or tongue base. Chondromas usually arise from the posterior lamina of the cricoid cartilage. Regardless of the specific histologic findings, benign pharyngeal tumors often appear on barium studies as smooth-surfaced hemispheric masses that protrude into the pharyngeal lumen [52] (Figure 6.25).

Squamous cell carcinoma

In the United States, squamous cell carcinoma of the head and neck (tongue, pharynx, larynx) is five times more common than squamous cell carcinoma of the esophagus. More than 20% of patients with squamous cell carcinomas of the head and neck have synchronous or metachronous carcinomas of the oral cavity, pharynx, larynx, esophagus, or lungs [53]. About 90% of malignant tumors in the oropharynx and hypopharynx are non-keratinizing squamous cell carcinomas. Almost all of these tumors are detected in moderate or heavy abusers of alcohol, tobacco, or both.

The signs, symptoms, prognosis, and treatment of pharyngeal cancer depend on the location of the tumor. Most patients have symptoms of short duration (less than 4 months), including sore throat, hoarseness, dysphagia, and odynophagia. The overall 5-year survival rate for these patients is 20–40% [52–54].

The radiographic findings of squamous cell carcinoma are those of any mucosal tumor in the gastrointestinal tract [55–58]. The normal contour of the involved structure is disrupted by a protrusion into the lumen or by an ulceration extending outside the expected luminal contour. Intraluminal tumor is manifested as an area of increased radio-opacity replacing the normally air-filled lumen or as a radiolucent filling defect in the barium pool [55] (Figure 6.26). The irregular mucosal surface of the tumor is manifested as a granular, nodular, ulcerated, or lobulated surface or as barium-etched lines in an unexpected configuration or location [57] (Figure 6.26). The mobility or distensibility of the involved structure may be compromised (Figure 6.27).

The palatine tonsil is the most common site of involvement of squamous cell carcinoma of the pharynx. Tonsillar tumors can spread to the posterior pharyngeal wall, soft palate, and base of the tongue. Lymph node metastases are seen in about one-half of these patients [52, 54]. Squamous cell carcinomas of the tongue base are usually advanced tumors that already have spread deep into the intrinsic or extrinsic muscles of the tongue [59] (Figure 6.26). These tumors can also invade the palatine tonsils, valleculae, or pharyngoepiglottic folds. Lymph node metastases are present in about 70% of cases at the time of presentation [52].

The supraglottic laryngeal structures (epiglottis, aryepiglottic folds, mucosa overlying the muscular process of the arytenoid cartilages, false vocal cords, and laryngeal ventricle) arise from pharyngobuccal anlage, forming a portion of the anterior wall of the hypopharynx [1]. Supraglottic cancers (Figures 6.27 and 6.28) are often classified as a subsite of "laryngeal" rather than pharyngeal tumors. These lesions frequently cause coughing and choking [60]. Hoarseness occurs in patients with supraglottic and laryngeal carcinomas as well as carcinomas of the medial piriform sinus infiltrating the arytenoid cartilage or cricoarytenoid joint [61]. The supraglottic region has an extensive lymphatic bed; supraglottic cancers therefore tend to spread throughout the supraglottic region and into the pre-epiglottic space. Cervical lymphadenopathy is detected in one-third to one-half of these patients [52, 54].

Squamous cell carcinomas of the piriform sinuses are usually bulky masses that already have spread to lymph nodes in 70–80% of patients at the time of presentation [52] (Figure 6.29). Tumors of the medial piriform sinus wall may invade the ipsilateral aryepiglottic fold, arytenoid and cricoid cartilage, and paraglottic space, often resulting in hoarseness [61]. Tumors of the lateral piriform sinus wall may invade the thyroid cartilage, thyrohyoid membrane, and neck, including the carotid sheath [52].

Squamous cell carcinomas of the posterior pharyngeal wall (Figure 6.30) are large, bulky tumors that cause few symptoms, often presenting as painless neck masses resulting from

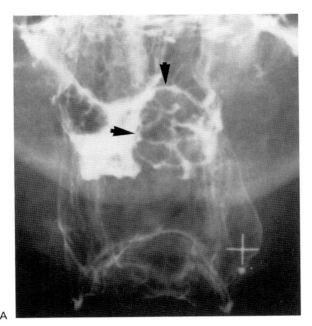

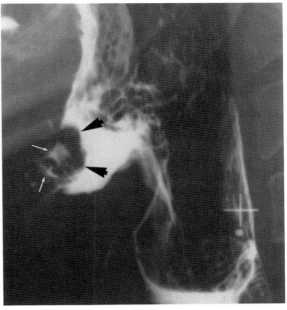

Figure 6.26 Polypoid squamous cell carcinoma of the base of the tongue. (A) Frontal view of the pharynx demonstrates that the barium pool in the left vallecula is replaced by a 1.5-cm nodular mass (arrows) with barium in its interstices. (B) Lateral view of the pharynx shows a

1.5-cm radiolucent filling defect (black arrows) in the barium pooling in the valleculae. Barium has entered the interstices of the tumor (white arrows) deep to the expected contour of the base of the tongue (reproduced from Rubesin and Glick [23], with permission).

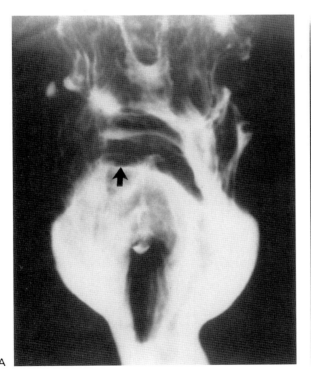

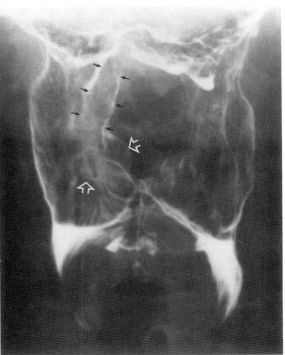

Figure 6.27 Infiltrative squamous cell carcinoma of right aryepiglottic fold. (A) Frontal view of the pharynx during drinking shows diminished epiglottic tilt on the right (arrow). (B) Spot radiograph after drinking demonstrates thickening of the right aryepiglottic fold (short arrows) and nodularity of the mucosa overlying the muscular process of the right arytenoid process (open arrows) (reproduced from Rubesin [10], with permission).

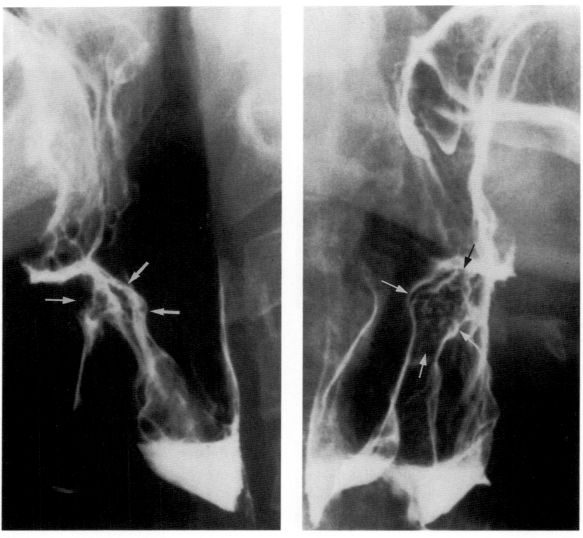

A   B

Figure 6.28 Ulcerative squamous cell carcinoma of the epiglottis. (A) Lateral view of the pharynx shows that the epiglottic tip is missing. Fine mucosal nodularity is seen on the superior anterior wall of the laryngeal vestibule (thin arrow) and aryepiglottic folds (thick arrows). (B) Left posterior oblique view of the pharynx demonstrates amputation of the epiglottic tip (black arrow) and nodularity of the mucosa (white arrows) (reproduced from Rubesin [31], with permission).

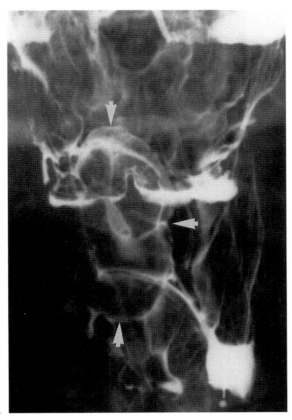

A

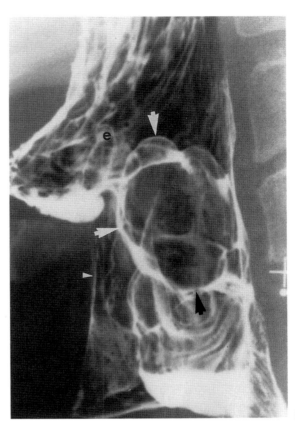

B

Figure 6.29 Polypoid squamous cell carcinoma of the right piriform sinus. (A) Frontal view of the pharynx demonstrates loss of the normal contour of the right piriform sinus and a barium-etched mass (arrows) protruding into the lumen. The valleculae and epiglottic tip are spared.

(B) Lateral view of the pharynx demonstrates a large, lobulated barium-etched mass (arrows). The epiglottic tip (e) and laryngeal vestibule (arrowhead) are spared (reproduced from Rubesin and Glick [23], with permission).

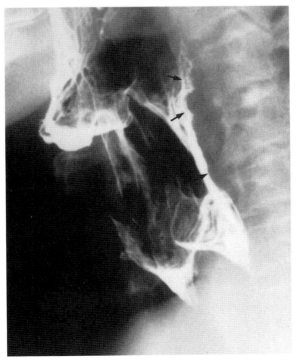

A

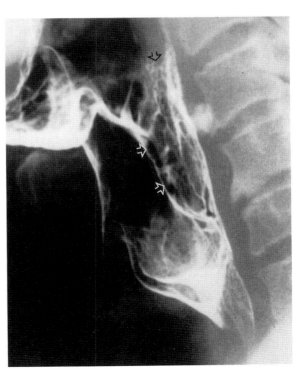

B

Figure 6.30 Plaque-like squamous cell carcinoma of the posterolateral pharyngeal wall. (A) Steep oblique view of the pharynx demonstrates focal mucosal nodularity and plaque-like elevation (arrows) of the posterior pharyngeal wall. (B) Lateral view of the pharynx demonstrates mucosal nodularity (arrows) *en face*.

metastases to cervical lymph nodes [62]. More than half of these patients have lymph node metastases at the time of diagnosis. These exophytic tumors may spread superiorly or inferiorly into the nasopharynx or cervical esophagus and posteriorly into the retropharyngeal space. These tumors are the pharyngeal cancers most frequently associated with a synchronous or metachronous squamous cell carcinoma of the oral cavity, pharynx, or esophagus [62].

Postcricoid carcinomas (Figure 6.31) are an uncommon form of pharyngeal squamous cell carcinoma, except in Scandinavia. These tumors may also spread superiorly or inferiorly into the hypopharynx or cervical esophagus.

Lymphoma

About 10% of pharyngeal malignancies are non-Hodgkin's lymphomas arising in the abundant lymphoid tissue of Waldeyer's ring: the adenoids, palatine tonsils, and lingual tonsil [63]. Hodgkin's disease involving the pharynx is uncommon, even though it is often first detected in cervical lymph nodes [64]. Patients with pharyngeal lymphoma frequently present with a neck mass, and cervical lymph nodes are initially involved in 60% of cases [63]. Other patients may present with nasal obstruction, sore throat, or dysphagia.

The palatine tonsil is the primary site of involvement by pharyngeal lymphoma in 40–60% of patients (Figure 6.32), the nasopharynx in 18–28%, and the lingual tonsil in 10% [40, 63]. Multiple sites are involved in about 25% of patients, but the hypopharynx is rarely involved by this tumor. Pharyngeal lymphomas typically appear on barium studies as large, bulky, lobulated masses (Figure 6.32). The mucosal surface may be smooth; however, because of the submucosal location of these tumors [31] (Figure 6.33).

Other rare tumors involving the pharynx include Kaposi's sarcoma, carcinoma of the minor salivary glands, synovial

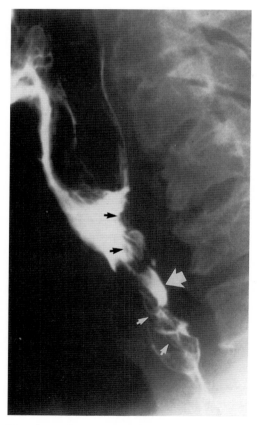

Figure 6.31 Ulcerated squamous cell carcinoma of the pharyngoesophageal segment. Lateral view of the pharynx shows a barium-filled ulcer (large arrow) at the pharyngoesophageal segment. The posterior pharyngeal wall is destroyed by tumor (small arrows) centered at the pharyngoesophageal segment but extending vertically into the distal hypopharynx and proximal cervical esophagus.

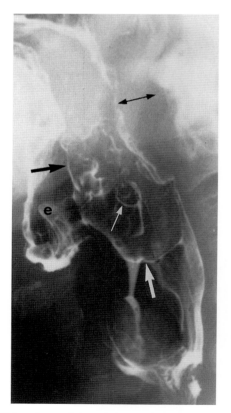

Figure 6.32 Lymphoma of the palatine tonsil. Lateral view of the pharynx after instillation of intranasal barium shows a large, smooth mass (thick arrows) filling the lateral hypopharynx. A barium-coated ring shadow (thin arrow) represents a central ulcer. The posterior pharyngeal wall is thickened (double arrow) and has a nodular surface. The epiglottic tip (e) is identified (reproduced from Levine MS, Rubesin SE. Radiologic investigation of dysphagia. *AJR Am J Roentgenol* 1990;154:1157–1163, with permission).

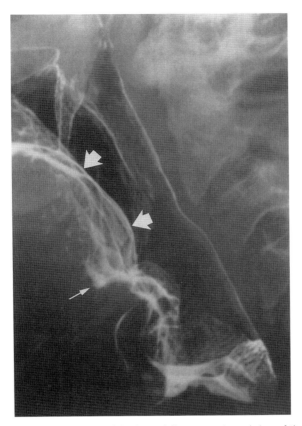

Figure 6.33 Lymphoma of the base of the tongue. Lateral view of the pharynx shows that the base of the tongue is enlarged (thick arrows) and protruding posteriorly. The valleculae are obliterated (thin arrow) (reproduced from Rubesin and Laufer [57], with permission).

sarcoma, and cartilaginous tumors of the larynx or cricoid cartilage.

Radiation change

The pharynx is irradiated when patients undergo radiation therapy for squamous cell carcinoma of the larynx or pharynx, lymphoma of the pharynx or cervical lymph nodes, or metastases to the neck. Historically, the pharynx was included in the radiation portal in patients who also underwent radiation therapy for thyrotoxicosis and tuberculous lymphadenitis. Chronic radiation injury to the pharynx is characterized by vascular damage with mucosal atrophy and fibrosis of muscle and submucosal tissue. Edema caused by lymphatic and venous obstruction is most marked in the epiglottis and mucosa overlying the muscular processes of the arytenoid cartilages. Osteomyelitis and chondronecrosis are more severe complications.

Radiation edema and fibrosis is manifested on barium studies by smooth, bulbous enlargement of the epiglottis, smooth thickening of the aryepiglottic folds, and elevation of the mucosa overlying the muscular processes of the arytenoid cartilages [31, 40, 65] (Figure 6.34). Other findings include flattening of the valleculae and atrophy of the soft palate, if this structure is included in the radiation portal [3]. Radiation fibrosis leads to diminished or absent epiglottic tilt and poor closure of the laryngeal vestibule with subsequent laryngeal penetration [66]. Constrictor muscle paresis may result in poor clearance from the hypopharynx with stasis and overflow aspiration. Nodularity or focal ulceration of the mucosal surface should suggest the possibility of persistent or recurrent tumor [65].

Esophagus

Technique

Barium studies of the esophagus are usually performed as biphasic examinations that include both upright double-contrast views with a high-density barium suspension and prone single-contrast views with a low-density barium suspension [67]. The patient first ingests an effervescent agent and then rapidly gulps the high-density barium in the upright, left posterior oblique (LPO) position in order to obtain double-contrast views of the esophagus. On such views, the esophagus normally has a smooth, featureless appearance *en face* and a thin white etching where it is seen in profile (Figure 6.35A). Occasionally, collapsed or partially collapsed views (also known as mucosal relief views) may show the normal longitudinal folds as thin, straight, delicate structures of no more than 1–2 mm in width (Figure 6.35B). The patient is then placed in a recumbent, right-side down position for double-contrast views of the gastric cardia and fundus. The cardia can often be recognized by the presence of three or four stellate folds that radiate to a central point at the gastroesophageal junction (GEJ), also known as the cardiac rosette [68] (Figure 6.35C). In some patients with tumor involving the cardia, these lesions may be manifested by distortion, effacement, or obliteration of this cardiac rosette.

After the double-contrast phase of the examination is completed, the patient is placed in the prone, right anterior oblique (RAO) position and asked to take discrete swallows of a low-density barium suspension in order to evaluate esophageal motility. Esophageal dysmotility is considered to be present when abnormal peristalsis is detected on two or more of five separate swallows [69]. The patient then rapidly gulps the low-density barium suspension to optimally distend the esophagus (particularly the distal esophagus) in order to rule out rings or strictures that could be missed on the double-contrast phase of the examination. Finally, the patient is turned from a supine to a right lateral position to assess for spontaneous gastroesophageal reflux or for reflux induced by a Valsalva maneuver.

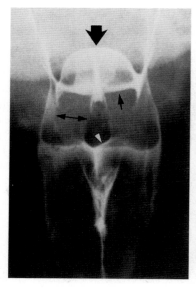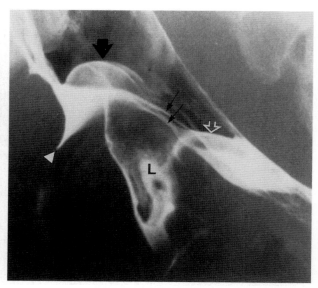

Figure 6.34 Diffuse radiation changes. (A) Frontal view of the pharynx shows that epiglottis (large arrow) is enlarged and has a smooth bulbous contour. The valleculae are flattened (left valleculae identified with a small arrow). The aryepiglottic folds are markedly but smoothly enlarged (right aryepiglottic fold identified by double arrow). The mucosa overlying the muscular processes of the arytenoids is elevated (white arrowhead identifies mucosa overlying muscular process of the left arytenoid cartilage). (B) Lateral view of the pharynx demonstrates a bulbous epiglottic tip (black arrow), elevated aryepiglottic folds (thin arrows), elevated mucosa overlying the muscular processes of the arytenoid cartilages (open arrow), and slit-like valleculae (arrowhead). Barium fills the laryngeal vestibule (L) (reproduced from Rubesin [31], with permission).

Gastroesophageal reflux disease

The purpose of barium studies in patients with reflux symptoms is not simply to document the presence of a hiatal hernia or gastroesophageal reflux, but rather to detect the morphologic sequelae of reflux, including reflex esophagitis, peptic strictures, Barrett's esophagus, and esophageal adenocarcinoma. These conditions are therefore considered separately in subsequent sections.

Reflux esophagitis

Reflux esophagitis is by far the most common inflammatory disease involving the esophagus. This condition is characterized on single-contrast esophagrams by thickened folds, marginal ulceration, and decreased distensibility, but such findings are detected only in patients with advanced disease. In contrast, double-contrast esophagrams have a sensitivity approaching 90% for the diagnosis of reflux esophagitis because of the ability to detect superficial ulcers or other findings that cannot be visualized on single-contrast studies [70, 71]. Thus, double-contrast esophagography is the radiologic technique of choice for patients with suspected GERD.

Early reflux esophagitis may be manifested on double-contrast studies by a finely nodular or granular appearance of the mucosa with poorly defined radiolucencies that fade peripherally as a result of mucosal edema and inflammation [72, 73] (Figure 6.36). In almost all cases, this nodularity or granularity extends proximally from the GEJ as a continuous area of disease. With more advanced disease, barium studies may reveal shallow ulcers and erosions in the distal esophagus. The ulcers may have a punctate, linear, or stellate configuration, and are frequently associated with surrounding halos of edematous mucosa, radiating folds, or sacculation of the adjacent esophageal wall [73] (Figure 6.37A). Other patients may have a solitary ulcer at or near the GEJ, often on the posterior wall of the distal esophagus [74] (Figure 6.37B). It has been postulated that the location of these ulcers is related to prolonged exposure to refluxed acid that pools posteriorly when patients sleep in the supine position [74]. Other patients may have widespread ulceration involving the distal third or even half of the thoracic esophagus. In such cases, however, the ulceration almost always extends distally to the region of the GEJ. Thus, the presence of ulcers that are confined to the upper or mid esophagus should suggest another cause for the patient's disease.

Reflux esophagitis may also be manifested on barium studies by thickened longitudinal folds as a result of edema and inflammation that extend into the submucosa [73] (Figure 6.38). These folds may have a smooth or irregular contour, occasionally mimicking the appearance of esophageal varices [75]. In general, thickened folds should be recognized as a non-specific finding of esophagitis as a result of a host of causes. Other patients with chronic reflux esophagitis may have a single prominent fold that arises in the

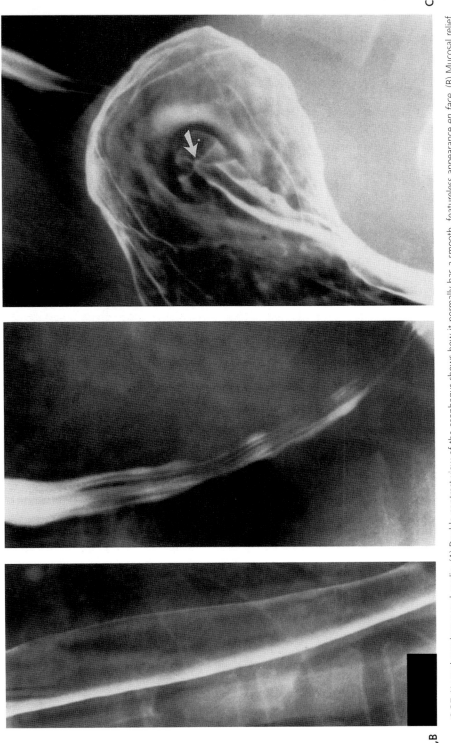

Figure 6.35 Normal esophagus and cardia. (A) Double-contrast view of the esophagus shows how it normally has a smooth, featureless appearance *en face*. (B) Mucosal relief view shows thin, straight longitudinal folds as a normal finding in the collapsed esophagus. (C) Recumbent right lateral view of the gastric fundus shows stellate folds radiating to a central point (arrow) at the gastroesophageal junction, also known as the cardiac "rosette."

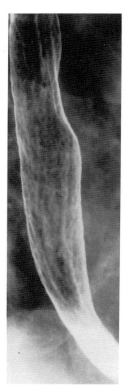

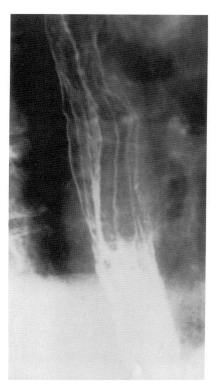

Figure 6.36 Reflex esophagitis with granular mucosa. Double-contrast view shows fine nodularity or granularity of the distal esophagus caused by edema and inflammation of the mucosa. Compare this image to the smooth, featureless appearance of the normal esophagus in Figure 6.35A.

Figure 6.38 Reflux esophagitis with thickened folds. Double-contrast view shows considerably thickened folds in the esophagus caused by edema and inflammation extending into the submucosa. Compare this image to the normal appearance of the longitudinal folds in Figure 6.35B (reproduced from Levine MS. *Radiology of the Esophagus*. Philadelphia: WB Saunders, 1989, with permission).

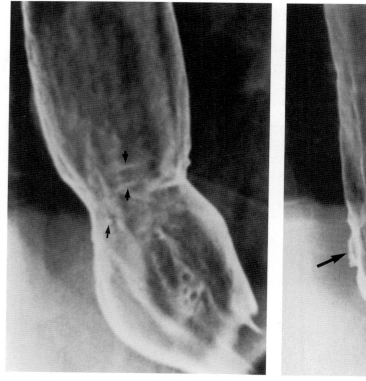

A

B

Figure 6.37 Reflux esophagitis with ulceration. (A) Double-contrast view shows shallow linear and punctate ulcers (arrows) in the distal esophagus above a hiatal hernia (reproduced from Levine [73], with permission.) (B) Double-contrast view in another patient shows a single flat ulcer (arrow) on the posterior wall of the distal esophagus (reproduced from Levine MS. *Radiology of the Esophagus*. Philadelphia: WB Saunders, 1989, with permission).

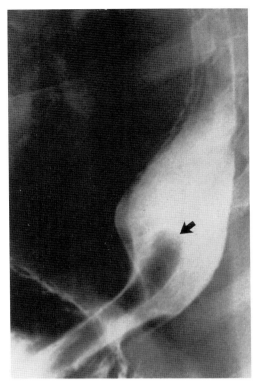

Figure 6.39 Reflux esophagitis with inflammatory esophagogastric polyp. Prone single-contrast view shows a prominent fold arising at the cardia and extending into the distal esophagus as a smooth polypoid protuberance (arrow). This appearance is characteristic of an inflammatory esophagogastric polyp.

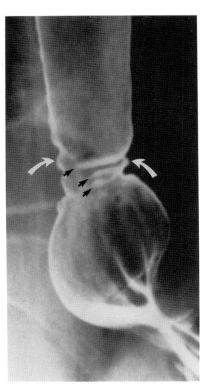

Figure 6.40 Scarring of distal esophagus with fixed transverse folds. Double-contrast view shows minimal narrowing of the distal esophagus above a hiatal hernia. Also note sacculation (white arrows) of the wall and pooling of barium between transverse folds (black arrows), producing a "stepladder" appearance (reproduced from Levine MS and Laufer I. The upper gastrointestinal series at a crossroads. *AJR Am J Roentgenol* 1993;161:1131–1137, with permission).

region of the gastric cardia and extends upward into the distal esophagus as a smooth, polypoid protuberance, also known as an inflammatory esophagogastric polyp [76, 77] (Figure 6.39). Because these lesions have no malignant potential, endoscopy is not warranted when barium studies reveal typical findings of an inflammatory esophagogastric polyp in the distal esophagus.

In advanced reflux esophagitis, extensive ulceration, edema, and spasm may cause the esophagus to have a grossly irregular contour with serrated or spiculated margins and loss of distensibility [73]. Occasionally, the narrowing and deformity associated with severe esophagitis can mimic the appearance of an infiltrating esophageal carcinoma, so endoscopy and biopsy may be required for a definitive diagnosis.

Scarring and strictures

As esophageal ulcers heal, localized scarring may be manifested on barium studies by flattening, puckering, or sacculation of the adjacent esophageal wall, often associated with the development of radiating folds [73] (Figure 6.40).

Further scarring can lead to the development of circumferential strictures (also known as "peptic" strictures) in the distal esophagus, almost always above a hiatal hernia [73, 78] (Figure 6.41). These strictures often appear as concentric areas of smooth, tapered narrowing, but asymmetric scarring can lead to asymmetric narrowing with focal sacculation or ballooning of the esophageal wall between areas of fibrosis. When there is marked irregularity, flattening, or nodularity of one or more walls of the stricture, endoscopy and biopsy should be performed to rule out a malignant stricture as the cause of these findings.

Scarring from reflux esophagitis can also lead to longitudinal shortening of the esophagus and the development of fixed transverse folds, producing a characteristic "stepladder" appearance caused by pooling of barium between the folds [79] (Figure 6.40). These fixed transverse folds should be differentiated on barium studies from the thin transverse folds (also known as the "feline" esophagus) often seen in patients with gastroesophageal reflux as a transient finding resulting from contraction of the longitudinally oriented muscularis mucosae [80, 81] (Figure 6.42).

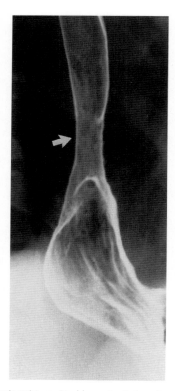

Figure 6.41 Peptic stricture. Double-contrast view shows a smooth, tapered area of concentric narrowing (arrow) in the distal esophagus above a hiatal hernia (reproduced from Gilchrist *et al.* [85], with permission).

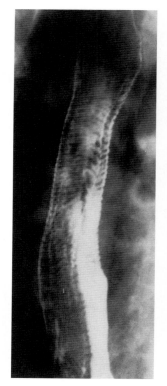

Figure 6.42 Feline esophagus. Double-contrast view shows delicate transverse folds as a transient finding in the esophagus. Compare this image to the fixed transverse folds in the distal esophagus in Figure 6.40.

Barrett's esophagus

Barrett's esophagus is characterized by progressive columnar metaplasia of the distal esophagus caused by chronic gastro-esophageal reflux and reflux esophagitis. The classic radiologic signs of Barrett's esophagus consist of a mid-esophageal stricture or ulcer occurring at a discrete distance from the GEJ [82] (Figure 6.43). In the presence of a hiatal hernia or gastroesophageal reflux, a mid-esophageal stricture or ulcer is thought to be highly suggestive, if not pathognomonic, of Barrett's esophagus. A distinctive reticular pattern of the mucosa has also been recognized as a relatively specific sign of Barrett's esophagus, particularly if adjacent to the distal aspect of a mid-esophageal stricture [83]. This reticular pattern is characterized by tiny barium-filled grooves or crevices resembling the areae gastricae on double-contrast studies of the stomach (Figure 6.44). However, the classic radiologic signs of Barrett's esophagus (a mid-esophageal stricture or ulcer, or a reticular mucosal pattern) are seen in only 5–10% of all patients with Barrett's esophagus [83, 84]. Other more common findings in Barrett's esophagus, such as reflux esophagitis and peptic strictures, are often present in patients with uncomplicated reflux disease who do not have Barrett's esophagus. Thus, those radiographic findings

that are more specific for Barrett's esophagus are not sensitive, and those findings that are more sensitive are not specific. As a result, many investigators have traditionally believed that esophagography has limited value in diagnosing Barrett's esophagus.

Even so, other investigators have shown that double-contrast esophagography can be a useful imaging test for Barrett's esophagus in patients with reflux symptoms when these individuals are classified as being either at high, moderate, or low risk for Barrett's esophagus based on specific radiologic criteria [85]. Patients who are classified at high risk for Barrett's esophagus because of a mid-esophageal stricture or ulcer or a reticular pattern are almost always found to have this condition, so endoscopy and biopsy should be performed for a definitive diagnosis. A larger group of patients are at moderate risk for Barrett's esophagus because of esophagitis or peptic strictures in the distal esophagus; so the decision for endoscopy should be based on the severity of symptoms, age, and overall health of the patient. However, most patients are at low risk for Barrett's esophagus because of the absence of esophagitis or strictures, and the risk of Barrett's esophagus is so small in this group that these individuals can be treated empirically for

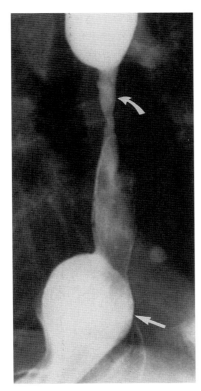

Figure 6.43 Barrett's esophagus with mid-esophageal stricture. Prone single-contrast view shows a large hiatal hernia (straight arrow) and a moderately long stricture (curved arrow) in the mid esophagus a considerable distance from the hernia. In the proper clinical setting, the presence of a mid-esophageal stricture should be highly suggestive of Barrett's esophagus, but this finding is seen on barium studies in only a small percentage of patients.

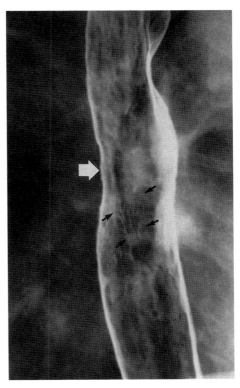

Figure 6.44 Barrett's esophagus with reticular pattern. Double-contrast view shows the earliest stage of a stricture in the mid esophagus with slight flattening of one wall (white arrow). Also note a distinctive reticular pattern of the mucosa (black arrows) just below the level of the stricture. This radiographic finding is thought to be highly suggestive of Barrett's esophagus (reproduced from Levine *et al.* [83], with permission).

their reflux symptoms without need for endoscopy. Thus, double-contrast esophagography can be used to separate patients into various risk groups for Barrett's esophagus to determine the relative need for endoscopy and biopsy in these patients.

Infectious esophagitis

Candida esophagitis

Candida albicans is the most common cause of infectious esophagitis. It usually occurs as an opportunistic infection in immunocompromised patients, particularly those with acquired immunodeficiency syndrome (AIDS), but *Candida* esophagitis may also result from local esophageal stasis caused by severe esophageal motility disorders such as achalasia and scleroderma [86]. In some patients with these motility disorders, a "foamy" esophagus may develop with innumerable tiny bubbles layering out in the barium column; this phenomenon presumably results from esophageal infection by the yeast form of the organism [87]. Single-contrast barium studies have limited value in detecting *Candida*

esophagitis because of the superficial nature of the disease. In contrast, double-contrast barium studies have a sensitivity of about 90% in diagnosing *Candida* esophagitis in relation to endoscopy [88, 89], primarily because of the ability to demonstrate mucosal plaques with this technique.

Candida esophagitis is usually manifested on double-contrast studies by discrete plaque-like lesions corresponding to the white plaques seen on endoscopy [88]. The plaques may appear as linear or irregular filling defects that are often oriented longitudinally in relation to the long axis of the esophagus and are separated by segments of normal intervening mucosa [88] (Figure 6.45). During the past two decades, a much more fulminant form of candidiasis has been encountered in patients with AIDS, who may present with a grossly irregular or "shaggy" esophagus caused by innumerable coalescent plaques and pseudomembranes with trapping of barium between the lesions [90] (Figure 6.46). Some of these plaques may eventually slough, producing one or more deep ulcers superimposed on a background of diffuse plaque formation (Figure 6.46). Occasionally, AIDS patients may present with the shaggy

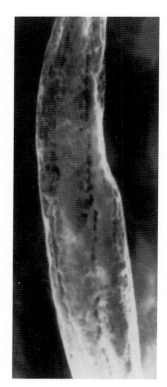

Figure 6.45 *Candida* esophagitis with plaques. Double-contrast view shows multiple discrete plaque-like lesions in the esophagus. Note how the plaques have a linear configuration and are separated by segments of normal intervening mucosa. This appearance is characteristic of *Candida* esophagitis (reproduced from Levine *et al.* [88], with permission).

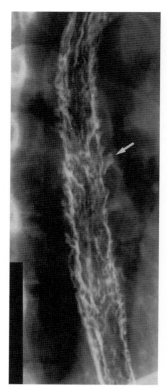

Figure 6.46 Advanced *Candida* esophagitis with "shaggy" esophagus. Double-contrast view shows a grossly irregular or shaggy esophagus caused by innumerable coalescent plaques and pseudomembranes with trapping of barium between the lesions. Also note a superimposed ulcer (arrow) due to sloughing of diseased mucosa. This patient had acquired immunodeficiency syndrome (reproduced from Levine *et al.* [90], with permission).

esophagus of candidiasis as the initial manifestation of their disease, so the radiologist performing the examination may be the first to suggest that the patient has AIDS. When typical findings of *Candida* esophagitis are encountered on double-contrast esophagography, these patients can be treated with antifungal agents such as fluconazole without need for endoscopic evaluation.

Herpes esophagitis

The herpes simplex virus is another frequent cause of infectious esophagitis. Most patients with this condition are immunocompromised, but herpes esophagitis may occasionally develop as an acute, self-limited disease in otherwise healthy patients who have no underlying immunologic problems [91]. Herpes esophagitis is initially manifested by small esophageal vesicles that subsequently rupture to form discrete, punched-out ulcers on the mucosa. Although some patients have associated herpetic lesions in the oropharynx, most do not have oropharyngeal disease, and others with herpetic infection of the oropharynx have *Candida* esophagitis.

Herpes esophagitis may be manifested on double-contrast studies by small, discrete ulcers on a normal background

mucosa [92, 93]. The ulcers can have a punctate, stellate, or volcano-like appearance and are often surrounded by radiolucent mounds of edema (Figure 6.47). Multiple discrete ulcers are found on double-contrast esophagography in about 50% of patients with herpes esophagitis [93]. In the appropriate clinical setting, the presence of small, discrete ulcers without plaques should be highly suggestive of herpes esophagitis on barium studies, because ulceration in candidiasis almost always occurs on a background of diffuse plaque formation. As the disease progresses, however, herpes esophagitis may be manifested by a combination of ulcers and plaques, mimicking the appearance of *Candida* esophagitis. Occasionally, herpes esophagitis in otherwise healthy patients may be manifested by innumerable tiny ulcers that tend to be clustered together in the mid esophagus below the level of the left main bronchus [91] (Figure 6.48). The ulcers are even smaller than those in immunocompromised patients with herpes esophagitis, presumably because these individuals have an intact immune system that can prevent the ulcers from enlarging.

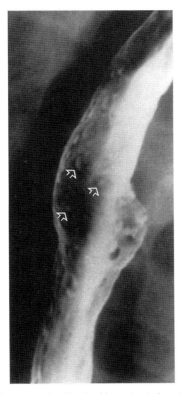

Figure 6.47 Herpes esophagitis. Double-contrast view shows multiple tiny ulcers (arrows) with surrounding mounds of edema in the mid esophagus. In an immunocompromised patient with odynophagia, this finding should be highly suggestive of herpes esophagitis (reproduced from Levine MS, Rubesin SE, Laufer I, eds. *Double Contrast Gastrointestinal Radiology*, 3rd edn. Philadelphia: WB Saunders, 2000, with permission).

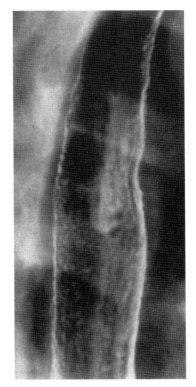

Figure 6.48 Herpes esophagitis in an otherwise healthy patient. Double-contrast view shows innumerable punctate ulcers clustered together in the mid esophagus below the level of the left main bronchus (reproduced from DeGaeta L, Levine MS, Guglielmi GE, *et al*. Herpes esophagitis in an otherwise healthy patient. *AJR Am J Roentgenol* 1985;244:1205–1206, with permission).

Cytomegalovirus esophagitis

Cytomegalovirus (CMV) is another cause of infectious esophagitis that occurs primarily in patients with AIDS. CMV esophagitis may be manifested on double-contrast studies by the development of one or more giant, flat ulcers that are several centimeters or more in length [94] (Figure 6.49). The ulcers may have an ovoid or diamond-shaped configuration and are often surrounded by a thin radiolucent rim of edematous mucosa. Because herpetic ulcers rarely become this large, the presence of one or more giant ulcers should suggest the possibility of CMV esophagitis in patients with AIDS. However, the differential diagnosis also includes giant human immunodeficiency virus (HIV) ulcers in the esophagus (see next section). Less commonly, CMV esophagitis may be manifested by small, superficial ulcers indistinguishable from those in herpes esophagitis [94]. Because CMV esophagitis is treated with relatively potent antiviral agents such as ganciclovir, which has associated bone marrow toxicity, endoscopy (with biopsy specimens, brushings, or cultures from the esophagus) is required to confirm the presence of CMV infection before treating these patients.

Human immunodeficiency virus esophagitis

HIV infection of the esophagus can lead to the development of giant esophageal ulcers indistinguishable from those caused by CMV esophagitis. Double-contrast esophagrams typically reveal one or more large, ovoid or diamond-shaped ulcers surrounded by a radiolucent rim of edema, sometimes associated with a cluster of small satellite ulcers [95, 96] (Figure 6.50). The diagnosis is established by obtaining endoscopy biopsy specimens, brushings, or cultures from the esophagus to rule out CMV esophagitis as the cause of the ulcers. Unlike CMV ulcers, HIV-related esophageal ulcers usually heal dramatically on treatment with oral steroids [95, 96]. Thus, endoscopy is required in HIV-positive patients with giant esophageal ulcers to differentiate esophagitis caused by HIV and CMV, so appropriate therapy can be instituted.

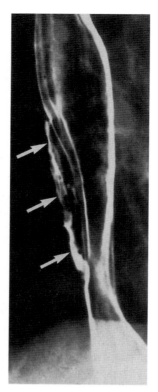

Figure 6.49 Cytomegalovirus (CMV) esophagitis in an acquired immunodeficiency syndrome (AIDS) patient. Double-contrast view shows a giant, flat ulcer (arrows) in the distal esophagus. Note the thin rim of edema abutting the ulcer. Because herpetic ulcers rarely become this large, the presence of one or more giant ulcers should be highly suggestive of CMV esophagitis in patients with AIDS (reproduced from Laufer I, Levine MS, eds. *Double Contrast Gastrointestinal Radiology*, 2nd edn. Philadelphia: WB Saunders, 1992, with permission).

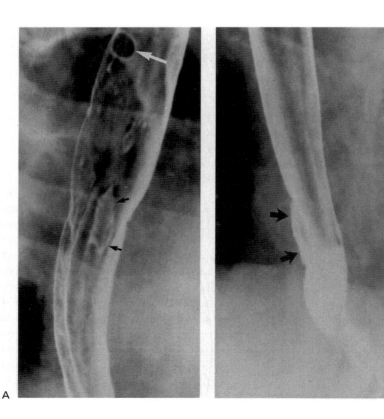

Figure 6.50 Human immunodeficiency virus (HIV) esophagitis in patients with acquired immunodeficiency syndrome (AIDS). (A) Double-contrast view shows a large diamond-shaped ulcer (black arrows) with a cluster of small satellite ulcers in the mid esophagus. The rounded filling defect (white arrow) proximally is an air bubble (reproduced from Levine *et al.* [95], with permission).
(B) Double-contrast view in another patient shows a large, flat ulcer (arrows) in profile in the distal esophagus. HIV ulcers are impossible to differentiate from cytomegalovirus ulcers on the basis of the radiographic findings, so endoscopy is required for a definitive diagnosis before treating these patients.

Drug-induced esophagitis

Tetracycline and its derivative, doxycycline, are two of the agents most commonly responsible for drug-induced esophagitis in the United States, but other offending medications include potassium chloride, quinidine, Aspirin or other non-steroidal anti-inflammatory drugs (NSAIDs), and alendronate [97]. Affected individuals typically ingest the medications with little or no water immediately before going to bed. The pills or capsules tend to become lodged in the upper or mid esophagus which is compressed by the adjacent aortic arch or left main bronchus. Prolonged contact of the esophageal mucosa with the pills presumably causes a focal contact esophagitis. These patients may present with severe odynophagia, but there is often marked clinical improvement after withdrawal of the offending agent.

The radiographic findings in drug-induced esophagitis depend on the nature of the offending medication. Tetracycline and doxycycline are associated with the development of small, superficial ulcers in the upper or mid esophagus indistinguishable from those in herpes esophagitis [98, 99] (Figure 6.51). Because of the superficial nature of the disease, these ulcers almost always heal without associated scarring or stricture formation. In contrast, potassium chloride, quinidine, and NSAIDs may cause more severe esophageal injury, sometimes leading to the development of much larger ulcers and subsequent strictures [100] (Figure 6.52). Alendronate may also cause a severe form of esophagitis with extensive ulceration and strictures, but these strictures are usually confined to the distal esophagus [101]. When drug-induced esophagitis is detected on barium studies, a repeat esophagram may be performed to document ulcer healing after withdrawal of the offending medication.

Idiopathic eosinophilic esophagitis

Idiopathic eosinophilic esophagitis (EoE) has been recognized as an increasingly common inflammatory condition of the esophagus, occurring predominantly in young men with long-standing dysphagia and recurrent food impactions, often associated with an atopic history and, occasionally, a peripheral eosinophilia [102]. The diagnosis of EoE can be confirmed on endoscopic biopsy specimens showing more

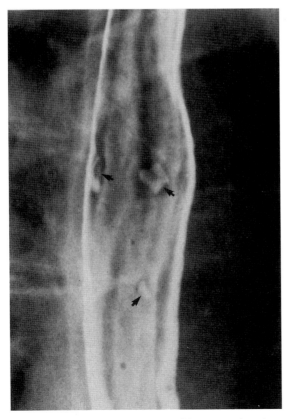

Figure 6.51 Drug-induced esophagitis. Double-contrast view shows several small, discrete ulcers (arrows) in the mid esophagus. This patient developed odynophagia after taking tetracycline. Herpes esophagitis could produce similar findings (reproduced from Levine MS. *Radiology of the Esophagus*. Philadelphia: WB Saunders, 1989, with permission).

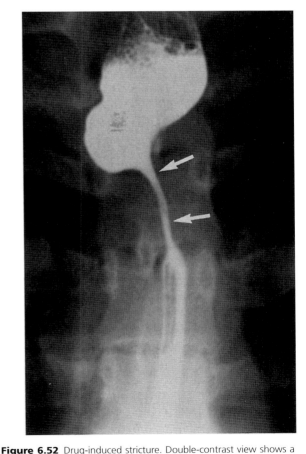

Figure 6.52 Drug-induced stricture. Double-contrast view shows a smooth, tapered stricture (arrows) in the upper thoracic esophagus caused by previous potassium chloride ingestion.

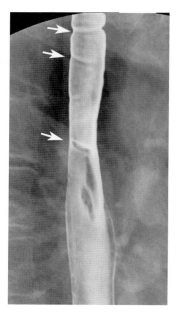

Figure 6.53 Idiopathic eosinophilic esophagitis with a "ringed esophagus." Double-contrast view shows a smooth, tapered stricture in the upper thoracic esophagus with distinctive ring-like indentations (arrows) in the region of the stricture.

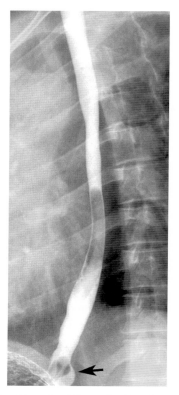

Figure 6.54 Idiopathic eosinophilic esophagitis with a "small-caliber esophagus." Prone single-contrast view shows a long segment of narrowing involving the entire thoracic esophagus with smooth contours and a mean diameter of less than 20 mm. Also note a small hiatal hernia (arrow).

than 20 eosinophils per high-power field [102, 103]. The etiology is uncertain, but many authors believe that EoE develops as an inflammatory response to ingested food allergens in predisposed individuals [102, 103]. As a result, symptomatic patients often have a marked clinical response to treatment with steroids or elemental diets.

The diagnosis of EoE may by suggested on barium studies by the presence of segmental esophageal strictures, sometimes associated with distinctive ring-like indentations, producing a so-called "ringed esophagus" [104] (Figure 6.53). The radiographic diagnosis may also be suggested by the development of a "small-caliber esophagus" manifested by a long but variable-length segment of narrowing in the thoracic esophagus that has smooth contours, tapered margins, and a mean diameter of 20 mm or less [105] (Figure 6.54), so 20 mm appears to be a useful threshold diameter for the diagnosis of EoE on barium studies.

Radiation esophagitis

A radiation dose of 5000 cGy or more to the mediastinum may cause severe injury to the esophagus. Acute radiation esophagitis usually occurs 2–4 weeks after the initiation of radiation therapy [106]. This condition may be manifested by ulceration or by a granular appearance of the mucosa and decreased distensibility resulting from edema and inflammation of the irradiated segment [106] (Figure 6.55A). The extent of disease conforms to the margins of the radiation

portal. Most cases of acute radiation esophagitis are self-limited, but some patients may have progressive dysphagia due to the development of radiation strictures 4–8 months after completion of radiation therapy [107]. These strictures typically appear as smooth, tapered areas of concentric narrowing within a pre-existing radiation portal (Figure 6.55B). Fistula formation is another uncommon complication of chronic radiation injury to the esophagus.

Caustic esophagitis

Whether accidental or intentional, ingestion of lye or other caustic agents can lead to a severe form of esophageal injury characterized by marked esophagitis and stricture formation. When esophagography is performed after a patient ingests a caustic agent, water-soluble contrast media should be used because of the risk of esophageal perforation. Such studies may reveal marked edema, spasm, and ulceration of the affected esophagus, and in some cases, esophageal disruption [108] (Figure 6.56). As the esophagitis heals, follow-up studies may reveal marked stricture formation, typically involving a long segment of the thoracic esophagus [108] (Figure 6.57). Patients with chronic lye strictures have an

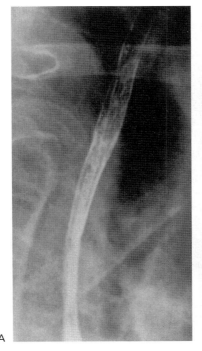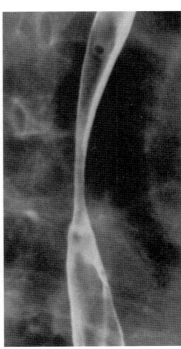

Figure 6.55 Radiation injury to the esophagus. (A) Double-contrast view shows decreased distensibility of the mid esophagus and a granular appearance of the mucosa caused by acute radiation esophagitis. (B) Double-contrast view from a follow-up study 6 months later shows a smooth, tapered area of narrowing in the mid esophagus due to the development of a radiation stricture (reproduced from Levine [108], with permission).

A

B

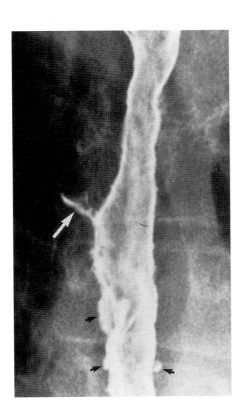

Figure 6.56 Acute caustic esophagitis. View of the esophagus with water-soluble contrast agent shows multiple ulcers (black arrows) and a sealed-off perforation with a small tract (white arrow) extending into the mediastinum. This patient ingested lye 2 days earlier.

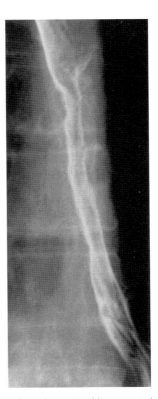

Figure 6.57 Chronic lye stricture. Double-contrast view shows a long stricture in the mid and distal esophagus caused by extensive scarring and fibrosis from lye ingestion many years earlier.

increased risk of developing squamous cell carcinoma of the esophagus [109], so a new area of mucosal irregularity or nodularity within a pre-existing lye stricture on barium studies should raise concern about the possibility of a superimposed carcinoma.

Other esophagitides

Alkaline reflux esophagitis is caused by reflux of bile or pancreatic secretions into the esophagus after partial or total gastrectomy [110]. The esophagitis is characterized on barium studies by mucosal nodularity or ulceration, or, in severe disease, by the development of distal esophageal strictures that may progress rapidly in length and severity over a short period of time [110]. The risk of developing alkaline reflux esophagitis can be decreased by performing a Roux-en-Y type of reconstruction to prevent or minimize reflux of bile or pancreatic secretions into the esophagus after partial or total gastrectomy.

Nasogastric intubation is an uncommon cause of esophagitis and stricture formation in the distal esophagus [108]. Most strictures develop after prolonged nasogastric intubation, but some patients have developed strictures from nasogastric tubes that were in place for as little as 48 h [108]. It has been postulated that these strictures result from severe reflux esophagitis caused by constant reflux of acid around the tube into the distal esophagus. Such strictures may progress rapidly in length and severity on follow-up barium studies [108].

Other uncommon causes of esophagitis include Crohn's disease, eosinophilic esophagitis, acute alcohol-induced esophagitis, chronic graft-versus-host disease, Behçet's disease, and, rarely, skin disorders involving the esophagus, such as epidermolysis bullosa dystrophica and benign mucous membrane pemphigoid [108].

Benign tumors

Papilloma

Squamous papillomas are uncommon benign mucosal tumors in the esophagus. These lesions consist histologically of a central fibrovascular core with multiple digit-like projections covered by hyperplastic squamous epithelium. Papillomas usually appear on double-contrast esophagography as small, sessile polyps with a smooth or slightly lobulated contour [111]. Occasionally, papillomas are difficult to distinguish from small esophageal cancers on the basis of the radiographic findings (Figure 6.58), so biopsy or resection of the lesions may be required. Some patients can have innumerable papillomas in the esophagus, a rare entity known as esophageal papillomatosis [112].

Adenoma

Esophageal adenomas are rare, benign lesions that usually arise in metaplastic columnar epithelium associated with

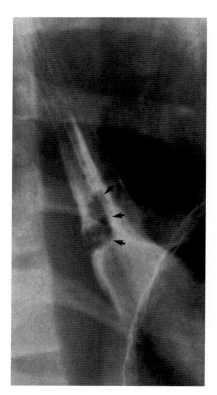

Figure 6.58 Squamous papilloma. Single-contrast view shows a small, lobulated mass (arrows) in the distal esophagus. A small esophageal cancer could produce similar findings.

Barrett's esophagus [112]. Because these lesions have the same potential for malignant degeneration as colonic adenomas, endoscopic or surgical resection is warranted. Adenomas typically appear on barium studies as sessile or pedunculated polyps in the distal esophagus at or near the GEJ [112]. Adenomatous polyps should be differentiated from inflammatory esophagogastric polyps, benign lesions in the distal esophagus that have no malignant potential (see above).

Glycogenic acanthosis

Glycogenic acanthosis is a benign condition in which there is accumulation of cytoplasmic glycogen in the squamous epithelial cells lining the esophagus, causing focal, plaque-like thickening of the mucosa [113]. It is a benign, degenerative condition, occurring primarily in elderly individuals. Glycogenic acanthosis can often be recognized on double-contrast studies by the presence of multiple small, rounded nodules or plaques in the mid or, less commonly, distal esophagus [114] (Figure 6.59). The major consideration in the differential diagnosis is *Candida* esophagitis. However, the plaques of candidiasis tend to have a more linear configuration and typically occur in immunocompromised patients with odynophagia, whereas glycogenic acanthosis

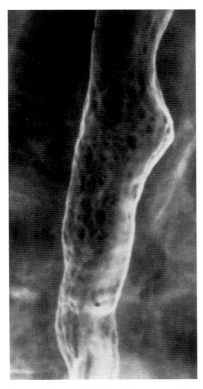

Figure 6.59 Glycogenic acanthosis. Double-contrast view shows multiple small, rounded plaques and nodules in the mid esophagus. Although *Candida* esophagitis could produce similar findings, this elderly patient was not immunocompromised and had no esophageal symptoms. The clinical history therefore is extremely helpful for differentiating these conditions (reproduced from Levine MS. *Radiology of the Esophagus*. Philadelphia: WB Saunders, 1989, with permission).

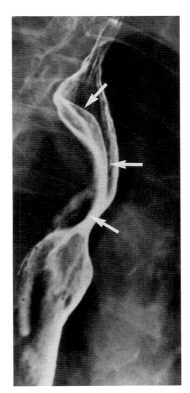

Figure 6.60 Leiomyoma. Double-contrast view shows a submucosal mass (arrows) in the upper thoracic esophagus. Note how the lesion has a smooth surface and forms slightly obtuse angles with the adjacent esophageal wall. These features are characteristic of a submucosal mass.

typically occurs in older individuals who are not immunocompromised and have no esophageal symptoms. Thus, it is usually possible to differentiate these conditions on the basis of the clinical and radiographic findings.

Leiomyoma

Leiomyomas are by far the most common benign submucosal tumors in the esophagus. Unlike gastrointestinal stromal tumors elsewhere, esophageal leiomyomas almost never undergo sarcomatous degeneration and, unlike gastrointestinal stromal tumors in the stomach, they are almost never ulcerated [112]. Patients with esophageal leiomyomas are usually asymptomatic but occasionally may present with dysphagia, depending on the size of the tumor and how much it encroaches on the lumen.

When esophageal leiomyomas grow exophytically into the mediastinum, they can sometimes be recognized on chest radiographs by the presence of a mass in the right superior mediastinum, occasionally containing punctate calcifications [112]. Esophageal leiomyomas are usually manifested on esophagography by a smooth submucosal mass, etched in white, that forms right angles or slightly obtuse angles with the adjacent esophageal wall when viewed in profile [112] (Figure 6.60). These lesions therefore may be indistinguishable on barium studies from other mesenchymal tumors such as granular cell tumors, lipomas, hemangiomas, fibromas, and neurofibromas, except that leiomyomas are more likely on empirical grounds. Occasionally, computed tomography (CT) may be helpful for differentiating submucosal esophageal masses from extrinsic tumors or lymphadenopathy in the mediastinum compressing the esophagus.

Fibrovascular polyp

Fibrovascular polyps are rare benign mesenchymal tumors characterized by the development of a pedunculated intraluminal mass that can grow to enormous sizes in the esophagus. These lesions consist histologically of varying amounts of fibrovascular and adipose tissue covered by

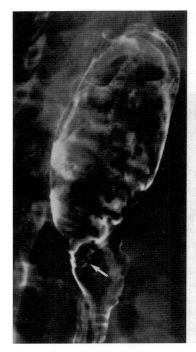
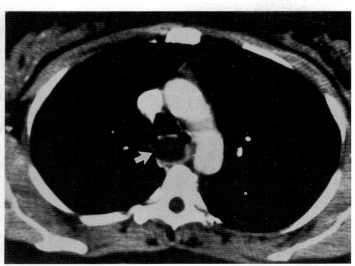

Figure 6.61 Giant fibrovascular polyp. (A) Double-contrast view shows a smooth, expansile, sausage-shaped mass in the upper thoracic esophagus (arrow denotes tip of polyp). (B) Computed tomography (CT) scan also shows an expansile mass (arrow) in the esophagus, with a thin rim of contrast surrounding the lesion, confirming its intraluminal location. Also note the predominantly fat density of the polyp. This CT finding is characteristic of fibrovascular polyps containing abundant adipose tissue (reproduced from Levine *et al.* [117], with permission).

normal squamous epithelium [115]. Fibrovascular polyps are almost always thought to arise near the level of the cricopharyngeus, gradually elongating over a period of years as they are dragged inferiorly by esophageal peristalsis [115]. Some of these polyps can become so large that they cause dysphagia or wheezing as a result of extrinsic compression of the trachea by the polyp. Rarely, these patients have a spectacular clinical presentation with regurgitation of a fleshy mass into the pharynx or mouth, or even asphyxia and sudden death if the regurgitated polyp occludes the larynx [116].

Fibrovascular polyps usually appear on esophagography as smooth, expansile, sausage-shaped masses that expand the lumen of the upper or mid esophagus [117] (Figure 6.61A). Occasionally, a discrete pedicle can be seen originating near the level of the cricopharyngeus. Fibrovascular polyps that contain a considerable amount of adipose tissue may appear as fat-density lesions on CT scan (Figure 6.61B), whereas fibrovascular polyps that contain varying amounts of fibrovascular and adipose tissue may have a heterogeneous appearance with areas of fat juxtaposed with areas of soft tissue density [117]. Thus, fibrovascular polyps may be manifested by a spectrum of findings on CT, depending on their predominant histologic components.

Duplication cyst

Duplication cysts are not true neoplasms, but they may also appear on esophagography as submucosal masses. Esophageal duplications cysts comprise about 20% of all duplication cysts in the gastrointestinal tract [112]. The cysts are development anomalies in which nests of cells are sequestered from the primitive foregut. Duplication cysts contain multiple layers of the bowel, including a mucosa, submucosa, and muscularis propria. Affected individuals are usually asymptomatic, but symptoms occasionally may be caused by bleeding or infection of the cyst. The cysts generally do not communicate with the esophageal lumen (so-called non-communicating cysts) and tend to be located in the right lower mediastinum. As a result, they can sometimes be recognized on frontal chest radiographs by the presence of a mass in the right lower mediastinum [112]. The cysts typically appear on barium studies as smooth submucosal masses indistinguishable from esophageal leiomyomas [112]. When duplication cysts do communicate with the esophageal lumen, they occasionally may be recognized as tubular, branching outpouchings from the esophagus that fill with barium [112] (Figure 6.62). These fluid-filled cysts usually appear as homogeneous low-attenuation structures on CT and as high-signal intensity structures on T2-weighted magnetic resonance imaging (MRI) [118].

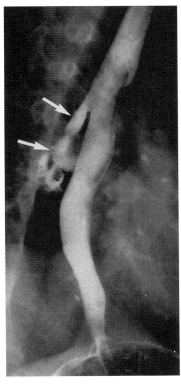

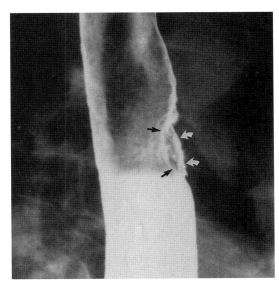

Figure 6.63 Early esophageal carcinoma. Double-contrast view shows a plaque-like lesion (black arrows) in the mid esophagus with a flat, central ulcer (white arrows).

Figure 6.62 Communicating esophageal duplication cyst. Single-contrast view shows a branching, tubular outpouching (arrows) from the midesophagus. This is a rare type of esophageal duplication cyst (reproduced from Levine [112], with permission).

Malignant tumors

Esophageal carcinoma

Esophageal carcinoma comprises about 1% of all cancers in the United States and 7% of all gastrointestinal tumors [119]. Patients with esophageal carcinoma usually present with dysphagia, but this is a late finding that generally develops only after the tumor has invaded periesophageal lymphatics or other mediastinal structures. As a result, most patients have advanced, unresectable lesions at the time of diagnosis, with overall 5-year survival rates of less than 10% [119]. Histologically, about 50% of these tumors are squamous cell carcinomas and the remaining 50% are adenocarcinomas [119].

Unlike squamous cell carcinomas of the esophagus, adenocarcinomas virtually always arise on a background of Barrett's mucosa in the esophagus. The reported prevalence of adenocarcinoma in patients with Barrett's esophagus is about 10% [119]. Studies using incidence rather than prevalence data indicate that the relative risk of adenocarcinoma developing in patients with Barrett's esophagus may be 30–40 times greater than that in the general population [120].

Early esophageal cancer is defined histologically as cancer limited to the mucosa or submucosa without lymph node metastases. Unlike advanced carcinoma, early esophageal cancer is a readily curable lesion with 5-year survival rates of about 90% [119]. As mentioned previously, early diagnosis of esophageal cancer is usually limited by the late onset of symptoms in patients with this disease. However, in a minority of patients, dysphagia or upper gastrointestinal bleeding develops while the tumor is still at an early stage. Patients with early adenocarcinoma arising in Barrett's mucosa may also seek medical attention because of their underlying reflux disease, so some early esophageal cancers may be detected fortuitously in patients with reflux symptoms [119].

Double-contrast esophagography has a sensitivity of greater than 95% in detecting esophageal cancer [121], a figure comparable to the reported endoscopic sensitivity of 95–100% when multiple brushings and biopsy specimens are obtained [119]. Early esophageal cancers are usually small, protruding lesions less than 3.5 cm in diameter. These tumors may be manifested on double-contrast studies by plaque-like lesions (often containing a flat central ulcer) (Figure 6.63), by sessile polyps with a smooth or slightly lobulated contour, or by focal irregularity of the esophageal wall [119, 122]. Early adenocarcinomas in Barrett's esophagus may also be manifested by a localized area of wall flattening or irregularity within a pre-existing peptic stricture [119] (Figure 6.64). Superficial spreading carcinoma is another form of early esophageal cancer characterized on double-contrast studies by a confluent area of poorly defined mucosal nodules or plaques that merge with one another [119, 122] (Figure

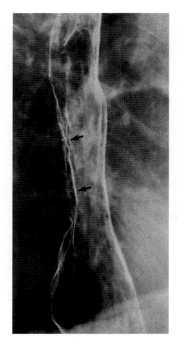

Figure 6.64 Early adenocarcinoma in Barrett's esophagus. Double-contrast view shows a long peptic stricture in the distal esophagus above a hiatal hernia. Also note irregular flattening (arrows) of one wall of the stricture. Endoscopic and surgical biopsy specimens revealed an early adenocarcinoma arising in Barrett's esophagus (reproduced from Levine *et al.* [125], with permission).

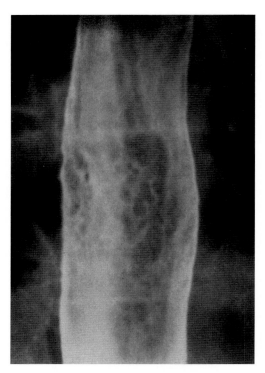

Figure 6.65 Superficial spreading carcinoma. Double-contrast view shows focal nodularity of the mucosa in the mid esophagus. Note how the nodules are poorly defined, producing a confluent area of disease. This appearance should be highly suspicious for a superficial spreading carcinoma (reproduced from Levine MS. *Radiology of the Esophagus*. Philadelphia: WB Saunders, 1989, with permission).

6.65). Although these lesions can sometimes be confused with focal *Candida* esophagitis, the plaques in candidiasis tend to be discrete lesions with normal intervening mucosa, whereas the nodules in superficial spreading carcinoma tend to coalesce, producing a continuous area of disease.

Advanced esophageal carcinomas usually appear on barium studies as infiltrating, polypoid, ulcerative, or, less commonly, varicoid lesions [119]. Infiltrating carcinomas are manifested by irregular luminal narrowing with mucosal nodularity or ulceration and abrupt, often shelf-like borders (Figure 6.66). Polypoid carcinomas appear as lobulated intraluminal masses (Figure 6.67). Primary ulcerative carcinomas are manifested by a giant, meniscoid ulcer surrounded by a radiolucent rind of tumor [123] (Figure 6.68). Finally, varicoid carcinomas are those in which submucosal spread of tumor produces thickened, tortuous longitudinal defects, mimicking the appearance of varices [124]. However, varicoid tumors have a fixed configuration, whereas varices tend to change in size and shape at fluoroscopy. Also, varices rarely cause dysphagia because they are soft and compressible. Thus, it is usually possible to differentiate varices from varicoid tumors on the basis of the clinical and radiographic findings.

Squamous cell carcinomas and adenocarcinomas of the esophagus cannot be reliably differentiated on esophagography. Nevertheless, squamous cell carcinomas tend to involve the upper or mid esophagus, whereas adenocarcinomas are located predominantly in the distal esophagus (Figure 6.69). Unlike squamous cell carcinomas, esophageal adenocarcinomas also have a marked tendency to invade the gastric cardia or fundus, comprising as many as 50% of all malignant tumors involving the GEJ [125, 126].

Esophageal carcinomas tend to metastasize to other parts of the esophagus via a rich network of submucosal lymphatic channels. These lymphatic metastases may appear as polypoid, plaque-like, or ulcerated lesions separated from the primary lesion by normal intervening mucosa [119]. Tumor may also spread subdiaphragmatically to the proximal portion of the stomach via submucosal esophageal lymphatic vessels. These metastases to the gastric cardia and fundus may appear as large submucosal masses, often containing central areas of ulceration [127].

Appropriate treatment strategies for esophageal carcinoma depend on accurate staging of the tumor. Various imaging techniques such as CT, MRI, and endoscopic sonography are used for staging esophageal carcinoma [119]. The

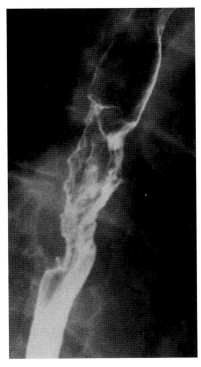

Figure 6.66 Infiltrating squamous cell carcinoma. Double-contrast view shows an irregular area of narrowing in the mid esophagus with nodularity and ulceration of the narrowed segment. Also note the abrupt, shelf-like margins of the lesion.

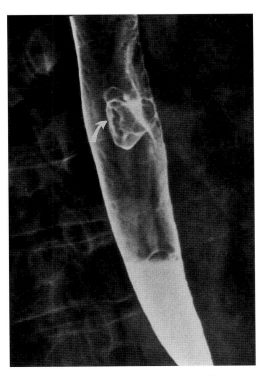

Figure 6.67 Polypoid squamous cell carcinoma. Double-contrast view shows a polypoid mass (arrow) in the mid esophagus.

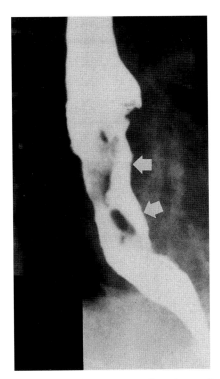

Figure 6.68 Primary ulcerative squamous cell carcinoma. Double-contrast view shows a large, meniscoid ulcer (arrows) surrounded by a thick rind of tumor in the distal esophagus (reproduced from Levine MS. *Radiology of the Esophagus*. Philadelphia: WB Saunders, 1989, with permission).

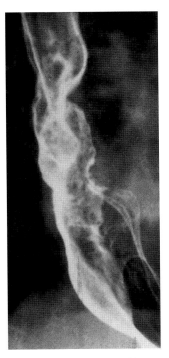

Figure 6.69 Infiltrating adenocarcinoma. Double-contrast view shows an irregular area of narrowing in the distal esophagus. Note how the lesion extends into proximal edge of hiatal hernia. This patient had an adenocarcinoma arising in Barrett's esophagus (reproduced from Levine MS. *Radiology of the esophagus*. Philadelphia: WB Saunders, 1989, with permission).

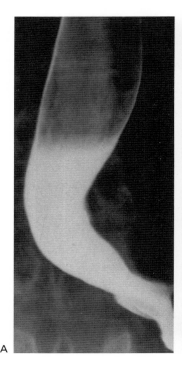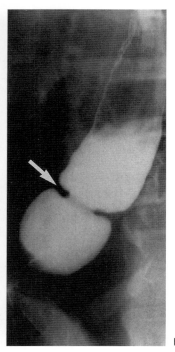

A B

Figure 6.70 Schatzki ring. (A) Double-contrast view shows no evidence of a ring in the distal esophagus, but the region abutting the gastroesophageal junction is not optimally distended. (B) Prone single-contrast view from the same examination shows a smooth, symmetric ring-like constriction (arrow) at the gastroesophageal junction above a hiatal hernia. This Schatzki ring caused intermittent dysphagia for solids.

tumor stage is assessed by evaluating the depth of esophageal wall invasion and the presence or absence of lymphatic or distant metastases.

Other malignant tumors

Non-Hodgkin's lymphoma and, rarely, Hodgkin's lymphoma may involve the esophagus. Esophageal lymphoma may be manifested on barium studies by submucosal masses, polypoid lesions, enlarged folds, or strictures [128]. Spindle cell carcinoma is another rare tumor characterized by a bulky, polypoid intraluminal mass that expands the lumen of the esophagus without causing obstruction [129]. Other rare malignant tumors involving the esophagus include leiomyosarcoma, malignant melanoma, and Kaposi's sarcoma [128].

Lower esophageal rings

Lower esophageal rings are a common finding on esophagography, but only a small percentage of patients are symptomatic. The term Schatzki ring should be reserved for symptomatic lower esophageal rings in patients who present with dysphagia. These rings almost always occur at the GEJ. Histologically, the superior surface of the ring is lined by stratified squamous epithelium and the inferior surface by columnar epithelium. The exact pathogenesis of Schatzki rings is uncertain, but some rings are thought to develop as a result of scarring from reflux esophagitis.

Symptomatic lower esophageal rings typically appear on barium studies as 2–3-mm high, symmetric, web-like constrictions (usually <13 mm in diameter) at the GEJ above a hiatal hernia (Figure 6.70). The rings can be missed if the distal esophagus is not adequately distended at fluoroscopy (Figure 6.70A), so it is important to obtain prone views of the esophagus during continuous drinking of a low-density barium suspension in order to visualize these structures (Figure 6.70B). Studies have shown that biphasic esophagography is a sensitive technique for the diagnosis of symptomatic lower esophageal rings, occasionally detecting rings that are missed on endoscopy [130].

Diverticula

Esophageal diverticula may be classified as pulsion or traction diverticula. The more common pulsion diverticula result from esophageal dysmotility with increased intraluminal pressures in the esophagus, whereas traction diverticula are caused by scarring in the soft tissues surrounding the esophagus. Diverticula most commonly occur in the region of the pharyngoesophageal junction (i.e. Zenker's diverticulum), mid esophagus, and distal esophagus above the GEJ (i.e. epiphrenic diverticulum). Other patients may develop tiny outpouchings from the esophagus, known as esophageal intramural pseudodiverticula.

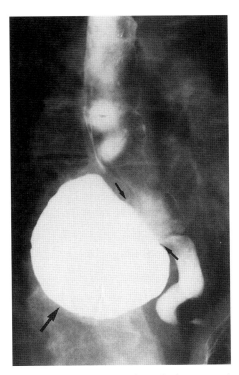

Figure 6.71 Giant epiphrenic diverticulum. Single-contrast view shows a large epiphrenic diverticulum (large arrow) arising from the right lateral wall of the distal esophagus. Note the wide neck (small arrows) of the diverticulum.

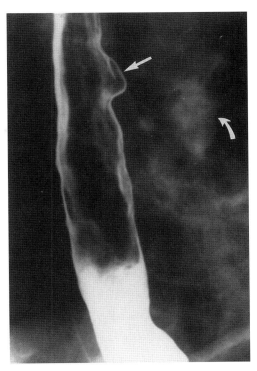

Figure 6.72 Traction diverticulum. Double-contrast view shows a triangular outpouching (straight arrow) from the left lateral wall of the mid esophagus. Also note a clump of calcified lymph nodes (curved arrow) in the adjacent pulmonary hilum. This traction diverticulum presumably was caused by scarring from old tuberculous disease in the mediastinum.

Pulsion diverticula

Pulsion diverticula tend to be located in the distal esophagus and are often associated with fluoroscopic or manometric evidence of esophageal dysmotility. The diverticula are usually detected as incidental findings in patients who have no esophageal symptoms. However, a large epiphrenic diverticulum adjacent to the GEJ may fill with debris, causing dysphagia, regurgitation, or aspiration (Figure 6.71). Pulsion diverticula appear on barium studies as rounded outpouchings from the esophageal lumen that have wide necks. They often do not empty completely when the esophagus collapses and may be associated with other radiologic findings of esophageal motor dysfunction.

Traction diverticula

Traction diverticula occur in the mid esophagus and are usually caused by scarring from tuberculosis or histoplasmosis involving perihilar or subcarinal lymph nodes. Traction diverticula are true diverticula containing all layers of the esophageal wall and therefore maintain their elastic recoil. As a result, they tend to empty their contents when the esophagus collapses at fluoroscopy. Traction diverticula often have a triangular or tented appearance resulting from traction on the diverticulum by the fibrotic process in the adjacent mediastinum (Figure 6.72). Thus, it is often possible to distinguish traction diverticula from pulsion diverticula on the basis of the radiographic findings.

Esophageal intramural pseudodiverticula

Esophageal intramural pseudodiverticula consist pathologically of dilated excretory ducts of deep mucous glands in the esophagus. The pseudodiverticula typically appear on esophagography as flask-shaped outpouchings in longitudinal rows parallel to the long axis of the esophagus [131] (Figure 6.73A). The pseudodiverticula classically have a diffuse distribution in the esophagus and are sometimes associated with strictures in the upper or mid esophagus [131]. However, it is more common to have an isolated cluster of pseudodiverticula in the distal esophagus in the region of a peptic stricture [131] (Figure 6.73B). In such cases, the pseudodiverticula most likely occur as a sequela of scarring from reflux esophagitis.

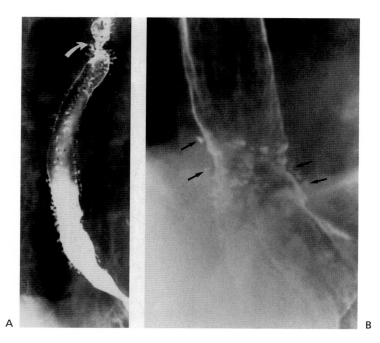

A

B

Figure 6.73 Esophageal intramural pseudodiverticulosis. (A) Double-contrast view shows multiple flask-shaped outpouchings throughout the esophagus in a patient with diffuse esophageal intramural pseudodiverticulosis. Also note a focal stricture (arrow) in the upper thoracic esophagus. (B) Double-contrast view in another patient shows a mild peptic stricture in the distal esophagus with multiple pseudodiverticula clustered together in the region of the stricture. When viewed *en face*, the pseudodiverticula could be mistaken for tiny ulcers. When viewed in profile, however, these structures (arrows) appear to be "floating" outside the esophagus without communicating with the lumen. This feature is characteristic of pseudodiverticula (reproduced from Levine MS. *Radiology of the Esophagus*. Philadelphia: WB Saunders, 1989, with permission).

When viewed *en face* on double-contrast esophagrams, esophageal intramural pseudodiverticula can sometimes be mistaken for tiny ulcers. When viewed in profile, however, they often appear to be "floating" or "levitating" outside the wall of the esophagus without any apparent communication with the lumen [131] (Figure 6.73B), whereas true esophageal ulcers are almost always seen to communicate directly with the lumen. This sign is extremely helpful for differentiating esophageal intramural pseudodiverticula from ulcers.

Esophageal motility disorders

Achalasia

Achalasia can be classified as primary when it occurs as an idiopathic condition involving the myenteric plexus of the esophagus or as secondary when it is caused by other underlying conditions, most commonly malignant tumor involving the GEJ (especially carcinoma of the gastric cardia and fundus). Primary achalasia is characterized by absent primary peristalsis in the body of the esophagus and incomplete relaxation of the lower esophageal sphincter, manifested on barium studies by tapered, beak-like narrowing of the distal esophagus directly adjacent to the GEJ [132] (Figure 6.74). In advanced disease, the esophagus can become massively dilated and tortuous distally (also known as a "sigmoid esophagus"). Because of the slow, insidious progression of symptoms, affected individuals typically have longstanding dysphagia when they seek medical attention.

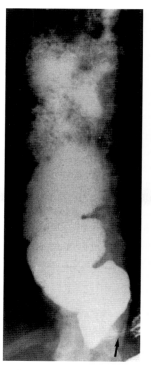

Figure 6.74 Primary achalasia. Single-contrast esophagram shows a markedly dilated esophagus filled with debris. Also note the beak-like narrowing (arrow) of the distal esophagus near the gastroesophageal junction in this patient with longstanding achalasia.

In contrast, secondary achalasia usually results from tumor at the GEJ that simulates the findings of primary achalasia because of destruction of ganglion cells in the distal esophagus. As a result, secondary achalasia is also characterized by absent peristalsis in the body of the esophagus and beak-like narrowing near the GEJ. In secondary achalasia, however, the length of the narrowed segment is often considerably greater than that in primary achalasia because of spread of tumor into the distal esophagus [133] (Figure 6.75). The narrowed segment also may be asymmetric, nodular, or ulcerated because of underlying tumor in this region. In some cases, barium studies may reveal other signs of malignancy in the region of the gastric cardia and fundus. The clinical history also is extremely helpful, as patients with primary achalasia almost always have longstanding dysphagia, whereas patients with secondary achalasia are usually older individuals (older than 60 years of age) with recent onset of dysphagia (<6 months) and weight loss [133]. Thus, it is often possible to differentiate these conditions on the basis of the clinical and radiographic findings.

Diffuse esophageal spasm

Patients with diffuse esophageal spasm typically present with recurrent chest pain, dysphagia, or both. Diffuse esophageal spasm is sometimes manifested on barium studies by intermittently absent or weakened primary esophageal peristalsis with simultaneous, lumen-obliterating, non-peristaltic contractions that compartmentalize the esophagus, producing a classic corkscrew appearance [132] (Figure 6.76A). In a study by Prabhakar *et al.*, however, most patients had non-peristaltic contractions of mild-to-moderate severity that did not obliterate the lumen [134], so the absence of a corkscrew esophagus on barium studies in no way excludes this diagnosis. It has also been found that the majority of patients with diffuse esophageal spasm have impaired opening of the lower esophageal sphincter on barium studies with the tapered, beak-like distal esophageal narrowing classically associated with achalasia [134] (Figure 6.76B). When these patients present with dysphagia, they may have a marked clinical response to treatment with the *Clostridium botulinum* toxin or endoscopic balloon dilatation [134]. Achalasia and diffuse esophageal spasm therefore may represent opposite ends of a spectrum of related esophageal motility disorders.

Presbyesophagus

Older patients often have intermittent weakening of primary peristalsis and multiple non-peristaltic contractions in the

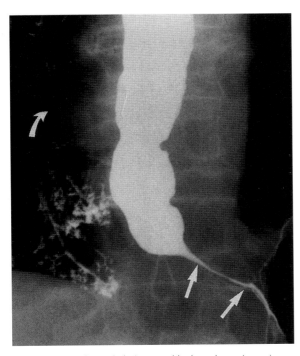

Figure 6.75 Secondary achalasia caused by bronchogenic carcinoma. Double-contrast view shows a mildly dilated esophagus with a beak-like distal narrowing (straight arrows). Unlike the patient with primary achalasia in Figure 6.74, however, the narrowed segment extends 4–5 cm above the gastroesophageal junction. Also note the large mass (curved arrow) abutting the right side of the mediastinum in a patient with bronchogenic carcinoma that had metastasized to the gastroesophageal junction. (Aspirated barium is seen in the right lung.) (reproduced from Levine MS. *Radiology of the esophagus*. Philadelphia: WB Saunders, 1989, with permission).

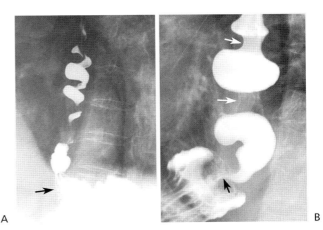

Figure 6.76 Diffuse esophageal spasm. (A) Prone single-contrast view shows multiple lumen-obliterating, non-peristaltic contractions that compartmentalize the esophagus, producing the classic corkscrew appearance associated with diffuse esophageal spasm. Note the presence of a small hiatal hernia (black arrow). (B) Prone single-contrast view in another patient shows multiple non-peristaltic contractions of mild-to-moderate severity (white arrows) with a tapered, beak-like narrowing of the distal esophagus (black arrow) secondary to lower esophageal sphincter dysfunction. This patient has diffuse esophageal spasm with impaired opening of the lower esophageal sphincter. Again note the presence of a small hiatal hernia.

absence of esophageal symptoms, a relatively common manifestation of aging known as presbyesophagus [132]. In other normal patients, there may be splitting of the barium column at or near the level of the aortic arch with retrograde flow of a portion of the bolus because of weakening of the amplitude of primary peristalsis at the transition zone between the striated and smooth muscle portions of the esophagus, a clinically trivial phenomenon known as "proximal escape" [132].

Varices

Esophageal varices may be classified as "uphill" or "downhill". Uphill varices are caused by portal hypertension with increased pressure in the portal venous system transmitted upward via dilated esophageal collaterals to the superior vena cava. In contrast, downhill varices are caused by superior vena cava obstruction with downward flow via dilated esophageal collaterals to the portal venous system and inferior vena cava. Uphill varices are much more common than downhill varices. Whether uphill or downhill, varices are important because of the risk of upper gastrointestinal bleeding.

Uphill varices

Uphill esophageal varices develop as a result of portal hypertension or other causes of portal venous obstruction. Varices appear on barium studies as serpiginous or tortuous longitudinal filling defects in the distal half of the thoracic esophagus [135] (Figure 6.77). They are best seen on mucosal

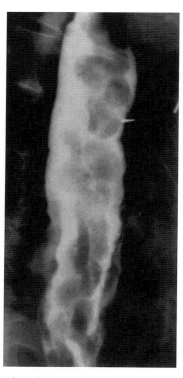

Figure 6.77 Esophageal varices. Single-contrast view shows multiple large serpiginous defects in the lower third of the esophagus in a patient with portal hypertension and uphill esophageal varices.

relief views of the collapsed or partially collapsed esophagus using a high-density barium suspension to increase mucosal adherence [135]. The differential diagnosis for varices includes submucosally infiltrating esophageal carcinomas (so-called varicoid carcinomas) and esophagitis with thickened folds caused by submucosal edema and inflammation.

Esophageal varices are characterized on CT by a thickened, lobulated esophageal wall containing tubular structures that enhance markedly after intravenous administration of contrast material [135]. Additional varices may be seen elsewhere in the abdomen at other sites of communication between the portal and systemic venous circulations. Angiography of the celiac or superior mesenteric arteries can be used to confirm the presence of varices in and around the distal esophagus. However, the need for portal venography for presurgical planning of portosystemic shunts has decreased with the widespread use of transjugular intrahepatic portosystemic shunting procedures.

Downhill varices

One of the most common causes of downhill varices is bronchogenic carcinoma with mediastinal metastases and superior vena cava obstruction [135]. Additional causes include other primary or metastatic tumors involving the mediastinum, mediastinal irradiation, sclerosing mediastinitis, substernal goiter, and central catheter-related thrombosis of the superior vena cava. Most patients with downhill varices present clinically with the superior vena cava syndrome.

Downhill varices typically appear as serpiginous longitudinal filling defects, which, unlike uphill esophageal varices, are confined to the upper or mid esophagus [135]. Venography may be performed to confirm the presence of superior vena cava obstruction, and chest radiographs or CT may be performed to determine the underlying cause.

Foreign body impactions

In adults, esophageal foreign body impactions most commonly are caused by inadequately chewed pieces of meat. Most of these foreign bodies pass spontaneously into the stomach, but 10–20% require some form of therapeutic intervention [136]. The risk of perforation is less than 1% during the first 24 h, but this risk increases substantially after 24 h because of ischemia and pressure necrosis at the site of impaction [136]. Affected individuals typically present with acute onset of dysphagia and substernal chest pain.

Contrast studies are often performed in patients with suspected food impaction to confirm the presence of obstruction, to determine its level, and to rule out esophageal perforation. An impacted food bolus typically appears as a

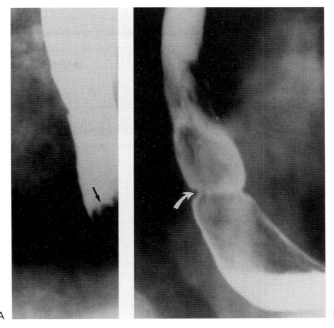

Figure 6.78 Esophageal food impaction. (A) On the initial barium study, an impacted bolus of meat in the distal esophagus appears as a polypoid defect (arrows) with complete obstruction at this level. (B) A repeat study 10 days after endoscopic removal of the bolus reveals a lower esophageal ring (arrow) as the cause of the impaction.

polypoid defect with an irregular meniscus superiorly [136] (Figure 6.78A). Because of the degree of obstruction, it may be difficult to assess the underlying esophagus at the time of impaction. It is therefore prudent to perform a follow-up barium study after the impaction has been relieved to determine whether the impaction was caused by a pathologic area of narrowing (Figure 6.78B). The most common causes are Schatzki rings and peptic strictures [136].

Intravenous glucagon may be used to relax the lower esophageal sphincter and facilitate passage of an impacted bolus from the distal esophagus into the stomach [137]. Effervescent agents may also help to distend the esophagus, promoting passage of the bolus [137]. Over time, however, pressure necrosis may develop at the site of impaction, so gas-forming agents should be avoided if the obstruction has been present more than 24 h because of an increased risk of perforation. Combination therapy with intravenous glucagon, an effervescent agent, and water has a success rate of 70% in relieving esophageal food impactions without need for endoscopic intervention [137].

Fistulae

Esophageal–airway fistulae most commonly result from direct invasion of the tracheobronchial tree by advanced esophageal carcinoma (Figure 6.79). Such fistulae have been reported in 5–10% of all patients with esophageal

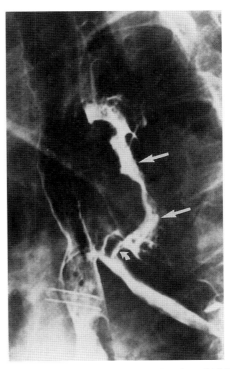

Figure 6.79 Esophageal carcinoma with esophagobronchial fistula. A barium study shows an advanced infiltrating squamous cell carcinoma of the mid esophagus (straight arrows) with an esophagobronchial fistula (curved arrow).

cancer, often occurring after treatment with radiation therapy [136]. Other causes of esophageal-airway fistulae include esophageal instrumentation, trauma, foreign bodies, and surgery. Affected individuals typically present with violent episodes of coughing and choking during deglutition. When an esophageal-airway fistula is suspected on clinical grounds, barium should be used instead of water-soluble contrast agents, because these hyperosmolar agents may cause severe pulmonary edema if a fistula is present [136].

Esophagopleural fistulae may be caused by esophageal carcinoma, radiation therapy, surgery, or instrumentation [136]. Such patients may present with a pleural effusion, pneumothorax, or hydropneumothorax. When an esophago-pleural fistula is suspected, the presence and location of the fistula can be confirmed by a study with water-soluble contrast agents.

Aortoesophageal fistulae are extremely rare but are associated with a high mortality rate. Such fistulae may be caused by a ruptured aortic aneurysm, aortic dissection, infected aortic graft, swallowed foreign body, or esophageal carcinoma [138]. Patients with aortoesophageal fistulae may present with an initial episode of arterial hematemesis followed by a variable latent period, before experiencing massive hematemesis, exsanguination, and death [138]. Oral studies with water-soluble contrast agents are unlikely to show the fistula because of high aortic pressures, whereas contrast aortography may fail to show the fistula because of occlusion of the fistulous tract by thrombus [138].

Perforation

If untreated, perforation of the thoracic esophagus is associated with a mortality rate of nearly 100% because of a fulminant mediastinitis that occurs in these patients [136]. Early diagnosis is therefore critical. Endoscopy is the most common cause of esophageal perforation, accounting for up to 75% of cases [136]. Other causes include foreign bodies, food impactions, penetrating and blunt trauma, and spontaneous esophageal perforation resulting from a sudden, rapid increase in intraluminal esophageal pressure (Boerhaave's syndrome).

Cervical esophageal perforation may be manifested on neck or chest radiographs by subcutaneous emphysema, retropharyngeal air, and pneumomediastinum [136]. Lateral radiographs of the neck may also show widening of the prevertebral space or a retropharyngeal abscess containing loculated gas or air–fluid levels. In contrast, thoracic esophageal perforation may be associated with pneumomediastinum, mediastinal widening, and a pleural effusion or hydropneumothorax [136]. In the proper setting, the presence of mediastinal gas on CT should be highly suggestive of esophageal perforation, whereas other findings such as pleural effusion

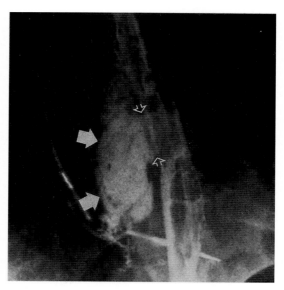

Figure 6.80 Esophageal perforation after traumatic endoscopy. A study with a water-soluble contrast agent shows focal extravasation of contrast from the right lateral wall of the mid esophagus (open arrows) into the right side of the mediastinum (closed arrows).

or mediastinal fluid are less specific [136]. However, CT is unreliable for determining the site of perforation.

Esophagography is often performed on patients with suspected esophageal perforation. Some patients may have free leaks into the mediastinum (Figure 6.80), whereas others may have small, sealed-off leaks. Although barium is the most sensitive contrast agent for detecting small leaks, it can potentially cause a granulomatous reaction in the mediastinum. In contrast, water-soluble agents do not incite a mediastinal reaction and are readily absorbed from the mediastinum if a leak is present. However, water-soluble contrast agents are less radio-opaque than barium and can miss a substantial percentage of esophageal perforations [136]. It is therefore recommended that the examination be repeated with barium to detect subtle leaks if the initial study with water-soluble contrast media shows no evidence of perforation [136].

References

1. DuBrul EL. *Sicher's Oral Anatomy*, 7th edn. St Louis: CV Mosby, 1980, pp. 319–350.
2. Rubesin SE, Jesserun J, Robertson D, *et al*. Lines of the pharynx. *RadioGraphics* 1987;7:217–237.
3. Rubesin SE, Rabischong P, Bilaniuk IT, *et al*. Contrast examination of the soft palate with cross-sectional correlation. *Radio-Graphics* 1988;4:641–665.

4. Pitman RG, Fraser GM. The post-cricoid impression of the esophagus. *Clin Radiol* 1965;16:34–39.

5. Donner MW, Bosma JF, Robertson DL. Anatomy and physiology of the pharynx. *Gastrointest Radiol* 1985;10: 196–212.

6. Rubesin SE. Pharynx: normal anatomy and techniques. In: Gore RM, Levine MS, Laufer I, eds. *Textbook of Gastrointestinal Radiology*. Philadelphia: WB Saunders, 1994, pp. 202–225.

7. Dodds WJ. The physiology of swallowing. *Dysphagia* 1989;3:171–178.

8. Dodds WJ, Stewart ET, Logemann JA. Physiology and radiology of the normal oral and pharyngeal phases of swallowing. *AJR Am J Roentgenol* 1990;154:953–963.

9. Rubesin SE, Stiles TD. Principles of performing a "modified barium swallow" examination. In: Balfe DM, Levine MS, eds. *Categorical Course in Diagnostic Radiology: Gastrointestinal*. Oak Brook, IL: RSNA Publications, 1997, pp. 7–20.

10. Rubesin SE. Pharyngeal dysfunction. In: Gore R, ed. *Syllabus for Categorical Course on Gastrointestinal Radiology*. Reston, VA: American College of Radiology, 1991, pp. 1–9.

11. Dodds WJ, Taylor AJ, Stewart ET, *et al*. Tipper and dipper types of oral swallows. *AJR Am J Roentgenol* 1989;153: 1197–1199.

12. Logemann JA. Effects of aging on the swallowing mechanism. *Otolaryngol Clin North Am* 1990;23:1045–1056.

13. Doty RW, Bosma JF. An electromyographic analysis of reflex deglutition. *J Neurophysiol* 1956;19:44–60.

14. Buchholz DW. Neurologic causes of dysphagia. *Dysphagia* 1987;1:152–156.

15. Buchholz DW. Dysphagia associated with neurological disorders. *Acta Otorhinolaryngol Belg* 1994;48:143–155.

16. Robbins J, Levine RL. Swallowing after unilateral stroke of the cerebral cortex; preliminary evidence. *Dysphagia* 1988;3:11–17.

17. Buchholz DW Clinically-probable brainstem stroke presenting primarily as dysphagia and non-visualized by MRI. *Dysphagia* 1993;8:235–238.

18. Leopold NA, Kagel MC. Pharyngo-esophageal dysphagia in Parkinson's disease. *Dysphagia* 1997;12:11–18.

19. Bosma JF, Brodie DR. Disabilities of the pharynx in ALS demonstrated by cineradiography. *Radiology* 1969;92:97–103.

20. Bosma JF. Studies of disability of the pharynx resultant from poliomyelitis. *Ann Otol Rhinol Laryngol* 1953;62:529–547.

21. Buchholz D, Jones B. Dysphagia occurring after polio. *Dysphagia* 1991;6:165–169.

22. Branski D, Levy J, Globus M, *et al*. Dysphagia as a primary manifestation of hyperthyroidism. *J Clin Gastroenterol* 1984;6: 437–440.

23. Rubesin SE, Glick SN. The tailored double-contrast pharyngogram. *Crit Rev Diagn Imaging* 1988;28:133–179.

24. Rubesin SE. Pharynx. In: Laufer I, Levine MS, eds. *Double Contrast Gastrointestinal Radiology*, 2nd edn. Philadelphia: WB Saunders, 1992, pp. 73–105.

25. Zaino C, Jacobson HG, Lepow H, *et al*. The pharyngoesophageal sphincter. *Radiology* 1967;89:639–645.

26. Zaino C, Jacobson HG, Lepow H, *et al*. *The Pharyngoesophageal Sphincter*. Springfield, IL: Charles C. Thomas, 1970.

27. Frieling T, Berges W, Lubke HJ, *et al*. Upper esophageal sphincter function in patients with Zenker's diverticulum. *Dysphagia* 1988;3:90–92.

28. Knuff TE, Benjamin SB, Castell DO. Pharyngoesophageal (Zenker's) diverticulum: a reappraisal. *Gastroenterology* 1982; 82:734–736.

29. Smiley TB, Caves PK, Porter DC. Relationship between posterior pharyngeal pouch and hiatus hernia. *Thorax* 1970;25: 725–731.

30. Delahunty JE, Margulies SE, Alonso UA, *et al*. The relationship of reflux esophagitis to pharyngeal pouch (Zenker's diverticulum). *Laryngoscope* 1971;81:570–577.

31. Rubesin SE. Structural abnormalities of the pharynx. In: Gore RM, Levine MS, eds. *Textbook of Gastrointestinal Radiology*, 2nd edn. Philadelphia: WB Saunders, 2000, pp. 227–255.

32. Shirazi KK, Daffner RH, Gaede JT. Ulcer occurring in Zenker's diverticulum. *Gastrointest Radiol* 1977;2:117–118.

33. Wychulis AR, Gunnulaugsson GH, Clagett OT. Carcinoma arising in pharyngoesophageal diverticulum. *Surgery* 1969;66: 970–979.

34. Brady AP, Stevenson GW, Somers S, *et al*. Premature contraction of the cricopharyngeus: new sign of gastroesophageal reflux disease. *Abdom Imaging* 1995;20:225–228.

35. Ekberg O, Nylander G. Lateral diverticula from the pharyngoesophageal junction area. *Radiology* 1983;146:117–122.

36. Rubesin SE, Levine MS. Killian-Jamieson diverticula: radiographic findings in 16 patients. *AJR Am J Roentgenol* 2001; 177:85–89.

37. Bachman AL, Seaman WB, Macken KL. Lateral pharyngeal diverticula. *Radiology* 1968;91:774–782.

38. Curtis DJ, Cruess DF, Crain M, *et al*. Lateral pharyngeal outpouchings: a comparison of dysphagic and asymptomatic patients. *Dysphagia* 1988;2:150–161.

39. Lindbichler F, Raith J, Uggowitzer M, *et al*. Aspiration resulting from lateral hypopharyngeal pouches. *AJR Am J Roentgenol* 1998;170:129–132.

40. Hyams VJ, Batsakis JG, Michaels L. Tumors of the upper respiratory tract and ear. In: *Atlas of Tumor Pathology*, second series, fascicle 25. Bethesda: Armed Forces Institute of Pathology, 1988.

41. Bosma JF, Gravkowski EA, Tryostad CW. Chronic ulcerative pharyngitis. *Arch Otolaryngol* 1968;87:85–96.

42. Gromet M, Homer MJ, Carter BL. Lymphoid hyperplasia at the base of the tongue. *Radiology* 1982;144:825–828.

43. Bachman AL. Benign, non-neoplastic conditions of the larynx and pharynx. *Radiol Clin North Am* 1978;16:273–290.

44. Clements JL, Cox GW, Torres WE, *et al*. Cervical esophageal webs-a roentgen-anatomic correlation. *AJR Am J Roentgenol* 1974;121:221–231.

45. Nosher JL, Campbell WL, Seaman WB. The clinical significance of cervical esophageal and hypopharyngeal webs. *Radiology* 1975;117:45–47.

46. Seaman WB. The significance of webs in the hypopharynx and upper esophagus. *Radiology* 1967;89:32–38.

47. Ekberg O. Cervical oesophageal webs in patients with dysphagia. *Clin Radiol* 1981;32:633–641.

48. Ekberg O, Nylander G. Webs and web-like formations in the pharynx and cervical esophagus. *Diagn Imaging* 1983;52: 10–18.

49. Gordon AR, Levine MS, Redfern RO, *et al.* Cervical esophageal webs: association with gastroesophageal reflux. *Abdom Imaging* 2001;26:574–577.

50. Shauffer IA, Phillips HE, Sequeira J. The jet phenomenon: a manifestation of esophageal web. *AJR Am J Roentgenol* 1977; 129:747–748.

51. Taylor AJ, Stewart ET, Dodds WJ. The esophageal jet phenomenon revisited. *AJR Am J Roentgenol* 1990;155: 289–290.

52. Balfe DM, Heiken JP. Contrast evaluation of structural lesions of the pharynx. *Curr Probl Diagn Radiol* 1986;15:73–160.

53. Goldstein HM, Zornoza J. Association of squamous cell carcinoma of the head and neck with cancer of the esophagus. *AJR Am J Roentgenol* 1978;131:791–794.

54. Kirchner JA, Owen JR. Five hundred cancers of the larynx and piriform sinus: results of treatment by radiation and surgery. *Laryngoscope* 1977;87:1288–1303.

55. Seaman WB. Contrast radiography in neoplastic disease of the larynx and pharynx. *Semin Roentgenol* 1974;9:301–309.

56. Ekberg O, Nylander G. Double contrast examination of the pharynx. *Gastrointest Radiol* 1985;10:263–271.

57. Rubesin SE, Laufer I. Pictorial review: principles of double contrast pharyngography. *Dysphagia* 1991;6:170–178.

58. Jing BS. Roentgen examination of the larynx and hypopharynx. *Radiol Clin North Am* 1970;8:361–386.

59. Apter AJ, Levine MS, Glick SN. Carcinomas of the base of the tongue: diagnosis using double-contrast radiography of the pharynx. *Radiology* 1984;151:123–126.

60. Mong A, Levine MS, Rubesin SE, *et al.* Epiglottic carcinoma as a cause of laryngeal penetration and aspiration. *AJR Am J Roentgenol* 2003;180:207–211.

61. Carpenter RJ III, DeSanto LW, Devine KD, *et al.* Cancer of the hypopharynx. *Arch Otolaryngol* 1976;102:716–721.

62. Cunningham MP, Catlin D. Cancer of the pharyngeal wall. *Cancer* 1967;20:1859–1866.

63. Banfi A, Bonadonna G, Carnevali G, *et al.* Lymphoreticular sarcomas with primary involvement of Waldeyer's ring. *Cancer* 1970;26:341–351.

64. Todd GB, Michaels L. Hodgkin's disease involving Waldeyer's lymphoid ring. *Cancer* 1974;34:1769–1778.

65. Quillen SP, Balfe DM, Glick SN. Pharyngography after head and neck irradiation: differentiation of postirradiation edema from recurrent tumor. *AJR Am J Roentgenol* 1993;161: 1205–1208.

66. Ekberg O, Nylander G. Pharyngeal dysfunction after treatment for pharyngeal cancer with surgery and radiotherapy. *Gastrointest Radiol* 1983;8:97–104.

67. Levine MS, Rubesin SE, Herlinger H, *et al.* Double-contrast upper gastrointestinal examination: technique and interpretation. *Radiology* 1988;168:593–602.

68. Herlinger H, Grossman R, Laufer I, *et al.* The gastric cardia in double-contrast study: its dynamic image. *AJR Am J Roentgenol* 1980;135:21–29.

69. Ott DJ, Chen YM, Hewson EG, *et al.* Esophageal motility: assessment with synchronous video tape fluoroscopy and manometry. *Radiology* 1989;173:419–422.

70. Koehler RE, Weyman PJ, Oakley HE Single- and double-contrast techniques in esophagitis. *AJR Am J Roentgenol* 1980; 135:15–19.

71. Creteur V, Thoeni RF, Federle MP, *et al.* The role of single- and double-contrast radiography in the diagnosis of reflux esophagitis. *Radiology* 1983;147:71–75.

72. Graziani L, Bearzi I, Romagnoli A, *et al.* Significance of diffuse granularity and nodularity of the esophageal mucosa at double-contrast radiography. *Gastrointest Radiol* 1985; 10:1–6.

73. Levine MS. Gastroesophageal reflux disease. In: Gore RM, Levine MS, eds. *Textbook of Gastrointestinal Radiology*, 2nd edn. Philadelphia: WB Saunders, 2000, pp. 329–349.

74. Hu C, Levine MS, Laufer I. Solitary ulcers in reflux esophagitis: radiographic findings. *Abdom Imaging* 1997;22:5–7.

75. Rabin M, Schmaman IB. Reflex oesophagitis resembling varices. *S Afr Med J* 1979;55:293–295.

76. Bleshman MH, Banner MP, Johnson RC, *et al.* The inflammatory esophagogastric polyp and fold. *Radiology* 1978;128: 589–593.

77. Styles RA, Gibb SP, Tarshis A, *et al.* Esophagogastric polyps: radiographic and endoscopic findings. *Radiology* 1985;154: 307–311.

78. Ho CS, Rodrigues PR. Lower esophageal strictures, benign or malignant? *J Can Assoc Radiol* 1980;31:110–113.

79. Levine MS, Goldstein HM. Fixed transverse folds in the esophagus: a sign of reflux esophagitis. *AJR Am J Roentgenol* 1984;143:275–278.

80. Gohel VK, Edell SI, Laufer I, *et al.* Transverse folds in the human esophagus. *Radiology* 1978;128:303–308.

81. Furth EE, Rubesin SE, Rose D. Feline esophagus. *AJR Am J Roentgenol* 1995;164:900.

82. Robbins AH, Hermos JA, Schimmel EM, *et al.* The columnar-lined esophagus: analysis of 26 cases. *Radiology* 1977;123:1–7.

83. Levine MS, Kressel HY, Caroline DF, *et al.* Barrett esophagus: reticular pattern of the mucosa. *Radiology* 1983;147: 663–667.

84. Chen YM, Gelfand DW, Ott DJ, *et al.* Barrett esophagus as an extension of severe esophagitis: analysis of radiologic signs in 29 cases. *AJR Am J Roentgenol* 1985;145:275–281.

85. Gilchrist AM, Levine MS, Carr RF, *et al.* Barrett's esophagus: diagnosis by double-contrast esophagography. *AJR Am J Roentgenol* 1988;150:97–102.

86. Gefter WB, Laufer I, Edell S, *et al.* Candidiasis in the obstructed esophagus. *Radiology* 1981;138:25–28.

87. Sam JW, Levine MS, Rubesin SE, *et al.* The "foamy" esophagus: a radiographic sign of *Candida* esophagitis. *AJR Am J Roentgenol* 2000;174:999–1002.

88. Levine MS, Macones AJ, Laufer I. *Candida* esophagitis: accuracy of radiographic diagnosis. *Radiology* 1985;154:581–587.

89. Vahey TN, Maglinte DDT, Chernish SM. State-of-the-art barium examination in opportunistic esophagitis. *Dig Dis Sci* 1986;31:1192–1195.

90. Levine MS, Woldenberg R, Herlinger H, *et al.* Opportunistic esophagitis in AIDS: radiographic diagnosis. *Radiology* 1987; 165:815–820.

91. Shortsleeve MJ, Levine MS. Herpes esophagitis in otherwise healthy patients: clinical and radiographic findings. *Radiology* 1992;182:859–861.

92. Levine MS, Laufer I, Kressel HY, *et al*. Herpes esophagitis. *AJR Am J Roentgenol* 1981;136:863–866.

93. Levine MS, Loevner LA, Saul SH, *et al*. Herpes esophagitis: sensitivity of double-contrast esophagography. *AJR Am J Roentgenol* 1988;151:57–62.

94. Balthazar EM, Megibow AJ, Hulnick D, *et al*. Cytomegalovirus esophagitis in AIDS: radiographic features in 16 patients. *AJR Am J Roentgenol* 1987;149:919–923.

95. Levine MS, Loercher G, Katzka DA, *et al*. Giant, human immunodeficiency virus-related ulcers in the esophagus. *Radiology* 1991;180:320–323.

96. Sor S, Levine MS, Kowalski TE, *et al*. Giant ulcers of the esophagus in patients with human immunodeficiency virus: clinical, radiographic, and pathologic findings. *Radiology* 1995;194:447–451.

97. Kikendall JW, Friedman AC, Oyewole MA, *et al*. Pill-induced esophageal injury: case reports and review of the medical literature. *Dig Dis Sci* 1983;28:174–182.

98. Creteur V, Laufer I, Kressel HY, *et al*. Drug-induced esophagitis detected by double contrast radiography. *Radiology* 1983;147:365–368.

99. Bova JG, Dutton NE, Goldstein HM, *et al*. Medication-induced esophagitis: diagnosis by double-contrast esophagography. *AJR Am J Roentgenol* 1987;148:731–732.

100. Teplick JG, Teplick SK, OMinsky SH, *et al*. Esophagitis caused by oral medication. *Radiology* 1980;134:23–25.

101. Ryan JM, Kelsey P, Ryan BM, *et al*. Alendronate-induced esophagitis: case report of a recently recognized form of severe esophagitis with esophageal stricture-radiographic features. *AJR Am J Roentgenol* 1998;206:389–391.

102. Fox VL, Nurko S, Furuta GT. Eosinophilic esophagitis: it's not just kid's stuff. *Gastrointest Endosc* 2002;56:260–270.

103. Munitiz V, Martinez de Haro LF, Ortiz A, *et al*. Primary eosinophilic esophagitis. *Dis Esophagus* 2003;16:165–168.

104. Zimmerman SL, Levine MS, Rubesin SE, *et al*. Idiopathic eosinophilic esophagitis in adults: the ringed esophagus. *Radiology* 2005;236:159–165.

105. White SB, Levine MS, Rubesin SE, *et al*. The small-caliber esophagus: a radiographic sign of eosinophilic esophagitis. *Radiology* 2010;256:127–134.

106. Collazzo LA, Levine MS, Rubesin SE, *et al*. Acute radiation esophagitis: radiographic findings. *AJR Am J Roentgenol* 1997;169:1067–1070.

107. Lepke RA, Libshitz HI. Radiation-induced injury of the esophagus. *Radiology* 1983;148:375–378.

108. Levine MS. Other esophagitides. In: Gore RM, Levine MS, eds. *Textbook of Gastrointestinal Radiology*, 2nd edn. Philadelphia: WB Saunders, 2000, pp. 364–386.

109. Appleqvist P, Salmo M. Lye corrosion carcinoma of the esophagus: a review of 63 cases. *Cancer* 1980;45:2655–2658.

110. Levine MS, Fisher AR, Rubesin SE, *et al*. Complications after total gastrectomy and esophagojejunostomy: radiologic evaluation. *AJR Am J Roentgenol* 1991;157:1189–1194.

111. Montesi A, Alessandro P, Graziani L, *et al*. Small benign tumors of the esophagus: radiological diagnosis with double-contrast examination. *Gastrointest Radiol* 1983;8:207–212.

112. Levine MS. Benign tumors of the esophagus. In: Gore RM, Levine MS, eds. *Textbook of gastrointestinal radiology*, second edition. Philadelphia: WB Saunders, 2000, pp. 387–402.

113. Rose D, Furth EE, Rubesin SE. Glycogenic acanthosis. *AJR Am J Roentgenol* 1995;164:96.

114. Glick SN, Teplick SK, Goldstein J, *et al*. Glycogenic acanthosis of the esophagus. *AJR Am J Roentgenol* 1982;139:683–688.

115. Avezzano EA, Fleischer DE, Merida MA, *et al*. Giant fibrovascular polyps of the esophagus. *Ann Thorac Surg* 1990;85:299–302.

116. Cochet B, Hohl P, Sans M, *et al*. Asphyxia caused by laryngeal impaction of an esophageal polyp. *Arch Otolaryngol* 1980;106:176–178.

117. Levine MS, Buck JL, Pantongrag-Brown L, *et al*. Fibrovascular polyps of the esophagus: clinical, radiographic, and pathologic findings in 16 patients. *AJR Am J Roentgenol* 1996;166:781–787.

118. Rafal RB, Markisz JA. Magnetic resonance imaging of an esophageal duplication cyst. *Am J Gastroenterol* 1991;86:1809–1811.

119. Levine MS, Halvorsen RA. Carcinoma of the esophagus. In: Gore RM, Levine MS, eds. *Textbook of Gastrointestinal Radiology*, 2nd edn. Philadelphia: WB Saunders, 2000, pp. 403–433.

120. Cameron AJ, Ott BJ, Payne WS. The incidence of adenocarcinoma in the columnar-lined (Barrett's) esophagus. *N Engl J Med* 1985;313:857–859.

121. Levine MS, Chu P, Furth EE, *et al*. Carcinoma of the esophagus and esophagogastric junction: sensitivity of radiographic diagnosis. *AJR Am J Roentgenol* 1997;168:1423–1426.

122. Levine MS, Dillon EC, Saul SH, *et al*. Early esophageal cancer. *AJR Am J Roentgenol* 1986;146:507–512.

123. Gloyna RE, Zornoza J, Goldstein HM. Primary ulcerative carcinoma of the esophagus. *AJR Am J Roentgenol* 1977;129:599–600.

124. Yates CW, LeVine MA, Jensen KM. Varicoid carcinoma of the esophagus. *Radiology* 1977;122:605–608.

125. Levine MS, Caroline D, Thompson JJ, *et al*. Adenocarcinoma of the esophagus: relationship to Barrett mucosa. *Radiology* 1984;150:305–309.

126. Keen SJ, Dodd GD, Smith JL. Adenocarcinoma arising in Barrett's esophagus: pathologic and radiologic features. *Mt Sinai J Med* 1984;51:442–450.

127. Glick SN, Teplick SK, Levine MS, *et al*. Gastric cardia metastasis in esophageal carcinoma. *Radiology* 1986;160:627–630.

128. Levine MS. Other malignant tumors of the esophagus. In: Gore RM, Levine MS, eds. *Textbook of Gastrointestinal Radiology*, 2nd edn. Philadelphia: WB Saunders, 2000, pp. 435–451.

129. Agha FP, Keren DF. Spindle-cell squamous carcinoma of the esophagus: a tumor with biphasic morphology. *AJR Am J Roentgenol* 1985;145:541–545.

130. Ott DJ, Chen YM, Wu WC, *et al*. Radiographic and endoscopic sensitivity in detecting lower esophageal mucosal ring. *AJR Am J Roentgenol* 1986;147:261–265.

131. Levine MS, Moolten DN, Herlinger H, *et al*. Esophageal intramural pseudodiverticulosis: a reevaluation. *AJR Am J Roentgenol* 1986;147:1165–1170.

132. Ott DJ. Motility disorders of the esophagus. In: Gore RM, Levine MS, eds. *Textbook of Gastrointestinal Radiology*, 2nd edn. Philadelphia: WB Saunders, 2000, pp. 316–328.

133. Woodfield CA, Levine MS, Rubesin SE, *et al*. Diagnosis of primary versus secondary achalasia: reassessment of clinical and radiographic criteria. *AJR Am J Roentgenol* 2000;175:727–731.

134. Prabhakar A, Levine MS, Rubesin SE, *et al.* Relationship between diffuse esophageal spasm and lower esophageal sphincter dysfunction on barium studies and manometry in 14 patients. *AJR Am J Roentgenol* 2004;183:409–413.

135. Levine MS. Varices. In: Gore RM, Levine MS, eds. *Textbook of Gastrointestinal Radiology*, 2nd edn. Philadelphia: WB Saunders, 2000, pp. 452–463.

136. Levine MS. Miscellaneous abnormalities of the esophagus. In: Gore RM, Levine MS, eds. *Textbook of Gastrointestinal*

Radiology, 2nd edn. Philadelphia: WB Saunders, 2000, pp. 465–483.

137. Robbins MI, Shortsleeve MJ. Treatment of acute esophageal food impaction with glucagon, an effervescent agent, and water. *AJR Am J Roentgenol* 1994;162:325–328.

138. Baron RL, Koehler RE, Gutierrez FR, *et al.* Clinical and radiographic manifestations of aortoesophageal fistulas. *Radiology* 1981;141:599–605.

7

Special Endoscopic Imaging and Optical Techniques

Babac Vahabzadeh and Prateek Sharma

Division of Gastroenterology and Hepatology, Veterans Affairs Medical Center and University of Kansas School of Medicine, Kansas City, KS, USA

Introduction

Endoscopy is an essential tool in the diagnosis and treatment of esophageal diseases, including but not limited to gastroesophageal reflux disease (GERD), esophageal strictures, Barrett's esophagus, and esophageal cancer. Imaging techniques such as mucosal staining, magnification and high-definition endoscopy, electronic chromoendoscopy, spectroscopy, and endoscopic ultrasound (EUS) have improved the ability to visualize the superficial mucosa and expanded visualization to include deeper tissue layers of the esophagus. The availability of advanced imaging techniques, EUS, and endoscopic eradication therapies (EET) has revolutionized the treatment of squamous dysplasia/cancer and Barrett's esophagus-associated high-grade dysplasia and early adenocarcinoma. The role of these special endoscopic techniques for esophageal diseases will be reviewed in this chapter.

History

Modern endoscopy is the end result of the cumulative contribution of multiple innovative individuals over the past 150 years. The modern videoendoscope has greatly evolved since the original steel tube that was first introduced by Kussmaul in 1868, to visualize the esophagus and stomach. The advent of optical fibers in 1954 by Hopkins and Kapany led to the development of modern flexible endoscopy [1]. This technology was later adapted to medical endoscopy by Hirschowitz in 1957 [2]. There have been several advances since, including the development of charged couple devices (CCDs) and videoendoscopy in 1983, followed by the introduction of endoscopic ultrasound by Hisanaga and DiMagno in 1980 [3, 4]. Through the years, the standard videoendo-scope has become increasingly compact, more maneuverable, with higher resolution images. More recently, the introduction of high-definition (HD) endoscopes with HDTV quality images has allowed for enhanced views, improving the diagnosis of mucosal diseases. A variety of spectroscopic technologies have advanced endoscopy beyond the visible-light wavelength. Significantly improved therapeutic capabilities were made available after the introduction of accessories, such as band ligation, mucosal resection, and mucosal ablation. These newer EETs have allowed the avoidance of more invasive therapies, including surgery.

Technique

The technique used for endoscopic evaluation of the esophagus has remained largely unchanged since the introduction of the modern endoscope, and while patient preparation may differ between centers, the examination is performed in the same general manner. It remains a procedure that is generally well tolerated by the majority of patients with proper sedation. Relative contraindications to upper endoscopy include a medically unstable patient, and patients with an unstable cervical spine, coagulopathy unresponsive to therapy, or known or suspected perforation of the gastrointestinal tract.

The procedure involves intubation of the esophagus with direct visualization of the mucosa to evaluate for abnormalities. The recognition and documentation of endoscopic landmarks is vital to a thorough examination. The gastroesophageal junction (GEJ) is identified as the proximal extent of the gastric folds or, alternatively, the distal end of the esophageal palisade vessels. Noting the site of the squamocolumnar junction (SCJ), which is the point where the mucosal lining changes from squamous to columnar type, is also essential. The diaphragmatic pinch should be identified as well. The

The Esophagus, Fifth Edition. Edited by Joel E. Richter, Donald O. Castell.
© 2012 Blackwell Publishing Ltd. Published 2012 by Blackwell Publishing Ltd.

proper identification of these landmarks allows for the correct diagnosis of hiatus hernias and Barrett's esophagus. A complete endoscopic examination of the esophagus should also include a retroflexed view of the GEJ area obtained from the stomach. Special caution is necessary in cases of dysphagia or suspected food impaction. These patients may have structural or motility abnormalities that may increase their risk of perforation. Specifically in patients with a known or suspected Zenker's diverticulum, intubating the esophagus may be difficult as it may be challenging to visualize the lumen of the esophagus. Blind forceful insertion of the endoscope should be avoided in these situations as this could result in a perforation.

The endoscopic description of esophageal mucosal diseases has become more standardized with the availability of reproducible and validated criteria. Erosive reflux esophagitis is commonly diagnosed as a manifestation of chronic GERD. The Los Angeles (LA) Classification was introduced in 1994 to provide endoscopists with a grading system (A–D) to describe and classify the appearance of erosive changes and mucosal breaks in the distal esophagus (Figure 7.1). The previously ambiguous and variable descriptions have now been largely replaced by this validated grading system (Table 7.1) [5, 6]. Another widely used classification is the Prague

C&M criteria, developed in 2004 for the endoscopic grading of Barrett's esophagus using the circumferential (C) and maximal (M) extent of the columnar-lined esophagus [7] (Figure 7.2). The diagnosis of Barrett's esophagus, a premalignant condition for esophageal adenocarcinoma (EAC), depends on the recognition of a columnar-lined esophagus [8, 9], and this grading system permits easier recognition and classification of this condition during screening and surveillance endoscopy.

Special endoscopic techniques

Diagnostic upper endoscopy and tissue sampling

Upper endoscopy is the primary modality for evaluating the esophageal mucosa in symptomatic patients. High-resolution images allow for visualization of subtle mucosal irregularities that may potentially lead to a specific diagnosis. However, many cases require that histologic or cytologic testing be performed; this can be achieved using tissue biopsies, brush cytology, or endoscopic mucosal resection (EMR). Standard biopsy forceps vary by size, style, and design; however, they generally allow for sufficient mucosal sampling. Specific techniques such as the "turn and suction" maneuver allow for larger mucosal sampling [10] in patients with Barrett's esophagus. This maneuver involves positioning of the open-jaw forceps flush with the end of the endoscope and turning the endoscope into the mucosa, followed by suctioning of air from the esophageal lumen, allowing the mucosa to collapse into the forceps before obtaining a biopsy. A specially designed sheathed disposable brush is used to obtain mucosal specimens for cytology [11]. The brush is vigorously rubbed against the mucosa causing cells to be captured by the bristles. Subsequently, the brush is removed and its contents are transferred to the surface of a glass slide by direct contact. The primary role of brush cytology is in the diagnosis of infectious esophagitis such as candidiasis [11, 12].

EMR is both a diagnostic and therapeutic approach that allows removal of large sections of tissue. It is performed in a variety of manners, but generally all describe separation of the superficial mucosa from deeper tissue layers by submucosal injection of fluid (saline, dilute epinephrine, etc.) followed by mucosal resection with the use of a snare device [13, 14] (Figure 7.3). Additional techniques have been described, such as cap-assisted EMR and multiband mucosectomy. Cap-assisted EMR involves the use of a transparent cap together with a single-use, crescent-shaped snare to suction mucosa for resection (Figure 7.4), while multiband mucosectomy uses a modified multiband variceal ligator that allows multiple resections without having to withdraw the endoscope [15, 16]. In patients with Barrett's esophagus and biopsy-proven high-grade dysplasia (HGD) or EAC, EMR has been proven to be superior to biopsy forceps for obtaining accurate pathologic staging and has been shown to upstage

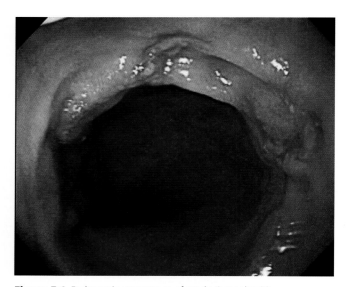

Figure 7.1 Endoscopic appearance of grade C esophagitis.

Table 7.1 LA grade classification of esophagitis.

Grade A	Mucosal break of ≤5 mm in length
Grade B	Mucosal break of ≥5 mm in length
Grade C	Mucosal break continuous between >2 folds but <75% of the esophageal circumference
Grade D	Mucosal break which involves ≥75% of the esophageal circumference

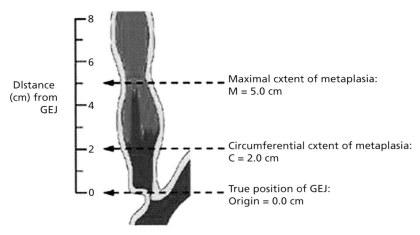

Figure 7.2 Endoscopic Barrett's esophagus demonstrating an area classified as C2M5. C, extent of circumferential metaplasia; M, maximal extent of the metaplasia (C plus a distal "tongue" of 3 cm); GEJ, gastroesophageal junction (reproduced from Sharma *et al.* [7], with permission).

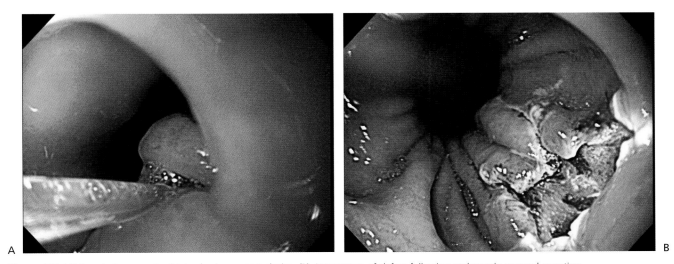

Figure 7.3 (A) Targeted mucosa is obtained using a snare device. (B) Appearance of defect following endoscopic mucosal resection.

or downstage the diagnosis of lesions in approximately 25% of patients [17]. In one study of 40 patients undergoing EMR (25 HGD and 15 EAC), 24% of the HGD patients were upgraded to mucosal EAC and 40% of the EAC patients were upgraded to invasive EAC [18]. As such, EMR assists in determining whether Barrett's esophagus with focal nodules or short-segment microscopic lesions are amenable to endoscopic therapy; if cancer has invaded into the submucosa, cure via EET is not possible [18]. A study of 49 Barrett's esophagus patients with HGD or intramucosal carcinoma (IMC) evaluated complete Barrett's eradication with EMR alone. Thirty-two patients underwent this therapy and complete eradication of IMC was achieved in 97% [19]. Another study evaluating 231 Barrett's esophagus patients with mucosal adenocarcinoma treated by EMR alone reported a complete eradication of dysplasia rate of greater than 97% [20]. A variety of complications have been reported following EMR therapy, including bleeding in approximately 10% and perforation in less than 1% of cases [20–23]. High rates of symptomatic esophageal stenosis have been documented (if circumferential EMR is preferred), ranging from 26% to 37%; however, most are managed successfully with endoscopic therapy [19, 23]. EMR has both an acceptable safety profile as well as successful eradication rates for Barrett's esophagus with HGD and mucosal carcinoma. Similarly, EMR plays a major role in patients with squamous dysplasia/cancer.

Endoscopic ultrasound

EUS has become increasingly utilized for imaging the deeper tissue layers of the esophagus as well as periesophageal structures. Ultrasound technologies, including radial and

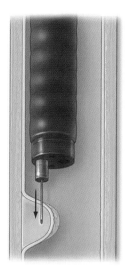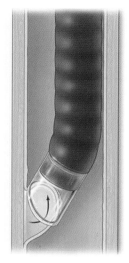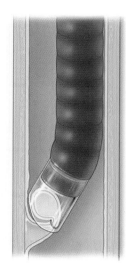

Figure 7.4 Removal of early cancer with the use of cap-assisted endoscopic mucosal resection in a patient with Barrett's esophagus (reproduced from Sharma P. Barrett's Esophagus. *N Engl J Med* 2009;361:2548–2556, with permission).

linear endoscope systems and through-the-scope mini-probes, are devices attached to an ultrasound processor, which includes a control panel allowing the ultrasound image to project onto a high-resolution monitor. The EUS endoscopes are larger (diameter 12–13 mm) than standard endoscopes; whereas EUS miniprobes, which are passed through the accessory channel of a standard endoscope and provide 360-degree imaging, can be used for superficial lesions of the esophagus. While miniprobes offer excellent resolution of the very superficial esophageal wall, they have a limited depth of penetration [24].

Several studies have evaluated the role of EUS in Barrett's esophagus with the finding that the esophageal wall appears thickened in these patients as compared to controls [25–27]. However, EUS was unable to reliably differentiate between dyplastic and non-dyplastic Barrett's esophagus and was not appropriate for routine screening or surveillance in these patients. Patients with Barrett's esophagus with dysphagia or the presence of a focal nodule or stricture have an increased likelihood of carcinoma. In one study, five of 12 patients with Barrett's esophagus and an associated nodule and/or stricture on endoscopy were found to have lesions that invaded into the submucosa or deeper, compared to none of the 10 patients without endoscopic visualization of a lesion (42% vs 0%, P = .04) [28]. As a result, this subset of patients may benefit from EUS to accurately evaluate disease stage and to deliver appropriate therapy.

EUS is widely used for the staging of esophageal cancer (Figure 7.5) and evaluation of submucosal lesions of the esophagus [29–33]. More recently, EUS has gained a predominant role as a safe and effective modality for the imaging and diagnosis of mediastinal masses [34]. Studies

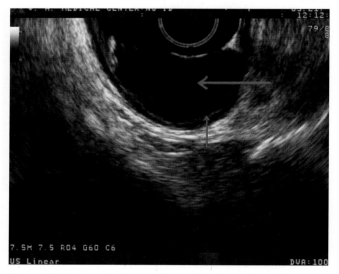

Figure 7.5 Endoscopic ultrasound image showing esophageal cancer (thick arrow) that has not invaded past the submucosa (thin arrow).

have demonstrated EUS to have an accuracy of 85% and 75% in T and N staging, respectively [35]. The addition of fine needle aspiration (FNA) and core biopsies improves the diagnostic accuracy of EUS, particularly in assessing lymph nodes for tumor spread [36]. Unfortunately, in approximately one-third of patients, luminal obstruction prevents complete staging via EUS. Advent of the narrow-diameter, non-optical wire-guided EUS scope has allowed for complete T staging in all patients [37]. However, its main limitations include inability to evaluate for celiac adenopathy, which is considered unresectable disease by most centers, as well as the lack of FNA capability. Curved linear-array transducers are primarily used for ultrasound guidance in FNA procedures for lymph node sampling and mediastinal lesions [34, 38]. Doppler ultrasound allows for the evaluation of portal hypertension, flow within the thoracic duct, identification of aberrant vascular anatomy, as well as guided resection of esophageal submucosal tumors [30, 33, 39–41].

Chromoendoscopy

Chromoendoscopy of the esophagus is the topical application of stains to enhance tissue characterization and aid diagnosis during endoscopy. Two commonly used stains include Lugol's solution and methylene blue. Lugol's solution is largely used in evaluating the GEJ and squamous cell neoplasia as its iodine component has an affinity for the glycogen present in normal squamous mucosa of the esophagus. After spraying a 1% solution during endoscopy, abnormal areas may become more easily visible and amenable to targeted biopsy and/or EMR. The normal squamous epithelium stains dark green–brown, while epithelium that does not contain glycogen, such as inflammation, dysplasia and carcinoma, appears unstained [42] (Figure 7.6). As a result, Lugol's solution may improve the sensitivity in the detection of dysplasia and early squamous cell cancer of the esophagus, as well as evaluating the extent of mucosal involvement in high-risk patients [43, 44]. Lugol's solution may cause local irritation and retrosternal pain, but these are generally self-limited side effects.

The methylene blue stain is absorbed by intestinal-type epithelial cells, such as small intestinal and colonic mucosa, as well as intestinal metaplasia of the esophagus, while not staining squamous or gastric mucosa. Initial application of a mucolytic agent, usually 10% N-acetylcysteine, is per-

formed, followed by methylene blue 0.5–1%, and finally the excess dye is washed away. It is thought to improve the detection of intestinal metaplasia and dysplasia of the esophagus. Methylene blue-directed biopsies were compared to standard white light endoscopy with four-quadrant random biopsies in a prospective randomized cross-over trial of 48 patients. Results were comparable for diagnosing intestinal metaplasia and dysplasia; however, the mean number of biopsies required was significantly lower in the methylene blue group (9.2 vs 18.9, $P < .001$) [45]. Overall, trials evaluating methylene blue have had discrepant results; this variability may be due to poor standardization of the application technique, and the subjective interpretation of staining intensity [46–52].

Electronic chromoendoscopy

Electronic chromoendoscopy has largely replaced traditional chromoendoscopy due to its ease of use and increasing availability. Narrow-band imaging (NBI) is a novel modality where the band-pass ranges of the green and blue components of the excitation light are narrowed and the relative intensity of the blue spectrum is increased, allowing for improved visualization of mucosal and vascular surface patterns. NBI can easily be activated and disabled manually during endoscopy by switching between standard white light and NBI mode.

NBI is being increasingly used for the evaluation of esophageal disease, specifically GERD and Barrett's esophagus, given its ease of use and its ability to evaluate a broad field. By highlighting specific characteristics of abnormal esophageal mucosa, NBI may improve the endoscopic diagnosis of GERD and Barrett's esophagus over standard endoscopy (Figure 7.7). For instance, it has been shown that the structure and organization of blood vessels undergo significant changes during inflammation and neoplasia [53]. In normal esophageal mucosa, submucosal vessels that traverse the muscle layer are connected to the arborescent vascular network [53]. Intrapapillary capillaries arise from this vascular network, forming intrapapillary capillary loops (IPCLs), and have been shown to dilate and elongate in mucosal squamous cancer. Similar changes have also been demonstrated in inflammatory states such as GERD [53]. A recent study evaluated the role of NBI in 50 GERD patients and 30 controls (without reflux symptoms). Results revealed that a significantly higher proportion of GERD patients had an increased number of IPCLs (66% vs 13%, $P < .0001$), tortuous IPCLs (80% vs 37%, $P < .0001$), and dilated IPCLs (80% vs 16.7%, $P < .0001$) when compared to controls [54]. NBI was also able to identify microerosions (52% vs 0%, $P < .0001$), which are definitive mucosal breaks not visible with standard endoscopy, and increased vascularity (40% vs 6.7%, $P = .001$), both of which are associated with GERD [54], while conventional endoscopy failed to detect these findings [54, 55].

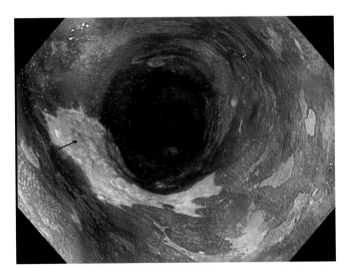

Figure 7.6 Endoscopic view of the esophagus following application of Lugol's solution identifying squamous cell cancer appearing as an area that is not stained (arrow).

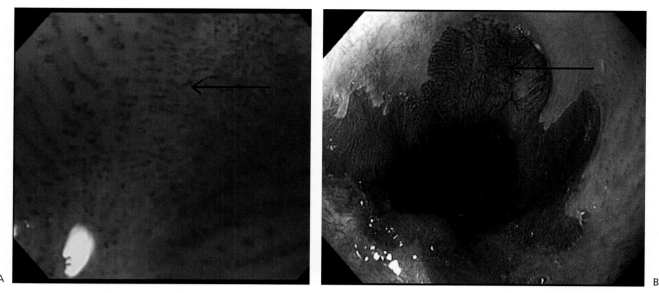

Figure 7.7 (A) Dilated intrapapillary capillary loops (arrow) with narrow-band imaging consistent with gastroesophageal reflux disease (GERD). (B) Mucosal changes consistent with Barrett's esophagus (arrow) visualized with NBI.

NBI has been extensively studied and may be useful in detecting subtle mucosal abnormalities, particularly in Barrett's esophagus and associated dysplasia [56–59]. Several classification systems have been proposed, one of which involves characterizing mucosal and vascular patterns as either regular or irregular; these descriptions have been shown to correlate with non-dysplastic Barrett's esophagus and HGD/cancer, respectively [60]. NBI enables identification of the irregular/distorted pattern with tortuous, abnormally branching, non-uniform vascular pattern that is seen in Barrett's esophagus patients, particularly those with HGD [61]. The very high correlation between various mucosal and vascular patterns with histology makes NBI ideal for the detection of Barrett's esophagus [61]. The use of NBI versus white light endoscopy (WLE) was investigated in 65 patients with Barrett's esophagus undergoing evaluation for previously detected dysplasia [62]. Higher grades of dysplasia were found by NBI (18%) vs WLE (0%), with a higher grade of histology detected by random biopsies ($P < .001$). NBI-directed biopsies detected dysplasia in more patients compared with WLE-directed biopsies (57% vs 37%). Furthermore, results showed that significantly more biopsies were taken using WLE versus NBI (mean 8.5 vs 4.7, $P < .001$) [62].

Confocal laser endomicroscopy

Confocal laser endomicroscopy (CLE) is a novel imaging modality that can aid in differentiating neoplastic from non-neoplastic tissue by allowing *in vivo* visualization of mucosal histology during endoscopy that usually involves the use of a fluorescent agent (fluorescein) (Figure 7.8). Currently there are two approved devices; one is integrated into the

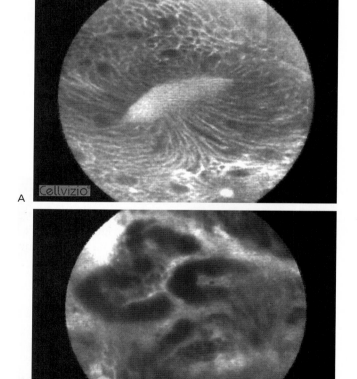

Figure 7.8 (A) Non-dysplastic Barrett's esophagus under confocal imaging. (B) Barrett's esophagus with dysplasia under confocal imaging.

endoscope (eCLE; Pentax, Fort Wayne, NJ, USA) and the other is probe based (pCLE; Cellvizio, Mauna Kea Technologies, Paris, France). These techniques use optical fibers with a distal lens and a proximal precision connector. A laser is emitted from either the endoscope or probe onto the mucosa, resulting in a fluorescent signal that is converted into an image with the use of a detector.

Initial studies using CLE for detecting neoplasia in Barrett's esophagus show promise. When compared with histologic specimens, CLE in a cohort of 63 patients detected intestinal metaplasia and associated neoplastic changes with a sensitivity of 98% and 93%, and specificity of 94% and 98%, respectively [63]. In another study, 39 patients were evaluated, 16 with suspected neoplasia and 23 for Barrett's esophagus surveillance. CLE-directed biopsies led to a 59% decrease in the number of biopsies needed per patient to detect dysplasia in comparison to standard endoscopy (9.8 vs 23.8 biopsies, $P = .002$) [64]. In Barrett's esophagus patients undergoing surveillance, the mean number of biopsies was 87% lower with CLE than standard endoscopy (1.7 vs 12.6, $P < .0001$) [64].

The *in vivo* histopathologic imaging makes CLE a unique technique to differentiate between normal and cancerous tissues, giving it great value as a potential tool for early detection of malignancy. However, its use requires specialized training by the endoscopist and provides visualization of small areas of the mucosa.

Tissue spectroscopy

Spectroscopy is another imaging technology being studied for the differentiation of neoplastic and non-neoplastic esophageal tissue. Spectroscopy can assist in evaluating a variety of tissue properties, including biochemical changes, extracellular matrix, nuclear size, and density of cells. The potential advantages of spectroscopy include the improved identification of dysplasia and the capability of immediate diagnosis and directed biopsy of "abnormal" areas during endoscopy.

Many types of spectroscopy have been investigated and used for the detection of esophageal neoplasia, including light (laser)-induced fluorescence (LIF), light scattering (LSS), and reflectance spectroscopy. LIF involves the use of fluorophores, which are biologic substances that produce fluorescent light when stimulated by laser light. Neoplastic tissues have varying concentrations and structures of fluorophores, leading to spectral differences. LSS involves measuring the extent to which light photons are elastically scattered by specific structures. The main determining factors in how light scatters include the size and number of structures in addition to the color of light used to illuminate the tissue. As a result, this method can characterize the number and the size of nuclei in Barrett's esophagus patients as a measure of dysplasia [65–67]. Reflectance spectroscopy is based on the premise that tissues either absorb or reflect light, and the measurement of the color and intensity of this light can

aid diagnosis. The use of white light, which contains multiple colors of the spectrum, results in some colors being absorbed while others are reflected. An important limitation of spectroscopy is that it only samples a limited area of the esophageal mucosa. Many of these current methods are still being studied and currently none is used in clinical practice.

Autofluorescence endoscopy

Autofluorescence imaging endoscopy (AFI) uses a high-resolution videoendoscope coupled with a fluorescence imaging modality. Standard white light is separated into red, green and blue (RGB) after being passed through an RGB filter, and is used to illuminate the mucosa. The resultant image is comprised of total autofluorescence after blue light excitation, green reflectance, and red reflectance. Separate CCDs for both WLE and AFI are at the tip of the endoscope. The endoscopist can easily switch manually between WLE and AFI mode by pressing a control on the endoscope.

When evaluating Barrett's esophagus during AFI mode, non-dysplastic Barrett's esophagus appears green, while dysplastic areas have a blue to violet color (Figure 7.9). Initial investigation has revealed that AFI improves both the number of patients and the number of lesions detected with HGD, and of early cancer when used in addition to WLE [68–70]. It was recently shown that, in comparison to standard endoscopy, AFI increased the detection of patients with HGD/early cancer from 45% to 90% [70]. The use of AFI also increased the total number of detected lesions containing HGD/early cancer from 21 to 40 when combined with high-resolution endoscopy [70]. Unfortunately, a limitation

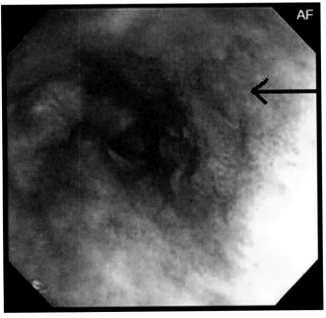

Figure 7.9 Autofluorescence endoscopic image highlighting non-dysplastic Barrett's esophagus (green) and dysplastic areas (violet; arrow).

of AFI is its exceedingly high false-positive rate of 81% [70]. AFI, while still in its initial stages of development, shows promise as a broad surface image modality to assist in the detection of dysplastic lesions.

Optical coherence tomography

Optical coherence tomography (OCT) is an imaging technology that uses the backscattering of light waves to provide two-dimensional cross-sectional images of the gastrointestinal tract and is capable of resolving the layers of the esophagus (mucosa, submucosa, muscularis, and serosa). This technique increases the resolution by up to tenfold that of high-frequency EUS and approaches that of light microscopy. One study evaluated 19 patients with reflux esophagitis, Barrett's esophagus, and Barrett's esophagus-related cancer with OCT [71]. OCT images revealed varying levels of edema, fibrinoid deposits, or loss of the epithelial layer, depending on the different stages of reflux esophagitis [71]. Furthermore, OCT images of Barrett's esophagus were characterized by an uneven mucosal surface which differed significantly from those of normal esophagus, reflux esophagitis, and esophageal cancer [71]. Although a number of other studies have shown promising results with OCT, it still remains in the investigational arena.

Conclusions

Significant advances have been made in endoscopic imaging to help diagnose and manage esophageal disease. These include methods to enhance endoscopic visualization of subtle lesions of the esophageal mucosa and other methods to obtain endoscopic imaging beyond the superficial layers. Validated criteria have been introduced which have simplified the classification and description of common esophageal diseases. These criteria and unique modalities have dramatically improved the description, as well as detection, surveillance, and endoscopic treatment of premalignant conditions such as Barrett's esophagus. While some techniques have already become widely used by endoscopists, many novel technologies remain under investigation. As new developments become available, they will play a vital role in esophageal imaging by allowing the endoscopist to evaluate tissue anatomy and function. New techniques will hopefully provide opportunities to improve the diagnosis and management of esophageal diseases and help in overcoming the limitations of random endoscopic biopsy.

References

1. Hopkins H, Kapany N. A flexible fiberscope using static scanning. *Nature* 1954;173:39–41.
2. Hirschowitz B. A personal history of the fiberscope. *Gastroenterology* 1979;76:864–869.
3. Hisanaga K, Hisanaga A, Nagata K, *et al.* High speed rotating scanner for transgastric sonography. *AJR Am J Roentgenol* 1980; 135:627–639.
4. DiMagno EP, Buxton JL, Regan PT, *et al.* Ultrasonic endoscope. *Lancet* 1980;22:629–631.
5. Armstrong D, Bennett JR, Blum AL, *et al.* The endoscopic assessment of oesophagitis: a progress report on observer agreement. *Gastroenterology* 1996;111:85–92.
6. Lundell LR, Dent J, Bennett JR, *et al.* Endoscopic assessment of oesophagitis: clinical and functional correlates and further validation of Los Angeles classification. *Gut* 1999;45:172–180.
7. Sharma P, Dent J, Armstrong D, *et al.* The development and validation of an endoscopic grading system for Barrett's esophagus: The Prague C & M criteria. *Gastroenterology* 2006; 131:1392–1399.
8. Mann NS, Tsal MF, Nair PK. Barrett's esophagus in patients with symptomatic reflux esophagitis. *Am J Gastroenterol* 1989;84: 1494–1496.
9. Winters C Jr, Spurling TJ, Chobanian, *et al.* Barrett's esophagus. A prevalent, occult complication of gastroesophageal reflux disease. *Gastroenterology* 1987;92:118–124.
10. Levine DS, Reid BJ. Endoscopic biopsy technique for acquiring larger mucosal samples. *Gastrointest Endosc* 1991;37:332–337.
11. Camp R, Rutkowski MA, Atkison K, *et al.* A prospective, randomized, blinded trial of cytological yield with disposable cytology brushes in upper gastrointestinal tract lesions. *Am J Gastroenterol* 1992;87:1439–1442.
12. Mendoza ML, Martin-Rabadan P, Carrion I, *et al. Helicobacter pylori* infection. Rapid diagnosis with brush cytology. *Acta Cytol* 1993;37:181–185.
13. Inoue H, Takeshita K, Hori H, *et al.* Endoscopic mucosal resection with a cap-fitted panendoscope for esophagus, stomach, and colon mucosal lesions. *Gastrointest Endosc* 1993;39:58–62.
14. Matsuda K. Introduction to endoscopic mucosal resection. *Gastrointest Endosc Clin North Am* 2001;11:439–443.
15. Peters FP, Kara MA, Rosmolen WD, *et al.* Endoscopic treatment of high-grade dysplasia and early stage cancer in Barrett's esophagus. *Gastrointest Endosc* 2005;61:506–514.
16. Soehendra N, Seewald S, Groth S, *et al.* Use of modified multi-band ligator facilitates circumferential EMR in Barrett's esophagus (with video). *Gastrointest Endosc* 2006;63:847–852.
17. Sayana H, Wani S, Keighley JD, *et al.* Endoscopic mucosal resection (EMR) as a diagnostic tool in Barrett's esophagus (BE) patients with high-grade dysplasia (HGD) and early esophageal adenocarcinoma (EAC): a systemic review. *Gastroenterology* 2008;134:A-724.
18. Larghi A, Lightdale CJ, Memeo L, *et al.* EUS followed by EMR for staging of high-grade dysplasia and early cancer in Barrett's esophagus. *Gastrointest Endosc* 2005;62:16–23.
19. Chennat J, Konda VJ, Ross AS, *et al.* Complete Barrett's eradication endoscopic mucosal resection: an effective treatment modality for high-grade dysplasia and intramucosal carcinoma—an American single-center experience. *Am J Gastroenterol* 2009;104:2684–2692.
20. Pech O, Behrens A, May A, *et al.* Long term results and risk factor analysis for recurrence after curative endoscopic therapies in 349 patients with high grade intraepithelial neoplasia and mucosal adenocarcinoma in Barrett's esophagus. *Gut* 2008;57:1200–1206.

21. Giovannini M, Bories E, Pesenti C, *et al.* Circumferential endoscopic mucosal resection in Barrett's esophagus with high-grade intraepithelial neoplasia or mucosal cancer. Preliminary results in 21 patients. *Endoscopy* 2004;36:782–787.

22. Seewald S, Akaraviputh T, Seitz U, *et al.* Circumferential EMR and complete removal of Barrett's esophagus containing high-grade intraepithelial neoplasia and intramucosal carcinoma. *Gastrointest Endosc* 2003;57:854–859.

23. Peters FP, Kara MA, Rosmolen WD, *et al.* Stepwise radical endoscopic resection is effective for complete removal of Barrett's esophagus with early neoplasia: a prospective study. *Am J Gastroenterol* 2006;101:1449–1457.

24. Chak A, Canto M, Stevens PD, *et al.* Clinical applications of a new through-the-scope ultrasound probe: prospective comparison with an ultrasound endoscope. *Gastrointest Endosc* 1997;45:291–295.

25. Srivastava AK, Vanagunas A, Kamel P, *et al.* Endoscopic ultrasound in the evaluation of Barrett's esophagus: a preliminary report. *Am J Gastroenterol* 1994;89:2191–2195.

26. Adrain AL, Ter HC, Cassidy MJ, *et al.* High-resolution endoluminal sonography is a sensitive modality for the identification of Barrett's metaplasia. *Gastrointest Endosc* 1997;46:147–151.

27. Kinjo M, Maringhini A, Wang KK, *et al.* Is endoscopic ultrasound (EUS) cost effective to screen for cancer in patients with Barrett's esophagus? *Gastrointest Endosc* 1994;40:205A.

28. Scotiniotis IA, Kochman ML, Lewis JD, *et al.* Accuracy of EUS in the evaluation of Barrett's esophagus and high grade dysplasia or intramucosal carcinoma. *Gastrointest Endosc* 2001; 54:689–696.

29. Mallery S, Van Dam J. EUS in the evaluation of esophageal carcinoma. *Gastrointest Endosc* 2000;52 (Suppl 6):S6–S11.

30. Waxman I, Saitoh Y, Raju GS, *et al.* High-frequency probe EUS assisted endoscopic mucosal resection: a therapeutic strategy for submucosal tumors of the GI tract. *Gastroinest Endosc* 2002; 55:44–49.

31. Takada N, Higashino M, Osugi H, *et al.* Utility of endoscopic ultrasonography in assessing the indications for endoscopic surgery of submucosal esophageal tumors. *Surg Endosc* 1999; 13:228–230.

32. Hino S, Kakutani H, Ikeda K, *et al.* Hemodynamic assessment of the left gastric vein in patients with esophageal varices with color Doppler EUS: factors affecting development of esophageal varices. *Gastrointest Endosc* 2002;55:512–517.

33. Miller LS. Endoscopic ultrasound in the evaluation of portal hypertension. *Gastrointest Endosc Clin North Am* 1999;9: 271–285.

34. Wallace MB, Silvestri GA, Sahai AV, *et al.* Endoscopic ultrasound-guided fine needle aspiration for staging patients with carcinoma of the lung. *Ann Thorac Surg* 2001;72:1861–1867.

35. Rosch T. Endosonographic staging of esophageal cancer: a review of literature results. *Gastrointest Endosc Clin North Am* 1995;5:537–547.

36. Vazquez-Sequeiros E, Norton ID, Clain JE, *et al.* Impact of EUS guided fine-needle aspiration on lymph node staging in patients with esophageal carcinoma. *Gastrointest Endosc* 2001; 53:751–757.

37. Mallery S, Van Dam J. Increased rate of complete EUS staging of patients with esophageal cancer using the nonoptical, wire-guided echoendoscope. *Gastrointest Endosc* 1999;50:53–57.

38. Eloubeidi MA, Wallace MB, Reed CE, *et al.* The utility of EUS and EUS-guided fine needle aspiration in detect celiac lymph node metastasis in patients with esophageal cancer: a single-center experience. *Gastrointest Endosc* 2001;54:714–719.

39. Parasher VK, Meroni E, Malesci A, *et al.* Observation of thoracic duct morphology in portal hypertension by endoscopic ultrasound. *Gastrointest Endosc* 1998;48:588–592.

40. De Luca L, Begmann JJ, Tytgat GN, *et al.* EUS imaging of the arteria lusoria: case series and review. *Gastrointest Endosc* 2000; 52:670–673.

41. Sun S, Wang M. Use of endoscopic ultrasound-guided injection in endoscopic resection of solid submucosal tumors. *Endoscopy* 2002;34:82–85.

42. Fennerty MB. Tissue staining. *Gastrointest Endosc Clin North Am* 1994;4:297–311.

43. Meyer V, Burtin P, Bour B, *et al.* Endoscopic detection of early esophageal cancer in a high-risk population: does Lugol staining improve videoendoscopy? *Gastrointest Endosc* 1997;45:480–484.

44. Dawsey SM, Fleischer DE, Wang GQ, *et al.* Mucosal iodine staining improves endoscopic visualization of squamous dysplasia and squamous cell carcinoma of the esophagus in Linxian, China. *Cancer* 1998;83:220–231.

45. Horwhat JD, Maydonovitch CL, Ramos F, *et al.* A randomized comparison of methylene blue-directed biopsy versus conventional four-quadrant biopsy for the detection of intestinal metaplasia and dysplasia in patients with long-segment Barrett's esophagus. *Am J Gastroenterol* 2008;103:546–554.

46. Canto MI, Setrakian S, Petras RE, *et al.* Methylene blue selectively stains intestinal metaplasia in Barrett's esophagus. *Gastrointest Endosc* 1996;44:1–7.

47. Canto MI, Setrakian S, Willis J, *et al.* Methylene blue-directed biopsies improve detection of intestinal metaplasia and dysplasia in Barrett's esophagus. *Gastrointest Endosc* 2000;51:560–568.

48. Sharma P, Topalovski M, Mayo MS, *et al.* Methylene blue chromoendoscopy for detection of short-segment Barrett's esophagus. *Gastrointest Endosc* 2001;54:289–293.

49. Kiesslich R, Hahn M, Herrmann G, *et al.* Screening for specialized columnar epithelium with methylene blue: chromoendoscopy in patients with Barrett's esophagus and a normal control group. *Gastrointest Endosc* 2001;53:47–52.

50. Wo JM, Ray MB, Mayfield-Stokes S, *et al.* Comparison of methylene blue-directed biopsies and conventional biopsies in the detection of intestinal metaplasia in Barrett's esophagus: a preliminary study. *Gastrointest Endosc* 2001;54:294–301.

51. Dave U, Shousha S, Westaby D. Methylene blue staining: Is it really useful in Barrett's esophagus? *Gastrointest Endosc* 2001;53:333–335.

52. Wong RK, Horwhat JD, Maydonovitch CL. Sky blue or murky waters: the diagnostic utility of methylene blue. *Gastrointest Endosc* 2001;54:409–413.

53. Kumagal Y, Tol M, Inoue H. Dynamism of tumour vasculature in the early phase of cancer progression: outcomes from oesophageal cancer research. *Lancet Oncol* 2002;3:604–610.

54. Sharma P, Wani S, Bansal A *et al.* A feasibility trail of narrow-band imaging endoscopy in patients with gastroesophageal reflux disease. *Gastroenterology* 2007;133:454–464.

55. Fock KM, Teo EK, Ang TL, *et al.* The utility of narrow band imaging in improving the endoscopic diagnosis of gastroesophageal reflux disease. *Clin Gastroenterol Hepatol* 2009;7:54–59.

56. Yosida T, Inoue H, Usui S *et al*. Narrow-band imaging system with magnifying endoscopy for superficial esophageal lesions. *Gastrointest Endosc* 2004;59:288–295.

57. Hamamoto Y, Endo T, Nosho K, et al. Usefulness of narrow-band imaging endoscopy for diagnosis of Barrett's esophagus. *J Gastroenterol* 2004;39(1):14–20.

58. Kara M, Peters F, Rosmolen W, et al. High-resolution endoscopy plus chromoendoscopy or narrow-band imaging in Barrett's esophagus: a prospective randomized crossover study. *Endoscopy* 2005;37:929–936.

59. Goda K, Tajiri H, Ikegami M, et al. Usefulness of magnifying endoscopy with narrow band imaging for the detection of specialized intestinal metaplasia in columnar-lined esophagus and Barrett's adenocarcinoma. *Gastrointest Endosc* 2007;65:36–46.

60. Singh R, Anagnostopoulos G, Yao K, et al. Narrow-band imaging with magnification in Barrett's esophagus: validation of a simplified grading system of mucosal morphology patterns against histology. *Endoscopy* 2008;40(6):457–463.

61. Sharma P, Bansal A, Mathur S, et al. The utility of a novel narrow band imaging endoscopy system in patients with Barrett's esophagus. *Gastrointest Endosc* 2006;64:167–175.

62. Wolfsen HC, Crook JE, Krishna M, et al. Prospective, controlled tandem endoscopy study of narrow band imaging for dysplasia detection in Barrett's Esophagus. *Gastroenterology* 2008;135:24–31.

63. Kiesslich R, Gossner L, Dahlmann A, et al. In vivo histology of Barrett's esophagus and associated neoplasia by confocal laser endomicroscopy. *Clin Gastroenterol Hepatol* 2006;8:979–987.

64. Dunbar KB, Okolo P 3rd, Montgomery E, et al. Confocal laser endomicroscopy in Barrett's esophagus and endoscopically inapparent Barrett's neoplasia: a prospective, randomized, double-blind, controlled, crossover trial. *Gastrointest Endosc* 2009;70:645–654.

65. Wallace M, Shields S, Perelman LT, et al. Fiber-optic detection of low-grade dysplasia in patients with Barrett's esophagus using reflectance spectroscopy. *Gastroenterology* 1998;114:A1336.

66. Perelman LT, Backman V, Wallace MB, et al. Observation of periodic fine structure in reflectance from biological tissue: a new technique for measuring nuclear size distribution. *Phys Rev Lett* 1998;80:627–630.

67. Backman V, Wallace MB, Perelman LT, et al. Detection of pre-invasive cancer cells. *Nature* 2000;406:35–36.

68. Kara MA, Peters FP, Ten Kate FJ, et al. Endoscopic video autofluorescence imaging may improve the detection of early neoplasia in patients with Barrett's esophagus. *Gastrointest Endosc* 2005;61:679–685.

69. Uedo N, Iishi H, Tatsuta M, et al. A novel videoendoscopy system by using autofluorescence and reflectance imaging for diagnosis of esophagogastric cancers. *Gastrointest Endosc* 2005;62:521–528.

70. Curvers WL, Singh R, Song LM, et al. Endoscopic tri-modal imaging for detection of early neoplasia in Barrett's oesophagus: a multi-centre feasibility study using high-resolution endoscopy, autofluorescence imaging and narrow band imaging incorporated in one endoscopy system. *Gut* 2008;57:167–172.

71. Jackle S, Gladkova N, Feldchtein F, et al. In vivo endoscopic optical coherence tomography of esophagitis, Barrett's esophagus, and adenocarcinoma of the esophagus. *Endoscopy* 2000;32:750–755.

8 Esophageal Manometry

Neeraj Sharma and Janice Freeman
Medical University of South Carolina, Charleston, SC, USA

Introduction

There has been increased interest in studies of esophageal function in the past several years, stimulated primarily by the growing use of laparoscopic antireflux surgery. Assessment of function includes complete evaluation of the lower esophageal sphincter (LES), esophageal body, and upper esophageal sphincter (UES). All this can be achieved by standard esophageal manometry.

Esophageal manometry is a diagnostic test that measures intraluminal pressures and coordination of pressure activity of the muscles of the esophagus (Figure 8.1). It provides both qualitative and quantitative assessment of the esophageal pressures and coordination of motility. Manometric studies are used in the assessment of patients with esophageal symptoms such as dysphagia and non-cardiac chest pain. A manometric study is also indicated before antireflux surgery to determine if a patient has adequate peristalsis (Table 8.1). Knowledge of standard esophageal manometry is essential if the newer high-resolution systems are to be understood.

Materials and equipment

The equipment and materials required to perform esophageal motility testing can be divided into a primary equipment group and a secondary materials group. The primary group consists of interconnected electronic equipment that makes up the permanent part of the motility system. The secondary group is made up of generally consumable materials required to assist in the performance of the motility study.

There are two types of esophageal motility systems within the primary equipment group: water perfusion and solid state. Both systems use esophageal motility catheters, a series of measuring instruments (transducers), and a recording and analysis device (physiograph or computer). In addi-

tion, a water perfusion pump is required for the former. Both systems measure strength and assess the coordination of the muscles of the esophagus and its sphincters, and they both transmit and convert this information into a permanent record that is easy to read and interpret. However, each system performs this function differently.

Primary equipment

The function of the primary equipment is to sense the pressure activity of the esophagus and to transmit and convert this to a permanent record that is easily read, measured, and stored. This equipment includes the manometry catheter system, transducers, and the physiograph or computer.

The motility catheter is inserted into the esophagus and measures the pressures of the esophageal contractions. It is a specially designed long, flexible tube. The water infusion system consists of a catheter made up of small capillary tubes that make up the manometry catheter and have an internal diameter of approximately 0.8 mm, and have an opening or port at a known point along the length of the catheter. One commonly used catheter has eight capillary tubes around a larger central tube with an overall diameter of 4.5 mm (Figure 8.2). The eight ports of this catheter are arranged so that the four distal ports have a radial orientation of 90 degrees and are either 1 cm apart or at the same level. The four proximal ports are 5 cm apart and are also radially oriented (Figure 8.3). Each lumen is connected to an external transducer. The infusion pump perfuses the capillary tubes with water at a rate of 0.5 mL/min. When a catheter port is occluded (e.g. by a muscular contraction), the water pressure builds within the catheter and exerts a force, which is transmitted to the external transducer.

The solid-state esophageal motility catheter is a soft, flexible tube with microtransducers contained within the catheter. These microtransducers measure esophageal contractions directly from the esophageal or sphincter wall (Figure 8.4). The type of transducer (circumferential or

The Esophagus, Fifth Edition. Edited by Joel E. Richter, Donald O. Castell.
© 2012 Blackwell Publishing Ltd. Published 2012 by Blackwell Publishing Ltd.

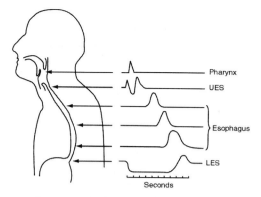

Figure 8.1 Schematic representation of the pressure sequence of a normal primary peristaltic wave. At the onset of the swallow, both the upper (UES) and lower esophageal sphincters (LES) relax. A peristaltic contraction begins at the pharynx and continues through the esophagus.

Table 8.1 Suggested clinical indications for manometric testing.

Evaluation of patients with dysphagia:
    Pharyngeal and upper esophageal sphincter abnormalities
    Primary esophageal motility disorders (e.g. achalasia)
    Secondary esophageal motility disorders (e.g. scleroderma)

Evaluation of patients with possible gastroesophageal reflux disease:
    Assistance in placement of pH probe
    Evaluation of lower esophageal sphincter pressure (e.g. poor treatment response)
    Evaluation of defective peristalsis (particularly before fundoplication)

Evaluation of patients with non-cardiac chest pain:
    Primary esophageal motility disorders
    Pain response to provocative testing

Exclusion of generalized gastrointestinal tract disease:
    Scleroderma
    Chronic idiopathic intestinal pseudoobstruction

Exclusion of esophageal etiology for suspected anorexia nervosa

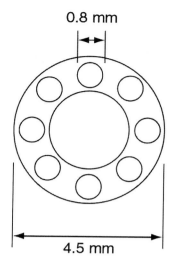

Figure 8.2 Cross-section of an eight-lumen water-perfused esophageal manometry catheter showing the internal diameter of individual catheters and the diameter of the entire catheter.

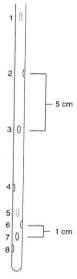

Figure 8.3 Distal end of an eight-lumen catheter showing placement and radial orientation of recording orifices.

unidirectional), and number, size, and placement of transducers vary among manufacturers(Figure 8.5). The diameter of the catheter used in our laboratory is 4.6 mm. Catheters or transducers of different diameter (water perfusion or solid state) measure different pressures, both in the two sphincters (LES and UES) and the esophageal body [1]. Small catheter diameter or transducer diameter yields lower pressures. Conversely, large diameter or larger transducer diameter yields higher pressures. When using catheters with smaller diameter, this should be an important consideration in the determination of normal values for minimum and maximum pressures.

Solid-state catheters have the advantage of measuring intraluminal pressures directly; in addition, measurements are unrelated to the relative position of the patient and the equipment. These features have made the development pos-

sible of special equipment for studies such as long-term ambulatory monitoring. The response time of solid-state catheters is much faster than that of the water-perfused system, making possible more accurate measurements of the cricopharyngeal region where the pressure rise rate exceeds the response time of water-perfused external transducers.

Development of a specialized solid-state transducer that senses pressures circumferentially over 360 degrees has simplified measurement of sphincter pressures (Figure 8.6). This is accomplished through the use of a polymeric silicone (silastic) circumferential anulus filled with a viscous fluid

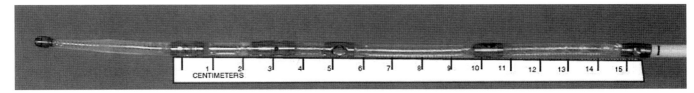

Figure 8.4 Esophageal motility catheter (solid state) alongside a centimeter ruler showing centimeter marks on catheter aligned with catheter marks on the ruler. Catheters are measured to the distal transducer.

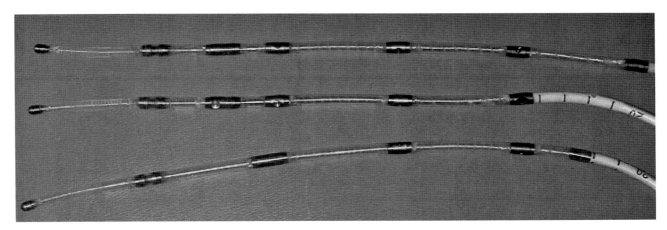

Figure 8.5 Examples of three catheter designs containing solid-state transducers.

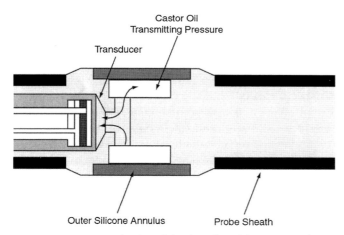

Figure 8.6 Schematic drawing of the circumferential pressure-sensing sphincter transducer showing the strain gauge surrounded by a fluid-filled chamber (USP grade castor oil) through which the pressure is transmitted.

(USP grade castor oil), which surrounds a single miniature titanium strain gauge. The oil-filled chamber surrounding the transducer produces an extremely noncompliant system. Studies by the manufacturer (Konigsberg Instruments Inc, Pasadena, CA, USA) reveal low hysteresis (0.40% of full scale) and low volumetric compliance ($7 \times 10^6 \text{mm}^3/\text{mmHg}$).

This transducer has a pressure rise rate greater than 2000 mmHg/s. The pressure-sensing portion of this transducer has an active length of 3.1 mm and a diameter range between 4.65 and 5.2 mm. The pressure-sensing diaphragm of the transducer is exposed to the fluid-filled anulus, whose the silicone rubber membrane makes direct contact with the sphincter wall. The pressure exerted by the sphincter is transmitted through the contained fluid to the strain gauge within the transducer. This transducer assembly provides a measure of circumferential squeeze, which is especially useful for pressure measurements in areas where pressure is not exerted symmetrically, such as the UES and LES [2–4].

Secondary equipment

In addition to the primary equipment, there are pieces of smaller equipment and consumable supplies that are needed for esophageal manometry. A mercury manometer attached to a calibration chamber (stoppered flask or test tube) should be available to calibrate the equipment. Necessary materials includes viscous lidocaine, lubricating jelly, tissue, tape, emesis basin, 20-mL syringe, 8-oz disposable cup, straw and container of room-temperature water, and cotton swab for applying lidocaine to the nares. During the study, we use the 20-mL syringe to give swallows of water (5 mL each).

At the completion of the study, a ready-to-use surface disinfectant is used to wipe down the wheeled cart and associated equipment. In our laboratory, motility catheters are washed with soap and water, dried, and then immersed in Cidex (glutaraldehyde) for approximately 20 min. It is important to note that the connectors must not be immersed in the cleaning solutions. The manufacturer's recommendations and the hospital's policy for proper cleaning and care should be followed.

Study technique

Careful attention to detail is essential for a successful manometric study. Manometry is performed while the patient is awake, alert, and in a supine position. Therefore, the cooperation and comfort of the patient are important for a good study outcome.

Patient preparation

The patient should have fasted for at least 6 h. Medications that might alter normal esophageal function should be discontinued at least 24 h before the study. These include nitrates, calcium channel blockers, anticholinergics, promotility agents, and sedatives. Patients who must take one or more of these medications for a serious, chronic medical condition may be studied while on the medication. All medications prescribed on an "as needed" basis should be discontinued.

Intubation and patient calibration

Intubation is the most uncomfortable part of the study for the patient and can be the most intimidating part for the clinician. It is important not to rush this part of the study. The patient should be informed of what to expect and how important cooperation is to the success of the study. The patient should be seated comfortably, and they should remove their glasses and any plates or dentures that are not strongly secured. The patient should be asked whether they have a preference as to which side of the nose to use. It should be explained that it is best to intubate through the nose instead of the mouth, because insertion through the later has a tendency to make patients gag. It should also be explained that the patient will be able to breathe with the tube in place. Gagging is a normal reflex. Passing a motility catheter is much like placing a nasal gastric tube.

The tip of the catheter is lubricated with 2% viscous xylocaine. If the patient feels the intubation is too uncomfortable, 0.5 mL of xylocaine can be injected in the nose and sniffed back into the nasal passage, or a cotton swab moistened with xylocaine may be used to apply the xylocaine to the nasal passage.

Intubation through the nasal route may be a little more uncomfortable than through the mouth, but it is much better tolerated during the procedure. An emesis basin should be close by; some patients have a sensitive gag reflex

and may vomit. The tip of the catheter is placed into the nose and advanced slowly straight back. There is some resistance as the tip of the catheter reaches the back of the nose and begins to make the bend into the throat. At this point, the patient should tip their chin down toward the chest to help the catheter slip into the esophagus. The patient should be instructed to sip water through the straw, and the catheter should be advanced as the patient swallows. Once through the UES, the catheter should be advanced fairly rapidly to a probe depth of 60 cm as the patient continues to swallow. If the patient coughs repeatedly and is unable to speak, the catheter may have slipped into the trachea instead of the esophagus. It should be withdrawn and an attempt made to reinsert it. The patient should be reassured throughout the intubation process. Once the catheter is down, the patient should be instructed to take some deep breaths to help calm them down. The catheter is secured in place with tape. At this point with most patients, the recording sites are in the stomach. The patient is then placed in the supine position and a "patient calibration" is performed. This procedure sets to zero all recording sites regardless of the pressure exerted against them. This allows gastric pressure to be used as a zero baseline when measuring LES pressures. The patient remains supine (head elevated no more than 30 degrees) during evaluation of the LES and esophageal body for two reasons: first, most published normal values for stationary manometry were obtained in the supine position; second, gravity is removed as a compounding factor. Once in the supine position, the patient should be reminded that it is important to be relaxed and to hold swallows until requested. In our laboratory, we use music to aid in patient relaxation.

Gastric baseline

In our laboratory, we begin the study by placing the two distal pressure transducers (the circumferential transducers) in the stomach. It is important to start the manometric study by measuring gastric pressure through a series of quiet respirations. A relatively flat, smooth tracing with small pressure changes with inspiration indicates proper gastric placement (Figure 8.7). Appropriate placement can be confirmed by having the patient take a deep breath and noting a rise in pressure with full inspiration. The gastric baseline pressure becomes the zero set for the subsequent LES pressure measurement. Thus, the LES pressure value is not an absolute pressure, but is a relative pressure related to the gastric baseline pressure. The study of the LES and the esophageal body are traditionally done with the patient in the supine position.

Lower esophageal sphincter

The LES is composed of tonically contracted smooth muscle, which relaxes with a swallow. The aim of the manometric assessment of the LES is to measure its resting pressure and

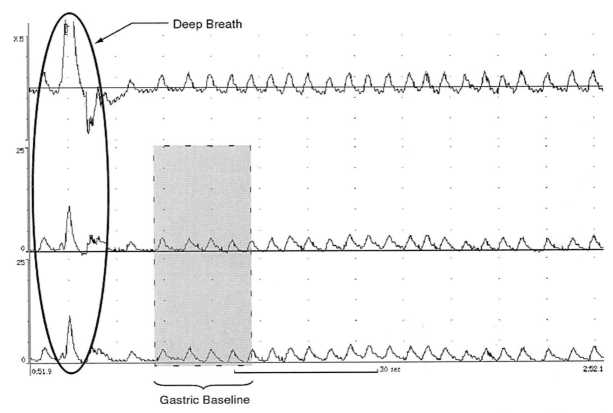

Figure 8.7 Tracing showing respiratory recording above and recordings from two transducers located in the stomach below. Note the increase in intragastric pressure with the deep inspiration. The gastric baseline pressure is obtained during a period of quiet respiration.

to assess its relaxation during swallowing. The LES resting pressure (LESP) is measured at the point of highest pressure. Assessment of the LES is best performed with a catheter containing distal averaging or circumferential sensors. This is important because of the asymmetric nature of the LES. The sensor is positioned in the high pressure zone (HPZ) of the LES, and LES relaxation is assessed by giving the patient a series of 5-mL water swallows. It is important to use water that is at room temperature. If the catheter contains directional sensors or water ports, the LES pressure must be measured with each port or sensor and the results averaged to get an accurate measurement of the LESP. Assessment of LES function is composed of two steps: profiling the LES and evaluation of sphincter relaxation.

Profiling the lower esophageal sphincter

The station pull-through technique for determining LES pressure involves a slow, stepwise withdrawal of the catheter through the LES. The catheter is moved in 0.5-cm increments and should remain at each position or "station" long enough to register a stable LESP. This usually requires waiting for a period of three to five respiratory cycles. This pull-through technique allows the identification of the LES

distal border, HPZ, pressure inversion point (PIP) or point of respiratory reversal, and proximal border of the LES.

The LES is first identified by increased respiratory pressure changes in the channel displaying waveforms from the proximal circumferential sensor, located directly above the distal sensor. This sensor is sometimes referred to as the scout, because it is used to identify the different landmarks in the LES. The increased respiratory pressure changes are followed by the rising of the bottom of the pressure tracing above the baseline (Figure 8.8). As the catheter is withdrawn, the pressure increases, and at the point where the transducer moves from the abdominal portion of the sphincter to the thoracic portion, the tracing shows a marked change in configuration, with a fall in pressure during inspiration instead of a rise in pressure. This is the PIP (Figure 8.8). The PIP is not the end of the sphincter, but rather a landmark within the sphincter that is used to calculate intra-abdominal LES length, because the PIP identifies the location of the diaphragm. The abdominal length of the LES is calculated by subtracting the probe depth where the PIP is located from the probe depth where the distal LES border is located (Figure 8.9). This measurement and the total LES length are used as important parameters in the assessment

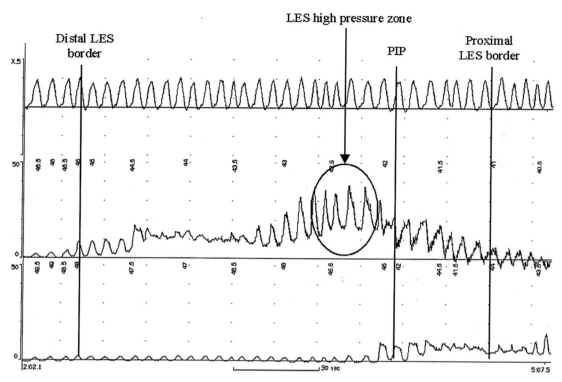

Figure 8.8 Pressure profile of the lower esophageal sphincter obtained by a station pull-through of a transducer from the stomach across the sphincter to the esophagus (middle tracing).

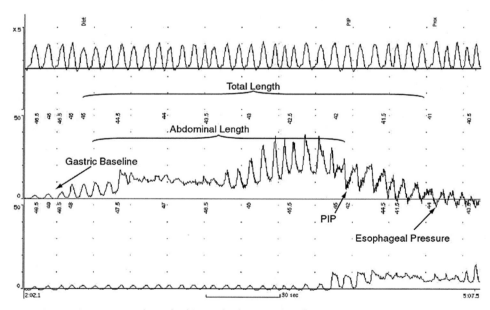

FIGURE 5.9. Lower esophageal sphincter (LES) pressure profile and calculation of the total LES length and the length of its abdominal portion.

Figure 8.9 Lower esophageal sphincter (LES) pressure profile and calculation of the total LES length and the length of its abdominal portion.

of the LES as a competent reflux barrier in some laboratories [5, 6]. As the catheter is further withdrawn, the pressure tracing drops and flattens. When the transducer leaves the LES, the pressure drops below the gastric baseline pressure, indicating that the transducer is then measuring esophageal baseline pressure. The proximal border of the LES is located at the probe depth where the pressure falls to or below the gastric baseline pressure (Figure 8.8). Subtracting this probe depth from that obtained for the distal border gives the total length of the LES (Figure 8.9).

Measurement of the LESP must take into account the changes in pressure resulting from respiration. As noted earlier, the LESP is not an absolute pressure but is a relative pressure related to the gastric baseline pressure. This is why LESP is always calculated as a pressure differential between the gastric baseline pressure and the highest LES pressure. There are two popular ways to measure LESP: from the gastric baseline to either the mid-respiratory or the end-expiratory pressure at the station with the highest overall pressure, i.e. the HPZ (Figure 8.10). There is some controversy concerning which of these methods is most accurate, but it is important to know which method was used when comparing results from different laboratories. One study suggested that end-expiratory pressure is more indicative of the true LESP, because it is at this point in the respiratory cycle that the diaphragmatic contribution to the observed pressure is at a minimum [7]. Other investigators have shown that the mid-respiratory pressure provides a LESP measurement that most reliably distinguishes patients with normal amounts of gastroesophageal reflux from those with abnormal reflux [8]. Thus, the pressure contributed by the diaphragm during respiration is an important component of the antireflux mechanism of the LES and should be included in the assessment of LESP.

The LESP measurement should include three or four respiratory cycles of level, even amplitude obtained at a fixed location (Figure 8.10). High pressure spikes are usually artifact and not a true representation of LESP; these should be disregarded. Also, pressure measurements should not be obtained after a swallow-induced relaxation because the pressure is often elevated for a while. In general, the highest pressure in the LES occurs on the abdominal side of the LES just distal to the PIP.

The results of any method must be compared with normal values obtained from using the same technique to test a cohort of age-matched normal subjects. The most comprehensive study of normal esophageal manometric parameters [9] established the following normal values (relative to gastric baseline pressure) in 95 healthy adult volunteers (mean age 43 years): end inspiration 39.7 ± 13.2 mmHg; mid respiration 24.4 ± 10.1 mmHg; and end expiration 15.2 ± 10.7 mmHg. All values are expressed as the mean ± 1 standard deviation.

Evaluation of sphincter relaxation

After the LES pull-through with the proximal transducer, the clinician continues to pull the catheter in 0.5-cm increments until the distal transducer is located in the HPZ of the LES (Figure 8.11). This placement allows evaluation of sphincter relaxation during swallowing. The catheter is

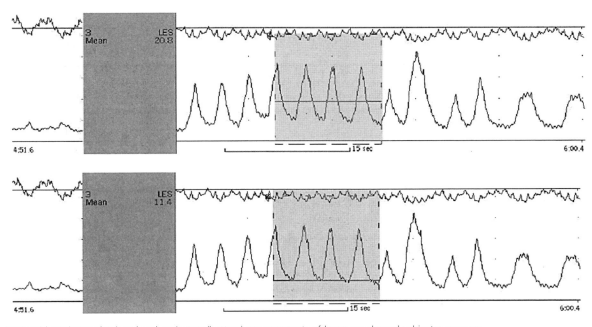

Figure 8.10 Mid-respiratory (top) and end-expiratory (bottom) measurements of lower esophageal sphincter pressure.

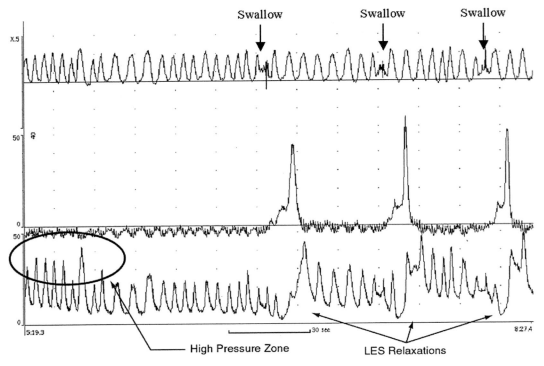

Figure 8.11 Lower esophageal sphincter (LES) high-pressure zone and LES relaxations.

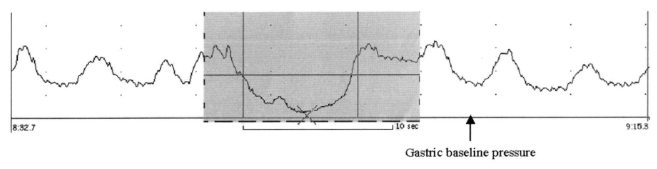

Figure 8.12 Normal swallow-induced lower esophageal sphincter relaxation showing measurement of residual pressure at the X.

taped in place and the LESP is recorded. Dry swallows often do not induce complete LES relaxation. Thus, in our laboratory, we give the patient a 5-mL bolus of room-temperature water. After a swallow, the LES pressure should drop to approximately the level of the gastric baseline. We observe the relaxation as the pressure falls, which allows the sphincter to open, and then the pressure returns to or exceeds the LESP as the sphincter contracts following the passage of the bolus. During the LES relaxation, the parameters that are usually evaluated are the duration of the relaxation and either the percentage relaxation or the residual pressure. The residual pressure is defined as the difference between the lowest pressure achieved during relaxation and the

gastric baseline pressure. This residual pressure is a better indicator of LES function than percentage relaxation because it is independent of the resting LES baseline pressure [10] (Figure 8.12). A normal residual pressure should be 8 mmHg or less.

Once the relaxation is complete, a 20–30-s interval passes before another water swallow is given. Five to ten relaxations should be repeated in this manner. Once the water swallows are completed, the catheter is pulled in 0.5-cm increments until the sensor exits the LES.

If using a catheter with directional sensors only, it is important that the sensors be rotated around the axis of the catheter so that the pressure in all four quadrants of the sphincter can be measured and averaged to produce an accurate measure of the resting pressures and relaxation. The foregoing procedure should be performed for each sensor, pulling it through the sphincter, assessing resting pressure and relaxation. The results for all sensors should be averaged. If a catheter with only a distal circumferential sensor is used, the directional sensor just proximal to the distal sensor may be used to profile the LES; it should not be used to assess resting pressure because of the asymmetry of the LES.

Manual interpretation of LES parameters, particularly the relaxation parameters, is highly subjective and qualitative. Attempts to provide a more objective and quantitative measure of these parameters have resulted in computer algorithms for an automated analysis [10, 11]. It is imperative, however, that the user reviews and, if necessary, adjusts the analysis provided by the computer (Figure 8.13). Most of these computer algorithms for LES evaluation have been adapted by manufacturers of motility equipment.

It is worth noting here that there is a second opportunity at the end of a manometric study to measure the LESP. This is significant when the initial measurement is not obtained due to artifact or technical difficulty. The technique used to obtain this second LESP reading is identical to that used to obtain the LESP at the beginning of the manometric study. After the final wet swallow, the catheter can be pulled back so that the distal sensor initially positioned in the distal LES is now in the HPZ. This will generate a HPZ reading similar to the one obtained prior to the wet swallows with similar results (Figure 8.14). A recent study showed good correlation between these two measurements (R value 0.71) [12]. If two adequate LESP readings are obtained, we generally report the average of the two measurements on our final report.

Body of the esophagus

The study of the body of the esophagus evaluates the esophageal body response to a water swallow. Contraction of the muscle normally begins at the proximal (top) portion of the esophagus and progresses in an orderly sequence to the distal (bottom) portion of the esophagus. This organized progression of the esophageal contractions represents a peristaltic wave. In the esophageal body, manometry measures amplitude, duration, and velocity of the esophageal contractions, allowing an assessment of the peristaltic activity and detection of possible motility abnormalities. A complete evaluation should include measurements of both the smooth muscle of the distal esophagus and the striated muscle of the distal esophagus. Special attention is directed to measurements made at 3 and 8 cm above the LES, because esophageal motility abnormalities occur more frequently in the distal segment of the esophagus comprised exclusively of smooth muscle. Dry swallows or double swallows are not measured.

When using catheters with two distal circumferential sensors, the distal sensor is usually placed in the HPZ of the LES. The sensors are 5 cm apart; thus censors are at 5, 10, 15, and 20 cm above the HPZ of the LES. This positioning allows simultaneous evaluation of the LES relaxation and the esophageal body contractions. Placing the distal sensor 3 cm above the proximal border of the LES is also a frequent positioning method. Most catheters have sensors or ports positioned 5 cm apart to allow assessment of the esophageal peristalsis. Usually, catheters have three to five sensors, with the most frequent spacing at 5 cm.

Once the catheter has been properly positioned and taped in place, a period of 10–15 s is allowed to elapse to establish the esophageal resting pressure as a baseline or reference

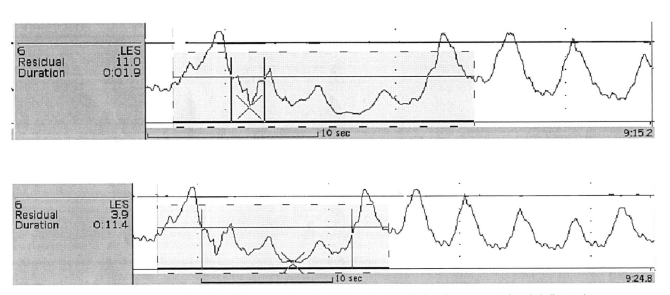

Figure 8.13 Incorrect computer-generated analysis of lower esophageal sphincter relaxation (top) and user-corrected analysis (bottom).

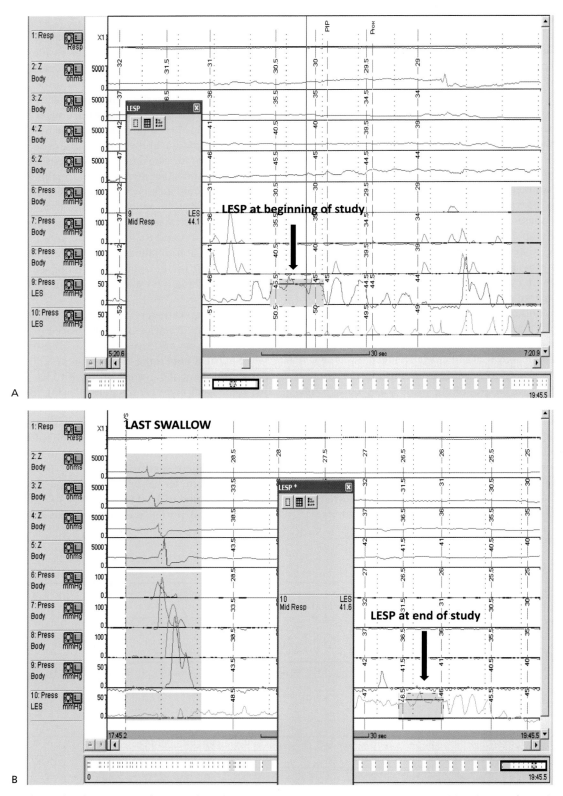

Figure 8.14 Similar results when measuring lower esophageal sphincter pressure (LESP) (A) at the beginning and (B) at the end of a study.

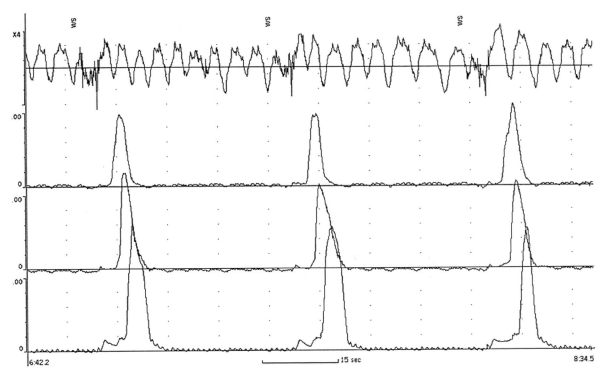

Figure 8.15 Esophageal body contractions.

point for assessing body contractions. The patient is then given a series of 5-mL boluses of room-temperature water with a 20–30-s interval between swallows (Figure 8.15). This allows time for the smooth muscle to repolarize. Each swallow should be annotated using the computer keys designated for swallow. If a strip chart is used, swallows should be marked on the graph to distinguish the water swallow from a dry swallow.

Usually, 10 wet swallows are assessed and parameters are based on the mean values. A study from our laboratory evaluated the reproducibility of swallow parameters and concluded that the mean values from five to eight swallows reliably characterize an individual's esophageal peristalsis [13]. Analysis of these parameters, especially those involving the identification of the onset of the peristaltic wave, can be subjective and time consuming. To obtain more objective and quantitative data, most laboratories use computer systems that collect, digitize, and analyze esophageal body pressure data [11, 13, 15]. Most manufacturers of manometric equipment have adapted and improved upon these programs for general use and they are commercially available.

In evaluating the esophageal body, we measure, at least, the following peristaltic parameters: amplitude, duration, and velocity. Amplitude is a measurement of how tightly the muscles of the esophagus are squeezing during a contraction and is expressed in mmHg. The baseline (0 mmHg) is the pressure in the body of the esophagus between swallows. Contraction amplitude is measured from the baseline to the peak of the pressure wave (Figure 8.16). The reported amplitude of each sensor location within the esophageal body is the mean value of the amplitude of 10 contractions in response to wet swallows. Mean values from the two most distal transducers can be averaged to obtain the distal esophageal amplitude, for which normal values of 10 swallows are 99 ± 49 mmHg.

Duration is a measurement of how long, in seconds, the muscles of the esophagus are squeezing during a contraction. The measurement is made from the onset of the major upstroke of the contraction to the point where the downstroke of the contraction returns to the baseline (Figure 8.17).

The esophageal baseline sometimes rises slightly before the actual contraction: this is called the intrabolus pressure and is due to the presence of the ingested water bolus (Figure 8.17). Normal duration values are 3.9 ± 0.9 s.

Velocity is the rate (cm/s) of progression of the contraction down the esophagus. It can be obtained between any two sites in the esophagus. The measurement is made by determining the time between the beginning of the upstroke of the contractions and dividing it by the centimeters separating the sensors. Normal values should be less than 8 cm/s (Figure 8.18).

Normal peristalsis in the distal esophagus is an orderly, sequential contraction down the esophagus, with amplitude, duration, and velocity in the normal range (Figure 8.15). In the striated muscle segment of the esophagus, the

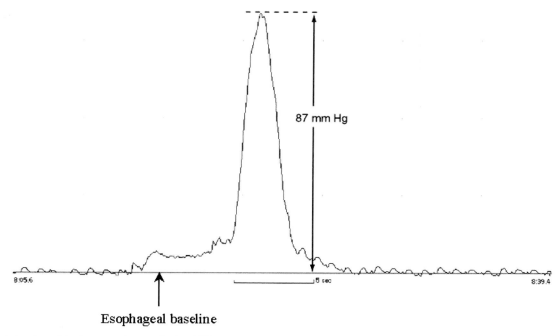

Figure 8.16 Esophageal body contraction amplitude of 87 mmHg.

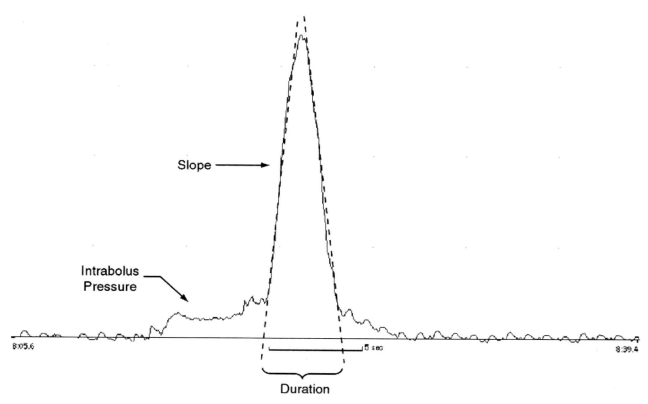

Figure 8.17 Esophageal body contraction showing the intrabolus pressure, slope of the pressure wave, and duration of the contraction.

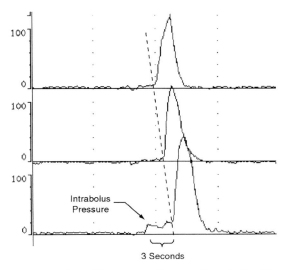

Figure 8.18 Esophageal body contractions showing velocity of the peristaltic wave.

Table 8.2 Normal esophageal pressure data from 95 healthy volunteers [10].

Parameter measured at given recording site	value
Amplitude (mmHg)	
At 18 cm above lower esophageal sphincter (LES)	62 ± 29
At 13 cm above LES	70 ± 32
At 8 cm above LES	90 ± 41
At 3 cm above LES	109 ± 45
Distal esophageal amplitude duration (s)	99 ± 40
At 18 cm above LES	2.8 ± 0.8
At 13 cm above LES	3.5 ± 0.7
At 8 cm above LES	3.9 ± 0.9
At 3 cm above LES	4.0 ± 1.1
Distal esophageal duration velocity (cm/s)	3.9 ± 0.9
Proximal	3.0 ± 0.6
Distal	3.5 ± 0.9

contractions are usually sharper than in the smooth muscle areas, with a shorter duration. If a transducer is placed in the transition zone between the striated and smooth muscle portions of the esophagus (usually around 6 cm below the UES), absent or very low amplitude contractions may be seen ("pressure trough"). The presence of a mid-esophageal pressure trough was confirmed by Clouse *et al.* [16–18], who recorded esophageal pressures at 1-cm intervals and generated isobaric contour plots for a detailed analysis of intraesophageal pressures. They also showed a difference in shape and peristaltic velocity between the distal and proximal esophagus. However, a study by Peghini *et al.* [19] determined that the striated muscle of the esophagus has manometric characteristics much closer to those of the smooth muscle portion than to those of the striated muscle in the pharynx. They also confirmed the presence of a pressure trough in the middle esophagus, although they found it in less than one-third of the subjects studied.

The definition of normal range comes from measurements of the contraction parameters in a large number of normal volunteers. The largest such study is the one by Richter *et al.* [9]. This study established normal values in 95 healthy volunteers (Table 8.2). When comparing studies done in patients with this or any other group of normal values, it is necessary to remember that these measurements are affected by the age of the subjects, body position, size of the bolus, size of the catheter, and location of the transducer.

Peristaltic contractions that have two pressure peaks are called double-peaked contractions and are considered a variant of normal. Each separate peak should be at least 10% of the overall wave amplitude and 1 s in duration (Figure 8.19). Contraction amplitude should be measured from the higher peak. Duration is measured from the upstroke of the first peak to the downstroke of the last. Triple peaked or

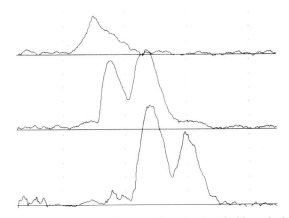

Figure 8.19 Esophageal body contractions showing double-peaked contraction waves.

more (Figure 8.20) peristaltic contractions are considered abnormal and usually indicate distal esophageal spasm.

The occurrence of a non-peristaltic contraction following a wet swallow is abnormal. Simultaneous and retrograde contractions constitute non-peristaltic contractions. Contractions are considered simultaneous when their velocity is more than 8 cm/s. A simultaneous contraction indicates that large portions of the esophagus are contracting at the same time, instead of in the normal, peristaltic sequence (Figure 8.21). In some cases, the entire esophagus contracts together, whereas in other cases, only the mid or distal esophagus contracts simultaneously. Twenty percent or more simultaneous contractions during water swallows is abnormal. Retrograde contractions may occur (Figure 8.22).

Sometimes, a wet swallow is followed by no activity in the distal esophagus (Figure 8.23) or a contraction failing to reach an amplitude of 30 mmHg (Figure 8.24). These are both examples of ineffective motility [20, 21]. The former is

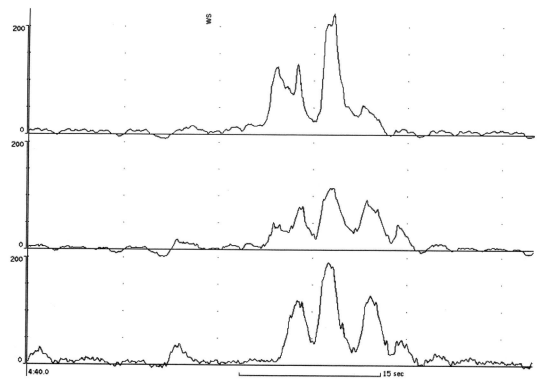

Figure 8.20 Triple-peaked (or more) peristaltic contractions.

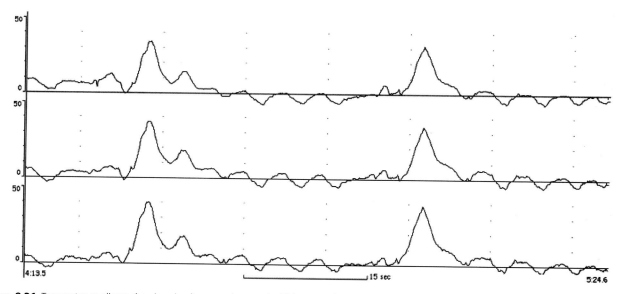

Figure 8.21 Two water swallows showing simultaneous (non-peristaltic) contractions.

known as a non-transmitted wave. A measurement of more than 50% ineffective waves after wet swallows is considered abnormal. Simultaneous comparisons of manometry with radiography [22] and scintigraphy [23] have shown that contractions with an amplitude of less than 30 mmHg may lack the necessary force to move a bolus through the esopha-

gus. However, the recent introduction of multichannel intraluminal impedance technology (see Chapter 10), which allows measurement of bolus transit simultaneously with pressure, suggests that a threshold lower than 30 mmHg may be needed because there appears to be frequent bolus transit with pressures between 25 and 30 mmHg.

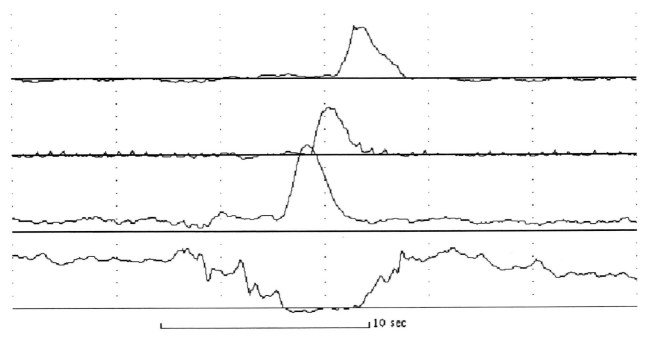

Figure 8.22 Water swallow showing a retrograde contraction.

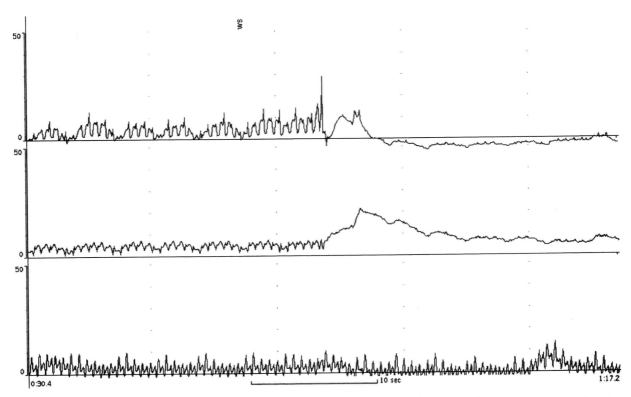

Figure 8.23 Example of non-transmitted contraction showing no activity in the distal esophagus when the distal esophagus contracts before the proximal esophagus (see Figure 8.21).

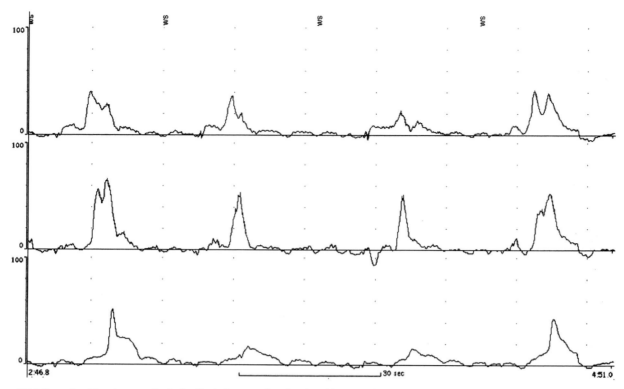

Figure 8.24 Example of two low-amplitude (ineffective) contractions bracketed by normal peristaltic waves.

In patients with a skeletal muscular disorder, it may be desirable to assess striated muscle function. To do this, the catheter is pulled orad until a pressure rise is noted in the proximal channel, indicating the sensor is entering the UES. The sensor is repositioned 1 cm lower, placing the sensor 1 cm below the distal border of the UES (Figure 8.25) to ensure that the proximal sensor is in striated muscle. Ten to 15 s of resting pressure establishes an esophageal baseline or reference point for the body contractions resulting from the water swallows. The patient makes five to 10 water swallows. It is not necessary to wait the 20–30 s required for assessing smooth muscle, because striated muscle does not require as long a recovery time.

Provocative testing

Provocative testing is an optional part of the esophageal manometry study. It elicits or reproduces symptoms that may be esophageal in origin. Interpretation is based on the patient's subjective complaints rather than on specific manometric change. The Bernstein test to assess acid sensitivity and the edrophonium (Tensilon) test for high-amplitude or simultaneous contractions have essentially become obsolete and will not be discussed further.

Upper esophageal sphincter

The final part of the study involves assessment of the UES, which includes a determination of the resting pressure of the UES, relaxation of the UES, pharyngeal contraction and peristalsis, and an assessment of the coordination between UES relaxation and pharyngeal contraction [24]. This study is best performed with the patient in a sitting position.

Like the LES, the UES is a sphincter that is tonically contracted and relaxes with swallowing. The UES and pharyngeal region differ from the body of the esophagus in several ways that markedly affect the manner in which manometry must be performed. First, the UES and pharynx are composed of striated muscle; therefore, the muscular contractions and responses are much more rapid than those in the smooth muscle distal esophagus. The rate of contraction of the striated muscle far exceeds the response time of low-compliance infusion systems, which substantially misrecord pharyngeal waveforms [25]. In addition to limitations imposed by the response of the transducer system, an analog recording system has a recording frequency that impacts the interpretation of the signal from the transducers. The mechanical recording pens of the polygraph generally record faithfully only to a frequency of 20–40 Hz [26]. A computerized manometry system allows more flexibility in recording frequencies. Although it is possible to collect data at much higher rates, practical considerations of memory and disk space utilization have kept those computer systems currently in use to a recording frequency of 100–128 Hz [8], which allows for a resolution of ±10 ms.

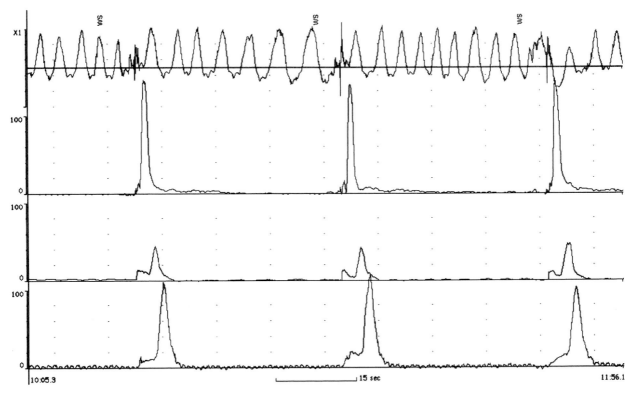

Figure 8.25 Upper esophageal body contractions.

The second difference that affects UES and pharyngeal manometry is inherent in the anatomy of the UES. The asymmetry of the UES pressure profile has been confirmed in humans by the use of an eight-lumen perfused manometry catheter in which the orientation of each orifice was known [27, 28]. The highest pressures are recorded from the anterior and posterior directions, and the lowest from the lateral direction. One possible solution to this dilemma is to use an oval catheter that ensures proper orientation within the sphincter and records only maximum and minimum pressures [29, 30]. Use of such a catheter instead of the round tube routinely used for esophageal manometry would present some practical problems. Green *et al.* reported on a comparison between a round and an oval catheter, each with four orifices spaced radially at 90 degrees [31]. They found that mean values for the oval and round catheters were not significantly different. Therefore, the recording of average sphincter pressures is independent of catheter shape. Thus, the development of a circumferential sphincter transducer has allowed for accurate sphincter measurements without the need to control catheter orientation [32].

The assessment of the UES begins by establishing a baseline or reference point in the body of the esophagus. The HPZ of the UES is usually found by the slow or station pull-through method. The UES is reactive to catheter move-

ment, so it is necessary to allow the recording device to remain in the HPZ for 15–20 s before measuring the pressure (Figure 8.26).

In addition to measuring the resting UES pressure, a manometric evaluation must also include an analysis of UES relaxation during swallowing. This analysis has been confounded by swallow-related movements of the sphincter [12]. If the sensor is positioned in the HPZ for the swallow, the pressure tracing produces what appears to be a prolonged relaxation (i.e. a relaxation without the elevation spike). This is due to the UES moving completely off the sensor as it moves orad with the swallow. The sensor actually drops into the body of the esophagus. When the UES returns to resting pressure, it moves back onto the sensor, giving the appearance that the UES has closed (Figure 8.27). A prolonged relaxation of more than 0.5 s (500 ms) should be an indication that the sensor may not be correctly positioned.

To properly assess UES relaxation, it is necessary to position the sensor above or proximal to the HPZ of the UES. If the sensor is properly positioned, the tracing seen during a swallow appears as an M-configuration (Figure 8.28). Initially, the pressure is well below that of the UES HPZ. However, as the UES moves orad with the initiation of the swallow, the pressure increases, corresponding to the movement of the HPZ onto the sensor. The pressure then

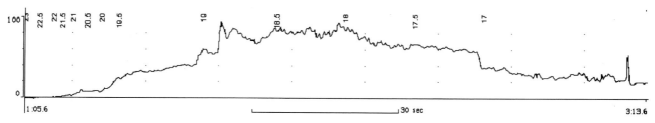

Figure 8.26 Upper esophageal sphincter pull-through localizing the high-pressure zone.

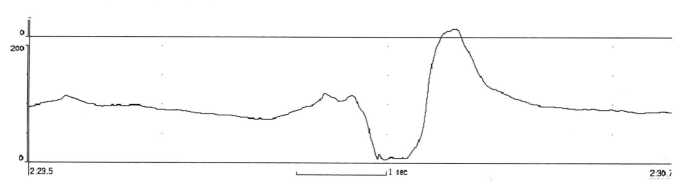

Figure 8.27 Artifactual apparent relaxation of upper esophageal sphincter with sensor improperly positioned within the high-pressure zone.

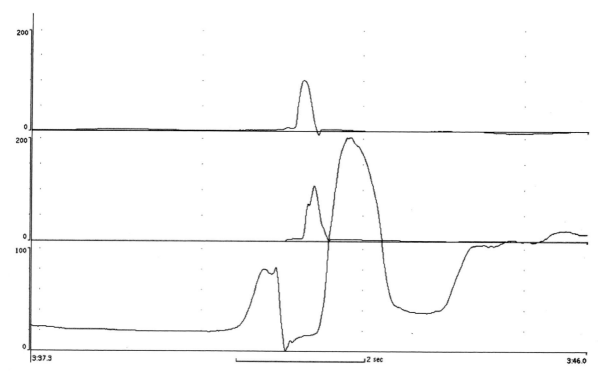

Figure 8.28 M configuration of upper esophageal sphincter relaxation.

drops and again increases as the sphincter relaxes and regains its resting tone. There is finally a slow drop in pressure as the HPZ returns to its original position distal to the sensor.

Once the sensor is properly positioned, it is possible to study both the UES function during swallowing and the coordination between the relaxation of the UES and the contraction of the pharynx. The pharynx, like the UES, is asymmetric with the highest pressures recorded in the anterior and posterior direction, and the lowest pressures laterally. A study using a special catheter with four solid-state transducers separated by 3 cm and oriented circumferentially at 90 degrees, measured pharyngeal pressures in four directions from the proximal edge of the UES through the hypopharynx and oropharynx [4]. There was statistically significant asymmetry in both the longitudinal and radial directions. Pressures varied from 365 ± 29 to 86 ± 13 mmHg.

To properly assess UES and pharyngeal contraction coordination, the catheter should contain three pressure sensors within a 5-cm total spacing. The best catheter configuration has two circumferential sensors spaced 3 cm apart, with a third unidirectional sensor positioned 2 cm above the secondary or proximal circumferential sensor. This configuration allows evaluation of the pharyngeal contractions with the two proximal sensors (one circumferential, one directional), while assessing UES relaxation with the distal circumferential sensor (Figure 8.28). There is no reason to wait between the swallows because the area being assessed is striated muscle which has rapid repolarization. Once a swallow is completed, the next one may be given as soon as the patient is ready.

The accurate evaluation of pharyngeal peristalsis and UES–pharyngeal coordination requires computer analysis. The sequence of events is so rapid (usually <1 s) that the higher resolution of computer-recorded data is necessary.

Conclusions

In the distant past, barium examination was the only useful technique for assessing patients with both oropharyngeal and esophageal dysphagia, because of its ability to assess actual bolus transfer and the possible presence of aspiration. However, using the technology described, manometric studies can also provide important information on the swallowing mechanism of the pharynx, UES, esophageal body, and LES. We believe that this information will augment that provided by the barium swallow and allow for a more complete assessment of the patient with dysphagia, in addition to delineating a treatment plan based on motor abnormalities. Though high-resolution manometry may eventually become the standard of care, basic manometry can still provide valuable information to a clinician.

References

1. Lydon SB, Dodds WJ, Hogan WJ, Arndorfer RC. The effect of manometric assembly diameter on intraluminal esophageal pressure recording. *Dig Dis Sci* 1975;20:968–670.
2. Castell JA, Dalton CB, Castell DO. Pharyngeal and upper esophageal sphincter manometry in humans. *Am J Physiol* 1990;258:G173–178.
3. Pursnani KG, Oeffner C, Gideon RM, Castell DO. Comparison of lower oesophageal sphincter pressure measurement using circumferential vs unidirectional transducers. *Neurogastroenterol Motil* 1997;9:177–180.
4. Sears VW, Castell JA, Castell DO. Radial and longitudinal asymmetry of the human pharynx. *Gastroenterology* 1991;101:1559–1563.
5. Bonavina L, Evander A, Demeester TR. Length of the distal esophageal sphincter and competency of the cardia. *Am J Surg* 1986;151:25–34.
6. O'Sullivan GC, Demeester TR, Joelsson BE, *et al.* Interaction of lower esophageal sphincter pressure and length of sphincter in the abdomen and determinants of gastroesophageal competence. *Am J Surg* 1982;143:40–47.
7. Castell JA, Castell DO. Modern solid state computerized manometry of the pharyngoesophageal segment. *Dysphagia* 1993;8:270–275.
8. Kraus BB, Wu WC, Castell DO. Comparison of lower esophageal sphincter manometries and gastroesophageal reflux measured by 24-hour pH recording. *Am J Gastroenterol* 1990;85:692–696.
9. Richter JE, Wu WC, Johns DN, *et al.* Esophageal manometry in 95 healthy adult volunteers. *Dig Dis Sci* 1987;32:583–592.
10. Castell JA, Dalton CB, Castell DO. On-line computer analysis of human lower esophageal sphincter relaxation. *Am J Physiol* 1988;255:G794–799.
11. Castell JA, Castell DO. Computer analysis of human esophageal peristalsis and lower esophageal sphincter pressure. II. An interactive system for on-line data collection and analysis. *Dig Dis Sci* 1986;31:1211–1216.
12. Roberts JR, Freeman J, Castell DO. Everyone deserves a second chance: validation of a double LESP profile technique [Abstract]. In: *American College of Gastroenterology Annual Scientific Meeting*, Oct 23–28, 2009, San Diego, p. 439.
13. De Vault K, Castell JA, Castell DO. How many swallows are required to establish reliable esophageal peristaltic parameters in normal subjects? An on-line computer analysis. *Am J Gastroenterol* 1987;82:754.
14. Tijskens G, *et al.* Validation of a fully automated analysis of esophageal body contractility and lower esophageal sphincter function: a study on the effect of the PGE, analogue rioprostil on human esophageal motility. *J Gastrointest Motil* 1989;1:21.
15. Wilson JA, *et al.* Computerized manometric recording: an evaluation. *Gullet* 1991;1:87.
16. Clouse RE, Staiano A. Topography of normal and high-amplitude esophageal peristalsis. *Am J Physiol* 1993;268:G1098–1107.
17. Clouse RE, Staiano A. Topography of the esophageal peristaltic pressure wave. *Am J Physiol* 1991;261:G677–684.
18. Clouse RE, Staiano A, Bickson SJ, Cohn SM. Characteristics of the propagating pressure wave in the esophagus. *Dig Dis Sci* 1996;41:2369–2376.

19. Peghini PL, Pursnani KG, Gideon MR, Castell JA, Nierman, J, Castell DO. Proximal and distal esophageal contractions have similar manometric features. *Am J Physiol* 1998;37:G325–330.

20. Kahrilas PJ, Dodds WJ, Hogan WJ. Effect of peristaltic dysfunction on esophageal volume clearance. *Gastroenterology* 1988; 94:73–80.

21. Leite LP, Johnston BT, Barrett J, Castell JA, Castell DO. Ineffective esophageal motility (IEM): the primary finding in patients with non-specific esophageal motility disorder. *Dig Dis Sci* 1997;42:1853–1865.

22. Hogan WJ, Dodds WJ, Stewart ET. Comparison of roentgenology and intraluminal manometry for evaluating oesophageal peristalsis. *Rend Gastroenterol* 1973:5:28.

23. Richter JE, Blackwell JN, Wu WC, Johns DN, Cowan RJ, Castell DO. Relationship of radionuclide liquid bolus transport and esophageal manometry. *J Lab Clin Med* 1987;109:217–224.

24. Castell JA, Castell DO. Stationary esophageal manometry. In: Scarpignato C, Galiche JP, eds. *Functional Investigation in Esophageal Disease.* Basel: Karger, 1994, pp. 109–129.

25. Dodds WJ, *et al.* Considerations about pharyngeal manometry. *Dysphagia* 1987;1:209.

26. Stef JJ, Dodds WJ, Hogan WJ, Linehan JH, Stewart ET. Intraluminal esophageal manometry :an analysis of variables affecting recording fidelity of peristaltic pressures. *Gastroenterology* 1974:67:221–230.

27. Welch RW, Luckman K, Ricks PM, Drake ST, Gates GA. Manometry of the normal upper esophageal sphincter and its alteration in laryngectomy. *J Clin Invest* 1979;63:1036–1041.

28. Winans CS. The pharyngoesophageal closure mechanism. A manometric study. *Gastroenterology* 1972;63:768–777.

29. Gergardt DC, *et al.* Esophageal dysfunction in esophagopharyngeal regurgitation. *Gastroenterology* 1980;78:893.

30. Knuff TE, Benjamin SB, Castell DO. Pharyngoesophageal (Zenker's) diverticulum, a reappraisal. *Gastroenterology* 1982; 82:734–736.

31. Green WE, Castell JA, Castell DO. Upper esophageal sphincter pressure recording: is an oval manometry catheter necessary? *Dysphagia* 1988;2:162–165.

32. Castell JA, Dalton CB, Castell DO. Effects of body position and bolus consistency on the manometric parameters and coordination of the upper esophageal sphincter and pharynx. *Dysphagia* 1990;5:179–186.

9 High-Resolution Manometry and Esophageal Pressure Topography

John E. Pandolfino and Peter J. Kahrilas
Department of Medicine, The Feinberg School of Medicine, Northwestern University, Chicago, IL, USA

Introduction

High-resolution manometry (HRM) is an adaptation of conventional manometry that employs an increased number of closely spaced pressure sensors so that the intraluminal pressure profile can be viewed as a continuum. To better visualize the data, Clouse and Staino devised a process of interpolation or averaging of pressure values between sensors to display the information in the form of seamless isobaric color regions on high-resolution esophageal pressure topography (HREPT) plots [1] (Figure 9.1). The HREPT or "Clouse plots" display manometric information as distinct patterns that illustrate the physiology of contractile coordination and the mechanics associated with bolus transit. This technique represents a major advance in manometric investigation and other pioneers in this technology, such as Cook and Brasseur should also be acknowledged for their pioneering work in describing the dynamics of bolus transit through the upper esophageal sphincter (UES) [2, 3]. Additionally, Geoff Hebbard deserves special mention in any discussion on HRM as he is responsible for developing one of the first analysis software packages focused on HREPT.

Although the utilization of HRM was initially limited to research centers, advances in the technology have now made it widely available and it is currently moving into mainstream clinical practice. The clinical indications for HRM are similar to those identified for conventional manometry as the technology provides similar, albeit enhanced, information. The goals of this review will be to examine how HRM differs from conventional manometry and to illustrate how this technology is being utilized to redefine esophageal motor function and categorize esophageal motor disorders.

High-resolution manometry

Definition

Conventional manometry typically incorporates 3–8 pressure sensors axially positioned along a recording assembly at 3–5-cm intervals. HRM simply implies that manometry is done with a multitude of closely spaced pressure sensors. By convention, this means spacing between sensors of 1 cm or less, based on the observation that with 1-cm spacing there is negligible loss of pressure data between sensors [1]. As such, HRM is not a new technology; instead, it represents a refinement in manometric methodology that provides greater resolution while improving data interpretation.

Data generated by HRM can be visualized using line tracings to depict the intraluminal pressure of the esophagus similar to conventional manometry. However, this can be quite cumbersome in terms of visualization and analysis (Figure 9.1). Pressure topography, on the other hand, is a method for viewing and analyzing manometric data that displays data in the format of isobaric contour plots or, in recognition of the investigator who first pioneered these, Clouse plots [1, 4] (Figure 9.1). These plots lay out a coordinate system of time on the x axis, sensor position on the y axis, and then localized pressure values represented by color, 3D elevation, or both (Figure 9.1) within that coordinate system. Pressure topography plots can be constructed with data from any number of manometric sensors; the more the better. Generally speaking, there is minimal data loss between sensors when utilizing a 1-cm spacing. However, special circumstances, notably recordings of the gastroesophageal junction (GEJ), may well benefit from the enhanced detail of even closer sensor spacing.

The Esophagus, Fifth Edition. Edited by Joel E. Richter, Donald O. Castell.
© 2012 Blackwell Publishing Ltd. Published 2012 by Blackwell Publishing Ltd.

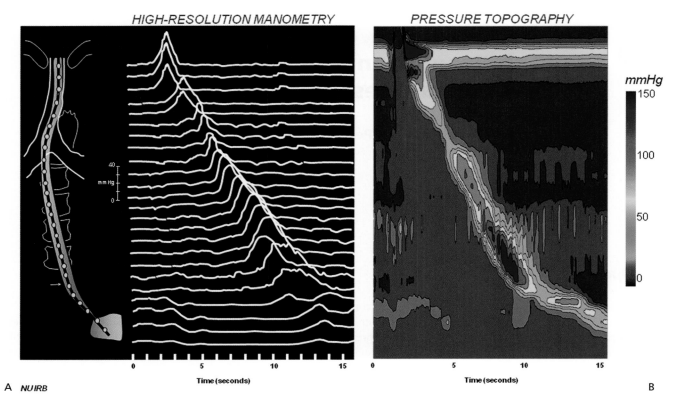

B

Figure 9.1 Typical swallow comparison of (A) high-resolution manometry and (B) esophageal pressure topography. The manometry catheter has closely spaced pressure sensors that record pressure and can display information in the line tracing format (A) or the pressure topography format (B). Note that the x axis (time) and y axis (location) are the same. The main difference is the reference for pressure, where it is the height of the tracing for the conventional line tracings (A) and a color scale for topography (B).

Technology

The concept of HRM is independent of the pressure transducer technology utilized; systems utilizing both water-perfused multilumen catheters with external pressure tranducers and solid-state microtransducers incorporated into the recording assemblies themselves are currently available. For esophageal studies, a desirable characteristic is for the recording assembly to span from the pharynx to the stomach, with sensor separation of no more than 1 cm within and around the sphincters and a temporal frequency response matched to the zone of the esophagus in which the sensors reside. Currently, there are three devices that fulfill these requirements (Medical Measurement Systems, Enschede, The Netherlands; Sandhill Scientific, Highlands Ranch, CO, USA; Sierra Scientific Instruments, Los Angeles, CA, USA). Each of these systems consists of 32–36 solid-state transducers spaced at 1-cm intervals, which is adequate to assess intraluminal activity from the pharynx to the stomach without the need to reposition the recording assembly.

There are also two sensor configurations currently available in solid-state HRM devices: unidirectional and circumferential. As the names infer, unidirectional sensors record pressure from just one side of the round recording assembly,

while circumferential sensors derive an average pressure from integration of multiple pressure-sensing elements around the circumference. In circumstances in which there is minimal asymmetry of the intraluminal contraction, such as in the intrasphincteric esophagus, sensor type makes little difference. However, within the UES and GEJ there is substantial radial asymmetry of intraluminal pressure during both contraction and relaxation, making circumferential sensors of theoretical benefit [5, 6].

Procedural advantages

Although the details of obtaining an HRM study are very similar to conventional manometry in terms of patient preparation and intubation, HRM offers several intuitive advantages over conventional manometry. With conventional manometry, a pull-through technique is necessary to locate the lower esophageal sphincter (LES) and position the pressure sensors relative to this landmark. With HRM, the multitude of closely-spaced pressure sensors simultaneously provides a comprehensive assessment of the entire esophagus, obviating the need for repositioning the assembly once it is in place. As a result, studies require less time to obtain and are easier to perform. Additionally, variability in the quality of studies attributable to errors in sensor placement is inherently eliminated, thus increasing the reproducibility of studies.

One failure of conventional manometry is the inability to account for anatomic changes in a dynamic esophagus, such as esophageal shortening or hiatus hernia, which may be lost in the intersensor "blind spots." Once again, the global esophageal assessment provided by HRM accommodates dynamic changes in the esophagus and permits the confident localization of pressure landmarks, such as the LES or crural diaphragm, regardless of their mobility during the study [4, 7]. Consequently, HRM studies have greater consistency and less artifact than does conventional manometry.

Although the new solid-state HRM systems come with many advantages, the systems are associated with some escalation in cost. The new catheters are expensive (ranging from US$8000 to US$10000) and have limited durability due to the intricate electronics required to support the increased number and reduced spacing of the solid-state sensors. Expected utilization can range up to 200–250 studies and thus, busy centers will require at least two catheters per year. Additionally, care must be taken when performing studies on difficult patients, such as those with a dilated esophagus or large hiatus hernia. As it can be very difficult to place the catheter across the GEJ or hiatal canal, endoscopy is often utilized to guide the catheter into the abdominal compartment. Care must be taken not to damage the catheter, and a closed snare or forceps should never be used as this can damage the protective barrier and expose the intricate hardware to the external environment. A gentle nudging or guiding with an open snare is preferred based on the above concerns.

Esophageal pressure topography

A description of the terms used in HREPT is given in Appendix 9.1.

Description

HREPT is not synonymous with HRM. Rather, EPT represents a new format for displaying manometric data that is inherently dependent on HRM. Any set of line tracing data can be converted to pressure topography plots that visualize pressure in a space–time continuum using color as a representative of pressure measurement. However, in order for these plots to appear smooth (as opposed to notched), the data must be enhanced both in the time dimension (between sampling times) and in the spatial dimension (between pressure recording sites) by interpolation or averaging between the pressure sensors. This interpolation is usually done using a cubic spline algorithm implemented on a finely resolved rectilinear space–time grid to generate intermediate data points [1] . Pressure topography plots can be constructed

from manometry data with sensors spaced 2 cm or more apart, but the validity of doing so is questionable because interpolating the intermediate values between two widely spaced pressure sensors assumes that a smooth pressure continuum exists between them and this simply may not be the case. Compared to conventional esophageal manometry utilizing pressure tracings, HREPT has the advantage of being more intuitive and more easily learned by trainees or practitioners naïve to esophageal manometry in any format [8].

Variables

Baseline gastroesophageal junction measurements

Because pressure events at the GEJ impact on more proximal pressure events within the esophagus, the first step in evaluating HREPT studies is focused on the GEJ, specifically the accurate identification of the location of the LES, its relative position to the crural diaphragm (CD), and the location of the respiratory inversion point (Figure 9.2). Localization of these parameters allows deglutitive relaxation to be confidently measured and also to assess whether the residual pressure measurement at the GEJ is a manifestation of impaired LES relaxation or elevated intrabolus pressure (IBP) associated with obstruction through the GEJ. Obstruction through the GEJ may occur as a consequence of rings, stricture, hiatus hernia or defects in the mechanical properties of the distal esophagus related to infiltrative processes (eosinophilic esophagitis, tumor).

Once the respiratory inversion point is localized, confirming that the manometric assembly has entered the intraabdominal compartment, the morphology of the GEJ is assessed by noting the relative positions of the LES contraction and the CD contraction. GEJ morphology is characterized by measuring the distance between the midpoint of the LES pressure zone and the midpoint of the crural diaphragm contraction during inspiration (Figure 9.2) [9]. Normally, these contractile elements should overlap and move in synchrony with respiration. A separation between the LES and CD of greater than 2 cm (type III morphology in Figure 9.2) suggests the presence of a hiatus hernia. Having said this, HREPT measurements of LES–CD separation greater than 2 cm may lose accuracy as hernia size increases because of the tendency for the manometric assembly to bend or curl within the hernia, falsely elevating the measurement. Type II GEJ morphology, characterized by a measurable LES–CD separation, but if less than 2 cm it probably represents an early stage in the development of hiatus hernia. Although this can be documented, its clinical significance is currently unclear. Consequently, the most clinically meaningful assessment of GEJ morphology is the documentation of either type I morphology indicative of a normal GEJ or type III morphology with clear LES–CD separation indicative of hiatus hernia.

Resting LES pressure is a highly variable quantity during manometric studies and the numeric value in and of itself

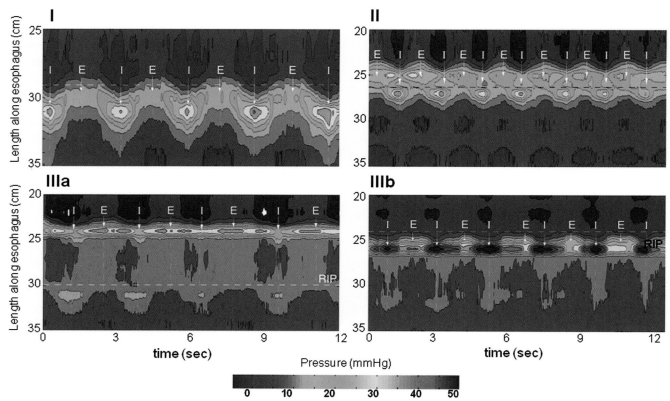

Figure 9.2 Pressure topography plots of gastroesophageal junction (GEJ) pressure morphology subtypes primarily distinguished by the extent of lower esophageal sphincter–crural diaphragm (LES–CD) separation during respiration. The pressure scale is shown at the bottom. Instants of peak inspiration are marked (I) with mid expiration (E) indicated midway between inspirations. The locus of the respiratory inversion point (RIP) is indicated by a horizontal dashed line. Type I is characterized by complete overlap of the CD and LES. The RIP lies at the proximal margin of the GEJ. Type II is characterized by minimal, but discernible, LES–CD separation. The RIP is within the GEJ at the proximal margin of the CD. GEJ type III is the high-resolution esophageal pressure tomography (HREPT) signature of a hiatus hernia. Two subtypes are discernible, IIIa and IIIb, with the distinction being that the respiratory inversion point was proximal to the CD with IIIa and proximal to the LES in IIIb. The shift in RIP is likely indicative of a grossly patulous hiatus, open throughout the respiratory cycle (modified from Pandolfino *et al.* [9]).

is not pathognomonic for any esophageal motor disorder. However, the detection of minimal LES pressure does provide supportive evidence for GERD, or esophageal involvement with connective tissue disease if it is extremely low. Additionally, there is the opposite extreme where LES pressure exceeds the 95th percentile of normal, and this may be associated with achalasia or a hypercontractile condition. Measurement of resting GEJ pressure must also specify the respiratory phase during which the measurement is made as this values is strongly influenced by pressure changes in the thoracic and intra-abdominal compartments related to respiration (Table 9.1) [10]. Values of resting LES pressure are minimally affected by body position.

Deglutitive gastroesophageal junction relaxation

Incomplete deglutitive LES relaxation is an essential criterion for the diagnosis of achalasia, making it one of the most important measurements made during esophageal manom-

etry. Despite this cardinal importance, there is no accepted convention for defining incomplete deglutitive LES relaxation in conventional manometry.

Several nuances of quantifying LES relaxation emerge in HREPT [10, 11]. First, as alluded to in the discussion of resting pressure, the CD is superimposed on the LES, making this a complex sphincter, and swallowing does not inhibit the CD. Consequently, other than in instances of hiatal hernia, GEJ relaxation, not LES relaxation, is actually being measured. Second, during swallowing the sphincter moves proximally by an average of 2 cm as a consequence of esophageal shortening with longitudinal muscle contraction during peristalsis; in extreme instances this can be by as much as 9 cm. Consequently, a point sensor positioned within the sphincter prior to swallowing can be distal to the sphincter during relaxation and subject to the artifact of "pseudorelaxation" [6]. Third, it is overly simplistic to think of GEJ relaxation pressure as solely indicative of LES relaxa-

Table 9.1 Gastroesophageal junction (GEJ), gastric, and esophageal pressure during normal respiration in a set of 75 normal volunteers (modified from Pandolfino *et al.* [7]).

Relative to atmospheric pressure

	Expiration[†]	Inspiration[†]	Inspiratory change[†]
GEJ pressure (mmHg)	23.9 (9.3)*	40.9 (12.3)	+16.9 (8.2)
Esophageal pressure (mmHg)	0.3 (2.3)*	−4.7 (2.3)	−5.0 (1.8)
Gastric pressure (mmHg)	5.5 (2.1)*	8.6 (2.3)	+3.1 (1.0)

Relative to gastric pressure

	Mean	2 SD range
Expiratory GEJ pressure (mmHg)	18.4	4.0–32.8
Inspiratory GEJ pressure (mmHg)	32.3	12.3–52.3

*$P < .05$ vs inspiration.
†All values expressed as mean (SD).

is of great clinical significance because failing to detect impaired GEJ relaxation in these patients has the result of giving them an alternative diagnosis, most commonly misclassifying them as ineffective esophageal motility or diffuse esophageal spasm (DES) [12].

Peristaltic integrity

Following the analysis of the GEJ morphology and relaxation, a swallow is next assessed for characteristics of the esophageal contraction. This analysis is greatly facilitated by creating a pressure topography plot highlighting the 20 and/or 30 mmHg isobaric contours and identifying characteristic patterns of peristalsis and IBP. Under circumstances of normal deglutitive GEJ relaxation, the 30 mmHg pressure threshold provides a reliable means of differentiating IBP from luminal closure pressure, thereby delineating the contractile front of the peristaltic contraction [13]. It is also the best-accepted threshold for peristaltic amplitude that is predictive of complete bolus clearance [14]. Threshold values for impaired bolus transit using the 30-mmHg isobaric contour have recently also been validated for HREPT. Using combined HRM and impedance, Bulsiewicz *et al.* reported that a break of 3 cm or more in the 30-mmHg isobaric contour is universally associated with impaired bolus transit [15]. Thus, swallows exhibiting an intact 30-mmHg isobaric contour or with breaks that are less than 3 cm in the region spanning from the transition zone to the proximal border of the LES are considered intact.

In addition to the size of the break in the 30-mmHg isobaric contour, the location of the break may have additional clinical relevance. Clouse originally described three regions subject to pressure troughs in the topography of peristalsis, labeled P (proximal), M (middle), and D (distal) in Figure 9.4. Although the clinical relevance and neuromuscular control of these segments and troughs is unclear, peristaltic contractions may exhibit exaggerated troughs resulting in breaks in the 30 mmHg isobaric contour at each location. Defects within the proximal trough deserve special emphasis as this location has also been referred to as the transition zone based on the hypothesis that it represents a transition in the neuromuscular control of the esophagus from extrinsically controlled striated muscle to intrinsically dominated smooth muscle [16, 17]. Transition zone defects that are greater than 2 cm in length measured on the 20-mmHg isobaric contour can be associated with impaired bolus transit and bolus retention at that locus.

Swallows can also be characterized by absent peristalsis, defects in the 30 mmHg isobaric contour that are so substantial that no propagating contractile activity is evident or only a short segment of contraction (<3 cm) is noted; these swallows should be categorized as failed peristalsis. An additional subtype of weak peristalsis exhibits a short segment of rapidly propagated contraction associated with a proximal defect. Rapidly propagated segmental contractions are of

tion. Actually, at any one instant the measured pressure is the greatest of three possible contributions: LES pressure, CD contraction, and IBP as the swallowed water traverses the GEJ [10] (Figure 9.3). For all of these reasons, the metric of nadir LES pressure is very inaccurate and insensitive for the detection of abnormal deglutitive GEJ relaxation. Hence, the development of the HREPT GEJ relaxation metric of the integrated relaxation pressure (IRP) [6]. The IRP is measured following UES relaxation within a 6-cm span, capturing the axial movement of the LES attributable to esophageal shortening and spanning from the time of UES relaxation until the arrival of the peristaltic contraction (or 10 s in the absence of peristalsis). Thus, the IRP is similar to measuring GEJ relaxation with a Dent sleeve, with the added stipulation that the relaxation pressure being reported is the lowest value persisting for a period of 4 s after the swallow, and the technique can distinguish between the LES and CD components of GEJ pressure in instances in which they are not superimposed (Figure 9.3). The 4-s period scored in computing the IRP does not need to be continuous and may be segmented to exclude CD contractions that may occur during deglutitive LES relaxation [11]. Table 9.2 illustrates the added yield of the IRP compared to the nadir LES or GEJ pressure in the detection of impaired GEJ relaxation in a series of well-defined achalasia patients. This improvement

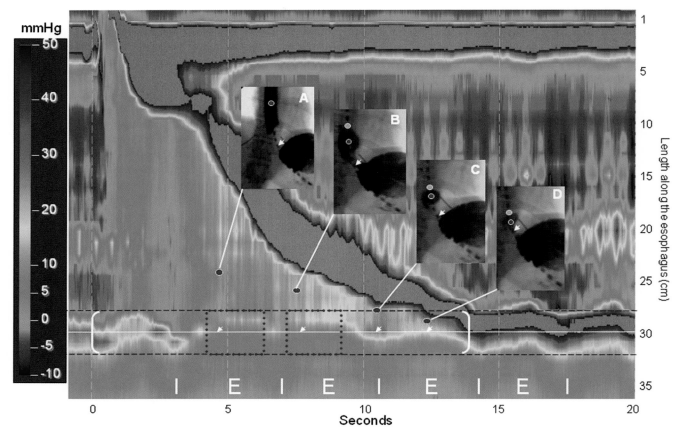

Figure 9.3 The integrated relaxation pressure (IRP) is a more complex metric of gastroesophageal junction (GEJ) relaxation than a simple end-expiratory measurement of GEJ pressure after a swallow. There are four fluoroscopic images correlating to the swallow with the hiatal canal location noted by the white arrow on the fluoroscopy image and the white horizontal line of the topography plot. Note that at the beginning of the swallow the GEJ is closed (A), and the relaxation here probably represents the best estimate of pure lower esophageal sphincter (LES) relaxation as it is not influenced by the crural diaphragm (CB) or intrabolus pressure (IBP) and flow through the GEJ. In contrast, panels B and D are associated with high IBP and bolus flow through the hiatal canal, while panel C is associated with a closed hiatus and no flow. The IRP requires persistence of GEJ relaxation for 4 s within the relaxation window (white brackets), but the actual time periods used in its calculation (dashed brown boxes) can be contiguous or, as in this example, non-contiguous. By finding the periods of lowest pressure within the relaxation window, the IRP reduces, but does not eliminate, the influences of IBP or CD contractions. The 4-s IRP was selected as the standard metric because it best differentiated the impaired GEJ relaxation in achalasia from non-achalasic individuals.

normal amplitude and duration, and should not grouped with spasm as they likely result from a localized defect in the contractile activity more akin to hypotensive peristalsis (Figure 9.4, lower right panel).

Contractile front velocity

With conventional manometry, the velocity of peristalsis is calculated based on the timing of the upstroke of the peristaltic contraction at two arbitrary locations in the distal esophagus with the assumption that this is a linear function. One obvious conclusion from HREPT studies is that such is not the case. Consequently, the methodology for measuring velocity of peristalsis has shifted to a more functional analysis based on the segmental architecture of peristalsis in EPT. The contractile front velocity (CFV) is one such metric measured along the 30-mmHg isobaric contour of the distal esophageal contraction (Figure 9.5). The CFV is measured at an isobaric contour pressure that exceeds IBP; by convention this is done at a default value of 30 mmHg, but in unusual instances, especially of impaired GEJ relaxation, this needs to be done at a threshold pressure that exceeds the abnormal IBP. Imaged fluoroscopically, the closure front velocity of the peristaltic stripping wave slows markedly in the distal esophagus with the shift from peristaltic transport through the tubular esophagus to phrenic ampullary emptying [18]. The correlate of this fluoroscopic phenomenon in HREPT is the contractile deceleration point (CDP), identified as the locus along the 30-mmHg isobaric contour at which an abrupt reduction in velocity occurs [19]. Although this point is readily identified by visual inspection, it can also be

Table 9.2 Comparison of gastroesophageal junction (GEJ) relaxation measures in 62 well-defined achalasia patients. The nadir pressure in conventional terms was the lowest pressure recorded from the sensor best centered on the GEJ, whereas the nadir pressure in high-resolution manometry (HRM) terms took the lowest value of any of the sensors placed in the region of the GEJ during the period of relaxation. Although the HRM method is marginally better because it at least accounts for the variability in GEJ movement among individuals, both of these methods exhibited very poor sensitivity for detecting impaired GEJ relaxation in achalasia because they fail to detect the subset of achalasia patients characterized by brief periods of GEJ relaxation to within the normal range. Of the two complex metrics that required persistence of GEJ relaxation, the integrated relaxation pressure (IRP) was marginally better than the 3-s nadir because it was less susceptible to crural diaphragm artifact during rapid respiration. Normal values were determined from 75 asymptomatic control subjects (adapted from Ghosh *et al.* [11]).

GEJ relaxation measure	Achalasia sensitivity (%)	False positives (%)	False negatives (%)
Nadir pressure, conventional (≥7 mmHg)	52	0	48
Nadir pressure, HREPT (≥10 mmHg)	69	0	31
HREPT, 3-s nadir (≥15 mmHg)	94	0	6
HREPT, IRP (≥15 mmHg)	97	0	3

HREPT, high-resolution esophageal pressure topography.

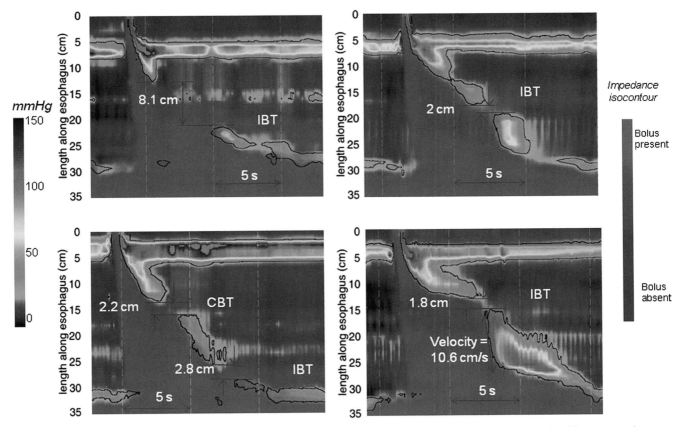

Figure 9.4 Examples of intrabolus transit (IBT) in high-resolution impedance manometry (HRIM) studies attributable to breaks in the 20-mmHg isobaric contour at the proximal (upper left), middle (upper right), and distal (lower left) pressure troughs. In the lower left panel, the minor proximal defect is associated with a complete bolus transit (CBT), whereas the distal defect is associated with IBT. IBT in the lower right panel occurs in conjunction with a segmental rapidly propagated contraction, a relatively rare occurrence seen only in seven swallows. Impedance data are displayed by overlaid pink colorization with the pink shading indicative of areas on the topography plots with retained bolus. The associated dimensions of the critical break in the isobaric contours are indicated on each panel.

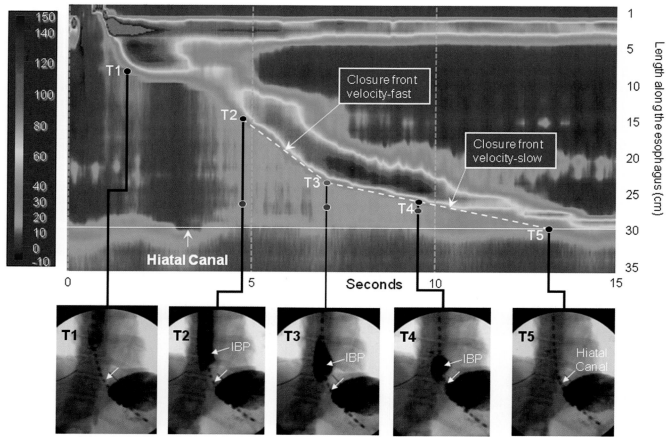

Figure 9.5 Methodology for measuring closure front velocity for the early and late phases of bolus transit. Times T1–T5 were the times at which five milestones of bolus transit occurred, identified by analysis of fluoroscopic swallow sequences (see text). Thereafter, the corresponding time and pressure at which luminal closure occurred was localized on the esophageal pressure topography (EPT) plots based on the encoded time on the fluoroscopy images and radio-opacity of the manometric sensors. The position of the hiatal canal is indicated on the fluoroscopic images by the white arrow and on the EPT plots by the white line at the 30-cm sensor. The white arrow (images) or dots (EPT plots) indicate the location at which intrabolus pressure (IBP) was measured. Note that the dominant determinant of bolus transit from T3 to T5 is descent of S4 back to its native position within the hiatus, which occurs as the esophageal shortening associated with peristalsis is reversed. In this swallow, T1 (bolus present) occurs immediately after the swallow and T2 (compartmentalized pressurization) occurs during the fast contractile front velocity (CFV$_{fast}$). Globular transformation (T3) occurs just after the contractile deceleration point (CDP) (pink dot). Most of emptying is associated with globular formation and/or formation of the phrenic ampulla (start of panel T4), and emptying finally ends as the esophagus elongates and the lower esophageal sphincter (LES) returns to its baseline position (T5).

localized objectively by fitting tangential lines to the initial and terminal portions of the 30 mmHg isobaric contour and noting the intersection of the lines. The first tangent skirts the 30 mmHg isobaric contour distal to the transition zone without intersecting it. The second tangent originates from the termination point at which the esophageal contraction intersects the post-swallow GEJ (be that the native position of the LES or GEJ depending on the individual's anatomy) and skirts the 30-mmHg isobaric contour in the retrograde direction without intersecting it. A horizontal line is then drawn through the intersection of these tangents to the 30-mmHg isobaric contour to localize the CDP (Figure 9.5). The fast contractile front velocity (CFV$_{fast}$) applies to the segment of esophagus distal to the transition zone and ending at the CDP. The slow contractile front velocity (CFV$_{slow}$) is the slope of the line connecting CDP to the leading edge of the post-swallow GEJ.

All measurements of CFV and CDP are made on the 30-mmHg isobaric contour as a default, with the caveats that lower or higher pressures should be used for hypotensive peristalsis and elevated IBP, respectively. In cases of peristaltic hypotension, the isobaric contour threshold is lowered to the magnitude at which a continuous contractile front is demonstrable and the deceleration point can then be localized similarly to with the standard 30-mmHg isobaric contour. In cases for whom no intact isobaric contour exists, measurement of CDP is not valid as these patients have failed or absent peristalsis. In instances in which there is elevated IBP and compartmentalization of pressure between the GEJ and the propagating contraction, the isobaric contour is set to a magnitude greater than IBP to differentiate contraction from pressurization.

Distal contractile integral

The distal contractile integral (DCI) is a measurement of the distal esophageal contraction that defines the vigor of contraction across the entire segment in a single number. The DCI integrates the length, amplitude, and duration of contraction occurring between the transition zone (proximal pressure trough, Figure 9.6) and the LES, expressed in mmHg•s•cm [20]. The DCI can be approximated using commercial analysis software by outlining a box encompassing the distal peristaltic contraction (Figure 9.6). The DCI is calculated by multiplying the mean pressure within the box (subtracting 20 to account for IBP) by the axial length of the box (cm) and duration of the box (s).

In data from 75 control subjects, a DCI value greater than 5000 mmHg•s•cm was considered elevated. Adopting the nomenclature "nutcracker esophagus" from conventional manometry, this is the HRM criterion defining hypertensive peristalsis and was seen in 9% of a 400-patient series [21]. However, there was substantial heterogeneity as to the locus of the hypertensive contraction within this group, potentially involving either or both of the subsegments within the distal esophageal contraction (segments 2 and 3). Similarly, the LES can exhibit a hypertensive after-contraction, defined as exceeding 180 mmHg. Furthermore, a particularly interesting subgroup, defined by having a higher threshold DCI (>8000 mmHg•s•cm), exhibited repetitive high-amplitude contractions and was clinically discernible by the uniform association with dysphagia or chest pain. Similar to distal esophageal spasm (DES), this "spastic nutcracker" pattern is rare, found in only 12 (3%) of this 400-patient series [21].

Upper esophageal sphincter

The UES is readily identified on pressure topography plots as a high-pressure band in the proximal esophagus separating the pharynx from the thoracic esophagus. UES pressure, referenced to atmospheric pressure, typically increases during inspiration and decreases with expiration. Normative data using HRM in both the supine and upright position are shown in Table 9.3. A recent study focused on globus patients reported an exaggerated inspiratory augmentation greater than 27 mmHg as a distinguishing feature of some patients with globus sensation [22].

Deglutitive UES relaxation is characterized by the nadir UES relaxation pressure following 5-mL water swallows quantified using the isobaric contour tool. The isobaric contour pressure value is progressively scaled down to the pressure at which it disappears, thereby defining the relaxa-

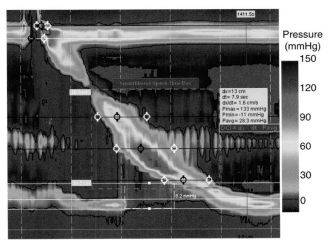

Figure 9.6 The Smart Mouse tool in ManoView™ analysis software can be used to calculate the distal contractile integral (DCI) by creating a space–time box starting at the transition zone and extending distal to the proximal aspect of the gastroesophageal junction (GEJ) and bound temporally at the end of peristalsis or 15 s if no peristaltic wave is noted. The values for distance of the esophageal segment (dx), time duration of the contraction measured (ds), and mean pressure (Pavg) over the entire space–time box are provided by the Smart Mouse tool (yellow box). DCI is calculated by multiplying these values together and is expressed in mmHg•s•cm. In this example, the mean pressure is 28.3 mmHg and the time and length of the space–time box are 7.9 s and 13 cm, respectively. Thus, the DCI is 2906.4 mmHg•s•cm.

tion minimum (Figure 9.7). A threshold value of 12 mmHg is considered the upper limit of normal and patients with higher values potentially attributable to UES obstruction disorders such as cricopharyngeal bars, cervical osteophytes, inflammation, and neoplasm. UES relaxation is most reproducibly defined in a sitting posture [23].

Classification scheme

One of the major challenges that arose with the widespread availability of HREPT instrumentation in the clinical arena was the absence of a validated method to interpret studies. Fortunately, HREPT studies encompass all of the information derived in conventional manometry studies, so at the very least, HREPT studies can be interpreted in terms of conventional manometry. However, adopting that approach fails to exploit the many advantages of HREPT as an evolutionary technology. In reaction to this void, the Chicago Classification of HREPT has been evolving. The overarching goal of the Chicago Classification working group, an international group of esophagologists, is to build a classification scheme for HREPT that parallels conventional manometric classification, but enhances it based on the strengths of the new technology. This classification was initially based on a comprehensive characterization of HREPT data from 75 normal subjects and 400 patients using analysis paradigms unique to pressure

Table 9.3 Upper esophageal sphincter (UES) pressure parameters in different subject groups.

	Average UES pressure (mmHg)	Respiratory augmentation of UES pressure (mmHg)	Nadir deglutitive UES relaxation pressure (mmHg)
Normal controls	55.7	10.6	6.2
	(26.3–85.1)	(1.6–27.0)	(0.1–11.9)
Patient controls (GERD without globus)	47.1	13.0	6.7
	(20.9–87.6)	(1.4–45.7)	(–2.1–12.5)
Globus patients	47.5	37.3*†	6.9
Normal distal esophageal motility	(18.6–106.2)	(1.6–93.0)	(0.6–13.8)
Globus patients	53.4	38.5*†	7.2
Abnormal distal esophageal motility	(18.8–112.0)	(4.4–89.4)	(1.0–19.2)

All data presented as median (5–95th percentile) and analyzed using the Kruskal-Wallis non-parametric test.

*$P < .05$ vs controls.

†$P < .05$ vs GERD patients.

GERD, gastroesophageal reflux disease.

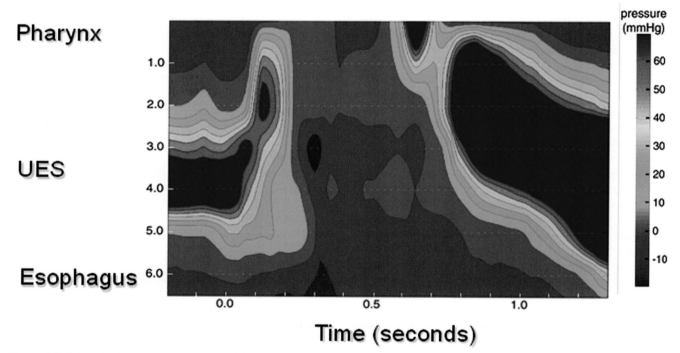

Figure 9.7 Color isobaric contour representation of the pressure variation within the upper esophageal sphincter (UES) during deglutitive relaxation. The horizontal axis denotes time, and the vertical axis denotes the axial position of the sensor spanning from the pharynx to the esophagus. Time 0 corresponds to the initiation of the swallow. The bar on the right shows the color scale for pressure magnitude. The rate of pressure increase within the UES often exceeded 1000 mmHg/s (modified from Ghosh *et al.* [23]).

topography interpretation [21, 24]. Following the original description of this classification scheme, major modifications have been made (and continue to be made) based on periodic discussion at workshops and also on new data as they emerge. The continuing goal of the Chicago Classification working group is to validate and refine the HREPT classifica-tion scheme with the intent of classifying functional abnor-malities with validated, reproducible metrics.

Currently, the Chicago Classification of HREPT is based on studies obtained using the HRM system developed by Sierra Scientific Instruments (Los Angeles, CA, USA). Normative data and all of the metrics described in the previous sections

Table 9.4 Chicago Classification of esophageal motility.

With *normal* GEJ relaxation (mean IRP < 15 mmHg)	
Absent peristalsis	100% swallows with failed peristalsis
Weak peristalsis	30% of swallows with any combination of:
	• Failed peristalsis
	• Diffuse hypotensive peristalsis (breaks in the 20-mmHg isobaric contour of >5 cm in length) subtyped by localization at proximal (P), middle (M) or distal (D) pressure troughs
	• Focal hypotensive peristalsis (breaks in the 20-mmHg isobaric contour of >2 cm in length) subtyped by localization at the proximal (P), middle (M) or distal (D) pressure troughs
	• Rapidly propagated segmental contractions between the proximal and distal pressure troughs in association with a small (<2 cm) break in the 20-mmHg isobaric contour
Hypertensive peristalsis	Normal CFV$_{fast}$, two swallows with average DCI between 5000 and 8000 mmHg•s•cm
Hypertensive LES	Two swallows with LES after-contraction > 180 mmHg
Spastic nutcracker	Normal CFV$_{fast}$, two swallows with average DCI > 8000 mmHg•s•cm
Diffuse esophageal spasm	Spasm (CFV$_{fast}$ > 10 cm/s and DCI ≥2000 mmHg•s•cm) with ≥20% of swallows

With *impaired* GEJ relaxation (IRP ≥ 15 mmHg)	
Achalasia	
Classic achalasia	100% absent peristalsis
Achalasia with esophageal compression	No intact peristalsis, pan-esophageal pressurization with ≥20% of swallows
Spastic achalasia	No intact peristalsis, spasm (CFV > 10 cm/s) with ≥20% of swallows
Functional GEJ obstruction*	Normal CFV$_{fast}$, IBP$_{esoph}$ ≥ 30 mmHg with ≥30% of swallows compartmentalized above GEJ with type I GEJ
Functional LES obstruction* (with LES–CD separation >2 cm)	Normal CFV$_{fast}$, IBP$_{esoph}$ ≥ 30 mmHg with ≥30% of swallows compartmentalized above the LES
Functional CD obstruction (with LES–CD separation >2 cm)	Normal CFV$_{fast}$, IBP$_{esoph}$ ≥ 30 mmHg with ≥30% of swallows compartmentalized above the CD

*May represent an achalasia variant.
CD, crural diaphragm; GEJ, gastroesophageal junction; LES, lower esophageal sphincter; CFV, contractile front velocity; IBP, intrabolus pressure; IRP, integrated relaxation pressure; DCI, distal contractile integral.

of this chapter were derived using the Manoscan™ 36-channel circumferential solid-state hardware and ManoView™ analysis software. Subsequently, all of the analysis paradigms described have been incorporated into the current version of ManoView™ software (version 2.0) and Solar GI HRM (Medical Measurement Systems). Although the numerical cut-offs defining normality may change with the use of alternative hardware, the principles of analysis described are intended to be generalizable to any HRM system since they are based on pressure topography patterns rather than strict numeric cut-offs. Table 9.4 summarizes the current Chicago Classification of esophageal motility.

Algorithm of analysis of studies

Intraluminal pressure within the esophagus after swallowing is strongly influenced by the resistance to flow though the esophagus. Consequently, the first step in the analysis of HREPT is focused on identifying abnormalities of the GEJ, the major contributor to downstream resistance. Particular emphasis is placed on the evaluation of deglutitive GEJ

relaxation because, as not only is this a cardinal abnormality of achalasia, but it is also the major determinant of IBP in the esophagus during peristalsis. Recognizing this fundamental importance, the first branch point in the classification outlined in Table 9.4 is normal versus abnormal deglutitive GEJ relaxation. Once GEJ relaxation has been characterized, each swallow is further categorized based on the ensuing contractile pattern, as outlined in Table 9.5. Although at first glance this categorization may seem complex, it is based on relatively few characteristics: the integrity of the 20 mmHg isobaric contour spanning from the UES to the GEJ, the CFV, and the DCI. The results of the 10-swallow analysis are then tallied to fit one of the HREPT classifications of Table 9.4.

Weak peristalsis

Establishing limits on what constitutes normal as opposed to abnormally weak peristalsis requires that some outcome be adopted defining the success of a peristaltic contraction. Conventionally, this has been that the contraction succeeds

Table 9.5 Classification of peristaltic contractions following individual swallows based on pressure topography criteria. Pressures are referenced to atmospheric pressure.

Normal	<2 cm defect in the 20-mmHg isobaric contour from the UES to the GEJ, CFV_{fast} < 10 cm/s, and DCI < 5000 mmHg•s•cm
Hypotensive peristalsis	• Diffuse hypotensive peristalsis defined by breaks in the 20-mmHg isobaric contour of >5 cm in length subtyped by localization at the proximal (P), middle (M) or distal (D) pressure troughs • Focal hypotensive peristalsis characterized by breaks in the 20-mmHg isobaric contour of >2 cm in length subtyped by localization at the proximal (P), middle (M) or distal (D) pressure troughs • Rapidly propagated segmental contractions between the proximal and distal pressure troughs in association with a defect of <2 cm in the 20-mmHg isobaric contour
Failed peristalsis	Minimal (<3 cm) integrity of the 20-mmHg isobaric contour distal to the proximal pressure trough
Hypertensive peristalsis	• Normal CFV_{fast} with DCI > 5000 mmHg•s•cm • Spastic nutcracker (DCI > 8000 mmHg•s•cm)
Hypertensive LES	LES after-contraction > 180 mmHg
Spasm	Rapidly propagated contraction (CFV_{fast} ≥ 10 cm/s), DCI > 2000 mmHg•s•cm
Pan-esophageal pressurization	Esophageal pressurization from the UES to the GeJ ≥ 30 mmHg

UES, upper esophageal sphincter; LES, lower esophageal sphincter; GEJ, gastroesophageal junction; CFV_{fast}, fast contractile front velocity; DCI, distal contractile integral.

in facilitating complete transit of swallowed liquid through the esophagus. Concurrent HREPT/fluoroscopy studies have demonstrated that swallows with an intact 20 mmHg isobaric contour or a break in that isobaric contour of less than 2 cm uniformly have normal bolus transit in the context of normal GEJ anatomy and relaxation. Given that impedance manometry studies analyzing bolus transit have found that the occurrence of incomplete bolus transit in up to 30% of test swallows is within the range of normal [15, 25], it is reasonable to accept that up to 30% of peristaltic contractions with incomplete bolus transit is also within the range of normal. Consistent with that, an analysis of peristalsis in 93 normal subjects revealed that the 95th percentile of normal for incomplete bolus transit attributable to failed peristalsis, major defects in the 20-mmHg isobaric contour, or minor defects in the 20-mmHg isobaric contour were each 30% or less. Thus, the HREPT criterion for the classification of weak peristalsis is greater than 30% of swallows exhibiting any combination of these subtypes of hypotensive peristaltic (Table 9.4). However, given that each mechanism of weak peristalsis has distinct implications with respect to pathophysiology or severity, they should be described qualitatively and quantitatively, stating the number of each contributing mechanistic subtype.

There are important qualifications to recognize in the analysis of weak peristalsis, as summarized in the preceding paragraph and in Table 9.4. Exceeding a normal range of incomplete bolus transit is not synonymous with defining a disorder and fitting within that range does not necessarily vindicate weak peristalsis as a cause of symptoms. The analysis that led to the summary data in Table 9.4 was based on 5-mL water swallows in a supine position in individuals with

normal GEJ relaxation, no hiatal hernia, and no obstructive process in the distal esophagus. Eliminating any of these qualifications (or others not identified) would necessarily impose increased demand on the peristaltic mechanism that it may or may not adapt to [26, 27]. Consequently, the clinical impact of weak peristalsis, regardless of subtype, is unclear other than being associated with poor bolus transit.

Absent peristalsis

Absent peristalsis in the context of normal GEJ relaxation is a separate entity from weak peristalsis in that these patients have failed peristalsis with 100% of their swallows [28]. This pattern is associated with negligible bolus transit in a supine posture and if the patient also exhibits a hypotensive resting GEJ pressure, they have a pattern that predisposes to GERD and is consistent with scleroderma (or other connective tissue disease) involvement of the esophagus. Care should be taken not to label this entity as "scleroderma pattern" as it is not pathognomonic for the disease and can be found outside of its association with collagen vascular disease.

Hypertensive peristalsis and spastic nutcracker

The upper limit of normal for contractile vigor of the esophageal segment between the proximal and distal pressure troughs in 75 control subjects was a DCI value greater than 5000 mmHg•s•cm. Adopting the nomenclature "nutcracker esophagus" from conventional manometry, this becomes the HRM criterion defining hypertensive peristalsis and this was seen in 9% of a 400-patient series [21]. However, there was substantial heterogeneity as to the locus of the hypertensive contraction within this group, potentially involving either

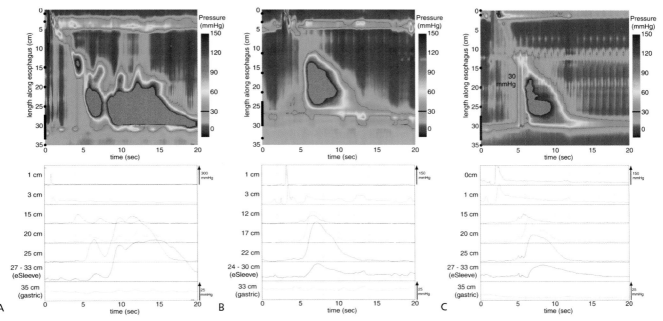

Figure 9.8 (A)Less common spastic variant of hypertensive peristalsis (spastic nutcracker) identifiable by a distal contractile integral value greater than 8000 mmHg•s•cm. In this example, the contraction does not meet contractile front velocity (CFV) criteria for spasm (>10 cm/s) and the contraction has a spastic component that occurs after the wavefront propagates to the gastroesophageal junction (GEJ). (B) Wwallow with rapid CFV due to a spastic contraction. In contrast, the swallow in (C) has a rapid CFV. However, this swallow is also associated with impaired GEJ relaxation and thus, is consistent with spastic achalasia. Clinically, patients with spastic achalasia share many similarities with the classic spasm depicted in B.

or both of the subsegments within the distal esophageal contraction. Furthermore, one particularly interesting subgroup that emerged from that series, defined by having a higher threshold DCI (>8000 mmHg•s•cm), exhibited repetitive high-amplitude contractions and was clinically characterized by the uniform association with dysphagia or chest pain. This "spastic nutcracker" pattern was rare, found in only 12 (3%) of the 400-patient series, but it was the most homogeneous symptomatic hypercontractile pattern, suggesting that it is an important HREPT subtype of esophageal spasm (Figure 9.8A).

Diffuse esophageal spasm

As a clinical syndrome, DES is manifest by episodes of dysphagia and chest pain attributable to abnormal esophageal contractions in the setting of normal LES function. However, beyond these entirely descriptive criteria, there is little to agree upon. The pathophysiology and natural history of the disorder are poorly defined. Radiographically, DES has been characterized by tertiary contractions or a "corkscrew esophagus," but in many instances these abnormalities are actually indicative of spastic achalasia. Manometrically, a variety of defining features have been proposed for DES. These include uncoordinated ("spastic") activity in the smooth muscle portion of the esophagus, spontaneous and repetitive contractions, or high amplitude and prolonged

contractions. Greatest consensus currently exists with the concept of simultaneous contractions, either with a minimum threshold amplitude of 30 mmHg or without a defining amplitude [4, 11]. However, similar to the problems with the conventional manometric definition of achalasia, there is no distinction between pressure waves within the esophageal body attributable to IBP, spasm, or peristalsis. Given all of these vagaries, it is likely that patients with a variety of contractile patterns have been defined as DES, irrespective of associated functional consequences. Similarly, a very heterogeneous group has been included in DES therapeutic trials. Not surprisingly, none of such trials has demonstrated efficacy. HREPT classification, based on homogeneous patterns of functional abnormalities, has the potential to substantially improve upon this.

Several nuances of defining DES emerge in HREPT. First, there is a very important distinction to be made between a simultaneous contraction in the distal esophagus and simultaneous pressurization in the setting of impaired GEJ relaxation (Figure 9.8B). Simultaneous contraction fits conceptually with the accepted descriptive criteria and conventional manometric definition of DES, while simultaneous pressurization is simply a consequence of impaired GEJ relaxation, most commonly in the setting of achalasia. Consequently, much of what would be labeled DES on the basis of simultaneous contractions in conventional manometry is really achalasia [12]. Similarly, instances of simultaneous contractions of low amplitude are almost invariably attributable to IBP in the setting of a failed peristaltic contraction due to a subtle obstructive phenomenon in the distal esophagus. Consequently, instances of DES defined by the criteria of normal GEJ relaxation and a spastic contraction in the distal esophagus, such as in Figure 9.5, are decidedly rare. Indeed, they are so rare that it may be speculated that these are usually variant expressions of achalasia in individuals who happen to also have a low resting LES pressure.

Achalasia

Apart from improving the sensitivity of manometry in the detection of achalasia by objectifying the definition of impaired deglutitive GEJ relaxation, HREPT has also defined a clinically relevant sub-classification of achalasia based on the pattern of contractility in the esophageal body [29]. The manometric criteria for the diagnosis of achalasia require both absent peristalsis and impaired deglutitive GEJ relaxation. However, absent peristalsis is not synonymous with an absence of pressurization or contractile activity within the intersphincteric esophagus. Rather, absent peristalsis accompanying impaired GEJ relaxation can occur in the setting of esophageal dilatation with negligible pressurization within the esophagus (Figure 9.9A); pan-esophageal pressurization, in which case there is a pressurized column of fluid within the esophagus (Figure 9.9B); or spastic contractions of the distal esophageal segment (Figure 9.8C). In HREPT classification these are referred to as classic achalasia, achalasia with esophageal compression, and spastic achalasia, respectively. In a series of 99 consecutive patients with newly diagnosed achalasia, 21 fitted criteria for classic achalasia, 49 had achalasia with esophageal compression, and 29 had spastic achalasia [29]. Emphasizing the added sensitivity of HREPT in the detection of achalasia, most of these patients would not be diagnosed as having achalasia with conventional manometric classification.

Ultimately, the significance of consistently identifying functionally distinct subtypes of achalasia is that it helps clarify patient management. Preliminary data suggest this to be the case, especially in the instance of achalasia with esophageal compression, a major subtype usually overlooked when evaluated with conventional manometry. Logistic regression analysis of predictors of treatment outcome in a large series of consecutive achalasia patients found that pan-esophageal pressurization (the defining feature of achalasia with esophageal compression; Figure 9.9B) to be a predictor of good treatment response, while spastic achalasia (Figure 9.8C) and pretreatment esophageal dilatation were predictive of a relatively poor treatment response [29]. Clearly, these nuances have not been utilized in the existing database of reports on achalasia treatment outcomes. Given that the mix of achalasia subtypes within any reported series likely impacts on the outcomes in that series, this calls into question the validity of the existing data on achalasia treatment in the era of HREPT. It is our suspicion that adopting these sub-classifications will likely strengthen future prospective studies of achalasia management. It is also likely that overall treatment efficacy will improve as more cases of achalasia are diagnosed early in the course of the disease, prior to the esophageal dilatation and stasis.

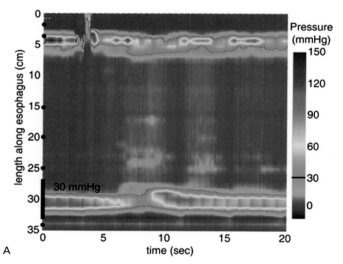

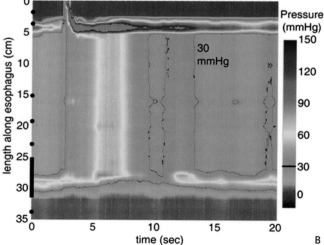

Figure 9.9 Achalasia subtypes are distinguished by distinct manometric patterns of esophageal body contractility. (A) Classic achalasia: there is no significant pressurization within the body of the esophagus and impaired gastroesophageal junction (GEJ) relaxation (integrated relaxation pressure [IRP] of 42 mmHg in this example). (B) A swallow in a patient with the "achalasia with compression" subtype exhibiting rapidly pan-esophageal pressurization (modified from Pandolfino et al. [29]).

Functional obstruction

As detailed above in the discussion of achalasia subtypes, many cases that would have been labeled "atypical disorders of LES relaxation" by conventional manometric classification are recognized as subtypes of achalasia with HREPT. However, even with HREPT there is still a group of patients with impaired GEJ relaxation failing to meet criteria for achalasia because they have some preserved peristalsis. Though not common, a series of 1000 consecutive patients studied with HREPT included 16 such individuals with functional GEJ obstruction exhibiting not only an IRP greater than 15 mmHg, but also preserved peristalsis and elevated IBP above the GEJ during peristalsis [30]. The finding of elevated IBP is important because it validates the determination of impaired GEJ relaxation; from a physiologic perspective, elevated IBP is the consequence of that impaired relaxation. Nonetheless, patients with functional GEJ obstruction are a heterogeneous group, with some individuals having a variant form or incomplete expression of achalasia and others likely having an undetected mechanical etiology of GEJ outflow obstruction. Consequently, it is a patient group that usually merits further evaluation prior to proceeding with achalasia therapy. Depending on the circumstances, such evaluation would likely include imaging studies to exclude inflammatory or malignant etiologies, be it with computerized tomography or endoscopic ultrasound.

Among the 16 patients with idiopathic functional obstruction described in the 1000 patient series alluded to above [30], three were noted to have hiatal hernias. In one of these patients, it was the CD rather than the LES that appeared to be the focus of deglutitive resistance to bolus transit evident from the extension of intraesophageal IBP through the LES to the CD, implicating the hernia itself as the cause of dysphagia in this individual. A subsequent patient series specifically focused on the GEJ relaxation characteristics of patients with a sliding hiatus hernia and dysphagia but without GERD symptoms, selectively restricting the deglutitive relaxation measurement to the LES and CD elements of the GEJ [31]. A subset of 10 patients was found to exhibit a relative obstruction at the CD with elevated IBP extending through the LES to the CD, supporting the concept that a sliding hiatus hernia, in and of itself, can be responsible for dysphagia (Figure 9.10). Consequently, patients presenting with elevated GEJ relaxation pressure in the context of a small sliding hiatus hernia require careful analysis of the LES and CD components of the GEJ before making a diagnosis of achalasia and proceeding with treatment.

High-resolution manometry and impedance

Intraluminal impedance monitoring allows for the assessment of the completeness of bolus transit through the esophagus. As such, it provides information that is

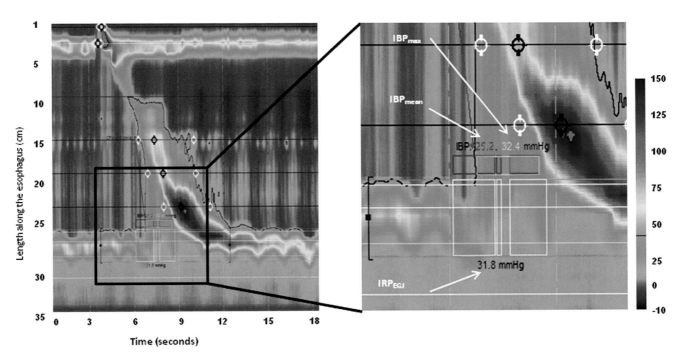

Figure 9.10 Representative example of a patient with functional gastroesophageal junction (GEJ) obstruction. Note that there is a propagating contraction that is associated with a compartmentalized intrabolus pressure (IBP) and an elavated integrated relaxation pressure (IRP). The black box on the right is the zoomed in region of interest for measuring elevated IBP. Max-IBP (yellow) is the greatest IBP obtained for a contiguous or non-contiguous 3-s period within the same 10-s temporal boundary used to calculate the IRP (white). Pressure is referenced to atmospheric with the 30 mmHg isobaric contour highlighted in black.

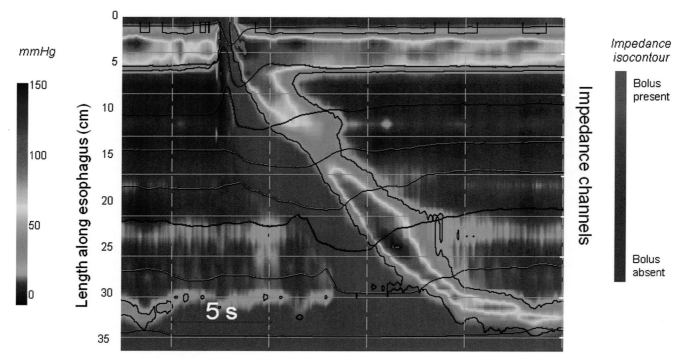

Figure 9.11 Example of intact peristalsis associated with complete bolus transit in an high-resolution impedance manometry (HRIM) study. Impedance tracings are superimposed to high-resolution esophageal pressure topography (HREPT) and impedance data are also displayed by overlaid pink colorization. The pink shading nearly corresponds to a 50% decrease of esophageal basal impedance and is indicative of areas on the topography plots with bolus. No bolus retention is observed following the contraction.

complimentary to that provided by HREPT, making it potentially advantageous for the two methods to be combined. Consistent with this, a recent report used a high-resolution impedance manometry (HRIM) catheter designed by Medical Measurement Systems to analyze HRM predictors of bolus transit [32] (Figure 9.11) following saline swallows in 16 asymptomatic volunteers and eight patients with dysphagia. Impedance data were used to determine complete or incomplete bolus transit, while peristaltic integrity and isobaric contour break size were ascertained using manometric data. Notably, none of the 24 patients had abnormal GEJ relaxation or evidence of hiatus hernia. Under these circumstances, a peristaltic contraction wave with an intact 20-mmHg isobaric contour along its entire course was associated with complete bolus transit in every instance. This represents a modification of the previously accepted minimal pressure threshold for normal peristalsis (30 mmHg) defined using conventional manometry [14, 33]. In cases in which the peristaltic integrity was compromised, the largest break in the 20- and 30-mmHg isobaric contour associated with complete bolus transit measured 1.7 cm and 3.0 cm in length, respectively. Conversely, the smallest break predictive of incomplete bolus transit measured 2.1 cm and 3.2 cm, respectively. It was thus concluded that aperistaltic contraction with breaks of less than 2 cm in the 20-mmHg isobaric contour or less than 3 cm in the 30-mmHg isobaric contour are associated with complete bolus transit, while defects of greater than 3 cm predict incomplete bolus transit [32].

Beyond research, the technology of HRIM may be clinically beneficial to the patients with anatomic or physiologic complexities that limit the applicability of normative data. As detailed above, investigations are in progress to improve our understanding of how such complexities may affect bolus transit. In such instances, impedance data are useful to define incomplete bolus transit and to localize its occurrence to specific features of HREPT recordings.

Acknowledgement

This work was supported by R01 DK56033 (PJK) and R01 DK079902 (JEP) from the Public Health Service.

References

1. Clouse RE, Staiano A. Topography of the esophageal peristaltic pressure wave. *Am J Physiol* 1991;261:G677–684.
2. Williams RB, Pal A, Brasseur JG, Cook IJ. Space-time pressure structure of pharyngo-esophageal segment during swallowing. *Am J Physiol Gastrointest Liver Physiol* 2001;281:G1290–1300.

3. Pal A, Williams RB, Cook IJ, Brasseur JG. Intrabolus pressure gradient identifies pathological constriction in the upper esophageal sphincter during flow. *Am J Physiol Gastrointest Liver Physiol* 2003;285:G1037–1048.

4. Clouse RE, Staiano A, Alrakawi A, Haroian L. Application of topographical methods to clinical esophageal manometry. *Am J Gastroenterol* 2000;95:2720–2730.

5. Castell JA, Dalton CB, Castell DO. Pharyngeal and upper esophageal sphincter manometry in humans. *Am J Physiol* 1990;258:G173–178.

6. Liu J, Parashar VK, Mittal RK. Asymmetry of lower esophageal sphincter pressure: is it related to the muscle thickness or its shape? *Am J Physiol* 1997;272:G1509–1517.

7. Pandolfino JE, Ghosh SK, Zhang Q, Jarosz A, Shah N, Kahrilas PJ. Quantifying EGJ morphology and relaxation with high-resolution manometry: a study of 75 asymptomatic volunteers. *Am J Physiol Gastrointest Liver Physiol* 2006;290:G1033–1040.

8. Grubel C, Hiscock R, Hebbard G. Value of spatiotemporal representation of manometric data. *Clin Gastroenterol Hepatol* 2008;6:525–530.

9. Pandolfino JE, Kim H, Ghosh SK, Clarke JO, Zhang Q, Kahrilas PJ. High-resolution manometry of the EGJ: an analysis of crural diaphragm function in GERD. *Am J Gastroenterol* 2007;102:1056–1063.

10. Pandolfino JE, Ghosh SK, Zhang Q, Jarosz A, Shah N, Kahrilas PJ. Quantifying EGJ morphology and relaxation with high-resolution manometry: a study of 75 asymptomatic volunteers. *Am J Physiol Gastrointest Liver Physiol* 2006;290:G1033–1040.

11. Ghosh SK, Pandolfino JE, Rice J, Clarke JO, Kwiatek M, Kahrilas PJ. Impaired deglutitive EGJ relaxation in clinical esophageal manometry: a quantitative analysis of 400 patients and 75 controls. *Am J Physiol Gastrointest Liver Physiol* 2007;293:G878–885.

12. Spechler SJ, Castell DO. Classification of oesophageal motility abnormalities. *Gut* 2001;49:145–151.

13. Massey BT, Dodds WJ, Hogan WJ, Brasseur JG, Helm JF. Abnormal esophageal motility. An analysis of concurrent radiographic and manometric findings. *Gastroenterology* 1991;101:344–354.

14. Kahrilas PJ, Dodds WJ, Hogan WJ. Effect of peristaltic dysfunction on esophageal volume clearance. *Gastroenterology* 1988;94:73–80.

15. Bulsiewicz WJ, Kahrilas PJ, Kwiatek MA, Ghosh SK, Meek A, Pandolfino JE. Esophageal pressure topography criteria indicative of incomplete bolus clearance: a study using high-resolution impedance manometry. *Am J Gastroenterol* 2009;104:2721–2728.

16. Fox M, Hebbard G, Janiak P, *et al.* High-resolution manometry predicts the success of oesophageal bolus transport and identifies clinically important abnormalities not detected by conventional manometry. *Neurogastroenterol Motil* 2004;16:533–542.

17. Pohl D, Ribolsi M, Savarino E, *et al.* Characteristics of the esophageal low-pressure zone in healthy volunteers and patients with esophageal symptoms: assessment by high-resolution manometry. *Am J Gastroenterol* 2008;103:2544–2549.

18. Lin S, Brasseur JG, Pouderoux P, Kahrilas PJ. The phrenic ampulla: distal esophagus or potential hiatal hernia? *Am J Physiol* 1995;268:G320–327.

19. Pandolfino JE, Leslie E, Luger D, Mitchell B, Kwiatek MA, Kahrilas PJ. The contractile deceleration point: an important physiologic landmark on oesophageal pressure topography. *Neurogastroenterol Motil* 2010;22:395–400.

20. Ghosh SK, Pandolfino JE, Zhang Q, Jarosz A, Shah N, Kahrilas PJ. Quantifying esophageal peristalsis with high-resolution manometry: a study of 75 asymptomatic volunteers. *Am J Physiol Gastrointest Liver Physiol* 2006;290:G988–997.

21. Pandolfino JE, Ghosh SK, Rice J, Clarke JO, Kwiatek MA, Kahrilas PJ. Classifying esophageal motility by pressure topography characteristics: a study of 400 patients and 75 controls. *Am J Gastroenterol* 2008;103:27–37.

22. Kwiatek MA, Mirza F, Kahrilas PJ, Pandolfino JE. Hyperdynamic upper esophageal sphincter pressure: a manometric observation in patients reporting globus sensation. *Am J Gastroenterol* 2009;104:289–298.

23. Ghosh SK, Pandolfino JE, Zhang Q, Jarosz A, Kahrilas PJ. Deglutitive upper esophageal sphincter relaxation: a study of 75 volunteer subjects using solid-state high-resolution manometry. *Am J Physiol Gastrointest Liver Physiol* 2006;291:G525–531.

24. Fox MR, Bredenoord AJ. Oesophageal high-resolution manometry: moving from research into clinical practice. *Gut* 2008;57:405–423.

25. Tutuian R, Vela MF, Balaji NS, *et al.* Esophageal function testing with combined multichannel intraluminal impedance and manometry: multicenter study in healthy volunteers. *Clin Gastroenterol Hepatol* 2003;1:174–182.

26. Pandolfino JE, Ghosh SK, Lodhia N, Kahrilas PJ. Utilizing intraluminal pressure gradients to predict esophageal clearance: a validation study. *Am J Gastroenterol* 2008;103:1898–1905.

27. Ghosh SK, Kahrilas PJ, Zaki T, Pandolfino JE, Joehl RJ, Brasseur JG. The mechanical basis of impaired esophageal emptying postfundoplication. *Am J Physiol Gastrointest Liver Physiol* 2005;289:G21–35.

28. Pandolfino JE, Fox MR, Bredenoord AJ, Kahrilas PJ. High-resolution manometry in clinical practice: utilizing pressure topography to classify oesophageal motility abnormalities. *Neurogastroenterol Motil* 2009;21:796–806.

29. Pandolfino JE, Kwiatek MA, Nealis T, Bulsiewicz W, Post J, Kahrilas PJ. Achalasia: a new clinically relevant classification by high-resolution manometry. *Gastroenterology* 2008;135:1526–1533.

30. Scherer JR, Kwiatek MA, Soper NJ, Pandolfino JE, Kahrilas PJ. Functional esophagogastric junction obstruction with intact peristalsis: a heterogeneous syndrome sometimes akin to achalasia. *J Gastrointest Surg* 2009;13:2219–2225.

31. Pandolfino JE, Kwiatek MA, Ho K, Scherer JR, Kahrilas PJ. Unique features of esophagogastric junction pressure topography in hiatus hernia patients with dysphagia. *Surgery* 2010;147:57–64.

32. Bulsiewicz WJ, Kahrilas PJ, Kwiatek MA, Ghosh SK, Meek A, Pandolfino JE. Esophageal pressure topography criteria indicative of incomplete bolus clearance: A study utilizing high resolution impedance manometry. *Am J Gastroenterol* 2009;104:2721–2728.

33. Ren J, Massey BT, Dodds WJ, *et al.* Determinants of intrabolus pressure during esophageal peristaltic bolus transport. *Am J Physiol* 1993;264:G407–413.

Appendix 9.1 Glossary of terms used in high-resolution esophageal pressure topography (HREPT)

High-resolution manometry plotting	*Pressure topography plots*: Pressure data displayed with time on the x-axis, location of the pressure sensors on the y-axis, and pressure magnitude on the z-axis, scaled by color intensity. To smooth the appearance, data are interpolated between sampling times and sensor positions. Pressure topography plots provide a quick assessment of peristalsis and sphincter relaxation.
	Isobaric contour: A line on a pressure topography plot where the pressure is equal to a specific value, e.g. 30 mmHg. The 30-mmHg isobaric contour circumscribes areas where pressure exceeds 30 mmHg and excludes areas of lesser pressure. Multiple isobaric contour lines, e.g. at 15-mmHg increments, can be used as an aid in scaling on pressure topography plots.
Gastroesophageal junction (GEJ) pressure morphology subtypes	*GEJ pressure morphology*: The GEJ derives pressure contributions from both the LES and the surrounding crural diaphragm (CD). The CD element is most evident during inspiration. GEJ pressure morphology subtypes are defined by relative localization of the lower esophageal sphincter (LES) and CD elements.
	LES–CD separation: When the location of maximal pressure is different during inspiration and expiration, the proximal (expiratory) peak is the LES and the distal (inspiratory) peak the CD. LES–CD measured during inspiration. To minimize sampling error, a mean of five consecutive values is derived.
	GEJ Type I: There is no discernible LES–CD separation because the CD is superimposed on the LES. In this case, neither LES nor CD pressure is independently quantifiable.
	GEJ Type II: There is minimal but discernible LES–CD separation, but the nadir pressure between the peaks is still positive. This represents an intermediate condition between normal and a hiatal hernia.
	GEJ Type III: LES–CD separation is >2 cm. This is the HREPT signature of hiatus hernia. Two subtypes are discernible (IIIa and IIIb) with the distinction being that the respiratory inversion point is proximal to the CD in IIIa and proximal to the LES in IIIb. Inspiratory augmentation is negative in type IIIa but positive in IIIb.
GEJ pressure (measured relative to gastric pressure)	*Basal pressure (inspiratory)*: Inspiratory GEJ pressure is defined as the maximal pressure occurring during the normal respiratory cycle. To minimize sampling error, a mean of five consecutive values is derived.
	Basal pressure (expiratory): Expiration is the lengthier portion of the respiratory cycle, and hence, not so easily isolated in time. Thus, expiratory GEJ pressure is defined as the pressure at the midpoint between adjacent inspiratory pressures during the normal respiratory cycle. Again, to minimize sampling error, a mean of five consecutive values is derived.
	Respiratory inversion point (RIP): The location at which the inspiratory GEJ pressure becomes less than the expiratory GEJ pressure. Conceptually, this is the position at which the external GEJ environment switches from intra-abdominal to intramediastinal.
	Inspiratory augmentation of GEJ pressure: The difference between basal inspiratory pressure and basal expiratory pressure. This can have a positive or negative value.
GEJ relaxation (measured relative to gastric pressure)	*Deglutitive relaxation window*: Deglutitive GEJ relaxation is measured within a 10-s period beginning with upper esophageal sphincter (UES) relaxation and ending either at 10 s or upon the arrival of the peristaltic contraction at the GEJ. Because the esophagus shortens and the LES is elevated during peristalsis, the relaxation window must also span a designated length (conventionally 6 cm) that is selected so as to accurately track the movement of the sphincter in the post-deglutitive period.
	eSleeve pressure: An electronic computation designed to detect maximal pressure across a span of several adjacent sensors. The *greatest* pressure among the sensors within this span is the eSleeve pressure.
	3-s nadir eSleeve relaxation pressure: An index of deglutitive GEJ relaxation derived from the eSleeve pressures expressed in mmHg. The 3-s nadir reports the lowest mean eSleeve pressure during a *contiguous* 3-s period of relaxation.
	Integrated relaxation pressure (IRP): An index of deglutitive GEJ relaxation derived from the eSleeve pressures expressed in mmHg. The IRP reports the lowest mean eSleeve pressure for four *contiguous or non-contiguous* seconds of relaxation.
Distal segment contractility (measured relative to gastric pressure)	*Distal contractile segment*: Peristalsis has distinct proximal and distal segments separated by a transition zone. The distal segment also has three less distinct sub-segments, the third of which is the LES (Figure 9.1). This analysis lumps together the two sub-segments extending from the transition zone to the proximal aspect of the GEJ.
	Intrabolus pressure (IBP): This is measured between the leading edge of the distal segment contraction and the GEJ and is a means of detecting functional GEJ obstruction. As the contractile wavefront nears the GEJ, the magnitude of IBP approximates the instantaneous GEJ relaxation pressure reflecting the pressure within the fluid compartmentalized between the two.
	Contractile front velocity (CFV): A measure derived from the 30-mmHg isobaric contour circumscribing the distal contractile segment designed to detect rapidly conducted contractions expressed in cm/s. Proximal and distal points are identified on the 30-mmHg isobaric contour and the slope of the line connecting the two is the CFV. Note that in instances of impaired GEJ relaxation, IBP will often exceed 30 mmHg, and in such instances the CFV is calculated from an isobaric contour line of magnitude greater than IBP.
	Distal contractile integral (DCI). A measure of contractile vigor. If the pressure topography plot of sub-segments 2 and 3 in the distal esophageal contraction is envisioned as a solid, it appears as a set of peaks with the height of the peaks corresponding to contractile pressure. The DCI is the entire volume of that solid spanning from 20 mmHg at the base to the top of the peak(s), and is expressed in mmHg•s•cm.

10 Esophageal Testing Using Multichannel Intraluminal Impedance

Marcelo F. Vela[1] and Amit Agrawal[2]

[1]Section of Gastroenterology & Hepatology, Baylor College of Medicine, Houston, TX, USA
[2]Medical University of South Carolina, Charleston, SC, USA

Introduction

Multichannel intraluminal impedance (MII) is a relatively new technique that enables detection of retrograde and antegrade bolus movement along the esophagus. This chapter reviews the basic principles of intraesophageal impedance measurement and its application to esophageal function testing (EFT) and gastroesophageal reflux (GER) monitoring. The clinical and research applications of impedance combined with manometry for EFT and impedance combined with pH-metry for GER monitoring are discussed in greater detail in Chapters 9 and 11.

Basic principles

The technique for assessing intraluminal bolus movement using impedance measurements was initially described by Silny *et al.* in the early 1990s [1]. Intraesophageal impedance is determined by measuring electrical conductivity across a pair of closely spaced electrodes within the esophageal lumen. Impedance in an esophageal measuring segment depends on the cross-sectional area of the organ and the conductivity of the material through which the electrical current must travel. Conductivity, in turn, is determined by the ionic content of the material surrounding the impedance measuring segment. Since the esophageal mucosa, air, and any given bolus material (i.e. swallowed food, saliva, or refluxed gastric contents) each has different ionic content and thus different electrical conductivity, they all produce a different change in impedance.

Combined videofluoroscopy–impedance measurements have validated changes observed with bolus entry, presence, and clearing in the impedance-measuring segment [1, 2] (Figure 10.1). In the absence of bolus, impedance is determined by the electrical conductivity of the esophageal lining. Upon arrival of bolus between the electrodes, impedance may increase abruptly as a result of the presence of a pocket of air in front of the head of the bolus. Intraluminal impedance then rapidly decreases as the high ionic content of the bolus provides good electrical conductivity. While the bolus is present in the impedance measuring segment, intraluminal impedance remains low. Esophageal contractions clearing the intraluminal content may increase the impedance, with a slight "overshoot" caused by a decrease in esophageal cross-section during contraction before returning to baseline.

By placing a series of conducting electrodes in a catheter that spans the length of the esophagus (Figure 10.2), changes in impedance at multiple segments (hence the term "multichannel intraluminal impedance," or MII) can be recorded in response to movement of intraesophageal material in either the antegrade or retrograde direction. Antegrade bolus movement (i.e. a swallow) is detected by impedance changes of bolus presence progressing from the proximal to the distal esophagus (Figure 10.3A). Retrograde bolus movement (i.e. reflux) is detected by changes in impedance progressing distal to proximal, followed by proximal to distal clearance of bolus (Figure 10.3B).

By incorporating impedance electrodes into classic manometry or pH catheters, MII now complements traditional esophageal motility and pH testing. Combined MII and manometry (MII–EM) provides simultaneous information on intraluminal pressure changes and bolus transit, whereas combined MII and pH (MII–pH) allows detection of reflux episodes regardless of their pH values, i.e. acid and non-acid (also called "weakly acidic") reflux.

The Esophagus, Fifth Edition. Edited by Joel E. Richter, Donald O. Castell.
© 2012 Blackwell Publishing Ltd. Published 2012 by Blackwell Publishing Ltd.

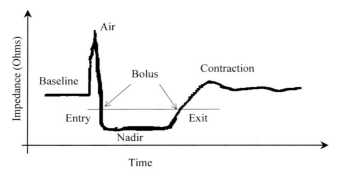

Figure 10.1 Impedance changes observed during bolus transit over a single pair of measurement rings separated by 2 cm. A rapid raise in impedance is noted when air travelling in front of the bolus head reaches the impedance measuring segment followed by a drop in impedance once higher conductive bolus material passes the measuring site. Bolus entry is considered at the 50% drop in impedance from baseline relative to nadir and bolus exit at the 50% recovery point from nadir to baseline. Lumen narrowing produced by the contraction transiently increases the impedance above baseline.

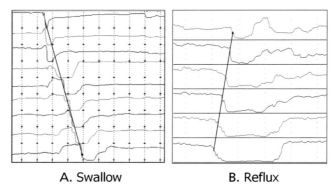

A. Swallow   **B. Reflux**

Figure 10.3 Movement of intraesophageal material detected by multichannel intraluminal impedance. (A) Antegrade bolus movement (i.e. a swallow) is characterized by sequential drops in impedance beginning at the proximal esophagus and progressing toward the distal esophagus. (B) Retrograde bolus movement (i.e. gastroesophageal reflux) is characterized by sequential drops in impedance beginning at the distal esophagus and moving upward toward the proximal esophagus.

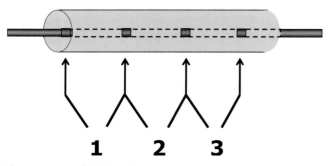

Figure 10.2 Multiple impedance measuring segments within the esophagus allow determination of direction of bolus movement within the esophagus; i.e. multichannel intraluminal impedance (MII).

Esophageal function testing using combined multichannel intraluminal impedance and manometry

MII–EM is a new technique using two complementary methods of EFT: (1) esophageal manometry (EM) provides information about intraluminal pressures generated during swallowing, and (2) MII assesses bolus movement during swallowing. Although it does not provide the anatomic details offered by radiographic barium swallow, MII has the advantage of not requiring radiation exposure in evaluating bolus movement. Furthermore, bolus transit and pressures are obtained during a single test procedure, and thus on the same swallows.

The indications for combined MII–EM are the same as for EM: evaluation of dysphagia, non-cardiac chest pain, and

gastroesophageal reflux disease (GERD), including preoperative evaluation before antireflux surgery or endoscopic antireflux procedures.

Initial studies on normal subjects indicated that MII could detect the presence of small volumes of swallowed liquid (i.e. 1 mL) and confirmed known pharmacologic effects of cholinergic medications on esophageal peristalsis and bolus movement [3].

There are catheters that enable combined impedance and manometry (both conventional and high resolution) measurements. These catheters incorporate a varying number of pressure transducers as well as multiple impedance measuring segments; an example of a combined MII–EM catheter is shown in Figure 10.4. Dedicated software programs are available for editing and analysis. Generally, these software programs facilitate the production of reports with details on manometric (contraction amplitude, duration and velocity, lower [LES] and upper esophageal sphincter [UES] characteristics), as well as impedance (bolus presence time, total and segmental bolus transit times) parameters. The clinical applications of combined impedance–manometry are described in greater detail in Chapter 9.

Multichannel intraluminal impedance for assessment of bolus transit in esophageal function tests

Bolus entry at a specific level measured by impedance is considered to occur at the 50% point between 3 s before swallow impedance baseline and impedance nadir during bolus presence. Bolus exit is determined as return to this 50% point on the impedance recovery curve (see Figure 10.1). These relationships have been validated by simultane-

Pressure | Impedance

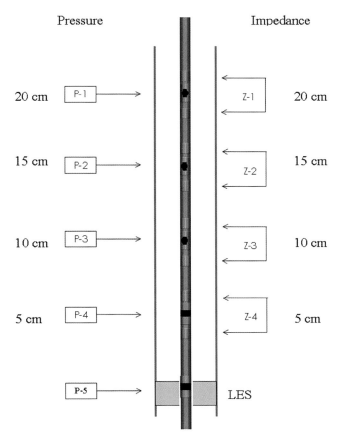

Figure 10.4 Nine-channel combined multichannel intraluminal impedance (MII) and manometry (EM) catheter. Circumferential solid-state pressure sensors located in lower esophageal sphincter (LES) high-pressure zone (P5) and 5 cm above it (P4); unidirectional solid-state pressure sensors located 10 cm (P3), 15 cm (P2), and 20 cm (P1) above LES. Impedance measuring segments centered at 5 cm (Z4), 10 cm (Z3), 15 cm (Z2), and 20 cm (Z1) above LES.

ous MII and videofluoroscopy with barium [1, 2]. Calculated impedance parameters are shown in Figure 10.5: total bolus transit time; bolus head advance time; bolus presence time; and segmental transit time [4].

Swallows are classified manometrically in standard fashion (see Chapter 8). Swallows are classified by MII as showing (1) complete bolus transit (Figure 10.6A), if bolus entry is seen at the most proximal site (20 cm above the LES) and bolus exit points are recorded at all three distal impedance measuring sites (i.e. 15, 10, and 5 cm above the LES); and (2) incomplete bolus transit (Figure 10.6B) if bolus exit is not identified at any of the three distal impedance measuring sites.

Normal EFT values for impedance parameters were proposed based on the 95th percentile in healthy volunteers (Table 10.1). Impedance parameters define a study as normal if at least 80% of liquid and at least 70% of viscous swallows

show complete MII-detected bolus transit [5]. When using liquid testing substances, a study is considered normal manometrically if it does not contain more than 20% ineffective and 10% simultaneous swallows [5].

Studies using MII–EM in patients with manometrically defined motility abnormalities have aimed to provide a better understanding of bolus transit in various categories of motility abnormalities. The effect of motility abnormalities on bolus transit (or lack thereof) has been clarified by MII–EM studies showing that more than half of patients with manometrically defined distal esophageal spasm (DES) or ineffective esophageal motility (IEM) have complete bolus transit measured by MII. Patients with nutcracker esophagus or isolated LES abnormalities (i.e. hypertensive or hypotensive LES, poorly relaxing LES) have complete bolus transit during swallowing, whereas patients with achalasia or scleroderma have incomplete bolus transit during swallowing (Figure 10.7) [6].

In summary, the addition of MII to manometry (MII–EM) incorporates two complementary techniques that, together, provide a more detailed evaluation of both aspects of esophageal function: esophageal contractile activity and bolus transit. The clinical applications of this approach are discussed in Chapter 5.

Combined multichannel intraluminal impedance and pH for detection of acid and non-acid gastroesophageal reflux

The pathophysiologic role of acid in GERD has been well established in studies in both animals and humans [7]. Until recently, measuring GER was based solely upon esophageal pH monitoring, which bases detection of reflux of acidic material into the esophagus on changes in hydrogen ion concentration (i.e. drops in esophageal pH to below 4.0) [8]. In a number of patients, reflux symptoms persist despite treatment with medications that decrease gastric acid secretion; recent studies have shown that these symptoms can be caused by reflux having pH greater than 4 (i.e. non-acid reflux or weakly acidic reflux) [9]. In fact, when the contents of the stomach are buffered (in the post-prandial period or during treatment with potent acid-suppressing medications like proton-pump inhibitors), a significant proportion of GER is non-acid and therefore not accurately detectable by conventional pH recording [10–13]. This is highlighted by the fact that the likelihood of a positive pH test in acid-suppressed patients is indeed very low [14].This limitation of pH-metry has created the need for a method that can accurately measure non-acid reflux.

Several techniques have been considered in the past for the study of non-acid or alkaline reflux, including aspiration, scintigraphy, ambulatory pH monitoring, and bilirubin monitoring (Bilitec) [15–19], all of which have certain limi-

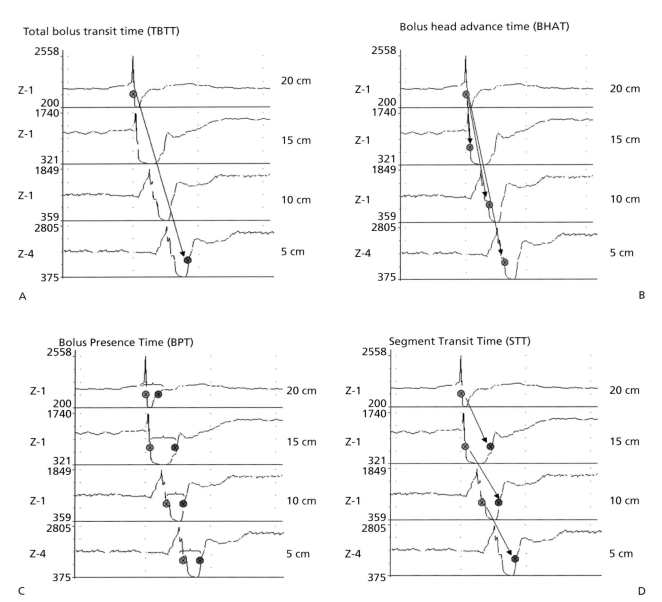

Figure 10.5 Definitions of impedance parameters. (A) Total bolus transit time (TBTT) as time elapsed between bolus entry at 20 cm above lower esophageal sphincter (LES) and bolus exit at 5 cm above LES. (B) Bolus head advance time as time elapsed between bolus entry at 20 cm above LES and bolus entry at 15, 10, and 5 cm above LES. (C) Bolus presence time (BPT) as time elapsed between bolus entry and bolus exit at each impedance measuring site (5, 10, 15, and 20 cm above LES). (D) Segmental transit time (STT) as time elapsed between bolus entry at a given level above LES and bolus exit at the next lower level.

tations. Aspiration studies allow for only short analysis periods, and the accuracy of enzymatic determination of the contents of the aspirates has been questioned [18, 20]. Scintigraphic studies are expensive, involve radiation exposure, and are usually limited to short monitoring periods [16]. During ambulatory pH monitoring, a pH of 7 or greater has been used as the definition of "alkaline" reflux, but increased saliva production or bicarbonate secreted by esophageal submucosal glands confounds measurements by increasing esophageal pH in the absence of reflux [21]. Some authors propose that reflux can be detected by pH-metry even when intraesophageal pH remains greater than 4.0 through measurement of pH decreases of greater than 1 unit [22]. However, ingestion of acidic foods can mimic reflux by provoking pH drops of greater than 1 unit [23]; furthermore, pH-metry is unable to detect non-acid reflux that occurs in the absence of pH changes or with small pH changes (<1 unit) [9]. Monitoring with the Bilitec probe is

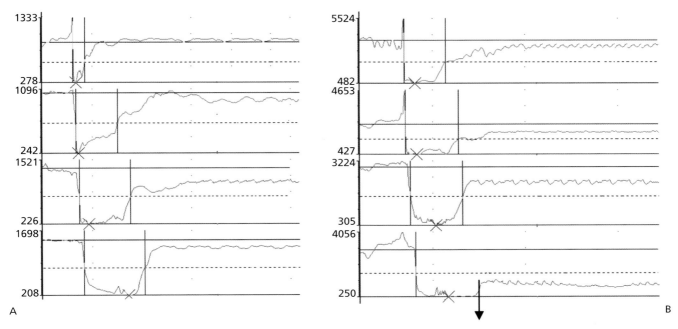

Figure 10.6 Classification of swallows by multichannel intraluminal impedance (MII) criteria. (A) Complete bolus transit if bolus entry is seen at the most proximal site (20 cm above lower esophageal sphincter (LES) and bolus exit points are recorded at all three distal impedance-measuring sites (i.e. 15, 10, and 5 cm above the LES). (B) Incomplete bolus transit if bolus exit is not identified at any one of the three distal impedance-measuring sites.

Table 10.1 Normative data of impedance (MII) parameters of esophageal function testing (EFT) for 10 liquid and 10 viscous swallows in 43 healthy volunteers. 95th percentile values can be considered the upper limit of normal for the given parameters [5].

	Liquid (n = 429)				Viscous (n = 425)			
	Median	Percentile			Median	Percentile		
		25th	75th	5–95th		25th	75th	5–95th
Bolus head advance time (s)								
20–15 cm	0.2	0.1	0.3	0.0–0.7	1.0	0.6	1.5	0.2–2.5
20–10 cm	0.6	0.4	0.9	0.1–1.7	3.3	2.4	4.0	0.9–5.1
20–5 cm	1.3	0.8	2.2	0.5–5.0	4.9	4.3	5.6	2.8–7.4
Bolus presence time (s)								
at 20 cm	1.7	1.1	2.7	0.6–5.9	1.9	1.2	2.9	0.8–5.0
at 15 cm	4.1	3.0	5.1	1.4–8.8	3.5	2.8	4.1	1.9–5.9
at 10 cm	5.3	4.5	6.3	3.5–9.9	3.4	2.6	4.3	1.9–7.6
at 5 cm	5.8	4.6	6.7	2.3–9.3	3.1	2.3	4.1	1.5–6.3
Segment transit time (s)								
20–15 cm	4.4	3.3	5.4	1.6–9.0	4.6	4.0	5.3	2.8–7.3
15–10 cm	5.7	5.0	6.7	3.9–10.5	5.3	4.5	6.3	3.8–10.1
10–5 cm	6.6	5.8	7.6	4.5–10.6	4.9	3.9	6.0	3.0–8.3
Total bolus transit time (s)	7.2	6.6	8.2	5.2–11.9	7.9	7.0	9.0	5.9–12.4

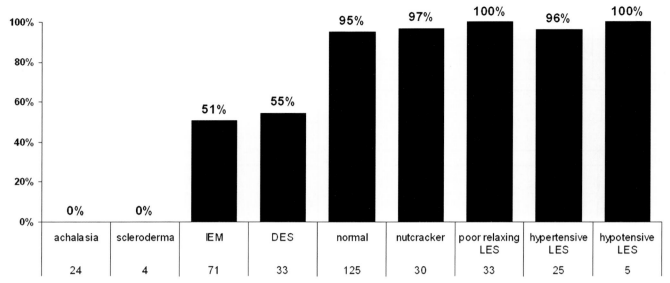

Figure 10.7 Percentage of patients with complete bolus transit in 350 patients with various manometric diagnoses. While all patients with achalasia and scleroderma have incomplete bolus transit, more than half of patients with distal esophageal spasm (DES) and ineffective esophageal motility (IEM) have complete bolus transit (51% and 55%, respectively). Almost all patients with nutcracker esophagus, normal esophageal manometry, and isolated lower esophageal sphincter (LES) abnormalities have complete bolus transit for liquid (Modified from Tutian and Castell [6]).

based on the presence of bilirubin and is therefore incapable of measuring bile-free non-acid reflux. Additionally, bilirubin monitoring requires a special diet to avoid false-positive readings [18].

MII–pH represents an important advance in GER testing because it enables accurate detection of GER at all pH levels: impedance detects retrograde bolus movement (i.e. reflux), while pH measurement establishes the acidity of the reflux episode (acid if pH < 4.0; non-acid otherwise). The technique has been validated fluoroscopically and manometrically to detect bolus movement in the esophagus, both in the oral and aboral direction [24], thus allowing measurement of and distinction between swallows and reflux. As discussed earlier, a catheter with multiple pairs of impedance electrodes can record impedance changes in response to movement of intraesophageal material in either antegrade or retrograde direction. As shown in Figure 10.3, this means that a swallow can be clearly distinguished from reflux, i.e. retrograde movement of gastric contents into the esophagus. Because MII records retrograde flow of gastric contents into the esophagus in a pH-independent fashion, combining the technique with pH-metry enables detection of acid as well as non-acid reflux. Some authors classify reflux with a pH above 4.0 as either weakly acidic (pH ≥ 4 but <7) or weakly alkaline (pH ≥ 7). In this chapter, non-acid reflux refers to any reflux with a pH of 4 or greater.

Because of its ability to measure GER at all pH levels, MII–pH monitoring has emerged as a useful diagnostic and research tool, particularly in patients with ongoing symp-

Table 10.2 Normative data for reflux using combined impedance–pH monitoring.

Study	n	Number of reflux episodes: upper limit of normal*		
		Total	**Acid**	**Non-acid**
United States (Shay et al. [27])	60	73	59	27
France–Belgium (Zerbib et al. [28])	72	75	50	48

*Upper limit of normal for the number of reflux episodes was based on the 95th percentile for the healthy volunteers in each study.

toms despite acid suppression [12]. Additionally, MII–pH provides very meticulous characterization of the reflux episode, including determination of the composition (gas, liquid, mixed), proximal extent (height reached), velocity, and clearance time [9]. Based on the very detailed information that MII–pH monitoring provides, a recently convened panel of experts concluded that it is the most sensitive tool for measuring GER [25]. Assessment of reflux with MII–pH has been found to be reproducible [26], and normal values for ambulatory 24-h MII–pH monitoring obtained by independent multicenter studies are similar (Table 10.2) [27, 28].

MII–pH catheter characteristics and placement

MII–pH monitoring can be performed with several different catheters (usually no more than 2 mm in diameter) that incorporate a varying number of impedance and pH electrodes in different configurations. The catheter is placed transnasally and is connected to a data logger that the patient carries for 24 h. Ordinarily, the catheter has a pH electrode for placement 5 cm above the LES (similar to conventional pH testing), with the possibility of additional pH sensors in the stomach or proximal esophagus. Catheters may incorporate six or more impedance measuring segments (each composed of two metal electrodes usually spaced 2 cm apart) to detect impedance changes along variable lengths of the esophagus. While there are no published studies comparing the accuracy of different catheter configurations, a catheter with six impedance measuring segments and one pH electrode (Figure 10.8) enables accurate detection of reflux episodes with an assessment of proximal extent of reflux, and it permits distinction between swallowing and reflux episodes; a smaller number of impedance measuring segments may compromise accuracy [29].

MII–pH interpretation

When MII is combined with pH, a distinction between acid and non-acid reflux can be made because MII detects the presence of the refluxate, whereas pH simply determines the acid or non-acid nature of the refluxate. Furthermore, MII–pH enables the measurement of additional reflux episodes during an ongoing acid reflux episode, so-called re-reflux. Examples of GER of three types (acid, non-acid, and re-reflux) recorded with a six-impedance/one-pH catheter are shown in Figure 10.9.

Assisted by the observation that air and gastric contents each produce a different change in impedance, reflux episodes can be characterized as containing gas, liquid, or both. Air conducts electricity poorly and therefore has high impedance, whereas liquid gastric contents have low impedance. As illustrated in Figure 10.10, gas increases intraluminal impedance, and liquid gastric contents decrease impedance.

Identification of reflux episodes requires visual analysis of changes in the multiple impedance measuring segments, making interpretation of MII–pH tracings more time-consuming compared to that of conventional pH which is fully automated. There is available software that enables automated detection of reflux episodes in the MII–pH tracing. However, the only published study evaluating automated analysis found that it tends to overestimate the number of reflux episodes [30]. Therefore, the recommended approach is to use the automated analysis software to mark the MII–pH tracing, and this is then reviewed and edited manually. Relying solely on the automated analysis software is not currently advised, but it is possible that software improvements will result in full automation in the future. It is important to mention that a low impedance baseline, which may be seen in patients with severe reflux or Barrett's esophagus, can make interpretation of the MII–pH tracings quite difficult.

In summary, MII–pH enables refined characterization of the reflux episode. Because it measures both volume presence (through MII) as well as changes in acidity (through pH), it enables detection of reflux of all types—acid, non-acid, and re-reflux—while providing details about the volume and acid clearance, as well as the composition and height reached by the refluxate.

Clinical applications

There is a growing body of work showing the clinical applications of MII–pH monitoring both in pediatric and adult patients, the details of which are discussed in Chapter 19. In short, with its ability to measure not only acid but also non-acid reflux, MII–pH monitoring shifts the GER testing paradigm: reflux events are no longer detected by pH alone. Instead, the presence, distribution, and clearing of refluxate is primarily detected by MII, and characterized as acid versus non-acid based on pH change and as liquid, gas, or mixed based on MII. Because of its enhanced ability to detect and characterize GER, MII–pH has evolved into a clinically useful tool, especially for the evaluation of persistent symptoms despite acid suppression, an increasingly frequent clinical problem.

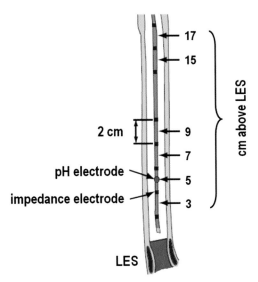

Figure 10.8 Schematic representation of the 2-mm diameter multichannel intraluminal impedance (MII)–pH catheter with impedance electrodes (4 mm in length) set in pairs at 2-cm intervals, allowing for six impedance measuring segments, as well as one pH electrode. Once properly positioned, this catheter allows recording of pH at 5 cm above the lower esophageal sphincter (LES) and impedance in six measuring segments, with their centers 3, 5, 7, 9, 15, and 17 cm above the LES (reproduced from Vela [9]).

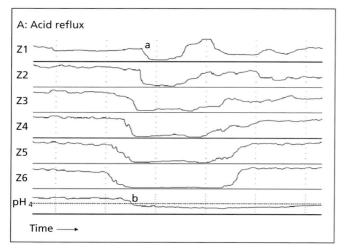

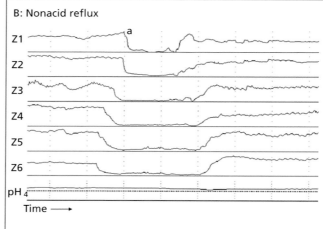

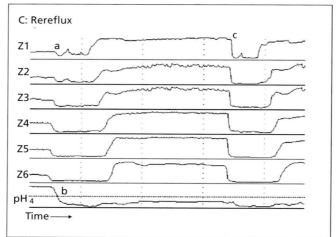

Figure 10.9 Impedance changes in ohms during three episodes of reflux. The six impedance measuring segments (Z1–Z6) and pH changes are shown on the "Y" axis. The dotted line marks a pH of 4.0. (A) Point a indicates the proximal extent of the reflux event. It is preceded by a sequential drop in impedance starting at the most distal measuring segment that proceeds toward the proximal esophagus. Arrival of the refluxate into the distal esophagus causes a fall in pH to below 4.0 (point b), an acid reflux episode. (B) The proximal extent is indicated by point a. This is not accompanied by a fall in pH to below 4.0 and is thus considered an episode of non-acid reflux. (C) Reflux detected by multichannel intraluminal impedance (MII) (point a) causes a fall in pH to below 4.0 (point b). A second MII-detected reflux episode (re-reflux, point c) occurs before the pH returns to 4.0.

A: gas reflux

B: liquid reflux

C: mixed reflux

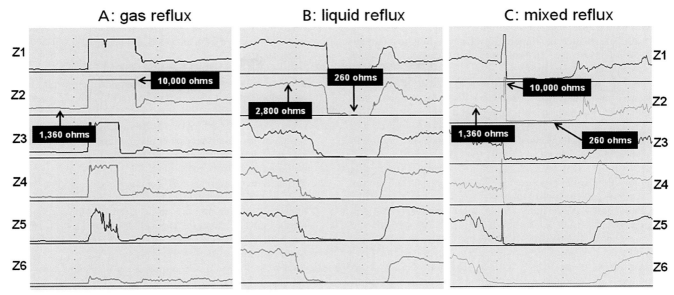

Figure 10.10 Impedance changes in ohms during reflux of gas, liquid, and mixed contents, obtained with a catheter incorporating six impedance measuring segments (Z1–Z6), which are shown on the "Y" axis. Impedance values for the second measuring segment (Z2) are shown for the three reflux episodes. (A) Reflux of gas is characterized by sharp increases in impedance beginning in the most distal recording segment and rapidly progressing upwards towards the proximal esophagus. In Z2, impedance rises from a baseline of 1360 ohms to a peak of 10 000 ohms. (B) Reflux of liquid is characterized by sequential impedance falls starting in the distal esophagus and moving upwards towards the mouth. In Z2, impedance falls from a baseline of 3600 ohms to a trough of 260 ohms. (C) Reflux of gas mixed with liquid. In Z2, impedance rises from a baseline of 2860 ohms to a peak of 10 000 ohms; this is followed by an impedance fall to a trough of 350 ohms.

References

1. Silny J. Intraluminal multiple electric impedance procedure for measurement of gastrointestinal motility. *J Gastrointest Motil* 1991;3:151–162.

2. Imam H, Shay S, Ali A, Baker M. Bolus transit patterns in healthy subjects: a study using simultaneous impedance monitoring, videoesophagram, and esophageal manometry. *Am J Physiol Gastrointest Liver Physiol* 2005;288:G1000–1006.

3. Srinivasan R, Vela MF, Katz PO, et al. Esophageal function testing using multichannel intraluminal impedance. *Am J Physiol Gastrointest Liver Physiol* 2001;280:G457–462.

4. Tutuian R, Vela MF, Shay SS, Castell DO. Multichannel intraluminal impedance in esophageal function testing and gastroesophageal reflux monitoring. *J Clin Gastroenterol* 2003;37:206–215.

5. Tutuian R, Vela MF, Balaji N, et al. Esophageal function testing using combined multichannel intraluminal impedance and manometry. Multicenter study in healthy volunteers. *Clin Gastroenterol Hepatol* 2003;1:174–182.

6. Tutuian R, Castell DO. Combined multichannel intraluminal impedance and manometry clarifies esophageal function abnormalities: study in 350 patients. *Am J Gastroenterol* 2004;99:1011–1019.

7. Vaezi MF, Singh S, Richter JE. Role of acid and duodenogastric reflux in esophageal mucosal injury: a review of animal and human studies. *Gastroenterology* 1995;108:1897–1907.

8. Hirano I, Richter JE. American College of Gastroenterology guidelines: esophageal reflux testing. *Am J Gastroenterol* 2007;102:668–685.

9. Vela M. Non-acid reflux: detection by multichannel intraluminal impedance and pH. Clinical significance and management. *Am J Gastroenterol* 2009;104:277–280.

10. Vela MF, Camacho-Lobato L, Srinivasan R, et al. Intraesophageal impedance and pH measurement of acid and nonacid reflux: effect of omeprazole. *Gastroenterology* 2001;120:1599–1606

11. Sifrim D, Holloway RH, Silny J, et al. Composition of the postprandial refluxate in patients with gastroesophageal reflux disease. *Am J Gastroenterol* 2001;96:647–655.

12. Mainie I, Tutuian R, Shay S, et al.. Acid and nonacid reflux in patients with persistent symptoms despite acid suppressive therapy: a multicenter study using combined ambulatory impedance-pH monitoring. *Gut* 2006;55:1398–1402.

13. Hila A, Agrawal A, Castell DO. Combined multichannel intraluminal impedance and pH esophageal testing compared to pH alone for diagnosing both acid and weakly acidic gastroesophageal reflux. *Clin Gastroenterol Hepatol* 2007;5:172–177.

14. Charbel S, Khandwala F, Vaezi MF. The role of esophageal pH monitoring in Symptomatic patients on PPI therapy. *Am J Gastroenterol* 2005;100:283–289.

15. Stein HJ, Feussner H, Kauer W, et al. Alkaline gastroesophageal reflux: assessment by ambulatory esophageal aspiration and pH monitoring. *Am J Surg* 1994;167:163–168.

16. Velasco N, Pope CE, Gannan RM, et al. Measurement of esophageal reflux by scintigraphy. *Dig Dis Sci* 1984;29:977–982.

17. Iftikhar SY, Ledingham S, Evans DF, *et al.* Alkaline gastrooesophageal reflux: dual probe pH monitoring. *Gut* 1995;37:465–470.

18. Vaezi MF, Richter JE. Importance of duodeno-gastro-esophageal reflux in the medical outpatient practice. *Hepatogastroenterology* 1999;46:40–47.

19. Stein HJ, Kauer WKH, Feussner H, *et al.* Bile acids as components of the duodenogastric refluxate: detection, relationship to bilirubin, mechanism of injury, and clinical relevance. *Hepatogastroenterology* 1999;46:66–73.

20. Girelli CM, Cuvello P, Limido E, *et al.* Duodenogastric reflux: an update. *Am J Gastroenterol* 1996;91:648–653.

21. DeVault KR, Georgeson S, Castell DO. Salivary stimulation mimics esophageal exposure to refluxed duodenal contents. *Am J Gastroenterol* 1993;88:1040–1043.

22. Smout AJPM. Ambulatory monitoring of esophageal pH and pressure. In: Castell DO, Richter JE, eds. *The Esophagus*, 3rd edn. Philadelphia: Lippincott Williams & Wilkins, 1999, pp. 119–133.

23. Agrawal A, Tutian R, Hila A, *et al.* Ingestion of acidic foods mimics gastroesophageal reflux during pH monitoring. *Dig Dis Sci* 2005;50:1916–1920.

24. Silny J, Knigge KP, Fass J, *et al.* Verification of the intraluminal multiple electrical impedance measurement for the recording of gastrointestinal motility. *J Gastrointest Motil* 1993;5:107–122.

25. Sifrim D, Castell D, Dent J, Kahrilas PJ. Gastro-oesophageal reflux monitoring: review and consensus report on detection and definitions of acid, nonacid, and gas reflux. *Gut* 2004;53:1024–1031.

26. Bredenoord AJ, Weusten BL, Timmer R, Smout AJ. Reproducibility of multichannel intraluminal electrical impedance monitoring of gastroesophageal reflux. *Am J Gastroenterol* 2005;100:265–269.

27. Shay S, Tutuian R, Sifrim D, *et al.* Twenty-four hour ambulatory simultaneous impedance and pH monitoring: a multicenter report of normal values from 60 healthy volunteers. *Am J Gastroenterol* 2004;99:1037–1043.

28. Zerbib F, des Varannes SB, Roman S, *et al.* Normal values and day-to-day variability of 24-h ambulatory oesophageal impedance-pH monitoring in a Belgian-French cohort of healthy subjects. *Aliment Pharmacol Ther* 2005;22:1011–1021.

29. Pandolfino JE, Vela MF. Esophageal reflux monitoring. *Gastrointest Endosc* 2009;69:917–930.

30. Roman S, Bruley des Varannes S, *et al.* Ambulatory 24-h oesophageal impedance-pH recordings: reliability of automatic analysis for gastro-oesophageal reflux assessment. *Neurogastroenterol Motil* 2006;18:978–986.

11 Ambulatory Monitoring for Reflux

Frank Zerbib and Pauline Roumeguère

CHU Bordeaux, Saint André Hospital, Gastroenterology and Hepatology Department, Bordeaux, Université Bordeaux Segalen, Bordeaux, France

Introduction

Gastroesophageal reflux disease (GERD) is a common disorder caused by the reflux of gastric contents into the esophagus. According to a recent global definition, GERD can cause esophageal and extraesophageal syndromes, which can be associated or not in the same individual [1]. The diagnosis of GERD can rely on typical symptoms, such as heartburn and regurgitation, as well as the on the presence of esophageal mucosal breaks at endoscopy. GERD management is primarily based on empiric therapy, with lifestyle modifications and medication, especially in general practice. However, many patients present with atypical symptoms (e.g. supraesophageal symptoms) and do not have any mucosal abnormalities at endoscopy, mainly because most of them have been prescribed proton pump inhibitors (PPIs) before being referred to gastrointestinal specialists. Moreover, available data from clinical trials with PPIs as GERD therapy suggest that up to 40% of included patients are considered to have inadequate symptom relief, especially when no esophagitis is present at endoscopy [2].

As a consequence, there has been an increasing need for objective tests of esophageal reflux. If pH monitoring has been for years the gold standard for esophageal reflux testing, combined esophageal impedance and pH monitoring is now considered to be the best technique to detect and characterize gastroesophageal reflux [3]. However, there is probably still room for pH monitoring alone, especially since a wireless technology has become available.

Esophageal pH monitoring

Esophageal pH monitoring systems use two electrodes, one acting as a reference electrode with a constant potential, and the other acting as an indicator electrode whose potential is sensitive to changes in H^+ concentration in the esophageal lumen. The electrodes are connected to a data logger with one (or more) event marker allowing ambulatory recordings. At completion of the recording, data stored in the data logger have to be downloaded into a computer and then automatically analyzed by dedicated software which also provides graphic display and printing of the report. Many devices are commercially available and will not be described in detail. Only the most relevant issues for clinical practice will be discussed.

Catheter-based pH monitoring

Electrodes

Antimony and glass electrodes are the two main types of pH electrodes (Figure 11.1) and they provide similar results for esophageal pH recordings. The performance of antimony electrodes is clearly inferior to that of glass electrodes: more frequent pH drifts, slower responses to pH changes, less linear response, and sensitivity to agents other than H^+. However, antimony electrodes are smaller, much less expensive, and more durable, and now have a built-in reference electrode which avoids the need for an external reference that was frequently responsible for artifacts. Finally, the availability of single-use antimony electrodes makes them very useful in the setting of clinical practice. Glass electrodes remain recommended for prolonged measurements of intragastric pH [4]. Calibration of the system is mandatory prior to each study using specific buffer solutions. A post-test calibration is recommended to correct calibration drift, but in practice is not often performed [5].

Practical aspects

The patient should be informed of the aims of the study and how to use the data logger, especially the event marker. Except for pharmacologic or research studies, no meal/activity standardization is needed. The recording should be performed under conditions as close as possible to the usual

The Esophagus, Fifth Edition. Edited by Joel E. Richter, Donald O. Castell.
© 2012 Blackwell Publishing Ltd. Published 2012 by Blackwell Publishing Ltd.

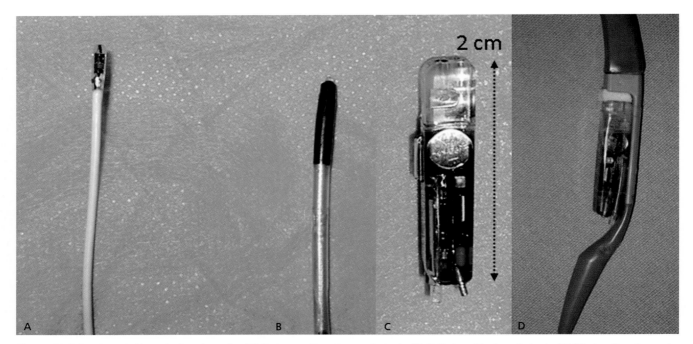

Figure 11.1 Esophageal pH monitoring electrodes. (A) Catheter with antimony electrode. (B) Catheter with glass electrode. (C) Wireless Bravo° capsule. (D) Wireless capsule with the delivery device (reproduced courtesy of S. Bruley des Varannes).

lifestyle and dietary habits of the patient. If patients have intermittent symptoms, they can be asked, if possible, to behave in manner that provokes symptoms.

Before starting the recording, it is important to check that the patient has fasted for at least 4 h beforehand and stopped any form of therapy which could interfere with the results. Whether the recording should be performed on or off PPIs will be discussed below.

The pH catheter is passed transnasally (with or without topical anesthesia) and by convention is positioned 5 cm above the proximal border of the lower esophageal sphincter (LES). For accurate positioning, LES should ideally be located by esophageal manometry, which may not be available in many centers. The step-up method is based on the pH profile recorded on withdrawal of the electrode from the stomach. This technique can be easily performed in patients studied off PPIs. The catheter is first introduced into the stomach. After confirmation of an acidic pH, the catheter is withdrawn gradually until an abrupt rise in pH to greater than 4.0 (pH step-up) is detected. The pH readings are used to indicate the proximal margin of the LES at the gastro-esophageal junction. To confirm this point, the catheter is withdrawn at least a further 10 cm and then reinserted into the stomach. The process is then repeated to confirm LES positioning. The accuracy of the pH step-up method has been determined in 50 subjects. Only one had a difference of more than 3 cm from the manometrically defined gastro-esophageal junction, thus confirming that it is an acceptable alternative [6].

It is now generally admitted that a 24-h recording is more accurate and reproducible than a shorter duration of recording (see below).

Interpretation: normal values

A correct interpretation of esophageal pH monitoring relies on qualitative and quantitative analysis, together with symptom-association analysis (see below). Qualitative analysis should determine whether the overall quality of the tracings is good, i.e. no pH drift, catheter displacement, loss of signal possibly related to disconnection, etc. (Figure 11.2). If necessary, some parts of the tracings should be excluded from the analysis since the software may take into account artifacts for determination of pH reflux parameters. In clinical practice, many patients are diagnosed as having very severe acid reflux based on low-quality pH recordings. These "false-positive" recordings may have important implications for patients' management. It is also recommended to exclude meal periods from the analysis to avoid artifacts related to food ingestion [7].

Analysis software provides the most relevant reflux parameters but has to be adequately set. A reflux is defined by a drop in pH below 4 for at least 10 s. For routine pH monitoring, most equipment uses 0.25 Hz as the sampling rate (one measurement every 4 s). When considering quantitative evaluation, i.e. evaluation of the amount of acid reaching the esophagus, the most relevant parameter to be determined is esophageal acid exposure, i.e. the proportion of time (in minutes or percentage of time) spent below pH

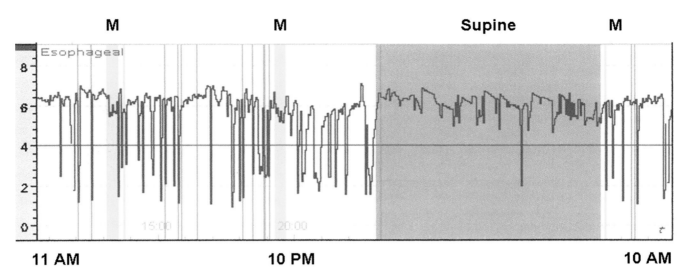

Figure 11.2 Example of 24-h esophageal pH monitoring in a patient with heartburn. The overall acid exposure is within the normal range (total 2.9%, upright 4.4%, supine 0%). The total number of reflux episodes is 57. Each red vertical line represents the activation of the event marker by the patient. Symptom association analysis can be performed as follows: a total of 15 heartburn episodes were reported, eight of which were associated with reflux; the symptom index (SI) is 8/15 = 53.3%. A total of eight of 57 reflux events were associated with symptoms; the symptom sensitivity index (SSI) is 14%. The software provides a symptom association probability of 99%, which is significant. This patient has a so-called "hypersensitive esophagus."

4. Other variables can be determined, but are less reproducible and/or have less discriminatory power. The sampling frequency does not affect the measuring of percentage time that the pH is below 4, but it does affect the number of reflux episodes. The number of reflux episodes, therefore, depends highly on the algorithm used for identification of a reflux and is much less correlated to the grade of esophagitis than esophageal acid exposure. The same holds true for acid clearance time, i.e. the mean duration of acid reflux episodes, and the number of reflux episodes lasting more than 5 min, which both reflect the esophageal clearance of acid. The clinical utility of composite scores, such as DeMeester's score, has not been clearly demonstrated.

Many sets of normal values for esophageal pH monitoring have been reported. The values vary widely because of various conditions of recordings (standardized or not), materials, age and definition of controls, analysis of data, and definitions of normal values (medians, 95th percentile, etc.). Ideally, each laboratory should determine its own normal values based on studies performed in a cohort of healthy asymptomatic subjects, but this is not done in most centers. Therefore, some experts have proposed cut-off points as acceptable upper limits for routine diagnosis of GERD (Table 11.1), the most important being the value of 5% for esophageal acid exposure [8]. These proposed values are very close to those used by many physicians. Esophageal acid exposure is the best discriminator between normal subjects and patients with GERD, although its accuracy is lower in patients with non-erosive disease compared to patients with esophagitis and Barrett's esophagus (Figure 11.3) [9].

Table 11.1 Upper limits of normal values of esophageal pH monitoring for the routine diagnosis of gastroesophageal reflux disease in centers which have not determined their own normal range (according to Galmiche and Scarpignato [8]).

Esophageal acid exposure (total)	5%
Esophageal acid exposure (upright)	8%
Esophageal acid exposure (supine)	3%
Number of reflux episodes	50
Number of reflux episodes >5 min	3

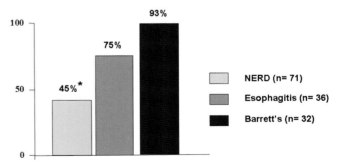

Figure 11.3 Proportion of patients with abnormal distal esophageal exposure according to the presence of esophagitis and Barrett's esophagus (*p < .001 vs esophagitis and Barrett's) (data from Martinez *et al.* [9]).

Proximal pH recordings

Proximal pH monitoring, i.e. in the proximal esophagus and/or the pharynx, has been proposed for the diagnosis of laryngopharyngeal reflux (LPR) [10]. Proximal esophageal recordings are often performed with a "dual-probe" pH catheter so that the distal probe can be positioned for monitoring distal esophageal reflux 5 cm above the LES, but this technique does not allow positioning of the proximal probe in a uniform location relative to the upper esophageal sphincter (UES) [11] and has a poor reproducibility [12]. Normal values for proximal esophageal acid reflux based on a sensor positioned 15 cm above the LES have been reported as less than 1.1% [12]. Pharyngeal pH recording can be done with a pH sensor positioned 2 cm above the UES using manometry, but this technique has many limitations mainly related to artifacts, which can be easily detected if a drop of pH in the pharynx occurs while no significant acidification of the distal esophagus is present. Most artifacts are related to swallowing and/or drying of the electrode. Several criteria have been proposed to define pharyngeal reflux: (1) magnitude of change of pH greater than 2 units; (2) nadir pH less than 4.0; (3) abrupt pH decrease (onset of pH decrease to nadir <30 s); and (d) pH decrease occurring during a period of distal esophageal acidification [13]. The 95th percentile for the upper limit of normal for total pharyngeal acid exposure time is probably less than 1% [14]. Recently, a novel pH device capable of measuring liquid and aerosolized acid levels has been developed and normal values established [15]. Whether this new device will represent a significant advance in the assessment of LPR remains to be determined and, for the time being, the clinical utility of proximal pH monitoring is a matter of debate; the recently published guidelines of the American College of Gastroenterology (ACG) stated that "available evidence does not support the routine use of proximal pH monitoring in clinical practice" [5].

Wireless pH monitoring

The use of a nasoesophageal pH catheter causes nasal, oral, and pharyngeal discomfort, and social embarrassment. Consequently, patients limit their activity and become more sedentary when monitored, which can result in less acid reflux and a false-negative test result. Wireless pH monitoring incorporates the antimony electrode into a wireless capsule that transmits pH data to an external receiver via radiofrequency telemetry (433 MHz), and allows a significant improvement in tolerability together with a 48-h recording (Figure 11.4).

Technical aspects

The Bravo® capsule measures 25 × 6 × 5.5 mm and contains a battery, radio transmitter, and an antimony pH electrode at its distal end (see Figure 11.1). The pH electrode samples esophageal pH every 6 s and data are transmitted every 12 s to a receiver unit clipped onto the patient's belt. Before use, the capsule's pH electrode is calibrated with buffer solutions. The delivery device and the capsule can be inserted either through an anesthetized nostril or transorally into the esophagus. The size of the device often makes nasal passage difficult and/or painful despite adequate topical anesthesia, such that oral passage of the delivery catheter is often necessary. A delivery system anchors the capsule to a fold of esophageal mucosa to maintain it at the appropriate level. Positioning of the capsule has been a matter of debate. It is currently recommended to position the capsule 6 cm above the squamocolumnar junction [5], based on the assumption that the proximal margin of the LES is approximately 1 cm above the squamocolumnar junction. This recommendation thereby implies that an endoscopy is performed just before

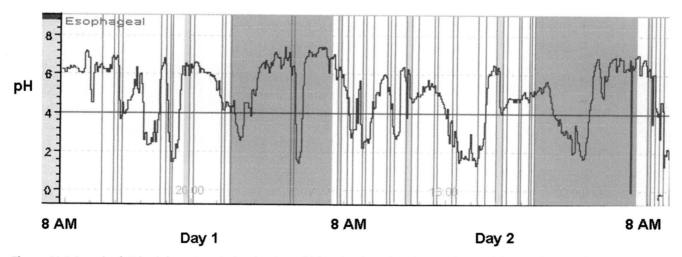

Figure 11.4 Example of 48-h wireless pH monitoring showing multiple and prolonged pH drops on day 1 and day 2. Each vertical line represents the activation of the event marker by the patient.

the capsule placement and increases the overall cost of the procedure. As an alternative option, LES position can be determined more accurately by manometry [16]; if the device cannot be inserted transnasally, a conversion factor of 4 cm permits accurate transoral placement of the capsule [17]. The technique is quite easy to learn and successful attachment of the capsule can be achieved in 90–95% of patients [18, 19]. During the recording, early detachment of the capsule may occur in approximately 10% of the subjects, resulting in premature transit of the capsule in the stomach and to a misinterpretation of the data as abnormal acid exposure [19, 20]. Loss of signal from the pH capsule can occur if the patient is too far away from the receiver, but missing data are usually of minimal importance and do not impact the overall results of the recording [18].

Comparison between catheter and capsule

Similarly to catheter-based systems, an upper normal value of approximately 5% of time spent at a pH below 4 for the 48-h period has been reported with the wireless pH system, whatever the method of LES positioning (Table 11.2) [16, 20]. Simultaneous recordings with wireless and catheter-based systems have been performed in both asymptomatic subjects and GERD patients. In asymptomatic subjects, Pandolfino et al. observed that catheter-based pH monitoring detected significantly more reflux events than the wireless system, which was in part related to a thermal calibration error for the catheter-based system used in their study [21]. After correction of this calibration error, there was still a higher number of reflux events detected by the catheter due to a higher detection of short reflux episodes, probably related to the lower sampling rate of the wireless system (Figure 11.5). These differences do not appear to be relevant regarding the diagnosis of GERD in symptomatic patients, since Bruley des Varannes et al. showed a good correlation

between the two devices for assessment of esophageal acid exposure [18]. Although esophageal acid exposure was significantly lower with the Bravo® capsule (2.4 vs 3.6%), thus justifying a modified cut-off of normal values in this study, the overall concordance for the diagnosis of GERD was 88% during the first 24 h. It is of note that short reflux episodes may be associated with symptoms and therefore affect the sensitivity/sensitivity of symptom-association analysis.

Tolerability and complications

The most prevalent symptoms related to capsule attachment are chest pain, dysphagia, and foreign body sensation, which are usually mild and only exceptionally require endoscopic removal of the capsule [18, 19]. Endoscopic removal of the capsule because of severe discomfort is required in fewer than 2% of subjects, usually by using a cold snare [22]. To date, only one case of esophageal perforation has been reported in the literature [23]. Failure of capsule detachment and prolonged retention requiring endoscopic removal is rare. Both randomized [24] and uncontrolled studies [20] have demonstrated that tolerability of wireless pH monitoring is better than catheter-based pH monitoring, regarding nasal, oral, and pharyngeal discomfort, as well as interference with daily activities, sleep, and eating.

Benefit of extended duration of recording

Several studies have shown that extending recording time to 48 h with the wireless pH monitoring system increases the likelihood of detecting reflux disease in patients undergoing symptom evaluation [16, 18, 20, 25]. There may be significant differences in acid exposure between the first and second 24-h recording periods, so that the diagnostic accuracy is highest when the "worst day" 24-h period is considered for diagnosis of GERD [16]. Prolongation of pH monitoring also increases the likelihood of establishing a positive symptom–reflux association, with an overall

Table 11.2 Normal values of wireless pH monitoring according to the modality of lower esophageal sphincter (LES) positioning.

	LES manometrically positioned [16]			LES endoscopically positioned [20]		
	First 24 h	Second 24 h	Combined 48 h	First 24 h	Second 24 h	Combined 48 h
pH < 4 total	1.08 (6.31)	1.21 (5.87)	1.40 (4.85)	2.30 (5.90)	1.80 (6.60)	2.00 (5.30)
pH < 4 upright	1.26 (7.99)	1.78 (7.47)	1.80 (7.29)	3.20 (5.80)	2.40 (7.30)	2.60 (6.90)
pH < 4 supine	0.00 (1.60)	0.00 (1.33)	0.00 (1.39)	0.10 (6.30)	0.20 (8.8)	0.50 (6.70)
Number of reflux episodes	15 (58)	18.5 (60)	37 (104)	40.9 ± 23*	NA	36.8 ± 20.1*
Number of reflux episodes ≥5 min	0 (4)	0 (3)	1 (5)	1.4 ± 1.3*	NA	1.2 ± 1.6*

Median values (95th percentile) except for * values, which are expressed as mean ± SD and are normalized to reflect what they would equal in 24-h recordings.
NA, not available.

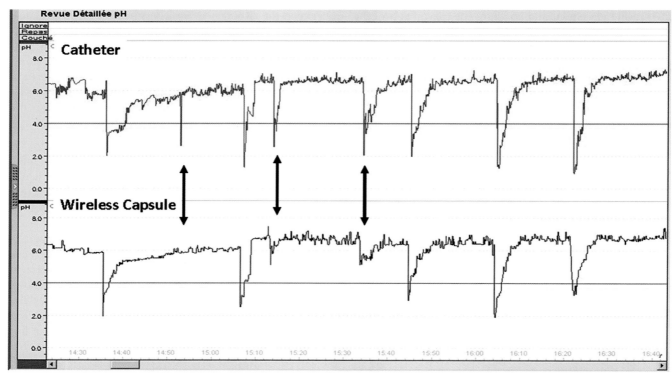

Figure 11.5 Example of simultaneous esophageal pH monitoring with catheter (top trace) and wireless capsule (bottom trace). Short reflux events detected by the catheter are not detected by the wireless system.

increased diagnostic yield as high as 31% [25] despite a lower number of short/very short reflux events detected by the wireless system. Extended recording time also offers the possibility of reflux testing both on and off therapy by using two separate receivers calibrated to a single Bravo® capsule. In a study of 60 patients studied off therapy for the first 48h and on rabeprazole 20mg bid on days 3 and 4, premature detachment of the capsule was observed in 20 patients [26]. Among patients who completed the whole study, acid exposure was abnormal off therapy in 35% and in 2% on therapy. Symptom index (SI) and symptom-association probability (SAP) were positive in 50% and 45% of patients off therapy, respectively, but only 9% and 10% on therapy, respectively. This study demonstrates the feasibility of 4-day pH monitoring, which, with a single procedure, may help to document the presence of acid reflux-related symptoms both off and on therapy.

Clinical relevance

pH monitoring off therapy
Determining 24-h esophageal acid exposure is the best method to discriminate between physiologic and pathologic GER [27]. Although considerable overlap can be observed among groups, esophageal acid exposure is associated with a graded increase in severity across the GERD spectrum [28]. There is a correlation between esophageal acid exposure and length of Barrett's mucosa [29]. However, up to 30% of

patients with reflux esophagitis, mainly those with mild esophagitis, may have normal esophageal acid exposure, and the proportion of false-negative studies is even higher in patients with non-erosive reflux disease (NERD) [9]. This lack of sensitivity may be due to day-to-day intraindividual variability of reflux, inclusion of patients with symptoms not related to GERD, and limitations of the technique of esophageal pH recording. It must be also kept in mind that false-positive results may occur related to artifacts such as pH drift, intragastric migration of the catheter, and ingestion of acidic food or beverages.

Abnormal esophageal acid exposure can help to predict response to medical and surgical therapy. Most patients with symptoms refractory to PPI therapy do not have either esophagitis or abnormal acid exposure [2], and normal esophageal acid exposure has been associated with worse outcome after fundoplication [30].

Esophageal pH monitoring also allows documentation of the association between reflux episodes and reported symptoms by using appropriate symptom-association analysis indices, i.e. SI and/or SAP (see below). Analysis of symptom-reflux association should be performed in all studies. A positive symptom reflux association is associated with a better response to PPIs [31]. An acid hypersensitive esophagus is defined by a normal esophageal acid exposure and a positive symptom association, thus reflecting an underlying visceral hypersensitivity [2]. These patients usually have NERD, very frequently dyspeptic associated symptoms [32, 33], and are probably less responsive to PPIs and fundoplication than patients with abnormal acid exposure [34], although prospective data are lacking.

To summarize, esophageal pH monitoring off therapy should be performed to document abnormal esophageal acid exposure and/or positive symptom reflux association in NERD patients being considered for surgery. A pH study off therapy could also be proposed in patients presenting with typical or atypical symptoms refractory to PPIs (see below).

pH monitoring on therapy

One of the most common indications for esophageal pH monitoring is refractory GERD. Patients with refractory symptoms are often tested on therapy to check whether acid reflux is controlled or not by the treatment. Whether such studies should be performed under a single or double dose of PPIs is not yet defined. Moreover, the definition of normal values of esophageal acid exposure on PPIs is still a matter of debate, since some authors have proposed a more stringent cut-off value of 1.6% for normal esophageal acid exposure on PPIs [35].

It is generally agreed that the diagnostic yield of esophageal pH monitoring on PPIs is low since, in this situation, most reflux events are weakly acidic and therefore not detected [5]. A study by Charbel et al. showed that approximately 30% of patients on PPI qid had persistent abnormal esophageal acid exposure [36]. However, among patients on double-dose PPIs, only 7% with typical symptoms and 1% presenting with atypical symptoms had an abnormal esophageal acid exposure and/or a positive SI, thus confirming that while on PPIs bid, the probability of having abnormal acid reflux is very low. In conclusion, the overall diagnostic yield of pH monitoring is relatively low in patients with persisting symptoms on PPI therapy, provided that refractoriness refers to patients taking PPIs bid In patients with a pretest low probability of GERD (e.g. atypical symptoms and/or no response to PPIs), pH monitoring should preferably be performed off therapy to rule out the presence of pathologic GER. By contrast, in patients with a higher probability of GERD (e.g. typical symptoms and/or incomplete response to PPIs), pH monitoring should be performed on therapy and will demonstrate abnormal esophageal acid exposure in only approximately 10% of them. Whether prolonged wireless pH monitoring, allowing both off and on PPI assessments [26], could be useful in clinical practice remains to be further determined.

Esophageal pH–impedance monitoring

Multichannel intraluminal impedance (MII) monitoring measures impedance from multiple intraluminal recording segments along the esophagus. This method allows detection of GER based on changes in resistance to electrical current flow between two electrodes, when a liquid and/or gas bolus moves between them [3]. Impedance is the opposite of conductivity. The impedance to the current flow delivered between two electrodes depends on the electrical conductivity of the environment surrounding the electrodes (luminal content, mucosa, wall thickness). When a liquid bolus with high electrical conductivity bridges two electrode rings, impedance decreases. In contrast, a gas bolus with very low electrical conductivity increases impedance. This technique, combined with pH monitoring, allows detection of GER of gas and acid or non-acid liquids.

Technical aspects

Esophageal impedance–pH monitoring systems include a portable data logger with impedance–pH amplifiers and a catheter containing at least one antimony pH electrode and six impedance electrodes (Figure 11.6). Each pair of adjacent electrodes represents an impedance measuring segment,

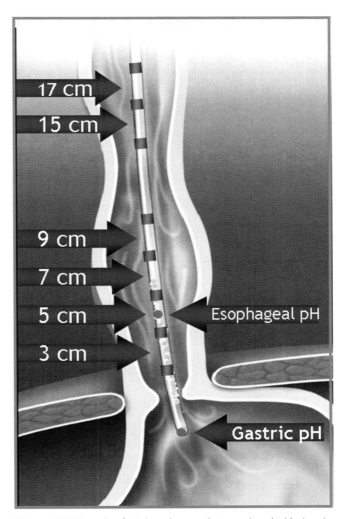

Figure 11.6 Example of pH–impedance catheter equipped with six pairs of impedance electrodes and two pH sensors (Sandhill Scientific, Highlands Ranch, CO, USA).

2 cm in length, corresponding to one recording channel. The impedance amplifier delivers AC voltage in a range of 1–2 kHz with resulting current flow variations in response to intraluminal impedance changes. The impedance and pH signals are recorded at a 50-Hz sampling rate and data are stored on a memory card for further analysis using dedicated software. As per pH monitoring alone, studies are preferably performed on an outpatient basis after an overnight fast. Before the start of the recordings, the pH recorder is calibrated using pH 4.0 and pH 7.0 buffer solutions. The pH–impedance catheter is passed transnasally under topical anesthesia and positioned in the esophageal body to record pH at 5 cm and impedance at six different levels proximal to the LES. Some catheters also have an antimony electrode for monitoring of gastric pH and/or pH at the level of the proximal esophagus. The center of the most distal impedance channel should be −3 cm above the proximal margin of the LES [3]. The catheter can be positioned by using the pH step-up technique (see above), but this cannot be performed in patient on PPIs. Therefore, LES should ideally be located by esophageal manometry. Subjects are encouraged to maintain normal activities and sleep schedule, and to eat their usual meals at their normal times. Between meals, patients are asked to abstain from frequent snacks and beverages out of the meal periods to avoid interpretation difficulties.

Interpretation

Meals have to be excluded for the analysis. Liquid reflux is defined as a retrograde 50% drop in impedance, starting distally (at the level of the LES) and propagating to at least the next two more proximal impedance measuring segments. Some experts have stated that 50% reduction is too stringent and that the pattern of reflux is as important [3]. If the impedance baseline values are abnormally low at the most distal levels (Barrett's esophagus, esophagitis), the recorded impedance drop may not be sufficient to reach the threshold. It is possible to use the more proximal channels, however, and a liquid reflux episode is proven when there is an abrupt reduction of impedance in the next two adjacent recording segments [3].

Gas reflux is defined as a rapid (3 kOhm/s) increase in impedance to greater than 5000 ohm, occurring simultaneously in at least two esophageal measuring segments, in the absence of swallowing. Mixed liquid–gas reflux is defined as gas reflux occurring immediately before or during a liquid reflux.

Reflux episodes are characterized by pH-metry as acid, weakly acidic, or weakly alkaline according to a consensus report (Figure 11.7) [3]: (1) *Acid reflux* is refluxed gastric juice with a pH less than 4 which can either reduce the pH of the esophagus to below 4 or occur when esophageal pH is already below 4; (2) *weakly acidic reflux* is reflux events that result in an esophageal pH between 4 and 7; and (3) *weakly*

alkaline reflux is reflux episodes during which nadir esophageal pH does not drop below 7. A slight modification of this definition has been used in some studies to differentiate weakly acidic from weakly alkaline reflux, considering pH 6.5 instead of pH 7 as the limit between them [37]. In the published literature, so-called "non-acid reflux" usually refers to any reflux event with a pH of 4 or greater. Although it is clearly a misnomer since chemical composition of the refluxate is of an acidic nature in most cases (pH < 7), it provides a better fit with the pH less than 4 threshold traditionally applied to acid reflux.

Analysis of pH–impedance recordings is time consuming and requires experience. The duration of manual analysis ranges from 20 min to 1 h, depending on the experience of the investigator and the number of reflux events to analyze. The Bioview® software developed by Sandhill® offers the possibility of an automatic analysis for reflux detection. A French study aimed to assess the accuracy of this automatic analysis as compared to visual analysis [38]: automatic analysis detected more reflux events, especially non-acid reflux events, as well as pure gas and proximal reflux episodes. These discrepancies were mostly related to swallow artifacts which were considered to be actual reflux episodes by the software. The diagnostic accuracy for acid GER was excellent in patients both off and on PPIs (97.6% and 100%, respectively). By contrast, because of an increased detection of non-acid reflux, the accuracy of automatic analysis for non-acid reflux was 82.9 and 75% in patients off and on therapy, respectively. This increased sensitivity may be considered a positive feature for a screening test for reflux; however, it clearly appears that this automatic analysis is not yet reliable, especially in patients on PPIs since 25% of them would have an incorrect final diagnosis. A more rapid analysis could be proposed to assess the temporal relationship between symptoms and GER detected by impedance: SI could be determined accurately by a visual analysis of the period preceding each reported symptom. However, this analysis cannot provide a reliable determination of the SAP. Although significant improvements can be expected in the future, visual analysis remains the gold standard to detect an association between symptoms and non-acid reflux events, especially in patients with persisting symptoms on PPIs.

In addition to the acid reflux parameters that are provided by the software, many additional parameters can be obtained regarding the so-called "bolus reflux," i.e. the reflux events detected by impedance: number of bolus reflux events according to their chemical composition, esophageal bolus exposure (time spent with bolus reflux within the esophageal lumen), bolus clearance time, and number of reflux events with extent to the proximal esophagus (i.e. 15 cm above the LES). Two sets of very similar normal values have been reported (Table 11.3) [37, 39]. Since most pH–impedance recordings are performed in patients taking antisecretory

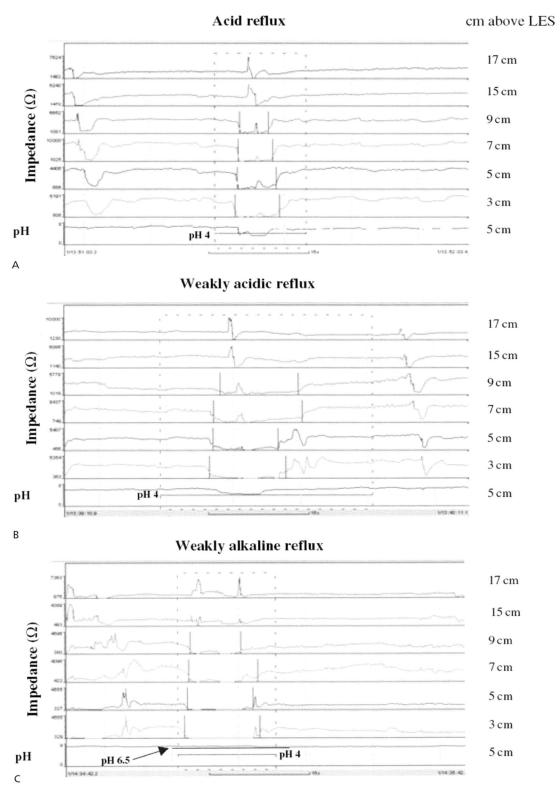

Figure 11.7 Combined impedance–pH recordings showing examples of the three types of reflux. Vertical bars on impedance channels indicate the beginning and end of bolus reflux. Horizontal bars on the pH channel indicate pH 4 and 6.5 values. (A) Liquid acid reflux: retrograde drop in impedance starting distally and propagated retrogradely up to 9 cm above the lower esophageal sphincter (LES), together with a pH fall below 4.

(B) Liquid weakly acidic reflux: retrograde drop in impedance starting distally and propagated retrogradely up to 9 cm above the LES, together with a pH fall below 6.5 but above 4. (C) Liquid weakly alkaline reflux: retrograde drop in impedance starting distally and propagated retrogradely up to 9 cm above the LES with pH values above 6.5.

Table 11.3 Median normal values of pH–impedance monitoring parameters in two cohorts of healthy subjects (95th percentile).

	Shay et al. [39] (n = 60)	Zerbib et al. [37] (n = 72)
Total number of reflux (n)	30 (73)	44 (75)
Acid reflux (n)	18 (55)	22 (50)
Weakly acidic reflux (n)	9 (26)	11 (33)
Weakly alkaline reflux (n)	0 (1)	3 (15)*
Esophageal bolus exposure (%)	0.5 (1.4)	0.8 (2.0)
Esophageal acid exposure (%)	1.2 (6.3)	1.6 (5.0)
Median bolus clearance time (s)	10.8	11.0

*Defined as nadir pH < 6.5.

Table 11.4 Normal values of reflux episodes in 20 healthy subjects on and off esomeprazole 40 mg bid [40].

		Off therapy		On therapy	
		Median	95th Percentile	Median	95th Percentile
5 cm above LES	Total	46.5	71.6	19.0	52.3
	Acid	26.5	45.0	0.0	20.5
	Non-acid	19.0	29.9	18.0	52.0
15 cm above LES	Total	12.5	35.6	6.0	22.6
	Acid	9.0	24.0	0.0	8.7
	Non-acid	4.0	12.9	5.0	22.6

LES, lower esophageal sphincter.

drugs, it is difficult to consider normal values obtained in subjects off PPIs; normal values have been reported in healthy subjects on therapy and these can be used in clinical practice (Table 11.4) [40]. Using the cut-off value of 48 reflux events/ day, Pritchett et al. have shown that an abnormal pH– impedance on therapy can predict pathologic acid reflux in patients tested off therapy [41]. However, for the time being, in the absence of prospective outcome studies, there are no data supporting the use of one specific parameter to consider the pH–impedance study as normal or not. Most investigators pay more attention to the symptom-association analysis than to the quantitative determination of excessive non-acid reflux on PPIs. The accuracy and clinical meanings of these indeces will be discussed below.

Pharyngeal impedance

Considering the drawbacks of proximal pH monitoring in patients with suspected LPR, pharyngeal impedance cathe-

ters have been developed and preliminary results are available. Kawamura et al. performed 24-h simultaneous ambulatory pharyngoesophageal impedance and pH recordings in 11 GERD patients, 10 patients with reflux-attributed laryngitis, and 10 controls [42]. They observed that pure liquid and mixed reflux into the pharynx were very uncommon compared to gas reflux, and were observed only in laryngitis patients. The number of gas reflux episodes accompanied by minor pH changes was higher in the laryngitis group than in the GERD group and controls. Oelschlager et al. conducted a similar study in 10 asymptomatic subjects in whom they observed a substantially higher amount of liquid and mixed reflux in the pharynx, which represented approximately 10% of the total number of reflux events in the distal esophagus [43]. The median number of pharyngeal reflux episodes was five, most of which were mixed and non-acidic. Although some technical issues need to be addressed, especially regarding the definition of pharyngeal reflux compared to swallow artifacts, these preliminary data suggest that, rather than liquid acidic reflux, most pharyngeal reflux events contain gas and are of non-acidic or weakly acidic composition. These results probably explain the lack of sensitivity of conventional pH monitoring. Whether pharyngeal impedance will be helpful in the management of patients with suspected LPR needs to be further evaluated.

Clinical relevance

Studies off therapy

As compared to pH monitoring alone, pH–impedance monitoring allows the detection of non-acid reflux, which may be responsible for symptoms. Most recent available data confirm that impedance monitoring adds little value to the diagnostic yield of pH monitoring alone in patients off therapy. Bredenoord et al. performed a pH–impedance study in 60 patients with typical GER symptoms off therapy [44]. Of these patients, 75% had a positive SAP when all types of reflux detected by impedance were taken into account (independent of pH value). The added value of impedance was less than 10%, since 66.7% of subjects had a positive SAP when reflux episodes were defined by a pH fall below 4. A French study reported consistent results in a cohort of 79 patients with either typical or atypical symptoms [45]. Forty-one of the symptomatic subjects (55.4%) had a positive SAP, but pH–impedance monitoring allowed a temporal association between reflux and symptoms to be established in only 4.1% of patients who would have been missed on a pH study alone. The results were very similar when symptom–reflux association was considered with the SI, which was positive for non-acid reflux in only 10.8% of patients. When the same patients are studied on and off therapy, conflicting results have been reported. Pritchett et al. observed that an abnormal number of weakly acidic reflux events on PPIs could predict the presence of abnormal acid reflux, since pH monitoring off therapy was found to be abnormal in 93% of these patients [41]. Hemmink *et al.* performed a similar study but analyzed the data according to the symptom-association analysis results [46]. They advocate performing pH–impedance monitoring after cessation of therapy, since this slightly increases the likelihood of establishing a positive relationship between symptoms and reflux episodes. These results are appear conflicting but it should be noted that they do not address the same issue. Abnormal reflux episode numbers on PPI therapy appear to be a good predictor of underlying abnormal acid reflux, while taking into account symptom-association analysis off therapy can confirm or exclude GERD as a cause of a patient's symptoms.

As a whole, combined pH–impedance study in patients off PPI allows the establishment of a temporal relationship between reflux and symptoms in only 5–10% more patients than conventional pH recording. Therefore, it appears that, if a patient is to be tested for reflux off therapy, a pH recording alone is sufficient as a first-line investigation, since pH–impedance is not available in many centers.

Studies on therapy

PPI therapy does not influence the total number of reflux episodes, but changes reflux patterns with a decrease in acid reflux events and an increase in weakly acidic reflux events, which represent the most prevalent type of reflux in this setting [46, 47]. Therefore, adding impedance to pH monitoring improves the diagnostic yield and allows better symptom analysis.

In the study by Mainie *et al.*, 168 patients with persisting symptoms despite adequate acid suppressive therapy (PPIs bid) underwent pH–impedance monitoring while on therapy [48]. As expected, only 17.3% of all reflux episodes were acidic, while 82.7% were non-acidic (mainly weakly acidic). In approximately one-half of the patients, no association between symptoms and any type of GER could be demonstrated with the SI, suggesting that the hypothesis of GER as a cause of their symptoms could be reasonably abandoned. By contrast, 11% had symptoms associated with acid reflux (which would had been detected by a pH study alone) and 37% had symptoms associated with non-acid reflux, mainly regurgitation, chest pain, and heartburn. In this study the proportion of atypical symptoms associated with reflux was only 22%, including 3% and 19% associated with acid and non-acid reflux, respectively. Very similar results were obtained in a cohort of 71 patients with persisting symptoms on PPIs bid [45]. A significant statistical association (SAP) between non-acid reflux and symptoms was found in 16.7% of patients who would have been missed on a pH study alone. Regurgitation and cough were the most prevalent symptoms associated with non-acid GER. When symptom–reflux association was considered with the SI, a positive association was found for non-acid reflux in 38.3%

of patients and for acid reflux in 8% of the symptomatic subjects.

The results of these two studies are concordant and can be summarized as follows: in unselected patients with persistent symptoms on double-dose PPIs, 50–60% do not have symptoms that can be associated with GER, 30–40% have symptoms associated with non-acid reflux, and approximately 10% have symptoms associated with acid reflux.

Esophageal bilirubin monitoring

Duodenogastroesophageal reflux (DGR) refers to the esophageal reflux of duodenal contents, i.e. biliary and pancreatic secretions. For years, many authors have paid attention to pH values greater than 7 as a marker of DGR, considered as "alkaline reflux." However, it is now generally admitted that most of these pH rises above 7 correspond to artifacts and that the term "alkaline reflux," at least based on pH measurements, is a misnomer. This assumption relies mainly on the results of studies performed with the Bilitec system, which is based on the detection of bile within the esophageal lumen by utilizing the optical properties of bilirubin [3]. Indeed, simultaneous esophageal recordings of pH and bile reflux have shown a poor correlation between bile reflux and time spent with a pH above 7 [49] and that, in fact, most bile reflux events occur concomitantly with acidic reflux [28, 49]. Similarly, simultaneous studies with impedance have shown that bile reflux and non-acid reflux are two distinct phenomena [50]. If esophageal pH–impedance monitoring can detect acid and non-acid reflux events, bilirubin concentration monitoring adds information about the chemical nature of the refluxate. A consensus of experts in the field of GERD stated that the term "esophageal bilirubin monitoring" should be applied to the use of continuous measurement of bilirubin concentration for recognition of reflux of duodenal contents into the esophagus" [3].

Technical aspects

The system consists of a miniaturized spectrophotometric probe of 1.5-mm diameter that carries light signals into the esophagus and back via a plastic fiberoptic bundle. Bilirubin is the principal pigment in bile and has a characteristic absorbance spectrum. The principle of the Bilitec system is based on the detection within the esophageal lumen of any absorption near 450 nm, thus suggesting the presence of bilirubin and therefore DGR. Validation studies using aspiration of esophageal content confirmed the good correlation between Bilitec measurements and concentration of bile acids and pancreatic enzymes [51].

Before each study, the probe has to be calibrated with water and positioned 5 cm above the LES. The conditions of ambulatory recordings are similar to those for other techniques, except for the need to avoid solid meals because food particles can be trapped at the end of the tip and therefore cause artifacts. It is also recommended not to drink colored liquids, such as coffee, tea or fruit juices, which may interfere with bilirubin detection. The sampling rate of the Bilitec probe is only once per 8 s and the software averages between absorbance values calculated over two successive samples. The sampling frequency has been considered to be too low to detect accurately the onset of a bilirubin reflux with the esophagus [3].

Bilirubin reflux is defined as an increase in bilirubin absorbance above 0.14 for more than 10 s (Figure 11.8) and data are expressed as the percentage of time bilirubin absorbance is higher than 0.14. Normal values have been established [52] (Table 11.5).

Clinical relevance

As for esophageal acid exposure, DGR shows a graded increase in severity across the GERD spectrum and probably plays a specific role in the development of Barrett's esophagus [28, 49]. Indeed, excessive amounts of esophageal bilirubin have been demonstrated in up to 50% of NERD patients, 79% of patients with esophagitis, and 95% of patients with Barrett's esophagus [28]. Most bile reflux events occur concomitantly with acid reflux and most of them are acidic in patients studied off therapy; moreover, PPI therapy markedly reduces the occurrence of both bile and acid reflux events [49, 53]. The group from Leuven has published the largest cohort of patients with persisting esophagitis and/or esophageal symptoms studied with simultaneous pH monitoring and Bilitec [54]. As a whole, 62% of patients with refractory GERD had abnormal DGR, while 40% had normal pH monitoring. However, when symptom association was analyzed, a positive SI for acid reflux, DGR, and mixed reflux was found in 19% 8%, and 5% of the patients, respectively. The relatively low contribution of DGR to the persistence of symptoms in refractory GERD has been further confirmed by Gasiorowska et al. who found that only 9% of symptoms reported by patients studied on single-dose PPIs correlated to DGR only [55].

Table 11.5 Upper limit of normal values of esophageal bilirubin monitoring in healthy subjects (95th percentile) [52].

Total number of reflux (n)	24.4
Upright reflux (n)	23.4
Supine reflux (n)	1.0
Post-prandial reflux (n)	6.1
Total time with reflux (%)	4.6
Time with reflux, upright (%)	7.8
Time with reflux, supine (%)	0.0
Time with reflux, post-prandial (%)	11.8

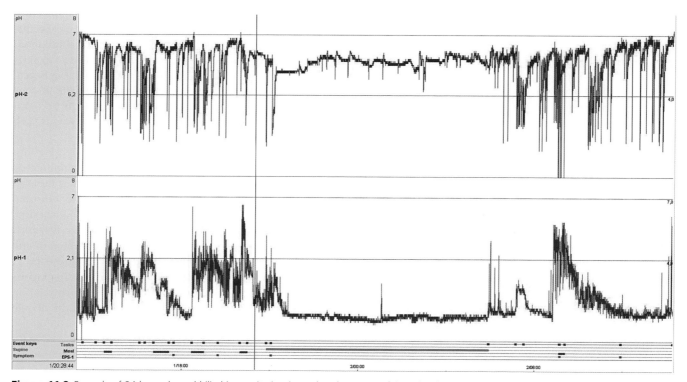

Figure 11.8 Example of 24-h esophageal bilirubin monitoring (reproduced courtesy of S. Bruley des Varannes).

Furthermore, this study also showed a similar degree of DGR in patients with refractory symptoms and those who were asymptomatic, suggesting that DGR plays a very limited role in symptom elicitation. Very few data are available about the putative role of DGR in atypical symptoms. The Leuven group observed that patients with ear, nose, and throat (ENT) symptoms requiring long-term PPI therapy had a higher level of DGR compared to those who could stop the treatment [56].

Therefore, when considering its relatively low diagnostic yield together with the limited commercial availability of the equipment, bilirubin esophageal monitoring does not appear to be a first choice for esophageal testing in patients with refractory GERD.

Symptom-association analysis

In addition to establishing whether a patient's reflux is within physiologic limits or not, esophageal testing for reflux allows the determination of a temporal relationship between the reflux events (whatever the method used to detect them) and the symptoms reported by the patient during the period of recording. This can be obtained provided the patient experiences symptoms during the recording, is aware of how to use the event marker, and reports the symptoms adequately. Most software currently available provide the three most popular indices to establish a correlation between symptoms and reflux events (Table 11.6).

The SI is defined as the percentage of symptoms related to reflux and is considered to be positive when equal to or above 50% [57]. The disadvantage of the SI is that it does not take into account the number of reflux episodes. The significance of an SI of 100% may be questionable in a patient with

one reflux-related symptom despite multiple reflux episodes and an association by chance cannot be ruled out.

The symptom sensitivity index (SSI) is obtained by dividing the total number of reflux episodes associated with symptoms by the total number of reflux episodes. This index is also limited and does not take into account the total number of symptom episodes [58].

The SAP determines the statistical validity of the reflux symptom association. It is obtained by constructing a 2 × 2 contingency table in which the numbers of 2-min segments of the whole 24-h period are tabulated according to the presence of reflux and/or symptoms [59]. The Fisher's exact test is then applied to calculate the probability that the observed association between reflux and symptoms occurred by chance. A SAP value of greater than 95% indicates that the probability that the observed association between reflux and the symptom occurred by chance is less than 5%.

These indices have been developed and validated in patients with typical GERD symptoms (heartburn and regurgitation) and chest pain, most of them having GERD-related symptoms. The clinical accuracy of these indices has been confirmed by outcome studies showing that a positive reflux symptom association was associated with a better response to antireflux therapy, especially in patients with normal esophageal acid exposure [31, 60, 61]. It is however difficult to extrapolate their accuracy in patients with atypical symptoms, since outcome studies are lacking. These indices are also frequently used in pH–impedance studies and can help to identify more patients with GERD-related symptoms. For example, Zerbib et al. found an abnormal number of reflux events in 20.2% and 8.4% of patients off and on PPI therapy, respectively, while a positive SAP was observed in 55.4% and 36.7% of them. However, there is to date only one outcome study based on the results of symptom indices [62].

Not surprisingly, the agreement between SI and SAP is poor, as shown in two impedance studies reporting kappa values of 0.26 [45] and 0.3 [48], respectively. While SAP is considered by some authors to be the best method to express the temporal relationship between symptoms and reflux episodes [63], SI is a simple, easy to determine and understand parameter, and describes the proportion of symptoms that are reflux related. SAP describes the probability that the observed relation between symptoms and reflux has not occurred by chance. For now, it cannot be stated which test should be used in clinical practice, and which should be taken into account if discrepancy exists between SI and SAP, but caution should be exercised in patients with a very low SI and a positive SAP.

The adequate time window before the onset of symptoms to determine temporal association is still a matter of debate. The 2-min time window was primarily adopted for symptom analysis as previous works had demonstrated that it was the most appropriate, at least in patients with chest pain [64], but some authors use a 5-min time window, which may be

---

Table 11.6 Main symptom correlation indices used in esophageal reflux testing.

Symptom index (SI): positive if ≥50%

$$\frac{\text{Number of reflux-related symptom episodes}}{\text{Total number of symptom episodes}} \times 100\%$$

Symptom sensitivity index (SSI): positive if ≥10%

$$\frac{\text{Number of symptom-associated reflux episodes}}{\text{Total number of reflux episodes}} \times 100\%$$

Symptom association probability (SAP): positive if ≥95%

$$SAP = (1.0 - P) \times 100\%$$

where P is the probability, determined by a Fisher's exact test, that the pobserved association between reflux and symptoms occurred by chance more appropriate for certain symptoms that lack sudden onset [48]. As an example, Mainie *et al.* used the SI with a 5-min time window in patients with refractory symptoms studied with pH–impedance on therapy [62]. Although relatively small and uncontrolled, this study showed that a positive SI for any type of reflux (acid or non-acid) could adequately select patients for surgery.

Despite all these unresolved issues, analysis of symptom–reflux association should be performed in all studies since it adds important information to the overall interpretation of the reflux testing. To date, these indices should be considered as complementary to the "quantitative" evaluation of reflux. They can help to identify more patients with symptoms possibly related to GERD; outcome studies comparing the different indices and the quantitative parameters are needed to identify the best way to predict response to therapy.

Clinical applications

Typical symptoms

It is generally admitted that pH monitoring in patients with typical GERD and adequate symptom relief is not useful. It has been proposed to check that acid reflux is adequately controlled by therapy in situations such as Barrett's esophagus, in which persistent abnormal esophageal acid exposure can be demonstrated in up to 60% of patients despite PPI therapy and absence of GERD symptoms. However, the benefit of this approach (especially regarding the development of dysplasia and/or cancer) is not demonstrated and pH monitoring is not recommended in asymptomatic patients with Barrett's esophagus [5]. By contrast, it has been recommended to perform esophageal pH monitoring off therapy in patients with NERD prior to surgery, to document abnormal esophageal acid exposure and/or significant association between GERD symptoms and acid reflux [5]. Although the sensitivity of pH monitoring is lower in NERD patients, a negative pH study should lead to reconsideration of surgery in these patients, since it is probably a predictive factor of poor outcome [34].

The most common indication for esophageal testing for reflux is refractory GERD. Patients can be tested off therapy to confirm the presence and pattern (day vs night) of abnormal acid reflux and/or positive symptom–reflux association; the added value of pH–impedance monitoring off therapy is limited and pH monitoring alone (catheter-based or wireless) can reasonably be proposed as the first-line investigation [5]. However, regarding the high specificity of typical symptoms, it seems more useful to perform studies on therapy. Whether these studies should be performed on single- or double-dose PPIs is still unknown. However, most patients referred for esophageal testing for refractory heartburn already have a double dose of PPIs and it seems logical to perform a study on double dose to check whether the persisting symptoms are related to GERD or not. Esophageal

pH monitoring on PPIs bid can demonstrate acid reflux-related symptoms and/or abnormal esophageal exposure in approximately 10% of patients with typical symptoms [36]. Whether prolonged wireless pH monitoring allowing both off and on PPI assessments [26] could be useful in clinical practice remains to be further determined.

It is now clear that in this situation, 24-h pH–impedance testing has a higher diagnostic yield [45, 48] and allows the establishment of a temporal relationship between symptoms and non-acid (mainly weakly acidic) reflux in 30–40% of patients who would have been missed with a pH study alone. The other important information provided by pH–impedance monitoring on therapy is that more than half of the patients do not have any symptom related to GERD [45, 48]. This technique may therefore prove to be useful in the future to select patients for antireflux medical or surgical therapy. Mainie *et al.* have reported favorable results of laparoscopic fundoplication in 18 of 19 patients with persistent symptoms despite PPI therapy and positive SI for non-acid reflux on esophageal pH–impedance monitoring [62]. It is currently the only available study suggesting that pH–impedance could have a significant impact on the management of GERD in patients who fail adequate acid suppressive therapy. Further controlled prospective studies are warranted to confirm these results.

Supraesophageal symptoms

Cough

GERD is one of the most frequent etiologies of chronic cough, probably accounting for approximately 20% of chronic cough cases [65]. However, only a minority of patients with chronic cough and GERD have typical digestive symptoms and/or clear evidence of esophagitis. The most convincing evidence linking reflux and cough comes from pH or pH–impedance monitoring studies, which can demonstrate a temporal relationship. As an example, a temporal relationship was demonstrated by a positive SAP in 35% of patients, those with pathologic acid exposure having a greater likelihood of a temporal correlation (57%) when not on acid-suppressive medications [66]. However, interpretation of pH data is not easy because there is no consensus as to how symptom analysis should be performed regarding criteria such as the time window between reflux episodes and the symptoms used to indicate that the correlation is present, or the type of symptom analysis required to demonstrate a positive correlation. Esophageal pH–impedance monitoring was used to investigate these patients and to establish the temporal relationship between cough bursts and reflux episodes in 100 patients with chronic cough (77 off and 23 on PPIs) [67]. Using esophagogastric manometry, cough was defined as a phasic, short duration, rapid pressure rise occurring simultaneously and with the same pressure configuration at both recording sites. With such stringent criteria, acid reflux was a potential mechanism of cough in 45 patients and weakly-acidic reflux in another group of 24 individuals. It is of note that cough-induced reflux events were observed, but this phenomenon had very little impact on esophageal acid exposure. However, several "cough–reflux–cough" sequences were observed, suggesting that a self-perpetuating mechanism may exist whereby acid reflux causes cough and the cough in turn amplifies reflux.

Whether esophageal testing can predict response to therapy is still unknown since outcome studies are scarce. In a randomized controlled study, only 35% of patients with a positive pH monitoring responded to PPI therapy [68]. Laparoscopic Nissen fundoplication led to disappearance of symptoms in six patients with cough associated with non-acid reflux (positive SI) during pH–impedance monitoring on therapy, with a median follow-up of 17 months [69]. Since most placebo-controlled studies showed no benefit of PPI as first-line therapy in unexplained chronic cough, the best option in patients without typical reflux symptoms appears to be to perform pH–impedance monitoring off therapy with careful analysis of the symptom–reflux temporal relationship in order to select the patients who can truly benefit from GERD treatment [65]. However, this approach requires further validation by appropriate controlled outcome studies.

Asthma

Asthma and GERD are very frequently associated [65]. A recent systematic review of 28 epidemiologic studies found a 59.2% weighted average prevalence of GERD symptoms in asthmatic patients compared to 38.1% in controls [70]. In patients with asthma, the average prevalence of abnormal esophageal pH monitoring, esophagitis and hiatus hernia was 50.9%, 37.3%, and 51.2%, respectively. Esophageal pH studies are particularly useful to establish the diagnosis of GERD, which cannot rely adequately on the observation of symptoms since a "clinically silent" acid reflux can be demonstrated in 25–60% of asthmatics without any typical reflux symptom [71, 72]. Furthermore, only 50% of asthmatics with typical reflux symptoms have a documented abnormal acid reflux on pH monitoring [73].

Theoretically, esophageal pH studies may help to identify patients with pathologic reflux as well as to evaluate the temporal association between reflux and respiratory symptoms. Although uncontrolled data have suggested that abnormal proximal acid reflux was associated with worse asthma [74], two recent controlled studies have shown that the results of pH monitoring could not predict the response to PPI therapy, for either asthma symptoms or pulmonary function [75, 76].

In clinical practice, despite these negative results, we propose that patients presenting with difficult-to-treat asthma and/or nocturnal symptoms without GERD symptoms should be offered an esophageal pH study off therapy to detect "silent GERD." Patients presenting with typical GERD symptoms and/or an abnormal pH study should be treated with a 3-month double-dose PPI therapy. Treatment efficacy should be assessed according to clinical (asthma symptoms, treatment needs) and functional (peak flow) endpoints. In patients who do not respond to this first therapeutic approach, ' pH–impedance monitoring performed on therapy may be useful to detect those with persistent reflux who need better therapeutic control [65]. Considering the results of the few controlled studies reported to date, great caution should be exercised before embarking on surgical antireflux procedures to improve asthma outcome. This approach could eventually be proposed in patients with documented reflux and clear temporal correlations between respiratory symptoms and reflux episodes during 24-h monitoring.

ENT symptoms

The so-called laryngopharyngeal reflux (LPR) is defined by the association of laryngeal symptoms with laryngeal inflammation at laryngoscopy [10]. However, the relationship between reflux and laryngeal symptoms is frequently difficult to establish with a high degree of certainty. The presence of esophagitis and/or abnormal distal esophageal acid exposure on pH monitoring can confirm the presence of pathologic GERD, but cannot provide any information on causality. Indeed, the link between reflux and laryngeal symptoms may not easily rely on symptom–reflux association analysis since these symptoms are often long lasting (or permanent) and do not have a sudden onset that could be easily perceived by the patient. Moreover, the presence of abnormal proximal and/or distal acid reflux on pH monitoring does not predict response to therapy [77]. In view of these difficulties, it is currently recommended to start with an empirical 3-month therapy with high doses of PPIs [78], but most placebo-controlled trials have failed to demonstrate any benefit of PPIs in patients with suspected reflux-related laryngeal symptoms [79, 80].

The diagnostic value of combined pH and impedance recordings has been established in some studies. In a cohort of 21 patients with persistent globus on PPI, Anandasabapathy *et al.* showed that non-acid reflux was not associated with symptoms but that proximal extent may play a role [81]. Therefore, it appears that a pathologic acid or non-acid GER can be demonstrated in a subgroup of patients with ENT symptoms on therapy. However, these results are quite difficult to interpret when no temporal relationship can be established between these symptoms and GER detected by impedance. Moreover, the populations studied are often very heterogeneous and present with symptoms that are difficult to characterize. Promising preliminary results have been reported with pharyngeal impedance [42, 43], but whether this technique will be further developed and prove to be helpful for the management of these difficult patients remains to be determined.

In clinical practice, it is recommended to take into account the presence of typical symptoms associated with ENT symp-

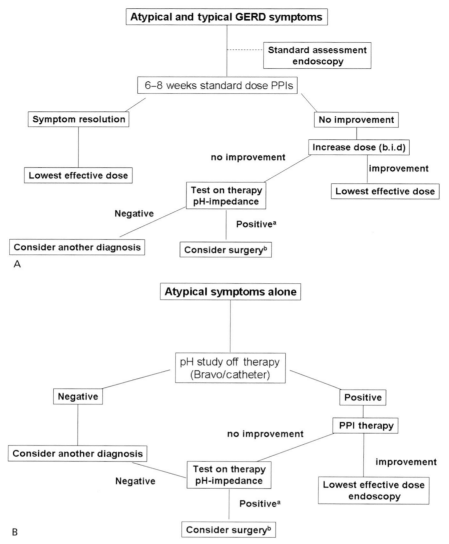

Figure 11.9 Algorithm for management of patients with suspected gastroesophageal reflux disease (GERD)-related symptoms according to (A) the presence or (B) absence of typical GERD symptoms. [a]The definition of a positive test on a proton pump inhibitor (PPI) is not currently known and may rely on either symptom association analysis or quantitative analysis. [b]There is virtually no outcome study to support the benefit of surgery in this situation.

toms [5]. The ACG recommendations suggest that the decision to test patients off or on therapy should be made according to the pretest probability of GERD: a low probability should favor a study off therapy to rule out GERD, while a study on therapy should be proposed if the probability of GERD is high. If heartburn and/or regurgitation are present, an empirical treatment with PPI can be proposed. In cases of refractory symptoms, esophageal testing should be proposed on therapy, ideally with pH–impedance. If ENT symptoms are not associated with typical symptoms, performing a pH monitoring off therapy could be proposed, although its usefulness is questionable (Figure 11.9). Nevertheless, it may help physicians, especially the gastroenterologist to whom the patient is referred, to rule out the diagnosis of

GERD in these patients with chronic difficult-to-treat symptoms, but considered by a majority of ENT physicians as having GERD-related symptoms [82].

References

1. Vakil N, van Zanten SV, Kahrilas P, Dent J, Jones R. The Montreal definition and classification of gastroesophageal reflux disease: a global evidence-based consensus. *Am J Gastroenterol* 2006;101:1900–1920; quiz 1943.

2. Fass R, Sifrim D. Management of heartburn not responding to proton pump inhibitors. *Gut* 2009;58:295–309.

3. Sifrim D, Castell D, Dent J, Kahrilas PJ. Gastro-oesophageal reflux monitoring: review and consensus report on detection

and definitions of acid, non-acid, and gas reflux. *Gut* 2004; 53:1024–1031.

4. Geus WP, Smout AJ, Kooiman JC, Lamers CB, Gues JW. Glass and antimony electrodes for long-term pH monitoring: a dynamic in vitro comparison. *Eur J Gastroenterol Hepatol* 1995; 7:29–35.

5. Hirano I, Richter JE. ACG practice guidelines: esophageal reflux testing. *Am J Gastroenterol* 2007;102:668–685.

6. Klauser AG, Schindlbeck NE, Muller-Lissner SA. Esophageal 24-h pH monitoring: is prior manometry necessary for correct positioning of the electrode? *Am J Gastroenterol* 1990;85: 1463–1467.

7. Agrawal A, Tutuian R, Hila A, Freeman J, Castell DO. Ingestion of acidic foods mimics gastroesophageal reflux during pH monitoring. *Dig Dis Sci* 2005;50:1916–1920.

8. Galmiche JP, Scarpignato C. Esophageal pH monitoring. In: Scarpignato C, Galmiche JP, eds. *Functional Investigation in Esophageal Disease*. Basel: Karger, 1994. pp. 71–108.

9. Martinez SD, Malagon IB, Garewal HS, Cui H, Fass R. Non-erosive reflux disease (NERD)–acid reflux and symptom patterns. *Aliment Pharmacol Ther* 2003;17:537–545.

10. Koufman JA, Aviv JE, Casiano RR, Shaw GY. Laryngopharyngeal reflux: position statement of the committee on speech, voice, and swallowing disorders of the American Academy of Otolaryngology-Head and Neck Surgery. *Otolaryngol Head Neck Surg* 2002;127:32–35.

11. McCollough M, Jabbar A, Cacchione R, Allen JW, Harrell S, Wo JM. Proximal sensor data from routine dual-sensor esophageal pH monitoring is often inaccurate. *Dig Dis Sci* 2004;49: 1607–1611.

12. Vaezi MF, Schroeder PL, Richter JE. Reproducibility of proximal probe pH parameters in 24-hour ambulatory esophageal pH monitoring. *Am J Gastroenterol* 1997;92:825–829.

13. Williams RB, Ali GN, Wallace KL, Wilson JS, De Carle DJ, Cook IJ. Esophagopharyngeal acid regurgitation: dual pH monitoring criteria for its detection and insights into mechanisms. *Gastroenterology* 1999;117:1051–1061.

14. Bove M, Ruth M, Cange L, Mansson I. 24-H pharyngeal pH monitoring in healthy volunteers: a normative study. *Scand J Gastroenterol* 2000;35:234–241.

15. Ayazi S, Lipham JC, Hagen JA, *et al*. A new technique for measurement of pharyngeal pH: normal values and discriminating pH threshold. *J Gastrointest Surg* 2009;13:1422–1429.

16. Ayazi S, Lipham JC, Portale G, *et al*. Bravo catheter-free pH monitoring: normal values, concordance, optimal diagnostic thresholds, and accuracy. *Clin Gastroenterol Hepatol* 2009;7: 60–67.

17. Lacy BE, O'Shana T, Hynes M, *et al*. Safety and tolerability of transoral Bravo capsule placement after transnasal manometry using a validated conversion factor. *Am J Gastroenterol* 2007; 102:24–32.

18. des Varannes SB, Mion F, Ducrotte P, *et al*. Simultaneous recordings of oesophageal acid exposure with conventional pH monitoring and a wireless system (Bravo). *Gut* 2005;54: 1682–1686.

19. Remes-Troche JM, Ibarra-Palomino J, Carmona-Sanchez RI, Valdovinos MA. Performance, tolerability, and symptoms related to prolonged pH monitoring using the Bravo system in Mexico. *Am J Gastroenterol* 2005;100:2382–2386.

20. Pandolfino JE, Richter JE, Ours T, Guardino JM, Chapman J, Kahrilas PJ. Ambulatory esophageal pH monitoring using a wireless system. *Am J Gastroenterol* 2003;98:740–749.

21. Pandolfino JE, Zhang Q, Schreiner MA, Ghosh S, Roth MP, Kahrilas PJ. Acid reflux event detection using the Bravo wireless versus the Slimline catheter pH systems: why are the numbers so different? *Gut* 2005;54:1687–1692.

22. Prakash C, Jonnalagadda S, Azar R, Clouse RE. Endoscopic removal of the wireless pH monitoring capsule in patients with severe discomfort. *Gastrointest Endosc* 2006;64:828–832.

23. Fajardo NR, Wise JL, Locke GR, 3rd, Murray JA, Talley NJ. Esophageal perforation after placement of wireless Bravo pH probe. *Gastrointest Endosc* 2006;63:184–185.

24. Wong WM, Bautista J, Dekel R, *et al*. Feasibility and tolerability of transnasal/per-oral placement of the wireless pH capsule vs. traditional 24-h oesophageal pH monitoring–a randomized trial. *Aliment Pharmacol Ther* 2005;21:155–163.

25. Prakash C, Clouse RE. Value of extended recording time with wireless pH monitoring in evaluating gastroesophageal reflux disease. *Clin Gastroenterol Hepatol* 2005;3:329–334.

26. Garrean CP, Zhang Q, Gonsalves N, Hirano I. Acid reflux detection and symptom-reflux association using 4-day wireless pH recording combining 48-hour periods off and on PPI therapy. *Am J Gastroenterol* 2008;103:1631–1637.

27. Kahrilas PJ, Quigley EM. Clinical esophageal pH recording: a technical review for practice guideline development. *Gastroenterology* 1996;110:1982–1996.

28. Vaezi MF, Richter JE. Role of acid and duodenogastroesophageal reflux in gastroesophageal reflux disease. *Gastroenterology* 1996;111:1192–1199.

29. Fass R, Hell RW, Garewal HS, *et al*. Correlation of oesophageal acid exposure with Barrett's oesophagus length. *Gut* 2001;48: 310–313.

30. Campos GM, Peters JH, DeMeester TR, *et al*. Multivariate analysis of factors predicting outcome after laparoscopic Nissen fundoplication. *J Gastrointest Surg* 1999;3:292–300.

31. Aanen MC, Weusten BL, Numans ME, de Wit NJ, Samsom M, Smout AJ. Effect of proton-pump inhibitor treatment on symptoms and quality of life in GERD patients depends on the symptom-reflux association. *J Clin Gastroenterol* 2008;42:441–447.

32. Savarino E, Pohl D, Zentilin P, *et al*. Functional heartburn has more in common with functional dyspepsia than with non-erosive reflux disease. *Gut* 2009;58:1185–1191.

33. Shi G, Bruley des Varannes S, Scarpignato C, Le Rhun M, Galmiche JP. Reflux related symptoms in patients with normal oesophageal exposure to acid. *Gut* 1995;37:457–464.

34. Thibault R, Coron E, Sebille V, et al. Antireflux surgery for non-erosive and erosive reflux disease in community practice. *Aliment Pharmacol Ther* 2006;24:621–632.

35. Kuo B, Castell DO. Optimal dosing of omeprazole 40 mg daily: effects on gastric and esophageal pH and serum gastrin in healthy controls. *Am J Gastroenterol* 1996;91:1532–1538.

36. Charbel S, Khandwala F, Vaezi MF. The role of esophageal pH monitoring in symptomatic patients on PPI therapy. *Am J Gastroenterol* 2005;100:283–289.

37. Zerbib F, des Varannes SB, Roman S, et al. Normal values and day-to-day variability of 24-h ambulatory oesophageal impedance-pH monitoring in a Belgian-French cohort of healthy subjects. *Aliment Pharmacol Ther* 2005;22:1011–1021.

38. Roman S, Bruley des Varannes S, Pouderoux P, *et al.* Ambulatory 24-h oesophageal impedance-pH recordings: reliability of automatic analysis for gastro-oesophageal reflux assessment. *Neurogastroenterol Motil* 2006;18:978–986.

39. Shay S, Tutuian R, Sifrim D, *et al.* Twenty-four hour ambulatory simultaneous impedance and pH monitoring: a multicenter report of normal values from 60 healthy volunteers. *Am J Gastroenterol* 2004;99:1037–1043.

40. Tutuian R, Mainie I, Agrawal A, Freeman J, Castell DO. Normal values for ambulatory 24-h combined impedance-pH monitoring on acid suppressive therapy. *Gastroenterology* 2006;130:A171.

41. Pritchett JM, Aslam M, Slaughter JC, Ness RM, Garrett CG, Vaezi MF. Efficacy of esophageal impedance/pH monitoring in patients with refractory gastroesophageal reflux disease, on and off therapy. *Clin Gastroenterol Hepatol* 2009;7:743–748.

42. Kawamura O, Aslam M, Rittmann T, Hofmann C, Shaker R. Physical and pH properties of gastroesophagopharyngeal refluxate: a 24-hour simultaneous ambulatory impedance and pH monitoring study. *Am J Gastroenterol* 2004;99:1000–1010.

43. Oelschlager BK, Quiroga E, Isch JA, Cuenca-Abente F. Gastroesophageal and pharyngeal reflux detection using impedance and 24-hour pH monitoring in asymptomatic subjects: defining the normal environment. *J Gastrointest Surg* 2006; 10:54–62.

44. Bredenoord AJ, Weusten BL, Timmer R, Conchillo JM, Smout AJ. Addition of esophageal impedance monitoring to pH monitoring increases the yield of symptom association analysis in patients off PPI therapy. *Am J Gastroenterol* 2006;101:453–459.

45. Zerbib F, Roman S, Ropert A, *et al.* Esophageal pH-impedance monitoring and symptom analysis in GERD: a study in patients off and on therapy. *Am J Gastroenterol* 2006;101:1956–1963.

46. Hemmink GJ, Bredenoord AJ, Weusten BL, Monkelbaan JF, Timmer R, Smout AJ. Esophageal pH-impedance monitoring in patients with therapy-resistant reflux symptoms: 'on' or 'off' proton pump inhibitor? *Am J Gastroenterol* 2008;103: 2446–2453.

47. Vela MF, Camacho-Lobato L, Srinivasan R, Tutuian R, Katz PO, Castell DO. Simultaneous intraesophageal impedance and pH measurement of acid and nonacid gastroesophageal reflux: effect of omeprazole. *Gastroenterology* 2001;120:1599–1606.

48. Mainie I, Tutuian R, Shay S, *et al.* Acid and non-acid reflux in patients with persistent symptoms despite acid suppressive therapy: a multicentre study using combined ambulatory impedance-pH monitoring. *Gut* 2006;55:1398–1402.

49. Champion G, Richter JE, Vaezi MF, Singh S, Alexander R. Duodenogastroesophageal reflux: relationship to pH and importance in Barrett's esophagus. *Gastroenterology* 1994;107: 747–754.

50. Pace F, Sangaletti O, Pallotta S, Molteni P, Porro GB. Biliary reflux and non-acid reflux are two distinct phenomena: a comparison between 24-hour multichannel intraesophageal impedance and bilirubin monitoring. *Scand J Gastroenterol* 2007;42:1031–1039.

51. Stipa F, Stein HJ, Feussner H, Kraemer S, Siewert JR. Assessment of non-acid esophageal reflux: comparison between long-term reflux aspiration test and fiberoptic bilirubin monitoring. *Dis Esophagus* 1997;10:24–28.

52. Cuomo R, Koek G, Sifrim D, Janssens J, Tack J. Analysis of ambulatory duodenogastroesophageal reflux monitoring. *Dig Dis Sci* 2000;45:2463–2469.

53. Netzer P, Gut A, Brundler R, Gaia C, Halter F, Inauen W. Influence of pantoprazole on oesophageal motility, and bile and acid reflux in patients with oesophagitis. *Aliment Pharmacol Ther* 2001;15:1375–1384.

54. Karamanolis G, Vanuytsel T, Sifrim D, *et al.* Yield of 24-hour esophageal pH and bilitec monitoring in patients with persisting symptoms on PPI therapy. *Dig Dis Sci* 2008;53:2387–2393.

55. Gasiorowska A, Navarro-Rodriguez T, Wendel C, *et al.* Comparison of the degree of duodenogastroesophageal reflux and acid reflux between patients who failed to respond and those who were successfully treated with a proton pump inhibitor once daily. *Am J Gastroenterol* 2009;104:2005–2013.

56. Poelmans J, Feenstra L, Tack J. Determinants of long-term outcome of patients with reflux-related ear, nose, and throat symptoms. *Dig Dis Sci* 2006;51:282–288.

57. Wiener GJ, Richter JE, Copper JB, Wu WC, Castell DO. The symptom index: a clinically important parameter of ambulatory 24-hour esophageal pH monitoring. *Am J Gastroenterol* 1988; 83:358–361.

58. Breumelhof R, Smout AJ. The symptom sensitivity index: a valuable additional parameter in 24-hour esophageal pH recording. *Am J Gastroenterol* 1991;86:160–164.

59. Weusten BL, Roelofs JM, Akkermans LM, Van Berge-Henegouwen GP, Smout AJ. The symptom-association probability: an improved method for symptom analysis of 24-hour esophageal pH data. *Gastroenterology* 1994;107:1741–1745.

60. Taghavi SA, Ghasedi M, Saberi-Firoozi M, *et al.* Symptom association probability and symptom sensitivity index: preferable but still suboptimal predictors of response to high dose omeprazole. *Gut* 2005;54:1067–1071.

61. Watson RG, Tham TC, Johnston BT, McDougall NI. Double blind cross-over placebo controlled study of omeprazole in the treatment of patients with reflux symptoms and physiological levels of acid reflux–the "sensitive oesophagus". *Gut* 1997;40: 587–590.

62. Mainie I, Tutuian R, Agrawal A, Adams D, Castell DO. Combined multichannel intraluminal impedance-pH monitoring to select patients with persistent gastro-oesophageal reflux for laparoscopic Nissen fundoplication. *Br J Surg* 2006;93:1483–1487.

63. Bredenoord AJ, Weusten BL, Smout AJ. Symptom association analysis in ambulatory gastro-oesophageal reflux monitoring. *Gut* 2005;54:1810–1817.

64. Lam HG, Breumelhof R, van Berge Henegouwen GP, Smout AJ. Temporal relationships between episodes of non-cardiac chest pain and abnormal oesophageal function. *Gut* 1994;35: 733–736.

65. Galmiche JP, Zerbib F, Bruley des Varannes S. Review article: respiratory manifestations of gastro-oesophageal reflux disease. *Aliment Pharmacol Ther* 2008;27:449–464.

66. Wunderlich AW, Murray JA. Temporal correlation between chronic cough and gastroesophageal reflux disease. *Dig Dis Sci* 2003;48:1050–1056.

67. Blondeau K, Dupont LJ, Mertens V, Tack J, Sifrim D. Improved diagnosis of gastro-oesophageal reflux in patients with unexplained chronic cough. *Aliment Pharmacol Ther* 2007;25: 723–732.

68. Ours TM, Kavuru MS, Schilz RJ, Richter JE. A prospective evaluation of esophageal testing and a double-blind, randomized study of omeprazole in a diagnostic and therapeutic

algorithm for chronic cough. *Am J Gastroenterol* 1999;94: 3131–3138.

69. Tutuian R, Mainie I, Agrawal A, Adams D, Castell DO. Nonacid reflux in patients with chronic cough on acid-suppressive therapy. *Chest* 2006;130:386–391.

70. Havemann BD, Henderson CA, El-Serag HB. The association between gastro-oesophageal reflux disease and asthma: a systematic review. *Gut* 2007;56:1654–1664.

71. Harding SM, Guzzo MR, Richter JE. The prevalence of gastro-esophageal reflux in asthma patients without reflux symptoms. *Am J Respir Crit Care Med* 2000;162:34–39.

72. Sontag SJ, O'Connell S, Khandelwal S, Miller T, Nemchausky B, Schnell TG, et al. Most asthmatics have gastroesophageal reflux with or without bronchodilator therapy. *Gastroenterology* 1990;99:613–620.

73. Kiljander TO, Laitinen JO. The prevalence of gastroesophageal reflux disease in adult asthmatics. *Chest* 2004;126:1490–1494.

74. DiMango E, Holbrook JT, Simpson E, *et al*. Effects of asymptomatic proximal and distal gastroesophageal reflux on asthma severity. *Am J Respir Crit Care Med* 2009;180:809–816.

75. Mastronarde JG, Anthonisen NR, Castro M, *et al*. Efficacy of esomeprazole for treatment of poorly controlled asthma. *N Engl J Med* 2009;360:1487–1499.

76. Kiljander TO, Harding SM, Field SK, *et al*. Effects of esomeprazole 40 mg twice daily on asthma: a randomized placebo-controlled trial. *Am J Respir Crit Care Med* 2006;173:1091–1097.

77. Vaezi MF, Richter JE, Stasney CR, *et al*. Treatment of chronic posterior laryngitis with esomeprazole. *Laryngoscope* 2006;116: 254–260.

78. Ford CN. Evaluation and management of laryngopharyngeal reflux. *JAMA* 2005;294:1534–1540.

79. Gatta L, Vaira D, Sorrenti G, Zucchini S, Sama C, Vakil N. Meta-analysis: the efficacy of proton pump inhibitors for laryngeal symptoms attributed to gastro-oesophageal reflux disease. *Aliment Pharmacol Ther* 2007;25:385–392.

80. Qadeer MA, Phillips CO, Lopez AR, *et al*. Proton pump inhibitor therapy for suspected GERD-related chronic laryngitis: a meta-analysis of randomized controlled trials. *Am J Gastroenterol* 2006;101:2646–2654.

81. Anandasabapathy S, Jaffin BW. Multichannel intraluminal impedance in the evaluation of patients with persistent globus on proton pump inhibitor therapy. *Ann Otol Rhinol Laryngol* 2006;115:563–570.

82. Ahmed TF, Khandwala F, Abelson TI, *et al*. Chronic laryngitis associated with gastroesophageal reflux: prospective assessment of differences in practice patterns between gastroenterologists and ENT physicians. *Am J Gastroenterol* 2006;101:470–478.

Role of Histology and Cytology in Esophageal Diseases

John R. Goldblum and Xiuli Liu
Department of Anatomic Pathology, Cleveland Clinic, Cleveland, OH, USA

Introduction

Histologic confirmation of the clinical and endoscopic impression is required in many patients with esophageal diseases, thereby necessitating the procurement of endoscopic biopsy specimens or cytologic brushings. While morphologic assessment of these specimens only helps to narrow down the diagnostic considerations in some cases, it can provide a specific diagnosis in many cases. As the incidence of gastroesophageal reflux disease (GERD) increases, Barrett's esophagus (BE) and BE-related dysplasia/neoplasm are more commonly encountered in daily pathology practice than before. In addition, endoscopic mucosal resection (EMR), a less invasive modality, has been increasingly used clinically to treat BE-related dysplasia and early cancer, and, as such, EMR specimens are also commonly encountered by pathologists.

We believe that the histologic evaluation of biopsy specimens and cytologic brushings is diagnostically complementary [1, 2] for both neoplastic and non-neoplastic conditions. Cytology may provide a definitive diagnosis of carcinoma when a biopsy specimen is inconclusive, and has the advantages of greater accessibility of stenotic or obstructive lesions and sampling of a larger area for screening. Cytologic examination of endoscopic fine-needle aspiration (FNA) specimens from periesophageal and celiac axis lymph nodes in patients with invasive carcinoma is commonly used for preoperative staging [3]. In addition, non-endoscopic, exfoliative cytology has been used to screen for squamous cell carcinoma in patients living in high-risk regions of the world [4, 5], for screening and surveillance of BE [6], and to identify infectious agents [7].

Normal esophagus

The esophagus has four concentric layers: the mucosa, submucosa, muscularis propria, and adventitia [8]. The esophageal mucosa is lined by non-keratinized, stratified squamous epithelium, which itself is composed of basal, intermediate, and superficial cell layers. The basal cell compartment comprises less than 15% of the thickness of the mucosa and is usually no more than two to three cell layers [8]. Mitotic figures are restricted to the basal cell zone under normal circumstances. The cells above the basal cell zone have more cytoplasm with a decrease in the nuclear-to-cytoplasmic (N/C) ratio. A basement membrane separates the epithelium from the lamina propria, which is composed of loose fibrovascular tissue (Figure 12.1A). Lymphatic channels are found within the esophageal mucosa. Infoldings of the lamina propria form papillae, which are generally evenly spaced and usually extend one-third to one-half of the thickness of the epithelium [8]. The muscularis mucosae separates the mucosa from the submucosa and is composed of slips of smooth muscle. The submucosa is composed of loose connective tissue containing nerves, lymphatic channels, blood vessels, and submucosal glands. The submucosal glands contain mucous cells surrounding a central lumen, in a radial fashion, and open to the lumen of the esophagus via squamous-lined ducts. The *submucosal glands* and *squamous-lined ducts* are significant esophageal landmarks as identification of these structures in esophageal biopsy or mucosal resection specimens confirms the tubular esophageal origin (Figure 12.1B). The composition of the muscularis propria changes throughout the esophagus; it is composed of skeletal muscle in the upper one-third, smooth muscle in the

The Esophagus, Fifth Edition. Edited by Joel E. Richter, Donald O. Castell.
© 2012 Blackwell Publishing Ltd. Published 2012 by Blackwell Publishing Ltd.

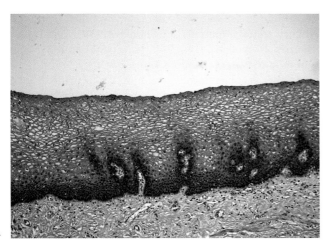
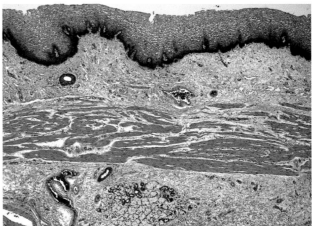

Figure 12.1 (A) Normal esophageal squamous mucosa with a thin basal epithelial zone and lamina propria papillae that are less than one-half of the total epithelial thickness. (B) Squamous epithelium-lined duct and submucosal mucous glands in the esophagus. The identification of these structures in a biopsy or an endoscopic mucosal resection (EMR) specimen indicates an esophageal origin.

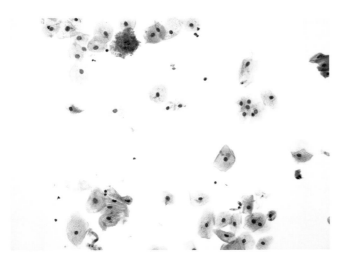

Figure 12.2 Normal esophageal brushing composed predominantly of mature squamous epithelial cells (Papanicolaou stain; reproduced courtesy of Longwen Chen).

lower one-third, and a mixture of skeletal and smooth muscle in the middle one-third. The myenteric plexus is found between the inner and outer layers of the muscularis propria and is composed of nerves, ganglion cells, and scattered inflammatory cells. The adventitia is composed of loose connective tissue.

Cytologic preparation obtained from a normal esophagus typically results in a cellular sample of squamous epithelial cells that are similar to those designated as "intermediate" and "superficial" cells in a cervical smear (Figure 12.2). Both intermediate and superficial squamous cells contain abundant cytoplasm with small, round, regular nuclei, resulting in cells with low N/C ratios. Intermediate nuclei contain finely granular chromatin with inconspicuous nucleoli. In

contrast, the superficial nuclei are dense and pyknotic without discernible chromatic structure. Both cell types can occur as individual cells, loosely cohesive cell aggregates, or large sheets. Glandular epithelial cells represent a normal finding if the gastroesophageal junction (GEJ) is sampled. These glandular cells occur as single cells or cohesive tissue fragments that appear as either flat, "honeycomb" sheets if viewed *en face* or as columnar cells with a small basally located nucleus containing a small nucleolus if oriented on edge. Often, ciliated columnar cells, pulmonary macrophages, or squamous cells with adherent bacterial or fungal colonies are also present because of contamination from the oral cavity, pharynx, or respiratory tract.

Esophagitis

Inflammation of the esophageal mucosa is common, and different etiologies may result in a similar histologic pattern. Thus, although clinical and radiologic findings may suggest a specific etiology, the histologic and cytologic alterations are often not specific. However, in some types of infectious esophagitis, histologic or cytologic evaluation can offer a specific diagnosis when the infectious organisms are identified [9].

Infectious esophagitis

Candida esophagitis
Infection caused by *Candida* species is the most frequently encountered, clinically significant infectious esophagitis. *Candida* esophagitis is a common disease in neutropenic cancer patients after chemotherapy as well as in patients infected with human immunodeficiency virus (HIV). Other conditions such as esophageal obstruction secondary to

neoplasm, benign stricture, or achalasia also predispose to *Candida* infection [10, 11]. Although *Candida albicans* is the main cause of fungal esophagitis, other species such as *C. tropicalis, C. (Torulopsis) glabrata,* and *C. lusitaniae* have also been implicated [12]. *C. tropicalis* is more virulent and has greater potential for tissue invasion than *C. albicans* [13].

Endoscopically, *Candida* esophagitis usually presents as slightly raised, white plaques on a background of erythematous squamous mucosa. Microscopically, a pseudomembrane composed of a mixture of pseudohyphae, necrotic squamous cells, and fibrinopurulent debris is often noted to be adherent to the underlying squamous mucosa, which frequently shows marked regenerative changes and intramucosal neutrophils [14] (Figure 12.3). Special stains (including silver-based stains or PAS stain) can highlight pseudohyphae and/or yeast forms invading the squamous epithelium. While *C. albicans* and *C. tropicalis* produce a mixture of budding yeasts and pseudohyphae, *C. (Torulopsis) glabrata* only produces tiny budding yeasts [15].

Cytologically, fungal pseudohyphae and yeasts are identified as red or pink structures within Papanicolaou-stained material (Figure 12.4), and may be more readily identified in cytologic brushings than in biopsy specimens [16]. Cytologic examination of the endoscopic brushings may provide a rapid and definitive diagnosis of *Candida* esophagitis in many cases.

Herpes esophagitis

Herpes esophagitis is the most common viral esophagitis. Herpes simplex virus (HSV) type 1, HSV type 2, and varicella-zoster virus (VZV) can cause herpes esophagitis, but HSV type 1 is by far the most common cause. While mucosal trauma, cancer, mucosal injury associated with chemoradia-

tion, immunosuppressive therapy, and other immunodeficiency states (especially infection with HIV) predispose to herpes esophagitis [17–19], this can also rarely occur in immunocompetent patients [20].

Herpes esophagitis most commonly affects the distal one-third of the esophagus and endoscopically is characterized by multiple shallow, small ulcers with sharply delineated borders [21]. The diagnostic viral cytopathic features are usually present in the squamous mucosa immediately adjacent to the ulcer, and, as such, the border of the ulcer is the optimal site of biopsy. Sometimes, herpes viral cytopathic features are also noted in the sloughed squamous cells in the exudate. The herpes virus infects the squamous epithelial cells and produces two types of viral cytopathic alterations. Cowdry's type A inclusion bodies are round, densely eosinophilic structures that are separated from a thickened nuclear membrane by a clear halo. So-called ground-glass nuclei result in a homogenous, faintly basophilic chromatin pattern (Figure 12.5). In both types of virocytes, the cell and nucleus are significantly enlarged. Multinucleated squamous cells with nuclear molding are also characteristic. Frequently, the mucosa adjacent to the characteristic inclusions is ulcerated, and the ulcer base is composed of necrotic cellular debris, acute inflammatory cells, granulation tissue, and sheets of macrophages [22]. The presence of significant mononuclear inflammatory cells in an ulcer bed should prompt a search for herpes virocytes in the adjacent squamous epithelium and the sloughed squamous cells in the exudate. In cases with only rare equivocal herpes virocytes, immunohistochemical staining can help detect those infected cells. Virocytes produced by HSV type 1, HSV type 2, and VZV are similar, and cannot be distinguished from each other morphologically.

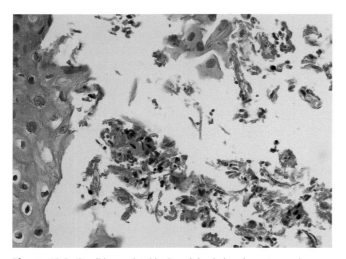

Figure 12.3 *Candida* esophagitis. Pseudohyphal and yeast organisms are identified in desquamated debris. Acute inflammatory cells are predominant within the mucosa (not pictured).

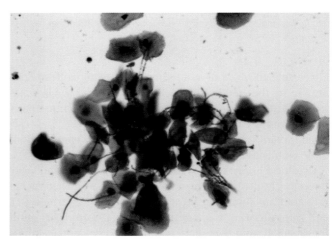

Figure 12.4 Esophageal brush cytology specimen with squamous epithelial cells and pseudohyphae consistent with candida esophagitis (Papanicolaou stain).

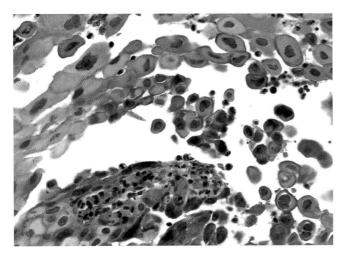

Figure 12.5 Herpes esophagitis. Squamous epithelial cells with ground-glass nuclei are prominent. A few multinucleated squamous cells with nuclear molding are also present.

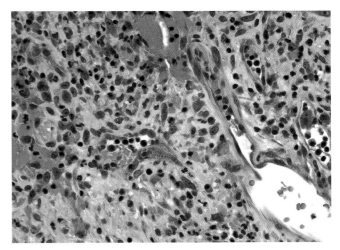

Figure 12.7 Cytomegalovirus (CMV) esophagitis. In the center of the field, there is an enlarged CMV-infected cell with a prominent intranuclear basophilic inclusion and many smaller cytoplasmic inclusions. This represents an infected endothelial cell.

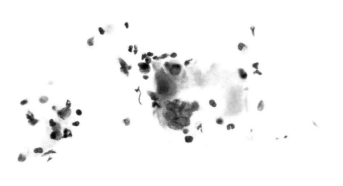

Figure 12.6 Esophageal brush cytology specimen showing multinucleation, molding of nuclei, and a ground-glass chromatin pattern in squamous epithelial cells (Papanicolaou stain).

Because herpes virus infects the squamous cells, their identification is possible by brush cytology. The infected squamous cells show characteristic nuclear changes, as described earlier, including nuclei with Cowdry's type A inclusions, ground-glass nuclei, and multinucleation with nuclear molding (Figure 12.6). Multinucleated glandular cells, a feature found in reactive glandular cells, may mimic infection with herpes. In many cases, the nature of the chromatin and the characteristic inclusions distinguish herpes infection from reactive changes.

Cytomegalovirus esophagitis

Cytomegalovirus (CMV) infection is the second most common cause of viral esophagitis. Like herpetic infection, CMV tends to affect immunocompromised patients [23–25].

Unlike herpes esophagitis, the endoscopic findings of CMV esophagitis are not characteristic. Also, unlike herpetic infection in which the characteristic alterations are found in the squamous cells, CMV tends to infect fibroblasts and capillary endothelial cells, which are often rich in the ulcer base, to produce the characteristic and diagnostic viral inclusions. Thus, the pathologist is more likely to be able to diagnose CMV esophagitis if the ulcer bed is sampled.

Histologically, CMV-infected cells show marked nuclear and cytoplasmic enlargement. Within the enlarged nucleus, a characteristic homogenous, basophilic inclusion that is separated from a thickened nuclear membrane by a halo is often present (Figure 12.7). In addition, some infected cells may contain small eosinophilic cytoplasmic inclusions. As with herpetic infection, sheets of macrophages are often seen at the base of the ulcer bed [26]. In equivocal cases, immunohistochemical staining may be used to confirm the diagnosis [27].

As discussed earlier, CMV does not typically infect the squamous epithelial cells, thereby making the diagnosis by cytology less likely. A cytologic diagnosis is more likely if the ulcer bed is vigorously brushed and a sample of the underlying granulation tissue produced. CMV inclusions are readily identified by the Papanicolaou stain (Figure 12.8). The intranuclear inclusions can be confused with prominent nucleoli seen with repair or carcinoma. Esophageal brushing smears also show a background of necrotic debris, acute inflammation, granulation tissue, and reparative epithelial cells [28].

Other types of infectious esophagitis

Other types of infectious esophagitis are only rarely encountered. Bacterial esophagitis is an uncommon clinical problem and typically affects immunocompromised patients [29] or

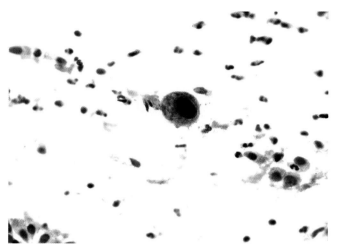

Figure 12.8 Esophageal brush cytology specimen showing a markedly enlarged cell with an intranuclear inclusion diagnostic of cytomegalovirus esophagitis (Papanicolaou stain; reproduced courtesy of Longwen Chen).

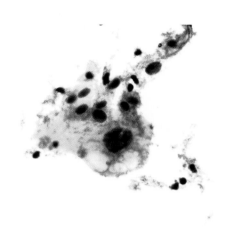

Figure 12.9 Atypical squamous epithelial cells following radiation therapy. Cellular and nuclear enlargement with cytoplasmic vacuolization is characteristic. Residual neoplasm is not identified (Papanicolaou stain).

patients who have been subjected to prolonged antibiotic therapy. Bacterial esophagitis may result in esophageal ulcers [30]. The bacterial organisms can be readily detected by Gram stain. In cytologic specimens, bacterial colonies are often admixed with necrotic debris, acute inflammatory cells, and reactive epithelial cells. However, it is often difficult to determine whether the bacterial colonies are causing the esophagitis, or represent a superimposed infection or simply colonization. Even less common than bacterial esophagitis, rare cases of esophagitis secondary to *Aspergillus*, *Mucor*, *Histoplasma*, and *Cryptococcus* have been described [31–34], and these usually occur in patients who are immunosuppressed. Special stains (including silver-based stains or periodic acid-Schiff [PAS] stain) highlight these fungal organisms and the diagnosis is usually straightforward.

Radiation- and chemotherapy-induced esophagitis

The esophagus is very sensitive to radiation and chemotherapeutic agents. Radiation-induced esophagitis is a common treatment-limiting acute side effect in patients who are treated for thoracic malignancies [35]. The severity of radiation-induced esophagitis appears to be related to the total radiation dose, fraction delivered per treatment, time period over which the radiation is given [36, 37], and concurrent chemotherapy [35].

While radiation-induced acute esophagitis is well characterized, the late effects of radiation on the esophagus are under-recognized and not well characterized [38, 39]; impairment of motility, stenosis and stricture, ulceration, and formation of pseudodiverticula may occur, and the risk is related to radiation dose.

Endoscopic findings for chemoradiotherapy-induced acute esophagitis usually include erythema, mucosal friability, hemorrhage, erosion/ulceration, and mucosal sloughing

[40]. Histologically, radiation esophagitis in the early phase is characterized by apoptotic bodies in the mucosal basal zone. Thereafter, within the first 4 weeks after therapy, a non-specific form of active, erosive/ulcerative esophagitis ensues. In the subacute and chronic phase of radiation-induced esophagitis, atypical mesenchymal cells and prominent vascular changes with intimal fibrosis or foam cells are commonly seen. The atypical mesenchymal cells have enlarged irregularly-shaped nuclei containing "smudgy" chromatin. Bizarre squamous epithelial cells with atypical nuclei associated with a commensurate increase in the cytoplasm are often seen. Multinucleated squamous cells, as well as prominent mitotic activity, including atypical mitotic figures, may be seen.

In cytologic preparations, highly atypical epithelial cells are characteristic of radiation-, chemotherapy-, and chemoradiotherapy-induced esophagitis [1, 41]. These atypical cells, however, have an increased amount of cytoplasm that is frequently vacuolated (Figure 12.9). Multinucleated squamous epithelial cells are also seen and are easily distinguished from herpetic virocytes by their significantly different nuclear features. Knowledge of treatment with chemotherapeutic agents or radiotherapy is the key to the diagnosis, although in patients with esophageal carcinoma who are treated with such therapies, it may be difficult to distinguish these alterations from persistent or recurrent carcinoma. In such cases, histologic evaluation of biopsy specimens is often more useful.

Pill/drug-induced and corrosive esophagitis

Pill/drug-related esophagitis

Esophagitis resulting from prolonged direct mucosal contact of ingested, particularly large-sized, tablets or capsules is quite common. Drugs commonly implicated in pill-associated esophagitis include antibiotics (particularly doxycycline), emepronium bromide, potassium chloride, ferrous sulfate, quinidine, and alendronate [42–47].

Endoscopically, pill-associated esophagitis manifests as discrete ulcers in a background of normal or only mildly inflamed esophageal mucosa. Ulcers are usually seen at the junction of the proximal and middle third of the esophagus, the area where the aortic arch compresses the esophagus, or in the middle third of the esophagus, the segment behind the left atrium [46]. Histologic features of pill-induced esophagitis are non-specific and include spongiosis, active inflammation with prominent eosinophilic infiltration, reactive changes with enlarged and hyperchromatic nuclei, and necrosis of squamous epithelium. In severe cases, inflammatory exudate and inflamed granulation tissue may be seen. In some cases, multinucleated squamous epithelial giant cells are also present [48, 49]. Foreign material may be seen in pill-induced esophagitis. For example, in cases of ferrous sulfate-induced esophagitis, crystalline stainable iron may be identified, and in alendronate-induced esophagitis, polarizable crystalline foreign material with or without multinucleated giant cells is seen [48].

Recently, a rare but unique form of sloughing esophagitis (esophagitis dissecans superficialis) has increasingly been reported in patients taking bisphosphonates (including alendronate) for osteoporosis. Endoscopically, sloughing esophagitis is characterized by cracking, peeling, and sloughing of a whitish membrane from the mucosa into the lumen [50], with cast formation in some cases. Histologically, the biopsy is usually superficial and the squamous mucosa may contain a layer of keratotic material, intraepithelial neutrophilic infiltration, and microabscess formation near the lamina propria papillae (Figure 12.10). Superficial bacterial and/or *Candida* colonization may be seen.

Corrosive esophagitis

Corrosive esophagitis may occur as a result of ingesting caustic material [51, 52]. The degree of esophageal injury depends on the type, physical state, concentration, and volume of the ingested material. Acid often produces coagulative necrosis with eschar formation, which usually limits the depth of injury. In contrast, alkali substances cause liquefactive necrosis without eschar formation; thus, the depth of injury is often greater. Endoscopically, in the acute phase, the esophagus may be normal or may show erythema, edema, hemorrhage, necrosis, mucosal sloughing, ulceration, or perforation [51]. Microscopically, in the early and acute phase, epithelial injury ranging from balloon degeneration, to acantholysis, and to necrosis predominates and is accompanied by congestion and thrombosis of vessels, bacterial colonization, and inflamed granulation tissue if the injury is severe. In the late phase, there may be fibrosis, which can lead to stricture formation in up to 20% of patients [52].

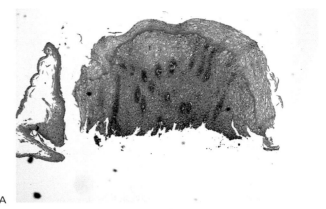

A

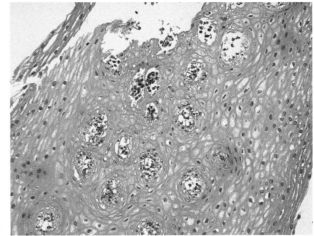

B

Figure 12.10 Esophagitis dissecans superficialis caused by alendronate. (A) Superficial biopsy shows hyperkeratosis. Apoptotic cells and a few neutrophils are also present in the biopsy (not pictured). (B) Neutrophilic microabscesses in the lamina propria papillae.

Primary eosinophilic esophagitis

Primary eosinophilic esophagitis is an increasingly recognized, distinctive, inflammatory disease of the esophagus. The recent American Gastroenterological Association (AGA)-sponsored review defines this disorder as "one in which more than 15 eosinophils per high power field (hpf) are identified in esophageal mucosal biopsies from patients who lack a positive response to proton pump inhibitor therapy, have normal pH monitoring value, or both" [53].

Endoscopically, the majority of the patients with eosinophilic esophagitis have mucosal abnormalities that are often described as concentric mucosal rings ("ringed" esophagus or "trachealization" of the esophagus), pinpoint white mucosal plaques/exudates, linear furrows/tears, "crêpe paper" mucosa, and narrow caliber of the esophagus [53, 54]. However, the esophagus may appear endoscopically normal in up to 25% of cases [54].

The histologic features of eosinophilic esophagitis are broadly divided into "major" and "minor" features. Major features are necessary to establish the diagnosis and include increased intraepithelial eosinophils (>15/hpf in areas of highest density), superficial layering of eosinophils (defined as distribution of eosinophils in the superficial layers of the squamous epithelium), eosinophilic microabscesses (defined as an organized collection of ≥4 eosinophils within the squamous epithelium), abundant eosinophils mixed with desquamated luminal debris, and marked degranulation of eosinophils [55]. Minor features are non-specific but useful features and include basal zone hyperplasia, elongation of lamina propria papillae, intercellular edema, increased intraepithelial lymphocytes and mast cells, and chronic inflammation and scarring in the lamina propria [55].

The diagnosis of eosinophilic esophagitis requires correlation with the patient's clinical, manometric, and endoscopic data, and the presence of a constellation of major features in the esophageal biopsies. Marked intraepithelial eosinophilia is not specific for eosinophilic esophagitis because severe GERD may produce pronounced eosinophilia in this range in a minority of cases. Histologic features in favor of eosinophilic esophagitis include the superficial layering of eosinophils, abundant eosinophils mixed with desquamated luminal debris, presence of eosinophilic microabscesses, and marked eosinophilic degranulation (Figure 12.11A). Further, the presence of intraepithelial eosinophilia in biopsies from the mid and proximal regions of the esophagus has greater diagnostic significance for eosinophilic esophagitis (Figure 12.11B), because GERD only rarely extends to the more proximal aspects of the esophagus.

Primary eosinophilic esophagitis often has a patchy distribution, and thus, multiple biopsies from the distal and mid/proximal esophagus and from normal and abnormal areas give the highest diagnostic yields [53]. Biopsies from the proximal/mid esophagus and the distal esophagus should be submitted separately. Biopsies should not be fixed in Bouin's solution because of the difficulty of assessing eosinophils in specimens fixed in this solution.

Other diagnostic considerations include Crohn's disease, collagen vascular disease, infectious esophagitis, pill/drug-induced esophagitis, esophageal involvement by eosinophilic gastroenteritis, and hypereosinophilic syndrome. While clinical correlation and histologic features often distinguish eosinophilic esophagitis from GERD and other conditions listed above, eosinophilic gastroenteritis with esophageal involvement is the most difficult one to differentiate if only the esophagus is biopsied since their histologic features are quite similar. Thus, biopsies from duodenal and gastric mucosa should always be obtained to help with this distinction [53, 55].

Esophageal involvement in systemic disease

Eosinophilic gastroenteritis

The esophagus may be involved by eosinophilic gastroenteritis. The histologic findings are non-specific, because intraepithelial eosinophilic infiltrates can be seen in many types of esophagitis, as described above. The diagnosis of esophageal involvement by eosinophilic gastroenteritis, therefore, is a diagnosis of exclusion. Other considerations include collagen vascular disease, pill/drug-induced esophagitis, infections including parasitic infestation, and, of course, GERD. Eosinophilia in peripheral blood and the presence of eosinophil-mediated injury in other parts (e.g. stomach and duodenum) of the gastrointestinal tract are helpful features.

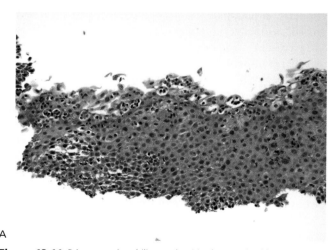
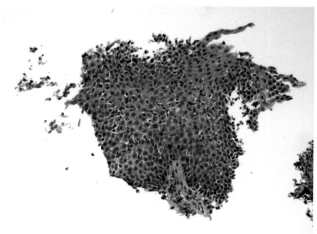

A   B

Figure 12.11 Primary eosinophilic esophagitis characterized by numerous intraepithelial eosinophils with a clustering of eosinophils near the surface of the squamous mucosa and eosinophilic microabscess formation. This pattern of intraepithelial eosinophilia is characteristic of primary eosinophilic esophagitis. Biopsy from (A) distal esophagus and (B) middle esophagus.

Crohn's disease

Crohn's disease may rarely involve the esophagus with a prevalence rate of less than 1%. The diagnosis is generally based on the presence of characteristic histologic features (stricture, deep ulcers, granulomas, mural fibrosis) in the esophagus in patients with known Crohn's disease elsewhere in the gastrointestinal tract. Lymphocytic esophagitis, a subtype of chronic esophagitis characterized by high numbers of intraepithelial lymphocytes (IELs) gathered mainly around peripapillary fields (>20 IELs/hpf), has been found by some [56], but not by others [57], to be associated with Crohn's disease elsewhere in the gastrointestinal tract.

Esophageal manifestations of dermatologic and collagen vascular diseases

Bullous diseases

Pemphigus vulgaris

Pemphigus vulgaris is the most common of the autoimmune mucocutaneous diseases characterized by the deposition of an autoantibody against the cell adhesion molecule, desmoglein 3, which is strongly expressed in the skin and esophagus. The interaction of antibody and antigen activates complement with resultant epithelial injury/necrosis and bulla formation. This condition occurs predominantly in middle-aged to elderly patients of Jewish or Mediterranean descent. Esophageal involvement may occur in 46.2–87.5% of patients with pemphigus vulgaris who undergo endoscopy with biopsy [58, 59]. Endoscopic findings include bullae, superficially erosive plaques, and ulcer [58, 59]. The middle and distal esophagus is primarily affected. Histologically, marked acantholysis is present [59]. In biopsies containing the blisters, a few acantholytic and degenerative cells are often present in the blister cavity and the basal cells may arrange themselves similar to a row of "tombstones" at the base of the blister with loss of their intercellular bridges. A mild, mixed inflammatory infiltrate including eosinophils both within and surrounding the bullae and in the lamina propria is often present. Direct immunofluorescence (DIF) study of esophageal biopsy specimens taken from both damaged and normal areas shows IgG and C3 deposits at the intercellular spaces [59].

Bullous pemphigoid

Bullous pemphigoid is a chronic autoimmune, subepidermal bullous dermatosis that can also affect the esophagus. Deposition of IgG autoantibodies to bullous pemphigoid antigen on the basement membrane activates complement and downstream inflammatory mediators, which leads to protease-mediated degradation of hemidesmosomal proteins and blister formation. Endoscopically, the esophagus may show tense, violaceous vesicular or bullous lesions protruding into the lumen, and extensive sloughing of the mucosa [60]. Histologically, subepithelial separation can be seen. DIF study of esophageal biopsy specimens taken from perilesional mucosa usually shows the presence of linear deposits of IgG and C3 at the level of the basement membrane [61].

Lichen planus

Lichen planus is an idiopathic mucocutaneous inflammatory disease; involvement of the esophagus appears to be underrecognized [62] and ranges from less than 1% to 26% in patients with mucocutaneous lichen planus [62, 63]. Unlike cutaneous lichen planus which often equally affects middle-aged men and women, esophageal lichen planus usually occurs in middle-aged or older women. Patients with esophageal lichen planus tend to have oral involvement, but the esophageal involvement may occur prior to mucocutaneous lesions [64]. The common symptoms include refractory or progressive odynophagia and dysphagia [64].

Endoscopically, lichen planus shows lacy white papules, pinpoint erosions, desquamation, pseudomembranes, and sometimes strictures [63, 64]. Although the proximal/mid esophagus is most commonly affected, rare cases involve the entire esophagus [63]. Lichen planus should always be considered for such lesions in patients on antireflux therapy. The mucosal biopsy should include the squamous epithelium, basement membrane, and lamina propria, and be submitted for routine histology and DIF study for the deposition of immunoglobulins, complement, and fibrinogen.

Histologic features of esophageal lichen planus differ from those seen in cutaneous lichen planus. The squamous epithelium usually shows parakeratosis rather than orthokeratosis and frequently lacks hypergranulosis [62]. The squamous epithelium may be atrophic rather than acanthotic, or it can show variable atrophy and acanthosis [62, 65]. The most characteristic finding is the band-like or lichenoid lymphocytic infiltrate involving the superficial lamina propria and basal epithelium [62, 66], predominantly composed of mature T cells and associated with basal keratinocyte degeneration, dyskeratotic epithelial cells, and Civatte bodies (anucleate remnants of necrotic keratinocytes) (Figure 12.12A). Concomitant candidal colonization in affected areas may occasionally occur. Although DIF study is routinely used for diagnosis of mucocutaneous lichen planus, its use in esophageal lichen planus is only rarely reported. In one case report, a shaggy deposition pattern of fibrinogen at the epithelial–lamina propria junction (Figure 12.12B), and globular deposition pattern of IgA, IgM, IgG, and C3 in the epithelium were noted [66].

Lichenoid lymphocytic infiltration and keratinocyte degeneration in an esophageal biopsy are characteristic of, but not specific for, lichen planus. This pattern of injury can be seen secondary to medication (including gold, thiazides, and antimalarial agents), esophageal mucosa near ulcers,

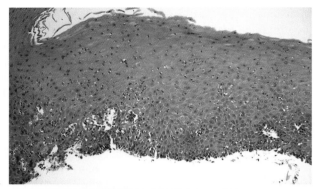

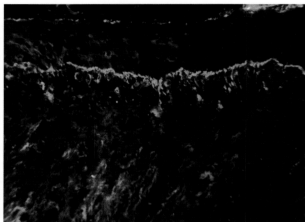

Figure 12.12 Esophageal involvement by lichen planus.
(A) Parakeratosis, intraepithelial lymphocytosis, and dyskeratotic cells are
seen. A lichenoid lymphoid interface infiltration is also present (not
pictured). (B) Direct immunofluorescence study shows a shaggy fibrinogen
deposition pattern at the epithelial-lamina propria junction.

viral esophagitis, stasis, graft-versus-host disease, and lymphocytic esophagitis.

Collagen vascular diseases

Scleroderma

Scleroderma, an idiopathic inflammatory disease mainly involving the skin and the smooth muscle, presents either as a localized disease or as a systematic disorder. The systematic form of scleroderma commonly involves the gastrointestinal tract [67] and the esophagus is the most commonly affected site (50–90% of cases) [67, 68]. In the late stage of scleroderma, the esophagus shows marked atrophy of smooth muscle and mural fibrosis in the distal two-thirds of the esophagus.

While the diagnosis of esophageal involvement by scleroderma is usually made by esophageal manometry [67], imaging study and endoscopic examination are commonly performed. Major endoscopic and imaging findings include those of reflux disease and esophagitis, stricture, and BE [69, 70]. Indeed, esophagitis is found in 33–63% of patients who

undergo endoscopic examination [67]. The incidence of BE in scleroderma varies from 0% to 37% [67, 69, 70]. The histologic findings in the esophageal mucosal biopsy from patients with scleroderma are mainly of those seen in reflux and BE, infection, and stasis.

Graft-versus-host disease

Graft-versus-host disease (GVHD) following allogeneic bone marrow transplantation, allogeneic hematopoietic stem cell transplantation, or blood transfusion in patients with severe immunodeficiency commonly affects the gastrointestinal tract including the esophagus. The National Institute of Health (NIH) consensus scheme recognizes two main categories of GVHD, each with two subcategories [71]. The broad category of acute GVHD includes classic acute GVHD occurring within 100 days post transplant and persistent, recurrent or late acute GVHD occurring beyond 100 days of transplantation. The broad category of chronic GVHD encompasses the classic chronic GVHD consisting only of manifestations that can be ascribed to chronic GVHD, and an acute and chronic overlap syndrome in which features of both acute and chronic GVHD coexist.

Endoscopically, in acute esophageal GVHD, the esophagus may display erythema, edema, erosion and ulceration, or casts in severe cases [72]; chronic esophageal GVHD often shows erosion and ulceration, web and stricture, and abnormal motility [73]. Multiple biopsies from lesional areas as well as the adjacent intact mucosa are needed to aid in the diagnosis, and at least 8–10 serial tissue sections are recommended to detect the minimal changes of GVHD [74].

Acute esophageal GVHD is characterized by apoptotic keratinocytes (dyskeratotic cells) within the squamous mucosa. A lichenoid lymphocytic inflammatory infiltrate is often present at the junction of the epithelium and lamina propria. Other non-specific findings include ballooning degeneration of keratinocytes, intercellular edema, non-specific erosion and ulceration, and intraepithelial eosinophilia. Major differential diagnoses for acute GVHD include infectious esophagitis, GERD, and medications including mycophenolic acid (cellcept or myofortic) [75]. The esophagitis caused by chemotherapy and/or radiation should always be considered, particularly in the early post-transplantation period (within 21 days post transplantation).

The histologic pattern of chronic esophageal GVHD is that of desquamative esophagitis with ulceration and submucosal fibrosis [73, 74]. As with acute GVHD, the presence of apoptotic squamous epithelial cells indicates ongoing activity [74].

Gastroesophageal reflux esophagitis

GERD is the most common chronic disorder of the esophagus and affects up to 40% of the general population in the

Western world [76, 77]. GERD-associated esophagitis is defined as esophageal mucosal injury caused by reflux of gastric acid or bile-containing duodenal contents into the esophagus. Although the etiology is multifactorial, the major risk factors include the presence of a hiatal hernia, a defective lower esophageal sphincter (LES), delayed gastric emptying, gastric acid overproduction, bile reflux, and obesity [77–81]. Significant discordance between clinical, endoscopic, and histologic findings exists [82, 83].

Reflux esophagitis can be non-erosive or erosive; complications include ulcers, strictures, BE, and carcinoma. Hiatal hernia, bile reflux, severely disturbed esophageal motility, and possibly obesity and genetic factors appear to be associated with the development of complications of GERD [80, 84, 85]. In symptomatic patients, esophageal mucosal biopsy is warranted not only to document the presence of esophagitis, but also to exclude other conditions including infectious esophagitis, BE, and neoplasm.

There are several important caveats with respect to the histologic diagnosis of reflux esophagitis. Reflux esophagitis may affect the mucosa in a patchy fashion, and, as such, multiple biopsies are warranted to document histologic abnormalities. Physiologic gastroesophageal reflux may cause minor histologic alterations in the most distal 2–3 cm of the esophageal mucosa [86]. Therefore, biopsies of the most distal esophagus are of limited value in diagnosing reflux esophagitis because it may not be possible to distinguish physiologic from pathologic alterations. Often, biopsies of this region are more useful in identifying other causes of esophagitis, BE, or neoplasm than for making a diagnosis of reflux esophagitis. Also of note, pinch biopsies obtained through standard endoscopes are usually inadequate for the evaluation of early histologic changes resulting from reflux [82]; use of jumbo biopsy forceps through an endoscope with a large-caliber biopsy channel is advocated [87].

No single or group of histologic features is entirely specific for GERD-related esophagitis. The major histologic components of reflux esophagitis include squamous epithelial injury and inflammation. Squamous epithelial injury includes basal hyperplasia, cell ballooning, intercellular edema (acantholysis), squamous cell necrosis, erosion, and ulceration. It has been suggested that squamous basal hyperplasia is among the earliest histologic manifestations of reflux-induced esophageal injury [88]. Johnson *et al.* have shown a strong correlation between the length of lamina propria papillae (an indirect indicator of basal hyperplasia) and severity of GERD as measured by the 24-h pH score [89]. Squamous hyperplasia should be evaluated in well-oriented sections containing at least three consecutive papillae. In squamous hyperplasia, the basal zone is thickened and usually occupies more than 15% of the mucosal thickness; lamina propria papillae typically exceed two-thirds of the thickness of the mucosa (Figure 12.13). Squamous hyperplasia is often accompanied by features such as

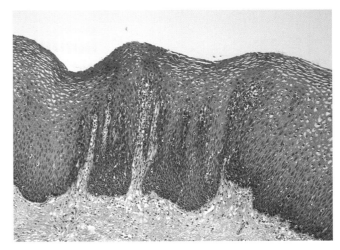

Figure 12.13 Early morphologic features in gastroesophageal reflux disease (GERD). The lamina propria papillae extend more than two-thirds of the full thickness of the epithelium. Squamous basal hyperplasia and an increased number of intraepithelial lymphocytes are present. These changes are not specific but are frequently seen in patients with GERD.

increased mitoses, slightly enlarged basal and parabasal nuclei, and prominent nucleoli. Cytoplasmic ballooning of squamous cells, acantholysis, erosions, ulceration, and granulation tissue may also be seen. In addition, regenerative features, including increased mitoses, decreased surface maturation, and multinucleated squamous cells, may be present. Not uncommonly, the exaggerated regenerative changes in the squamous cells may cause diagnostic difficulties; multinucleated squamous cells may mimic virally infected cells and the decreased surface maturation may appear similar to squamous dysplasia.

Inflammation is also a histologic component of reflux esophagitis. The principal inflammatory cells include neutrophils, eosinophils, and lymphocytes. In adult patients, intraepithelial eosinophils are only considered to be significant when there are more than six eosinophils present in a biopsy section [90–92] (Figure 12.14). In contrast, any degree of eosinophilia is considered to be pathologic in children because intraepithelial eosinophils are not normally present in the esophageal mucosa of pediatric patients [93–95]. In addition, eosinophils in the lamina propria are considered an even more sensitive indicator of reflux disease in infants [93]. Other conditions in which intraepithelial eosinophils are seen include primary eosinophilic esophagitis [53, 96, 97], pill-induced esophagitis, eosinophilic gastroenteritis, and drug reactions [98]. Intraepithelial neutrophils are present in less than one-third of patients with GERD (Figure 12.15), but this histologic feature lacks specificity because anything that causes erosion or ulceration in the esophagus can result in neutrophilic infiltration in the

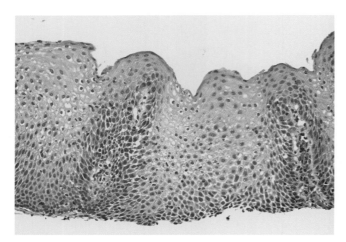

Figure 12.14 Intraepithelial eosinophilia in a patient with gastroesophageal reflux disease.

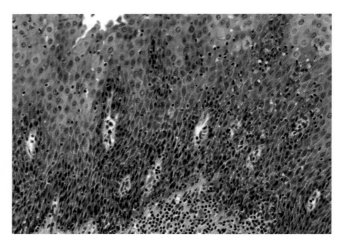

Figure 12.16 Lymphocytic esophagitis in a patient with gastroesophageal reflux disease.

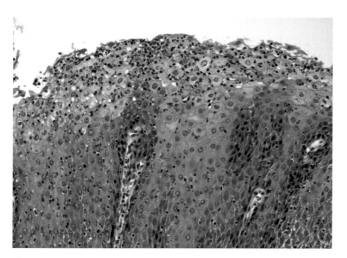

Figure 12.15 Intraepithelial neutrophils in a patient with gastroesophageal reflux disease.

adjacent, intact, squamous mucosa and the presence of neutrophils is a common feature of infectious esophagitis. Scattered lymphocytes, particularly T lymphocytes, are normal within the esophageal squamous mucosa [99, 100]. These lymphocytes typically have irregular nuclear contours and often appear to be squeezed between squamous cells. Although an increased number of lymphocytes are frequently seen in patients with reflux (Figure 12.16), this finding alone has no independent diagnostic value, because normal control subjects may also reveal increased numbers [100]. In addition, an increased number of intraepithelial lymphocytes can be seen in a variety of conditions, including esophageal stasis, achalasia, diverticulum, Crohn's disease, celiac disease, pill/drug-related esophagitis, primary eosinophilic esophagitis, GVHD, esophageal involvement by

certain dermatologic diseases, and lymphocytic esophagitis [56, 57].

Other non-specific histologic features can also be seen in reflux esophagitis. For example, marked dilatation of capillaries within the lamina propria is often seen [101], but similar histologic findings may be seen as a biopsy artifact in normal patients [102]. In long-term reflux esophagitis, mucosal scarring, variable degree of muscular proliferation, and submucosal fibrosis may also be present.

The cytologic abnormalities resulting from GERD are similar to those noted with any inflammatory process involving the esophagus. Specifically, basal cell hyperplasia results in numerous cells with a high N/C ratio in cytologic preparations. An inflammatory background containing neutrophils or eosinophils and degenerating squamous cells are present when frank ulcers are found. Caution must be taken not to overinterpret reparative epithelial changes as dysplastic or neoplastic. Although there is considerable overlap in the cytologic features between repair and carcinoma, reparative epithelial cells usually contain vesicular nuclei with single large nucleoli and delicate nuclear membranes, and do not demonstrate diffuse nuclear hyperchromasia or marked nuclear membrane abnormalities, features typically seen in squamous dysplasia (Figure 12.17).

Barrett's esophagus

BE is a complication of chronic GERD and is defined as "a change in the distal esophageal epithelium of any length that can be recognized as columnar-type mucosa at endoscopy and is confirmed to have intestinal metaplasia by biopsy of the tubular esophagus" in the recently updated Guidelines 2008 for the Diagnosis, Surveillance and Therapy of BE provided by the American College of Gastroenterology (ACG). The prevalence of BE in the general population in the Western world is 1.6% [77]. The importance of diagnosing this condi-

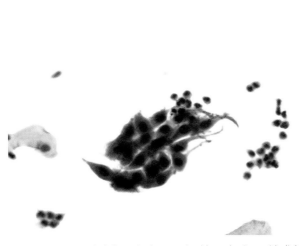

Figure 12.17 Epithelial repair characterized by cohesive epithelial cells arranged in a monolayered streaming sheet (Papanicolaou stain; reproduced courtesy of Longwen Chen).

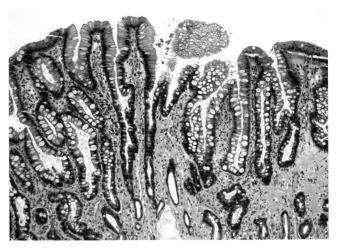

Figure 12.18 Low-magnification view of Barrett's esophagus. Goblet cells are easily identified. The base of the mucosa shows nuclear stratification, a feature that is characteristically found in the basal portion of Barrett's mucosa.

tion is related to its association with the development of esophageal adenocarcinoma [103], the frequency of which has rapidly increased over the past several decades [104].

Diagnosis in esophageal mucosal biopsy

In order to establish a definitive diagnosis of BE, the endoscopist should procure biopsies from the columnar-lined tubular esophagus and inform the pathologist of the tubular esophageal origin of the biopsies; the pathologist should document the presence of intestinal metaplasia in these biopsies [105].

Histologically, BE is characterized by the presence of acid mucin-containing goblet cells in a background of columnar mucosa in the tubular esophagus. Thus, the presence of acid mucin-containing goblet cells (specialized columnar epithelium) is the histologic *sine qua non* for making this diagnosis, regardless of the precise site of the biopsy within the tubular esophagus (Figures 12.18 and 12.19). Cytologically, goblet cells are barrel-shaped and have distended, mucin-filled, often slightly blue-tinged cytoplasm. The nuclei of the goblet cells are often eccentrically displaced and sometimes compressed by the abundant cytoplasmic mucin. The goblet cells may locate in the crypts and surface epithelium, and may be few in number to diffuse and numerous. Goblet cells contain both sialo- and sulfated mucin that stains positively with Alcian blue at pH 2.5; this stain can be used to aid the identification of goblet cells in cases with only rare goblet cells; caution should be taken when interpreting this stain because the columnar cells between the goblet cells may also contain some Alcian blue-positive mucin (so-called columnar blue cells), although the staining intensity is not as great as seen in the goblet cells [106]. The identification of such cells is not sufficient to render a definitive diagnosis of BE. Also, because Alcian blue stain is costly and time consuming

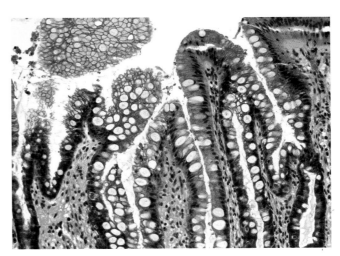

Figure 12.19 Higher magnification view of Barrett's esophagus, characterized by acid mucin-containing goblet cells.

and goblet cells can be readily recognized in H&E-stained tissue sections, routine use of Alcian blue stains is not recommended.

The columnar cells in the crypts and surface epithelia between the goblet cells may resemble either intestinal absorptive cells (complete intestinal metaplasia) (Figure 12.20) or gastric foveolar cells (incomplete intestinal metaplasia) (Figure 12.21). The glandular compartment of BE often has a higher portion of fundic-type glands in the distal portion of the columnar-lined esophagus, or mixed cardiac- and fundic-type glands, compared with the more proximal regions of columnar-lined esophagus [107, 108]. If only cardiac- or fundic-type mucosa is identified in a biopsy specimen in the absence of intestinal metaplasia (goblet cells), the

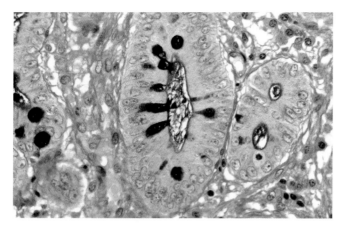

Figure 12.20 Barrett's esophagus with complete intestinal metaplasia. The Alcian blue portion of this combined Alcian blue and periodic acid-Schiff (PAS) stain highlights the goblet cells. The PAS portion of the stain highlights the luminal aspect of the glands, suggestive of a primitive brush border.

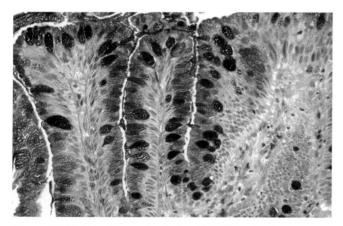

Figure 12.21 Alcian blue and periodic acid-Schiff (PAS) stain highlighting incomplete intestinal metaplasia in Barrett's esophagus. The Alcian blue portion of the stain highlights the goblet cells. The cells between the goblet cells are stained by PAS, indicating that they are filled with neutral mucins reminiscent of foveolar-type cells.

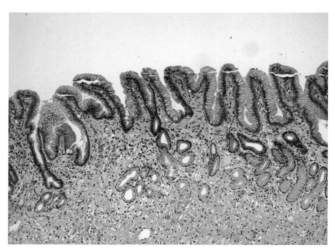

Figure 12.22 Atrophic cardiac-type mucosa in a biopsy obtained from this distal esophagus. Because goblet cells are not present, this would not be diagnostic of Barrett's esophagus.

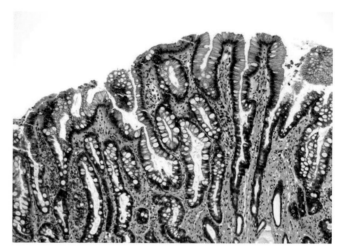

Figure 12.23 Intestinal metaplasia in a biopsy specimen obtained near the esophagogastric junction. Although this could represent short-segment Barrett's esophagus, it could just as easily represent intestinal metaplasia of the gastric cardia.

biopsy specimen would not be considered sufficient evidence for a diagnosis of BE (Figure 12.22). However, this problem becomes exceedingly rare with long segments of columnar epithelium; representing less than 1% of 250 cases of BE in which columnar epithelium extended more than 2 cm into the lower esophagus [109]. Thus, the longer the segment of columnar epithelium, the higher the likelihood of identifying goblet cells, such that virtually all columnar-lined segments of 3 cm or more have goblet cells (if adequately sampled) and are diagnostic of BE. Based on a recent retrospective study, eight random biopsies obtained from the columnar-lined esophagus [110] or four targeted biopsies that straddle the neo-squamocolumnar junction (SCJ) are adequate for assessment of the presence of intestinal metaplasia [108].

Given the difficulties in accurately and reproducibly recognizing the anatomic landmarks of the GEJ, it may not be possible to be sure whether the biopsy specimen comes from above (within the most distal esophagus) or below the GEJ (within the cardia, the most proximal portion of stomach) in some cases. Thus, there are problems equating intestinal metaplasia near the GEJ to BE in all cases [111] (Figure 12.23). The prevalence of intestinal metaplasia near the GEJ ranges from 9% to as high as 18% [112, 113]. Some investigators have found intestinal metaplasia in this location to be more strongly associated with GERD [114], while others have shown it to be more closely associated with *Helicobacter pylori* infection and intestinal metaplasia in other parts of the stomach [115–117]. Several studies have suggested a much

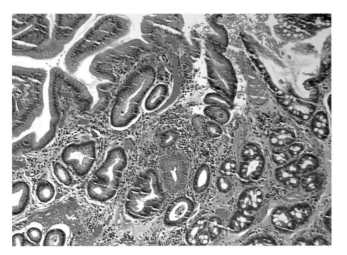

Figure 12.24 Presence of squamous epithelium-lined duct in the mucosa indicates the esophageal origin of this biopsy and therefore, is diagnostic of Barrett's esophagus.

lower risk of progression to dysplasia and carcinoma of intestinal metaplasia of the cardia when compared with either short- or long-segment BE [118, 119]. If these risks are truly different, as the evidence would suggest, then it is important to distinguish intestinal metaplasia of esophageal from proximal gastric origin (cardia intestinal metaplasia [CIM]). Srivastava *et al.* have reported several morphologic features including crypt disarray and atrophy, incomplete and diffuse intestinal metaplasia, multilayered epithelium, squamous epithelium overlying columnar crypts with intestinal metaplasia, hybrid glands, and esophageal glands/ducts, are associated with intestinal metaplasia of esophageal origin (a diagnosis of BE) [120]; the latter three features are observed exclusively in BE biopsies (Figure 12.24).

In addition, several studies have shown that a characteristic CK7/20 immunoreactivity pattern may help differentiate short-segment BE from CIM [121–123]. In virtually all cases of BE, there is superficial and deep CK7 staining in the intestinalized mucosa, with only superficial CK20 staining in the areas of intestinal metaplasia. In contrast, intestinal metaplasia of gastric origin, including the proximal stomach, virtually never shows such a Barrett's CK 7/20 immunoreactivity pattern [121–123]. In a few cases of CIM with this Barrett's CK7/20 immunoreactivity pattern, there is a strong association with acid reflux and some of these cases eventually progress to BE and even dysplasia [124]. However, routine use of these markers to diagnose BE is not recommended.

Barrett's esophagus-related dysplasia and neoplasm

Patients with a diagnosis of BE undergo surveillance, the goal of which is to detect dysplasia or early adenocarcinoma; surveillance has been shown to render a survival advantage for these patients [125, 126]. Although all patients with BE

are at an increased risk for developing adenocarcinoma, some are at higher risk than others [127]. Most patients with BE-associated adenocarcinoma are elderly Caucasian males, have BE-related dysplasia (particularly high-grade dysplasia), and long-segment BE [127–129]. The most recently updated ACG guidelines for BE clearly define an essential role of histologic assessment of dysplasia in the surveillance and therapy of BE because low-grade dysplasia (LGD) requires more frequent endoscopy and biopsy and high-grade dysplasia (HGD) represents a threshold for intervention [105]. If a patient with BE is a suitable surveillance candidate, surveillance endoscopy should be performed after reflux symptoms are controlled with appropriate antireflux treatment, because the presence of erosive esophagitis interferes with visual recognition [130] as well as histologic assessment of dysplasia.

Diagnosis in esophageal mucosal biopsies

Dysplasia is defined as the presence of neoplastic epithelium that is confined above the basement membrane of the gland from which it arises [131]. Histologic criteria for dysplasia in BE were well described in 1988 by Reid *et al.* [132]. Both cytologic and architectural alterations are components in making the diagnosis [129, 133]. In every biopsy with BE, a comment should be made as to the presence or absence of dysplasia; BE with dysplasia, LGD; BE with dysplasia, HGD; BE with changes indefinite for dysplasia.

Negative for dysplasia

A diagnosis of "negative for dysplasia" is typically applied to cases of BE that show metaplastic but otherwise unremarkable columnar epithelium, or metaplastic columnar epithelium with regenerative changes due to persistent reflux injury. The metaplastic columnar epithelium in BE usually does not have an evenly spaced, "test-tube–like" glandular arrangement. Instead, the metaplastic crypts often show a mild degree of architecture abnormality and cytologic atypia. Architecturally, the crypts often show budding, variable degree of branching, or atrophy (Figure 12.25). Cytologically, the cells often demonstrate loss of mucin, slightly increased N/C ratio, increased mitotic activity in the bases of the crypts and mild hyperchromasia, although there is characteristically surface maturation. Regenerative changes due to persistent reflux can be challenging; regenerative cells show loss of mucin, relatively high N/C ratio and mild hyperchromasia. Occasionally, regenerative epithelial cells may contain bizarre, multinucleated cells but without stratification. The updated ACG guidelines for BE recommend that patients with two consecutive endoscopies with biopsies that are negative for dysplasia should be followed up by endoscopic surveillance at an interval of 3 years [105].

Indefinite for dysplasia

A diagnosis of "indefinite for dysplasia" is a legitimate histologic interpretation, as it may be difficult to distinguish

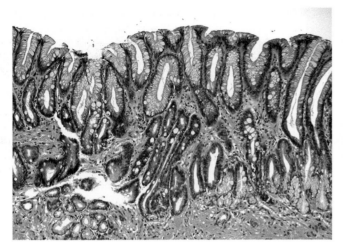

Figure 12.25 Non-dysplastic Barrett's esophagus. The base of the mucosa shows glands with hyperchromasia and sight nuclear stratification. However, this is the "baseline atypia" characteristic of Barrett's esophagus. There is cellular maturation toward the surface.

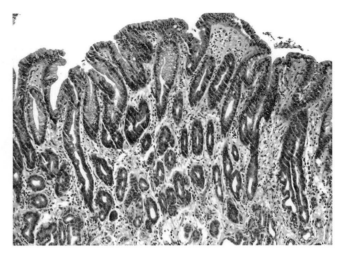

Figure 12.26 Barrett's esophagus with low-grade dysplasia. The glands show nuclear hyperchromasia and nuclear pseudostratification. There is no cellular maturation toward the surface.

marked regenerative changes from dysplasia. Caution should be exercised in making a diagnosis of dysplasia in the face of active inflammation. In addition, the mucosa in BE always displays a certain degree of "baseline architectural abnormality and cytologic atypia" [133], most pronounced at the base of the mucosa. In well-oriented biopsy specimens, it is usually easy to assess surface maturation, one of the most important criteria used to distinguish dysplasia from negative for dysplasia. However, in tangentially sectioned biopsy specimens, this evaluation may be challenging, and in such cases a diagnosis of "indefinite for dysplasia" may be rendered. Following this diagnosis, it is recommended to treat with antireflux medications in order to decrease reflux-associated injury and inflammation, and then to rebiopsy in 3–6 months [105].

Positive for dysplasia
Dysplasia is defined as the presence of neoplastic epithelium that is confined above the basement membrane of the gland from which it arises [131]. After determining the presence of dysplasia in BE, the dysplasia is further arbitrarily assigned with a grade, either LGD or HGD, according to the degree of architecture and cytologic abnormality.

Low-grade dysplasia: In LGD, the crypt architecture is largely preserved or minimally distorted (Figure 12.26). However, the epithelial cells in LGD typically have enlarged, crowded, and dark nuclei, which are often pencil-shaped, stratified, but for the most part, basally located. The epithelial cell nuclei may or may not have multiple, small, inconspicuous nucleoli [129]. There is a lack of surface maturation. Dysplastic epithelial cells are often mucin poor and show a marked decrease in or diminished goblet cell differentiation, but in some cases, significant numbers of dystrophic goblet

cells may be seen. In contrast to HGD, the epithelial cells in LGD usually have preserved polarity, or only mild loss of polarity limited to the bases of the crypts; show slightly increased N/C ratio; do not show significant pleomorphism; and the mitoses, both typical and atypical, are usually limited to the bases of the crypts. Very often, the dysplastic epithelium shows an abrupt transition to non-dysplastic epithelium. The finding of LGD warrants follow-up endoscopy within 6 months to ensure that no dysplasia higher than LGD is present in the esophagus. The patient can be followed annually endoscopically until no dysplasia is present on two consecutive annual endoscopic examinations [105].

High-grade dysplasia: HGD shows more severe cytologic atypia and architectural complexity than LGD, although in some cases, this distinction is difficult and somewhat arbitrary [129]. Architecturally, HGD is characterized by the presence of crowded and disorganized crypts or glands, including cribriform and branching ones of variable sizes and irregular shapes [129]. In addition, villiform mucosal configuration is also a common finding in HGD. Cytologically, the cells show more nuclear pleomorphism and hyperchromasia, and there is usually nuclear stratification extending from the epithelial basement membrane to the luminal aspects of the crypts and involving the full length of the crypts without surface maturation. Significant loss of polarity is also one of the most reliable features of HGD (Figure 12.27). In addition, the cells in HGD have prominent mitotic figures, including atypical ones, and even in the surface epithelium. Other important features include loss of mucin, decrease or complete absence of goblet cells, and prominent nucleoli. Although crypts in HGD can show intraluminal papillae or bridges, features of intramucosal adenocarcinoma such as extensive intraluminal bridges, intraluminal

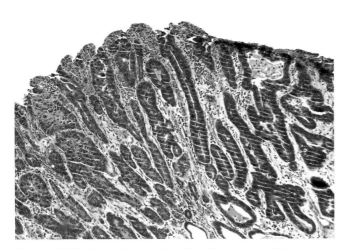

Figure 12.27 High-grade dysplasia in Barrett's esophagus. There is marked cytologic atypia and architectural complexity that exceeds that seen in low-grade dysplasia.

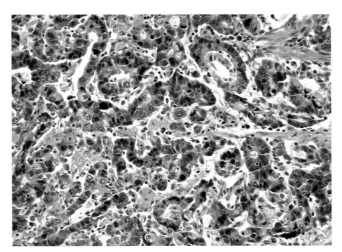

Figure 12.28 Intramucosal adenocarcinoma arising in Barrett's esophagus. There is an apparent infiltration of glands and individual cancer cells into the lamina propria.

necrosis, and back-to-back crypt pattern should not be present.

Although HGD is the strongest risk factor for development of BE-associated adenocarcinoma, the overall cancer incidence in patients with HGD followed by surveillance endoscopy appears to be lower than previously reported [134]. In a meta-analysis including a total of 236 patients with HGD followed for 1241 patient-years, esophageal adenocarcinoma was reported in 69 patients with a crude incidence rate of 5.57 per 100 patient-years [134]. Similarly, another meta-analysis including a total of 441 patients undergoing esophagectomy for HGD reported that for HGD without a visible lesion, the rate of concomitant invasive adenocarcinoma was 3% [135].

The diagnosis of HGD should be confirmed by at least one experienced gastrointestinal pathologist, and BE patients with HGD should have an immediate repeat endoscopy with special attention to mucosal abnormalities and more intense mucosal sampling to rule out synchronous adenocarcinoma [105]. Four quadrant biopsies should be spaced every 1 cm [136]. In addition, any visible lesions (including nodularity, ulcer, stricture, mucosal friability) within the BE segment should undergo endoscopic resection to obtain adequate tissue for more accurate diagnosis, as mucosal visible lesions have been shown to be associated with a much higher frequency of malignancy [105, 135, 137]. If the immediate repeat endoscopy with biopsies and/or endoscopic mucosal resection does not reveal a synchronous adenocarcinoma, patients with focal HGD may be followed by endoscopic surveillance at an interval of 3 months; patients with multifocal or diffuse HGD are treated with endoscopic mucosal ablation in conjunction with acid suppression, endoscopic mucosal resection, or esophagectomy [105].

Intramucosal adenocarcinoma

Intramucosal adenocarcinoma (IMAC) is defined as the presence of neoplastic cells that have penetrated through the basement membrane into the lamina propria or muscularis mucosae but not below [132]. Given the presence of lymphatic channels within the esophageal mucosa, there is a small but definite risk of regional lymph node metastasis in patients with IMAC alone (<5%) [138]. The criteria for IMAC include: (1) individual malignant cells infiltrating the lamina propria and lacking a connection to the crypts; (2) sheets of malignant cells in the lamina propria without gland formation; (3) markedly angulated and abortive glands infiltrating the lamina propria; (4) a complex anastomozing glandular pattern within the lamina propria; and (5) neoplastic glands or cells arranged in a back to back or highly irregular architectural pattern that cannot be explained by the presence of pre-existing BE [139, 140] (Figure 12.28). IMAC can be extremely difficult to distinguish from HGD on small biopsies.

Adenocarcinoma with submucosal invasion

Esophageal adenocarcinoma with submucosal invasion is associated with significant regional lymph node metastatic rate (approximately 30%). In superficial biopsies, the diagnosis of submucosal invasion can be challenging because the presence of "entrapped" dysplastic glands within the newly formed spaces between the superficially located, duplicated muscularis mucosae and the original muscularis mucosae, can mimic submucosal invasion. The most reliable feature indicating submucosal invasion is the presence of a desmoplastic stroma.

Diagnostic challenges

Significant diagnostic difficulty exists in the upper end of the dysplasia spectrum (HGD, IMAC, and submucosally invasive adenocarcinoma) in pretreatment BE biopsies [139, 140], and thus strongly challenges the "conventional" assumption that the upper end of the dysplasia spectrum can reliably be distinguished from each other in BE biopsies to direct therapeutic decision-making. Recently, a two-tiered system (HGD and HGD with features "suspicious" for carcinoma [HGD/S]) was reported to better stratify patients in pretreatment BE mucosal biopsies [141]. Using a set of histologic features, including solid or cribriform growth, dilated tubules/necrotic debris, ulceration occurring within the HGD mucosa, marked neutrophilic infiltration in HGD epithelium, and invasion of the squamous epithelium, the researchers redefined an HGD category that had only a 5% chance of having an unrecognized carcinoma in the subsequent esophagectomy, compared to a 17% rate of unrecognized adenocarcinoma associated with the original "HGD" diagnosis. This retrospective study suggests that there may be a category of true HGD associated with a relatively low risk for a concomitant carcinoma.

Evaluation of endoscopic mucosal resection specimens

EMR has been increasingly utilized to treat superficial BE-related neoplasms [142]; endoscopists perform EMR to excise discrete esophageal mucosal nodules or lesions that are small, flat, or polypoid, not invading deeper than the submucosa. EMR removes the lesion at the submucosal level and produces a specimen that allows more accurate histologic diagnosis [143]. EMR specimens should be marked with ink at their deep and circumferential margins, well mounted, and fixed for at least 12 h [144]. Tissue sections from fixed EMR specimens should be performed at 2-mm intervals and radial sections submitted if the specimen is wide enough.

Histologic evaluation should include determination of the nature of the lesion, status of the margins, and presence or absence of angiolymphatic invasion in cases where carcinoma is present. A resection is considered as *complete* if deep and lateral/circumferential margins are negative (2 mm from the neoplasm), *incomplete* when neoplastic epithelium (with or without electrodiathermic burn artifact) is present at the deep and lateral/circumferential margin(s), or *indefinite* when neoplastic epithelium is located within 2 mm from the margins.

Problems may arise with the determination of the depth of carcinoma. More specifically, the space between the superficial layer of muscularis mucosae and the original layer of muscularis mucosae may look like submucosa; the entrapment of dysplastic glands within proliferated muscularis mucosae can mimic invasive adenocarcinoma; and the thickened muscularis mucosae may be interpreted as muscularis propria [145]. In addition, hemorrhage, electrodiathermic burn, and tissue fragmentation present in EMR specimens may also limit histologic interpretation, particularly of the margin status [144, 146, 147].

Evaluation of esophageal mucosal biopsy following mucosal ablation therapy

Photodynamic therapy (PDT), radiofrequency ablation (RFA), and cryoablation have also been used to eradicate either BE-related dysplasia or BE. The replacement of BE by newly developed squamous epithelium (referred to as neosquamous epithelium [NSE] or re-epithelialization), occurs in 100% patients treated with PDT or RFA [144]. Sometimes, however, NSE can bury the metaplastic or dysplastic epithelium and the frequency of this phenomenon varies depending upon the type of ablation technique used. In post-PDT follow-up biopsies, the frequency of buried BE ranges from 6% to 51.1% and the frequency of buried dysplasia from 0% to 27.3% [148, 149]. Unlike PDT, the rate of buried BE following RFA is relatively low, ranging from 0% to 5.1% [150–153].

The endoscopic brush cytology is a valuable technique in BE and BE-related dysplasia [6, 154–156]. Endoscopic brushing of non-dysplastic BE usually produces a cellular sample of columnar cells. These cells typically occur as large tissue fragments with sharp or smooth edges. These sheets of cells have evenly distributed nuclei with distinct cell borders, producing a "honey-comb" arrangement when reviewed *en face*. Large villiform structures, small acini and rosette formations, and occasional single cells can also be encountered. Non-dysplastic nuclei have an oval shape with smooth external contours, uniform nuclear membrane thickness, only mild size variation, and small or inconspicuous nucleoli. The chromatin is fine and evenly distributed. In the tissue fragments on edge, the nuclei are basally located. Goblet cells contain a single, large apical mucin vacuole that displaces the nucleus, resulting in a crescent rather than a round/oval nuclear configuration. Goblet cell differentiation results in a "Swiss cheese" appearance on the tissue fragments when viewed *en face*.

Endoscopic brushing of dysplastic BE usually produce cell groups smaller than those obtained from BE without dysplasia [155, 157, 158]. These cell groups frequently occur as three-dimensional clusters and usually show frayed edges with cells falling away from the group. In addition, flat sheets, acini, and isolated single cells may be found. The dysplastic cells show indistinct cell borders, high N/C ratio, loss of nuclear polarity, nuclear overlap, irregular nuclear contours, and nuclear membrane thickening and notching. The distinction between LGD and HGD may be subtle, with the latter showing greater degrees of abnormalities (Figure 12.29). Large numbers of atypical aggregates and single atypical cells as well as giant nuclei have been reported as features favoring the diagnosis of adenocarcinoma [157] (Figure 12.30).

Non-endoscopic cytologic techniques have also been evaluated in the context of BE. While balloon cytology is not sensitive in detecting goblet cells [6, 159] or abnormal cells in LGD [6], it may be a valuable technique for the detection of HGD and adenocarcinoma [6].

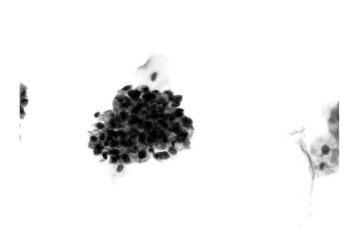

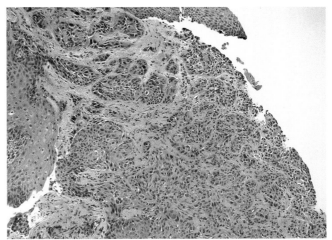

Figure 12.29 Brush cytology specimen of Barrett's esophagus with high-grade dysplasia. Nuclear pleomorphism, nuclear membrane irregularity, and hyperchromasia are present in a sheet of irregularly arranged cohesive cells (Papanicolaou stain).

Figure 12.31 Superficially invasive esophageal squamous cell carcinoma. Small nests of infiltrating cells with obvious squamous differentiation are seen.

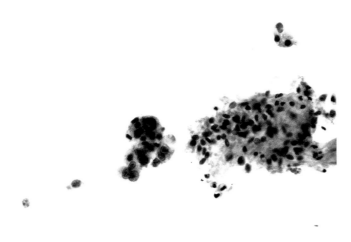

Figure 12.30 Adenocarcinoma arising in Barrett's esophagus, characterized by the presence of large numbers of atypical aggregates with haphazardly arranged and crowded tumor cells, and single atypical cells (not pictured; Papanicolaou stain).

Other carcinomas and malignancies

Squamous cell carcinoma

Although the incidence of squamous cell carcinoma has been steadily decreasing in Western countries, including the United States, and is now far surpassed by BE-related adeno-carcinoma, squamous cell carcinoma still comprises the vast majority of esophageal cancers worldwide. Many patients present at an advanced stage of disease, and the prognosis is generally poor [160, 161].

Histologically, esophageal squamous cell carcinoma resembles squamous cell carcinomas that arise in other ana-

tomic sites (Figure 12.31). Most arise from an adjacent identifiable *in situ* component. These tumors may be keratinizing or non-keratinizing and are classified as well, moderately, and poorly differentiated neoplasms. Well-differentiated squamous cell carcinoma is characterized by infiltrative nests of cells that are generally surrounded by a desmoplastic stroma. Occasionally, tumor may invade as nests of cells with an expanding as opposed to infiltrative growth pattern. Cytoplasmic keratinization and keratin pearls as well as intracellular bridges (desmosomes) are easily identified. As the degree of tumor differentiation decreases, it becomes more difficult to immediately recognize the neoplastic cells as having squamous differentiation. As such, poorly differentiated squamous cell carcinomas lack easily identifiable features of squamous differentiation. In such tumors, the cells show considerable nuclear pleomorphism and easily identifiable mitotic figures, including atypical forms. Basaloid squamous cell carcinoma, a morphologically and molecularly distinctive variant, occurs rarely in the esophagus and usually contains variably sized nests or sheets of tumor cells with scant cytoplasm and hyperchromatic, high-grade nuclei [162]. Verrucous carcinoma, an uncommon form of squamous cell carcinoma, by definition, does not exhibit malignant cytologic features but shows a pushing infiltrating border into the underlying stroma [163, 164].

The histologic grade of the squamous cell carcinoma should be based on the least differentiated portion of the neoplasm, even if it only comprises a small component of the tumor. In addition, the relationship of the tumor to the surgical resection margins should be noted, because the risk of local recurrence is significantly increased with positive surgical margins. Tumor stage is a major prognostic factor as well. Vascular invasion may also be present and should be specifically noted.

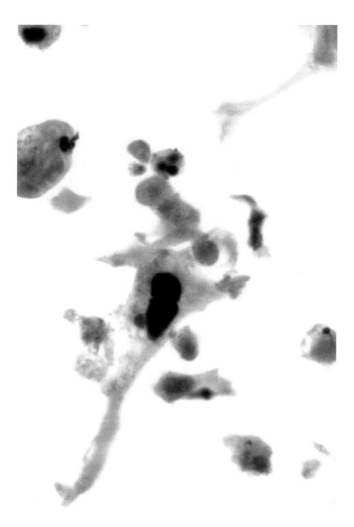

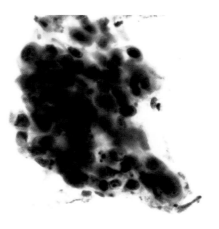

Figure 12.33 Brush cytology specimen of a poorly differentiated squamous cell carcinoma. The neoplastic cells are haphazardly arranged and show marked nuclear pleomorphism and abnormal chromatin distribution without clear evidence of squamous differentiation (Papanicolaou stain).

Figure 12.32 Well-differentiated squamous cell carcinoma. Spindle–shaped malignant cells with orangeophilic cytoplasm indicative of keratin production (Papanicolaou stain; reproduced courtesy of Longwen Chen).

The cytologic features of esophageal squamous cell carcinoma are dependent on the degree of differentiation. Well-differentiated squamous cell carcinomas produce numerous individual atypical keratinizing cells. The production of keratin causes the cytoplasm to be dense, refractile, and orange with a Papanicolaou stain (Figure 12.32). Difficulties may arise in distinguishing carcinoma from a hyperkeratotic reactive process and biopsy may be required to document stromal invasion because, in some cases, this may be the only feature that allows the distinction of carcinoma from a reactive process. Poorly differentiated tumors are composed of cells with classic malignant cytologic features but without obvious squamous differentiation (Figure 12.33). The malignant cells show increased N/C ratios with nuclei containing coarse, clumped chromatin and often prominent nucleoli. The malignant cells may occur as cohesive tissue fragments or as individual neoplastic cells. Poorly differentiated squamous cell carcinoma may be difficult to distinguish from poorly differentiated adenocarcinoma, lymphoma, and melanoma. Spindled or sarcomatoid squamous cell carcinoma yield spindle-shaped tumor cells with sarcomatous features as well as more conventional keratinizing or non-keratinizing polygonal cells. Basaloid squamous cell carcinoma of the esophagus usually contains cohesive clusters of small cells that are hyperchromatic with irregularly distributed coarse chromatin, and must be distinguished cytologically from small cell carcinoma. In difficult cases, special studies, particularly immunohistochemical studies, are often required to make a definitive diagnosis.

Preinvasive lesions of the squamous mucosa result in a spectrum of cytologic abnormalities. Western pathologists have applied the classification scheme commonly used in the cervix as a result of the relative lack of experience with esophageal cytology specimens. For example, Roth *et al.* devised a modification of the Bethesda system used for the evaluation of cervical cytology and this classification scheme uses categories such as atypical squamous cells of undetermined significance, LGD, and HGD [165]. The use of cytology to screen for esophageal squamous cell carcinoma in high-risk regions of the world has been attempted. Esophageal balloon cytology has been used in China for many years to identify patients with early stage disease or preinvasive lesions [4, 5, 165] to provide the potential for improved long-term survival over that typically seen in other parts of the world without screening programs. Although cytology is highly sensitive in detecting carcinoma in symptomatic patients, the ability to detect significant lesions in asymptomatic patients has been less impressive

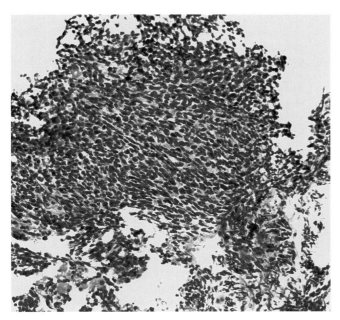

Figure 12.34 Esophageal small cell carcinoma. At low magnification, the cells are markedly hyperchromatic.

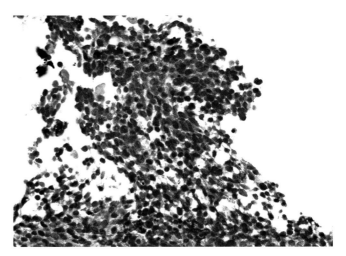

Figure 12.35 High-magnification view of an esophageal small cell carcinoma. The cells are marked hyperchromatic and have high N/C ratio. A finely granular chromatin pattern suggests neuroendocrine differentiation. Single cell necrosis is also present (not pictured).

with a sensitivity of 18–44% in specimens obtained by a balloon or a sponge device for the detection of biopsy-proven squamous cell carcinoma [165].

Small cell carcinoma

Esophageal small cell carcinoma is an exceedingly rare neoplasm and accounts for less than 5% of all esophageal malignancies [166, 167]. This tumor typically occurs in middle-aged or elderly patients and usually arises in the middle or distal portion of the esophagus [167]. Histologically, esophageal small cell carcinoma is identical to that seen in other sites and is composed of varying sized nests of small and highly malignant cells with significant crush artifact. The tumor cells have dark nuclei and an extremely high N/C ratio and exhibit nuclear molding without prominent nucleoli (Figures 12.34 and 12.35). These tumors are typically deeply invasive at the time of initial diagnosis [167].

The cytologic features of small cell carcinoma are identical to those of the more commonly encountered small cell carcinoma of the lung. The tumor is composed of cells with prominent nuclear molding and nuclei with finely stippled chromatin without prominent nucleoli [168]. The high N/C ratio is reminiscent of lymphocytes when the cells are scattered individually. A necrotic background is frequently conspicuous and significant crush artifact may exist.

The differential diagnosis of esophageal small cell carcinoma includes metastatic small cell carcinoma from another site, basaloid squamous cell carcinoma, and lymphoma. Given the rarity of primary esophageal small cell carcinoma and the proximity of the esophagus to the lung, the possibil-

ity of a pulmonary metastasis should always be excluded. On occasion, it may be difficult to establish the diagnosis of small cell carcinoma, and, in such cases, immunohistochemical findings of neuroendocrine differentiation are useful.

Malignant melanoma

Primary melanoma of the esophagus is exceedingly rare with an age-adjusted rate of 0.03 per million [169]. Primary esophageal malignant melanoma does occur and characteristically exhibits an exophytic growth pattern producing an intramucosal polypoid mass. The presence of atypical junctional melanocytic activity, *in situ* melanoma, radial growth phase, melanocytosis, and mixed epithelioid and spindle cell morphology, in the absence of history of melanoma, is useful in distinguishing primary from metastatic melanoma [170]. Atypical junctional melanocytic activity and/or *in situ* melanoma are often only observed at the tumor periphery. The submucosal portion of the tumor is composed of nests of loosely cohesive, large epithelioid to spindle-shaped cells with abundant granular cytoplasm and eccentric vesicular nuclei with prominent nucleoli [170] (Figure 12.36). Cytoplasmic pigmentation may be present. Scattered multinucleated cells and intranuclear cytoplasmic inclusions are also seen.

In cytologic brushings or aspirates, the specimens are usually highly cellular and composed of large obviously malignant cells with vesicular nuclei, macronucleoli, and abundant granular cytoplasm. The cells may be in loosely cohesive aggregates or they may occur singly in the specimen. Nuclei are typically eccentrically located and may have intranuclear cytoplasmic inclusions. If present, cytoplasmic melanin appears as finely dispersed dark brown granules. In

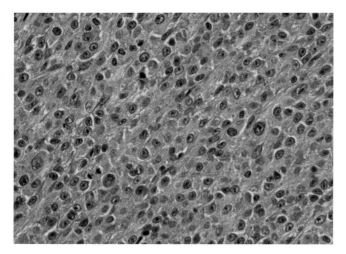

Figure 12.36 High-magnification view of an esophageal melanoma. The tumor is composed of sheets of large epithelioid cells with abundant cytoplasm and vesicular nuclei with prominent nucleoli and rare intranuclear cytoplasmic inclusions. The presence of atypical junctional melanocytic activity (not pictured) is strong evidence that the melanoma is primary to this site.

difficult cases, immunohistochemical stains for S-100 protein and melanocytic antigens (HMB-45 and MART-1) are useful in confirming the diagnosis.

References

1. Geisinger KR. Endoscopic biopsies and cytologic brushings of the esophagus are diagnostically complimentary. *Am J Clin Pathol* 1995;103:295–299.
2. Geisinger KR. Alimentary tract (esophagus, stomach, small intestine, colon, rectum, anus, biliary tract). In: Bibbo M, ed. *Comprehensive Cytopathology*, 2nd edn. Philadelphia: WB Saunders, 1997, pp. 413–444.
3. Lightdale CJ, Kulkarni KG. Role of endoscopic ultrasonography in the staging and follow-up of esophageal cancer. *J Clin Oncol* 2005;23:4483–4489.
4. Liu SF, Shen Q, Dawsey SM, *et al*. Esophageal balloon cytology and subsequent risk of esophageal and gastric-cardia cancer in a high-risk Chinese population. *Int J Cancer* 1994;57:775–780.
5. Dawsey SM, Shen Q, Nieberg RK, *et al*. Studies of esophageal balloon cytology in Linxian, China. *Cancer Epid Biomark Prev* 1997;6:121–130.
6. Falk GW, Chittajallu R, Goldblum JR, *et al*. Surveillance of patients with Barrett's esophagus for dysplasia and cancer with balloon cytology. *Gastroenterology* 1997;112:1787–1797.
7. Brandt LJ, Coman E, Schwartz E, *et al*. Use of a new cytology balloon for diagnosis of symptomatic esophageal disease in acquired immunodeficiency syndrome. *Gastrointest Endosc* 1993;39:559–561.
8. DeNardi FG, Riddell RH. Esophagus. In: Mills SE, ed. *Histology for Pathologists*, 3rd edn. Philadelphia; Lippincott Williams & Wilkins, 2007, pp. 565–588.
9. Baehr PH, McDonald GB. Esophageal infections: risk factors, presentation, diagnosis and treatment. *Gastroenterology* 1994; 106:509–532.
10. Gefter WB, Laufer I, Edell S, *et al*. Candidiasis in the obstructed esophagus. *Radiology* 1981;138:25–28.
11. Kodsi BE, Wickremeisinghe PC, Kozinn PJ, *et al*. Candida esophagitis. A prospective study of 27 cases. *Gastroenterology* 1976;71:715–719.
12. Kliemann DA, Pasqualotto AC, Falavigna M, *et al*. Candida Esophagitis: species distribution and risk factors for infection. *Rev Inst Med Trop Sao Paulo* 2008;50:261-263.
13. Walsh TJ, Merz WG. Pathologic features in the human alimentary tract associated with invasiveness of Candida tropicalis. *Am J Clin Pathol* 1986;85:498–502.
14. Mathieson R, Dutta SK. Candida esophagitis. *Dig Dis Sci* 1983;28:365–370.
15. Fidel PL Jr, Vazquez JA, Sobel JD. *Candida glabrata*: review of epidemiology, pathogenesis, and clinical diseases with comparison to *Candida albicans*. *Clin Microbiol Rev* 1999;12:80–96.
16. Wang HH, Jonasson JG, Ducatman BS. Brushing cytology of the upper gastrointestinal tract: obsolete or not? *Acta Cytol* 1991;35:195–198.
17. Buss DH, Scharyj M. Herpes virus infection of the esophagus and other visceral organs in adults. Incidence and clinical significance. *Am J Med* 1979;66:457–462.
18. McDonald GB, Sharma P, Hackman RC, *et al*. Esophageal infection in immunosuppressed patients after marrow transplantation. *Gastroenterology* 1985;88:1111–1117.
19. McBane RD, Gross JB. Herpes esophagitis: clinical syndrome, endoscopic appearance and diagnosis in 23 patients. *Gastrointest Endosc* 1991;37:600–603.
20. Kirsch M. Herpes esophagitis in an immunocompetent host. *Am Fam Phys* 1998;57:1778.
21. Amaro R, Poniecka AW, Goldberg RI. Herpes esophagitis. *Gastrointest Endosc* 2000;51:68.
22. Greenson JK, Beschorner WE, Boitnott JK, *et al*. Prominent mononuclear cell infiltrate is characteristic of herpes esophagitis. *Hum Pathol* 1991;22:541–549.
23. Chetty R, Roskell DE. Cytomegalovirus infection in the gastrointestinal tract. *J Clin Pathol* 1994;47:968–972.
24. Wilcox CM, Straub RF, Schwartz DA. Prospective endoscopic characterization of cytomegalovirus esophagitis in AIDS. *Gastrointest Endosc* 1994;40:481–484.
25. Hackman RC, Wolford JL, Cleaves CA, *et al*. Recognition and rapid diagnosis of upper gastrointestinal cytomegalovirus infection in bone marrow transplant recipients. *Transplantation* 1994;57:231–237.
26. Greenson JK. Macrophage aggregates in cytomegalovirus esophagitis. *Hum Pathol* 1997;28:375–378.
27. Theise ND, Rotterdam H, Dieterich D. Cytomegaloviral esophagitis in AIDS: diagnosis by endoscopic biopsy. *Am J Gastroenterol* 1991;86:1123–1126.
28. Teot LA, Ducatman BS, Geisinger KR. Cytologic diagnosis of cytomegaloviral esophagitis. A report of three acquired immunodeficiency syndrome-related cases. *Acta Cytol* 1993;37: 93–96.
29. Walsh TJ, Belitsos NJ, Hamilton SR. Bacterial esophagitis in immunocompromised patients. *Arch Intern Med* 1986;146: 1345–1348.

30. Miller JT Jr, Slywka SW, Ellis JH. Staphylococcal esophagitis causing giant ulcers. *Abdom Imaging* 1993;18:225–226.

31. Mineur PH, Ferrant A, Walton J, *et al*. Bronchoesophageal fistula caused by pulmonary Aspergillosis. *Eur J Respir Dis* 1985;66:360–366.

32. Jenkins DW, Fisk DE, Byrd RB. Mediastinal Histoplasmosis with esophageal abscess. *Gastroenerology* 1976;70:109–111.

33. Lamps LW, Molina CP, West AB, *et al*. The pathologic spectrum of gastrointestinal and hepatic Histoplasmosis. *Am J Clin Pathol* 2000;113:64–72.

34. Jacobs DH, Macher AM, Handler R, *et al*. Esophageal cryptococcosis in a patient with hyperimmunoglobulin E-recurrent infection (Job's syndrome). *Gastroenterology* 1984;87:201–203.

35. Werner-Wasik M. Treatment-related esophagitis. *Semin Oncol* 2005;32 (2 Suppl 3):S60–66.

36. Berthrong M, Fajardo LE. Radiation injury in surgical pathology: II. Alimentary tract. *Am J Surg Pathol* 1981;5:153–178.

37. Novak JM, Collins JT, Donowitz M, *et al*. Effects of radiation on the human gastrointestinal tract. *J Clin Gastroenterol* 1979; 1:9–39.

38. Pavy JJ, Bosset JF. Late effects of radiation on the esophagus. *Cancer Radiother* 1997;1:732–734.

39. Mahboubi S, Silber JH. Radiation-induced esophageal strictures in children with cancer. *Eur Radio* 1997;7:119–122.

40. Hirota S, Tsujino K, Hishikawa Y, *et al*. Endoscopic findings of radiation esophagitis in concurrent chemoradiotherapy for intrathoracic malignancies. *Radiother Oncol* 2001;58:273–278.

41. O'Morchoe PJ, Lee DC, Korak CA. Esophageal cytology in patients receiving Cytoxan drug therapy. *Acta Cytol* 1983; 27:630–634.

42. Kadayifci A, Gulsen MT, Koruk M, *et al*. Doxycycline-induced pill esophagitis. *Dis Esophagus* 2004;17:168–171.

43. Bott S, Prakash C, McCallum RW. Medication-induced esophageal injury: survey of the literature. *Am J Gastroenterol* 1987;82:758–763.

44. Jaspersen D. Drug-induced oesophageal disorders: pathogenesis, incidence, prevention and management. *Drug Saf* 2000;22:237–249.

45. de Groen PC, Lubbe DF, Hirsch LJ, *et al*. Esophagitis associated with the use of alendronate. *N Engl J Med* 1996;335: 1016–1021.

46. Zografos GN, Georgiadou D, Thomas D, *et al*. Drug-induced esophagitis. *Dis Esophagus* 2009;22:633-637.

47. Teplick JG, Teplick SK, Ominsky SH, *et al*. Esophagitis caused by oral medication. *Radiology* 1980;134:23-25.

48. Abraham SC, Cruz-Correa M, Lee LA, *et al*. Alendronate-associated esophageal injury: pathologic and endoscopic features. *Mod Pathol* 1999;12:1152–1157.

49. Singh SP, Odze RD. Multinucleated epithelial cell changes in esophagitis: a clinicopathologic study of 14 cases. *Am J Surg Pathol* 1998;22:93–99.

50. Hokama A, Ihama Y, Nakamoto M, *et al*. Esophagitis dissecans superficialis associated with bisphosphonates. *Endoscopy* 2007; 39:E91.

51. Symbas PN, Vlasis SE, Hatcher CR Jr. Esophagitis secondary to ingestion of caustic material. *Ann Thorac Surg* 1983;36:73–77.

52. de Jong AL, Macdonald R, Ein S, *et al*. Corrosive esophagitis in children : a 30-year review. *Int J Pediatr Otorhinolaryngol* 2001;57:203–211.

53. Furuta GT, Liacouras CA, Collins MH, *et al*. Eosinophilic esophagitis in children and adults: a systemic review and consensus recommendations for diagnosis and treatment. *Gastroenterology* 2007;133:1342–1363.

54. Müller S, Pühl S, Vieth M, *et al*. Analysis of symptoms and endoscopic findings in 117 patients with histological diagnoses of eosinophilic esophagitis. *Endoscopy* 2007;39:339–344.

55. Odze RD. Pathology of eosinophilic esophagitis: what the clinician needs to know. *Am J Gastroenterol* 2009;104:485–490.

56. Rubio CA, Sjödahl K, Lagergren J. Lymphocytic esophagitis: a histologic subset of chronic esophagitis. *Am J Clin Pathol* 2006; 125:432–437.

57. Purdy JK, Appelman HD, Golembeski CP, *et al*. A chronic or recurring pattern of esophagitis resembling allergic contact dermatitis. *Am J Clin Pathol* 2008;130:508–513.

58. Calka Ö, Akdeniz N, Tuncer I, *et al*. Oesophageal involvement during attacks in pemphigus vulgaris patients. *Clin Exp Dermatol* 2006;31:515–519.

59. Gomi H, Akiyama M, Yakabi K, *et al*. Oesophageal involvement in pemphigus vulgaris. *Lancet* 1999;354:1794.

60. Eng TY, Hogan WJ, Jordon RE. Oesophageal involvement in bullous pemphigoid. *Br J Dermatol* 1978;99:207–210.

61. Egan CA, Hanif N, Taylor TB, *et al*. Characterization of the antibody response in oesophageal cicatricial pemphigoid. *Br J Dermatol* 1999;140:859–864.

62. Chandan VS, Murray JA, Abraham SC. Esophageal lichen planus. *Arch Pathol Lab Med* 2008;132:1026–1029.

63. Dickens CM, Heseltine D, Walton S, *et al*. The oesophagus in lichen planus: an endoscopic study. *Br Med J* 1990;300:84.

64. Harewood GC, Murray JA, Cameron AJ. Esophageal lichen planus: the Mayo Clinic experience. *Dis Esophagus* 1999;12:309–311.

65. Keate RF, Williams JW, Connolly SM. Lichen planus esophagitis: report of three patients treated with oral tacrolimus or intraesophageal corticosteroid injection or both. *Dis Esophagus* 2003;16:47–53.

66. Liu X, McMahon J, Lai KK. Direct immunofluorescence in esophageal lichen planus. *Arch Pathol Lab Med* 2009;133:1627.

67. Ebert EC. Esophageal disease in Scleroderma. *J Clin Gastroenterol* 2006;40:769–775.

68. Cozzi F, Zucchetta P, Durigon N, *et al*. Changes in esophageal peristalsis in diverse clinical forms and antibody specificity in scleroderma: a scintigraphic study in 100 cases. *Reumatismo* 2003;55:86–92.

69. Weston S, Thumshirn M, Wiste J, *et al*. Clinical and upper gastrointestinal motility features in systemic sclerosis and related disorders. *Am J Gastroenterol* 1998;93:1085–1089.

70. Recht MP, Levine MS, Katzka DA, *et al*. Barrett's esophagus in scleroderma: increased prevalence and radiographic findings. *Gastrointest Radiol* 1988;13:1–5.

71. Pavletic SZ, Lee SJ, Socie G, *et al*. Chronic graft-versus-host disease: implications of the National Institutes of Health consensus development project on criteria for clinical trial. *Bone Marrow Transplant* 2006;38:645–651.

72. Nakshabendi IM, Maldonado ME, Coppola D, *et al*. Esophageal cast: a manifestation of graft-versus-host disease. *Dig Dis* 2000; 18:103–105.

73. McDonald GB, Sullivan KM, Schuffler MD, *et al*. Esophageal abnormalities in chronic graft-versus-host disease in humans. *Gastroenterology* 1981;80:914–921.

74. Shulman HM, Kleiner D, Lee SJ, *et al.* Histopathologic diagnosis of chronic graft-versus-host disease: National Institutes and Health Consensus Development Project on Criteria for Clinical Trials in Chronic Graft-versus-Host disease: II. Pathology Working Group Report. *Biol Blood Marrow Transplant* 2006; 12:31–47.

75. Nguyen T, Park JY, Scudiere JR, *et al.* Mycophenolic acid (cellcept and myofortic) induced injury of the upper GI tract. *Am J Surg Pathol* 2009;33:1355–1363.

76. Pettit M. Gastroesophageal reflux disease: clinical features. *Pharm World Sci* 2005;27:417–420.

77. Ronkainen J, Aro P, Storskrubb T, *et al.* High prevalence of gastroesophageal reflux symptoms and esophagitis with or without symptoms in the general adult Swedish population: A Kalixanda study report. *Scand J Gastroenterol* 2005;40:275–285.

78. Pope CE. Acid-reflux disorders. *N Engl J Med* 1994;331: 656–660.

79. Mittal RK, Balaban DH. The esophagogastric junction. *N Engl J Med* 1997;336:924–932.

80. Vaezi MF, Richter JR. Role of acid and duodenogastroesophageal reflux in gastroesophageal reflux disease. *Gastroenterology* 1996;111:1192–1199.

81. Wilson LJ, Ma W, Hirschowitz BI. Association of obesity with hiatal hernia and esophagitis. *Am J Gastroenterol* 1999;94: 2840–2844.

82. Knuff TE, Benjamin SB, Worsham GF, *et al.* Histologic evaluation of chronic gastroesophageal reflux: an evaluation of biopsy methods and diagnostic criteria. *Dig Dis Sci* 1984;29: 194–201.

83. Frierson HF. Histology in the diagnosis of reflux esophagitis. *Gastroenterol Clin North Am* 1990;19:631–644.

84. Hampel H, Abraham NS, El-Serag HB. Meta-analysis: obesity and the risk for gastroesophageal reflux disease and its complications. *Ann Intern Med* 2005;143:199–211.

85. MacDonald K, Porter GA, Guernsey DL, *et al.* A polymorphic variant of the insulin-like growth factor type 1 receptor gene modifies risk of obesity for esophageal adenocarcinoma. *Cancer Epidemiol* 2009;33:37–40.

86. Weinstein WM, Bogoch ER, Bowes KL. The normal human esophageal mucosa: a histological reappraisal. *Gastroenterology* 1975;68:40–44.

87. Levine DS, Blount PL, Rudolph RE, *et al.* Safety of a systemic endoscopic biopsy protocol in patients with Barrett's esophagus. *Am J Gastroenterol* 2000;95:1152–1157.

88. Ismail-Beigi F, Horton PF, Pope CE, *et al.* The histological consequences of gastroesophageal reflux in man. *Gastroenterology* 1970;58:163–174.

89. Johnson LF, DeMeester TR, Haggitt RC. Esophageal epithelial response to gastroesophageal reflux: a quantitative study. *Am J Dig Dis* 1978;23:498–509.

90. Haggitt RC. Histopathology of reflux-induced esophageal and supraesophageal injuries. *Am J Med* 2000;108 (Suppl 4A): 109S–111S.

91. Brown LF, Goldman H, Antonioli DA. Intraepithelial eosinophils in endoscopic biopsies of adults with reflux esophagitis. *Am J Surg Pathol* 1984;8:899–905.

92. Tummala V, Barwick KW, Sontag SJ, *et al.* The significance of intraepithelial eosinophils in the histologic diagnosis of gastroesophageal reflux. *Am J Clin Pathol* 1987;87:43–48.

93. Orenstein SR. Gastroesophageal reflux. *Curr Probl Pediatr* 1991;21:193–241.

94. Black DD, Haggitt RC, Orenstein SR, *et al.* Esophagitis in infants: morphometric histological diagnosis and correlation with measures of gastroesophageal reflux. *Gastroenterology* 1990;98:1408–1414.

95. Winter HS, Madara JL, Stafford RJ, *et al.* Intraepithelial eosinophils: a new diagnostic criterion for reflux esophagitis. *Gastroenterology* 1982;83:818–823.

96. Kelley K, Lazenby AJ, Rowe PC, *et al.* Eosinophilic esophagitis attributed to gastroesophageal reflux: improvement with an amino acid-based formula. *Gastroenterology* 1995;109:1503–1512.

97. Walsh SV, Antonioli DA, Goldman H, *et al.* Allergic esophagitis in children: a clinicopathologic entity. *Am J Surg Pathol* 1999; 23:390–396.

98. Lee RG. Marked eosinophilia in esophageal biopsies. *Am J Surg Pathol* 1985;9:475–479.

99. Mangano MM, Antonioli DA, Schnitt SJ, *et al.* Nature and significance of cells with irregular nuclear contours in esophageal mucosal biopsies. *Mod Pathol* 1992;5:191–196.

100. Wang HH, Mangano MM, Antonioli DA. Evaluation of T-lymphocytes in esophageal mucosal biopsies. *Mod Pathol* 1994;7:55–58.

101. Geboes K, Desmet V, Vantrappen G, *et al.* Vascular changes in the esophageal mucosa. An early histologic sign of esophagitis. *Gastrointest Endosc* 1980;26:29–32.

102. Collins BJ, Elliott H, Cloan JM, *et al.* Oesophageal histology in reflux esophagitis. *J Clin Pathol* 1985;38:1265–1272.

103. Haggitt RC, Tryzelaar J, Ellis FH, *et al.* Adenocarcinoma complicated columnar epithelial-lined (Barrett's) esophagus. *Am J Clin Pathol* 1978;7:1–5.

104. Pohl H, Welch HG. The role of overdiagnosis and reclassification in the marked increase of esophageal adenocarcinoma incidence. *J Natl Cancer Inst* 2005;97:142–146.

105. Wang KK, Sampliner RE. Updated guidelines 2008 for the diagnosis, surveillance and therapy of Barrett's esophagus. *Am J Gastroenterol* 2008;103:88–797.

106. Offner FA, Lewin KJ, Weinstein WM. Metaplastic columnar cells in Barrett's esophagus: a common and neglected cell type. *Hum Pathol* 1996;27:885–889.

107. Paull A, Trier JS, Dalton MD, *et al.* The histologic spectrum of Barrett's esophagus. *N Engl J Med* 1976;295:476–480.

108. Chandrasoma PT, Der R, Dalton P, *et al.* Distribution and significance of epithelial types in columnar-lined esophagus. *Am J Surg Pathol* 2001;25:1188–1193.

109. Weinstein WM, Ippoliti AF. The diagnosis of Barrett's esophagus. Goblets, goblets, goblets. *Gastrointest Endosc* 1996;44: 91–94.

110. Harrison R, Perry I, Haddadin W, *et al.* Detection of intestinal metaplasia in Barrett's esophagus: an observational comparator study suggests the need for a minimum of eight biopsies. *Am J Gastroenterol* 2007;102:1154–1161.

111. Goldblum JR. The significance and etiology of intestinal metaplasia of the esophagogastric junction. *Ann Diagn Pathol* 2002; 6:67–73.

112. Johnston MH, Hammond AS, Laskin W, *et al.* The p-revalence and clinical characteristics of short segments of specialized intestinal metaplasia in the distal esophagus on routine endoscopy. *Am J Gastroenterol* 1996;91:1507–1511.

113. Spechler SJ, Zeroogian JM, Antonioli DA, *et al.* Prevalence of metaplasia at the gastroesophageal junction. *Lancet* 1994;344: 1533–1536.

114. Oberg S, Peters JH, DeMeester TR, *et al.* Inflammation and specialized intestinal metaplasia of cardiac mucosa is a manifestation of gastroesophageal reflux disease. *Ann Surg* 1997;26: 522–532.

115. Hirota WK, Loughney TN, Lazas DJ, *et al.* Specialized intestinal metaplasia, dysplasia and cancer of the esophagus and esophagogastric junction: prevalence and clinical data. *Gastroenterology* 1999;116:277–285.

116. Morales TG, Sampliner RE, Bhattacharyya A. Intestinal metaplasia of the gastric cardia. *Am J Gastroenterol* 1997;92: 414–418.

117. Goldblum JR, Vicari JJ, Falk GW, *et al.* Inflammation and intestinal metaplasia of the gastric cardia: the role of gastroesophageal reflux and *H. pylori* infection. *Gastroenterology* 1998; 114:633–639.

118. Sharma P, Weston AP, Morales T, *et al.* Relative risk of dysplasia for patients with intestinal metaplasia in the distal oesophagus and in the gastric cardia. *Gut* 2000;46:9–13.

119. Morales TG, Camargo E, Bhattacharyya A, *et al.* Long-term follow-up of intestinal metaplasia of the gastric cardia. *Am J Gastroenterol* 2000;95:1677–1680.

120. Srivastava A, Odze RD, Lauwers GY, *et al.* Morphologic features are useful in distinguishing Barrett esophagus from carditis with intestinal metaplasia. *Am J Surg Pathol* 2007;31: 1733–1741.

121. Ormsby AH, Goldblum JR, Rice TW, *et al.* Cytokeratin subsets can reliably distinguish Barrett's esophagus from intestinal metaplasia of the stomach. *Hum Pathol* 1999;30:288–294.

122. Ormsby AH, Vaezi MF, Richter JE, *et al.* Cytokeratin immunoreactivity patterns in the diagnosis of short-segment Barrett's esophagus. *Gastroenterology* 2000;119:682–690.

123. Couvelard A, Cauvin J-M, Goldfain D, *et al.* Cytokeratin immunoreactivity of intestinal metaplasia of the normal oesophagogastric junction indicates its aetiology. *Gut* 2001;49: 761–766.

124. White N, Gabril M, Ejeckam G, *et al.* Barrett's esophagus and cardiac intestinal metaplasia: two conditions within the same spectrum. *Can J Gastroenterol* 2008;22:369–375.

125. Corley DA, Levin TR, Habel LA, *et al.* Surveillance and survival in Barrett's adenocarcinoma: a population-based study. *Gastroenterology* 2002;122:633–640.

126. Incarbone R, Bonavina L, Saino G, *et al.* Outcome of esophageal adenocarcinoma detected during endoscopic biopsy surveillance for Barrett's esophagus. *Surg Endosc* 2002;16: 263–266.

127. Weston AP, Badr AS, Hassanein RS. Prospective multivariate analysis of clinical, endoscopic, and histological factors predictive of the development of Barrett's multifocal high-grade dysplasia or adenocarcinoma. *Am J Gastroenterol* 1999;94: 3413–3419.

128. Smith RR, Hamilton SR, Boitnoit JK, *et al.* The spectrum of carcinoma arising in Barrett's esophagus: a clinicopathologic study of 26 patients. *Am J Surg Pathol* 1984;8:563–573.

129. Montgomery E, Bronner MP, Goldblum JR, *et al.* Reproducibility of the diagnosis of dysplasia in Barrett esophagus: a reaffirmation. *Hum Pathol* 2001;32:368–378.

130. Hanna S, Rastogi A, Weston AP, *et al.* Detection of Barrett's esophagus after endoscopic healing for erosive esophagitis. *Am J Gastroenterol* 2006;101:1416–1420.

131. Riddell RH, Goldman H, Ransohoff DF, *et al.* Dysplasia in inflammatory bowel disease: standardized classification with provisional clinical applications. *Hum Pathol* 1983;14:931–968.

132. Reid BJ, Haggitt RC, Rubin CE, *et al.* Observer variation in the diagnosis of dysplasia in Barrett's esophagus. *Hum Pathol* 1988; 19:166–178.

133. Goldblum JR, Lauwers GY. Dysplasia arising in barrett's esophagus: diagnostic pitfalls and natural history. *Semin Diagn Pathol* 2002;19:12–19.

134. Rastogi A, Puli S, El-Serag HB, *et al.* Incidence of esophageal adenocarcinoma in patients with Barrett's' esophagus and high-grade dysplasia: a meta-analysis. *Gastrointest Endosc* 2008; 67:394–398.

135. Konda V, Ross AS, Ferguson MK, *et al.* Is the risk of concomitant invasive esophageal cancer in high grade dysplasia in Barrett's esophagus overestimated? *Clin Gastroenterol Hepatol* 2008;6:159–164.

136. Reid BJ, Blount P, Feng Z, *et al.* Optimizing endoscopic biopsy detection of early cancers in Barrett's high-grade dysplasia. *Am J Gastroenterol* 2000;95:3089–3096.

137. Buttar NS, Wang KK, Sebo TJ, *et al.* Extent of high-grade dysplasia in Barrett's esophagus correlates with risk of adenocarcinoma. *Gastroenterology* 2001;120:1630–1639.

138. Sabik JF, Rice TW, Goldblum JR, *et al.* Superficial esophageal carcinoma. *Ann Thorac Surg* 1995;60:896–901.

139. Ormsby AH, Petras RE, Henricks WH, *et al.* Observer variation in the diagnosis of superficial esophageal adenocarcinoma. *Gut* 2002;51:671–676.

140. Downs-Kelly E, Mendelin JE, Bennett AE, *et al.* Poor interobserver agreement in the distinction of high-grade dysplasia and adenocarcinoma in pretreatment Barrett's esophagus biopsies. *Am J Gastroenterol* 2008;103:2333–2340.

141. Zhu W, Appelman HD, Greenson JK, *et al.* A histologically defined subset of high-grade dysplasia in Barrett mucosa is predictive of associated carcinoma. *Am J Clin Pathol* 2009;132: 94–100.

142. Fernando HC, Murthy SC, Hofstetter W, *et al.* The Society of Thoracic Surgeons practice guideline series: Guidelines for the management of Barrett's esophagus with high-grade dysplasia. *Ann Thorac Surg* 2009;87:1993–2002.

143. Nijhawan PK, Wang KK. Endoscopic mucosal resection for lesions with endoscopic features suggestive of malignancy and high–grade dysplasia within Barrett's esophagus. *Gastrointest Endosc* 2000;52:328–332.

144. Odze RD, Lauwers GY. Histopathology of Barrett's esophagus after ablation and endoscopic mucosal resection therapy. *Endoscopy* 2008;40:1008–1015.

145. Lewis JT, Wang KK, Abraham SC. Muscularis mucosae duplication and the musculo-fibrous anomaly in endoscopic mucosal resections for barrett esophagus: implications for staging of adenocarcinoma. *Am J Surg Pathol* 2008;32: 566–571.

146. Peters FP, Brakenhoff KP, Curvers WL, *et al.* Histologic evaluation of resection specimens obtained at 293 endoscopic resections in Barrett's esophagus. *Gastrointest Endosc* 2008;67: 604–609.

147. Mino-Kenudson M, Brugge WR, Puricelli WP, *et al.* Management of superficial Barrett's epithelium–related neoplasms by endoscopic mucosal resection: clinicopathologic analysis of 27 cases. *Am J Surg Pathol* 2005;29:680–686.

148. Gossner L, Stolte M, Sroka R, *et al.* Photodynamic ablation of high-grade dysplasia and early cancer in Barrett's esophagus by means of 5-aminolevulinic acid. *Gastroenterology* 1998;114:448–455.

149. Ban S, Mino M, Nishioka NS, *et al.* Histopathologic aspects of photodynamic therapy for dysplasia and early adenocarcinoma arising in Barrett's esophagus. *Am J Surg Pathol* 2004;28:1466–1473.

150. Sharma VK, Wang KK, Overholt BF, *et al.* Balloon–based, circumferential, endoscopic radiofrequency ablation of Barrett's esophagus: 1-year follow–up of 100 patients. *Gastrointest Endosc* 2007;65:185–195.

151. Sharma VK, Kim HJ, Das A, *et al.* A prospective pilot trial of ablation of Barrett's esophagus with low–grade dysplasia using stepwise circumferential and focal ablation (HALO system). *Endoscopy* 2008;40:380–387.

152. Gondrie JJ, Pouw RE, Sondermeijer CM, *et al.* Stepwise circumferential and focal ablation of Barrett's esophagus with high-grade dysplasia: results of the first prospective series of 11 patients. *Endoscopy* 2008;40:359–369.

153. Shaheen NJ, Sharma P, Overholt BF, *et al.* Radiofrequency ablation in Barrett's esophagus with dysplasia. *N Engl J Med* 2009;360:2277–2288.

154. Robey SS, Hamilton SR, Gupta P, *et al.* Diagnostic value of cytopathology in Barrett esophagus and associated adenocarcinoma. *Am J Clin Pathol* 1988;89:493–498.

155. Geisinger KR, Teot LA, Richter JE. A comparative cytopathologic and histologic study of atypia, dysplasia and adenocarcinoma in Barrett's esophagus. *Cancer* 1992;69:8–16.

156. Wang HH, Sovie S, Zeroogian JM, *et al.* Value of cytology detecting intestinal metaplasia and associated dysplasia at the gastroesophageal junction. *Hum Pathol* 1997;28:465–471.

157. Shurbaji M, Erozan YS. The cytopathologic diagnosis of esophageal adenocarcinoma. *Acta Cytol* 1991;35:189–194.

158. Wang HH, Doria MI, Purohit-Buch S, *et al.* Barrett's esophagus: the cytology of dysplasia and comparison to benign and malignant lesions. *Acta Cytol* 1992;36:60–64.

159. Fennerty MB, Ditomasso J, Morales T, *et al.* Screening for Barrett's esophagus by balloon cytology. *Am J Gastroenterol* 1995;90:1230–1232.

160. Trivers KF, Sabatino SA, Stewart SL. Trends in esophageal cancer incidence by histology, United States, 1998–2003. *Int J Cancer* 2008;123:1422–1428.

161. Ruol A, Castoro C, Portale G, *et al.* Trends in management and prognosis for esophageal cancer surgery: twenty five years of experience at a single institution. *Arch Surg* 2009;144:247–254.

162. Bellizzi AM, Woodford RL, Moskaluk CA, *et al.* Basaloid squamous cell carcinoma of the esophagus: assessment for high-risk human papillomavirus and related molecular markers. *Am J Surg Pathol* 2009;33:1608–1614.

163. Tajiri H, Muto M, Boku N, *et al.* Verrucous carcinoma of the esophagus completely resected by endoscopy. *Am J Gastroenterol* 2000;95:1076–1077.

164. Malik AB, Bidani JA, Rich HG, *et al.* Long-term survival in a patient with verrucous carcinoma of the esophagus. *Am J Gastroenterol* 1996;91:1031–1033.

165. Roth MJ, Liu SF, Dawsy SM, *et al.* Cytologic detection of esophageal squamous cell carcinoma and precursor lesions using balloon and sponge samplers in asymptomatic adults in Linxian, China. *Cancer* 1997;84:2047–2059.

166. Briggs JC, Ibrahim NBN. Oat cell carcinoma of the esophagus: a clinicopathologic study of 23 cases. *Histopathology* 1983;7:261–277.

167. Bennouna J, Bardet E, Deguiral P, *et al.* Small cell carcinoma of the esophagus: analysis of 10 cases and review of the published data. *Am J Clin Oncol* 2000;23:455–459.

168. Chen KTK. Cytology in small-cell carcinoma arising in Barrett's esophagus. *Diagn Cytopathol* 2000;23:180–182.

169. Coté TR, Sobin LH. Primary melanomas of the esophagus and anorectum: epidemiologic comparison with melanoma of the skin. *Melanoma Res* 2009;19:58–60.

170. Sanchez AA, Wu TT, Prieto VG, *et al.* Comparison of primary and metastatic malignant melanoma of the esophagus: clinicopathologic review of 10 cases. *Arch Pathol Lab Med* 2008;132:1623–1629.

III

Motility Disorders

13 Achalasia

Joel E. Richter[1] and Jason R. Roberts[2]

[1]Division of Digestive Diseases and Nutrition,University of South Florida, Tampa, FL, USA
[2]Division of Gastroenterology and Hepatology, Medical University of South Carolina, Charleston, SC, USA

Introduction

Achalasia is an esophageal disorder of unknown cause characterized by aperistalsis of the esophageal body and impaired relaxation of the lower esophageal sphincter (LES). Although uncommon, any individual specializing in esophageal diseases sees this disease with some frequency. The history is usually classic and the diagnosis easily made with a combination of barium esophagram and esophageal manometry. These patients generally have few comorbid illnesses, and their dysphagia and bland regurgitation respond well to a number of treatment modalities, including pneumatic dilatation, surgical myotomy, or drugs.

Historical perspectives

The first case of achalasia was described in 1674 by Sir Thomas Willis, an English anatomist, who described a network of arteries at the base of the brain (circle of Willis) and the 11th cranial nerve (spinal accessory nerve, or nerve of Willis). In his description of a patient with achalasia, he noted, "the mouth of the stomach (i.e. cardia) being always closed either by tumour or palsie, nothing could be admitted into the ventricle (i.e. stomach) unless it was violently opened." The patient was treated with a primitive but effective dilator made from a whale bone with a small sponge at the tip. Over the next 15 years, the patient did well while performing post-prandial dilations to force his food into the stomach [1].

Achalasia has been known by a variety of names, including simple ectasia, cardiospasm, megaesophagus, diffuse dilatation of the esophagus without stenosis, and idiopathic dilatation of the esophagus. In 1881, Von Mikulicz suggested that spasm of the esophagus (i.e. cardiospasm) was the etiologic cause of achalasia [2]. Hurst and Rake in 1929, aware of the ease with which bougies could be passed into the stomach of patients with achalasia, questioned the spasm concept. Instead, they coined the term achalasia, derived from a Greek word for "lack of relaxation" because they believed the LES was unable to open normally [3].

It is humbling to admit that the current treatments of achalasia, balloon dilation and surgical myotomy, are techniques that, although extensively modified, have nevertheless been used for more than a century. In 1898, Russel was the first to report success using a bag, or pneumatic, dilator made from a sausage-shaped silk bag containing a rubber bag. The rubber bag was connected to a hollow tube, which was inserted into the esophagus across the LES and inflated with air or water [4]. Nearly all the surgical techniques for treating achalasia were developed in 20th century Germany. The most important operation, the long cardiomyotomy, was first described by Ernst Heller in 1914 when he was a senior surgical assistant at the University Surgical Clinic in Leipzig, Germany. His first patient was a 49-year-old man with a 30-year history of dysphagia, whose distal esophagus and cardia, at operation, reminded him of the multiple cases of pyloric stenosis that he had so often fixed with a simple pyloromyotomy. Heller's technique involved mobilizing the distal half of the esophagus completely and incising the muscular coat through to the mucosa. His incision was 8 cm in length and distally went just over the gastroesophageal junction (GEJ), and omentum was placed into the defect to maintain separation of the muscle layers. Seven years after the original procedure, his patient continued to do well [5].

Epidemiology

Achalasia is a disease that occurs with equal frequency among men and women. Case studies show an age

The Esophagus, Fifth Edition. Edited by Joel E. Richter, Donald O. Castell.
© 2012 Blackwell Publishing Ltd. Published 2012 by Blackwell Publishing Ltd.

distribution between birth and the ninth decade of life, but it occurs rarely during the first two decades of life. The mean ages for achalasia patients in case studies range between 30 and 60 years, with some studies suggesting an increased incidence with age, particularly after the seventh decade [6]. In children, achalasia is part of the Triple A syndrome, characterized by achalasia, alacrima, and adrenocorticotrophic hormone-resistant adrenal insufficiency.

Achalasia is an uncommon disease, but it is frequent enough to be encountered at least yearly by most gastroenterologists and esophageal surgeons. The disease prevalence is approximately 10 cases per 100 000 population. Its incidence has been fairly stable over the last 50 years at about 0.5 cases per 100 000 population per year. There are, however, striking international differences: achalasia is more common in North America, north-western Europe, and New Zealand, with a reported incidence between 0.6 and 1.0, and it is rare in Singapore and Zimbabwe, where its incidence is fewer than 0.3 per 100 000 population per year [7, 8]. There is some evidence from human leukocyte antigen (HLA) studies that whites are at a greater risk than blacks [9, 10]. However, these data are relatively crude, with most published studies being retrospective, based on hospital records, and using less than optimal methods for diagnosing achalasia, such as X-ray studies rather than esophageal manometry—all these techniques are likely to underestimate the true frequency of the disease [7]. The only prospective review of the epidemiology of achalasia was performed in Edinburgh, Scotland [11]. This study was conducted over a 5-year period and included only cases in which a manometric diagnosis of achalasia was made. Twenty men and 18 women presented throughout adult life with a mean age at the time of diagnosis of 44 years (range 17–76 years). The annual incidence was 0.8 cases per 100 000 population, comparable to other retrospective studies from the British Isles. Although associated with complications, the one available study shows that the causes of death and general life-expectancy of patients with achalasia do not differ from those of the average population [12].

Pathophysiology

Neuropathology

A wide variety of pathologic abnormalities have been described in patients with achalasia [13]. Some of these changes may be primary (i.e. loss of ganglion cells and myenteric inflammation), whereas others (i.e. degenerative changes in the vagus nerve and dorsal motor nucleus of the vagus as well as mucosa and muscle changes) are likely secondary phenomena caused by long-standing esophageal obstruction and stasis. Probably as a result of vagal damage, other organs outside the esophagus may be involved in achalasia.

Abnormalities of extrinsic innervation

The vagal efferent nerves, with their cell bodies in the dorsal motor nucleus (DMN) of the vagus, initiate and modulate LES relaxation and esophageal peristalsis in response to swallows [14]. By light microscopy, vagal fibers from the esophagus appear normal in achalasia patients. However, Cassella *et al.* performed electron microscopic studies and found evidence of wallerian degeneration of the vagus nerve with disintegration of the axoplasm changes in Schwann cells, and degeneration of the myelin sheath, which are characteristic of experimental nerve transection [15]. In meticulous dissection studies of the brain, both Kimura *et al.* [16] and Cassella *et al.* [17] described degeneration and absolute reduction of the number of DMN neurons in four patients with advanced achalasia. It is plausible that these lesions in the DMN or vagus nerve are pathologic, because bilateral lesions in the cat DMN can produce dysfunction resembling achalasia [18]. However, these changes were not invariably present (absent in one patient), and, unlike the pathologic changes in the myenteric plexus, were not associated with an inflammatory cell infiltration. It is likely that these changes in the vagus nerve and DMN are secondary phenomena, and as such they are not required for expression of the disease.

Abnormalities of intrinsic innervation

Nitrergic neurons within the myenteric plexus mediate inhibition along the esophageal body and LES that occurs at the onset of swallowing. This inhibition is crucial in producing an aborally increasing latency of contractions along the esophagus, resulting in peristalsis and relaxation of the LES. In classic achalasia, the intrinsic inhibitory esophageal nervous system is selectively damaged with inflammation and loss of ganglion cells within the myenteric (Auerbach's) plexus. This was first reported by Lendrum in a detailed autopsy study of 13 patients with cardiospasm and marked esophageal dilatation; he reported a 20-fold decrease in the number of ganglion cells per plexus [19]. In the most comprehensive study to date, Goldblum *et al.* examined 42 resected esophagi from patients with advanced disease [20]. In all cases, myenteric ganglion cells were markedly diminished in number, with 20 specimens having none. Inflammation of varying intensity was present in the myenteric nerves of all specimens, consisting primarily of lymphocytes and eosinophils, with a small number of plasma and mast cells. In addition, all cases had collagen deposition within the myenteric plexus. Subsequently, Goldblum *et al.* reported on the histopathologic features in esophagomyotomy specimens from 11 patients with less advanced disease [21]. As in the endstage cases, myenteric plexus inflammation was present in all cases, with most cells staining positive with Leu-22, a pan T-cell lymphocyte marker. Ganglion cells were absent or markedly decreased in eight of the 11 patients (all with classic achalasia by manometry), and the extent of ganglion cell loss correlated inversely with the degree of

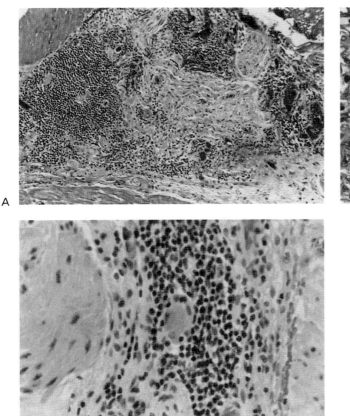

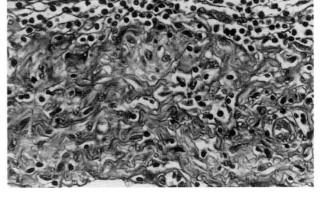

Figure 13.1 (A) Myenteric plexus from patient with classic achalasia showing rare ganglion cells and increased lymphocytic inflammation. (B) High-magnification view of a trichome-stained section from a patient with classic achalasia. This nerve is markedly scarred and a small amount of residual lymphocytic inflammation is seen both within and surrounding the residual nerve (reproduced courtesy of John Goldblum MD).

(C) High-magnification view of myenteric plexus from a patient with vigorous achalasia showing moderate degree of inflammation, predominantly lymphocytic, surrounding both myenteric nerves (left) and ganglion cells (center). In this case, a normal number of ganglion cells was seen and there was minimal fibrous scarring (reproduced courtesy of John Goldblum MD).

myenteric fibrosis (Figure 13.1A, B). Interestingly, the three patients with normal ganglion cell numbers all had manometric criteria of vigorous achalasia with minimal esophageal dilatation (Figure 13.1C). Two earlier studies had also noted a small number of patients with early-stage disease, characterized by non-dilated esophagus or short symptom duration, and a normal number of ganglion cells within the myenteric plexus [17, 22]. A complimentary study by Gockel *et al.* showed a greater reduction in CD117-staining interstitial cells of Cajal (ICC) in patients with longer duration of symptoms and fewer neuronal nitric oxide synthase (NOS) cells in patients with more severe dysphagia scores [23]. Taken together, these studies suggest that an inflammatory process involving the myenteric plexus is present in the early stages of achalasia, and only later over years is there a loss of ganglion cells and myenteric fibrosis. Along with the destruction of ganglion cells, there is also reduction in intermediary ICC, and in the nerve fibers within the walls of the achalasia esophagus [24].

Immunohistochemical studies have provided insight into the neurotransmitter content of affected myenteric plexus nerves in achalasia. Nitric oxide (NO) is the primary esophageal inhibitory neurotransmitter with subsequent studies confirming that intrinsic nitrergic neurons are either lost or markedly diminished in achalasia [25, 26] (Figure 13.2). Perhaps an earlier phenomenon is down regulation of NOS in nitrergic neurons. This idea was proposed after observing that incubating sera from achalasia patients on *ex vivo* human fundic tissue resulted in a significant reduction in the immunoreactivity of NOS compared to controls. This phenotypic change was accompanied by altered electrical field stimulation-induced relaxation, reported as a decrease in the area under the curve [27]. They also found an increase in the immune reactivity of acetylcholinesterase neurons in the same fundic specimens following incubation with sera from achalasia patients. Loss of intrinsic neuropeptide Y immunoreactive nerves has also been reported in achalasia [25], but the functional significance of this is unknown.

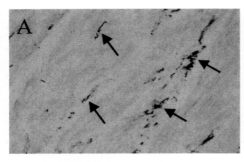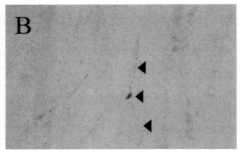

Figure 13.2 Immunostaining for NADPH diaphorase (which stains NO synthase) from the lower esophageal sphincter in (A) a control subject and (B) patients with achalasia. There is abundant labeling of NADPH diaphorase nerve profiles in the control section (arrows), but near absence of labeling in achalasia patients (arrowheads) (reproduced from DeGiorgio et al. [25], with permission).

In addition to ganglion cells in the myenteric plexus, other cell bodies are affected in achalasia. ICC are stellate mesenchymal cells located within the circular and longitudinal muscle layers of the gastrointestinal tract. First described by Spanish neuroanatomist Santiago Ramon y Cajal in the early 20th century, these cells have dentritic processes that allow for communication with smooth muscle cells [28]. Experiments by Ward et al. using a murine model concluded that ICC play an important role in facilitating NO-dependent hyperpolarization and relaxation of the LES [29]. The intermediary function of ICC in smooth muscle is further supported by the structural arrangement of smooth muscle cells, ICC, and NO containing inhibitory nerve terminals [30]. Using immunohistochemical staining for CD117 (ICC) and n-NOS (NO nerve terminals), Gockel et al. demonstrated a strong correlation (r = 0.781; $P < .0001$) in the reduction of these two cell types in the LES specimens from patients with achalasia [23]. Whether reduced numbers of ICC in achalasia is a primary or secondary phenomenon and the pathophysiologic impact remain unclear (see Figure 13.1).

Abnormalities of esophageal smooth muscle

The muscularis propria, especially the circular smooth muscle, is usually thickened in patients with achalasia. Goldblum et al. described in detail the various muscular abnormalities in patients with advanced achalasia undergoing esophagectomy [21]. Muscular hypertrophy was present in all cases, and 79% of specimens had evidence of muscle degeneration, usually involving fibrosis but also including liquefactive necrosis, vacuolar changes, and dystrophic calcification. Nearly half of the specimens also had eosinophilia of the muscularis propria. The authors speculated that the degenerative changes were caused by the muscles outgrowing their blood supply due to long-standing obstruction and esophageal dilatation. Another possibility was that muscle hypertrophy is a reaction to loss of innervation [31]. In a complimentary paper by Gockel et al., the muscular pathology, including hypertrophy, was more commonly found in patients with symptoms for more than 10 years and

advanced disease requiring esophagectomies [32] (see Figure 13.2).

Abnormalities of esophageal mucosa

Mucosal abnormalities, presumably secondary to chronic luminal stasis, have been described in achalasia. In another series from Goldblum's group, squamous alterations in 35 esophagectomy specimens from patients with endstage achalasia were compared with the squamous mucosa near the GEJ from pediatric autopsies (younger than 18 years of age) and from patients with no esophageal disease [33]. In all cases, the squamous mucosa from the achalasia patients was markedly hyperplastic with papillomatosis and basal cell hyperplasia. In addition, p53 staining in the squamous mucosa was seen in nearly all specimens and CD3+ cells (pan T-cell marker) always far outnumbered CD20+ cells (pan B-cell markers). These latter changes have clinical significance in that chronic inflammation may be related to the increased risk of squamous cell carcinoma in these patients. A series by Kjellin et al. analyzed distal esophageal biopsies obtained from non-consecutive patients with achalasia as part of their routine clinical care [34]. Thirty-eight percent of patients (10 of 26) had abnormal findings on biopsies with only four reporting heartburn. Six patients with abnormal biopsies had previously been treated with either Heller myotomy or balloon dilation, which is known to increase the frequency of gastroesophageal reflux disease (GERD). These data bring into question when in the natural history of achalasia do mucosal changes occur, if at all, and by what mechanism. Certainly the answers to these questions could impact the management of the disease, as endoscopy and histologic examination of the mucosa are not routinely recommended.

Abnormalities outside the smooth muscle esophagus

Striated muscle function in the proximal esophagus and upper esophageal sphincter (UES) may be impaired in achalasia patients. Although peristalsis is intact in the striated muscle, the amplitude of contractions may be diminished [35]. Massey *et al.* reported that the belch reflex was impaired in achalasia patients with an increase, rather than decrease, in UES pressure and rapid infusion of air into the esophagus [36]. This impairment may contribute to the massive esophageal dilatation and acute airway obstruction occasionally reported in patients with achalasia [37].

Motility abnormalities in the gallbladder [38], small intestine [39], and sphincter of Oddi [40] have rarely been reported in achalasia patients, but their clinical significance is unknown. On the other hand, abnormalities of stomach function have been reported in up to 50% of achalasia patients. Reported pathologic abnormalities include decreased myenteric ganglion cells [20], a loss of NADPH diaphorase (a marker for NO synthase) neural staining [25] in the proximal stomach, and loss of ganglion cells and myenteric plexus inflammation in the mid stomach [22]. These findings are consistent with the loss of inhibitory innervation to the proximal stomach, which, in some achalasia patients, has been associated with rapid gastric emptying of liquid [41] and abnormal fundic relaxation [42]. Lastly, sensory and extrinsic autonomic nervous system dysfunction has been described in some patients with achalasia [43].

Neurophysiologic abnormalities

Studies from isolated LES muscle strips from achalasia patients suggest that the absence of ganglionic inhibitory stimulation results in unopposed LES contractions [44]. Similarly, during electrical field stimulation, Tottrup *et al.* observed contractions rather than relaxation of circular muscle strips from achalasia patients, whereas stimulation of the longitudinal muscle in these patients and in control subjects resulted in relaxation [45]. Further evidence of denervation is supported by the abnormal response to various drugs in achalasia patients when compared with healthy volunteers. For example, cholecystokinin, which normally causes LES relaxation, produces a paradoxical increase in sphincter pressure in achalasia patients [46]. This can be explained by the observation that cholecystokinin receptors are present on both intrinsic inhibitory nerves (to cause relaxation) and circular smooth muscle of the LES (to cause contractions). Normally, activation of inhibitory neurons predominates, promoting LES relaxation, but if they are destroyed or dysfunctional, the direct excitatory effect on the muscle predominates. Also, in keeping with the loss of intrinsic inhibitory innervation, the LES in achalasia patients has been reported to be supersensitive (i.e. denervation hypersensitivity) to intravenous gastrin [47], intravenous vasoactive intestinal polypeptide (VIP) [48], or an NO donor [49], and intravenous acetylcholine [44, 50]. The latter drug, in the form of the Mecholyl test, was used in the past to help diagnose achalasia with an injection, which resulted in a marked increase in esophageal and LES baseline pressure with spontaneous contractions and retrosternal pain [50].

On the other hand, morphine and secretin decrease LES pressure in achalasia patients, although the degree may be greater than that noted in healthy control subjects [51]. Finally, consistent with the muscle strip studies, Holloway *et al.* found evidence *in vivo* that post-ganglionic cholinergic innervation was either normal or only minimally impaired in achalasia patients [52]. These conclusions were based on the observations that atropine significantly decreased resting LES pressure in achalasia patients similar to that in control subjects, and edrophonium, by promoting the availability of acetylcholine, increased LES pressure.

Several novel human studies give a better understanding of the abnormalities in peristalsis seen in achalasia patients and the important role of NO. Using a partially inflated esophageal balloon to measure esophageal inhibition during primary peristalsis, Sifrim *et al.* noted absent or impaired initial inhibition in patients with achalasia [53]. It is known from animal studies that this initial inhibition is mediated by intrinsic nitrergic innervation. The generation of secondary peristalsis in response to balloon distention is also impaired in patients with achalasia. In healthy subjects, balloon distention in the mid esophagus produces contractions above the balloon and inhibition in both the esophageal body below and the LES. In achalasia patients, balloon distention-induced relaxation is markedly impaired and paradoxical contractions are often recorded below the balloon in the esophageal body, but contractions in the smooth muscle esophagus above the balloon are maintained [54]. From animal studies, the distal esophageal response is consistent with a loss of intrinsic inhibitory neurons, whereas the proximal contractions are maintained because they involve vagal cholinergic mechanisms [55]. Finally, Murray *et al.*, in a serendipitous experiment, noted that the infusion of synthetic recombinant human hemoglobin, which is known to bind and inactivate NO, caused impairment in LES relaxation, simultaneous swallow-induced contractions, and sometimes chest pain when infused in human volunteers [56]. This pattern was identical to the manometric findings in achalasia, confirming the critical role of NO in promoting normal LES relaxation and peristalsis.

Lastly, Singarum *et al.* have created an opossum model of achalasia by destroying the esophageal myenteric plexus using benzalkonium compounds [57]. The LES of these esophagi were unresponsive to infused arginine and showed a decrease in NADPH diaphorase activity, but an increase in cholinergic nerve bundles, suggesting greater cholinergic input in the face of a markedly damaged NO system, which resulted in a hypertensive LES [57, 58].

Etiology

Pathologic and pathophysiologic studies strongly point to an inflammatory injury to the myenteric plexus as the crucial insult in achalasia. The underlying cause is unknown and remains an area of intense interest and speculation. Available data have suggested hereditary, infectious, autoimmune, and degenerative factors as possible causes of achalasia.

Genetic theory

Reports of achalasia occurring in family members has led to the suggestion that achalasia might be inherited. Familial achalasia probably accounts for only 1–2% of the achalasia population [59, 60]. Fewer than 100 familial achalasia cases have been reported, with many being linked to consanguinity. Most reported familial cases are horizontally transmitted, occurring in the pediatric age group, and between siblings and even monozygotic twins [59–62]. With an early childhood presentation, usually before age 5 years, associated anomalies can occur, including adrenocorticotropic hormone insensitivity, alacrima (lack of tears), microcephaly, Sjögren's syndrome, short stature, nerve deafness, vitiligo, hyperlipoproteinemia, and autonomic and motor neuropathy [61]. The mode of inheritance is most likely autosomal recessive, with full penetrance in the homozygote form. In a linkage study, the gene for the triple A syndrome was localized to chromosome 12q13 near the type II keratin gene cluster [63]. Five vertically transmitted cases of achalasia have been reported, with these being in children of both sexes and their father or mother [2, 64–66]. Unlike the horizontally transmitted cases, these cases present at an older age (range 37–72 years, mean age 56 years). On the other hand, the rarity of a hereditary form of achalasia was noted in a survey of 1012 first-degree relatives of 159 patients with achalasia, including 447 siblings and 247 children, among whom not a single case was found [67]. According to mendelian principles, if achalasia were an autosomal recessive disorder, 112 of the 447 siblings would be affected.

Infectious theory

Epidemiologic studies demonstrate geographic variations in the prevalence of achalasia that might be caused by infectious or environmental factors. Implicated factors include bacteria (diphtheria pertussis, clostridia, tuberculosis, and syphilis), viruses (herpes, varicella zoster, polio, and measles), toxic agents (combat gas), esophageal trauma, and ischemic esophageal damage *in utero* during gut rotation [68]. The strongest evidence to date suggests that a neurotropic infectious agent could be the involved etiologic factor. First, the specific localization of the disease to the esophagus and the fact that the esophagus is the only part of the gut where a smooth muscle is covered by squamous epithelium make it plausible that certain infectious agents with an affinity for squamous mucosa could be involved [69]. The herpes viruses, for example, have a predilection for squamous mucosa but rarely involve the columnar mucosa of the gastrointestinal tract [69, 70]. Furthermore, an infectious agent, *Trypanosoma cruzi*, can cause a form of achalasia that has

many of the features seen in idiopathic achalasia [71]. Second, the T-cell lymphocytic infiltrate seen in achalasia could be explained by an infectious process, particularly those caused by neurotropic viruses [72]. Third, serologic studies in achalasia patients, compared with age- and gender-matched control subjects, show an association with measles and varicella zoster viruses [70, 73]. Additionally, a case report identified a patient with varicella infection who soon afterward developed achalasia [74].

The major argument against an infectious etiology has been the general failure to demonstrate an infectious agent in tissue samples from achalasia patients. Robertson *et al.*, using *in situ* DNA hybridization, demonstrated varicella zoster virus—DNA in esophageal tissue obtained at cardiomyotomy, in three of nine achalasia patients but in none of the 20 controls [70]. However, using more advanced methodology, including polymerase chain reaction techniques, the Cleveland Clinic group and others failed to find evidence of DNA or RNA from a variety of human viruses, including herpes simplex, measles, cytomegalovirus, Epstein–Barr, varicella zoster, and human papilloma virus [75–77]. On the other hand, looking for viral nuclear elements may be an insensitive approach in linking remote viral infection to the immunologic insult in achalasia. An illustrative example of this principle is a study where trigeminal neuritis induced in rabbits resulted in recovery of HSV-1 DNA in only 10% of ganglion cells [78]. The number of myenteric ganglion cells in achalasia specimens is known to be significantly reduced or absent by the time patients present with clinical symptoms. If the number of ganglion cells harboring latent virus is similar to that of trigeminal neuritis following an immune reaction, recovery of viral DNA may be a difficult endeavor. In experiments carried out by Castagliuolo *et al.*, lymphocytes from patients with achalasia showed a 3.4-fold increased proliferation in response to HSV-1 antigen and secretion of interferon-gamma (IFN-γ) compared to controls [77]. If an immune-mediated ganglionitis is triggered by HSV-1, the mere presence of the virus is perhaps neither necessary nor sufficient. However, the antigen-specific activation of clonal T cells gives both a link and a mechanism for the disease. One of the more informative investigations to date in supporting HSV-1 as an etiologic candidate of achalasia is the study by Facco *et al.* [79]. They analyzed and compared the T-cell receptor RNA from lymphocytes isolated from the LES of both patients with achalasia and controls with their respective, peripherally circulating lymphocytes. Their findings included a greater lymphocytic infiltration in patients, and lymphocytes from achalasia patients had a greater proliferation index and released significantly more IFN-γ with exposure to HSV-1 antigen [79].

Autoimmune theory

Evidence of an autoimmune etiology for achalasia comes from several sources. First, the inflammatory response in the esophageal myenteric plexus is usually dominated by T lymphocytes, which are known to be involved in autoimmune diseases [20]. Second, a higher prevalence of certain class II histocompatibility antigens, which are known to be associated with other autoimmune disorders, have been reported in achalasia. Wong *et al.* reported a higher than expected prevalence of the DQw1 antigen [9], whereas subsequent investigators, using molecular techniques to subtype alleles, reported an association with HLA-DQA1*0101 [80] and DQB1*0602 [10]. These associations were present in white but not black patients. Finally, several reports have found autoantibodies to myenteric plexus neurons in some achalasia patients. Storch *et al.* found IgG antibodies directed against the cytoplasm of the myenteric plexus in 37 of 58 patients with achalasia with variable stages of disease, but in only four of 54 healthy subjects and two of 48 disease control subjects [81]. Using a double-label, indirect immunofluorescence technique, Verne *et al.* found that the sera from seven of 18 achalasia patients stained neurons within the myenteric plexus from rat esophagus and intestine; this was not observed in 22 disease-free control subjects [82]. In a Spanish population, Ruiz-De-Leon *et al.* found that patients with achalasia and the HLA heterodimer DQA1*0103-DQB1*0603 had antibodies against the myenteric plexus in 81.8% of cases compared to 45.7% of patients with other heterodimers (OR = 5.34; *P* = .003) [83]. When compared by gender, the associations are stronger in women, with 100% antibody association as compared to 66.7% in men. Overall, this heterodimer was increased in patients compared to controls (OR = 2.57; *P* = .013). In a geographically and ethnically distinct study, Latiano *et al.* determined a previously unreported association with the HLA-DQB1-0502/0601 allelic subtypes, but the authors failed to find a correlation with antineuronal antibodies and any of the other HLA alleles found in their population [84]. In their study, Latiano *et al.* detected antineuronal antibodies in only 24% of patients compared to 54% in the Ruiz-De-Leon *et al.* study, and only one of 60 patients exhibited the heterodimer DQA1*0103-DQB1*0603. Although neuron-specific autoantibodies targeted at ganglion cell proteins have been associated with various paraneoplastic syndromes resulting in achalasia, antineuronal antibodies in the idiopathic form of the disease have yet to be characterized in any detail [85]. These autoantibodies and HLA markers are only reported in at most half of achalasia patients. Furthermore, they may be a non-specific reaction to neurons that have been altered by some other causative agent.

Degenerative theory

An epidemiologic study from the United States suggested that achalasia was associated with older subjects having various neurologic or psychiatric diseases, such as Parkinson's disease and depression [86]. Case reports have associated achalasia with neurologic disorders such as hereditary cerebellar ataxia and neurofibromatosis [87, 88]. Additionally, some studies have demonstrated Lewy bodies in the myenteric plexus and dorsal motor nucleus of the vagus in achalasia patients as well as in patients with Parkinson's disease having dysphagia [89]. These studies suggest that a small population of elderly patients may have achalasia secondary to degenerative neurologic disorders.

Figure 13.3 summarizes the pathogenesis of idiopathic achalasia suggested by Paterson [13]. He conceptualizes that achalasia is a disease that initially and primarily affects the nitrergic myenteric plexus neurons of the LES and esophageal body of the smooth muscle esophagus. An initiating

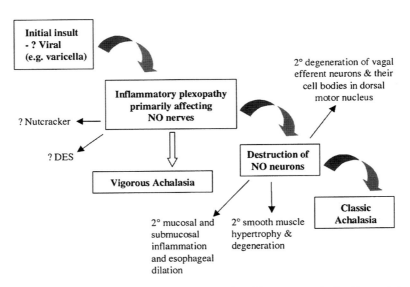

Figure 13.3 Overview of possible etiopathogenesis of idiopathic achalasia (reproduced from Paterson [13], with permission.)

insult, be it viral infection, a toxin, or some other unknown factor, likely occurs long before the patient comes to clinical attention. This injury triggers a chronic inflammatory response within the myenteric plexus, damaging but not destroying primarily NO-containing neurons. At this stage, a functional motility disorder of variable severity may be produced, including diffuse esophageal spasm, nutcracker esophagus, and vigorous achalasia, all of which have been rarely reported to progress to achalasia [90, 91]. Over time, probably measured in years, the inflammation results in death and destruction of the myenteric ganglion cells with fibrous tissue replacement, producing the classic manometric features of achalasia associated with progressive esophageal dilatation. Secondary muscle hypertrophy may occur as a result of chronic obstruction and dilatation, and eventually muscle degeneration evolves. Secondary inflammatory changes within the esophageal mucosa occur because of chronic stasis. Finally, in some patients, degeneration of vagal efferent neurons and their cell bodies in the DMN of the vagus may occur. This may be a consequence of loss of functional contact of these extrinsic nerves with their myenteric plexus effector neurons, but a primary insult to these neurons cannot be excluded. In fact, it is possible in this model that idiopathic achalasia may be the end result of more than one etiologic and pathophysiologic mechanism.

Clinical presentation

The most common symptoms for achalasia are summarized in Table 13.1 [68]. Most patients are symptomatic for years before seeking medical attention, probably because they learn to adapt to their slowly worsening symptoms, but some patients present early with severe symptoms. The mean duration of symptoms in 12 studies involving more than 1200 patients was 4.6 years [11, 92–99]. The duration of symptoms ranged from as short as 1 month to as long as 67 years. Many patients see several physicians before the correct diagnosis is made, sometimes because their com-

Table 13.1 Symptoms in achalasia patients (from Birgisson and Richter [68]).

Symptom	Number of patients studied	Mean %	Mean % range
Dysphagia	1930	97	82–100
Regurgitation	1892	75	56–97
Weight loss	1675	58	30–91
Chest pain	1894	43	17–95
Heartburn	127	36	27–42
Cough	732	30	11–46

plaints are vague, but more likely because many physicians lack an appreciation of functional esophageal disorders [100]. Common antecedent misdiagnoses include gastroesophageal reflex, peptic stricture, esophageal spasm, presbyesophagus, allergies, and eating disorder [100]. Others are misdiagnosed because improper tests are done, especially the initial use of endoscopy as a diagnostic tool in all patients with dysphagia. On the other hand, a study from Scotland found that the current widespread use of esophageal manometry resulted in more cases of early achalasia and milder symptoms being diagnosed and treated [11].

Dysphagia

Dysphagia is reported by most patients with achalasia. In many patients, the dysphagia is initially more for solids than liquids, but by the time of presentation as many as 70–97% of patients have troubling dysphagia for liquids [11, 92–99]. In contrast to patients with anatomic obstructing esophageal lesions, those with achalasia report their symptoms not only during the intake of solid food, but perhaps more frequently when drinking liquids between meals. The onset of dysphagia is usually gradual, being described initially as an infrequent "fullness in the chest" or "sticking sensation," but usually occurs daily or with every meal by the time of presentation to a physician. Some patients correctly locate their dysphagia to the xiphoid area, but in our personal experience many complain of dysphagia referred to the region of the cervical esophagus. In many patients, the dysphagia seems to increase in severity, reaching a plateau over time, whereas other patients note increasing symptoms that lead to significant weight loss. Occasionally, the patient does not complain of dysphagia, although family members note the prolonged time required to complete a meal. Patients over the years learn to accommodate their dysphagia using various maneuvers, including throwing the shoulders back, lifting the neck or using the headback position and simultaneously performing the Valsalva maneuver in an upright position to help empty the esophagus [98]. Other patients may try to increase intraesophageal pressure by using slow deliberate swallowing during a meal or by drinking large volumes of liquids, especially carbonated beverages. All of these maneuvers attempt to increase intraesophageal pressure by 10–20 mmHg, thereby encouraging esophageal emptying [99]. Other remedies reported to improve dysphagia include drinking alcohol, warm liquids, or smoking marijuana, all of which relax the patient or the LES [98].

Regurgitation

Regurgitation of undigested, retained food or accumulated saliva occurs in about 75% of patients with achalasia [11, 92–99, 101]. The material brought up is often recognized as food that has been eaten many hours previously. It tends to be non-bilious and not to have an acid taste. However, fermented intraesophageal contents may taste and become acidic over time [102]. Unprovoked regurgitation often occurs during or shortly after a meal. It is not unusual for some patients to induce vomiting manually to relieve chest discomfort. Other patients complain of thick white phlegm in their mouth, the result of regurgitated swallowed saliva. This sometimes leads to the initial misdiagnosis of allergies or sinus problems. Typically, patients note food or saliva backing up in the mouth while asleep. Nocturnal regurgitation can be annoying or severe. Regurgitated food or saliva may end up on the pillow case, cause audible gurgling sounds, or sometimes be aspirated into the trachea, producing severe bouts of coughing and choking. Respiratory complications, such as aspiration pneumonia or lung abscess, may occur, particularly in older patients [86, 103]. Many achalasia patients learn to adapt to these problems by elevating the head of the bed at night and not eating large meals for several hours before bedtime. Occasionally in young women, these symptoms of regurgitation may be confused with those of an eating disorder, such as anorexia nervosa or bulimia [104].

Chest pain

Chest pain or retrosternal discomfort is reported by nearly 40% of patients with achalasia; however, it is rarely the major complaint [11, 92–99, 101]. Pain episodes mainly affect younger patients [105] and are usually described as cramping in nature and radiating to the back and lower jaw, sometimes mimicking angina pectoris. Symptoms can last for minutes to all day. Chest pain frequently awakens the patient at night, can be precipitated by eating and may be so severe as to cause decreased food intake and weight loss. Prominent pain occurs more frequently early in the course of achalasia, usually when the esophagus is only minimally dilated. As the esophagus dilates, the pain usually lessens and sometimes resolves [105]. The mechanism of chest pain is unknown, but it is not simply repetitive episodes of simultaneous contractions causing the esophageal lumen to be occluded [105]. Some patients practice self-induced vomiting to relieve their pain, whereas others believe cold beverages help. Smooth muscle relaxants, nitrates, and acid suppressive medications do not predictably relieve the chest pain [98]. Whereas pneumatic dilatation or surgery usually relieves dysphagia and regurgitation, the chest pain in achalasia responds much more unpredictably. In the first few weeks following dilatation, some patients even describe an increase in chest pain frequency and fewer than 20% notice a major improvement in this symptom [105]. Other causes of chest pain in achalasia are pill-induced esophagitis, candidal esophagitis, and impairment of the belch reflex, causing increased intraesophageal pressure from trapped air [36].

Heartburn

Heartburn is not an uncommon complaint in achalasia patients (see Table 13.1), although the contrary would be expected based on the high LES pressure and impaired relaxation [11, 92–99, 101]. Characteristically, the heartburn is not immediately post-prandial and responds poorly to acid-suppressing medications, including proton pump inhibitors (PPIs) [11]. The etiology of heartburn in achalasia is controversial and unresolved. Some have reported patients with well-defined GERD progressing to diffuse esophageal spasm and achalasia [106]. Smart *et al.* noted that four of their five patients had hiatal hernias and postulated that the progression from gastroesophageal reflux to achalasia may be secondary to acid damage to the autonomic nervous system [107]. Spechler *et al.* noted that achalasia patients complaining of heartburn had lower LES pressures than those without heartburn and that in some patients, heartburn disappeared with the onset of dysphagia, suggesting that GERD was present before the development of achalasia [108]. On the other hand, these isolated cases do not explain the patients with current symptoms of heartburn. Several studies using prolonged pH monitoring found evidence of excessive acid exposure, but the pattern was characterized by a slow steady drift to a pH of less than 4, rather than the abrupt pH decreases with slow clearance seen in classic GERD [102, 109]. This abnormal acid response is likely secondary to the slow clearance of exogenous ingested acidic materials, such as carbonated drinks, or *in situ* production of lactic acid from retained food in a dilated esophagus [110].

Weight loss

More than half of patients with achalasia report weight loss (see Table 13.1). The weight loss is usually mild and occurs over several months to years, but some patients have marked weight loss of up to 100–150 lb. In the latter group, significant weight loss over a short period of time associated with progressive dysphagia should raise the suspicion of secondary achalasia [111, 112]. On the other hand, many patients do not lose weight and some are obese.

Miscellaneous symptoms

Although most presentations of achalasia are typical, important complications of achalasia can occur in patients with megaesophagus and long-standing disease. These complications are associated with three major physiologic processes: (1) displacement of mediastinal structures by the esophagus; (2) esophageal ulcerations and perforation through the esophageal wall; and (3) aspiration of esophageal contents [98] (Table 13.2). Approximately 10% of achalasia patients have significant bronchopulmonary complications as a result of regurgitation of material from the esophagus [92]. Patients with esophageal symptoms of long duration may actually come to medical attention because of pulmonary complications. Organisms involved most commonly are aerobic and anaerobic oropharyngeal flora, which are aspirated, leading to bronchitis, pneumonia, or lung abscess. There is also an

Table 13.2 Complications of achalasia (modified from Wong and Maydonovitch [98]).

Aspiration pneumonia
Bezoar of the esophagus
Bronchitis
Distal esophageal diverticulum
Esophagocardiac fistula
Esophageal bleed
Esophagobronchial fistula
Esophageal foreign body
Esophageal perforation
Esophageal squamous cell cancer
Esophageal varices
Gastroesophageal intussusceptions
Hiccups
Lung abscess
Neck mass (bullfrog neck)
Pneumopericardium
Post-myotomy Barrett's esophagus
Pulmonary *Myocobacterium fortuitum*
Small cell carcinoma
Stridor with upper airway obstruction
Sudden death
Suppurative pericarditis

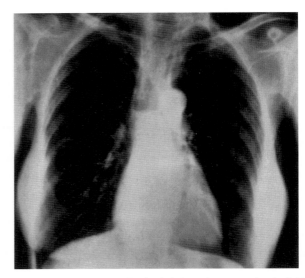

Figure 13.4 Chest X-ray study of achalasia patient. Note the air–fluid level from retained secretions across from the aortic arch and the widened mediastinum from esophageal dilation.

apparent increased incidence of pulmonary infection with mycobacteria in achalasia [103]. Rarely, the dilated, fluid-filled esophagus can lead to hypopharyngeal displacement (bull frog neck) and acute obstruction of the airway, usually the trachea [113]. Such patients may be difficult to intubate endotracheally, requiring decompression of the esophagus by a nasogastric tube or rarely by pharyngotomy. Some achalasia patients have hiccups, which usually occur during meals and disappear after ingestion of liquids or following forced regurgitation. It has been speculated that hiccups are the consequence of esophageal distention and stimulation of afferent vagal fibers [114]. Bleeding is rare in achalasia, although there has been one report of massive bleeding from an esophagopericardial fistula [115].

Diagnostic evaluation

Achalasia is suspected from a compatible history and the diagnosis usually is not difficult. Early cases may be misdiagnosed because screening barium X-ray studies fail to reveal esophageal dilatation and peristalsis is not evaluated, or endoscopy is used as the sole test for the patient presenting with dysphagia. However, the diagnosis is made correctly in virtually all cases if a systematic approach, including esophageal manometry, is taken for patients with symptoms suggestive of this motility disorder.

Radiographic studies

The plain chest X-ray film may suggest achalasia. The classic sign of an absent gastric air bubble in the upright position, present in almost all healthy individuals, may be found in 50% of achalasia patients [92, 116, 117]. The plain chest film may also show an air–fluid level in the posterior mediastinum from retained secretions, widened mediastinum from esophageal dilation and chronic parenchymal lung changes, and lung abscesses from chronic aspiration [118] (Figure 13.4).

A barium esophagram with fluoroscopy may be the single best diagnostic test for achalasia (Figure 13.5A). The classic features are esophageal dilation, aperistalsis, impaired esophageal emptying in the upright position, and symmetric tapering at the GEJ (bird's beak appearance). Aperistalsis results in failure to clear the barium bolus from the esophagus in the supine position, and subsequent barium boluses cause to-and-fro movement with esophageal dilation [119]. In the upright position, retained food and saliva cause a heterogeneous air–fluid level at the top of the barium column. This upright position also can be used to assess barium emptying [120]. Healthy subjects should empty a barium bolus challenge of 150–250 mL within 1–2 min. Most patients with achalasia have residual barium in the esophagus at the end of 5 min. Early in the disease, the esophagus may be minimally dilated and, with the distal tapering at the GEJ, confused for a peptic stricture (Figure 13.5B). However, a careful fluoroscopic evaluation of esophageal peristalsis always finds evidence of simultaneous contractions and failure of the primary esophageal wave to clear the esophagus of barium [118, 119]. As the disease progresses, the

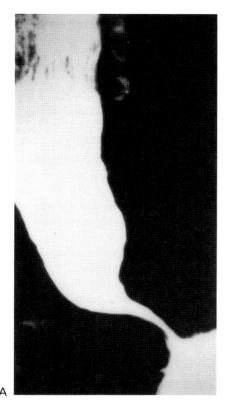 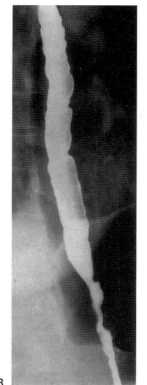 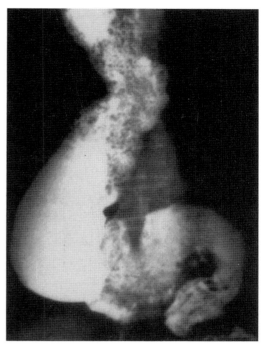

A   B   C

Figure 13.5 Barium esophagrams in patients with achalasia. (A) Classic features of esophageal dilation, retention of liquids and secretions, and symmetric smooth tapering at the gastroesophageal junction (GEJ) known as a bird's beak. (B) In early disease, the esophagus may not be dilated and the distal tapering at the GEJ may be confused for a peptic stricture. However, on fluoroscopy, aperistalsis is usually present. This patient was originally referred for antireflux surgery. (C) Chronic endstage achalasia with marked dilation and sigmoid-like left angle distortion.

esophagus becomes more dilated generally in the range of 3–8 cm, sometimes with a sigmoid-like left angle deviation of the distal esophagus. In chronic endstage cases, the esophagus becomes massively dilated (>9 cm) and may resemble a sigmoid colon with stool (the inhomogeneous barium from the residual food) (Figure 13.5C). In classic achalasia, the distal esophagus has a smooth tapering resembling a bird's beak. On spot films, this may appear to be a fixed obstruction, but fluoroscopy reveals intermittent partial opening of the GEJ, allowing the barium to trickle or sometimes spurt into the stomach.

We and others have found that these classic radiologic features of achalasia show some correlation with symptoms [121, 122]. The height of the barium column in the upright position is related to the degree of regurgitation, whereas chest pain is inversely correlated with esophageal dilation [121]. The severity of dysphagia may parallel the decline of esophageal emptying over 5 min in the upright position [121]. The overall degree of esophageal dilation and the development of a sigmoid esophagus show little relationship to the severity of symptoms or the presence of weight loss. In fact, rare patients with massive esophageal dilation present serendipitously with no esophageal symptoms and only because of their cough or pneumonia from silent aspiration.

Other less common radiologic abnormalities in achalasia include an epiphrenic diverticulum and hiatal hernia. The unexpected presence of an epiphrenic diverticulum in the distal esophagus strongly suggests the associated diagnosis of achalasia [123]. Hiatal hernias are infrequently found in achalasia patients (1.2–14%) compared with a higher prevalence (20–50%) in the general population [124–126]. These hernias are generally small (<2 cm), although in elderly patients they can be large. Some believe the presence of a hiatal hernia increases the chance of perforation during dilatation [124]. Spot films of the gastric cardia should always be done to look for a tumor of the cardia or GEJ. However, compiled data from five studies found that the barium X-ray studies detected tumors of the GEJ in only 28% of patients (10 of 36) with pseudoachalasia [99, 100].

Esophageal manometry

Esophageal manometry is the gold standard for diagnosing achalasia. Table 11.3 reviews the manometric findings in

Table 13.3 Manometric findings in achalasia.

Lower esophageal sphincter:
Elevated resting pressure
Abnormal relaxation:
  Absent
  Incomplete
  Short but complete
  Mean integrated relaxation pressure >15 mmHg

Esophageal body:
Aperistalsis:
  Isobaric simultaneous waves
  Simultaneous contractions
  Pan-esophageal pressurization
Repetitive waves
Increased intraesophageal baseline pressure > gastric pressure

Upper esophageal sphincter:
Elevated resting pressure
Shortened duration of relaxation
Spontaneous repetitive contractions
Abnormal belch reflex

achalasia. Although the diagnosis of achalasia is often suggested by the barium esophagram or sometimes endoscopy, the diagnosis is confirmed by esophageal manometry. It is an essential test before pneumatic dilatation or surgical myotomy, in which there are potential treatment risks for the patient. Manometry may not be necessary when the symptoms and X-ray findings are classic, and less invasive treatments such as botulinum toxin (BTX) or drug therapies are planned. Placement of the manometry catheter may be difficult in the very dilated or tortuous esophagus. We have found that these patients can have manometry completed by passing a water-perfused motility catheter over a guidewire endoscopically placed in the stomach. The decision to perform endoscopy for manometric catheter placement is based on the appearance of the barium esophagram.

Although occasional peristaltic and retrograde contractions may be seen on prolonged ambulatory manometry studies [127], standard manometric studies in achalasia always show aperistalsis in the distal smooth muscle portion of the esophagus. This means that all swallows in response to a water bolus are followed by simultaneous contractions. The contractions (or more correctly waves) are classically identical to each other (isobaric or mirror images) as a result of a common cavity or closed chamber phenomena (Figure 13.6A). The contractile pressures are typically low (10–40 mmHg), and repetitive, prolonged waves are frequently observed [128]. Physiologically, the low-amplitude waves represent simultaneous fluid movement in a fluid-filled dilated esophagus, rather than true lumen occluding contractions. In contrast, the term vigorous achalasia is

sometimes used when there is aperistalsis with higher than normal contraction amplitudes (usually defined as >37–40 mmHg) [129–131]. These simultaneous contractions can be high, sometimes reaching 100–200 mmHg [128, 131]. These contractions are usually not mirror images of each other (Figure 13.6B), because the esophagus is actually contracting and occluding the lumen of the minimally dilated esophagus. Patients with vigorous achalasia have less esophageal dilatation on barium esophagram, but otherwise do not differ from patients with classic achalasia [129, 130]. In several series, including our own experience, the diagnosis of vigorous achalasia is made in up to one-third of patients with achalasia [129–131]. Several other variations of aperistalsis may be seen. In the usual patient, aperistalsis is confined to the distal two to three manometric sites recording from the smooth muscle esophagus. In patients with a markedly dilated esophagus to the level of the UES, recording sites throughout the esophagus show aperistalsis as lumen occluding waves cannot be generated. A patient with classic symptoms of achalasia and a poorly relaxing hypertensive LES was reported with aperistalsis confined to the distal 3 cm of the esophagus [128]. The patient did well with a surgical myotomy. It has been reported that peristaltic contractions may be restored in some (up to 15%) patients with achalasia after treatment by myotomy or pneumatic dilatation [132]. In future, impedance studies may help to define whether this represents the actual return of peristalsis with intermittent normal bolus clearance. If true, then it suggests that functional obstruction of the LES may play a role in the esophageal aperistalsis seen in some achalasia patients. This would be similar to the model of an achalasia-like syndrome generated in animals by tying off the GEJ [133] or in patients with a pseudoachalasia-like syndrome after a tight antireflux fundoplication [134]. Lastly, intraesophageal pressure exceeds intragastric pressure in some achalasia patients, probably because of retained food and saliva, because the pressure gradient returns to normal with evacuation of the esophagus.

Manometric abnormalities of the LES are always present in achalasia. The LES resting pressure is normal (10–45 mmHg) in up to 40% of achalasia patients; therefore, an elevated resting pressure is not required for the diagnosis [53, 129]. It has been speculated that the subset of achalasia patients with GERD preceding the onset of dysphagia may have normal resting LES pressure, especially those who experience cessation of heartburn as their dysphagia progresses [108]. A low LES pressure is never seen in untreated achalasia patients. The constellation of a low LES pressure and aperistalsis should raise the question of scleroderma or severe GERD.

Abnormal LES relaxation is seen in all achalasia patients [135–137]. About 70–80% of patients have absent or incomplete LES relaxation with wet swallows [136] (Figure 13.6D). Normally, LES relaxation exceeds 90% but averages only

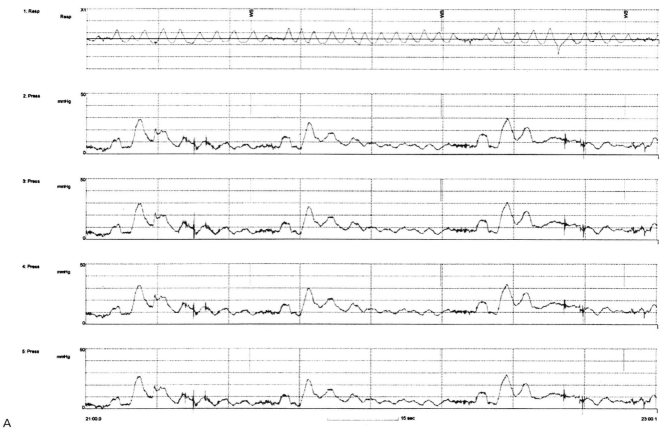

A

Figure 13.6 Manometric features of achalasia. (A) Classic achalasia with aperistalsis and low-amplitude isobaric waves after all wet swallows. (B) Vigorous achalasia with aperistalsis and simultaneous high-amplitude (some >200 mmHg) contractions. Note that these contractions do not have the mirror-image quality seen in classic achalasia. (C) Achalasia with intraesophageal pressure exceeding intragastric pressure best seen in the fourth tracing from the top. There is also evidence of incomplete lower esophageal sphincter (LES) relaxation. (D) Achalasia with incomplete LES relaxation and increased residual pressure of 30 mmHg. In this lead, LES pressure is also elevated measuring 60–80 mmHg. (E) Complete but short duration LES relaxation in achalasia. Relaxation to baseline for only 3–4 s duration is not adequate for normal esophageal emptying.

40% in achalasia patients [136]. Incomplete relaxation can be seen in normal individuals after dry swallows, so wet swallows should be used to evaluate LES relaxation [138]. Studies using the Dent sleeve [128] or computerized assessment of LES relaxation [138] suggest that residual or nadir LES pressure may be the best manometric indicator of impaired relaxation, with values exceeding 8–10 mmHg being abnormal. In the elderly achalasia patient (older than 75 years), resting LES pressure and esophageal body contraction amplitudes do not differ from those in younger patients, but residual LES pressure may be significantly lower, possibly confusing the diagnosis [139]. On the other hand, complete LES relaxation does not exclude achalasia and can be seen in 20–30% of these patients [137]. These relaxations are complete to the gastric baseline but of short duration (usually <6 s) and functionally inadequate as assessed by nuclear emptying studies (Figure 13.6E). They are probably artifacts related to the small diameter of the

manometry catheter or movement allowing the manometry orifice to drop into the stomach. Patients with apparent complete LES relaxation usually have early-stage achalasia in that their duration of symptoms and esophageal dilatation are less than in patients with classic achalasia [137]. Other reports have found evidence of intermittent transient LES relaxation but absence of swallow-induced LES relaxation [127, 128, 140]. This finding suggests the possibility that transient LES relaxations and deglutitive LES relaxation may involve distinct neuropathways. Finally, a rare patient has been reported with aperistalsis and complete LES relaxation as the earliest stage of achalasia. At myotomy, preservation of the myenteric ganglions was seen, but there was myenteric inflammation involving some of the ganglion cells and the patient's symptoms improved after myotomy [128].

UES and striated muscle function can be abnormal in achalasia. Although peristalsis is intact in the striated muscle, the amplitude of contractions may be diminished [35]. Using

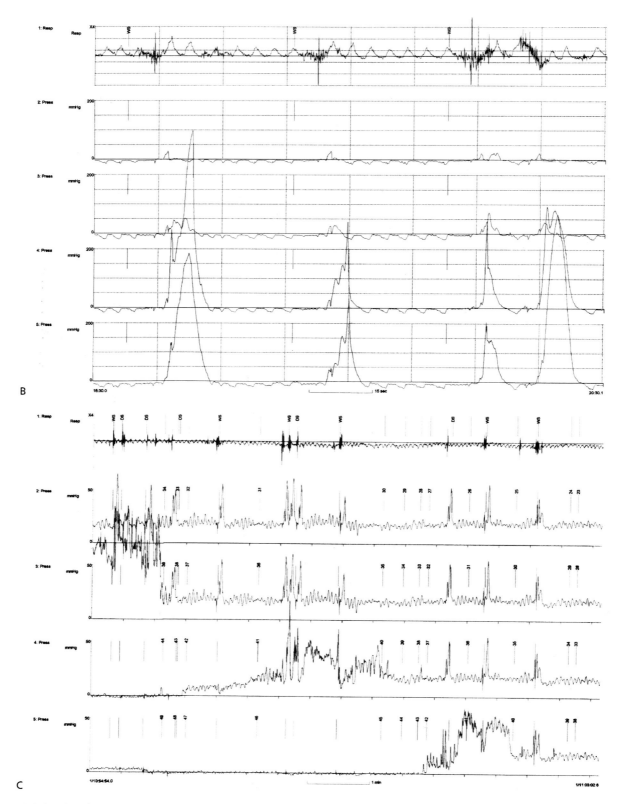

Figure 13.6 (continued)

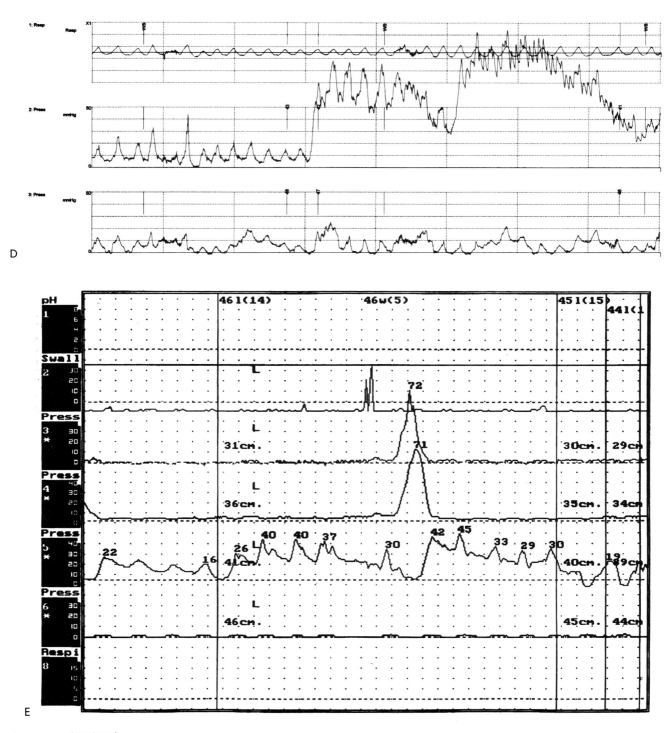

Figure 13.6 (*continued*)

solid-state or sleeve techniques, increased UES residual pressure, shortened duration of relaxation, repetitive spontaneous UES contractions, and impaired belch reflex have been recorded in some achalasia patients [36, 141]. UES changes may represent a reflex measure to prevent aspiration.

The new technique of high-resolution manometry has improved the sensitivity of manometry for detecting achalasia. It allows a more careful evaluation of LES and more appropriately, GEJ relaxation using the integrated relaxation pressure (IRP). Recently, the Northwestern group reported in a series of achalasia patients a false-negative rate of 48% for the traditional LES nadir pressure, while an IRP of greater than 15 mmHg was seen in all but 3% of patients with achalasia [142]. In addition, high-resolution manometry defined a clinically relevant subclassification of achalasia based on the pattern of contractility in the esophageal body [143]. This technology shows that absent peristalsis accompanying impaired GEJ relaxation can occur in the setting of esophageal dilation with negligible esophageal pressurization (classic achalasia) (see Chapter 9, Figure 9.9A), pan-esophageal pressurization, in which case there is a pressurized column of fluid within the esophagus (achalasia with esophageal compressions) (see Chapter 9, Fig 9.9B), or spastic contractions of the distal esophageal segment (spastic–vigorous achalasia) (see Chapter 9, Figure 9.8C). In a series of 99 patients with newly diagnosed achalasia, the Northwestern group found that 21 met the criteria for classic achalasia, 49 had achalasia with esophageal compression, and 29 had spastic achalasia [143].

Endoscopy

Endoscopic examination of the esophagus is required to exclude neoplastic processes at the level of the GEJ and evaluate the esophageal mucosa before therapeutic manipulations [98, 112, 144]. Practically, it is usually done immediately before pneumatic dilatation unless there is a high suspicion of associated tumor. Patients with a markedly dilated esophagus may need to be lavaged or kept on a clear liquid diet for several days before endoscopy to avoid aspiration and allow complete visualization of the esophagus. The esophageal body usually appears dilated, atonic, and often tortuous with normal-appearing mucosa. Sometimes the mucosa is reddened, friable, thickened, or even superficially ulcerated as a result of chronic stasis, pills, or candidal esophagitis (Figure 13.7A, B). White plaques may suggest the presence of a fungal infection and, if confirmed by mucosal biopsies, topical antifungal therapy before pneumatic dilatation is recommended as prophylaxis against mediastinal contamination in case perforation occurs. The LES appears puckered and remains closed with air insufflation; however, the endoscope usually passes into the stomach with gentle pressure (Figure 13.7C). In some patients a "pop" is noted but this is uncommon. If excessive pressure is required, the presence of pseudoachalasia should be highly suspected [144], although benign strictures, usually from pills, are another possible etiology. In four studies involving 20 patients with pseudoachalasia resulting from tumors of the GEJ, difficulty in passing the endoscope through to the LES was noted in 55% of patients [111, 112, 144, 145]. Retroflex view of the cardia and GEJ should always be done and biopsy samples obtained from suspicious areas to exclude a malignancy before treatment (Figure 13.7D). Endoscopy is not infallible in that tumors of the GEJ can be missed in about 35% of patients with pseudoachalasia [111, 112, 144, 145].

Endoscopic ultrasound and computed tomography scan

Both endoscopic ultrasound (EUS) and computed tomography (CT) scan may be helpful in evaluating the patient with suspected pseudoachalasia. Using a 20-MHz probe, EUS reveals a thickened LES muscle in achalasia patients, measuring 31 mm rather than 22 mm for normal subjects [146]. In patients with cancer of the distal esophagus or cardia causing secondary achalasia, EUS may show thickening of the second and third hypoechoic layers (mucosa and submucosa) as well as enlargement of adjacent lymph nodes [147]. Thoracic CT may detect asymmetric esophageal wall thickening or nodularity, extrinsic masses, or lymphadenopathy in addition to esophageal dilation in pseudoachalasia [148]. However, EUS is better for evaluating a submucosal etiology of achalasia and CT scan may have difficulty in differentiating a mass from a hiatal hernia or tortuous redundant sigmoid esophagus. Neither can be recommended as a routine test in achalasia [149], and EUS is preferred to CT scanning for the initial evaluation of a patient with suspected pseudoachalasia [150].

Differential diagnosis

As shown in Table 13.4, a number of disorders are associated with achalasia-like syndromes, with esophageal manometry and barium esophagram being indistinguishable from primary achalasia [100, 111, 112, 144]. The most common disorders mimicking primary achalasia are malignancies [112, 145, 151–160] and Chagas' disease [71], with the other disorders being rare case reports [161–166].

Secondary achalasia related to malignancies, "pseudoachalasia," represents about 3% of all achalasia cases and about 9% of achalasia patients older than 60 years of age[100, 111, 112, 144]. Most commonly, these tumors are adenocarcinomas of the GEJ, but reports exist of pancreatic, oat cell, squamous cell of the esophagus, prostate, and lymphoma invading the region of the LES [153–157]. These tumors usually produce achalasia as a result of one or two mechanisms: (1) the tumor mass encircles or compresses the distal esophagus producing a constricting segment or (2) malignant cells infiltrate the esophageal myenteric plexus [167]. However, there are other reports of apparently non-neurogenic involvement by tumors such as Hodgkin's disease, poorly differentiated bronchogenic carcinoma, small cell carcinoma, and hepatoma that cause achalasia from a distance, probably as a result of a paraneoplastic syndrome [151, 152, 156, 161]. In 1978, Tucker *et al.* identified three clinical criteria that could distinguish pseudoachalasia from primary achalasia: age older than 50 years, duration of symptoms less than 1 year, and weight loss greater than 6.8 kg [111]. However, others found that the positive predictive value of these symptoms was only 18%, with the sen-

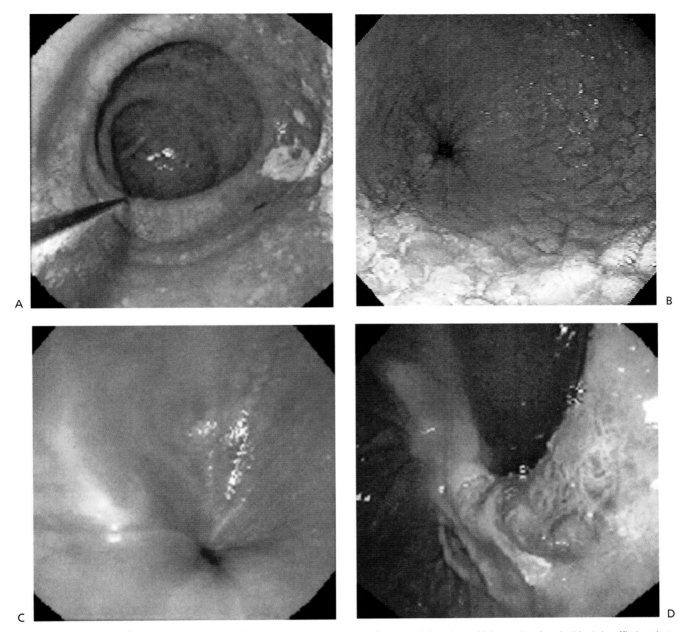

Figure 13.7 Endoscopic findings in achalasia. (A) Dilated atonic esophagus with normal appearing mucosa. Savary wire has been placed in the stomach to aid in esophageal manometry catheter placement. (B) Reddened, friable, thickened, and cracked mucosa in a patient with megaesophagus from longstanding achalasia. (C) Puckered esophagogastric junction, which remains closed with air insufflations but opens easily, sometimes with a "pop," with gentle pressure from the endoscope. (D) Pseudoachalasia from an adenocarcinoma of the gastric cardia noted at retroflexion of the endoscope.

sitivity and specificity being 100% and 55–85%, respectively [145]. Clinically, this symptom triad is not very helpful because four of five cases of older patients with achalasia would be mistaken for pseudoachalasia [145]. Barium studies reveal classic findings of secondary achalasia with an eccentric, nodular, or shoulder segment of distal esophageal narrowing in about 40% of patients with this condition. In the remaining patients, the narrowed segment is smooth and symmetric with tapered proximal borders. A report identified two additional radiologic findings seen in more than 80% of patients with pseudoachalasia and not in patients with idiopathic achalasia. These findings included a narrowed distal esophageal segment that was longer than 3.5 cm and a minimal degree of esophageal dilatation of 4 cm or less [168]. Additionally, amyl nitrate inhaled during barium examination may aid in distinguishing

Table 13.4 Secondary causes of achalasia (modified from Birgisson and Richter [68]).

Malignancies (pseudoachalasia) involving the gastroesophageal junction (GEJ):
Adenocarcinomas (breast, gastric, prostate, lung)
Esophageal squamous cell carcinoma
Lymphoma (gastric, esophageal)
Esophageal lymphangioma
Remote from the GEJ
Brainstem metastasis
Hodgkin's disease
Hepatocellular carcinoma
Gastric adenocarcinoma
Poorly differentiated lung cancer
Reticular cell sarcoma
Peritoneal mesothelioma
Retroperitoneal B-cell lymphoma

Non-malignant esophageal infiltrative disorders:
Amyloidosis
Leiomyomatosis
Eosinophilic esophagitis
Sarcoidosis
Sphingolipidiosis (Anderson–Fabry's disease)

Miscellaneous:
Chagas' disease
Congenital lower esophageal diaphragmatic web
Diabetes mellitus
Familial adrenal insufficiency with alacrima
Multiple endocrine neoplasia, type IIB
Pancreatic pseudocysts
Post vagotomy
Laparoscopic Nissen fundoplication
Laparoscopic banding operation for obesity

pseudoachalasia from primary achalasia [169]. Amyl nitrate does not affect LES diameter in pseudoachalasia, but usually causes a 2 mm or greater increase in diameter in patients with primary achalasia. Endoscopy with biopsies results in the diagnosis of pseudoachalasia in most patients. Ominous endoscopic findings include mucosal ulcerations or nodularity, reduced compliance of the GEJ, or the inability to pass the endoscope into the stomach. However, as many as 25% of patients with pseudoachalasia have a normal endoscopic examination because of submucosal involvement by the malignancy [100, 111, 112, 144]. EUS is helpful in selected cases [136], but CT scans usually find only non-diagnostic features unless massive tumor involvement is present. Successful treatment of the underlying tumor sometimes cures the pseudoachalasia [153, 154, 156].

Chagas' disease (American trypanosomiasis) is a multisystem infectious disease caused by the protozoan *Trypanosoma cruzi* and transmitted by bites from reduviid (kissing) bugs. The disease is endemic in Central and South America, affect-

ing millions of people [170]. Latin American immigrants and travelers to endemic areas are increasingly seen with this disease [171]. Ganglion cells are destroyed throughout the body, resulting in megaesophagus, megaduodenum, megacolon and rectum, in addition to cardiac involvement, the leading cause of death in Chagas' patients [170]. The clinical presentation, radiographic and manometric features, and treatment for Chagas' disease are no different from those for primary achalasia [172]. The clinical suspicion of Chagas' disease is confirmed with a positive serologic complement fixation or hemagglutination reaction [172; see Chapter 18 for more details].

The advent of laparoscopic foregut surgery has been associated with secondary cases of achalasia after Nissen fundoplication and lap banding surgery for obesity [173, 174]. The proposed contributing factors may be outflow obstruction at or just below the GEJ or unsuspected injury to the vagus nerve.

Treatment

The degenerative neural lesion of achalasia cannot be corrected. Therefore, treatment is directed at palliation of symptoms and prevention of complications. This is mainly accomplished by reducing LES pressure, because peristalsis rarely, if ever, returns with therapy [132]. LES pressure can be reduced by three modalities: drug therapy, forceful pneumatic dilation, and surgical myotomy. These therapies intend to overcome the obstructing LES pressure by improving gravitational esophageal emptying through reduction of sphincter tone while maintaining an adequate barrier against gastroesophageal reflux. Abnormal LES relaxation is not improved by any form of therapy. In most patients, swallowing can return to near normal quality and regurgitation is eliminated. Improvement and normalization of esophageal emptying in the upright position usually parallels symptom relief and may predict long-term success. Adequate decompression of the esophagus is key to preventing the development of complication, especially megaesophagus.

Assessment of treatment success

Traditionally, the success of medical and surgical treatments for achalasia is based on the patient's report of improved symptoms after therapy [68]. This type of follow-up relies on subjective symptoms and not objective evaluation of esophageal function. Proponents of symptom follow-up argue that objective evaluation is not important if treatment relieves the complaints of dysphagia and regurgitation, the driving force in the initial presentation to the physician. Furthermore, it can be argued that the complications associated with treatment may preclude pushing for improvement other than symptom relief. However, these arguments are only valid if symptom relief parallels improvement in esophageal emptying. Data show that 30% of patients who

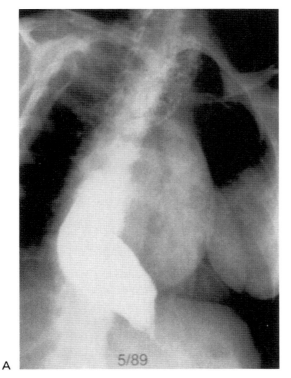
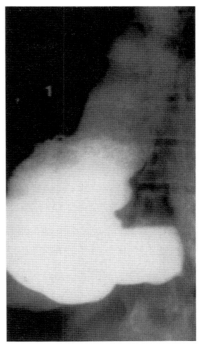

Figure 13.8 Progressive esophageal dilation with development of megaesophagus over nearly 10 years. (A) Initial barium esophagram in May 1989 with early sigmoid deviation. The patient was treated with single pneumatic dilation and was lost to follow-up. (B) Nearly 10 years later, the patient presented primarily with symptoms of regurgitation and recurrent pneumonias. Laparoscopic Heller myotomy gave only minimal relief and esophagectomy was finally required.

experience complete or near-complete resolution of symptoms with a pneumatic dilation still have poor esophageal emptying as suggested by barium X-ray studies [175]. This group of patients is likely to have symptom recurrence earlier than those who have both subjective and objective improvement after therapy [176]. More importantly, ignoring poor esophageal emptying in the setting of improved symptoms can result in worsening of esophageal function with the development of megaesophagus (Figure 13.8).

The esophageal tests most commonly used for assessing treatment success include esophageal manometry and barium esophagram. Manometric studies have reported a correlation between symptom improvement, especially in those patients experiencing at least a 40–50% reduction in baseline LES pressure [177, 178] or in those with a post-treatment LES pressure less than 10–15 mmHg [179–181]. The latter criterion was shown to be the single most valuable predictor ($P < .005$) of long-term clinical success over 5 years in a large study of 54 achalasia patients treated with pneumatic dilation by Eckardt *et al.* [179]. Similarly, several surgical series found that post-myotomy LES pressures of less than 10 mmHg favored long-term success [182, 183]. However, pneumatic dilation studies using the Rigiflex balloons failed to identify any manometric predictors of symptom response [184, 185].

Additionally, patients do not like serial manometric studies, and manometry may be difficult and requires repeat endoscopy in patients with megaesophagus.

Assessment of barium emptying in the upright position is simple, widely available, inexpensive, acceptable to the patient for serial testing, and associated with very little radiation exposure. Although emptying of liquids is usually assessed, foods and pills can also be evaluated. Early studies reported that post-treatment predictors of success included an esophageal diameter of less than 3 cm, barium height of less than 1 cm at 5 min, or an esophagogastric diameter of 8–10 mm [186–188]. However, other studies have not shown a good correlation between symptom improvement and barium findings [184, 185, 189, 190]. The conflicting data may be because of measurement of esophageal emptying at varying time intervals after pneumatic dilation, the use of different dilators for pneumatic dilation, or differences in radiographic techniques. For example, barium emptying results may be affected if patients are tested only 1 day after therapy, as performed by Cohen [187] and Lee *et al.* [189], because considerable edema and spasm may still be present. A standardized approach may clarify the role of barium esophagram in the objective assessment of achalasia after therapy.

We developed a timed-barium esophagram, which is a simple and reproducible means of assessing esophageal function before and after treatment of achalasia [191]. The technique is as follows:

1. The patient stands and ingests 100–200 mL of low-density barium (45% weight and volume) over 30–45 s. The volume ingested is based on patient tolerance.

2. Three-on-one spot films (35 × 35 cm) are obtained at 1, 2, and 5 min after ingestion, with the patient in a left posterior oblique position. The distance of the fluoroscope carriage from the patient is kept constant for all spot films. The 2-min film is optional, but fluoroscopy at 2 min is performed to determine the state of emptying. Healthy subjects all empty their esophagi by 2 min.

3. The degree of emptying is estimated qualitatively by comparing the 1- and 5-min films. The degree of emptying may also be estimated by measuring the height and width for films, calculating the surface area for both periods, and determining the percentage of change in the area. A recent study suggests the surface area of barium retention at 5 min is the best predictor of resting LES pressure [192].

4. On subsequent follow-up studies, the same volume of barium is used for accurate serial assessment.

We routinely follow-up patients at 1 month after pneumatic dilation and surgery with an assessment of symptoms and objective measurements of esophageal diameter and emptying by barium esophagram (Figure 13.9). This test is better tolerated than repeat esophageal manometry. It is more physiologic because it allows assessment of both changes in diameter and improvement of esophageal emptying (both measures of decreased LES resistance) and can be performed easily in small clinics and hospitals where esophageal manometry may not be available.

Using this method, we have shown that both short- and long-term clinical response after pneumatic dilations have good correlation with esophageal barium emptying. This was accomplished by evaluating the symptom response and barium esophagram results of 61 pneumatic dilations in 37 achalasia patients who were treated using Rigiflex pneumatic balloons [175]. There was a significant association (r = .61; $P < .001$) between improvement in patient's symptoms and barium emptying. Short-term symptom improvement at 1 month and esophageal barium emptying were similar in 44 of 61 patients (72%). Ten of 34 patients (30%), however, who reported almost complete symptom resolution, had barium esophagram emptying that was less than 50% improved as assessed by barium height (Figure 13.10). The latter group was older than their successfully treated colleagues, suggesting a possible disturbance in esophageal sensation. Importantly, we followed these two groups of patients for several years, finding that patients with both symptomatic and objective improvement at 1 month were significantly ($P < .001$) more likely to be in remission long term than those who had poor objective emptying 1 month after pneumatic dilatation [176]. Eighteen of 22 (82%) of the former group and only one of 10 (10%) of the latter group were in remission on follow-up. The patients doing well at follow-up usually continued to have good esophageal emptying. Subsequently, several other groups have confirmed the utility of the timed barium swallow in predicting both short- and long-term improvement after surgery or pneumatic dilation [193, 194]. We believe the results of these studies emphasize the need for objective assessment of achalasia patients after treatment rather than reliance solely on the patient's reported improvement in symptoms.

Pharmacologic and other medical treatment
Smooth muscle relaxants

The two most common drug classes used in treating achalasia are nitrates and calcium-channel blockers. Nitrates

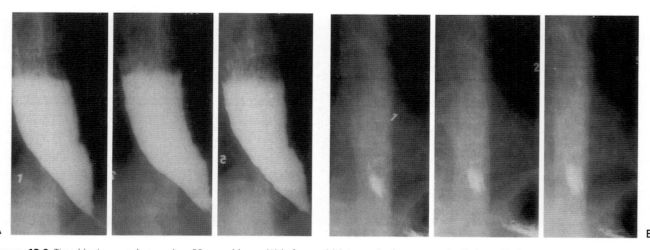

Figure 13.9 Timed barium esophagram in a 33-year-old man (A) before and (B) 1 month after pneumatic dilation with the 3.0-cm Rigiflex balloon. He had complete symptom relief and excellent esophageal emptying at 5 min.

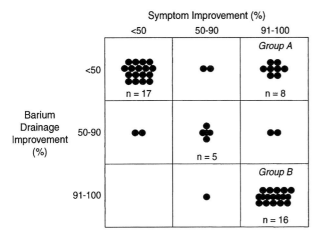

Symptom Improvement (%)

Figure 13.10 Association between degree of symptom improvement and barium drainage after 61 pneumatic dilations in 37 achalasia patients. Note that 10 of 34 patients (30%; group A) reporting complete symptoms relief had barium esophagram emptying that was less than 50% improved as assessed by barium height. In subsequent follow-up, group A patients were much more likely to relapse than group B patients, who had concordance between symptoms and esophageal emptying (reproduced from Vaezi *et al.* [175], with permission).

increase the nitric oxide concentration in smooth muscle cells, which subsequently increases cyclic guanosine monophosphate (GMP) levels and results in muscle relaxation. Calcium is necessary for esophageal smooth muscle contractions and its action is blocked by calcium antagonists [195]. Both drug classes are effective in reducing LES pressure and temporarily relieving dysphagia, but do not improve LES relaxation or improve peristalsis. These drugs are best used sublingually 15–45 min before meals with doses ranging from 10 to 30 mg for nifedipine, the most effective calcium-channel blocker, and 5–20 mg for isosorbide dinitrate (Isordil) [195]. Nitrates and calcium-channel blockers decrease LES pressure in a dose-dependent manner with a maximum effect of approximately 50%, with the long-acting nitrates having a shorter time to maximum effect (3–27 min) compared with sublingual nifedipine (30–120 min) [196–200]. Overall, sublingual nitrates result in symptom improvement in 53–87% of patients with achalasia [196, 199, 201], whereas calcium-channel blockers improve symptoms in 53–77% of similar patients [197, 199, 200–202]. Comparative studies suggest that sublingual isosorbide dinitrate (5 mg) is more effective than 20 mg of sublingual nifedipine (85% vs 50%) [199]. On the other hand, nifedipine has been shown to be more effective than both diltiazem and verapamil [203, 204]. The clinical responses to these drugs are short-lived and usually do not provide complete relief, and efficacy decreases with time. For example, Bortolotti and Labo published their 20-year experience with nifedipine 10–20 mg [197]. Thirty-nine of 56 patients with achalasia were selected

for long-term treatment based on a good manometric response to nifedipine administration (defined by a decrease in LES pressure >30% for at least one episode of 10 min). Even in this select group of patients, only one-third were still on therapy after an average follow-up of about 4 years. Both nitrates and calcium-channel blockers are associated with frequent side effects, including headaches, dizziness, and pedal edema. This is a major factor limiting the use of these drugs as is the frequent development of tolerance to their beneficial effects.

Other medications that have been used to decrease LES pressure in achalasia patients include anticholinergics (cimetropium), β-adrenergic agonists (terbutaline and carbuterol), and peripheral opioid agonists (loperamide) [205–208]. Most of these reports are small short-term studies without placebo controls, and route of administration and side effects have often limited their widespread application in patients. Cimetropium bromide was evaluated in a double-blind, placebo-controlled trial and was found to reduce LES pressure by 70% for a duration of about 40 min [205]. This was accompanied by improvement in esophageal transit time and few cardiovascular side effects. Improvement in achalasia symptoms was not evaluated. Most recently, sildenafil (Viagra), best known for its use in impotence, was evaluated in achalasia patients. Sildenafil blocks phosphodiesterase-type 5 (the enzyme responsible for degradation of cyclic GMP), which results in increased cyclic GMP levels within the muscles, resulting in relaxation. In a placebo-controlled study involving 14 achalasia patients, sildenafil 50 mg by mouth significantly decreased LES pressure, residual pressure, and wave amplitude with its maximum inhibitory effect (about 50%) reached in 15–20 min after ingestion and lasting for up to 1 h [209].

Other intriguing methods to relax LES pressure have included transcutaneous electrical nerve stimulation (TENS) and behavioral pain management. It has been suggested that the response to low-frequency TENS stimulation may be mediated by a non-adrenergic, non-cholinergic pathway in which the release of VIP is responsible for smooth muscle relaxation. In a study of six achalasia patients, Guelrud *et al.* observed that after 1 week of TENS therapy there was a significant decrease in LES pressure by 28%, improved LES relaxation, and increased VIP plasma levels, but symptom relief was not assessed [199, 210]. Shabsin *et al.* reported complete relief of chest pain in a patient with vigorous achalasia following behavioral pain management, suggesting that psychophysiologic mechanisms can be recruited to improve esophageal symptoms and emptying [211].

Botulinum toxin

BTX is a potent inhibitor of acetylcholine release from nerve endings. The inactive form of BTX is synthesized by the *Clostridium botulinum* species as a single-chain polypeptide. The active form is a protein that consists of a light chain and a heavy chain, linked by a disulfide bond. It cleaves SNAP-25, a cytoplasmic protein involved in the fusion of acetylcholine-containing presynaptic vesicles with the neuronal plasma membrane. Once BTX cleaves SNAP-25, exocytosis of acetylcholine is inhibited and paralysis of the innervated muscle occurs [212]. Because the pathophysiologic derangement underlying achalasia results in relatively unopposed stimulation of the LES by cholinergic neurons, BTX helps restore the LES to a lower resting pressure by blocking the release of acetylcholine.

Recognizing the pharmacologic attributes of BTX, Pasricha *et al.* were the first to describe the successful use of BTX in reducing the LES pressure by 60% in piglets [213]. Subsequently, the same investigators performed a pilot study on 10 achalasia patients using 80U of BTX endoscopically injected into the LES [214]. One week after injection, there was a significant reduction in symptom scores (87%), LES pressure (43%), esophageal diameter (17%), and esophageal retention (25%). Later, Pasricha *et al.* published a double-blind, placebo-controlled trial in 21 achalasia patients. BTX was significantly more effective than placebo at 1 week in 82% (nine of 14) of the drug-treated patients compared to 10% (one of 10) of the placebo group [215]. Long-term follow-up (median 18 months) found that 70% of their 21 patients had symptomatic and objective improvement [216]. However, 40% needed more than one injection.

Similar results had been reported in a number of other studies in which the overall efficacy of one BTX injection was evaluated from 1 month to more than 24 months [217–228] (Table 13.5). Overall, 76% of achalasia patients initially responded to BTX, but symptoms recurred in more than 50% of patients within 6 months, possibly because of regen-

eration of the affected receptors [212]. In those responding to the first injection, 75% responded to a second BTX injection, but some reported a decreased response to further injections, probably from antibody production to the foreign protein [212]. Fewer than 20% of patients failing to respond to the initial injection responded to a second BTX injection [219]. Many patients in the aforementioned studies were treated with BTX after failing pneumatic dilation or Heller myotomy. In some reports, patients older than 60 years [216, 219, 228] and those with vigorous achalasia [216, 217, 223] were found more likely to have a sustained response (up to 1.5 years) to BTX injections. Most studies assessing both subjective symptoms and esophageal function tests (i.e. LES pressure, esophageal emptying by barium or nuclear scintigraphy) found that symptom relief of dysphagia and regurgitation was much more striking than the improvement in esophageal function [215–225]. This raises the possibility that BTX is also affecting sensory neurons and raises concerns that its chronic use for symptom relief may obscure a marginal improvement in esophageal function [223]. BTX has also been reported to help some patients with pseudoachalasia [219, 229] and may be used as a diagnostic test in patients with achalasia-like symptoms but atypical manometric features [230].

BTX (Allergen Inc, Irvine, CA, USA) is injected during a routine outpatient endoscopy. It is kept at −5°C prior to reconstitution and is gently diluted with 5mL of preservative-free, sterile saline, being careful not to agitate the solution by forming bubbles during the mixing process, which could decrease the potency of the toxin [98]. Once reconstituted, the toxin should be kept at 2–8°C and used within 4h. Injections are contraindicated in patients allergic to egg

Table 13.5 Botulinum toxin treatment for achalasia (modified from Hoogerwerf and Pasricha [195], with permission).

Study	Number of patients	Symptomatic improvement after one injection				% Responding to repeat injections
		1 month or less	6 months	12 months	24 months	
Pasricha *et al.* [215, 216]	31	90	55			27
Cuillere *et al.* [217]	55	75	50			33
Rollan *et al.* [218]	3	100	66			
Fishman *et al.* [219]	60	70		36		86
Annese *et al.* [220]	8	100	13			100
Gordon and Eaker [221]	16	75	44			
Muehldorfer *et al.* [222]	12	75	50	25	10	
Vaezi *et al.* [223]	22	63	36	32		
Annese *et al.* [224]	118	82		64		100
Kolbasnik *et al.* [225]	30	77	57	39	25	100
Mikaeli *et al.* [226]	20	65	25	15		60
Allescher *et al.* [227]	23	74		45	30	
Neubrand *et al.* [228]	25	65			36	0

proteins and should be administered cautiously to patients receiving aminoglycosides because these medications may potentiate the effect of the toxin [98]. The average total dose used per session ranges between 80 and 100 U, with a concentration of 20–25 U/mL injected into each quadrant of the LES. Endoscopically, BTX is injected using a sclerotherapy needle inserted at a 45-degree angle into the esophageal wall, entering the mucosa approximately 1–2 cm above the squamocolumnar junction. This location places the needle just above the proximal margin of the LES with the toxin injected caudad into the sphincter. EUS may help identify the LES and allow for more precise injection of the BTX, but there is no evidence that this approach improves efficacy [231]. BTX dose and dosing schedule may be important in prolonging the duration of response. In a study of nearly 200 patients receiving one of three doses of BTX (50, 100, or 200 U), those receiving 100 U followed by a second injection of 100 U 30 days later did the best. After 12 months, patients who received this two-dose regimen were more likely to be in remission (80% vs 55% for the other two groups) [224].

Complications after BTX injections are mild and infrequent, usually consisting of chest pain in 16–25% of patients [98]. There is some concern regarding the effects of prior BTX treatments on the success of subsequent Heller myotomy. Three surgical series [232–234] report difficulty in the dissection of the submucosal plane with increased intraoperative mucosal perforation rate in patients receiving prior BTX treatment. However, there was no difference in time of hospitalization or postoperative symptom improvement, although two patients in one series had persistent dysphagia [234].

Pneumatic dilation

Balloon dilation is considered the most effective non-surgical therapy for achalasia. The aim is to produce a controlled tear of the LES, resulting in relief of the distal esophageal obstruction and clinical improvement without perforating the esophagus. The first reported case of achalasia was treated with self-bougienage using a whale bone attached to a sponge [1]. Although bougie dilation with a large Hurst or Maloney dilator can transiently relieve symptoms [235], pneumatic dilation has become the dilation procedure of choice for treating patients with achalasia.

Older dilators

Early metal dilators (Starck) were modified in the early 1900s such that expanding bags and balloons were incorporated onto flexible shafts so that they could be placed across the LES to dilate it forcefully. The first balloon was the Plummer hydrostatic dilator, which used water to expand it [236]. Subsequent dilators replaced the water with air and were called pneumatic dilators [237, 238]. The Browne–McHardy and Hurst–Tucker pneumatic dilators consisted of a mercury-filled tube with a rubber-covered silk bag at the distal end. The Mosher bag contained barium strips impregnated into the wall of the bag for easy visualization at fluoroscopy. The Rider–Mueller dilator contained a dumbbell-shaped bag that could be positioned across the GEJ by a guidewire and was the first dilator available in variable sizes. The Sippy pneumatic dilator had two latex balloons covered by a nylon bag to limit expansion of the balloon. Progressively larger balloons were used until symptom relief was obtained. All these dilators required fluoroscopy for proper positioning before dilation, and balloon size, when expanded, ranged from 2.5 to 4.5 cm [238].

There is a significant experience reported in the literature using the older dilators. Results of five prospective studies in 235 achalasia patients using the older type of dilators reported a good to excellent symptomatic response (defined as >50% improvement in dysphagia) varying between 61% and 100%, with a cumulative mean of 85% [179, 239–242]. The follow-up of these studies ranged from a few months to more than 9 years with a mean of nearly 3 years. The overall perforation rate when reported was 2%. Results of 15 retrospective studies in nearly 2200 patients found a similar overall good-to-excellent symptomatic response averaging 71% (range 34–96%) [238]. The mean follow-up in these studies was 5 years with an esophageal perforation rate of 3%. However, this information is only of historical interest because most of these older dilators are no longer in use. The Browne–McHardy dilator, once the most commonly used dilator in the United States, is no longer manufactured.

Newer dilators

Two newer type pneumatic dilators are available worldwide. The most commonly used balloon is the Rigiflex dilator (Boston Scientific Corporation, Boston, MA, USA), which is made of a modified polyethylene polymer mounted on a flexible catheter similar in design to the Gruentzig angioplasty catheter. The Rigiflex balloon is 10 cm long and comes in three diameters, 3.0, 3.5, and 4.0 cm (Figure 13.11). It is not visible under fluoroscopy but has several radio-opaque markers on the shaft that define the upper, middle, and distal borders of the balloon. The Rigiflex balloon is non-compliant, meaning that it inflates maximally to its designated diameter only. Further inflation pressure increases the pounds per square inch (psi) within the lumen but not the balloon diameter. Once the maximum psi for any balloon is exceeded, it simply ruptures without ever increasing the diameter. The other pneumatic dilator is the Witzel dilator (U.S. Endoscopy, Mentor, OH, USA), which is made of a 20-cm long polyvinyl tube surrounded by a 15-cm long polyurethane balloon, which is passed in a retrograde fashion over an endoscope (Figure 13.12). The Witzel dilator has the advantage of direct endoscopic visualization of the

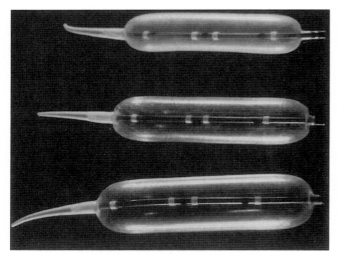

Figure 13.11 Rigiflex pneumatic balloons with three diameter sizes: 3.0, 3.5, and 4.0 cm.

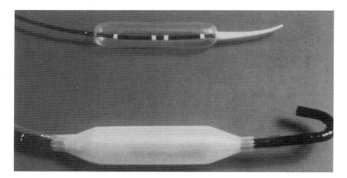

Figure 13.12 Rigiflex pneumatic balloon (3.0-cm diameter) compared to the Witzel over-the-scope pneumatic balloon, which comes in only the 4.5-cm diameter size.

Table 13.6 Technique for pneumatic dilation using Rigilex balloons.

1. Fasting for at least 12 h before endoscopy
2. Esophageal lavage with Ewald tube (if needed)
3. Standard conscious sedation and upper endoscopy in left lateral position
4. Savary guidewire placed in stomach and Rigiflex balloon passed over it
5. Accurate placement of the balloon with it centered across the gastroesophageal junction by fluoroscopy with the patient in the supine position (this is key to a successful dilation)
6. Balloon distended, usually to 7–12 psi, enough to obliterate the waist and maintained for 60 s
7. Patient repositioned in the left lateral position and the balloon carefully removed after deflating
8. Patient sent for Gastrografin followed by barium swallow after recovery from conscious sedation to exclude esophageal perforation
9. Observation for 4 h for chest pain or fever. Patient discharged home after drinking fluids without difficulty
10. Clinic follow-up in 1 month to assess symptoms and esophageal emptying with timed barium esophagram
11. If symptoms and/or barium emptying not improved, then repeat dilation with the next larger size balloon

balloon position during dilation; however, its utility is limited because it comes in only one size, a 4.0-cm balloon diameter. In the United States, the vast majority of dilations are done with the Rigiflex balloons.

Technique

The technique used for pneumatic dilation varies at different institutions depending on the experience of the individuals performing the procedure. Most pneumatic dilations done in the United States are single events, although the balloon may be distended several times. Some of our European colleagues perform serial sessions over several days, until the manometrically measured LES pressure is below 10–15 mmHg [181, 243]. For the last 30 years, one of us (JER) has used the Rigiflex balloon dilators exclusively, using the

technique outlined in Table 13.6. Several additional points regarding the procedure are:
• Screening endoscopy to exclude cancer is usually performed at the same time as pneumatic dilation unless there is a high suspicion of malignancy.
• Graded pneumatic dilation is performed traditionally, starting all patients with the smallest 3.0-cm balloon [184]. However, based on recent experience, the smallest balloon is used initially for most women and older men, and the middle balloon (3.5 cm) is now used initially for younger men and symptomatic patients after Heller myotomy [244, 245].
• The positioning of the Rigiflex balloon may be difficult, especially if a good waist caused by the hypercontracting LES is not easily seen. Partial inflation and repositioning may be required to get the balloon in proper position, i.e. with half of the partially inflated balloon above the waist and half below the waist. This is the "key" step in the dilation procedure.
• As the balloon is inflated, there is a tendency for the dilator to be pulled down into the stomach. Therefore, the individual holding the balloon must apply appropriate upward traction at the mouthpiece to keep the balloon in proper position.
• The duration of balloon inflation does not appear to be as important as making sure the waist is obliterated. This was confirmed in a study comparing the efficacy of 6- or 60-s balloon distention times [246]. Some authors suggest repeat inflation for up to 3 min, but none of these variables has been prospectively studied.

• Blood on the balloon indicates a mucosal tear but does not always indicate a successful dilatation.

• The Gastrografin swallow is followed by the heavier barium swallow if no perforation is noted. This study may not show good esophageal emptying secondary to edema and LES spasm; it is done solely to identify early esophageal perforation [189, 190]. Some, however, do not recommend obtaining barium X-ray films unless clinically indicated [247].

• Before 1994, we used to observe all our achalasia patients overnight in the hospital after dilation, but since the report of Barkin et al. [248], most patients are discharged after 4 h of outpatient observation.

Efficacy: short and long term

There are no clinical trials that compare pneumatic dilation to placebo (i.e. sham dilation). The efficacy and complication rates with the two pneumatic dilators are not comparable. The results of the six studies using the Witzel dilator for the treatment of achalasia in 266 patients only reported good to excellent symptomatic response in 66% of the subjects with an average follow-up of 11 months [180, 188, 245–251]. In the largest series, Ponce et al. reported symptom improvement in 59% of 157 patients, which is the lowest response among all six studies (others ranged from 78% to 94% improvement) [180]. Furthermore, the perforation rate was high in five of the six series (mean 6% with a range from 0% to 13%). This perforation rate is two to three times higher than reported for the older dilators and the Rigiflex balloons.

Table 13.7 summarizes the results of 24 uncontrolled studies of Rigiflex pneumatic dilation for the treatment of achalasia, usually with a follow-up of less than 5 years [177, 185, 189, 241, 248, 252–268]. The degree of heterogeneity of these studies is not known. The pooled result of 1144 patients followed for a mean of 37 months found an excellent-to-good symptom response in 78% of patients, with an esophageal perforation rate of only 1.9%. Among these studies, the clinical response improved in a graded fashion with increasing size of the balloon diameter. However, it should be emphasized that uncontrolled studies tend to exaggerate the benefits of intervention and the criteria to determine the response to treatment varies across studies. For example, while a graded approach to pneumatic dilation

Table 13.7 Rigiflex pneumatic balloon dilation for achalasia.

Study	Number of patients	Study design	Dilator size (cm)	% with excellent/ good response	Follow-up (mean months)	Perforation rate (%)
Cox et al. [252]	7	P	3	86	9	0
Gelfand and Kozarek [177]	24	P	3, 3.5	93	NR	0
Barkin et al. [248]	50	P	3, 3.5, 4	90	20	2
Stark et al. [241]	10	P	3.5	74	6	0
Markela et al. [253]	17	R	3, 3.5, 4	75	6	5.9
Levine et al. [254]	62	R	3, 3.5, 4	85	NR	0
Kim et al. [185]	14	P	3, 3.5	75	4	0
Lee et al. [189]	28	P	3, 3.5, 4	87	NR	0
Abid et al. [255]	36	P	3, 3.5, 4	88	27	6.6
Wehrmann et al. [256]	40	R	3, 3.5	87	NR	2.5
Lambroza and Schuman [257]	27	P	3, 3.5, 4	89	21	0
Muehldorfer et al. [258]	12	R	3.5	83	18	8.3
Bhatnager et al. [259]	15	R	3, 3.5	84	14	0
Gideon et al. [260]	24	R	3, 3.5	NR	6	4
Khan et al. [261]	9	P	3.5	85	NR	0
Kadakia et al. [184, 238]]	56	P	3, 3.5, 4	88	59	0
Chan et al. [262]	66	R	3, 3.5, 4	62	55	4.5
Dobrucali et al. [263]	43	P	3, 3.5	54	29	2.3
Kostic et al. [264]	26	P	3, 3.5	87	12	NR
Vela et al. [244]	106	R	3, 3.5, 4	78	36	1.9
Mikaeli et al. [265]	200	P	3, 3.5, 4	65	36	1.5
Ghoshal et al. [266]	125	R	3, 3.5, 4	78	15	0.8
Boztas et al. [267]	50	R	3, 3.5, 4	67	38	0
Chuah et al. [268]	30	P	3	62	84	3.3
24 studies	**1144 patients**			**78**	**37**	**1.9**

P, prospective; R, retrospective; NR, not recorded.

is considered standard, in some studies a repeat procedure within a graded dilation program is considered a failure.

Long-term outcome studies with pneumatic dilation are limited, but suggest that most patients do well, while requiring periodic "touch up" dilations over their lifetime. Zerbid *et al.* used an iterative approach with pneumatic dilation, repeating the procedure when symptoms recurred [269]. In their protocol, graded dilations were performed every 2–3 weeks until remission occurred. Initial remission was achieved in 137 of 150 (91.3%) patients. The probability of being in remission without further dilations at 5 and 10 years was 67% and 50%, respectively. Performing repeat pneumatic dilations when symptoms recurred increased the 5- and 10-year remission rate to 96.8% and 93.4%, respectively. Similar results were reported recently by the Leuven group who performed graduate dilations over 1–3 consecutive days until the resting LES pressure was less than 15 mmHg [181]. With an average follow-up of 6 years, 66% of patients required no additional treatment, whereas 23% underwent repeat pneumatic dilations. Repeat dilation increased the long-term success rate to 77%. Other studies using Rigiflex balloons found similar rates of initial success, deteriorating over time with excellent-to-good responses of 58% and 51% at 9 and 15 years, respectively. The success of repeated dilations was not discussed in these two studies [270, 271].

The group at the Academic Medical Center in Amsterdam has reported the longest symptomatic follow-up of 125 achalasia patients from a cohort of 249 patients treated at their Center over the last 30 years [243]. The mean follow-up was 12 years with a success rate of 50%, obtained after a median of four dilations. For the groups treated for 5–9 years, the success rate was 60%; in the group treated for 10–14 years, the rate was 50%; and in the 25 patients treated for more than 15 years, the success rate was only 40%. Most of the patients with the longest follow-up were treated with homemade pneumatic dilators, the Rigiflex balloon only being used over the last 10 years.

The need for repeat pneumatic dilations was confirmed in a retrospective longitudinal study using linked administrative health databases for the entire province of Ontario, Canada from July 1991 to December 2002 [272]. Among the 1181 patients initially treated with pneumatic dilation, the cumulative need for subsequent treatment, usually repeat dilation, after 1, 5, and 10 years was 36.8%, 56.2% and 63.5%, respectively.

Predictors of success
Pneumatic dilation does not improve LES relaxation but decreases LES pressure by 39–68% [135, 177, 184, 185, 256]. Partial return of peristalsis is reported in 20% of patients [273–275], but does not correlate with symptom improvement or esophageal emptying. Over time, LES pressure seems to increase to a varying degree [177].

Table 13.8 Pneumatic dilation predictors of relapse.

Related to patient:
Younger age (<40 years)
Male gender
Wide esophagus

Related to procedure:
Single dilation
Small size balloon (<30 mm)
Lower esophageal sphincter pressure >10–15 mmHg
Poor esophageal emptying post treatment

Related to manometry:
Type I and III pattern on high-resolution manometry

With the standardization of balloon systems, we are beginning to define the risk factors for relapse after pneumatic dilation (Table 13.8). These are mainly young age (<40 years), male gender, single dilation with a 3.0-cm balloon, post-treatment LES pressure above 10–15 mmHg and poor esophageal emptying on a timed barium swallow. The effects of age on the success of pneumatic dilation are most reproducible [96, 179, 180, 244, 276] from as far back as 1971 [277], even with the older balloons. For example, Eckhardt *et al.* using a 4-cm Brown–McHardy dilator, demonstrated a 5-year remission rate of 16% for patients younger than 40 years, compared with 58% for those older than 40 years [278]. Studies suggest young men do not do as well as young women with pneumatic dilation. In a study of 126 patients, Ghosal *et al.* found that male gender, but not age, was independently associated with poor outcome after dilation [266]. Another large study from the Cleveland Clinic (106 patients, 51 women) confirmed the importance of age, but also found gender to be equally important [244]. Men up to age 50 years did not do well with a single 3.0-cm Rigiflex pneumatic dilation. However, only young women (<35 years of age) did poorly with pneumatic dilation, while most older women had sustained relief over at least 5 years with a single pneumatic dilation.

Physiologic studies can also predict the long-term success rate of pneumatic dilation. Eckhardt *et al.* reported that all patients with post-procedure LES pressure of 10 mmHg or lower were in remission after 2 years compared with 71% for pressures between 10 and 20 mmHg and 23% for pressures over 20 mmHg [179]. More recently, the Leuven group observed that 66% of their patients with post-procedure LES pressures of less than 15 mmHg were in symptomatic remission after an average of 6 years [181]. Using the timed barium swallow, we found that patients with complete symptom relief correlating with marked improvement in esophageal emptying were more likely to do well at 3 years than those with symptom relief but poor esophageal emptying (82% vs 10%, respectively) [176]. A randomized clinical trial of pneumatic dilation versus surgery found that patients with a less than 50% improvement in the height of the barium column at 1 min post-treatment had a 40% risk of treatment failure during follow-up [265]. Most recently, the Northwestern group observed that patients with a Type II achalasia pattern (panesophageal pressurization) on high-resolution manometry were more likely to respond to any therapy (BTX 71%, pneumatic dilation 91%, Heller myotomy 100%) compared to Type I (56% overall) and Type III (29% overall) [143]. This was a single-center study enthusiastic about high-resolution manometry; therefore, confirmation by other centers of excellence is needed.

Complications

Complications after pneumatic dilation are reported in up to 33% of patients, with most complications being minor [278]. In a prospective study with long-term follow-up by Eckhardt et al., prolonged post-dilation chest pain was reported in 15% of patients. The intensity and long duration of chest pain in this study, however, may be caused by lack of routine use of conscious sedation [278]. This has not been our experience or that of others [238] when conscious sedation is administered for pneumatic dilation. Other usually minor complications after pneumatic dilation include aspiration pneumonia, hematemesis without a decrease in hemoglobin, fever that resolves spontaneously, esophageal mucosal tear without perforation, esophageal hematoma, and angina [278, 279].

The most significant and serious complication after pneumatic dilation is esophageal perforation. Although the perforation rate varies from 0% to 16%, the overall perforation rate of 1.9% with the new Rigiflex balloon dilators is acceptable (see Table 13.7). Some researchers have suggested that patients with vigorous achalasia, associated epiphrenic diverticulum or hiatal hernia, malnutrition, or more than one previous dilation may have an increased risk of perforation [90, 280]. However, a retrospective study of 237 patients by Metman et al. found no difference in clinical, endoscopic, manometric, or radiographic characteristics among seven patients who had perforations and 230 patients who did not [281]. Furthermore, one of us (JER) has performed pneumatic dilation on all these subsets of achalasia patients without perforation and found the only contraindications to pneumatic dilation to be patients who cannot undergo safely the anesthesia required to perform the procedure comfortably or who cannot tolerate surgery if a perforation occurs.

After pneumatic dilation, all our patients undergo a Gastrografin X-ray study followed by a more careful barium study to exclude obvious and subtle perforations. Others suggest a more selected approach [247], obtaining X-ray films only if patients have prolonged chest pain, tachycardia, dyspnea, or fever [279]. Patients with free perforation into the mediastinum, pleural or peritoneal space should undergo surgery to close the perforation, preferably through an open

posterior thoracotomy. If performed within the first 8–12 h, a myotomy on the contralateral esophageal wall also can be done. Perforations that appear to be contained within the muscle wall can be treated medically with nasogastric suction, parenteral alimentation, and intravenous antibiotics for 10–14 days [90, 282, 283]. When the perforation was recognized early, Schwartz et al. found no difference in the duration of the operation, intensive care stay, hospitalization days, or the long-term outcome in seven patients who had surgical repair for pneumatic perforation compared with those outcomes in five patients undergoing elective myotomy during the same period [284]. However, surgical myotomy in these patients was an open operation through the chest, rather than laparoscopic abdominal myotomy, which has become more common in recent years.

The incidence of gastroesophageal reflux after pneumatic dilation has been poorly studied. Older reports suggest this is a minor problem, with fewer than 20% of patients experiencing symptomatic heartburn, with rare cases of esophagitis or peptic stricture [237, 240, 277]. Two studies evaluated patients before and after pneumatic dilation, finding that 25–33% had abnormal pH values not noted before treatment, but most were asymptomatic [285, 286]. The importance of this asymptomatic reflux is unknown. In our recent follow-up of 106 patients undergoing pneumatic dilation, 26% had heartburn symptoms requiring PPIs with an average follow-up of nearly 4 years [244].

Surgical cardiomyotomy

The first successful surgery for achalasia was performed in 1913 by the German surgeon Ernest Heller [5]. Until the mid-1990s, the Heller myotomy, usually performed via a left posterior thoracotomy, was the primary surgical operation for achalasia. Good-to-excellent results were obtained in about 83% (range 60–94%) of achalasia patients followed up for 1–36 years [287]. In 1992, Pellegrini et al. reported the first series of achalasia patients who underwent minimally invasive Heller myotomy via the thorascopic approach [288]. The benefits of a shorter hospital stay with decreased morbidity and earlier resumption of normal activity compared with the open operation has led to the widespread popularity of minimally invasive Heller myotomy, especially performed laparoscopically over the last decade. Chapter 15 reviews the surgical treatments of esophageal motility disorders in detail. In this section, we highlight some of these areas and help position laparoscopic Heller myotomy in the gastroenterologist's armamentarium of treatments for achalasia.

Esophageal myotomy lowers LES pressure more consistently than pneumatic dilation [240, 289, 290]. Depending on the distal extent of the myotomy onto the cardia, LES pressure is lowered by 55–75%, with the remaining residual pressure usually being less than 10 mmHg. Partial return of peristalsis is reported in up to 20% of patients after myotomy

[291–293], with one report [293] suggesting key predictors were shorter duration of dysphagia, less esophageal dilation, and greater contractile activity. Myotomy also lowers intraesophageal pressure but does not improve LES relaxation [240]. Solid esophageal emptying studies are markedly improved, LES maximal diameter increases significantly, and esophageal diameter measured by the barium esophagram decreases after a successful myotomy [121, 240, 294].

Laparoscopic Heller myotomy

The first laparoscopic Heller myotomy was performed in 1989 by Cuschieri *et al.* [295]. Over the next 10 years, this operation became the preferred surgical approach for achalasia because it is less invasive, the hospital stay is shorter (usually 2–5 days), there is less incisional pain, and most patients can return to nearly normal activity in about 2

weeks [296, 297]. Furthermore, it is a less demanding and better operation because there is excellent mobilization of the cardioesophageal junction, allowing instruments to work parallel to the axis of the esophagus, the longer intra-abdominal LES is more accessible through the abdomen, complex anesthesia is not required, there is no need for an uncomfortable chest tube postoperatively, and the abdominal approach is easier for adding an effective antireflux procedure [298].

As summarized in Table 13.9, 30 studies containing at least 10 patients each found that laparoscopic Heller myotomy has a cumulative good-to-excellent symptom improvement rate of 87.5% in 924 patients (range 52–100%) [244, 264, 297–322]. Three of the more recent studies found that improvement in esophageal symptoms was associated with improvement in patient quality of life

Table 13.9 Surgical myotomy for achalasia: the laparoscopic approach in series with more than 10 patients.

Study	Number of patients	Antireflux procedure	% Symptoms improve good/excellent	Follow-up (mean months)	% complication GERD
Rosati *et al.* [297]	25	Yes	96	12	—
Ancona *et al.* [298]	17	Yes (Dor)	100	8	6
Mitchell *et al.* [299]	14	Yes (Dor)	86	—	7
Swanstrom and Pennings [300]	12	Yes (Toupet)	100	16	16
Morino *et al.* [301]	18	Yes (Dor)	100	8	6
Robertson *et al.* [302]	10	No	88	14	13
Bonovina *et al.* [303]	33	Yes (Dor)	97	12	—
Delgado *et al.* [304]	12	Yes (Dor)	83	4	—
Hunter *et al.* [305]	40	Yes (Dor/Toupet)	90	13	18
Kjellin *et al.* [306]	21	No	52	22	38
Ackroyd *et al.* [307]	82	Yes (Dor)	87	24	5
Yamamura *et al.* [308]	24	Yes (Dor)	88	17	0
Patti *et al.* [309]	102	Yes (Dor)	89	25	—
Pechlivanides *et al.* [310]	29	Yes (Dor)	90	12	10
Sharp *et al.* [311]	100	No	87	10	14
Donahue *et al.* [312]	81	Yes (Dor)	84	45	26
Zaninotto *et al.* [313]	113	Yes (Dor)	92	12	5
Ramacciato *et al.* [314]	17	Yes (Dor)	94	18	6
Luketich *et al.* [315]	62	Yes (Toupet/Dor)	92	19	9
Decker *et al.* [316]	73	Yes (Toupet/Dor)	83	31	11
Mineo and Pompeo [317]	14	Yes (Dor)		85	14
Gockel *et al.* [318]	108	Yes (Dor)	97	55	22
Wright *et al.* [319]	52	Yes (Dor)	83	46	19
Wright *et al.* [319]	63	Yes (Toupet)	95	45	50
Khajanchee *et al.* [320]	121	Yes (Toupet)	84	9	33
Kostic *et al.* [264]	25	Yes (Toupet)	96	12	
Zaninotto *et al.* [321]	40	Yes (Dor/F*)	88	38	3
Vela *et al.* [244]	73	Yes (Dor/Toupet)	57	72	56
Csendes *et al.* [322]	67	Yes (Dor)	73	190	33
Total	**1487**		**86.7%**	**32**	**18%**

GERD, gastroesophageal reflux disease.
*Floppy Nissen.

comparable to that of control populations in the United States and Europe [310, 313, 314]. Another advantage of the laparoscopic approach is the ability to perform a partial fundoplication (Dor or Toupet). The addition of an antireflux procedure demonstrated favorable outcomes with less postoperative GERD and no difference in postoperative dysphagia [323, 324]. In the three studies without a partial fundoplication, the symptomatic improvement rate (52–88%) tended to be lower than for the operations adding an antireflux procedure, and the GERD rate was higher (13–38%) [302, 306, 311]. The average follow-up of these patients in the 30 series was 32 months. Only one of the studies addressed the learning curve for this procedure. Sharp *et al.* observed that most of the complications occurred in the first 50 operations and the operative time decreased significantly in the last 20 procedures in a series of 100 operations compared with the first 20, from 144 ± 7 min to 110 ± 5 min [311]. No study or society identifies the number of procedures to be performed yearly to maintain competency with laparoscopic Heller myotomy.

Failure of primary myotomy and need for esophagectomy

Recurrence of dysphagia after laparoscopic myotomy is reported to range from 8% to 31% [309, 313, 325, 326], with more than half of these patients requiring more surgery. Early postoperative dysphagia is usually the result of incomplete myotomy, periesophageal scarring, obstructing fundoplication, or megaesophagus, and usually manifests within 3 years after surgery [325]. Incomplete myotomy may be prevented by extending the incision by at least 1.5–3 cm onto the stomach to ensure transection of the gastric sling fibers, and separating the cut edges of the myotomy by at least 30% of the esophageal circumference [319]. An obstructing fundoplication may be almost impossible to distinguish from an incomplete myotomy by either manometry, barium esophagram, or endoscopy. For this reason, some experts suggest using intraoperative manometry to help guide the completeness of the myotomy and the snugness of the fundoplication [327, 328]. BTX injection or pneumatic dilation can be performed postoperatively with prolonged improvement of symptoms favoring the diagnosis of an incomplete myotomy [234, 329]. A non-randomized retrospective analysis by Guardino *et al.* compared the safety and efficacy of graded pneumatic balloon dilations in untreated patients and 12 patients with failed myotomies [245]. Only 20% in the surgical group had an initial response to the first dilation, usually with a 3.0-cm diameter balloon, and 50% overall, whereas the untreated group had a 51% initial response and 74% response after the last dilation. After the last dilation, 10% of surgical patients had complete timed barium swallow emptying compared to 52% of the untreated patients. Despite a theoretically increased risk of perforation during balloon dilation in post-myotomy patients, none were reported in this study. If dilation is not available or if it fails to resolve the dysphagia, 70–80% of patients respond to a repeat myotomy, which, in many cases, can be done laparoscopically [240, 326].

Late recurrences of dysphagia are usually secondary to GERD or the recurrence of achalasia, with the latter reported to occur from 8% to 13% of the time [313, 330]. As Table 13.9 shows, 5–56% (mean 18%) of patients after surgical myotomy suffer from troubling heartburn requiring H_2-receptor antagonists or PPIs. These values may be a gross underestimation as the group from the University of Washington reported [317] (see Chapter 15). After a laparoscopic Heller–Dor or Heller–Toupet procedure, 19% of patients had heartburn more than once a week, but of the subset of patients undergoing postoperative 24-h pH studies, more than twice that number (35%) had abnormal acid reflux values. This chronic gastroesophageal reflux over time can potentially cause esophagitis, peptic stricture, and even Barrett's esophagus with adenocarcinoma. Jaakkola *et al.* found that Barrett's esophagus developed in four of 46 patients following Heller's myotomy after an average follow-up of 13 years [331]. In a review of the literature, Guo *et al.* reported 30 cases of Barrett's esophagus in patients with achalasia; 73% (22 cases) were after Heller myotomy. In 20% of the cases (six subjects), dysplasia and adenocarcinoma developed in the Barrett's esophagus [332]. For these reasons, some authorities are suggesting routine 24-h pH testing after surgical myotomy with chronic medical antireflux therapy if abnormal gastroesophageal reflux is identified (see Chapter 15).

Some patients with achalasia and a megaesophagus may require esophagectomy to relieve their symptoms of dysphagia and regurgitation [333, 334]. The definition of a megaesophagus varies, but it is suggested by a sigmoid configuration, especially when the maximum esophageal diameter exceeds 6–9 cm [305, 335]. Several series have suggested that many of these patients will not do well after a surgical myotomy [310, 313]. However, Patti *et al.* reported that 19 patients with megaesophagus (<6 cm), some with sigmoid deviation, did as well after Heller myotomy as those with mild esophageal dilation [335]. Therefore, we recommend initial treatment with a laparoscopic myotomy with either no or minimal (Dor) fundoplication in all our patients with untreated achalasia and a megaesophagus, reserving esophagectomy for the failures.

Comparison of medical and surgical treatment of achalasia
Pneumatic dilation versus Heller myotomy

Multiple studies, including a randomized study, have compared pneumatic dilation with older balloon systems (Brown–McHardy, Mosher or Rider–Mueller) and open surgical myotomy. In 1989, Csendes *et al.* reported a single-center study comparing surgery and pneumatic dilation with a Mosher bag [240]. They found that 95% of the 41 patients undergoing Heller myotomy were improved with a mean follow-up of 62 months, which was significantly better ($P < .01$) than the 65% improvement rate observed in the 39 patients undergoing pneumatic dilation with an average 58-month follow-up. This small study was supported by a review of 12 other studies, mostly retrospective, comparing 1199 patients undergoing pneumatic dilation and 2549 being treated with surgery [336]. All surgical cases were classic Heller myotomies by either a thoracotomy or laparotomy. The cumulative success rate, defined as good-to-excellent symptom response, was 65% (range 38–89%) for pneumatic dilation, compared with 86% (range 63–95%) for surgical myotomy with an average follow-up for both groups of about 4 years. In these comparative studies, the perforation rate for pneumatic dilation was 5%, whereas GERD developed in nearly 25% of surgical patients.

Studies comparing pneumatic dilation with the Rigiflex balloon and laparoscopic Heller myotomy have been reported. These studies began to appear at a critical time when many gastroenterologists had stopped performing pneumatic dilations and the laparoscopic technique had made Heller myotomy the more favored treatment for achalasia.

A large study from the Cleveland Clinic compared 106 patients treated with Rigiflex balloons by a single gastroenterologist and 73 patients undergoing primarily laparoscopic Heller myotomy (20 had failed pneumatic dilation and crossed over to surgery) by a single esophageal surgeon [244]. The success of graded pneumatic dilation and myotomy, defined as dysphagia/regurgitation less than three times a week or freedom from alternative treatment, was similar: 90% versus 89% at 6 months decreasing to 44% versus 57% at 6 years. Causes of symptom recurrence were incompletely treated achalasia (96% after pneumatic dilation vs 64% after myotomy) and complications of GERD (4% after dilation vs 36% after surgery).

To date, two randomized studies have been reported comparing Rigiflex balloon dilation and laparoscopic myotomy. The first series (26 dilations, 25 surgeries) with follow-up for at least 12 months observed six failures in the dilation group and one with surgery [264]. This difference reached statistical significance ($P = .04$) in the per protocol analysis but not the intention-to-treat analysis ($P = .09$). Most recently, an achalasia trial involving five European countries randomized 94 patients to Rigiflex pneumatic dilation (3.0 and 3.5 cm) and 106 patients to laparoscopic Heller myotomy with Dor fundoplication [337]. After 2-year follow-up, both treatments had comparable success rates—92% for pneumatic dilation and 87% for laparoscopic myotomy. Barium swallow emptying and LES pressures were similar for both groups. Four perforations occurred after pneumatic dilation compared to 11 perioperatively recognized perforations (one

converted to open operation) during laparoscopic Heller myotomy.

Another method to address this issue is to investigate large population-based databases comparing outcomes of these two procedures in typical practice settings. This was reported by Lopushinskey and Urbach in a retrospective longitudinal study in Ontario, Canada, from July 1991 to December 2002 [272]. A total of 1461 persons aged 18 years or older received treatment for achalasia: 1181 (80.8%) had pneumatic dilation and 280 (19.2%) had surgical myotomy as their first procedure. The cumulative risk of any subsequent intervention for achalasia (pneumatic dilation, myotomy or esophagectomy) after 1, 5, and 10 years, respectively, was 36.8%, 56.2%, and 63.5% after initial dilation treatment as compared to 16.4%, 30.3%, and 37.5% after initial myotomy (hazard risk 2.37; CI 1.86–3.02, $P < .001$). As shown in Table 13.10, the differences in risk were observed only when repeat pneumatic dilation was recorded as an adverse outcome. Since "on-demand" pneumatic dilation is the accepted approach to treating achalasia, this cannot logically be viewed as failure of this treatment modality. Interestingly, the 33% need for subsequent pneumatic dilation and 18% risk of repeat surgery following myotomy were much higher than the current surgery literature suggests, probably defining the more realistic surgical experience in the clinical community.

Heller myotomy versus botulinum toxin

Two studies have compared surgical myotomy with endoscopic injections of BTX, finding the same results. In the study by Andrews et al., 22 achalasia patients were given a choice of treatment: laparoscopic Heller myotomy or 100 U of BTX. Eighteen patients chose BTX as the initial treatment; 78% required a second or further injections [338]. Over time, the interval between each BTX injection decreased (i.e. 324-day mean intervals between the first and second injection vs 130 days between the third and fourth injections). Both treatments significantly improved symptoms to the same degree; however, only laparoscopic Heller myotomy significantly decreased basal LES pressure and improved esophageal emptying by barium esophagram. Overall, five

Table 13.10 Cumulative risk of subsequent intervention for achalasia after 10 years according to initial treatment (reproduced from Lopushinsky and Urbach [272], with permission).

Subsequent intervention	Surgical myotomy	Pneumatic dilation	*P*-value
Pneumatic dilation (%)	33.6	60.5	<.001
Surgical myotomy (%)	11.4	16.0	0.10
Esophagectomy (%)	6.8	2.1	0.16
Any of the above (%)	37.5	63.5	<.001

Table 13.11 Botulinum toxin versus pneumatic dilation for achalasia: prospective studies.

Study	Pneumatic dilation symptom improvement (%)					Botulinum toxin symptom improvement (%)					
	Number of patients	Initial	6 months	12 months	>30 months	Number of patient	Dose (U)	Initial	6 months	12 months	>30 months
Annese et al. [220]	8	100	—	—	—	8	100	100	13	—	—
Vaezi et al. [223]	20	75	75	70	—	22	100	64	36	32	—
Muehldorfer et al. [222]	12	83	75	66	50	12	80	75	50	25	0
Mikali et al. [226]	20	90	75	53		20	200	65	25	15	—
Allescher et al. [227]	14	78	—	65	50	23	100	74		45	15
Bansal et al. [339]	18	100	89	89	—	16	80	75	63	38	—
Ghosal et al. [340]	10	80	80	70	—	7	60–80	86	29	29	—
Total	**102**	**86**	**76**	**69**	**50**	**108**		**77**	**31**	**31**	**15**

of 18 (28%) patients in the BTX group switched to Heller myotomy after an average of 1.5 years because of treatment failure. There were no treatment failures in the laparoscopic Heller myotomy group. In a large study by Zaninotto et al., 40 patients each received BTX or Heller myotomy [321]. After 6 months, symptom improvement was comparable, but at 2 years the probability of being symptom free was 87.5% after surgery and 34% after BTX.

Botulinum toxin versus pneumatic dilation

Table 13.11 summarizes the seven prospective published studies comparing endoscopic injection of BTX with pneumatic dilation in the treatment of achalasia [220, 222, 223, 226, 227, 339, 340]. All seven reports were randomized studies involving about 100 patients in each treatment arm. In four studies, one or two BTX injections were given and the responders were followed up until symptoms relapsed [222, 223, 339, 340]. Repeat injections were administered in the three other studies [220, 226, 227], but subset analysis allowed determination of response rates for single injections versus serial injections. All but two studies used the Rigiflex balloons [222, 340] with pneumatic dilation performed once or twice, and then the patients were followed up until symptoms relapsed. As Table 13.11 shows, the initial response to BTX and pneumatic dilation are similar, but a single successful injection of BTX does not have the durability of pneumatic dilation, with the effects of the average injection lasting about 6–7 months. Whereas the success after pneumatic dilation gradually deteriorates over

the 30-month follow-up from 86% to 50%, BTX showed a dramatic deterioration in success by 6 months (31%), with only 15% of the remaining patients having symptom relief after 30 months. Two of these studies permitted a critical assessment of pneumatic dilation versus BTX when retreatment of relapses was allowed, but here again pneumatic dilation seems superior. Mikaeli et al. observed that all 12 patients in the pneumatic dilation group requiring retreatment were in symptomatic remission at 12 months versus 12 of 20 BTX patients (60%) [226]. In the study by Allescher et al., there was no significant difference at 1 year among those treated once or requiring retreatment in either the pneumatic dilation or BTX groups [227]. However, after 24, 36, and 48 months, a single pneumatic dilation was significantly superior to a single BTX injection, and after 36 and 48 months, a single pneumatic dilation was even superior to repeat BTX injections.

Cost analysis and quality of life comparisons between treatments

Six studies addressing some form of cost analysis in the treatment of achalasia are summarized in Table 13.12 [276, 341–346]. Three studies are true cost analyses] [276, 343, 344] in an actual series of patients, whereas the other studies are decision models.

Parkman et al. attempted to address the direct and indirect costs of pneumatic dilation versus open Heller myotomy in a large series of patients treated at the University of Pennsylvania from 1976 to 1986 [276]. Direct medical costs

Table 13.12 Cost analysis for achalasia treatment.

	Pneumatic dilation (US$)	Myotomy (US$)	Botulinum toxin (US$)	Time horizon (years)
Parkman et al. [276]	8474	20064[a]	—	7
Panaccione et al. [341])	2345	—	3271	10
Imperiale et al. [342])	3111	10792	3723	5
Kostic et al. [343]	2669	10229	—	1
Zaninotto et al. [344]	—	5074	4811	2
Karanicolas et al. [345]	7335	11089	—	10
O'Conner et al. [346]	7069	21407	7011	5

[a]Open myotomy; other studies laparoscopic Heller myotomy.

as determined from financial records and indirect non-medical costs estimated from patient surveys were compared at the time of first intervention and over a 7-year follow-up period. The initial cost of Heller myotomy was five times greater than the cost of pneumatic dilation and 2.4 times greater after 7 years (US$20064 vs US$8474).

Kostic et al. collected cost data in a prospective randomized controlled study comparing the efficacy of pneumatic dilation with the Rigiflex balloon dilator to laparoscopic Heller myotomy [343]. The initial costs of pneumatic dilation (two dilations within 10 days) and total costs over 12 months were significantly less than the costs of laparoscopic Heller myotomy (US$1418/$2669 vs $9910/$10229; P = .0002 and .0019, respectively). There was no difference in the follow-up costs between the two treatments, indicating the higher costs associated with surgical myotomy are due to the initial surgical intervention and longer hospital stay (0 vs 3 days, P = .023). The limitation of this study is the limited time horizon of 12 months, which places a disproportionate share of the total costs on the initial costs. The authors estimated costs for each initial treatment strategy over 3 years, assuming a failure rate of 20% for pneumatic dilation and 4% for Heller myotomy, with the alternative treatment performed in failures. Using this model, the cost estimates are similar for both treatment strategies.

In the Italian study by Zaninotto et al., 37 patients with achalasia were randomized to either laparoscopic Heller myotomy or BTX injections [344]. Patients treated with BTX were given two injections a month apart and those with recurrent symptoms were considered failures and treated with Heller myotomy. Only the direct medical costs were analyzed in this study, and as expected BTX injections were more cost-effective at 6 months (US$1688 vs US$4820) as both treatments were equally efficacious in the short term. However, after 2 years the total costs nearly tripled for patients initially treated with BTX, whereas the costs in the myotomy group were largely unchanged. The probability of remaining asymptomatic at 30 months was 90% for Heller myotomy and 22% for BTX. Because of the decreased efficacy over time, the advantage in cost-effectiveness for BTX versus Heller myotomy was negated with time, going from a ratio of 2.8:1 at the beginning of the study to 1.2:1 after 2 years. The cost-effectiveness of BTX as a short-term treatment was further supported by the observations of Panaccione et al. in a cost minimization analysis where BTX was less costly for patients with a life-expectancy of less than 2 years [341].

A decision model by Karanicolas et al. compared the costs accrued by an initial treatment strategy of pneumatic dilation or laparoscopic Heller myotomy over a 5- and 10-year horizon [345]. The pneumatic dilation treatment strategy resulted in 5- and 10-year costs of US$5198 and US$7560, respectively, compared to US$10445 and US$11429 for Heller myotomy. The probability estimates used in this study were systematically derived by two investigators after a comprehensive literature review. The lower difference in incremental costs between the two treatments at 10 years compared to 5 years may indicate that myotomy may become more cost-effective over a longer period of time. Longer term follow-up of ongoing patient series may help answer this question.

The second decision model by O'Connor et al. compared BTX injections, pneumatic dilation using a Rigiflex balloon, and laparoscopic Heller myotomy over a 5-year horizon [346]. This model analyzed the cost-effectiveness of these treatments as a product of quality-adjusted life-years (QALYs). QALYs are calculated as the time spent in a particular state of health multiplied by the quality of life assigned to that health state. In this study the utility was determined using the time trade-off technique in an interview of five patients with achalasia. The utility could range from 0 (death) to 1 (perfect health), and in the patients interviewed, the mean utility was 0.862. This value was assumed to be 1 following successful treatment. Over the 5-year time horizon, pneumatic dilation was more cost-effective than the other two treatment modalities (see Table 13.11). Compared to BTX and Heller myotomy, the incremental cost-effectiveness ratio per QALY for pneumatic dilation was US$1348 and US$5376750, respectively. Surgical myotomy would need to have an initial cost of US$2150 before it would be more cost-effective than pneumatic dilation. Similarly to the Karanicolas *et al.* study, myotomy may become the preferred treatment option from a cost standpoint when the time horizon is extended, in this case to 50 years. One of the limitations of this study is the small number of patients interviewed to obtain the utility for the QALY analysis.

Other authors have recently used decision-analysis modeling to address the gain in quality-adjusted life-expectancy, the product of the duration of survival in a particular health state and the quality of life (0, dead to 1, perfect health) associated with state of health, to compare treatments for achalasia. Urbach *et al.* calculated that laparoscopic Heller myotomy with a partial fundoplication was associated with the longest QALYs, but this only occurred after 10 years [347]. However, the differences between this strategy and pneumatic dilation were small, with pneumatic dilation becoming the preferred strategy when the effectiveness of

laparoscopic surgery was less than 90%, the operative mortality greater than 0.7%, or the probability of reflux after pneumatic dilation less than 19%.

Limitations of these studies are similar and include relatively short follow-up periods in the life of a patient with achalasia, modeled data rather than actual cost analysis for BTX injections and laparoscopic Heller myotomy, and no consideration for patient preference. Nevertheless, all these cost analyses find pneumatic dilation to be the most economic approach to treating achalasia.

General recommendations and the Cleveland Clinic experience

For the newly diagnosed patient with achalasia, a suggested treatment algorithm is shown in Figure 13.13 [348]. Symptomatic healthy patients with achalasia should be

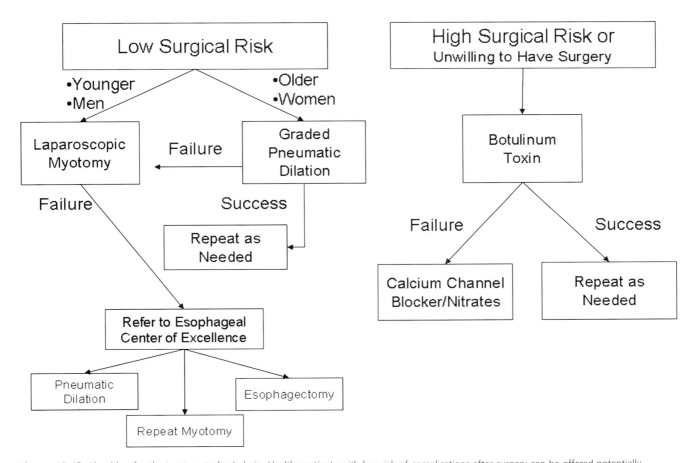

Figure 13.13 Algorithm for the treatment of achalasia. Healthy patients with low risk of complications after surgery can be offered potentially definitive therapy with either pneumatic dilation or laparoscopic myotomy. High-risk patients, especially the elderly, are best treated with botulinum toxin injections (reproduced from Vaezi and Richter [348], with permission).

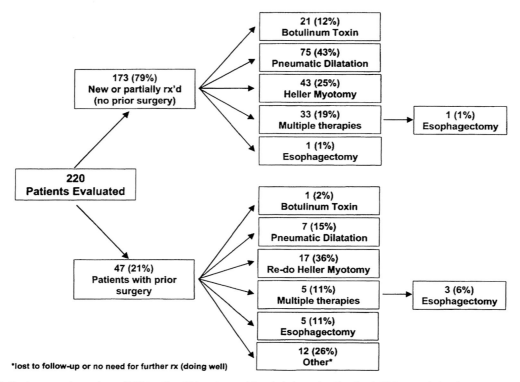

Figure 13.14 Author's personal experience (JER) treating 220 patients with achalasia at the Cleveland Clinic Foundation from 1994 to 2002. Note the multiple therapies required in the treatment of many of these achalasia patients.

given the option of graded pneumatic dilation or laparoscopic Heller myotomy (see Tables 13.7 and 13.9) and experience suggests relatively similar efficacies in the hands of experienced gastroenterologists and surgeons. Pneumatic dilation has the advantage of being an outpatient procedure, pain is minimal, GERD is an infrequent problem, it can be performed in any age group (children to 90 years of age) and during pregnancy [349], it does not hinder the performance of a future myotomy, and all cost analyses find it to be less expensive than Heller myotomy over 5–10 years. On the other hand, laparoscopic Heller myotomy has the advantage of being a single procedure, dysphagia relief may be greater at the cost of more troubling heartburn, and it may be a more effective treatment than pneumatic dilation in adolescents and young adults, especially men. Myotomy is definitely the treatment of choice in uncooperative patients and patients in whom pseudoachalasia cannot be excluded. In healthy subjects, we do not offer BTX as an option, because the treatment is not definitive and the duration of relief is short term. On the other hand, BTX injections are the treatment of choice in patients who are poor surgical candidates or older than 80 years, because it is safe, improves symptoms, and generally elderly patients require retreatment no more frequently than once a year. Nifedipine or isosorbide dinitrate are at best second-line treatments, being rarely used because of drug side effects. If medical therapy

fails, a "gentle" pneumatic dilatation can be performed with a 3.0-cm Rigiflex balloon.

Figure 13.14 summarizes the personal experience of one of us (JER) in treating 223 achalasia patients at the Cleveland Clinic from 1994 to 2002 [350]. Nearly 80% of these patients (173 subjects) had newly diagnosed achalasia or were diagnosed and treated unsuccessfully elsewhere with drugs, BTX, or pneumatic dilation. Very old patients or those with severe comorbid illnesses (21 patients [12%]) received BTX injections as initial treatment. Healthy patients were offered either graded pneumatic dilation by Dr. Richter or laparoscopic Heller myotomy by an experienced senior esophageal surgeon, Thomas Rice. Seventy-six patients (44%) were successfully treated with pneumatic dilatation and 43 patients (25%) underwent successful Heller myotomy. Overall, good-to-excellent symptom relief at last follow-up for pneumatic dilation and surgical myotomy were remarkably similar (82% vs 80%, respectively). The esophageal perforation rate was 2%; 15% of patients undergoing pneumatic dilation had troubling heartburn requiring PPIs, and 15 patients eventually required myotomy to relieve their dysphagia. In the patients treated with laparoscopic myotomy, two (3%) required repeat myotomy, four (6%) required subsequent pneumatic dilations, and 51% had troubling heartburn requiring PPIs. The high rate of GERD is bothersome but is representative of personal evolution with the technique of laparoscopic Heller myotomy. Initially, the operation was done with a Toupet fundoplication, but several patients required wrap modification or takedown because of dysphagia. Next, the myotomy was performed without a fundoplication with minimal dissection of the hiatus and a gastropexy. As a result of the high rate of heartburn, we have added a Dor fundoplication, which has resulted in fewer gastroesophageal reflux problems. Forty-seven patients (21%) with achalasia were referred after failing surgery; 93% had prior Heller myotomy (>60% via the thoracic approach) and 7% were initially misdiagnosed with GERD and underwent antireflux surgery. The success rate for either pneumatic dilation (67%) or repeat Heller myotomy (65%) was significantly less in this group of patients than for untreated achalasia patients. In the patients with prior surgery, eight patients (17%) eventually needed an esophagectomy with gastric pull up, and in the entire 223-patient experience, 10 patients (4.5%) ultimately required esophagectomy.

This experience with complicated achalasia patients confirms our recommendation in the algorithm [350] that patients failing initial laparoscopic myotomy need referral to specialized esophageal centers with expertise in pneumatic dilation, repeat myotomy, and esophagectomy. Furthermore, our ongoing long-term follow-up of these patients, both symptomatically and objectively with the timed barium esophagram, suggests that the vast majority of individuals can be helped with general relief of their dysphagia and good quality of life. However, as others have reported [181, 243], few patients are "cured" with a single procedure, and intermittent "tune-up" procedures (especially pneumatic dilation and occasionally repeat myotomy) may be required.

Esophageal cancer

In 1872, Fagge first described the relationship between achalasia and esophageal cancer in an 84-year-old patient suffering from dysphagia for more than 40 years [351]. Over the past 30 years, 16 studies have addressed this issue, showing an overall prevalence rate of 0–6.7% with a mean of 3%. Among these studies, five found no correlation but the remainder had incidences that ranged from 1% to 20% (mean 7.5%), with the average risk being 197 cases per 100 000 achalasia patients [352]. In the most careful endoscopic follow-up of achalasia, Meijssen *et al.* prospectively studied 195 patients with surveillance endoscopy at 3 months and at 1, 2, 7, and 10 years after dilation [353]. Squamous cell carcinoma was discovered in the mid esophagus in three patients at 5, 19, and 28 years following the onset of dysphagia, with the age of the patients being 89, 37, and 77 years, respectively. In a German study of 124 patients with achalasia followed by endoscopy after their initial treatment at intervals of 1–2 years, the incidence of carcinoma was 1 for 174 patient-years of follow up [354].

The four patients with carcinoma were diagnosed 14.5, 12.0, 7.7, and 5.1 years, respectively, following their initial presentation. The intervals of time between the onset of symptoms and the diagnosis of carcinoma were 17.8, 27.5, 38.6, and 42.5 years (mean 31.6 years).

Achalasia patients with esophageal cancer are on average 60 years of age. They are four times more likely to be men, despite the prevalence of achalasia being equal between genders [352]. Compared with the general population presenting with esophageal cancer, achalasia patients have a poorer prognosis and have more unresectable disease (50% vs 80%) [353]. This difference is most likely related to the more dilated esophagi and large tumor mass necessary to produce symptoms, as well as a lack of patient and physician alarm when new dysphagia complaints present. Cancer presents in the mid esophagus in 50% of cases, lower third in 38%, and upper esophagus in 12% of patients, with more than 90% having a predominant histologic type of squamous cell carcinoma. Adenocarcinoma more commonly occurs following myotomy and comprises fewer than 10% of cases [352]. Most cancers occur in patients with a megaesophagus [355]. The malignancy rarely occurs at the stenotic area and is more common in the dilated esophagus. It is theorized that stasis of esophageal contents causes chronic esophagitis, which progresses to chronic ulcerations. Over time, the ulcerations can heal to form epithelial hyperplasia and benign papillomas. As the irritation continues in the poorly emptying esophagus, the opportunity for malignant degeneration occurs [356]. This theory has been confirmed in two large esophageal resection studies [20, 357].

The diagnosis of esophageal cancer in an achalasia patient is best made by careful endoscopy after the subject has been on a clear liquid diet for several days. The right wall of the lower third of the esophagus should be inspected carefully, because this area is most susceptible to malignant changes [358]. Lugol staining to help direct biopsies [359] and brush cytology may help in patients without obvious masses. Overall survival in achalasia patients after the diagnosis of esophageal cancer generally is not good because of the large tumor burden with extensive regional and distant spread. Only 20% of these patients are suitable for surgery [353]. In a study of 167 cases of achalasia and cancer, only five of 38 subjects undergoing surgery could be resected and no patient was alive beyond 5 years [358]. Over the past 30 years, 5-year survival rates for esophageal cancer in the general population have significantly improved, varying from 25% to 40% [360], whereas the mean survival for achalasia patients with cancer is approximately 10 months, with most patients living less than 6 months [352].

Because the data confirming the risk of squamous cell carcinoma in achalasia are overwhelming, the key is prevention and early detection. Although Ronald Belsey in 1958 suggested that "procrastination and the extended trial of less than satisfactory procedures, such as repeated attempts at dilation, can only increase the risk of malignant generation" [361], there are many examples in the literature of squamous cell cancer after myotomy [352]. Because most patients have megaesophagus, this suggests the need for careful follow-up of patients, monitoring esophageal diameter and emptying time, perhaps with a timed barium swallow [191], independent of the patient's complaints about dysphagia or regurgitation. Despite this cancer risk, the most recent guidelines from the American Society of Gastrointestinal Endoscopy do not recommend routine endoscopic surveillance for squamous cell cancer in achalasia patients [362]. Without guidelines, this is an area of debate and further intervention studies are unlikely because the disease (cancer in achalasia) is rare and would require long-term and probably multicenter studies. We agree with others that older patients with long-standing disease and megaesophagus are the best candidates for a surveillance program [271, 350, 351]. The endoscopy interval is unknown but probably should be every 2–3 years.

References

1. Willis T. *Pharmaceutic Rationalis: Sive Diatriba de Medicamentorum; Operatimibus in Humano Corpore*. London, Hagae-Comitis, 1674.

2. Von Mikulicz J. Ueber Gastroskopic and Oesophagoskopic. *Miu Ver Aeszte Niedes Orst Wein*. 1882;8:41–44.

3. Hurst AF. Achalasia of the cardia. *Q J Med* 1915;8:200–202.

4. Russel JC. Diagnosis and treatment of spasmodic strictures of the esophagus. *Br Med J* 1898;1:1450–1454.

5. Heller E. Extramukoese cardinplastik bein chronischen cardiopsasmus mit dilation des oesophagus. *Mitt Grenzgeb Med Chir* 1914;27:141–145.

6. Mayberry JF, Atkinson M. Variations in the prevalence of achalasia in Great Britain and Ireland: an epidemiological study based on hospital admissions. *Q J Med* 1987;62:67–71.

7. Mayberry JF. Epidemiology and demographics of achalasia. *Gastrointest Endosc Clin North Am* 2001;11:235–247.

8. Birgisson S. Richter, JE. Achalasia in Iceland, 1952–2002: An epidemiologic study. *Dig Dis Sci* 2007;52(8):1855–1860.

9. Wong RK, Maydonovitch CL, Metz SJ, *et al*. Significant DQw1 association in achalasia. *Dig Dis Sci* 1989;34: 349–354.

10. Verne GN, Hahn AB, Pineau BC, *et al*. Association of HLADR and -DQ alleles with idiopathic achalasia. *Gastroenterology* 1999;117:26–31.

11. Howard PJ, Maker L, Pryde A, *et al*. Five year prospective study of the incidence, clinical features, and diagnosis of achalasia in Edinburgh. *Gut* 1992;33:1011–1015.

12. Eckard VF, Hoischen T, Bernhard G. Life expectancy, complications and causes of death in patients with achalasia: results of a 33-year follow-up investigation. *Eur J Gastroenterol Hepatol* 2008;20:956–960.

13. Paterson WG. Etiology and pathogenesis of achalasia. *Gastrointest Endosc Clin North Am* 2001;11:249–265.

14. Goyal RK, Paterson WG. Esophageal motility. In: Woods JD, ed. *Handbook of Physiology*. New York: Oxford Press, 1989, pp. 865–882.

15. Cassella RR, Ellis FH, Brown AL. Fine structure changes in achalasia of the esophagus. I. Vagus nerves. *Am J Pathol* 1965; 279:46–54.

16. Kimura K. The nature of idiopathic esophagus dilatation. *Jpn J Gastroenterol* 1929;1:199–201.

17. Casella RR, Brown AL, Sayre GP, *et al*. Achalasia of the esophagus: pathologic and etiologic observations. *Ann Surg* 1964; 160:474–480.

18. Higgs B, Kerr FWL, Ellis FH. The experimental production of esophageal achalasia by electrolytic lesions in the medulla. *J Thorac Cardiovasc Surg* 1965;50:613–617.

19. Lendrum FC. Anatomic features of the cardiac orifice of the stomach with special reference to cardiospasm. *Arch Intern Med* 1937;59:474–478.

20. Goldblum JR, Whyte RI, Orringer MB, *et al*. Achalasia: a morphologic study of 42 resected specimens. *Am J Surg Pathol* 1994;18:327–337.

21. Goldblum JR, Rice TW, Richter JE. Histopathologic features in esophagomyotomy specimens from patients with achalasia. *Gastroenterology* 1996;111:648–654.

22. Csendes A, Smok G, Braghetto I, *et al*. Histological studies of Auerbach's plexuses of the oesophagus, stomach, jejunum, and colon in patients with achalasia of the esophagus: correlation with gastric acid secretion, presence of parietal cells and gastric emptying of solids. *Gut* 1992;33:150–155.

23. Gockel I, Juergen RE, Junginger T, *et al*. Reduction of interstitial cells of Cajal (ICC) associated with neuronal nitric oxide synthase (n-NOS) in patients with achalasia. *Am J Gastroenterol* 2008;103:856–864

24. Friesen DL, Henderson RD, Hanna W. Ultrastructure of the esophageal muscle in achalasia and diffuse esophageal spasm. *Am J Clin Pathol* 1983;79:319–322.

25. DeGiorgio R, Di Simone MP, Stanghellini V, *et al*. Esophageal and gastric nitric acids synthesizing innervation in primary achalasia. *Am J Gastroenterol* 1999;94:2357–2362.

26. Mearin F, Mourelle M, Guarner F, *et al*. Patients with achalasia lack nitric oxide synthase in the gastro-oesophageal function. *Eur J Clin Invest* 1993;23:724–728.

27. Varannes SB, Chevalier J, Pimont S. Serum from achalasia patients alters neurochemical coding in the myenteric plexus and nitric oxide mediated motor response in normal human fundus. *Gut* 2006;55:319–326.

28. Cajal SR. *Histologie du Ssystéme Nnerveux de l'homme et des Vvertébrés, Vol. 2: Grand Ssympathique*. Paris: Maloine, 1911, pp. 891–942.

29. Ward SM, Morris G, Reese L, *et al*. Interstitial cells of Cajal mediate enteric inhibitory neurotransmission in the lower esophageal and pyloric sphincters. *Gastroenterology* 1998;115:314–329.

30. Daniel EE, Posey-Daniel V. Nneuromuscular structures in opossum esophagus; role of interstitial cells of Cajal. *Am J Physiol* 1984;246:G305–315.

31. Blennerhassett MG, Lourenssen S. Neural regulation of intestinal smooth muscle growth. *Am J Physiol* 2000;279:6511–6517.

32. Gockel I, Bohl JRE, Junginger T, *et al*. Spectrum of histopathologic findings in patients with achalasia reflexts different etiologies. *J Gastroenterol Hepatol* 2006;21:727–733.

33. Lehman MB, Clark SB, Ormsby AH, *et al*. Squamous mucosal alterations in esophagectomy specimens from patients with end-stage achalasia. *Am J Surg Pathol* 2001;25:1413–1418.

34. Kjellin AP, Ost AIE, Pope CE II. Histology of esophageal mucosa from patients with achalaia. *Dis Esophagus* 2005;18:257–261.

35. Dunaway PM, Maydonovitch CL, Wong RKH. Characterization of esophageal muscle in patients with achalasia. *Dig Dis Sci* 2000;45:285–290.

36. Massey BT, Hogan WJ, Dodds WJ, *et al*. Alteration of upper esophageal sphincter belch reflex in patients with achalasia. *Gastroenterology* 1992;103:1574–1579.

37. Ali GN, Hunt DR, Jorgensen JO, *et al*. Esophageal achalasia and coexistent upper esophageal sphincter relaxation disorder presenting with airway obstruction. *Gastroenterology* 1995; 109:1328–1332.

38. Annese V, Caruso N, Accadia L, *et al*. Gallbladder function and gastric liquid emptying in achalasia. *Dig Dis Sci* 1991; 36:1116–1120.

39. Schmidt T, Pfeiffer A, Hachelsberger N, *et al*. Dysmotility of the small intestine in achalasia. *Neurogastroenterol Motil* 1999; 11:11–15.

40. Hagenmuller F, Classen M. Motility of Oddi's sphincter in Parkinson's disease, progressive systemic sclerosis and achalasia. *Endoscopy* 1988;20 (Suppl 1):189–192.

41. Eckardt WF, Krause I, Belle D. Gastrointestinal transit and gastric acid secretion in patients with achalasia. *Dig Dis Sci* 1989;34:665–670.

42. Mearm F, Papo M, Malagelda JR. Impaired gastric relaxation in patients with achalasia. *Gut* 1995;36:363–368.

43. Olk W, Kiesewalter B, Aver P, *et al*. Extraesophageal autonomic dysfunction in patients with achalasia. *Dig Dis Sci* 1999; 44:2088–2092.

44. Misiewicz J, Waller SC, Anthony PP, *et al*. Pharmacology and histopathology of isolated cardiac sphincter muscle from patients with and without achalasia. *Q J Med* 1969;38:17–20.

45. Tottrup A, Forman A, Funch-Jensen P, *et al*. Effects of postganglionic nerve stimulation in oesophageal achalasia: an *in vitro* study. *Gut* 1990;31:17–20.

46. Dodds WJ, Dent J, Hogan WJ, *et al*. Paradoxical lower esophageal sphincter contraction induced by cholecystokininoctapeptide in achalasia. *Gastroenterology* 1981;80:27–33.

47. Cohen S, Fisher R, Tuch A. The site of denervation in achalasia. *Gut* 1972;13:556–559.

48. Guelrud M, Rossiter A, Souney E, *et al*. The effect of vasoactive intestinal polypeptide on the lower esophageal sphincter in achalasia. *Gastroenterology* 1992;103:377–382.

49. Gonzales M, Mearin F, Vasconez JR, *et al*. Oesophageal tone in patients with achalasia. *Gut* 1997;41:291–296.

50. Kramer P, Ingelfinger FJ. Esophageal sensitivity to Mecholyl in achalasia. *Gastroenterology* 1951;19:242–244.

51. Penagini R, Bartesaghi B, Zannini P, *et al*. Lower esophageal sphincter hypersensitivity to opioid receptor stimulation in patients with idiopathic achalasia. *Gut* 1993;34:16–20.

52. Holloway RH, Dodds WJ, Helm JF, *et al*. Integrity of cholinergic innervation to the lower esophageal sphincter in achalasia. *Gastroenterology* 1986;90:924–929.

53. Sifrim D, Janssen J, Vantrappen G. Failing deglutitive inhibition in primary esophageal motility disorders. *Gastroenterology* 1994;106:875–882.

54. Paterson WG. Esophageal and lower esophageal sphincter response to balloon distention in patients with achalasia. *Dig Dis Sci* 1997;42:106–110.

55. Paterson WG. Neuromuscular mechanisms of esophageal response at and proximal to a distending balloon. *Am J Physiol* 1991;42:106–110.

56. Murray JA, Ledlow A, Launspach J, *et al*. The effects of recombinant human hemoglobin on esophageal motor function in humans. *Gastroenterology* 1995;109:1241–1248.

57. Singarum C, Snipes RL, Bass P, *et al*. Evaluation of early events in the creation of amyenteric opossum model of achalasia. *Neurogastroenterol Motil* 1996;8:351–357.

58. Gaumnitz EA, Bass P, Osinski M, *et al*. Electrophysiological and pharmacological responses of chronically denervated LES of the opossum. *Gastroenterology* 1995;109:789–799.

59. Zimmerman FH, Rosenzweig NS. Achalasia in a father and son. *Am J Gastroenterol* 1984;79:506–508.

60. Bosher LP, Shaw A. Achalasia in siblings. Clinical and genetic aspects. *Am J Dis Child* 1981;135:709–710.

61. Ehrich E, Aranoff G, Johnson WG. Familial achalasia associated with adrenocortical insufficiency, alacrima, and neurological abnormalities. *Am J Med Genet* 1987;26:637–644.

62. Stein DT, Knauer M. Achalasia in monozygote twins. *Dig Dis Sci* 1982;27:636–640.

63. Weber A. Linkage of the gene for the triple A syndrome to chromosome 12q13 near the type 11 keratin gene cluster. *Hum Mol Genet* 1996;5:2061–2067.

64. Chawla K, Chawla SK, Alexander LL. Familial achalasia of the esophagus in mother and son: a possible pathogenic relationship. *J Am Geriatr Soc* 1979;27:519.

65. Kilpatrick ZM, Milles S. Achalasia in mother and daughter. *Gastroenterology* 1972;62:1042–1046.

66. Machler D, Schneider R. Achalasia in a father and son. *Dig Dis Sci* 1978;23:1042–1045.

67. Mayberry JF, Atkinson M. A study of swallowing difficulties in first-degree relatives of patients with achalasia. *Thorax* 1985;40:391–393.

68. Birgisson S, Richter JE. Achalasia: what's new in diagnosis and treatment. *Dig Dis* 1997;15 (Suppl):1–27.

69. Atkinson M. Antecedents of achalasia. *Gut* 1994;35:861–862.

70. Robertson CS, Martin BA, Atkinson M. Varicella-zoster virus DNA in the oesophageal myenteric plexus in achalasia. *Gut* 1993;34:299–302.

71. Oliveira RB, Filho RJ, Dantas RO, *et al*. The spectrum of esophageal motor disorders in Chagas' disease. *Am J Gastroenterol* 1995;90:119–124.

72. Koelle DM, Abbo H, Corey L, *et al*. Direct recover of herpes simplex virus specific T-lymphocyte clones from recurrent genital HSV-2 lesions. *J Infect Dis* 1994;169:956–961.

73. Jones DB, Mayberry JF, Rhodes J, *et al*. Preliminary report of an association between measles virus and achalasia. *J Clin Pathol* 1983;36:655–657.

74. Castex F, Guillemot F, Talbode N, *et al*. Association of an attack of varicella and achalasia. *Am J Gastroenterol* 1995;90:1188–1189.

75. Niwamoto H, Okamoto E, Fujmoto J, *et al*. Are human herpes viruses or measles virus associated with esophageal achalasia? *Dig Dis Sci* 1995;40:859–864.

76. Birgissen S, Galinski MS, Goldblum JR, *et al*. Achalasia is not associated with measles as known herpes or human papilloma viruses. *Dig Dis Sci* 1997;42:300–306.

77. Castagliuolo I, Brun P, Aninotto G, *et al*. Esophageal achalasia: Is the herpes simplex virus really innocent? *J Gastrointest Surg* 2004;8:24–30.

78. Hill JM, Gebhardt BM, Kaufman HE, *et al.* Quantitation of herpes simplex virus type 1 DNA and latency-associated transcripts in rabbit trigeminal ganglia demonstrates a stable reservoir of viral nucleic acids during latency. *J Virol* 1996;70:3137–3141.

79. Facco M, Brun P, Zaninotto G, *et al.* T cells in the myenteric plexus of achalasia patients show a skewed TCR repertoire and react to HSV-1 antigens. *Am J Gastroenterol* 2008;103:1598–1609.

80. de la Concha EG, Fernandez-Arquero M, Mendoza JL, *et al.* Contribution of HLA class II genes to susceptibility in achalasia. *Tissue Antigens* 1998;52:3812–3815.

81. Storch WB, Eckardt VF, Wienbeck M, *et al.* Autoantibodies to Auerbach's plexus in achalasia. *Cell Mol Biol* 1995;41:1033–1038.

82. Verne GN, Sallustio JE, Eaker EY Anti-myenteric neuronal antibodies in patients with achalasia. *Dig Dis Sci* 1997;42: 302–313.

83. Ruiz-De-Leon A, Mendoza J, de la Concha EG, *et al.* Myenteric antiplexus antibodies and class II HLA in achalasia. *Dig Dis Sci* 2002;47:15–19.

84. Latiano A, De Giorgia R, Annese V, *et al.* HLA and enteic antineuronal antibodies in patients with achalasia. *Neurogastroenterol Motil* 2006;18:520–525.

85. Kraichely RE, Farrugia G, Lennon VA, *et al.* Neural autoantibody profile of primary achalasia. *Dig Dis Sci* 2010;55:307-311.

86. Sonnenberg A, Massey BT, McCarty DJ, *et al.* Epidemiology of hospitalization for achalasia in the United States. *Dig Dis Sci* 1993;38:233–244.

87. Murphy MS, Gardner-Medwin D, Eastham EJ. Achalasia of the cardia associated with hereditary cerebellar ataxia. *Am J Gastroenterol* 1989;84:1329–1330.

88. Foster PN, Stewart M, Lowe JS, *et al.* Achalasia-like disorder of the oesophagus in von Recklinghausen's neurofibromatosis. *Gut* 1987;28:1522–1526.

89. Qualman SJ, Hupt HM, Yang P, *et al.* Esophageal Lewy bodies associated with ganglion cell loss in achalasia. Similarity to Parkinson's disease. *Gastroenterology* 1984;87:848–856.

90. Vantrappen G, Janssen J, Hellemans J, *et al.* Achalasia, diffuse spasm and related motility disorders. *Gastroenterology* 1979;76:450–459.

91. Paterson WG, Beck IT, DaCosta TR. Transition from nutcracker esophagus to achalasia. A case report. *J Clin Gastroenterol* 1991;13:554–555.

92. Vantrappen G, Hellemans J, Deloof W, *et al.* Treatment of achalasia with pneumatic dilatation. *Gut* 1971;12:268–275.

93. Black J, Vorbach AW, Collis J. Results of Heller operation for achalasia of the esophagus: the importance of hiatal hernia. *Br J Surg* 1976;63:649–653.

94. Menzies-Gow N, Gummes WP, Edward DAW. Results of Heller's operation for achalasia of the cardia. *Br J Surg* 1978; 65:483–485.

95. Sawyer JG, Foster JH. Surgical consideration in the management of achalasia of the esophagus. *Ann Surg* 1967;165:780–783.

96. Fellows IW, Ogilivie AL, Atkinson M. Pneumatic dilation in achalasia. *Gut* 1983;24:1020–1023.

97. Clouse RE, Abramson BK, Todorszuk JR. Achalasia in the elderly. Effect of aging on clinical presentation and outcome. *Dig Dis Sci* 1991;36:225–228.

98. Wong RKH, Maydonovitch CL. Achalasia. In: Castell DO, Richter JE, eds. *The Eesophagus*, 3rd edn. Philadelphia: Lippincott Williams and Wilkins, 1999, pp. 185–404.

99. Eckardt VF. Clinical presentation and complications of achalasia. *Gastrointest Endosc Clin North Am* 2001;11:281–292.

100. Rosenzweig S, Traube M. The diagnosis and misdiagnosis of achalasia. *J Clin Gastroenterol* 1989;11:147–153.

101. Reynolds JC, Parkman HE. Achalasia. *Gastroenterol Clin North Am* 1989;18:223–255.

102. Crookes PF, DeMeester TF, Corkill S. Gastroesophageal reflex in achalasia. When is reflux really reflux? *Dig Dis Sci* 1997;42:1354–1359.

103. Aronchick JM, Miller WT, Epstein DM, *et al.* Association of achalasia and pulmonary *Mycobacterium fortuitum* infection. *Radiology* 1986;160:85–86.

104. Stacher G, Kiss A, Wiesnagrotzki S, *et al.* Oesophageal and gastric motility disorders in patients categorized as having primary anorexia nervosa. *Gut* 1986;27:1120–1126.

105. Eckardt VF, Stauf B, Bernhard G. Chest pain in achalasia: patient characteristics and clinical course. *Gastroenterology* 1999;116:1300–1304.

106. Robson K, Rosenberg S, Lembo T. GERD progressing to diffuse esophageal spasm and then achalasia. *Dig Dis Sci* 200;45: 110–113.

107. Smart HC, Mayberry JF, Atkinson M. Achalasia following gastro-oesophageal reflux. *J R Soc Med* 1986;79:71–73.

108. Spechler SJ, Souza RF, Rosenberg SJ, *et al.* Heartburn in patients with achalasia. *Gut* 1995;37:305–308.

109. Shoenut JP, Micflikier AB, Yaffe CS, *et al.* Reflux in untreated achalasia patients. *J Clin Gastroenterol* 1995;20:6–11.

110. Smart HL, Foster PN, Evans DF, *et al.* Twenty-four hour oesophageal acidity in achalasia before and after pneumatic dilation. *Gut* 1987;28:883–887.

111. Tucker HJ, Snape WJ, Cohen S. Achalasia secondary to carcinoma: manometric and clinical features. *Ann Intern Med* 1978;89:315–318.

112. Rozman RW, Achkar E. Features distinguishing secondary achalasia from primary achalasia. *Am J Gastroenterol* 1990; 85:1327–1330.

113. Becker DJ, Castell DO. Acute airway obstruction in achalasia: possible role of defective belch reflex. *Gastroenterology* 1989; 97:1323–1326.

114. Seeman H, Traube M. Hiccups and achalasia. *Ann Intern Med* 1991;115:711–712.

115. Breatnach E, Han SY. Pneumopericardium occurring as a complication of achalasia. *Chest* 1986;90:292–294.

116. Siriser F, Bardaxaglow E, Lebeau S, *et al.* A long-term clinical study of the effectiveness of myotomy for achalasia. *Gullet* 1992;2:124–128.

117. Orlando RC, Call DL, Beam CA. Achalasia and absent gastric air bubble. *Ann Intern Med* 1978;88:60–61.

118. Stewart ET. Radiographic evaluation of the esophagus and its motor disorders. *Med Clin North Am* 1981;65:1173–1190.

119. Schima W, Ryan JM, Harisinghani M, *et al.* Radiographic detection of achalasia: diagnostic role of video fluoroscopy. *Clin Radiol* 1998;53:372–375.

120. DeOliveira JMA, Birgisson S, Doinoff C, *et al.* Timed-barium swallow: a simple technique for evaluating esophageal emptying in patients with achalasia. *AJR Am J Roentgenol* 1997;169:473–479.

121. Kostic SV, Rice TV, Baker ME, *et al.* Timed barium esophagram: a simple physiologic assessment for achalasia. *J Thorac Cardiovasc Surg* 2000;120:935–946.

122. Meshkinpour H, Kaye L, Elias A, *et al*. Manometric and radiologic correlations in achalasia. *Am J Gastroenterol* 1992;87:1567–1570.

123. Debas HT, Payne WS, Cameron AJ, *et al*. Physiopathology of the lower esophageal diverticulum and its implications for treatment. *Surg Gynecol Obstet* 1980;151:593–600.

124. Taub W, Achkar E. Hiatal hernia in patients with achalasia. *Am J Gastroenterol* 1987;82:1256–1258.

125. Goldenberg SP, Vos C, Burrell M, *et al*. Achalasia and hiatal hernia. *Dig Dis Sci* 1992;37:528–531.

126. Ott DJ, Hodge RG, Chen MYM, *et al*. Achalasia associated with hiatal hernia: prevalence and potential implications. *Abdom Imaging* 1993;18:7–9.

127. Herwaarden MAV, Samson M, Smout AJPM. Prolonged manometric recordings of oesophagus and lower oesophageal sphincter in achalasia patients. *Gut* 2001;49:813–821.

128. Hirano I, Tatum RP, Shi G, *et al*. Manometric heterogeneity in patients with idiopathic achalasia. *Gastroenterology* 2001; 120:789–798.

129. Goldenberg SP, Burell M, Fette GG, *et al*. Classic and vigorous achalasia: a comparison of manometric, radiographic, and clinical findings. *Gastroenterology* 1991;101:743–748.

130. Todorczuk JR, Aliperti G, Staiano A, *et al*. Reevaluation of manometric criteria for vigorous achalsia. Is this a distinct clinical disorder? *Dig Dis Sci* 1991;36:274–278.

131. Camacho-Lobato L, Katz PO, Eveland J, *et al*. Vigorous achalasia. Original description requires minor change. *J Clin Gastroenterol* 2001;33:375–377.

132. Vantrappen G, Hellemans J. Treatment of achalasia and related motor disorders. *Gastroenterology* 1980;79:144–154.

133. Schneider JH, Peters JH, Kirkman E, *et al*. Are the motility abnormalities of achalasia reversible? An experimental outflow obstruction in the feline model. *Surgery* 1999;125:498–503.

134. Parilla P, Aguayo JR, Martinex DHL, *et al*. Reversible achalasia-like motor pattern of esophageal body secondary to postoperative stricture of gastroesophageal junction. *Dig Dis Sci* 1992; 37:1781–1784.

135. Vantrappen G, Van Goidsenhoven GE, Verbekke S, *et al*. Manometric studies in achalasia of the cardia, before and after pneumatic dilation. *Gastroenterology* 1963;45:317–325.

136. Cohen S, Lipschutz W. Lower esophageal sphincter dysfunction in achalasia. *Gastroenterology* 1971;61:814–820.

137. Katz PO, Richter JE, Cowan R, *et al*. Apparent complete lower esophageal sphincter relaxation in achalasia. *Gastroenterology* 1986;90:978–983.

138. Castell JA, Dalton CB, Castell DO. On-line computer analysis of human lower esophageal sphincter relaxation. *Am J Physiol* 1988;255:G794–799.

139. Clouse RE, Abramson BK, Todorczuk JR. Achalasia in the elderly. Effects of age on clinical presentation and outcome. *Dig Dis Sci* 1991;36:225–228.

140. Holloway RH, Wyman JB, Dent J. Failure of transient lower oesophageal sphincter relaxation in response to gastric distension in patients with achalasia: evidence for neural mediation of transient lower oesophageal sphincter relaxation. *Gut* 1989;30:762–767.

141. Dudnick RS, Castell JA, Castell DO. Abnormal upper esophageal sphincter function in achalasia. *Am J Gastroenterol* 1992; 87:1712–1715.

142. Ghosh SK, Pandolfino JE, Rice J, *et al*. Impaired deglutitive EGJ relaxation in clinical manometry: a quantitative analysis of 400 patients and 75 controls. *Am J Physiol Gastrointest Liver Physiol* 2007;293:G878–885.

143. Pandolfino JE, Kwiatek MA, Nealis T, *et al*. Achalasia: a new clinically relevant classification by high resolution manometry. *Gastroenterology* 2008;135:1526–1533.

144. Gockel I, Eckhard VF, Schmitt T, Junginger T. Pseudoachalasia: A case series and analysis of the literature. *Scand J Gastroenterol* 2005;40:378–385.

145. Sandler RS, Bozymski EM, Orlando RC. Failure of clinical criteria to distinguish between primary achalasia and achalasia secondary to tumor. *Dig Dis Sci* 1982;27:209–213.

146. Liu JB, Miller LS, Goldberg BB, *et al*. Transnasal ultrasound of the esophagus: preliminary morphologic and function studies. *Radiology* 1992;184:721–727.

147. Miller LS, Liu JB, Menn PJ, *et al*. High-resolution endoluminal sonography in achalasia. *Gastrointest Endosc* 1995;42:545–549.

148. Carter M, Deckmann RC, Smith RC, *et al*. Differentiation of achalasia from pseudoachalasia by computed tomography. *Am J Gastroenterol* 1997;92:624–628.

149. Van Dam J, Falk GW, Sivak MV, *et al*. Endosonographic evaluation of the patient with achalasia: appearance of the esophagus using the echoendoscope. *Endoscopy* 1995;27:185–190.

150. Deviere J, Dunham F, Rickaert F, *et al*. Endoscopic ultrasonography in achalasia. *Gastroenterology* 1989;96:1210–1213.

151. Benjamin SB, Castell DO. Achalasia and Hodgkin's disease. A chance association. *J Clin Gastroenterol* 1981;3:175–178.

152. Roark G, Shabot M, Patterson M. Achalasia secondary to hepatocellular carcinoma. *J Clin Gastroenterol* 1983;5:255–258.

153. Kline MM. Successful treatment of vigorous achalasia associated with gastric lymphoma. *Dig Dis Sci* 1980;25:311–213.

154. Goldin NR, Butud TW, Ferrante WA. Secondary achalasia: association with adenocarcinoma of the lung and reversal with radiation therapy. *Am J Gastroenterol* 1983;78:203–205.

155. Eaves R, Lambert J, Rees J, *et al*. Achalasia secondary to carcinoma of the prostate. *Dig Dis Sci* 1983;28:278–284.

156. Davis JA, Kantrowitz PA, Chandler HL, *et al*. Reversible achalasia due to reticulum-cell sarcoma. *N Engl J Med* 1975; 293:130–132.

157. Rock LA, Latham PS, Hankins JR, *et al*. Achalasia associated with squamous cell carcinoma of the esophagus. *Am J Gastroenterol* 1985;80:526–528.

158. Goldschmiedt M, Peterson WL, Spielberger R, *et al*. Esophageal achalasia secondary to mesothelioma. *Dig Dis Sci* 1989; 34:1285–1288.

159. Herrera JL. Esophageal metastasis from breast carcinoma presenting as achalasia. *Am J Med Sci* 1992;303:321–323.

160. Manela FD, Quiqley EMM, Paustian FF, *et al*. Achalasia of the esophagus in association with renal cell carcinoma. *Am J Gastroenterol* 1991;86:1812–1816.

161. Lefkowitz JR, Brand DL, Schuffler MD, *et al*. Amyloidosis mimics achalasids effect on lower esophageal sphincter. *Dig Dis Sci* 1989;34:630–635.

162. Dufresne CR, Jeyasingham K, Baker RR. Achalasia of the cardia associated with pulmonary sarcoidosis. *Surgery* 1983;94:32–35.

163. Roberts DH, Gilmore IT Achalasia in Anderson-Fabry's disease. *J R Soc Med* 1984;77:430–431.

164. Hollis JR, Castell DO, Braddom RL. Esophageal function in diabetes mellitus and its relation to peripheral neuropathy. *Gastroenterology* 1977;73:1098–1102.

165. Woods CA, Foutch PG, Waring JP, *et al*. Pancreatic pseudocyst as a cause for secondary achalasia. *Gastroenterology* 1989;96:235–239.

166. Duntemann TJ, Dresner DM. Achalasia-like syndrome presenting after highly selective vagotomy. *Dig Dis Sci* 1995;40:2081–2083.

167. Liu W, Fackler W, Rice TW, *et al*. The pathogenesis of pseudoachalasia: a clinicopathologic study of 13 cases of a rare entity. *Am J Surg Pathol* 2002;26:784–788.

168. Woodfield CA, Levine MS, Rubesin SE, *et al*. Diagnosis of primary versus secondary achalasia: reassessment of clinical and radiographic criteria. *AJR Am J Roentgenol* 2000;175:727–731.

169. Dodds WJ, Stewart ET, Kishk SM, *et al*. Radiologic amyl nitrite test for distinguishing pseudoachalasia from idiopathic achalasia. *AJR Am J Roentgenol* 1986;146:21–23.

170. Koberle F., Chagas' disease and Chagas' syndrome: the pathology of American trypanosomiasis. *Adv Parasitol* 1968;6:63–73.

171. Kirchoff LV. American trypanosomiasis (Chagas' disease): a tropical disease now in the United States. *N Engl J Med* 1993;329:639–644.

172. Herbella FAM, Aquino JLB, Stefani-Nakano S, *et al*. Treatment of achalasia: lessons learned from Chagas' disease *Dis Esophagus* 2008;21:461–467.

173. Stylopoulos N, Bunker CJ, Rattner DW. Development of achalasia secondary to laparoscopic Nissen fundoplication. *J Gastrointest Surg* 2002;6:368–378.

174. Weisner W, Hauser M, Schob O, *et al*. Pseudo achalasia following laparoscopically placed adjustable gastric banding. *Obesity Surgery* 2001;11:513–518.

175. Vaezi MF, Baker ME, Richter JE. Assessment of esophageal emptying post-pneumatic dilation: use of timed barium esophagram. *Am J Gastroenterol* 1999;94:1802–1807.

176. Vaezi MF, Baker MF, Achkar E, *et al*. Timed barium esophagram: better predictor of long-term success after pneumatic dilation than symptoms assessment. *Gut* 2002;50:765–770.

177. Gelfand MD, Kozarek RA. An experience with polyethylene balloon for pneumatic dilation for achalasia. *Am J Gastroenterol* 1989;84:924–927.

178. Alonso P, Gonzalez-Conde B, Macenille R, *et al*. Achalasia: the usefulness of manometry for evaluation of treatment. *Dig Dis Sci* 1999;44:536–541.

179. Eckardt VF, Aignherr C, Bernhard G. Predictors of outcome in patients with achalasia treated by pneumatic dilation. *Gastroenterology* 1992;103:1732–1738.

180. Ponce J, Garrigues V, Pertejo V, *et al*. Individual prediction of response to pneumatic dilation in patients with achalasia. *Dig Dis Sci* 1996;41:2135–2141.

181. Hulselmans M, Vanuytsel T, Degreef T, *et al*. Long-term outcome of pneumatic dilation in the treatment of achalasia. *Clinical Gastroenterol and Hepatoll* 2010;8:30–35.

182. Rosati R, Fumagolli U, Bona S, *et al*. Evaluating results of laparoscopic surgery for esophageal achalasia. *Surg Endosc* 1998;12:270–273.

183. Anselmino M, Zaniotto G, Costantini M. One year follow-up after laparoscopic Heller-Dor operation for esophageal achalasia. *Surg Endosc* 1997;11:3–7.

184. Kadakia SC, Wong RKH. Graded pneumatic dilation using Rigiflex achalasia dilators in patients with primary esophageal achalasia. *Am J Gastroenterol* 1993;88:34–38.

185. Kim CH, Cameron AJ, Hsu JJ, *et al*. Achalasia: prospective evaluation of relationship between lower esophageal sphincter pressure, esophageal transit, and esophageal diameter and symptoms in response to pneumatic dilation. *Mayo Clin Proc* 1993;68:1067–1073.

186. Sultan M, Norton RA. Esophageal diameter and the treatment of achalasia. *Am J Dig Dis* 1969;14:611–618.

187. Cohen NN. An endpoint for pneumatic dilation of achalasia. *Gastrointest Endosc* 1975;22:29.

188. Agha FP, Lee HH. The esophagus after endoscopic pneumatic balloon dilation for achalasia. *Am J Roentgenol* 1986;146:25–29.

189. Lee JD, Cecil BD, Brown PE, *et al*. The Cohen test does not predict outcome in achalasia after pneumatic dilation. *Gastrointest Endosc* 1992;39:157–160.

190. Ott DJ, Donati D, Wu WC, *et al*. Radiographic evaluation of achalasia immediately after pneumatic dilation with the Rigiflex dilator. *Gastrointest Radiol* 1991;16:279–282.

191. DeOliveira JMA, Birgisson S, Doinoff C, *et al*. Timed-barium swallow: a simple technique for evaluating esophageal emptying in patients with achalasia. *AJR Am J Roentgenol* 1997;169:473–479.

192. Montazeri G, Nouri N, Estakhri A, *et al*. Surface area: a better predictor of disease severity than the height and volume of the barium column in patients with achalasia. *Eur J Gastroenterol Hepatol* 2006;18:1203–1208.

193. Chuah SK, Hu TH, Wu KL, *et al*. The role of barium esophagram measurements in assessing achalasia patients after endoscope-guided pneumatic dilation. *Dis Esophagus* 2009;22:163–168.

194. Andersson M, Lundell L, Kostic S, *et al*. Evaluation of the response to treatment in patients with idiopathic achalasia by the timed barium esophagram: results of a randomized clinical trial. *Dis Esophagus* 2009;22:264–273.

195. Hoogerwerf WA, Pasricha PJ. Pharmacologic therapy in treating achalasia. *Gastrointest Endosc Clin North Am* 2001;11:311–323.

196. Gelfand M, Rozen P, Keren S, *et al*. Effect of nitrates on LOS pressure in achalasia: a potential therapeutic aid. *Gut* 1981;22:312–318.

197. Bortolotti M, Labo G. Clinical and manometric effects of nifedipine in patients with esophageal achalasia. *Gastroenterology* 1981;80:39–44.

198. Berger K, McCallum RW. Nifedipine in the treatment of achalasia. *Ann Intern Med* 1982;96:61–62.

199. Gelfand M, Rozen P, Gilat T. Isosorbide dinitrate and nifedipine treatment of achalasia: a clinical, manometric and radionuclide evaluation. *Gastroenterology* 1982;83:963–969.

200. Traube M, Dubovik S, Lange RC, *et al*. The role of nifedipine therapy in achalasia: results of a randomized, double-blind, placebo-controlled study. *Am J Gastroenterol* 1989;84:1259–1262.

201. Rozen P, Gelfand M, Salzman S, *et al*. Radionuclide confirmation of the therapeutic value of isosorbide dinitrate in relieving dysphagia in achalasia. *J Clin Gastroenterol* 1982;4:17–22.

202. Coccia G, Bortolotti M, Michetti P, *et al*. Prospective clinical and manometric study comparing pneumatic dilation and sublingual nifedipine in the treatment of oesophageal achalasia. *Gut* 1991;32:604–606.

203. Becker BS, Burakoff R. The effect of verapamil on the lower esophageal sphincter pressure in normal subjects and in achalasia. *Am J Gastroenterol* 1983;78:773–776.

204. Triadafilopoulos G, Aaronson M, Sackel S, et al. Medical treatment of esophageal achalasia. Double-blind crossover study with oral nifedipine, verapamil and placebo. *Dig Dis Sci* 1991; 36:260–267.

205. Marzio L, Grossi L, DeLaurentilis MF, et al. Effect of cimetropium bromide on esophageal motility and transit in patients affected by primary achalasia. *Dig Dis Sci* 1994;39:1389–1394.

206. DiMarino AJ, Cohen S. Effect of an oral beta 2-adrenergic agonist on lower esophageal sphincter pressure in normals and in a patient with achalasia. *Dig Dis Sci* 1982;27:1063–1066.

207. Wong RKH, Maydonovitch C, Garcia JE, et al. The effect of terbutaline sulfate, nitroglycerin, and aminophylline on lower esophageal sphincter pressure and radionuclide esophageal emptying in patients with achalasia. *J Clin Gastroenterol* 1987;9:386–340.

208. Penagini R, Bartesaghi B, Negri G, et al. Effect of loperamide on lower esophageal sphincter pressure in idiopathic achalasia. *Scand J Gastroenterol* 1994;29:1057–1060.

209. Bortolotti M, Mari C, Lopilato C, et al. Effects of sildenafil on esophageal motility of patients with idiopathic achalasia. *Gastroenterology* 2000;118:253–257.

210. Guelrud M, Rossiter A, Souney PF, et al. Transcutaneous electrical nerve stimulation decreases lower esophageal sphincter pressure in patients with achalasia. *Dig Dis Sci* 1991;36:1029–1033.

211. Shabsin HS, Katz PO, Schuster MM. Behavioral treatment of intractable chest pain in a patient with vigorous achalasia. *Am J Gastroenterol* 1988;83:970–973.

212. Tsai JKC. Botulinum toxin as a therapeutic agent. *Pharmacol Ther* 1996;72:13–24.

213. Pasricha PJ, Ravich WJ, Kalloo AN. Effects of intrasphincteric botulinum toxin on the lower esophageal sphincter in piglets. *Gastroenterology* 1993;105:1045–1049.

214. Pasricha PJ, Ravich WJ, Hendrix TR, et al. Treatment of achalasia with intrasphincteric injection of botulinum toxin. A pilot trial. *Ann Intern Med* 1994;121:590–591.

215. Pasricha PJ, Ravich WJ, Hendrix TR, et al. Intrasphincteric botulinum toxin for the treatment of achalasia. *N Engl J Med* 1995;322:774–778.

216. Pasricha PJ, Rai R, Ravich WJ, et al. Botulinum toxin for achalasia: Long-term outcome and predictor of response. *Gastroenterology* 1996;110:1410–1415.

217. Cuilliere C, Ducrotte P, Zerbib F, et al. Achalasia: outcome of patients treated with intrasphincteric injection of botulinum toxin. *Gut* 1997;41:87–92.

218. Rollan A, Gonzales R, Carvajal S, et al. Endoscopic intrasphincteric injection of botulinum toxin for the treatment of achalasia. *J Clin Gastroenterol* 1995;20:189–191.

219. Fishman VM, Parkman HP, Schiano TD, et al. Symptomatic improvement in achalasia after botulinum toxin injection of the lower esophageal sphincter. *Am J Gastroenterol* 1996;91:1724–1723.

220. Annese V, Basciani M, Perri F, et al. Controlled trial of botulinum toxin injection versus placebo and pneumatic dilation in achalasia. *Gastroenterology* 1996;111:1418–1424.

221. Gordon JM, Eaker EY. Prospective study of esophageal botulinum toxin injection in high-risk achalasia patients. *Am J Gastroenterol* 1997;92:1812–1816.

222. Muechldorfer SM, Schneider TH, Hochberger J, et al. Esophageal achalasia: intrasphincter injection of botulinum toxin versus balloon dilation. *Endoscopy* 1999;31:517–521.

223. Vaezi MJ, Richter JE, Wilcox CM, et al. Botulinum toxin versus pneumatic dilation in the treatment of achalasia: a randomized trial. *Gut* 1999;44:231–239.

224. Annese V, Bassotti G, Coccia G, et al. A multicenter randomized study of intrasphincteric botulinum toxin in patients with oesophageal achalasia. *Gut* 2000;46:597–600.

225. Kolbasnik J, Waterfall WE, Fachnie B, et al. Long-term efficacy of botulinum toxin in classical achalasia; a prospective study. *Am J Gastroenterol* 1999;94:3434–3439.

226. Mikaeli J, Fazel A, Montazeri G, et al. Randomized controlled trial comparing botulinum toxin injection to pneumatic dilatation for the treatment of achalasia. *Aliment Pharmacol Ther* 2001;15:1389–1396.

227. Allescher HD, Storr M, Seige M, et al. Treatment of achalasia: botulinum toxin injection vs pneumatic balloon dilation. A prospective study with long-term follow-up. *Endoscopy* 2001;33:1007–1017.

228. Neubrand M, Scheurlen C, Schepke M, et al. Long-term results and prognostic factors in the treatment of achalasia with botulinum toxin. *Endoscopy* 2002;34:519–523.

229. Vallera RZ, Brazer SR. Botulinum toxin for suspected pseudoachalasia. *Am J Gastroenterol* 1995;90:1319–1321.

230. Katzka DA, Castell DO. Use of botulinum toxin as a diagnostic/therapeutic trial to help clarify and indication for definitive therapy in patients with achalasia. *Am J Gastroenterol* 1999;94:637–642.

231. Hoffman BJ, Knapple WL, Bhutani MS, et al. Treatment of achalasia by injection of botulinum toxin under endoscopic ultrasound guidance. *Gastrointestinal Endosc* 1997;45:77–79.

232. Bonavina L, Incarbone R, Antoniazzi L, et al. Previous endoscopic treatment does not affect complication rate and outcome of laparoscopic Heller myotomy and anterior fundoplication for achalasia. *Ital J Gastroenterol Hepatol* 1999;31:827–830.

233. Horgan S, Hudda K, Eubanks T, et al. Does botulinum toxin injection make esophagomyotomy a more difficult operation? *Surg Endosc* 1999;13:576–579.

234. Fergunson MK, Reeder GB, Olak J. Results of myotomy and partial fundoplication after pneumatic dilation for achalasia. *Ann Thorac Surg* 1996;62:327–330.

235. McJunkin B, McMillian WO, Duncan HE, et al. Assessment of dilation methods in achalasia: large diameter mercury bougienage followed by pneumatic dilation as needed. *Gastrointest Endosc* 1991;37:18–21.

236. Olsen AM, Harrington SW, Moersch HJ, et al. Treatment of cardiospasm: analysis of a twelve-year experience. *J Thorac Surg* 1951;22:164–169.

237. Bennett JR, Hendrix TR. Treatment of achalasia with pneumatic dilatation. *Mod Treat* 1970;7:1217–1228.

238. Kadakia SC, Wong RKH. Pneumatic balloon dilation for esophageal achalasia. *Gastrointest Endosc Clin North Am* 2001; 11:325–345.

239. Heimlich HU, O'Connor TW, Fiores DC. Case for pneumatic dilation for achalasia. *Ann Otol* 1978;87:519–522.

240. Csendes A, Braghetto I, Henriques A, et al. Late results of a prospective randomized study comparing forceful dilatation and esophagomyotomy in patients with achalasia. *Gut* 1989;30:299–305.

241. Stark GA, Castell DO, Richter JE, et al. Prospective randomized comparison of Browne-McHardy and Microvasive balloon

dilator in the treatment of achalasia. *Am J Gastroenterol* 1990;85:1322–1326.

242. Wong RKH, Maydonovitch C. Utility of parameters measured during pneumatic dilation as predictors of successful dilation. *Am J Gastroenterol* 1996;91:1120–1129.

243. West RC, Hirsch DP, Bartelsman JFWM, *et al*. Long term results of pneumatic dilation in achalasia followed for more than 5 years. *Am J Gastroenterol* 2002;97:1346–1351.

244. Vela M, Richter JE, Khandwala E, *et al*. The long-term efficacy of pneumatic dilation and Heller myotomy for the treatment of achalasia. *Clin Gastroenterol Hepatol* 2006;4:580–587.

245. Guardino J, Vela M, Connor J, Richter JE. Pneumatic dilation for the treatment of achalasia in untreated patients and patients with failed Heller myotomy. *J Clin Gastroenterol* 2004;38:855–860.

246. Khan AA, Shah SWH, Alam A, *et al*. Pneumatic balloon dilation in achalasia: a prospective comparison of balloon distention time. *Am J Gastroenterol* 1998;93:1064–1067.

247. Ciarolla DA, Traube M. Achalasia. Short-term clinical monitoring after pneumatic dilation. *Dig Dis Sci* 1993;38:1905–1908.

248. Barkin JS, Guelrud M, Reiner DK, *et al*. Forceful balloon dilation: an outpatient procedure for achalasia. *Gastrointest Endosc* 1990;36:123–125.

249. Elta GH, Nostrant TT, Wilson JAP. Treatment of achalasia with the Witzel pneumatic dilator. *Gastrointest Endosc* 1987;33:101–103.

250. Barnett JL, Eisenman R, Nostrant TT, *et al*. Witzel pneumatic dilation for achalasia: safety and long-term efficacy. *Gastrointest Endosc* 1990;36:482–485.

251. Johnston BT, Collins BJ, Collins JSA, *et al*. Perendoscopic pneumatic dilatation in achalasia: assessment of outcome using esophageal scintigraphy. *Dysphagia* 1992;7:201–204.

252. Cox J, Buckton GK, Bennett JR. Balloon dilatation in achalasia: a new dilator. *Gut* 1986;27:986–989.

253. Makela J, Kiviniemi H, Laitinen S. Heller's cardiomyotomy compared with pneumatic dilation for the treatment of oesophageal achalasia. *Eur J Surg* 1991;157:411–414.

254. Levine ML, Moskowitz GW, Dorf BS, *et al*. Pneumatic dilation in patients with achalasia with a modified Gruntzig dilator (Levine) under direct endoscopic control. Results after 5 years. *Am J Gastroenterol* 1991;86:1581–1584.

255. Abid S, Champion G, Richter JE, *et al*. Treatment of achalasia: the best of both worlds. *Am J Gastroenterol* 1993;89:979–985.

256. Wehrmann T, Jacobi V, Jung M, *et al*. Pneumatic dilation in achalasia with a low-compliance balloon. Results of a 5 year prospective evaluation. *Gastrointest Endosc* 1995;42:31–36.

257. Lambroza A, Schuman RW. Pneumatic dilation for achalasia without fluoroscopic guidance: safety and efficacy. *Am J Gastroenterol* 1995;90:1226–1229.

258. Muehldorfer SM, Hahn EG, Eli C. High- and low-compliance balloon dilators in patients with achalasia: a randomized prospective comparison trial. *Gastrointest Endosc* 1996;44:398–403.

259. Bhatnager MS, Nanivadekar SA, Sawant P, *et al*. Achalasia cardia dilation using polyethylene balloon (Rigiflex) dilator. *Ind J Gastroenterol* 1996;15:49–51.

260. Gideon RM, Castell DO, Yarze J. Prospective randomized comparison of pneumatic dilation techniques in patients with idiopathic achalasia. *Dig Dis Sci* 1999;44:1853–1857.

261. Khan AA, Shah WH, Alam A, *et al*. Massively dilated esophagus in achalasia: response to pneumatic balloon dilation. *Am J Gastroenterol* 1999;94:2363–2366.

262. Chan KC, Wong SKH, Lee DWH, *et al*. Short-term and long-term results of endoscopic balloon dilation for achalasia: 12 years' experience. *Endoscopy* 2004;36:690–694.

263. Dobrucali A, Erzin Y, Tuncer M, Dirican A. Long-term results of graded pneumatic dilation under endoscopic guidelines in patients with primary esophageal achalasia. *World J Gastroenterology* 2004;10:3322–3327.

264. Kostic S, Kjellin A, Ruth M, *et al*. Pneumatic dilation or laparoscopic myotomy in the management of newly diagnosed idiopathic achalasia. *World J Surgery* 2007;31:470–478.

265. Mikaeli J, Bishehsari F, Montazeri G, *et al*. Pneumatic balloon dilation in achalasia: a prospective comparison of safety and efficacy with different balloon diameters. *Aliment Pharmacol Ther* 2004;20:431–436.

266. Ghoshal UC, Kumar S, Saraswat VA, *et al*. Long-term follow-up after pneumatic dilation for achalasia of the cardia: Factors associated with treatment failure and recurrence. *Am J Gastroenterol* 2004;99:2304–2310.

267. Boztas G, Mungan Z, Ozdil S, *et al*. Pneumatic dilation in primary achalasia: the long-term follow-up results. *Hepatogastroenterology* 2005;52:475–480.

268. Chuah SK, Hu TH, Wu KL, *et al*. Clinical remission in endoscope-guided pneumatic dilation for the treatment of esophageal achalasia: 7 year follow-up of a prospective intervention. *J Gastrointest Surg* 2009;13:862–867.

269. Zerbid F, Thetiot V, Richy F, *et al*. Repeated pneumatic dilations as long-term maintenance therapy for esophageal achalasia. *Am J Gastroenterol* 2006;101:692–697.

270. Karamanolis G, Sgouros S, Karatzias G, *et al*. Long-term outcome of pneumatic dilation in the treatment of achalasia. *Am J Gastroenterol* 2005;100:270–274.

271. Katsinelos P, Kountouras J, Paroutglou G, *et al*. Long-term results of pneumatic dilation for achalasia: a 15 year experience. *World J Gastroenterol* 2005;11:5701–5705.

272. Lopushinsky SR, Urbach DR. Pneumatic dilation and surgical myotomy for achalasia. *JAMA* 2006;296:2227–2233.

273. Lamet H, Fleshler B, Achkar E. Return of peristalsis in achalasia after pneumatic dilation. *Am J Gastroenterol* 1985; 80:602–604.

274. Mellow MH. Return of esophageal peristalsis in idiopathic achalasia. *Gastroenterology* 1976;70:1148–1151.

275. Bielefeldt K, Enck P, Erckenbrecht E. Motility changes in primary achalasia following pneumatic dilation. *Dysphagia* 1990;5:152–158.

276. Parkman HP, Reynolds JC, Ouyang A, *et al*. Pneumatic dilatation or esophagomyotomy treatment for idiopathic achalasia: clinical outcome and cost analysis. *Dig Dis Sci* 1993;38:75–85.

277. Vantrappen G, Hellemans J, Deloof W, *et al*. Treatment of achalasia with pneumatic dilation. *Gut* 1971;12:268–275.

278. Eckardt VF, Kanzler G, Westermeier T. Complications and their impact after pneumatic dilation for achalasia: prospective long-term follow-up study. *Gastrointest Endosc* 1997;45:349–353.

279. Nair LA, Reynolds JC, Parkman HP, *et al*. Complications during pneumatic dilation for achalasia and diffuse esophageal spasm: analysis of risk factors, early clinical characteristics and outcome. *Dig Dis Sci* 1993;38:1893–1904.

280. Borotto E, Gaudric M, Daniel B, *et al*. Risk factors of oesophageal perforation during pneumatic dilation for achalasia. *Gut* 1996;39:9–12.

281. Metman EH, Lagasse JP, Alteroche L, *et al*. Risk factors for immediate complications after progressive pneumatic dilation for achalasia.. *Am J Gastroenterol* 1999;94:1179–1185.

282. Michel L, Grillo HC, Malt RA. Operative and non-operative management of esophageal perforation. *Ann Surg* 1981;194:57–63.

283. Swedlund A, Traube M, Siskind BN, *et al*. Nonsurgical management of esophageal perforation from pneumatic dilation in achalasia. *Dig Dis Sci* 1989;34:379–384.

284. Swartz AM, Cahow CE, Traube M. Outcome after perforation sustained during pneumatic dilation for achalasia. *Dig Dis Sci* 1993;38:1409–1413.

285. Shoenut JP, Duerksen D, Yaffe CS. A prospective assessment of gastroesophageal reflux before and after treatment of achalasia patients: Pneumatic dilation vs transthoracic limited myotomy. *Am J Gastroenterol* 1997;92:1109–1112.

286. Burke CA, Achkar EA, Falk GW. Effect of pneumatic dilation on gastroesophageal reflux in achalasia. *Dig Dis Sci* 1997;42:998–1002.

287. Vaezi MF, Richer JE. Current therapies for achalasia. Comparison and efficacy. *J Clin Gastroenterol* 1998;27:21–35.

288. Pelligrini C, Wetter LA, Patti M, *et al*. Thoracoscopic esophagomyotomy. Initial experience with a new approach for achalasia. *Ann Surg* 1992;216:291–296.

289. Ellis FH, Crozier RE, Watkins E. Operation for esophageal achalasia. Result of esophagomyotomy without an antireflux operation. *J Thorac Cardiovas Surg* 1984;88:344–351.

290. Little AG, Soriano A, Fergusson MK, *et al*. Surgical treatment of achalasia: results with esophagomyotomy and Belsey repair. *Ann Thorac Surg* 1988;45:489–494.

291. Ponce J, Miralbes M, Garriques V, *et al*. Return of esophageal peristalsis after Heller's myotomy for idiopathic achalasia. *Dig Dis Sci* 1986;31:545–547.

292. Bianco A, Cagossi M, Scrimieri D, *et al*. Appearance of esophageal peristalsis in treated idiopathic achalasia. *Dig Dis Sci* 1986;31:40–48.

293. Parilla P, Martinez de Haro LF, Ortiz A, *et al*. Factors involved in the return of peristalsis in patients with achalasia of the cardia after Heller's myotomy. *Am J Gastroenterol* 1995;90:713–717.

294. Csendes A, Larrain A, Strauszer R, *et al*. Long-term clinical, radiological and manometrical follow-up of patients with achalasia of the esophagus treated with esophagomyotomy. *Digestion* 1975;13:27–32.

295. Shimi S, Nathanson LK, Cuschieri A. Laparoscopic cardiomyotomy for achalasia. *J R Coll Surg Edinburgh* 1991;36:152–154.

296. Ali A, Pellegrini CA. Laparoscopic myotomy. Technique and efficacy in treating achalasia. *Gastrointest Endosc Clin North Am* 2001;11:347–357.

297. Rosati R, Fumagalli U, Bonavina L, *et al*. Laparoscopic approach to esophageal achalasia. *Am J Surg* 1995;169:424–427.

298. Ancona E, Anselmino M, Zaninotto G, *et al*. Esophageal achalasia: laparoscopic vs conventional open Heller-Dor operation. *Am J Surg* 1995;170:265–270.

299. Mitchell PC, Watson DI, Devitt PG, *et al*. Laparoscopic cardiomyotomy with a Dor patch for achalasia. *Can J Surg* 1995;38:445–449.

300. Swanstrom LL, Pennings J. Laparoscopic esophagomyotomy for achalasia. *Surg Endosc* 1995;9:286–292.

301. Morino M, Rebecchi F, Festa V, *et al*. Laparoscopic Heller cardiomyotomy with intraoperative manometry in the management of oesophageal achalasia. *Int Surg* 1995;80:332–335.

302. Robertson GSM, Lloyd DM, Wicks ACB, *et al*. Laparoscopic Heller's cardiomyotomy without an antireflux procedure. *Br J Surg* 1995;82:957–959.

303. Bonovina L, Rosati P, Segalin A, Peracchia A. Laparoscopic Heller-Dor operation for the treatment of oesophageal achalasia: technique and early results. *Ann Chir Gynaecol* 1995;84:165–168.

304. Delgado F, Bolufer JM, Martinex-Abad M, *et al*. Laparoscopic treatment of esophageal achalasia. *Surg Laparosc Endosc* 1996;2:83–90.

305. Hunter JG, Trus TL, Branum GD, *et al*. Laparoscopic Heller myotomy and fundoplication for achalasia. *Ann Surg* 1997;225:655–665.

306. Kjellin AP, Granquist S, Ramel S, *et al*. Laparoscopic myotomy without fundoplication in patients with achalasia. *Eur J Surg* 1999;165:1162–1166.

307. Ackroyd R, Watson DI, Devitt PG, *et al*. Laparoscopic cardiomyotomy and anterior partial fundoplication for achalasia. *Surg Endosc* 2001;15:683–686.

308. Yamamura MS, Gilster JC, Myers BS, *et al*. Laparoscopic Heller myotomy and anterior fundoplication for achalasia results in a high degree of patient satisfaction. *Arch Surg* 2000;135:902–906.

309. Patti MG, Molena D, Fisichella PM, *et al*. Laparoscopic Heller myotomy and Dor fundoplication for achalasia. Analysis of successes and failures. *Arch Surg* 2001;136:870–877.

310. Pechlivanides G, Chryos E, Athanasakis E, *et al*. Laparoscopic Heller cardiomyotomy and Dor fundoplication for esophageal achalasia. *Arch Surg* 2001;136:1240–1243.

311. Sharp KW, Khaitan L, Scholz S, *et al*. 100 consecutive minimally invasive Heller myotomies: lessons learned. *Ann Surg* 2002;235:631–639.

312. Donahue PE, Horgan S, Liu KJM, *et al*. Floppy Dor fundoplication after esophagocardiomyotomy for achalasia. *Surgery* 2002;132:716–722.

313. Zaninotto G, Costantini M, Portale G, *et al*. Etiology, diagnosis and treatment of failures after laparoscopic Heller myotomy for achalasia. *Ann Surg* 2002;235:186–192.

314. Ramacciato G, Mercantini P, Amodio PM, *et al*. The laparoscopic approach with antireflux surgery is superior to the thoracoscopic approach for the treatment of esophageal achalasia. *Surg Endosc* 2002;16:1431–1437.

315. Luketich JD, Fernando HC, Christie, *et al*. Outcome after minimally invasive esophagomyotomy. *Ann Thorac Surg* 2001;72:1909–1913.

316. Decker G, Borie F, Bouamirrene D, *et al*. Gastrointestinal quality of life before and after laparoscopic Heller myotomy with partial posterior fundoplication. *Surgery* 2002;236:750–758.

317. Mineo T, Pompeo E. Long-term outcome of Heller myotomy in achalasia sigmoid esophagus. *J Thoracic Cardiovascular Surgery* 2004;128:402–407.

318. Grockel I, Junginger T, Eckhardt V. Long-term results of conventional myotomy in patients with achalasia: a prospective 20 year analysis. *Society Surg Alimentary Trackt* 2006;10:1400–1408.

319. Wright AS, Williams CW, Pellegrini CA, Oelschlager BK. Long-term outcome confirms the superior efficacy of extended Heller myotomy with Toupet fundoplication for achalasia. *Surg Endoscopy* 2007;21:713–718.

320. Khajanchee Y, Kanneganti S, Leatherwood A, *et al*. Laparoscopic Heller myotomy with Toupet fundoplication. *Arch Surg* 2005;140:827–834.

321. Zanninotto G, Annese V, Costantino, *et al.* Randomized controlled trial of botulinum toxin vs laparoscopic Heller myotomy for achalasia. *Ann Surg* 2004;239:364–370.

322. Csendes A, Braghetto I, Burdiles P, Korn O, *et al.* Very late results of esophagomyotomy for patients with achalasia. *Ann Surg* 2006;243:196–203.

323. Rice T, McKelvey A, Richter J, *et al.* A physiologic clinical study of achalasia: Should Dor fundoplication be added to Heller myotomy? *J Thorac Cardiovasc Surg* 2005;130: 1593–1600.

324. Richards W, Torquati A, Holzman M, *et al.* Heller myotomy versus Heller myotomy wWith Dor fundoplication for achalasia: A prospective randomized double-blind clinical trial. *Ann Surg* 2004;240:405–415.

325. Di Simone MP, Felice V, D'Errico A, *et al.* Onset timing of delayed complications and criteria of follow-up after operation for esophageal achalasia. *Ann Thorac Surg* 1996; 61:1106–1111.

326. Gorecki PJ, Hinder RA, Libbey JS, *et al.* Redo laparoscopic surgery for achalasia. Is it feasible? *Surg Endosc* 2002; 16:772–776.

327. Nussbaum MS, Jones MP, Pritts TA, *et al.* Intraoperative manometry to assess the esophagogastric junction during laparoscopic fundoplication and myotomy. *Surg Laparosc Endosc Percutan Tech* 2001;11:294–300.

328. Tatum RP, Kahrilas PJ, Manka M, *et al.* Operative manometry and endoscopy during laparoscopic Heller myotomy. An initial experience. *Surg Endosc* 1999;13:1015–1020.

329. Ponce J, Juan M, Garriques V, *et al.* Efficacy and safety of cardiomyotomy in patients with achalasia after failure of pneumatic dilatation. *Dig Dis Sci* 1999;44:2277–2282.

330. Johnson O. Achalasia of the cardia: experience of extramucosal cardiomyotomy during a ten-year period. *Ethiopian Med J* 1994;32:89–91.

331. Jaakkola A, Reinikainen P, Ovaska J, *et al.* Barrett's esophagus after cardiomyotomy for esophageal achalasia. *Am J Gastroenterol* 1994;89:165–169.

332. Guo JP, Gilman PB, Thomas RM, *et al.* Barrett's esophagus and achalasia. *J Clin Gastroenterol* 2002;34:439–443.

333. Miller DL, Allen MS, Trastek VF, *et al.* Esophageal resection for recurrent achalasia. *Ann Thorac Surg* 1995;60:922–928.

334. Banbury MK, Rice TW, Goldblum JR, *et al.* Esophagectomy with gastric reconstruction for achalasia. *J Thorac Cardiovasc Surg* 1997;117:1077–1085.

335. Patti MG, Feo CV, Diener U, *et al.* Laparoscopic Heller myotomy relieves dysphagia in achalasia when the esophagus is dilated. *Surg Endosc* 1999;13:843–846.

336. Richter JE. Comparison and cost analysis of different treatments. *Gastrointest Endosc Clin North Am* 2001;11:359–369.

337. Boeckxstaens GE, Annese V, des Varannes SB; European Achalasia Trial Investigators. Pneumatic dilation versus laparoscopic Heller's myotomy for idiopathic achalasia. *N Engl J Med* 2011;364:1807–1816.

338. Andrews CN, Anvari M, Dobranowski J. Laparoscopic Heller's myotomy or botulinum injection for management of achalasia. *Surg Endosc* 1999;13:742–746.

339. Bansal R, Nostrant TT, Chey WD, *et al.* Intrasphincteric botulinum toxin versus pneumatic balloon dilation for treatment of primary achalasia. *J Clin Gastroenterol* 2003; 36:209–214.

340. Ghosal UC, Chaudhuri S, Banerjee PK, *et al.* Randomized controlled trial of intrasphincteric botulinum toxin A injection versus balloon dilation for achalasia. *Dis Esophagus* 2001; 14:227–231.

341. Panaccione R, Gregor JC, Reynolds RPE, *et al.* Intrasphincteric botulinum toxin versus pneumatic dilatation for achalasia: a cost minimization analysis. *Gastrointest Endosc* 1999; 50:492–498.

342. Imperiale TF, O'Connor B, Vaezi ME *et al.* A cost-minimization analysis of alternative treatment strategies for achalasia. *Am J Gastroenterol* 2000;95:2737–2745.

343. Kostic S, Johnsson E, Lundell L, *et al.* Health economic evaluation of therapeutic strategies in patients with idiopathic achalasia: results of a randomized trial comparing pneumatic dilatation with laparoscopic cardiomyotomy. *Surg Endosc* 2007;21:1184–1189.

344. Zaninotto G, Vergadoro V, Ancona E, *et al.* Botulinum toxin injection vs laparoscopic myotomy for the treatment of esophageal achalasia. *Surg Endosc* 2004;18:691–695.

345. Karanicolas PJ, Smith SE, Gafni A, *et al.* The cost of laparoscopic myotomy versus pneumatic dilatation for esophageal achalasia. *Surg Endosc* 2007;21:1198–1206.

346. O'Connor JB, Singer ME, Richter JE, *et al.* The cost-effectiveness of treatment strategies for achalasia. *Dig Dis Sci* 2002; 47:1516–1525.

347. Urbach DR, Hansen PD, Khajanchee YS, *et al.* A decision analysis of the optimal initial approach to achalasia: laparoscopic Heller myotomy with partial fundoplication, thoracoscopic Heller myotomy, pneumatic dilatation, or botulinum toxin injection. *J Gastrointest Surg* 2001;5:191–205.

348. Vaezi MF, Richter JE. American College of Gastroenterology practice guidelines: diagnosis and management of achalasia. *Am J Gastroenterol* 1999;94:3406–3412.

349. Fiest TC, Foong A, Chokhavatia S. Successful balloon dilation of achalasia during pregnancy. *Gastrointest Endosc* 1993;39: 810–812.

350. Vela MF, Richter JE. Management of achalasia at a tertiary center-a complicated disease. *Gastroenterology* 2003;124:S1635.

351. Fagge CH. A case of simple stenosis of the oesophagus, followed by epithelioma. *Guys Hosp Report* 1872;108:75–77.

352. Dunaway PM, Wong RKH. Risk and surveillance intervals for squamous cell carcinoma in achalasia. *Gastrointest Clin North Am* 2001;11:425–433.

353. Meijssen MAC, Tilanus HW, Blakenstein MV, *et al.* Achalasia complicated by oesophageal squamous cell carcinoma: a prospective study in 195 patients. *Gut* 1992;33:155–158.

354. Brucher BLDM, Stein HJ, Siewert JR, *et al.* Achalasia and esopahagel cancer: incidence, prevalence, and prognosis. *World J Surg.* 2001;25:745–749.

355. Barrett NR. Achalasia of the cardia: Reflections upon a clinical study of over 100 cases. *Br Med J* 1964;1:1135–1138.

356. Rake G. Epithelioma of the oesophagus in association with achalasia of the cardia. *Lancet* 1931;2:262–267.

357. Camara-Lopes LK. Carcinoma of the esophagus as a complication of megaesophagus: an analysis of seven cases. *Am J Dig Dis* 1961;6:741–746.

358. Just-Viera JO, Haight C. Achalasia and carcinoma of the esophagus. *Surg Gynecol Obstet* 1969;128:1081–1084.

359. Loviscek LF, Cenoz MC, Badaloni AE, *et al*. Early cancer in achalasia. *Dis Esophagus* 1998;11:239–243.

360. Lerut T, Coosemans W, DeLeyn P, *et al*. Treatment of esophageal carcinoma. *Chest* 1999;116:463–465.

361. Belsey RHR. Discussion. In: Tuttle WM, Crowley RT, Barrett RJ, eds. Achalasia of the esophagus. Further thoughts on surgical management. *J Thorac Surg* 1958;36:453–455.

362. American Society of *Gastrointestinal Endosc*opy Guidelines. The role of endoscopy in surveillance of premalignant conditions of the upper gastrointestinal tract. *Gastrointest Endosc* 1998;48:663–668.

14 Non-Achalasia Esophageal Motility Abnormalities

Daniel Pohl,[1,3] Radu Tutuian,[2] and Donald O. Castell[3]

[1]Division of Gastroenterology and Hepatology, University Hospital Zurich, Zurich, Switzerland
[2]Division of Gastroenterology, University Clinics of Visceral Surgery and Medicine, Bern University Hospital, Switzerland
[3]Division of Gastroenterology, Department of Internal Medicine, Medical University of South Carolina, Charleston, SC, USA

Introduction

Patients with dysphagia that is not explained by endoscopic or radiologic finding (i.e. non-obstructive dysphagia) and patients with chest pain that is not explained by heart disease (i.e. non-cardiac chest pain [NCCP]) are regularly referred for esophageal motility studies. Esophageal manometry often finds abnormalities, but the clinical relevance of these findings remains controversial. Recent technical developments, including combined impedance–manometry and high-resolution manometry (HRM), provide additional insight and novel classification schemes of detected abnormalities have been proposed. The aim of this chapter is to review conventional and high-resolution manometry abnormalities, in particular esophageal spasm, nutcracker esophagus, hypertensive lower esophageal sphincter (LES), and ineffective esophageal motility (IEM).

Definition of esophageal motility abnormalities

Conventional manometry

Esophageal motility abnormalities (EMAs) are esophageal manometry findings deviating to a meaningful degree from findings in normal individuals [1]. The steps to identify EMAs include classification of individual esophageal contractions and LES dynamics, followed by a summary of the information for individual swallows to provide an overall finding. Performance of esophageal manometry is described in Chapter 8. Esophageal body contractions are classified as being: (1) normal peristaltic if the contraction amplitude in the distal part of the esophagus exceeds 30 mmHg and the onset velocity in the distal esophagus is not greater than 8 cm/s; (2) simultaneous contractions if the contraction amplitude in the distal part of the esophagus exceeds 30 mmHg and distal onset velocity is greater than 8 cm/s; and (3) ineffective contractions if the contraction amplitude in the distal part of the esophagus is less than 30 mmHg. Conventional manometric criteria further classify normal peristaltic contractions as hypercontractile if the distal esophageal amplitude exceeds 220 mmHg. With regards to the LES residual pressure, a contraction is considered to be accompanied by complete LES relaxation if the LES residual pressure is less than 8 mmHg, or by incomplete LES relaxation if the LES residual pressure exceeds 8 mmHg. Normal esophageal manometry features are summarized in Table 14.1.

Information from individual swallows is then summarized into a finding of normal esophageal motility or EMAs. Thus, esophageal spasm is defined by the presence of an increased number (i.e. 20% or more) of simultaneous contractions, nutcracker esophagus by the presence of high-amplitude, peristaltic contractions [i.e. average distal contraction amplitude (DEA) exceeding 220 mmHg] and IEM by the presence of an increased number (i.e. 50% or more) of low-amplitude contractions. Hypertensive LES is characterized by the presence of an LES resting pressure above the upper limit of normal (i.e. >45 mmHg) and hypotensive LES is defined by the presence of a LES resting pressure below the lower limit of normal (i.e. <10 mmHg). A poorly relaxing LES is defined as an elevated LES residual pressure in the presence of esophageal peristalsis. EMAs can be grouped into hypercontractile (esophageal spasm, nutcracker esophagus, and hypertensive LES) and hypocontractile (IEM, hypotensive LES) dysmotilities in order to assist with proposing management options for these patients. The criteria for EMAs defined by Spechler and Castell [2] are summarized in Table 14.2.

Table 14.1 Normal esophageal manometric features (adapted from Spechler and Castell [2]).

Parameter	Normal
Basal LES pressure	10–45 mmHg (mid-respiratory pressure measured by station pull-through technique)
LES relaxation with swallow	Complete (to a level <8 mmHg above gastric pressure)
Wave progression	Peristalsis progressing from UES through LES at a rate of 2–8 cm/s
Distal wave amplitude	30–220 mmHg (average of 10 swallows at two recording sites positioned 3 and 8 cm above the LES0

LES, lower esophageal sphincter; UES, upper esophageal sphincter.

Table 14.2 Original classification of esophageal motility abnormalities based on conventional manometry findings (adapted from Spechler and Castell [2]).

Motility abnormality	Features
Inadequate LES relaxation	
Classic achalasia	Complete (100%) esophageal aperistalsis
	Elevated LES residual pressure (>8 mmHg)
	Elevated LES resting pressure (>45 mmHg)
Atypical disorders of LOS relaxation	Normal esophageal peristalsis
	Elevated LES residual pressure (>8 mmHg)
Uncoordinated contraction	
Distal esophageal spasm	20% or more manometric simultaneous contractions
Hypercontraction	
Nutcracker esophagus	Normal esophageal peristalsis
	Elevated distal esophageal amplitude (>220 mmHg)
Isolated hypertensive LES	Normal esophageal peristalsis
	Elevated LES resting pressure (>45 mmHg)
Hypocontraction	
Ineffective esophageal motility	50% or more manometric ineffective contractions

High-resolution manometry

HRM collects data from pressure sensors that are 1–1.5 cm apart, and the software constructs pressure topography plots using complex algorithms including interpolation. Details on performing HRM recordings are presented in Chapter 9. While HRM is promoted as quicker to perform, providing

Table 14.3 Classification of individual esophageal contractions based on high-resolution manometry findings (adapted from Pandolfino JE, Fox MR, Bredenoord AJ, Kahrilas PJ. High-resolution manometry in clinical practice: utilizing pressure topography to classify oesophageal motility abnormalities. *Neurogastroenterol Motil* 2009;21:796–806).

Classification	Criteria
Normal	<3 cm defect in the 30 mmHg isobaric contour distal to the TZ CFV <8 cm/s, IBP <15 mmHg, and DCI <5000 mmHg/s/cm
Hypotensive peristalsis	Normal appearing wavefront propagation with a ≥3 cm defect in the 30 mmHg isobaric contour distal to the TZ
Absent peristalsis	No propagating contractile wavefront and minimal (<3 cm) contractile activity or pressurization greater than the 30 mmHg isobaric contour
Hypertensive peristalsis	Normal appearing wavefront propagation with a DCI > 5000 mmHg/s/cm
Spasm	Rapidly propagated contraction (CFV ≥8 cm/s)
Elevated IBP	IBP > 15 mmHg compartmentalized between the GEJ and the peristaltic wavefront
Pan-esophageal pressurization	Esophageal pressurization from the UES to the GEJ with >30 mmHg IBP

TZ, transition zone; CFV, contractile front velocity; DCI, distal contractile integral; IBP, intrabolus pressure; UES, upper esophageal sphincter; GEJ, gastroesophageal junction.

more standardized recordings, and being more intuitive and easier to learn compared to conventional manometry [3], diagnosing EMAs follows the same procedure as during conventional manometry: classification of individual contractions followed by a summary of individual findings into normal or abnormal categories.

The isocontour representation of esophageal contractions includes information on the position of the proximal and distal border of the upper esophageal sphincter (UES) and LES, and the position of the transition zone (TZ) between the striated and smooth muscle portions of the esophagus. Integrating pressure data from the pressure sensors located in the distal esophagus provides information on the distal contractile integral (DCI), intrabolus pressure (IBP), and contraction front velocity (CFV). Rather than trying to identify optimal individual levels for assessing normal esophageal peristaltic contraction, the HRM approach defines normal contractions based on the length of isobaric (most commonly 30 mmHg) contour plots. Data from pressure sensors located in the LES are used to calculate the integrated relaxation pressure (IRP).

Classification of individual esophageal contractions based on HRM findings are summarized in Table 14.3. Novel to the classic classification is the elevated intrabolus pressure (IBP) and the use of DCI instead of the DEA.

The classification of EMAs from HRM findings is based on data collected in 75 healthy volunteers and 400 patients with various abnormalities [4]. The Chicago classification distinguishes between abnormalities with impaired gastroesophageal junction (GEJ) relaxation (IRP > 15 mmHg) and/or elevated IBP (>15 mmHg) and those with normal GEJ relaxation and normal IBP (Table 14.4). The first group includes patients with achalasia (classic or spastic) and functional GEJ obstruction, while the second includes patients with hypotensive and absent peristalsis, hypertensive peristalsis (at its extreme, called spastic nutcracker), and esophageal spasms.

Given the relatively new introduction of HRM into clinical practice, most studies evaluating EMAs have been performed using conventional manometry. We prefer to use the conventional classification of EMAs, while awaiting the results of future studies revealing the added value of HRM and the new classification in the diagnosis and management of these patients [5].

Esophageal spasm

Distal or diffuse esophageal spasm (DES) is an uncommon EMA with an estimated prevalence of 1.5–5% [6–8] and it may present at any age [9, 10]. The symptoms may mimic those of coronary artery disease and may also respond to nitrates (by relaxing the esophageal smooth muscle), reinforcing the importance of a cardiac work-up. Dysphagia and chest pain are the symptoms invariably connected to esophageal spasm. However only 3–4% of patients with the diagnosis of a motility disorder present features of esophageal spasm, and recent data suggest that its overall prevalence is less than 1.5% [11].

The currently accepted concept attributes this manometric abnormality to an altered endogenous nitric oxide (NO) synthesis and/or degradation. Chakder *et al.* reported the effects of the NO scavenger human recombinant hemoglobin (rHb) in anesthetized opossums [12]. Esophageal manometry recordings before and following the administration of rHb showed significant impairment in swallowing-induced LES relaxation and a significant increase in the speed of esophageal peristalsis. Similar data in the opossum were reported by Conklin *et al.* in studies monitoring intraluminal pressures in the esophagus and transmembrane potential differences of circular smooth muscle from the esophagus [13]. In addition to an increased velocity of esophageal peristalsis, decreased amplitudes of these contractions and diminished LES relaxation, the authors also found that rHb diminished the inhibitory junction potential and shortened the latency of the off response. Following these animal studies, Murray *et al.* investigated the effect of rHb in nine healthy human male volunteers [14]. Esophageal manometric studies performed before, during, and up to 6 h

Table 14.4 Chicago classification of esophageal motility abnormalities based on high-resolution manometry findings (adapted from Pandolfino JE, Fox MR, Bredenoord AJ, Kahrilas PJ. High-resolution manometry in clinical practice: utilizing pressure topography to classify oesophageal motility abnormalities. *Neurogastroenterol Motil* 2009;21:796–806).

Motility abnormality	Criteria
With impaired GEJ relaxation (IRP ≥ 15 mmHg) and/or elevated IBP (mean ≥ 15 mmHg)	
Achalasia:	
Classic achalasia	Mean IRP ≥ 15 mmHg, absent peristalsis
Achalasia with esophageal compression	Mean IRP ≥ 15 mmHg, absent peristalsis, and pan-esophageal pressurization with ≥20% of swallows
Spastic achalasia	Mean IRP ≥ 15 mmHg, absent peristalsis, and spasm (CFV > 8 cm/s) with ≥20% of swallows
Functional GEJ obstruction	Normal CFV, max IBP > 15 mmHg with ≥30% of swallows compartmentalized above GEJ
With normal GEJ relaxation (mean IRP < 15 mmHg) and normal IBP	
Absent peristalsis	100% swallows with absent peristalsis
Hypotensive peristalsis:	
Intermittent	>30% of swallows with hypotensive or absent peristalsis
Frequent	≥70% of swallows with hypotensive or absent peristalsis
Hypertensive peristalsis	Normal CFV, mean DCI > 5000 and <8000 mmHg/s/cm or LES after contraction >180 mmHg
Spastic nutcracker	Normal CFV, mean DCI > 8000 mmHg/s/cm
Distal esophageal spasm:	Spasm (CFV > 8 cm/s) with ≥20% of swallows
Segmental	Spasm limited to mid or distal esophageal segment
Diffuse	Spasm involving both mid and distal segment

IRP, integrated relaxation pressure; CFV, contractile front velocity; DCI, distal contractile integral; IBP, intrabolus pressure; LES, lower esophageal sphincter; GEJ, gastroesophageal junction.

after the intravenous infusion of rHb found that this NO scavenger increased the velocities of peristaltic contractions to produce simultaneous contractions in six (67%) subjects; spontaneous, simultaneous high-pressure contractions in eight (89%); and even lower retrosternal chest pain during swallowing in four (44%).

Xue *et al.* evaluated the role of the NO control of esophageal peristalsis and LES function in cats [15]. Measuring pressures at the LES and 2, 4, and 6 cm above the LES (smooth muscle), and 12 and/or 14 cm above the LES (striated muscle) in anesthetized cats before and during the intravenous administration of L-Ng-nitro-arginine (L-NNA), they observed that L-NNA increased the velocity of swallow-induced peristalsis and decreased the amplitude of peristaltic contractions in the smooth muscle esophagus, which was associated with the appearance of repetitive contractions. Investigating the influence of the NO synthase blocker, NG-monomethyl-L-arginine (L-NMMA) on esophageal motility, Konturek et al. noted that L-NMMA led to a significant and dose-dependent reduction in the latency period between swallows and the onset of contractions, and this phenomenon was most pronounced in the distal esophagus [16].

In summary, these animal and human experiments support the hypothesis that NO plays an important role in maintaining esophageal peristalsis, and are consistent with prior observations that nitrates provide some benefit in the treatment of patients with esophageal spasm [17, 18].

Before esophageal manometry became widely available, esophageal spasm was largely a clinical and radiologic diagnosis. It was defined by its typical symptoms (chest pain and dysphagia) and the presence of tertiary (purposeless) con-tractions of the esophagus noted during esophageal fluoro-scopic recordings. In the 1930s the first case series including radiographic images of esophageal spasms were reported. However, radiologic examinations were later shown to be primarily complimentary tests that correlate poorly with symptoms and offer only limited sensitivity and specificity [19, 20]. Manometric patterns were described as manometry was introduced into clinical practice [21, 22].

Definitions of spasm have changed over the years with variable cut-off values used for amplitude, frequency, and propagation velocity. Initially esophageal manometry testing was performed using dry swallows. Under these circum-stances, spastic contractions occurred frequently, as shown in a study of 95 healthy adult volunteers of whom 37% exhibited simultaneous spastic contractions during dry swal-lows [1]. The currently accepted definition of simultaneous contractions requires the presence of a contraction onset velocity exceeding 8 cm/s with an amplitude of greater than 30 mmHg in the distal esophagus (Figure 14.1A). When at least 20% of swallows are accompanied by simultaneous contractions, a patient may be diagnosed with esophageal

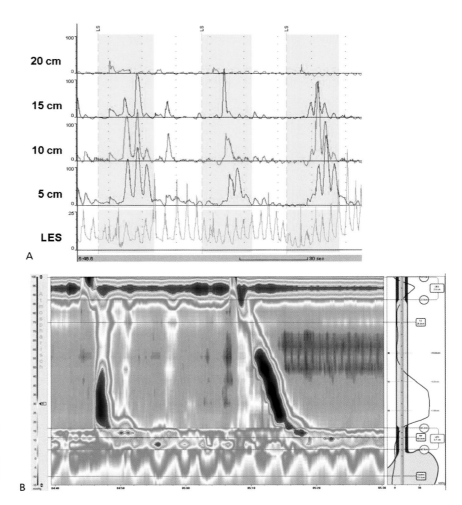

Figure 14.1 (A) Conventional manometry tracings featuring intermittently manometric simultaneous (onset velocity >8 cm/s) multipeaked contractions diagnostic for esophageal spasm. (B) High-resolution manometry recording showing simultaneous contractions alternating with normal peristaltic contractions.

spasm [23]. More recent studies indicate that esophageal spasm exclusively affects the distal esophageal smooth muscle portion in more than 90% of cases, which lead us to rename the entity distal rather than diffuse esophageal spasm [24]. In addition to the contraction onset criteria, other commonly described but not defining manometric findings in patients with esophageal spasm are multipeaked contractions (>2), prolonged contractions, and abnormalities in LES function [1]. In HRM recordings the simultaneous onset of the contraction in the distal esophagus can be readily appreciated (Figure 14.1B).

Before embarking on specific treatments for DES physicians should rule out a cardiac or pulmonary origin of the chest pain and/or obstructive or neoplastic origin of the dysphagia. Treating esophageal spasm is rarely easy. Based on the heterogeneity of symptoms and bolus transit impairments in patients with esophageal spasm, the rarity of this condition, and results of treatment interventions being reported from studies with a small number of patients, minimal data are available on the optimal treatment of this disorder. Once the above mentioned life-threatening conditions have been ruled out, the patient can be reassured that DES is a benign condition and therapies are aimed at decreasing the frequency of simultaneous contractions and control of symptoms. Endoscopic or surgical therapies should be used with great caution. Treatment options for DES are summarized in Table 14.5.

One of the first reports on the use of nitroglycerine in patients with esophageal spasms was published by Orlando and Bozymski in 1973 [25]. Subsequently Swamy reported on the effect of nitroglycerine and long-acting nitrites in a group of 12 patients with esophageal spasm, seven of whom were found to have gastroesophageal reflux as well [26]. The response to nitroglycerine in these seven patients was unpredictable. In contrast, the other five patients with spasm and no reflux responded well to treatment with nitroglycerine. Furthermore, the initial response to nitroglycerine could be maintained with long-acting nitrates from 6 months to 4 years. Unfortunately, these initial observations were not followed by controlled studies to systematically evaluate the long-term benefits of nitrates in the treatment of esophageal spasm.

Nashrallah *et al.* compared the effects of nifedipine 10 mg and placebo tid in a 4-week placebo-controlled, cross-over study in 20 patients with primary esophageal motor disorders [27]. This group included 10 patients with hypertensive LES, four with DES, three with vigorous achalasia, one with achalasia, and two with nutcracker esophagus. While overall the patients responded better to nifedipine compared to placebo, the improvement was most marked in patients with hypertensive LES.

Drenth *et al.* compared the effects of diltiazem to placebo in a 10-week double-blind cross-over study in eight patients with DES presenting with chest pain and/or dysphagia [28].

Table 14.5 Treatment options for patients with esophageal spasm.

Category	Medications
Reassurance that the condition is not life threatening	
Acid suppressive therapy for GERD:	
Proton pump inhibitors	Omeprazole 20–40 mg qid/bid
	Lansoprazole 15–30 mg qid/bid
	Pantoprazole 20–40 mg qid/bid
	Rabeprazole 20 mg qid/bid
	Esomeprazole 20–40 mg qid/bid
Smooth muscle relaxants:	
Nitrates	Nitroglycerine 0.4 mg sl prn
	Isosorbide dinitrate 10–30 mg bid/tid
Calcium-channel blockers	Diltiazem 60–90 mg tid/qid
	Nifedipine 10–30 mg tid/qid
Phosphodiesterase 5 (PD5) inhibitors	Sildenafil 50 mg qhs
	Vardenafil 10 mg qhs
	Tadalafil 10 mg qd
Antimuscarinics	Dicyclomine 10–20 mg qid
Psychotropic medications	Trazodone 100–150 mg qid
	Imipramine 50 mg qid
Botulinium toxin injection	Endoscopic injection Botox 100 U in 4 quads
Long myotomy	

Using visual analog scales to assess the severity of chest pain and dysphagia, the authors found that diltiazem lead to a reduction in the dyphagia (four of six patients) and chest pain (six of eight patients) scores. Compared to placebo though, the differences in chest pain and dysphagia scores were statistically not significant, most likely due to the small number of patients included in this study.

Approaching symptomatic esophageal dysmotilities from a different perspective, investigators have evaluated the role of tricyclic antidepressants or serotonin reuptake inhibitors (SSRIs) in influencing esophageal perception [29]. Clouse *et al.* reported on the beneficial effect of low-dose trazodone (100–150 mg/day) to improve symptoms in patients with symptomatic esophageal contraction abnormalities in a 6-week double-blind, placebo-controlled trial [30]. At the end of the trial period, patients receiving trazodone (n = 15) had a significantly greater global improvement of symptoms compared to those receiving placebo (n = 14). In addition, the authors noted that the active treatment did not change the manometric findings during the study. In a subsequent study, Handa *et al.* evaluated the role of antidepressant treatment of patients with DES and compared the results in patients with those recorded in a group of healthy volunteers [31]. Nine patients with DES initially underwent treatment with isosorbide dinitrate (ISDN) for 1 month and were then prescribed SSRIs for an additional month. The authors noted symptomatic improvement in one patient during treatment with ISDN and in eight patients during treatment with SSRIs, and concluded that antidepressant treatment may be effective in patients with DES.

Storr *et al.* evaluated the short- and long-term effects of botulinum toxin (Botox) injection in nine symptomatic patients with esophageal spasm [32]. Patients who were asked to rate their symptoms before, 1 day after, and 1, 4, and 6 months after the injection of 100 IU of Botox reported a decrease in the total symptom scores 1 day and 1 month after the injection compared to baseline. At the 1-month post-treatment evaluation, eight of nine patients were in remission and the remission lasted for another 6 months in eight of these patients. Four patients required Botox reinjection at 8, 12, 15 or 24 months after the initial treatment and similarly good results were reported for them during follow-up. Based on these results, the authors concluded that Botox injections represent an effective treatment for symptomatic esophageal spasm and that they can be repeated when symptoms relapse.

The effect of Botox in patients with NCCP was reported by Miller *et al.* [33]. The authors grouped 18 patients with esophageal spasm, five with hypertensive LES, one with nutcracker esophagus, and five with IEM as having "non-achalasia, non-reflux-related spastic esophageal motility disorders." Patients were asked to rate the severity of chest pain, dysphagia, regurgitation, and heartburn before and 1 month after the injection of 100 IU of Botox at the GEJ. The clinical evaluation also included the duration of response, defined as the time period between the injection and the time at which the severity of symptoms returned to the preinjection level. One month after the injection of Botox 14 of 18 (77%) patients with esophageal spasm reported a reduction of at least 50% in the chest pain score. In the entire group the mean duration of response for chest pain was 7.3 (range 1–18) months. Both this and the study by Storr *et al.* report favorable responses to the treatment with Botox, but unfortunately lacked a placebo/non-intervention or medical treatment arm.

Given the limited benefit of pharmacologic interventions for esophageal spasms, Eypash *et al.* evaluated the effect of long esophageal myotomy with antireflux procedure in 15 patients with severe chest pain and/or dysphagia attributed to esophageal spasm [34]. Evaluating the severity of dysphagia, chest pain, regurgitation, and heartburn before and at a mean of 2 years after the operation, the authors noted a symptomatic improvement. When performed after the myotomy, manometry identified a significant reduction in the amplitude of esophageal contractions, LES pressure, and frequency of simultaneous and triple-peak contraction. In addition to these 15 patients, the group evaluated the symptomatic response in four patients who underwent esophagectomy after having failed multiple previous esophageal procedures, and noted the same favorable

outcome. Based on these results, the authors concluded that long esophageal myotomy is a valid treatment alternative in appropriately selected patients with esophageal spasm.

A similar experience with myotomies of the esophagus in 42 patients with NCCP attributed to esophageal spasms or other related disorders was reported by Ellis [35]. In contrast to the previous study, Ellis performed only a restricted myotomy of the affected portion of the esophagus as identified by manometry. At follow-up at up to 5 years and 8 months, Ellis observed an overall improvement rate of 70%.

In summary, treatment of esophageal spasm should include reassuring the patient of the benign nature of this condition, exclusion or treatment of gastroesophageal reflux disease (GERD) as one of the most common underlying causes, use of smooth muscle relaxants or visceral analgesics, and careful selection of patients to whom endoscopic and/or surgical therapies should be offered.

Nutcracker esophagus

The initial description of high-amplitude peristaltic contractions came from the laboratory of Charles Pope, and used the term "super squeezer" when referring to patients with chest pain and excessively large peristaltic waves [36]. The term "nutcracker esophagus" was first proposed by Benjamin *et al.* to describe patients with a distal esophageal amplitude exceeding 180 mmHg (i.e. the mean + 2 SD reported in healthy volunteers) [37]. As the concept of the nutcracker esophagus as a clinical entity has evolved, there has been considerable discussion concerning its possible clinical relevance. Whether it is a true primary motility disorder has been the subject of much debate and controversy over the past 20 years. Strong support for recognizing this motility abnormality comes from the reports of many laboratories showing that many patients being evaluated for chest pain will have this manometric finding. A study in 910 patients with NCCP found that nutcracker esophagus was the most common EMA in this group of patients, suggesting that it is a manometric marker of NCCP [38]. The overall prevalence of Nutcracker esophagus in patients referred for esophageal function testing in a tertiary referral center is approximately 7–10% [10, 39].

The pathophysiology of nutcracker esophagus is debated in the literature. Recognizing the association between nutcracker esophagus and gastroesophageal reflux, some investigators opened the debate whether nutcracker esophagus might not be a result of gastroesophageal reflux [40], while others even challenged its meaning [41], leading to fiery discussions in the literature [42]. High-frequency endoscopic ultrasound (HFIUS) studies found an increased thickness of the esophageal musculature in patients with nutcracker esophagus compared to healthy volunteers,

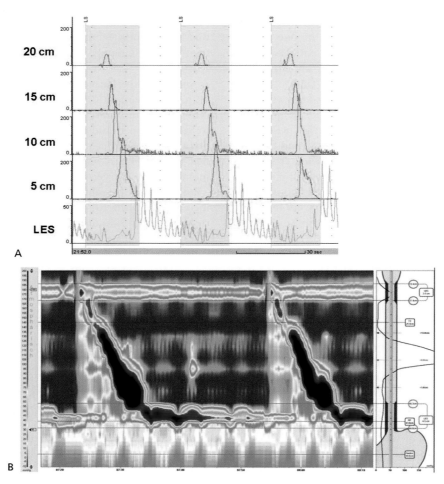

Figure 14.2 (A) Conventional manometry tracings featuring high amplitude contractions (distal contraction amplitude [DEA] >220 mmHg) diagnostic for nutcracker esophagus. (B) High-resolution manometry recording showing high-amplitude contractions diagnostic for nutcracker esophagus.

indicating a structural correlate of the high-amplitude contractions [43, 44]. Sifrim *et al*. proposed that the increase in contraction amplitude might be due to an imbalance between excitatory and inhibitory innervation, and that patients with spastic disorders of the esophagus have impaired inhibitory innervations [45, 46]. Conversely, Brito *et al*. documented that physiologic events such as deglutitive inhibitions are preserved in patients with nutcracker esophagus [47]. In addition, recent observations indicate that high-amplitude contractions characteristic for the nutcrackers esophagus do not impair bolus transit [10]. The debate on the clinical relevance of nutcracker esophagus is further fueled by monitoring the "natural history" of this abnormality. Dalton *et al*. found that on repeated testing, only 54% of patients diagnosed with nutcracker esophagus had similar findings on subsequent studies and only four of 17 (23%) patients always had high-amplitude pressures.

Nutcracker esophagus is often suspected in patients with NCCP, although many patients with this manometric diagnosis do not complain of chest pain, resulting in questions regarding the clinical relevance of nutcracker esophagus. Manometric criteria to diagnose nutcracker esophagus include an average DEA exceeding 220 mmHg (Figure 14.2A) or average DCI exceeding 5000 mmHg/cm/s (Figure 14.2B). On reviewing the presenting symptoms and reflux parameters in a group of 56 patients with nutcracker esophagus, we observed that patients with DEA between 180 and 220 mmHg had a more heterogeneous presentation (i.e. chest pain, dysphagia, reflux symptoms) and were more likely to have an abnormal distal esophageal acid exposure as an expression of GERD, whereas patients with contraction amplitudes greater than 260 mmHg had a more homogeneous clinical presentation (i.e. all being evaluated for chest pain) and normal distal esophageal acid exposure [48].

Therapeutic approaches to nutcracker esophagus are similar to those used for distal esophageal spasm (see Table 14.5). The only difference is the consideration of a calcium-channel blocker before nitrates as the therapy should be aimed at reducing contraction amplitudes rather than trying to re-establish esophageal peristalsis.

In a comprehensive evaluation of various calcium-channel blockers, Konrad-Dalhoff *et al.* reported on the effects of nifedipine, nitrendipine, nimodipine, and nisoldipine on esophageal smooth muscle function in healthy male volunteers [49]. Compared to placebo, LES pressure was significantly decreased by 24% by nifedipine and 17% by nimodipine, whereas the effects of nitrendipine (decreased by 15%) and nisoldipine (9%) were not significant. In addition, the authors noted that the decrease in sphincter pressure correlated with the plasma drug levels of nifedipine (r = 0.92), nitrendipine (r = 0.80), and nisoldipine (r = 0.79).

Ehrer *et al.* reported on the effects of sildenafil 50 mg on symptoms and manometric parameters in 11 patients with hypercontractile esophageal motility disorders [50]. During treatment with sildenafil nine (81%) of these patients showed manometric improvement after sildenafil, but only four (36%) reported a symptomatic response to this treatment. Unfortunately, two of the four patients experienced side effects and did not continue the treatment. In another study, Lee *et al.* evaluated a group of nine patients with nutcracker esophagus before and 1 h after sildenafil [51]. Measuring the intraluminal pressure in the LES and at 3, 8, 13, and 18 cm above the LES, the authors found that sildenafil decreased the LES resting pressure and prolonged LES relaxation. In addition, they observed a decrease in pressure in the distal part of the esophagus (i.e. 3–13 cm above the LES) after the ingestion of sildenafil. Our group has also reported on one patient with hypercontractile esophageal dysmotility who had a sustained positive response while being treated with phosphodiesterase 5 (PD5) inhibitors [52]. Of note is the positive manometric and symptomatic response with all three currently available PD5 inhibitors (i.e. sildenafil, vardenafil, and tadalafil).

Hypertensive lower esophageal sphincter

Hypertensive LES was described by Code *et al.* in the early 1960s [53] and is currently defined as a resting LES pressure exceeding 2 SD the average measured in healthy volunteers [1]. Hypertensive LES can be present alone or in combination with high-amplitude esophageal contractions (i.e. nutcracker esophagus), in which case it is grouped under the umbrella of hypercontractile esophageal dysmotility. Hypertensive LES has been associated with gastroesophageal reflux even though at first this association appears paradoxical because of the original association of GERD and decreased LES pressures [54]. Other investigators reported an increased intrabolus pressure and impaired bolus transit in patients with hypertensive LES, suggesting that this motility abnormality might be a form of outflow obstruction [55]. Our experience using combined multichannel intralu-minal impedance and manometry to evaluate esophageal contractions and bolus transit showed that almost all patients with isolated hypertensive LES had a normal bolus transit [11].

Treatment for hypertensive LES includes the same options as for esophageal spasms and nutcracker esophagus (see Table 14.5). Katada *et al.* reported on the association of GERD and hypertensive LES in a group of 53 patients with hypertensive LES. Among these patients 19% had evidence of GERD and 82% responded to symptom-directed medical therapy [56]. In the study by Katzka *et al.*, which included 18 patients with hypertensive LES, the authors found a wide range of distal esophageal acid exposure from slightly above normal to an esophageal pH of less than 4 for 25% of the time[19]. Of 16 patients, 12 responded to antireflux treatment, including the three patients who required fundoplication [19]. The four patients who did not respond to treatment had poor correlation of reflux episodes to symptoms on pH monitoring, displayed markedly elevated LES pressures, and did not present with heartburn.

Bortolotti *et al.* evaluated the effects of sildenafil in 14 patients with hypertensive LES [57]. The authors found that compared to placebo sildenafil decreased sphincter tone and wave amplitude. The inhibitory effect reached its maximum 10 min after the infusion and lasted approximately 1 h.

Tamhankar *et al.* reported on the benefits of myotomy plus fundoplication in a group of 16 patients with hypertensive LES [58]. The fundoplication was tailored to the presence of reflux and hiatus hernia: patients with hypertensive LES and reflux or grade III hiatus hernia underwent a complete wrap (Nissen fundoplication) in addition to the myotomy, while patients with isolated hypertensive LES underwent a partial fundoplication. After a median follow-up of 3.6 years, 10 (62.5%) patients had a excellent outcome, three (18.8%) a good one, and three (18.7%) a fair one. The authors reported that all but one patient were satisfied with the surgical outcome.

Ineffective esophageal motility

IEM is characterized by distal esophageal contractions of less than 30 mmHg (Figure 14.3) and/or non-transmitted proximal contractions in 50% or more of wet swallows [59]. This definition is based on the concept that pressure waves in the distal esophagus with amplitudes lower than 30 mmHg are associated with ineffective bolus movement. IEM was first described under the term "non-specific esophageal motility disorders" (NEMD), which was used to describe manometric patterns that did not fit specific categories [60, 61].

Leite *et al.* reviewed the manometric patterns of patients with NEMD over a 2.5-year period. In this study, 60 of 61 patients previously described as NEMD had contraction amplitudes of less than 30 mmHg in the failed or incomplete

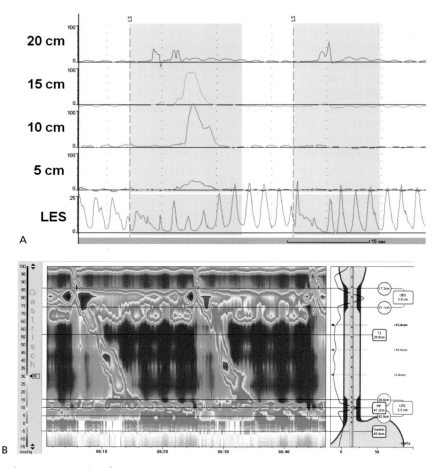

Figure 14.3 (A) Conventional manometry tracings featuring manometric low amplitude (i.e. <30 mmHg in at least one distal channel) peristaltic contraction diagnostic for ineffective esophageal motility. (B) High-resolution manometry recording showing low amplitude contractions diagnostic for ineffective esophageal motility.

contractions [31]. On the basis of these findings, the authors recommended that NEMD be replaced by the more accurate term IEM.

Between 21% and 49% of patients with IEM also have GERD [62, 63]. IEM seems to be particularly common in GERD patients with respiratory symptoms [64]. Although some studies have suggested that IEM could be a marker for GERD, Vinjirayer *et al.* showed no difference in the prevalence of IEM in patients with and without abnormal esophageal acid exposure [65]. When GERD is linked with esophagitis, the association with IEM has been well documented in animal models [66] and in clinical studies [67, 68]. Studies suggest that proinflammatory cytokines, such as interleukin-1β and interleukin-6, may be involved in reducing esophageal muscle contractility by reducing acetylcholine release from excitatory myentric neurons to circular smooth muscle [69, 70]. Interestingly, esophageal hypomotility associated with acute esophagitis can be reversed [71, 72]. However, patients with chronic esophagitis do not

experience complete recovery of esophageal dysmotility [73],suggesting that the development of chronic inflammation may result in permanent alteration in neuromotor function.

The clinical significance of IEM remains unclear. The minimum threshold of the wave amplitude to clear liquids from the esophagus (on 80% or more occasions) is 30 mmHg [74]. However, abnormal bolus transit is present in only approximately 45% of patients with IEM undergoing multichannel intraluminal impedance measurement [11][11]. A possible explanation for this discrepancy may concern the length of esophagus affected by hypocontractility. Several studies have found that the longer the segment of distal esophagus affected by hypocontractility, the greater the likelihood of impaired bolus transit [75, 76].

On the basis of the limited data currently available on IEM, its clinical significance remains unclear. Further functional studies are needed to determine whether manometric findings are clinically relevant.

Treatment of IEM has been difficult because of the lack of promotility agents that have a definite effect on esophageal function. Primary cholinergic agents need to be considered in order to achieve a measurable effect on esophageal peristaltic pressure and bolus transit. We have used either bethanechol as a direct cholinergic agent or pyridostigmine as a cholinesterase inhibitor to stimulate cholinergic activity in the esophagus. Both of these agents given orally can be shown to significantly increase esophageal amplitude and improve bolus transit. In addition, buspirone has been shown to have a similar esophageal promotility effect [77].

In the patient with dysphagia who also has IEM, it is reasonable to try one of the above esophageal promotility agents. We have used bethanechol in a dose of 25–50 mg before meals [78] or pyridostigmine in a dose of 30 mg orally before meals [79]. There have been a number of cases in which these drugs have dramatically improved the dysphagia, objectively increased the esophageal contraction amplitudes, and speeded bolus transit. There is, to date, no controlled observation with these drugs, but clinically we believe they are worth trying in IEM patients, particularly when dysphagia is a troublesome and persisting symptom.

Conclusions

EMAs are esophageal manometry findings that differ to a meaningful degree from findings in asymptomatic, normal individuals. Diagnostic criteria are available for both conventional esophageal manometry as well as HRM. While the pathophysiology of EMAs is still subject to investigations, these findings provide certain explanations for patients' symptoms (most commonly dysphagia and/or chest pain) and guide the therapeutic approach. Given its high prevalence, GERD should always be regarded as a potential cause of EMAs and investigated and/or treated appropriately. Patients with hypercontractile EMAs (i.e. esophageal spasms, nutcracker esophagus, hypertensive LES) might benefit from calcium-channel blockers, long-acting nitrates or Botox injection in the distal esophagus. Patients with hypocontractile EMAs (i.e. IEM) might benefit from maximized acid suppression and/or cholinergic medications. EMAs should be regarded as a valuable piece of the puzzle in the management of patients with esophageal symptoms.

References

1. Richter JE, Wu WC, Johns DN, *et al*. Esophageal manometry in 95 healthy adult volunteers. Variability of pressures with age and frequency of "abnormal" contractions. *Dig Dis Sci* 1987;32:583–392.
2. Spechler S, Castell DO. Classification of oesophageal motility abnormalities. *Gut* 2001;49:145–151.
3. Grübel C, Hiscock R, Hebbard G. Value of spatiotemporal representation of manometric data. *Clin Gastroenterol Hepatol* 2008;6:525–530.
4. Pandolfino JE, Ghosh SK, Rice J, Clarke JO, Kwiatek MA, Kahrilas PJ. Classifying esophageal motility by pressure topography characteristics: a study of 400 patients and 75 controls. *Am J Gastroenterol* 2008;103:27–37.
5. Castell DO. High resolution esophageal manometry: devils and dinosaurs. *Neurogastroenterol Motil* 2010;22:600–601.
6. Dalton CB, Castell DO, Hewson EG, Wu WC, Richter JE. Diffuse esophageal spasm. A rare motility disorder not characterized by high-amplitude contractions. *Dig Dis Sci* 1991;36:1025–1028.
7. Katz PO, Dalton CB, Richter JE, Wu WC, Castell DO. Esophageal testing of patients with noncardiac chest pain or dysphagia. Results of three years' experience with 1161 patients. *Ann Intern Med* 1987;106:593–597.
8. Pandolfino JE, Kahrilas PJ. AGA technical review on the clinical use of esophageal manometry. *Gastroenterology* 2005;128:209–224.
9. Millaire A, Ducloux G, Marquand A, Vaksmann G. [Nitroglycerin and angina with angiographically normal coronary vessels. Clinical effects and effects on esophageal motility]. *Arch Mal Coeur Vaiss* 1989;82:63–68.
10. Milov DE, Cynamon HA, Andres JM. Chest pain and dysphagia in adolescents caused by diffuse esophageal spasm. *J Pediatr Gastroenterol Nutr* 1989;9:450–453.
11. Tutuian R, Castell DO. Combined multichannel intraluminal impedance and manometry clarifies esophageal function abnormalities: study in 350 patients. *Am J Gastroenterol* 2004;99:1011–1019.
12. Chakder S, Rosenthal GJ, Rattan S. In vivo and in vitro influence of human recombinant hemoglobin on esophageal function. *Am J Physiol* 1995;268:G443–450.
13. Conklin JL, Murray J, Ledlow A, Clark E, Hayek B, Picken H, Rosenthal G. Effects of recombinant human hemoglobin on motor functions of the opossum esophagus. *J Pharmacol Exp Ther* 1995;273:762–767.
14. Murray JA, Ledlow A, Launspach J, Evans D, Loveday M, Conklin JL. The effects of recombinant human hemoglobin on esophageal motor functions in humans. *Gastroenterology* 1995;109:1241–1248.
15. Xue S, Valdez D, Collman PI, Diamant NE. Effects of nitric oxide synthase blockade on esophageal peristalsis and the lower esophageal sphincter in the cat. *Can J Physiol Pharmacol* 1996;74:1249–1257.
16. Konturek JW, Thor P, Lukaszyk A, Gabryelewicz A, Konturek SJ, Domschke W. Endogenous nitric oxide in the control of esophageal motility in humans. *J Physiol Pharmacol* 1997;48:201–209.
17. Orlando RC, Bozymski EM. Clinical and manometric effects of nitroglycerin in diffuse esophageal spasm. *N Engl J Med* 1973;289:23–25.
18. Swamy N. Esophageal spasm: clinical and manometric response to nitroglycerine and long acting nitrites. *Gastroenterology* 1977;72:23–27.
19. Hewson EG, Ott DJ, Dalton CB, Chen YM, Wu WC, Richter JE. Manometry and radiology. Complementary studies in the assessment of esophageal motility disorders. *Gastroenterology* 1990;98:626–632.
20. Tutuian R, Castell DO. Review article: oesophageal spasm—diagnosis and management. *Aliment Pharmacol Ther* 2006;23:1393–1402.

21. Creamer B, Donoghue E, Code CF. Pattern of esophageal motility in diffuse spasm. *Gastroenterology* 1958;34:782–796.

22. Roth HP, Fleshler B. Diffuse Esophageal spasm; clinical, radiological, and manometric observations. *Ann Intern Med* 1964;61:914–923.

23. Pandolfino JE, Kahrilas PJ. AGA technical review on the clinical use of esophageal manometry. *Gastroenterology* 2005;128:209–224.

24. Sperandio M, Tutuian R, Gideon RM, Katz PO, Castell DO. Diffuse esophageal spasm: not diffuse but distal esophageal spasm (DES). *Dig Dis Sci* 2003;48:1380–1384.

25. Orlando RC, Bozymski EM. Clinical and manometric effects of nitroglycerin in diffuse esophageal spasm. *N Engl J Med* 1973;289:23–25.

26. Swamy N. Esophageal spasm: clinical and manometric response to nitroglycerine and long acting nitrites. *Gastroenterology* 1977;72:23–27.

27. Nasrallah SM, Tommaso CL, Singleton RT, Backhaus EA. Primary esophageal motor disorders: clinical response to nifedipine. *South Med J* 1985;78:312–315.

28. Drenth JP, Bos LP, Engels LG. Efficacy of diltiazem in the treatment of diffuse oesophageal spasm. *Aliment Pharmacol Ther* 1990;4:411–416.

29. Peghini PL, Katz PO, Castell DO. Imipramine decreases oesophageal pain perception in human male volunteers. *Gut* 1998;42:807–813.

30. Clouse RE, Lustman PJ, Eckert TC, Ferney DM, Griffith LS. Low-dose trazodone for symptomatic patients with esophageal contraction abnormalities. A double-blind, placebo-controlled trial. *Gastroenterology* 1987;92:1027–1036.

31. Handa M, Mine K, Yamamoto H, *et al.* Antidepressant treatment of patients with diffuse esophageal spasm: a psychosomatic approach. *J Clin Gastroenterol* 1999;28:228–232.

32. Storr M, Allescher HD, Rosch T, Born P, Weigert N, Classen M. Treatment of symptomatic diffuse esophageal spasm by endoscopic injections of botulinum toxin: a prospective study with long-term follow-up. *Gastrointest Endosc* 2001;54:754–759.

33. Miller LS, Pullela SV, Parkman HP, *et al.* Treatment of chest pain in patients with noncardiac, nonreflux, nonachalasia spastic esophageal motor disorders using botulinum toxin injection into the gastroesophageal junction. *Am J Gastroenterol* 2002;97:1640–1646.

34. Eypasch EP, DeMeester TR, Klingman RR, Stein HJ. Physiologic assessment and surgical management of diffuse esophageal spasm. *J Thorac Cardiovasc Surg* 1992;104:859–868.

35. Ellis FH Jr. Esophagomyotomy for noncardiac chest pain resulting from diffuse esophageal spasm and related disorders. *Am J Med* 1992;92:129S–131S.

36. Brand DL, Martin D, Pope CE. Esophageal manometrics in patients with angina-like chest pain. *Dig Dis* 1977;22:300–304.

37. Benjamin SB, Gerhardt DC, Castell DO. High amplitude, peristaltic esophageal contractions associated with chest pain and/or dysphagia. *Gastroenterology* 1979;77:478–483.

38. Katz PO, Dalton CB, Richter JE, Wu WC, Castell DO. Esophageal testing of patients with noncardiac chest pain or dysphagia. Results of three years' experience with 1161 patients. *Ann Intern Med* 1987;106:593–597.

39. Cho YK, Choi MG, Park JM, *et al.* Evaluation of esophageal function in patients with esophageal motor abnormalities using multichannel intraluminal impedance esophageal manometry. *World J Gastroenterol* 2006;12:6349–6354.

40. Achem SR, Kolts BE, Wears R, Burton L, Richter JE. Chest pain associated with nutcracker esophagus: a preliminary study of the role of gastroesophageal reflux. *Am J Gastroenterol* 1993;88:187–192.

41. Kahrilas PJ. Nutcracker esophagus: an idea whose time has gone? *Am J Gastroenterol* 1993;88:167–169.

42. Castell DO. The nutcracker and the ostrich. *Am J Gastroenterol* 1993;88:1287–1288.

43. Melzer E, Ron Y, Tiomni E, Avni Y, Bar-Meir S. Assessment of the esophageal wall by endoscopic ultrasonography in patients with nutcracker esophagus. *Gastrointest Endosc* 1997;46:223–225.

44. Pehlivanov N, Liu J, Kassab GS, Beaumont C, Mittal RK. Relationship between esophageal muscle thickness and intraluminal pressure in patients with esophageal spasm. *Am J Physiol* 2002;282:G1016–1023.

45. Sifrim D, Janssens J, Vantrappen G. Failing deglutitive inhibition in primary esophageal motility disorders. *Gastroenterology* 1994;106:875–882.

46. Sifrim D, Janssens J, Vantrappen G. A wave of inhibition precedes primary peristaltic contractions in the human esophagus. *Gastroenterology* 1992;103:876–882.

47. Brito EM, Camacho-Lobato L, Paoletti V, Gideon M, Katz PO, Castell DO. Effect of different swallow time intervals on the nutcracker esophagus. *Am J Gastroenterol* 2003;98:40–45.

48. Agrawal A, Tutuian R, Hila A, Mainie I, Castell DO. Clinical relevance of the nutcracker esophagus: suggested revision of criteria for diagnosis. *J Clin Gastroenterol* 2006;40:504–509.

49. Konrad-Dalhoff I, Baunack AR, Ramsch KD, *et al.* Effect of the calcium antagonists nifedipine, nitrendipine, nimodipine and nisoldipine on oesophageal motility in man. *Eur J Clin Pharmacol* 1991;41:313–316.

50. Eherer AJ, Schwetz I, Hammer HF, *et al.* Effect of sildenafil on oesophageal motor function in healthy subjects and patients with oesophageal motor disorders. *Gut* 2002;50:758–764.

51. Lee JI, Park H, Kim JH, Lee SI, Conklin JL. The effect of sildenafil on oesophageal motor function in healthy subjects and patients with nutcracker oesophagus. *Neurogastroenterol Motil* 2003;15:617–623.

52. Agrawal A, Tutuian R, Hila A, Castell DO. Successful use of phosphodiesterase type 5 inhibitors to control symptomatic esophageal hypercontractility: a case report. *Dig Dis Sci* 2005;50:2059–2062.

53. Code CF, Schlegel JF, Kelley ML Jr, Olsen AM, Ellis FH Jr. Hypertensive gastroesophageal sphincter. *Proc Staff Meet Mayo Clin* 1960;35:391–399.

54. Katzka DA, Sidhu M, Castell DO. Hypertensive lower esophageal sphincter pressures and gastroesophageal reflux: an apparent paradox that is not unusual. *Am J Gastroenterol* 1995;90:280–284.

55. Gockel I, Lord RV, Bremner CG, Crookes PF, Hamrah P, DeMeester TR. The hypertensive lower esophageal sphincter: a motility disorder with manometric features of outflow obstruction. *J Gastrointest Surg* 2003;7:692–700.

56. Katada N, Hinder RA, Hinder PR, *et al.* The hypertensive lower esophageal sphincter. *Am J Surg* 1996;172:439–442.

57. Bortolotti M, Pandolfo N, Giovannini M, Mari C, Miglioli M. Effect of Sildenafil on hypertensive lower oesophageal sphincter. *Eur J Clin Invest* 2002;32:682–685.

58. Tamhankar AP, Almogy G, Arain MA, *et al*. Surgical management of hypertensive lower esophageal sphincter with dysphagia or chest pain. *J Gastrointest Surg* 2003;7:990–996.

59. Leite LP, Johnston BT, Barrett J, *et al*. Ineffective esophageal motility (IEM): the primary finding in patients with nonspecific esophageal motility disorder. *Dig Dis Sci* 1997;42: 1859–1865.

60. Kaye MD. Dysfunction of the lower esophageal sphincter in disorders other than achalasia. *Am J Dig Dis* 1973; 18:734–745.

61. Clouse RE, Staiano A. Contraction abnormalities of the esophageal body in patients referred to manometry. A new approach to manometric classification. *Dig Dis Sci* 1983;28:784–791.

62. Ho SC, Chang CS, Wu CY, Chen GH. Ineffective esophageal motility is a primary motility disorder in gastroesophageal reflux disease. *Dig Dis Sci* 2002;47:652–656.

63. Diener U, Patti MG, Molena D, Fisichella PM, Way LW. Esophageal dysmotility and gastroesophageal reflux disease. *J Gastrointest Surg* 2001;5:260–265.

64. Fouad YM, Katz PO, Hatlebakk JG, Castell DO Ineffective esophageal motility: the most common motility abnormality in patients with GERD-associated respiratory symptoms. *Am J Gastroenterol* 1999;94:1464–1467.

65. Vinjirayer E, Gonzalez B, Brensinger C, *et al*. Ineffective motility is not a marker for gastroesophageal reflux disease. *Am J Gastroenterol* 2003;98:771–776.

66. Eastwood GL, Castell DO, Higgs RH. Experimental esophagitis in cats impairs lower esophageal sphincter pressure. *Gastroenterology* 1975;69:146–153.

67. Kahrilas PJ, Dodds WJ, Hogan WJ, Kern M, Arndorfer RC, Reece A. Esophageal peristaltic dysfunction in peptic esophagitis. *Gastroenterology* 1986;91:897–904.

68. Timmer R, Breumelhof R, Nadorp JH, Smout AJ. Oesophageal motility and gastro-oesophageal reflux before and after healing of reflux oesophagitis. A study using 24 hour ambulatory pH and pressure monitoring. *Gut* 1994;35:1519–1522.

69. Cao W, Cheng L, Behar J, Fiocchi C, Biancani P, Harnett KM. Proinflammatory cytokines alter/reduce esophageal circular muscle contraction in experimental cat esophagitis. *Am J Physiol Gastrointest Liver Physiol* 2004;287:G1131–1139.

70. Rieder F, Cheng L, Harnett KM, *et al*. Gastroesophageal reflux disease-associated esophagitis induces endogenous cytokine production leading to motor abnormalities. *Gastroenterology* 2007;132:154–165.

71. Shirazi S, Schulze-Delrieu K, Custer-Hagen T, Brown CK, Ren J. Motility changes in opossum esophagus from experimental esophagitis. *Dig Dis Sci* 1989;34:1668–1676.

72. Zhang X, Geboes K, Depoortere I, Tack J, Janssens J, Sifrim D. Effect of repeated cycles of acute esophagitis and healing on esophageal peristalsis, tone, and length. *Am J Physiol Gastrointest Liver Physiol* 2005;288:G1339–1346.

73. Fibbe C, Layer P, Keller J, Strate U, Emmermann A, Zornig C. Esophageal motility in reflux disease before and after fundoplication: a prospective, randomized, clinical, and manometric study. *Gastroenterology* 2001;121:5–14.

74. Kahrilas PJ, Dodds WJ, Hogan WJ. Effect of peristaltic dysfunction on esophageal volume clearance. *Gastroenterology* 1988;94:73–80.

75. Tutuian R, Castell DO. Clarification of the esophageal function defect in patients with manometric ineffective esophageal motility: studies using combined impedance-manometry. *Clin Gastroenterol Hepatol* 2004;2:230–236.

76. Nguyen NQ, Tippett M, Smout AJ, *et al*. Relationship between pressure wave amplitude and esophageal bolus clearance assessed by combined manometry and multichannel intraluminal impedance measurement. *Am J Gastroenterol* 2006; 101:2476–2484.

77. Di Stefano M, Vos R, Sifrim D, Tack J. Effect of buspirone, a 5 HT1A receptor agonist, on oesophageal peristalsis and lower esophageal sphincter function in healthy volunteers. *Gastroenterology* 2004;126:A-638

78. Agrawal A, Hila A, Tutuian R, Mainie I, Castell DO. Bethanechol improves smooth muscle function in patients with severe ineffective esophageal motility. *J Clin Gastroenterol* 2007;41: 366–370.

79. Blonski W, Vela MF, Freeman J, Sharma N, Castell DO. The effect of oral buspirone, pyridostigmine, and bethanechol on esophageal function evaluated with combined multichannel esophageal impedance-manometry in healthy volunteers. *J Clin Gastroenterol* 2009;43:253–260.

Surgery for Esophageal Motor Disorders

Roger P. Tatum, Brant K. Oelschlager, and Carlos A. Pellegrini
Department of Surgery, University of Washington, Seattle, WA, USA

Introduction

In general, those esophageal motor disorders amenable to surgical treatment are those in which the muscular activity is either too great, is poorly coordinated, or some combination thereof. Fundamentally, treatment is based on transecting the appropriate muscle. For some of these problems it is necessary to also treat associated sequelae, such as resecting esophageal diverticula, or adding an antireflux procedure to a lower esophageal sphincter (LES) myotomy. In extreme cases, for patients who have failed all other forms of medical and surgical treatment, and present with lengthy, convoluted, wide, non-emptying esophagi, an esophageal resection and reconstruction may be necessary. For most patients, minimally invasive surgical techniques have been developed and are now the first line for treatment of these disorders. In this chapter, the motor disorders of the esophagus are discussed in relation to their anatomic location, starting from the upper esophageal sphincter (UES) and working toward the gastroesophageal junction (GEJ). A summary of each disease is presented, followed by the assessment and surgical treatment. The controversial issues for each topic are discussed at the end of each section.

Upper esophageal sphincter

Swallowing consists of oral, pharyngeal, and esophageal phases. The UES plays a role in the pharyngeal phase and in the transition from the pharyngeal to the esophageal phase. Pharyngoesophageal diverticulum (Zenker's diverticulum) and cricopharyngeal bar, also referred to as cricopharyngeal achalasia, have been identified as pathologic entities of the UES. Understanding the anatomy and function of the UES is essential to planning an operation to treat these maladies.

The pharynx meets the esophagus where the inferior pharyngeal constrictor joins the cricopharyngeus muscle. The inferior constrictor takes origin from the thyroid and cricoid cartilage, and its fibers run obliquely and horizontally to insert on the median raphe (posterior aspect) of the pharynx. The cricopharyngeus muscle arises from the cricoid cartilage, passes posteriorly to the pharyngoesophageal junction, and inserts on the contralateral side of the cricoid cartilage. Some anatomists view the cricopharyngeal muscle as simply the most inferior segment of the inferior constrictor, differing from the other muscle fibers in that they do not insert into the median raphe [1]. However, the structures are seen as distinctly separate in the surgical approach to the UES. The interlacing of muscle fibers at the posterior aspect of the pharynx leaves areas of potential weakness where herniation of the mucosa may occur, especially when intraluminal pressures are elevated. The triangle of Killian is one of these areas and is found between the inferior constrictor and the cricopharyngeus muscle [2, 3]. Two additional areas where the relative paucity of muscle fibers creates a relative weakness in the pharyngeal wall are the Killian–Jamieson's area between the fibers of the cricopharyngeus, and Laimer's triangle between the junction of the cricopharyngeus and the first circular fibers of the esophagus [4] (Figure 15.1). The purpose of the inferior constrictor is to compress the pharynx during swallowing, displacing the food bolus downward. The cricopharyngeus muscle maintains tonic contraction, closing the inlet to the esophagus between swallows, and relaxes during swallowing to allow bolus entry into the esophagus. The cricopharyngeus muscle generates most of the pressure at the manometrically identified UES, because the physiologic high-pressure zone is often found to be of greater length than the anatomically identified muscle fibers. The function of the UES is to prevent the entrance of air into the esophagus and to prevent high gastroesophageal reflux from entering the larynx [5].

The Esophagus, Fifth Edition. Edited by Joel E. Richter, Donald O. Castell.
© 2012 Blackwell Publishing Ltd. Published 2012 by Blackwell Publishing Ltd.

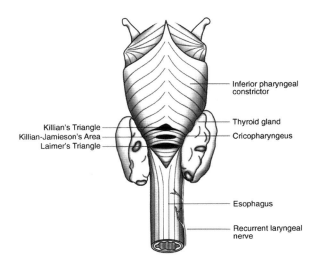

Figure 15.1 Posterior aspect of the pharyngoesophageal junction with areas of weakness identified.

When a swallow is initiated, the UES relaxes while the oral and pharyngeal phases of deglutition proceed. As the tongue propels the bolus posteriorly, the larynx is elevated and compressed to prevent the bolus from entering the trachea. The bolus passes into the pharynx and the constrictors then contract to propel the bolus into the esophagus. The tonic contraction of the UES is inhibited and the bolus proceeds into the esophagus. This is a conceptually simple interpretation of deglutition. However, extensive study of the physiology of the UES and the pathophysiology of the diseases that affect the UES have revealed the complexity of UES activity. A more concise description may be found elsewhere in this book.

Pharyngoesophageal diverticulum (Zenker's)

Since all reported cases of pharyngoesophageal diverticulum have occurred in elderly patients, it is assumed to be an acquired disease. The diverticulum is not a true one, in that it consists of only mucosa, which escapes the pharynx between the areas of weakness in the muscle fibers described earlier. It is classified as a pulsion diverticulum because it is thought to arise from increased pressure within the pharynx. The reason for this increase in intraluminal pressure within the pharynx is not known, but at least four hypotheses have been advanced as an explanation [6]. The early explanation was that the UES was maintaining tonic contraction during swallowing in response to lower esophageal disease, such as gastroesophageal reflux. Then, the concept of achalasia of the UES, a failure to relax, was put forward as the explanation for the high resistance at the pharyngoesophageal junction. As manometric evaluation of the UES became available,

it was found that the UES was capable of relaxing, but that lack of coordination between bolus propagation and sphincter relaxation was the primary cause of the increased pressure in the pharynx. Finally, evidence suggests that the muscles of the cricopharyngeus and the proximal esophagus are fibrosed and therefore do not function as they normally would.

The last two theories have the greatest support, and both contribute conceptually to understanding the dysfunction of the UES. Manometry of the UES shows some degree of incoordination in more than two-thirds of patients [7]. The dysfunction occurs most frequently during the UES closure after relaxation and the initiation of the proximal esophageal peristaltic wave [8]. The precise nature of the dysfunction can be difficult to assess with stationary manometry because the UES is relatively narrow compared with the vertical distance it moves during normal deglutition. The combination of manometry with simultaneous fluoroscopy has helped resolve this problem. By ensuring proper placement of the manometry catheter at the UES, it was found that the sphincter was not relaxing completely and that its baseline pressure was also decreased [9]. Further investigation of the sphincter muscles showed that they were replaced by fibrotic tissue, which explained the abnormal response of the sphincter to swallowing [10–12]. It is not known whether the fibrosis is a cause or effect of the disease.

Clinical evaluation

Pharyngoesophageal diverticulum usually occurs in the seventh or eighth decade of life. Cervical esophageal dysphagia and regurgitation are the most common complaints. Dysphagia may occur as a result of the dysfunctional UES. It may also be due to displacement or obstruction of the pharyngoesophageal junction caused by a large diverticulum and its contents. As the diverticulum enlarges, regurgitation of undigested food particularly during recumbence becomes more prevalent. Aspiration, halitosis, excessive salivation, and a sensation of fullness in the neck may also occur. The physical examination is usually not helpful but may reveal a palpable mass, most commonly on the left side of the neck, and a foul odor may be detected on the breath.

A contrast esophagogram should be obtained. It usually reveals the diverticulum and helps exclude a high esophageal tumor (Figure 15.2). Although a videoesophagram also demonstrates abnormal movement of the contrast during deglutition, it is probably not necessary to obtain one. Other studies that can confirm the diagnosis include esophagoscopy and manometry. A 24-h pH study has been used to determine whether there is associated gastroesophageal reflux, which is believed by some to contribute to the pathogenesis of the disease. None of the last three tests is likely to alter the therapy, and they are probably not necessary in the average patient with a pharyngoesophageal diverticulum. Recently, high-resolution esophageal manometry (HRM), in which a catheter employing many pressure

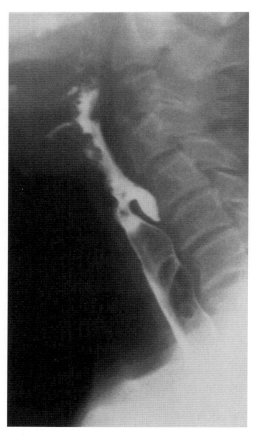

Figure 15.2 Lateral view of an esophagogram demonstrating a Zenker's diverticulum projecting downward posterior to the cricopharyngeus muscle.

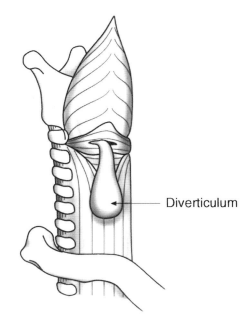

Figure 15.3 Diverticulum relative to the surgical landmarks of the posterior pharynx.

sensors, typically circumferential and spaced 1 cm apart, has been applied to the evaluation of the UES. A study by Ghosh *et al.* on 75 normal patients demonstrated that using the HRM technique, the challenges of the manometric evaluation of the LES, including axial movement of the sphincter relative to the manometry catheter and accurate capture of the very rapid relaxation interval, can be overcome [13]. This has resulted in the generation of better normative data not only for pressure and relaxation parameters of the UES but also for UES intrabolus pressure, which could be quite relevant in the evaluation of patients with cervical dysphagia. This should allow better characterization of the UES in disease states including Zenker's diverticulum and cricopharyngeal bar. To date, however, a study using HRM in patients with these problems has not been performed.

Treatment

Currently, both the more traditional open approach for diverticulectomy and cricopharyngeal myotomy and the endoscopic technique are commonly employed. Both are described below.

Open technique

Before operative treatment of the diverticulum, the patient should be on a liquid diet for 1 or 2 days to minimize the amount of retained food particles in the diverticulum. Although the preoperative contrast study helps decide which side of the neck will provide the best exposure for the procedure, the left side is usually preferred. Most diverticula originate in the posterior aspect of the pharynx. As they grow, about 25% project to the left side and 10% project to the right side; thus, the left side is used in 90% of cases. The approach from the left is easier from an anatomic standpoint. The tracheoesophageal groove and the recurrent laryngeal nerve are more accessible because of the slight rightward shift of the trachea relative to the esophagus in the neck.

Access to the area is gained through a low cervical incision along the anterior border of the sternocleidomastoid muscle. The dissection proceeds along the avascular plane anterior to the sternocleidomastoid muscle, which is retracted laterally. The carotid sheath is retracted laterally as well, and the thyroid gland medially. Often, the middle thyroid vein is ligated and transected, as is the omohyoid muscle to improve exposure. As the tracheoesophageal groove is approached, care must be taken to avoid injuring the recurrent laryngeal nerve. With the posterolateral aspect of the esophagus exposed, a bougie may be carefully passed into the esophagus. The surgeon should guide the bougie to prevent it from entering the diverticulum. With the bougie in place, a circumferential dissection of the esophagus is performed. The esophagus is then dissected cephalad along the posterior midline toward its junction with the pharynx. During this dissection, the diverticulum is encountered (Figure 15.3).

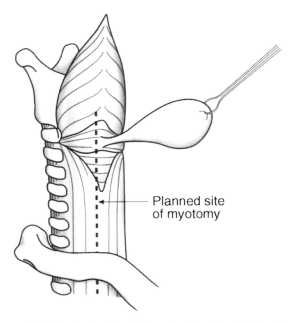

Figure 15.4 Diverticulum elevated from the dissection site. The site of the planned myotomy is marked by the dotted line.

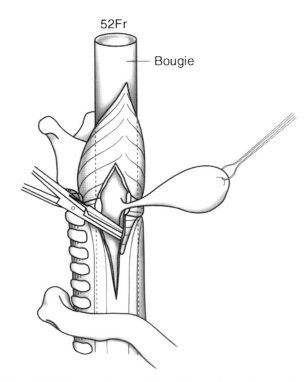

Figure 15.5 Myotomy is extended onto the esophagus for several centimeters.

The diverticulum is grasped with a Babcock forceps, dissected free from adjacent structures, and elevated into the wound (Figure 15.4). The neck of the diverticulum is cleared of the surrounding tissues. This should reveal the triangle of Killian. At this point, a myotomy is performed. The cricopharyngeus muscle and the proximal few centimeters of the longitudinal and circular muscle of the esophagus are also transected, so that the mucosa protrudes through the myotomy site (Figure 15.5). The diverticulum should be excised when possible to reduce the amount of redundant mucosa at the pharyngoesophageal junction. To accomplish this, a linear stapler is placed across the neck of the diverticulum with a bougie inside the esophagus to prevent narrowing of the lumen (Figure 15.6). Notably, when the diverticulum is less than approximately 1.5 cm in size, it is often left in place, as these small diverticula tend to essentially disappear after correction of the relative cricopharyngeal obstruction [14]. The platysma is closed loosely and the skin is approximated. Drainage of the wound is not necessary. The patient is allowed a liquid diet on the first postoperative day, and if no evidence of a leak is present, the diet may be advanced.

Outcome
Resolution of dysphagia and regurgitation may be expected and has been reported in 82–100% of patients treated with this approach [7, 15, 16]. Despite the symptomatic improvement, the mechanism of deglutition is not entirely restored to normal. For example, postoperative video contrast studies show abnormalities in pharyngeal peristalsis, a visible

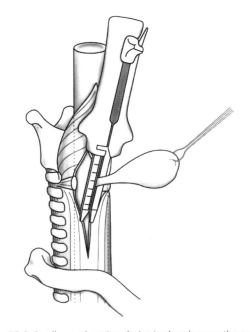

Figure 15.6 Stapling and cutting device is placed across the neck of the diverticulum. Note that the bougie is in place before transecting the diverticulum.

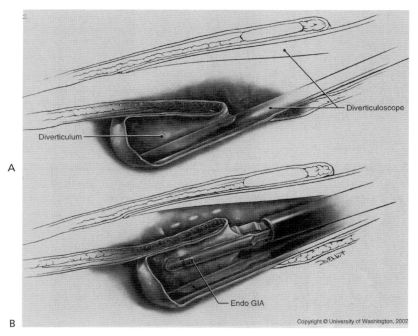

Figure 15.7 (A) Exposure of the esophagus and diverticulum is gained with a diverticuloscope placed perorally. (B) The linear stapler is across the cricopharyngeus muscle by placing a blade in the esophagus and the diverticulum (reproduced courtesy of the University of Washington, Seattle, WA, with permission.)

cricopharyngeus, premature closure of the cricopharyngeus, and, occasionally, a residual diverticulum [17].

Complications

Mortality from this procedure should be less than 1%. The most disturbing complication, esophagocutaneous fistula, occurs in 6–20% of cases but heals spontaneously [16]. Other potential complications include soft tissue infection, mediastinitis, recurrent laryngeal nerve injury, hematoma, and late stenosis. The frequency of these complications ranges between 1% and 6% [10]. Some authors feel that mucosal injury and recurrent laryngeal nerve injury may be reduced by operating with loupe magnification [18]. Recurrence rates are low, and if the diverticulum is excised while a bougie is in the esophagus, postoperative stenosis is rare.

Endoscopic technique

The minimally invasive, transoral approach to Zenker's diverticulum dates back to Mosher's first description in 1917 [19]. The technique was improved significantly by Dohlman and Matson in 1960 [20], and variations on this are now in common use. The most common technique in use today is based on that described by Collard *et al.* in 1993 [21]. This involves the use of a specialized rigid endoscope ("diverticuloscope") to gain exposure to the pharynx and expose the mouth of the diverticulum. With the patient under general anesthesia, the diverticuloscope is inserted transorally. This has two blades, one of which is placed in the esophageal lumen while the other is positioned within the diverticulum. The intervening muscle between the lumen of the esophagus and the pouch of the diverticulum is then divided with a linear cutting stapling device, which fires four rows of staples and then cuts between the inner two rows (Figure 15.7). At this point the diverticulum is no longer a blind-ended pouch, in that the anterior wall of the diverticulum communicates with the esophageal lumen. Importantly, the cricopharyngeus muscle is divided as a result of this technique.

Limitations and contraindications to the procedure include restrictions in exposure (small oral cavity, prominent dentition, or cervical spine disease) and a relatively small diverticulum. A diverticulum smaller than 3 cm is problematic because in these cases the stapler will not extend far enough distally to fully divide the cricopharyngeus, resulting in inadequate treatment. For this reason, in patients for whom the preoperative esophagram demonstrates a diverticulum smaller than 3 cm, the open approach is recommended [22]. Additionally, endoscopic stapling may not be adequate for extremely large diverticula, in that there is often persistent bolus pooling in the diverticulum.

Another endoscopic technique involves the use of a CO_2 laser to divide the septum between the cricopharyngeus and the diverticulum; the laser also accomplishes coagulation of the edges of the divided septum, rendering suturing or stapling unnecessary. This was first described in 1984 by van Overbeek *et al.* [23], and numerous other reports have indicated that it is safe and generally successful [24–29].

Outcome

To date, many series have shown the stapled technique to be a safe and effective procedure with satisfaction rates in the 90% range [22, 30–34]. The advantages of this technique include shorter operative times [35], shorter hospital stay (typically 1 day), avoidance of an incision, and potentially less morbidity. This is an important consideration because Zenker's diverticulum most commonly presents in the seventh or eighth decade of life.

Several recent series have demonstrated similar rates of symptomatic relief and durability to those for the open technique [22, 33, 34]. The largest series to date to compare the two approaches was reported by Bonavina *et al.*, involving 181 patients treated via the endoscopic approach and 116 who underwent open diverticulectomy with cricopharyngeal myotomy. Complete symptom relief was achieved in 92% and 94%, respectively, and 82% and 84% of a smaller subset of patients with a 10-year follow-up [22].

Complications

The most serious complication of the transoral stapled technique is esophageal or pharyngeal perforation, which occurs up to 10% in some series [30]. Inadequate cricopharyngeal transection may also occur, leading to persistent or recurrent symptoms and requiring surgical revision.

Controversies in treatment

All patients with symptomatic pharyngoesophageal diverticula who are able to tolerate an operation should probably be treated, because the natural history of the disease is one of progression leading to complications [6]. No medical therapy has been shown to be effective at treating these diverticula. Several elements of the surgical treatment have been topics of debate.

Diverticulectomy versus diverticulopexy

In an effort to decrease the incidence of soft tissue infection and mediastinitis, the diverticulum may be sutured to the precervical fascia so that the apex is cephalad to the neck (Figure 15.8). By not breaching the esophageal mucosa, the incidence of infection would theoretically be decreased. In a non-randomized study of 43 patients approached by a transcervical route, all patients had myotomies performed; 14 had diverticulectomy, and 29 had diverticulopexy [18]. Neck infection developed in two patients in both groups, and mediastinitis developed in one patient in the diverticulectomy group. There was no statistical difference in the incidence of wound infection or mediastinitis between the two groups. It may be argued that the study did not have enough patients to detect a difference in infectious complications. This may obscure the theoretical benefit of the diverticulopexy procedure. However, diverticulopexy was the procedure of choice in the most recent patients, in that the authors discarded the use of diverticulectomy for treatment. Thus,

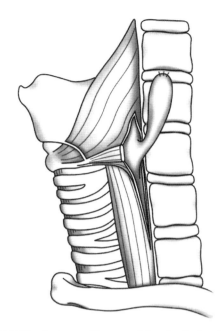

Figure 15.8 Diverticulopexy. The apex of the diverticulum is sutured to the precervical fascia.

no known difference exists between the two procedures with respect to outcome or complications.

The most important point is that whether a diverticulectomy or diverticulopexy is performed, it is essential to proceed with a cricopharyngeal myotomy. Although in the past some have advocated diverticulectomy alone, the incidence of recurrence was so high that it is now inadvisable to treat the diverticulum without performing a myotomy [36].

Treating associated foregut pathology

Other abnormalities of esophageal and gastric function may be found in up to 60% of patients with pharyngoesophageal diverticula [37]. The most common finding is gastroesophageal reflux disease (GERD). As with cricopharyngeal bar (discussed later), the association between the two is thought to stem from an attempt by the UES to prevent gastric contents from reaching the pharynx. The issue of addressing both entities simultaneously has waxed and waned over time depending on the accepted explanation of the pathophysiology of pharyngoesophageal diverticulum [38]. Some surgeons believe that if abnormal gastroesophageal reflux is demonstrated preoperatively, it should be treated surgically during the same procedure as the pharyngoesophageal diverticulum, or as a subsequent follow-up procedure. The rationale behind this approach is the assumption that once the cricopharyngeal myotomy is performed, the refluxed contents from the stomach may more easily enter the larynx, causing laryngitis, hoarseness, and even aspiration. However, not all patients with Zenker's diverticulum have concomitant foregut pathology. The best approach is to address each pathologic entity based on its severity and the discomfort it creates for the patient. If heartburn, regurgitation of digested food, and esophagitis are the predominant findings in a patient who has a small Zenker's diverticulum on a contrast study, the reflux should be treated first, because some relief from both may be gained [5]. Similarly, if the patient has cervical dysphagia, regurgitation of undigested food, and a mildly abnormal 24-h pH study, the pharyngoesophageal diverticulum should be treated alone.

Conclusions

Zenker's diverticula are the result of a dysfunctional UES and a weakness in the posterior muscular fibers of the pharyngoesophageal junction. Regurgitation and cervical dysphagia are the most common symptoms. Diagnostic work-up may be limited to a contrast study of the pharynx and the esophagus. Concurrent foregut pathology should be addressed on its own merit. No medical therapy is effective in the treatment of pharyngoesophageal diverticula. Surgical treatment, including resection of the diverticulum and cricopharyngeal myotomy, by either an open or endoscopic approach as dictated by the patient's overall status as well as the size of the diverticulum, relieves symptoms and has excellent results.

Cricopharyngeal bar

A cricopharyngeal bar is identified radiographically by a persistent posterior indentation of contrast in the pharyngoesophageal segment. This is seen on a lateral view during a videoesophagram or barium swallow (Figure 15.9). In addition, residual contrast may be seen above the cricopharyngeus well after the UES has closed (Figure 15.10). Despite the presence of such a finding, no consistent clinical symptoms have been identified in these patients. In fact, the etiology and significance of a cricopharyngeal bar are unknown.

Based on the concept that the UES relaxes during swallowing, the persistent indentation has been described as either a failure to relax (thus the term UES achalasia) or incoordination of the constrictors and cricopharyngeus muscle. Dantas *et al.* examined six patients with cricopharyngeal bars and eight control subjects without this finding on barium swallow [39]. The subjects were assessed using videofluoroscopy and UES manometry. The patients were found to have normal contraction of the pharynx, UES pressure, and bolus flow rate. When compared with control subjects, the patients with cricopharyngeal bars had reduced UES relaxation during swallowing and increased upstream bolus pressures. From these data, it appears that cricopharyngeal bars arise as a result of failure of the muscle to completely relax. Others have found that resting, relaxation, and contraction pressures are normal in patients with cricopharyngeal bar [40]. In fact, these authors claim that the cricopharyngeal muscle is the only normal portion of the pharyngoesophageal segment and that the inferior constrictor and proximal esophagus are abnormally dilated.

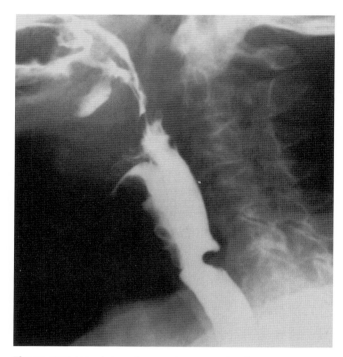

Figure 15.9 Lateral view of an esophagogram showing a cricopharyngeal bar. The persistent indentation posteriorly is caused by the cricopharyngeus muscle.

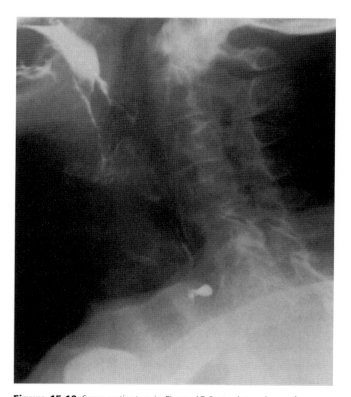

Figure 15.10 Same patient as in Figure 15.9 at a later phase of swallowing, showing the persistent contrast above the cricopharyngeus muscle. Note how the relative position of the cricopharyngeus muscle has descended back toward the clavicle.

Even when a cricopharyngeal bar can be demonstrated, the clinical significance of this finding is difficult to discern. Patients who are asymptomatic may have the same degree of narrowing as patients being evaluated for cervical esophageal dysphagia [39]. Furthermore, cricopharyngeal bar is seen in greater than 50% of patients with gastroesophageal reflux [41]. Because of the ambiguity of the finding and the lack of symptoms attributable to this dysfunction, surgical intervention for cricopharyngeal bar is only appropriate for selected patients. The patients should not have a medical condition known to affect motility (myopathy, Parkinson's disease, or myasthenia gravis), neoplasia must be excluded, and gastroesophageal reflux should be eliminated as a cause of the cricopharyngeal bar [42]. If these requirements are satisfied and the patient has symptoms referable to the cervical esophagus, a cricopharyngeal myotomy may provide some relief. Alternatively, endoscopic dilation has been reported to provide long-term relief in approximately 50% of patients [43]. Botulinum toxin injection has also been used in cases of hypertonicity of the cricopharyngeus in order to potentially predict the success of myotomy; additionally, it can provide temporary relief of symptoms for up to 4 months [44].

Achalasia

Achalasia is the most common esophageal motor disorder that warrants surgical intervention. This disease is characterized by incomplete LES relaxation and absent esophageal peristalsis. As a consequence, esophageal emptying is impaired, which causes progressive dilation and lengthening of the organ. Both medical and surgical treatments are geared toward decreasing resistance to flow through the GEJ. Although this improves emptying and relieves symptoms of the disease, it does not directly affect the underlying etiology of the pathologic process.

Despite multiple attempts at defining the pathophysiology of achalasia, little is known about the etiology of the disease. Chagas disease does provide some insight into achalasia, because the symptoms, anatomic findings, and physiologic aspects of the two diseases are similar. In Chagas disease, *Trypanosoma cruzi* destroys the myenteric plexus of the esophagus, which is thought to be the cause of altered motor dysfunction and LES relaxation. Patients with achalasia also have a decreased number of neural cells in their myenteric plexus.

Because most cases occur between the fourth and sixth decades of life, there is little suspicion of a congenital cause. However, familial achalasia has been reported in up to six siblings in a single family [45]. Robertson *et al.* reported finding varicella zoster virus DNA in the esophageal muscular wall of 33% of patients with achalasia [46]. A recent study by Facco *et al.* suggest that HSV-1 exposure may trigger a specific T-cell mediated immune-inflammatory reaction within the myenteric plexus of the LES to produce this dis-

order in certain susceptible individuals [47]. Other investigators have reported no correlation between viral infections and the incidence of achalasia [48].

The one pathologic finding that is agreed upon in achalasia is the relative paucity of the myenteric plexus in the esophageal wall. Whether this is a cause or an effect of achalasia is unknown. The lack of LES relaxation is thought to be related to impaired non-adrenergic, non-cholinergic inhibitory control and the lack of nitric oxide (NO) synthase [49]. Despite the lack of NO, the LES is still sensitive to other enteric hormones such as secretin [50]. More investigation is needed to determine the etiology of achalasia and, therefore, for the chance to halt progression or prevent the disease. For now, palliation of the symptoms is all physicians have to offer.

Clinical evaluation

Achalasia usually presents with symptoms of progressive dysphagia and regurgitation of undigested food. Other symptoms may include substernal chest pain, heartburn, and, rarely, abdominal pain. As the esophagus becomes more dilated, patients tend to complain less about dysphagia and more about regurgitation. Weight loss is common, and, occasionally, patients are malnourished. Dysphagia is primarily related to the ingestion of solid food. Most patients relate a "need to push food down with liquids" and frequent episodes of complete occlusion of the esophagus leading to "vomiting." Because progression of the disease is insidious, most patients do not seek medical attention for quite some time. The average length of time between the onset of symptoms and operative intervention is 60 months [51].

Whenever a patient presents with these complaints, other etiologies must be considered, such as tumors of the GEJ, neurologic diseases, and connective tissue disorders. Pseudoachalasia, also called secondary achalasia, may be caused by neoplasms, paraneoplastic syndromes, pseudocysts, and postoperative obstruction of the GEJ after a perihiatal operation [52, 53]. These patients present with manometric and radiologic signs of achalasia and may be difficult to distinguish from patients with achalasia. A careful history and physical examination often aids in identifying patients with pseudoachalasia. Tumors generally occur in older patients, and the progression of dysphagia and weight loss is more rapid. Thus, the physician should be wary when the diagnosis of achalasia is entertained in a patient older than 70 years, particularly when the duration of symptoms is less than 6 months and the weight loss is greater than 20 lb. These patients should be carefully examined in search of palpable supraclavicular lymphadenopathy and other signs of a neoplastic process. In addition, their diagnostic evaluation should include an accurate assessment of the morphology of the esophageal wall. The test of choice is a transesophageal endoscopic ultrasound. If this is not available, a computed tomography scan may provide useful information.

Achalasia is rare in children, and a timely diagnosis is difficult. The time lapse between symptoms and correct diagnosis is between 6 months and 9 years. Children may manifest the disease by recurrent episodes of pneumonia, failure to thrive, coughing, and hoarseness [54]. Some teenagers have even been given a diagnosis of anorexia nervosa [55].

Diagnostic tests

Evaluation of patients suspected of having achalasia should include manometry, an esophagogram, and upper endoscopy. If possible, a 24-h pH study should also be performed.

Manometry

Manometry is the gold standard for diagnosing achalasia. The criteria for diagnosis are aperistalsis of the esophageal body, incomplete relaxation of the LES, and normal or hypertonic LES pressure (see Chapter 8). Disorganized contractions of the esophageal body usually have normal or less than normal amplitudes. The waves are not propagated throughout the length of the esophagus and are often simultaneous. The LES pressure fails to drop to the gastric baseline as it does in the normal state. The need for preoperative manometry when contemplating a functional procedure on the esophagus is unquestionable. It is necessary to prevent performing an improper operation, such as a total fundoplication on untreated achalasia [56].

In some patients, chest pain is a predominant symptom. Many patients have high-amplitude contractions. In this variant of the disease, called vigorous achalasia, the high-amplitude waves are thought to cause pain. Thus, dilation or myotomy limited to the GEJ, although enough to relieve dysphagia, may not be adequate to relieve pain in these patients. Parrilla *et al.*, however, reported excellent pain relief following a standard myotomy in patients with vigorous achalasia [57]. To help understand the origin of these high-amplitude contractions, Stuart *et al.* performed manometry on 13 patients with achalasia while they were consuming a standard meal [58]. Elevated baseline esophageal pressures developed and peak contractile pressures ranged from 65 to 120 mmHg in all patients [58]. Although none of these patients had a diagnosis of vigorous achalasia on stationary manometry, all developed high contractile pressures when their esophagus became distended. The results of this study question the diagnosis of vigorous achalasia on stationary manometry alone.

Recently, HRM (described above) has become widely available, and may facilitate the identification of achalasia. Because of the color-contour display of the entire esophageal body and LES, it is possible to better characterize a non-relaxing LES in cases in whom there is sphincter movement in relation to the manometry catheter. The simultaneous contractions that are frequently seen on conventional manometry most typically appear as pan-esophageal pressurizations, a continuous pressure event from the UES to the LES, on HRM (Figure 15.11).

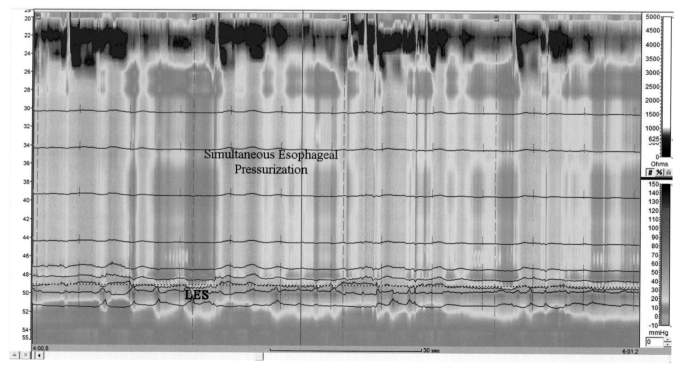

Figure 15.11 High-resolution manometry tracing of achalasia; note failure of lower esophageal sphincter (LES) relaxation and simultaneous esophageal pressurization (rather than true contractions).

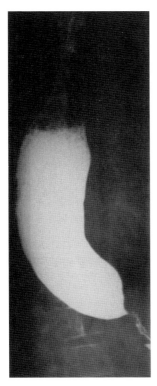

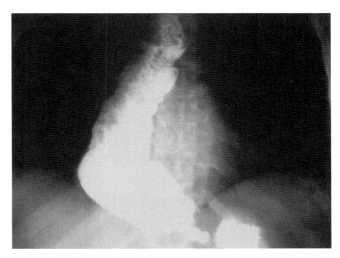

Figure 15.13 Patient with more advanced achalasia demonstrating a sigmoid esophagus.

Figure 15.12 Esophagogram demonstrating achalasia. The patient has a smooth, abrupt tapering of the distal esophagus and an air–fluid level proximally.

Esophagogram

The esophagogram defines the anatomy of the esophageal body and may help exclude tumor. The esophageal body is dilated and the lumen is smooth without evidence of peristaltic waves. Often, an air–fluid level is visible. A discrete narrowing at the GEJ is noted, often referred to as a "bird's beak" (Figure 15.12). The tapering of the distal esophagus should be concentric, without evidence of a mass effect. Advanced disease often reveals a tortuous esophagus or a "sigmoid esophagus" (Figure 15.13). A diverticulum may be an associated finding.

Some have used contrast studies to evaluate the degree of esophageal dilation and the height of the contrast column before and after intervention [59]. Although improvement in these measures can be seen after treatment of achalasia, the correlation with clinical outcome is not clear.

Endoscopy

Upper endoscopy is essential in patients with dysphagia to exclude intraluminal esophageal neoplastic processes. It may also identify other pathology in the stomach and duodenum. The expected findings in a patient with achalasia are a dilated proximal esophagus, retained food or liquid, and no evidence of esophagitis. The endoscope should pass the LES with minimal effort in patients with achalasia; if stubborn

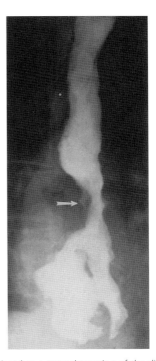

Figure 15.14 Patient has a ragged tapering of the distal esophagus, which is suspicious for malignancy.

resistance is met, other causes of esophageal obstruction must be suspected. Endoscopic ultrasound is useful in these situations, because it provides a detailed view of the entire wall and may help identify tumors at the GEJ (Figures 15.14 and 15.15). It can also identify the proximal extent of hypertrophic muscle in the esophageal wall.

24-H pH monitoring

The pH study usually shows little, if any, reflux in classic achalasia. The pH in both the proximal and distal channels should remain greater than 4. If, however, gastroesophageal reflux does occur, it cannot be cleared by the aperistaltic esophagus. For this reason, preoperative episodes of gastroesophageal reflux are important to document.

Interpreting the pH data may be difficult and requires some degree of experience with achalasia. A computer program that receives the data directly from a digital record-ing device often analyzes the data. The automated analysis can be misleading because achalasia patients may have an acidic environment (pH < 4.0) without any reflux. This phenomenon has been demonstrated by Crookes *et al.* [60], who showed that fermentation of bland food can generate a pH of less than 4.0 when mixed with saliva. Careful inspection of the graphic tracing reveals a gradual decrease in pH over several hours as opposed to the rapid decline in pH seen with episodes of reflux (Figure 15.16). The distinction is important for clinical assessment in both preoperative and postoperative studies [61].

Other studies

Stationary manometry may not be possible in some patients because the GEJ cannot be negotiated by the catheter. In this case, esophageal function may be determined using radionuclide transit and videofluoroscopic studies. Using manometry as the standard, these studies have a sensitivity of 68% and 41%, respectively [62].

Surgical treatment

The aim of treatment is to decrease LES pressure and improve esophageal emptying. Both medical and surgical approaches are available. The decision to proceed with one or the other is discussed later. The standard surgical treatment is a myotomy with or without an antireflux procedure. The myotomy should be extended onto the cardia because 45% of the LES pressure is maintained by the stomach [63]. The principles of operative therapy are to transect completely the longitudinal and circular muscle fibers of the esophagus and the sling fibers of the cardia. The cut edges

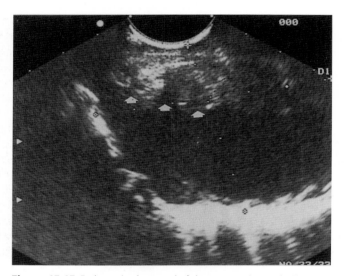

Figure 15.15 Endoscopic ultrasound of the same patient as in Figure 15.13. Arrows show the tumor of the distal esophagus disrupting the normal tissue planes.

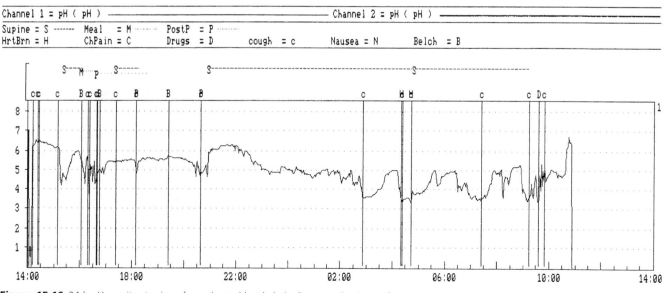

Figure 15.16 24-h pH monitor tracing of a patient with achalasia. Between the times of 22:00 and 04:00, there is a gradual decrease in the pH consistent with fermentation.

of the muscle must be separated widely and prevented from reapproximating. The length of the myotomy should be great enough to extend onto the stomach for 3 cm and to extend up the esophagus until normal muscle thickness is encountered [64].

Minimally invasive surgical techniques provide an excellent approach to this operation. Both laparoscopic and thoracoscopic approaches may be used [65–68], although currently the laparoscopic approach is more commonly employed. For the average patient with achalasia, an abdominal approach is recommended because there is less pain, better access to the GEJ, no need to collapse the lung during the operation, and better results. The preparation and operation are carried out as described in the following paragraphs.

Preparation

The patient should be restricted to a liquid diet for at least 2 days before the operation. This helps clear solid material from the dilated body of the esophagus and prevents aspiration of food into the airway at the time of intubation. Use of a lighted bougie dilator and esophagoscopy should be available during the operation to facilitate transection of the muscle fibers and to determine the adequacy of the myotomy [69].

Operation

The patient is placed in a low lithotomy position with the surgeon standing between the patient's legs and the assistant standing on the patient's left. A laparoscope holder may be used to secure the instrument, which retracts the liver. Five trocars are used during the procedure. The assistant operates the laparoscope with the left hand and provides retraction with the right (Figure 15.17).

After retracting the left lobe of the liver anteriorly, the peritoneum overlying the left crus is divided. The short gastric vessels are divided and the phrenoesophageal membrane is opened anteriorly. The right crus is then dissected so that the lateral and anterior attachments of the abdominal esophagus are freed. Posterior mobilization of the esophagus is required only when a Toupet fundoplication is planned after completion of the myotomy. The anterior aspect of the esophagus should be dissected well into the mediastinum. At this time, the lighted bougie (number 52F) is introduced into the esophagus transorally. The fat overlying the GEJ should be removed, and the anterior vagus dissected free from the esophageal wall. The cardiomyotomy site is marked with cautery in a straight line along the anterior portion of the esophagus and stomach (Figure 15.18). The distal esophageal muscle fibers are usually the most difficult to dissect, especially if previous dilation or botulinum toxin injection has been performed [70]. For this reason, the initial dissection is started on the stomach or an area of less fibrosed esophagus. Cautery is used to divide the muscle

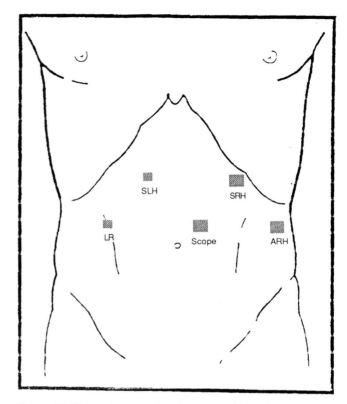

Figure 15.17 Port placement for a laparoscopic Heller–Toupet procedure. SLH and SRH mark the ports for the surgeon's left and right hands, respectively. Scope and ARH mark the ports for the assistant's left and right hands, respectively. LR marks the port for the liver retractor.

fibers down to the submucosa (Figure 15.19). When the proper plane is identified, the cardiomyotomy is extended cephalad approximately 6 cm until normal esophageal muscle is identified and caudad until the sling fibers of the cardia are divided (Figure 15.20). Intraoperative endoscopy may be performed to identify the GEJ and to ensure the myotomy is of sufficient length. This may be confirmed by adequate distention of the esophagus with insufflation. Since we began extending our myotomy 3 cm onto the stomach, we have had no concerns about insufficient length [64].

Once the cardiomyotomy is sufficient, a partial posterior fundoplication (Toupet) is performed (Figure 15.21). The posterior fundus is placed around the esophagus, and the top is fixated to the esophagus and diaphragm. The leading edge of the stomach is sutured to the edge of the myotomy and is separately secured to the right crus. The same is done with the anterior fundus on the left side. Alternatively, an anterior fundoplication (Dor) may be performed (Figure 15.22), and is recommended to buttress an intraoperative perforation if it occurs. With the bougie or the flexible endoscope in the esophagus, the fundus of the stomach is

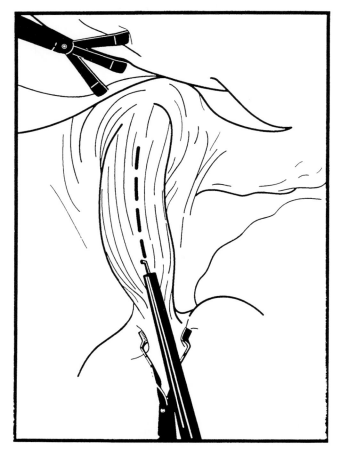

Figure 15.18 Planned myotomy site is marked along the anterior surface of the esophagus with electrocautery.

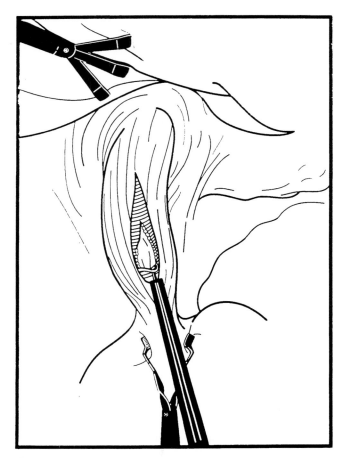

Figure 15.19 Longitudinal and circular muscle fibers are transected with a combination of electrocautery and blunt dissection.

positioned anterior to the myotomy. Sutures are placed to anchor the fundus to the right and left crura as well as to the transected edges of the esophageal muscle. When the wrap is completed, the liver retractor is removed, and the incisions are closed.

A nasogastric tube is not used postoperatively. The patient is allowed a liquid diet on the night of the operation and begins a graduated solid diet the next morning. Most patients may be discharged from the hospital within 2 days. All patients are strongly encouraged to have manometry and pH studies 6–8 weeks after surgery.

Postoperative evaluation of the esophagus is important because the most common cause for late failure is likely to be GERD. As discussed later in this section, it is often asymptomatic, so patients do not seek treatment. If pathologic reflux is present on the 24-h pH study, the patients should be treated with a proton pump inhibitor to help prevent peptic stricture formation at a later date.

Outcome

At the University of Washington, we converted from a thoracoscopic approach to a laparoscopic Heller myotomy in

1994. The impetus for this was the recognition that a limited gastric myotomy did not protect the patient from gastroesophageal reflux and that many patients required an extension of the myotomy for relief of their dysphagia. The laparoscopic approach still allowed for a long esophageal myotomy, but it could be extended onto the stomach (1.5–2.0 cm). Over the next 4 years, 52 patients were operated on using this approach, with the majority having excellent improvement in their dysphagia (>90%). Still there was the occasional patient who had inadequate relief or recurrence of dysphagia, some of whom improved with reoperation to extend the myotomy. Therefore, in 1998 we changed our approach, extending the myotomy 3 cm on the gastric side. We also began performing a Toupet fundoplication rather than a Dor, both because an anterior fundoplication was difficult to do with such a long myotomy and in the hope that a Toupet might provide better control of reflux. A comparison of the two approaches confirmed that an extended myotomy with Toupet (EM/Toupet) more effectively obliterated the LES than the shorter myotomy with Dor fundoplication (SM/Dor) as evidenced by the residual LES pressure (9.5 vs 15.8 mmHg). This translated into improved clinical

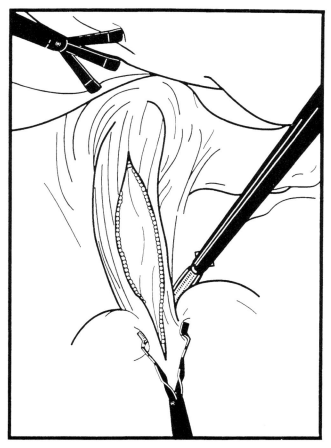

Figure 15.20 Completed myotomy extending onto the stomach.

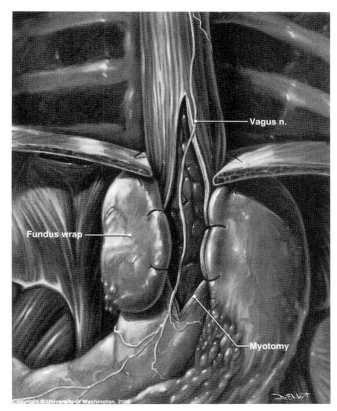

Figure 15.21 Posterior fundoplication (Toupet) is performed by suturing the fundus to the cut edges of the myotomy and securing the stomach to the diaphragm (reproduced courtesy of University of Washington, Seattle, WA, with permission.)

outcomes, in that dysphagia was both less frequent (once a month vs once a week on average) and less severe (3.2 vs 5.3 on a 10-point visual analog scale) in the EM/Toupet group; overall, 17% of patients in the SM/Dor group experienced recurrent dysphagia, compared with only 3% among the EM/Toupet patients. This improvement in the EM/Toupet approach was not at the expense of more reflux, in that the mean distal esophageal acid exposure was equivalent (EM/Toupet 6.0% vs SM/Dor 5.9%) [64]. Longer term follow-up of up to 8 years in 30 patients from the EM/Toupet group indicates the durability of this approach [71].

These results are similar to those reported by others. Relief from dysphagia is between 85% and 95% at 5 years, weight gain is common, and overall satisfaction with the operation is high [60, 72, 73]. Because the obstruction to flow is relieved, regurgitation is reduced. Relief from chest pain may occur in 60–75% of patients who had the symptom preoperatively.

Improved esophageal motility has been demonstrated after cardiomyotomy for achalasia [74, 75]. The return of peristalsis to some degree has been demonstrated in up to 63% of achalasia patients after surgery, although typically it never returns to normal [76]. This finding implies that LES contributes to the esophageal body dysfunction, but is not solely responsible for the disorganized peristalsis. Others argue that this finding does not represent an intrinsic change in the motility of the esophagus, but is an artifact of manometry and that an apparent improvement in peristalsis is only a function of the decreased caliber of the esophagus after surgery [11].

Complications

Complications of the procedure are uncommon. In our experience at the University of Washington, perforations occur in less than 5% of cases. Perforations are more common when patients are treated with one or more botulinum toxin injections. The overall complication rate is around 5%, and we have experienced no mortality.

Esophageal perforation is repaired intraoperatively using a laparoscopic intracorporeal suturing technique. The mucosa is closed primarily, then buttressed with the serosa of the stomach by performing an anterior partial fundoplication (Dor). Pneumothorax, bleeding, wound infection, and intra-abdominal abscess are other complications that have

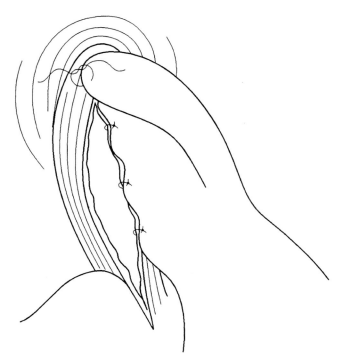

Figure 15.22 Anterior hemifundoplication (Dor) is performed by suturing the fundus to the cut edges of the myotomy site.

been reported in fewer than 3% of cases [77]. Most early complications can be avoided by careful dissection. However, previous operations or botulinum toxin injections distort the natural tissue planes and thus increase the likelihood of one of these complications.

Late complications of myotomy are related mostly to the recurrence of the initial symptoms, particularly dysphagia. Postoperative dysphagia may be caused by several discrete entities: incomplete myotomy, perihiatal scarring, progressive dysmotility of the esophagus, peptic stricture, and tumor. Some clinical clues may help distinguish among these, but physiologic and anatomic information must be obtained to confirm the diagnosis.

In 129 patients followed up for an average of 12 years, 40 were identified as having postoperative dysphagia [78]. Symptoms of incomplete myotomy occurred early and rarely caused dysphagia after 3 years. Postoperative scarring caused dysphagia 1–2 years after surgery. Gastroesophageal reflux caused dysphagia after 6 years. The authors were 100% accurate in diagnosing the cause of dysphagia using esophagogram, endoscopy, and manometry in the 12 patients whose diagnosis was confirmed by reoperation.

Incomplete myotomy may be prevented by extending the incision onto the stomach to ensure transection of the sling fibers. The cut edges of the myotomy must be separated by at least 30% of the esophageal circumference. Perihiatal scarring may be prevented by minimizing the amount of electrocautery injury to the crura.

Pathologic gastroesophageal reflux may be detected in almost 50% of patients if 24-h pH studies are performed [79]. Most authors believe that the incidence of abnormal gastroesophageal reflux in a patient undergoing a myotomy and an antireflux procedure to be about 10% [72, 79]. The trade-off between relieving dysphagia and limiting reflux is clear—the greater the improvement of dysphagia, the higher is the incidence of reflux. This is clearly shown in a study by Pandolfo *et al.* [73]. In 11 patients, the authors used intraoperative manometry to assess the extent of LES relaxation during an open cardiomyotomy and anterior hemifundoplication via an abdominal approach. Manometric readings of the LES pressure were performed before the myotomy and again after the myotomy was completed. The myotomy was not considered complete until the LES pressure was less than 5 mmHg. The results were compared with 16 patients who underwent the same procedure without the intraoperative study. Patients with intraoperative manometry had a 0% dysphagia rate but an 18.2% reflux rate. This compared with a 21.5% dysphagia rate and a 7.3% reflux rate in those who did not have intraoperative manometry. A more thorough myotomy leads to less dysphagia but more reflux.

Besides peptic stricture, postoperative reflux may lead to other complications including esophagitis and Barrett's esophagus. Although some patients have pathologic reflux, many do not have symptoms. Jaakkola *et al.* found that Barrett's esophagus developed in four of 46 patients after cardiomyotomy after an average follow-up of 13 years [80]. Others found dysplasia and intramucosal adenocarcinoma in patients with reflux after myotomy [78]. In a series of 100 patients undergoing myotomy, cancer developed in three [74]. This stresses two points: the need to know which patients have reflux after the operation and the importance of following these patients with endoscopy.

The management of patients with postoperative dysphagia is not well defined. An attempt at conservative treatment using dilation is appropriate as long as no evidence of tumor is present. Parkman *et al.* successfully managed six patients with peptic stricture using multiple dilations (average 3.6 per patient) and acid suppression [81]. Conservative management is a reasonable strategy in that reoperation for dysphagia has a lower success rate than the initial operation [82].

Recurrent achalasia

Recurrence after operative treatment is reported to range from 8% to 13% [83, 84]. Late recurrence must be assessed carefully, because dysphagia may develop from other causes mentioned earlier. The diagnosis of recurrence must be confirmed by manometry, which should show a normal or elevated LES pressure and incomplete relaxation. Manometry may also reveal another motor disorder, which may explain the symptoms and affect the treatment. Endoscopy and a contrast esophagogram should also be obtained to exclude other diseases such as a tumor or paraesophageal hernia. If recurrence is confirmed, there are several options available depending on the findings, overall health of the patient, and available expertise. Some patients may be treated with dilation. The endoscopist must be skilled in the use of pneumatic dilation because only the mucosa stands between the balloon and the mediastinum or the peritoneal cavity. If dilation is not available or if it fails to resolve the symptoms, a repeat myotomy may be considered. Between 70% and 80% of patients respond to a repeat operation for recurrent or persistent achalasia [85, 86] and most of these patients can be approached laparoscopically [87]. If the preoperative manometry reveals a diffuse esophageal abnormality, then a thoracic approach may be beneficial, especially if the first approach was by way of the abdomen. Otherwise, there is little evidence to support one approach over the other. If repeat myotomy is not helpful, then esophageal resection may be the only surgical alternative. The patient must be informed that this is a more extensive procedure and has a mortality rate between 2% and 8% [84, 88]. If esophageal resection is performed, the results can be expected to be good to excellent in 78–90% of patients [53, 84]. The choice of conduit for the operation is discussed later.

Emergent operation after perforation

Esophageal perforation occurs approximately 3% of the time after pneumatic dilation in the treatment of achalasia. The management of the perforation depends on clinical assessment and the interpretation of the esophagogram. In a stable patient, a small contained perforation that does not communicate with other mediastinal structures or the pleural space may be treated with antibiotics and cessation of oral intake. If the patient has clinical manifestations or if radiographic studies show free communication with either the pleural cavity or the mediastinum (Figure 15.23), then

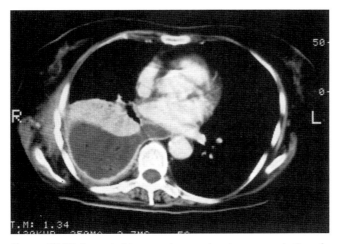

Figure 15.23 Computed tomography scan showing communication of esophageal perforation with right pleural space.

urgent operative intervention is indicated. Regardless of the initial management plan, a surgical evaluation should be obtained as soon as a perforation is expected.

The principles of operative intervention include debridement and irrigation to remove injured and necrotic tissue, closure of the perforation site, and myotomy. A posterolateral thoracic approach through the seventh intercostal space is used. The mediastinum is exposed and cleansed of all esophageal contamination. After the perforation is debrided, a two-layered closure is used. The mucosa is sutured with an absorbable polyglyconate-based 3-0 suture, and the muscularis is closed with a permanent suture. A myotomy should be performed on the opposite side of the perforation. Occasionally, the diaphragm may be enlarged and the cardia of the stomach used to place a serosal patch over the repair. In general, this is not feasible or advisable, because it creates a hiatal hernia. Two chest tubes are placed for drainage, and the incision is closed.

If the degree of soiling is extensive or if delay to operative intervention is prolonged, Schwartz *et al.* recommend diversion [89]. This would consist of esophagostomy, gastrostomy, and interruption of the gastroesophageal continuity. Rarely is it necessary to divert a patient, because esophageal resection or wide drainage of the perforated area can be safely performed in such situations [90]. Although a myotomy is usually performed during the emergent operation, one group has reported six patients in whom they simply repaired the perforation without performing a myotomy [91]. They found that none of their patients had recurrent symptoms of dysphagia after an average follow-up of 5 years. Others have approached perforation after dilation using minimally invasive surgery. These authors performed a primary repair using videoendoscopy and then drained the thorax with chest tubes [92].

The outcome of emergent surgery for perforation is often said to be the same as with elective surgery. Ferguson *et al.* reported six patients treated emergently for perforation and compared them with 54 patients undergoing elective treatment for achalasia [93]. They found all six patients had good or excellent results based on symptom scoring, whereas 88% of the elective cases had the same score. Postoperative endoscopy, pH studies, and manometry were not reported for either group.

Controversies in treatment

The approach to surgical management of achalasia may appear to be straightforward, but many issues in the management of this disease process remain topics of some debate.

Medical versus surgical treatment

Medical therapy with calcium-channel blockers or nitrates is clinically ineffective and has been relegated to a role as a temporizing measure before or a supplemental treatment after definitive therapy [94–97]. Another therapeutic modality involves injecting botulinum toxin into the LES. The effect of this treatment is also temporary, with only 66% of patients experiencing symptomatic relief at 6 months [96]. Although this may be appropriate therapy for patients who are at risk for operative intervention because of age or comorbid conditions, its long-term efficacy is unproven.

The two types of definitive therapy include pneumatic dilation and surgical myotomy, as described in detail above. Each approach has advantages and disadvantages. When the two are compared, the following issues arise: symptom resolution, immediate morbidity, degree of reflux as a result of therapy, and cost. Although many studies over the last two decades have been performed in an attempt to resolve the quandary, a consensus has not been reached, and ultimately the decision as to which treatment to pursue is commonly based on a combination of patient-specific factors and practice preferences. Many retrospective studies comparing the results of surgery and forceful dilation are inconclusive because of selection bias, use of historical controls, and small sample size [98–100]. A 1989 trial prospectively randomized patients to either pneumatic dilation or open surgical myotomy [85, 101]. In this study, 39 patients were treated by dilation and 42 by surgery. After 5 years of follow-up, excellent or good results were present in 65% of patients undergoing dilation and 95% of patients treated surgically. Interestingly, the authors performed both surgery and dilation on their study patients. The specific surgical procedures performed were an open abdominal cardiomyotomy extending onto the stomach for 5–10 mm and an anterior (Dor) fundoplication. Pneumatic dilation was accomplished using a Mosher bag inflated to 12– 15 psi for 10–20 s. Two patients underwent emergency surgery for perforation of the esophagus after dilation. Post-procedure "acid reflux tests" were performed in both groups, and reflux was documented in 8% of the dilation patients and 28% of the surgery patients. The authors concluded that surgery offered better clinical results than did dilation. A more recent randomized trial comparing pneumatic dilation in 25 achalasia patients to laparoscopic Heller myotomy with Toupet fundoplication in 26 patients found that treatment failures over 12 months were significantly more common after pneumatic dilation [102]. In a cohort analysis with 6-year follow-up, Vela *et al.*, reporting on 106 patients treated by pneumatic dilation and 73 treated by surgical myotomy, observed that the long-term outcomes of each treatment were statistically similar [103]. Though each treatment was associated with an approximately 90% success rate at 6 months, at 6 years only 44% of patients who underwent dilation and 57% of those after myotomy were either relatively symptom free or had not required any additional treatment. Interestingly, the causes for symptom recurrence were due to incompletely treated achalasia in 96% of the patients in the pneumatic dilation group, while in the myotomy group symptoms were more associated with the occurrence of postoperative gastro-

esophageal acid reflux in 36%; only 4% of the dilation group had recurrence secondary to reflux.

The question of the optimal initial treatment for achalasia remains unanswered. Aggressive pneumatic dilation may be able to attain similar results as operative therapy. However, because it is an uncontrolled disruption of the LES, the number of perforations is proportional to the aggressiveness of the dilation technique. Currently, both options are quite acceptable, and in many cases a combined approach, using one after failure of the other, is advisable. Given the refinements in and recent favorable long-term results of minimally invasive surgical myotomy, surgery can be recommended to most individuals who are fit for an operation as the first approach.

Operative approach

The first operative treatment of achalasia was described in 1913 by the procedure's namesake, Ernest Heller. His approach was via a laparotomy and consisted of a double myotomy. The open thoracic approach was championed in the United States by E. Henry Ellis in the 1950s. These two approaches were the only methods available to the surgeon until 1991, when Cuschieri *et al.* first described a successful laparoscopic myotomy [68]. Shortly after that, Pellegrini *et al.* described a thoracoscopic approach for achalasia and reported their experience with 17 patients [66]. Since then, many authors have addressed the issues of open and videoendoscopic surgery.

The outcomes with the open and videoendoscopic abdominal approach appear to be similar [104–107]. The benefits of minimally invasive surgery for the patient are to be found in the decreased hospital stay and recuperation.

Cuschieri *et al.* were the first to point out the potential advantages of reduced trauma and quicker recovery using a videoendoscopic technique [68]. Others supported their observation by demonstrating decreased recovery time, less pain, and improved aesthetic appearance of the incisions with laparoscopic myotomy [108]. In one study, the authors compared a matched group of laparotomy and laparoscopy Heller–Dor procedures [109]. Seventeen patients in each group were analyzed retrospectively for operative time, hospital stay, and return to normal activity. Although the operative time was greater for the minimally invasive group (178 vs 125 min), the patients were discharged from the hospital earlier (4 vs 10 days) and returned to normal activity earlier (14 vs 30 days). Based on charges at the authors' institution, the cost of a laparoscopic myotomy compared with that of an open myotomy was about US$400 lower. The largest component of cost in the laparoscopic procedure was the surgical supplies, and the largest component of cost in the open procedure was the length of stay. As experience has evolved, it has become clear that the use of an imaging system that allows for substantial magnification of the images and the excellent view of the field inherent in a videoendoscopic approach probably enhances the ability of surgeons to perform the operations with greater accuracy.

Chest versus abdomen

As videoendoscopic procedures replaced the open techniques, the issue of whether the myotomy should be performed through the chest or the abdomen was raised. The same question existed during the era of open surgery, wherein the discussion focused on outcome/response to treatment, postoperative gastroesophageal reflux, and recurrence. Those who employ the thoracic approach point out that the esophagus and the GEJ are more accessible from the chest. They also note that less mobilization of the structures that support the competency of the cardia is necessary, and, therefore, an antireflux procedure is not needed [110, 111]. The laparoscopic approach, although requiring a larger mobilization of the cardioesophageal junction, allows instruments to be parallel to the axis of the esophagus, as opposed to being perpendicular during thoracoscopy. Also, the majority of the LES is intra-abdominal and thus easier to approach laparoscopically, particularly with respect to the need to extend the myotomy 3 cm distally onto the gastric cardia [112]. The anesthetic management is simplified because there is no need to use single-lung ventilation and a chest tube postoperatively. Finally, another advantage of the abdominal approach is the ease of adding an antireflux procedure. Thus, most surgeons who treat achalasia using minimally invasive techniques use this approach [112, 113–116].

Adding an antireflux procedure

The issue of adding an antireflux procedure to a cardiomyotomy was previously controversial. It was reasoned in the past that if the cardiomyotomy extends too far onto the stomach, it may disrupt all the physiologic and anatomic contributions to the lower esophageal sphincter, thereby allowing gastroesophageal reflux to occur. If the cardiomyotomy does not extend too far onto the stomach, then no reflux occurs; however, the results of the operation may be inferior in terms of relieving dysphagia. In an attempt to solve both problems, the cardiomyotomy may be extended onto the stomach for a distance and then the LES mechanism may be reconstructed with an antireflux procedure. As previously noted, clinical assessment of reflux status underestimates the amount of reflux when compared with 24-h pH studies in patients treated for achalasia. This holds true for patients treated operatively or by pneumatic dilation [117]. Therefore, all patients who undergo a myotomy should be evaluated postoperatively by 24-h pH monitoring to determine objectively whether pathologic reflex is occurring. Whether subclinical reflux causes late failure in the treatment of achalasia is not known. Notably, because gastroesophageal reflux was identified so frequently after thoracic myotomy, many surgeons moved to an abdominal approach where it is easier (and necessary) to perform some type of antireflux procedure.

Two types of fundal wraps are available to the surgeon using an abdominal approach to the esophagus: a complete wrap (Nissen) or some variation of a partial wrap (Dor or Toupet). Most surgeons perform a partial fundoplication because a total fundoplication causes too much resistance and more commonly results in dysphagia. There is controversy, however, regarding which type of fundoplication should be used. An anterior fundoplication (Dor) eliminates the need to perform a posterior esophageal dissection, preserving some attachment of the esophagus to the hiatus, and helps to maintain an intra-abdominal segment of distal esophagus. The second advantage of the Dor is that it allows the wall of the stomach to buttress the myotomy site. The cardia helps seal any injury to the esophageal mucosa, prevents adhesion of the esophagus to the left lobe of the liver, and allows the myotomy edges to be sutured in an open position. A posterior fundoplication (Toupet), on the other hand, may provide better control of reflux. In addition, it naturally separates the edges of the myotomy, theoretically keeping it from joining and causing recurrent dysphagia. Rosetti *et al.* have reported success in using total fundoplication in conjunction with Heller myotomy, with resolution of dysphagia in 167 of 182 (92%) patients and no abnormal acid exposure in any of them postoperatively [118]. However, many surgeons are reluctant to adopt this approach because of the typical absence of peristaltic activity seen in patients with achalasia.

The amount of gastroesophageal reflux is less with the addition of an antireflux procedure. Peracchia *et al.* reported only an 8% pathologic gastroesophageal reflux rate based on pH studies after laparoscopic Heller–Dor procedures [67]. Similarly, Parrilla *et al.* reported a 12% reflux rate after open Heller–Toupet procedures using 24-h pH studies [59]. Another study reported no gastroesophageal reflux by pH studies in patients undergoing laparoscopic myotomies with partial fundoplications [113]. Most significantly, in 2004, Richards *et al.* published the results of a randomized controlled trial comparing 21 patients with Heller myotomy alone to 22 patients undergoing Heller myotomy with Dor anterior fundoplasty. The incidence of abnormal gastroesophageal reflux, defined as a pH of less than 4.0 for more than 4.2% of the 24-h pH study, was 48% in patients after Heller myotomy alone versus 9% in those who also had the antireflux procedure. They concluded that the addition of an antireflux procedure, in this case Dor anterior fundoplasty, provided superior control of post-myotomy acid reflux [79]. Which type of fundoplication is the most efficacious while resulting in the least postoperative dysphagia, however, warrants further comparative investigation.

Conclusions

The symptoms of achalasia may be effectively treated by operative therapy. The principles of the operation include sufficient length of the myotomy, adequate separation of the transected muscle, and a plan to prevent postoperative gastroesophageal reflux. The operation may be performed using minimally invasive techniques. Postoperative assessment of gastroesophageal reflux should be performed in all patients to prevent late failure resulting from peptic stricture.

Hypercontractile and spastic disorders

The use of stationary and ambulatory esophageal manometry in the evaluation of patients with non-cardiac chest pain has led to the identification of several uncommon esophageal dysmotility syndromes. Although criteria have been developed to aid in the diagnosis of these syndromes, the relative paucity of cases has hindered the development of standard treatment. All are considered together in this section because the experience with each is limited and the surgical treatments are similar.

Diffuse esophageal spasm (DES) is characterized by simultaneous contractions and intermittent normal peristalsis on manometry. Repetitive contractions, prolonged wave duration, high-amplitude contractions, spontaneous contractions, and an elevated LES pressure may also be observed (Figure 15.24). Nutcracker esophagus is diagnosed in patients who have a distal esophageal contraction amplitude greater than 180 mmHg. An elevated LES pressure and prolonged wave duration (longer than 6 s) may also be encountered, but are not necessary for the diagnosis. In essence, this condition appears to be an "exaggeration" in the amplitude and duration of otherwise normal peristaltic waves. Hypertensive lower esophageal sphincter (HLES) is a condition diagnosed when the LES pressure is greater than 45 mmHg on solid-state manometry together with normal LES relaxation, and there is an absence of any other disorders of the esophageal body, which may account for the elevated sphincter pressure. More than 50% of patients with elevated LES pressures have other disorders of peristalsis [119]. When more than 20% of swallow sequences result in hypotensive or dropped peristaltic contractions, the pattern is referred to as ineffective esophageal motility (IEM); previously, this fell under the general term, non-specific esophageal dysmotility, which was essentially a catchall category for patients with abnormal manometric findings that do not conform to the criteria of the other dysmotility syndromes. By itself, IEM is not amenable to surgical therapy and will not be discussed further here (see Chapter 14).

Epiphrenic diverticula are considered in this section because they are associated with some type of esophageal dysmotility in about 60% of patients, most commonly with hypertensive disorders of the LES [120]. When an operation is indicated, treatment of the disease is similar to the treatment of other motility disorders.

Clinical evaluation

Most patients present with the complaint of dysphagia and chest pain. Some may also complain of heartburn and regur-

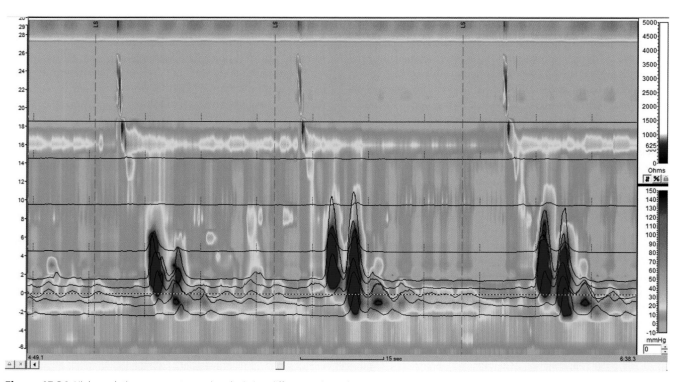

Figure 15.24 High-resolution manometry tracing depicting diffuse esophageal spasm.

gitation, especially if a diverticulum is present. Most often, patients have undergone some form of cardiac evaluation for their chest pain. If this is not the case, the patient should be evaluated by the appropriate clinician to ensure this more common, life-threatening etiology is not the cause of the chest pain.

The clinical evaluation of a patient with non-cardiac chest pain is similar to that of achalasia (see above). It should include manometry, a contrast study of the esophagus, and upper endoscopy. Manometry is necessary to define the type of motility disorder. The esophagogram and endoscopy are necessary to exclude other etiologies of abnormal motility such as benign and malignant neoplasms.

Gastroesophageal reflux should always be considered when evaluating patients with spastic dysmotility, because it has been hypothesized to be a contributing factor to different esophageal disorders, such as HLES and high-amplitude peristaltic contractile disorders such as nutcracker esophagus [119]. Therefore, 24-h pH monitoring is an essential test for anyone with such a disorder. Traditional surgical management for spastic dysmotility included an esophageal myotomy, but for some patients gastroesophageal reflux may be the primary disorder and the spastic dysmotility secondary. In such cases, therapy directed toward reflux may be more appropriate, including possibly a Nissen fundoplication [121]. Thus, GERD should be investigated in all patients with dysphagia or chest pain. A hypercontractile esophagus in patients with GERD should not be considered a contraindication to antireflux therapy; instead it may be the treatment of choice rather than esophageal myotomy in such situations.

Another consideration in the preoperative evaluation of patients with spastic dysmotility is the indication for 24-h manometry. Although experience with this technique is limited to a few centers, the information gained may be helpful in guiding therapy and predicting prognosis [122]. Ambulatory manometry is particularly useful in patients with daily symptoms who have been diagnosed with nutcracker esophagus and IEM on stationary manometry, because it may change the diagnosis in up to 30% of cases [123]. Ambulatory manometry allows the physician to correlate symptoms as reported by the patient in an event diary with the manometric measurements. Although the diagnosis may change with nutcracker esophagus and IEM, ambulatory manometry disagrees less often with stationary manometry when the diagnosis is DES. In this case, 24-h manometry need not be performed. In difficult situations, endoscopic ultrasonography may define the area of the esophagus that is most affected, because the thickness of the muscularis can be accurately estimated by this study. Hypertrophy of the LES and the muscularis of the distal esophagus has been reported in patients with nutcracker esophagus and DES using high-frequency intraluminal ultrasound (HFIUS) imaging [124]. It has also been reported

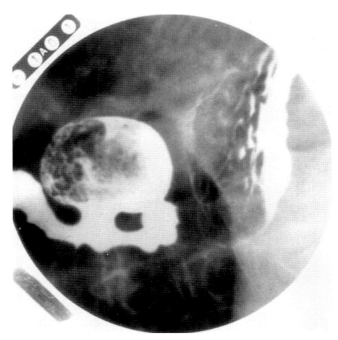

Figure 15.25 Lateral view of an esophagogram revealing an anterior esophageal diverticulum.

that HFIUS combined with esophageal manometry demonstrates an asynchrony between longitudinal and circular muscle contraction during peristalsis in patients with nutcracker esophagus [125]. The implications of this latter finding on a potential surgical target for this disorder are unclear, however.

Occasionally, an epiphrenic diverticulum is found in a patient who has an upper gastrointestinal contrast study for an unrelated problem (Figure 15.25). If the patient is clearly asymptomatic, then they may not need an operation. A follow-up esophagogram in 1–2 years helps gauge the progression of the diverticulum and reveals associated disease. Most asymptomatic diverticula do not progress into clinical problems [120]. If, however, the patient has symptoms referable to the diverticulum, operative treatment is recommended. In this case, it is imperative to have a reliable manometric evaluation before operation because it affects the surgical approach and the procedure.

Treatment

Spastic dysmotility disorders of the esophagus have been infrequently treated by surgical therapy. The reason for this is based partly on the fact that some reports have shown an 80% response to medical therapy [119] and partly on the reluctance of physicians to eliminate all peristaltic activity in the body of the esophagus with an operation. As with achalasia, spastic disorders are well suited to a minimally invasive operative approach. The procedure performed in most cases consists of a myotomy with or without an antireflux procedure. If a diverticulum is present, a diverticulectomy is also performed.

It is important to point out that even if the LES pressure is normal, it should be transected. After an extensive myotomy of the esophageal body, the ability to transmit a bolus of food normally is lost. Even a normal LES pressure presents a challenge to a myotomized esophagus. Therefore, a laparoscopic myotomy, as described in the previous section, is our preferred initial approach. In these cases, the myotomy may be extended higher on the esophagus than in patients with achalasia. In the relatively infrequent situation where the patient has persistent or recurrent symptoms, then a thoracoscopic revision, typically through the right chest, may be performed, with extension further proximally on the esophagus.

A description of the thoracoscopic approach to long esophageal myotomy is described here. The patient should be placed on a liquid diet for 2 days before the operation if esophageal emptying is inhibited. This decreases the amount of solid debris in the lumen of the esophagus. A bougie, preferably lighted, is needed for the operation. The bougie should be placed under direct vision during the operation, especially if a diverticulum is present. This prevents injury to the esophagus. A double-lumen endotracheal tube is necessary to allow single-lung ventilation.

A lateral decubitus position is used. Access to the lower esophagus, cardioesophageal junction, and upper stomach can only be achieved through a left-sided approach. Because most pathologic processes described earlier require ablation of the LES, the majority of myotomies are performed from the left. The right-sided approach is best if the patient needs a myotomy of the entire esophagus, except its most inferior aspect. This approach is also useful for a mid-esophageal diverticulum located on the right side. An antireflux procedure cannot be performed easily from this approach. The working ports are placed to allow maximum vision of the inferior thoracic esophagus and the superior esophagus if needed. The ports are placed in an equilateral triangle, notably much closer than what is normally done in the abdomen, with the videoendoscope located in the fifth intercostal space, just inferior to the scapular tip. The working ports should be located in the posterior axillary line. A fourth port in the anterior axillary line is used by the assistant to retract the lung (Figure 15.26). Both the surgeon and the assistant stand on the same side of the operating table, which is the ipsilateral side of the chosen approach. Thus, both are standing at the patient's back, while the video cart monitor is in front of the patient. Carbon dioxide insufflation is not necessary for the procedure, because single-lung ventilation usually suffices.

The lung is retracted anteriorly after it is deflated (Figure 15.27). The inferior pulmonary ligament is divided with cautery and blunt dissection, avoiding the inferior pulmo-

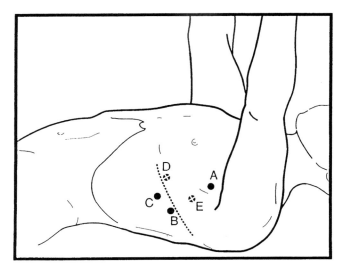

Figure 15.26 Port placement for a thoracoscopic myotomy. (A) Optional lung retraction port. (B) Scope port. (C) Surgeon's left hand. (D) Lung retractor. (E) Surgeon's right hand.

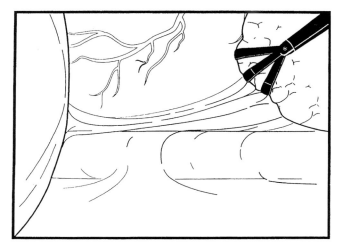

Figure 15.27 Lung is retracted anteriorly, exposing the pleural reflection over the esophagus.

nary vein. Once this is accomplished, the pleural reflection over the esophagus is taken down with cautery dissection so that the longitudinal muscle fibers of the esophagus may be identified (Figure 15.28). At this point, the lighted bougie is passed into the esophagus by the anesthesiologist. By splaying the muscle fibers of the esophagus over the bougie with one instrument, cautery dissection down to the submucosa is performed. A combination of blunt dissection, spreading, and cauterization is used to divide the muscular layers of the esophagus for the length of the myotomy (Figures 15.29 and 15.30). Flexible endoscopy should be used to verify the adequacy of the myotomy (Figure 15.31).

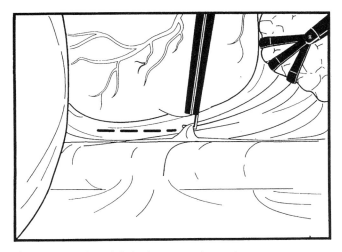

Figure 15.28 Pleura is incised to expose the esophagus.

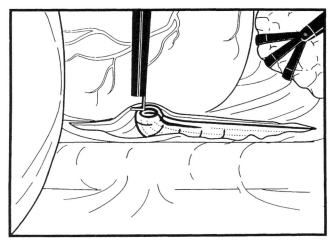

Figure 15.31 Flexible endoscopy is performed to inspect the myotomy.

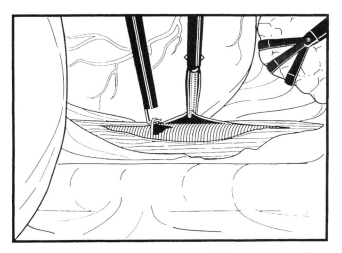

Figure 15.29 Longitudinal and circular muscle fibers are transected.

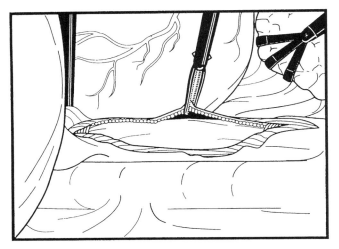

Figure 15.30 Completed myotomy.

The vagus nerves should be avoided during this dissection. If a left-sided approach is used, a partial wrap (Dor or Belsey) may be added. If the right-sided approach is used, then the antireflux procedure is not possible. If a diverticulum is present, it may be dissected to its neck and transected by an automatic stapling and cutting device.

One chest tube is placed through trocar sites, and the remaining sites are closed. The patient is allowed to consume a liquid diet on the day of the operation, unless a diverticulum has been resected, in which case the diet is started on the third postoperative day. Hospital stay varies, but patients are usually discharged within 2 days of starting a diet.

The length of the myotomy varies with each of the disease processes and with the findings of the preoperative evaluation. If HLES without concomitant esophageal body dysmotility is being treated, the myotomy is confined to the distal esophagus, LES, and cardia. If NE is being treated and preoperative manometry revealed high-amplitude contractions in the proximal esophagus, an extended myotomy should be performed, perhaps through a right thoracoscopic approach.

Outcome

The surgical approach to patients with spastic motility disorders is based mostly on transferred principles from achalasia. Because the number of patients with these disorders is so small, and even fewer of them come to surgical therapy, only limited experience is available. Most information comes from case reports and technique articles [126–129], and the outcomes among these are quite variable [130]. Although no prospective, randomized studies are available comparing medical with surgical therapy, one study prospectively compared the outcome of the two treatments in patients with esophageal motility disorders [131]. In this study, patients with achalasia, DES, and nutcracker esophagus were treated by medical therapy, including dilation, or operative therapy based on the request of the referring physician. The operation was performed via left thoracoscopy. Eight of 10 patients with DES or nutcracker esophagus had good or excellent relief with surgical treatment. Only eight of 30 patients had the same level of relief with medical therapy. Although this study was not randomized, it did show the benefits of operative therapy over medical therapy. No long-term studies are available to assess the outcome of surgically treated patients.

A report by Patti *et al.* describes the outcomes of surgical myotomy for DES and nutcracker esophagus and compares the laparoscopic to the thoracoscopic approach [129]. In patients with DES, dysphagia was relieved in 86% of patients undergoing the laparoscopic myotomy, and in 80% of those with the thoracoscopic approach; chest pain improved in 80% and 75%, respectively. On the basis of these data, the authors recommend laparoscopic myotomy as the preferred approach. The results for patients with nutcracker esophagus were less encouraging, with 80% relief of dysphagia overall but with 50% of patients continuing to experience chest pain postoperatively. This prompted the authors to suggest that laparoscopic myotomy be only performed in those nutcracker esophagus patients for whom dysphagia is the dominant symptom and who also have a manometrically hypertensive LES.

Complications

The operative complications are similar to those of myotomy performed for achalasia, except if a diverticulectomy is added. In this case, additional morbidity may be expected from opening the esophageal mucosa. Esophageal leak rates have been reported to be as high as 18% using an open technique [120], and range from 8% to 23% in series of patients undergoing a laparoscopic approach [132–134].

Conclusions

Operative intervention for spastic motility is not common. The myotomy should include division of the muscular fibers of the LES. The laparoscopic approach is preferred as this facilitates complete myotomy of the LES; if necessary for persistent or recurrent symptoms, a thoracoscopic myotomy may be performed to extend the myotomy further proximally along the esophagus. After surgical intervention, dysphagia improves more often than chest pain.

Esophageal resection

Resection of the esophagus is usually performed for malignant disease; however, this procedure is contemplated in esophageal motility disorders when certain conditions exist.

If the esophagus is severely dilated and elongated after years of untreated disease, some authors have recommended resection as an initial therapy. Over the years, however, there

has been a tendency in the surgical community to use total esophagectomy less and less. There is no question that whenever the problem can be corrected, even if the correction is not perfect, while preserving the natural conduit, this is better. Our philosophy has been to reoperate as needed, to use dilation and other means, and to prevent, whenever possible, a total esopahagectomy for patients with achalasia. On the other hand, patients with benign stricture, occurring as a result of previous intervention or as a natural sequelae of untreated disease, which cannot be treated by dilation is another indication for esophageal resection. Failure of previous operative therapy to relieve symptoms associated with motility disorders is another. Indeed after two or three operations on the esophagus to treat a stricture, esophagectomy is the best alternative. Some have used esophageal resection as treatment for a perforation occurring after dilation, particularly when the esophagus has other underlying pathology.

Patients must be aware of the technical challenge the operation poses. They should be aware of the significant morbidity (20–30%) and mortality (1–8%) accompanying the operation. Given the information, they may decide their symptoms are more acceptable than the risk of the procedure.

The principles of esophageal resection center on safe, effective removal of the esophagus and replacement using a conduit that allows for adequate nutritional intake. The most common approach to this procedure for benign disease is a transhiatal approach from the abdomen, using the stomach as the conduit to anastomose to the cervical esophagus.

Operative approach

Patients requiring esophagectomy for esophageal motor disorders are often nutritionally depleted. If preoperative nutritional supplementation is possible with high-calorie, high-protein liquids, some advantage in postoperative healing may be gained. The patient should be on a liquid diet 2 days before the operation to minimize the amount of solid debris present in the esophagus.

The patient is placed in the supine position on the operating table with the head turned to the right. A roll is usually placed across the lumbar area elevating the costal margin. This position facilitates exposure to the cervical esophagus, abdomen, and distal thoracic esophagus. The abdominal portion of the operation is performed first.

Generous mobilization of the duodenum is performed, elevating the second and third portions to the patient's left. The stomach is then mobilized along the greater curvature taking care to preserve the gastroepiploic artery. All short gastric vessels are ligated and transected to free the cardia. Division of the lesser omentum and the left gastric artery is performed next. The right gastric artery is carefully preserved. This frees the lesser curvature down to the previously mobilized duodenum. Any posterior attachments of the stomach are freed at this time.

Dissection of the lower esophagus requires a 2–3-cm opening of the hiatus. This is performed anteriorly after incising the phrenoesophageal ligament. After the anterior and lateral hiatal attachments are freed, circumferential dissection of the esophagus is completed. The GEJ and the distal 5 cm of the esophagus can be dissected sharply from the abdomen.

Posterior mediastinal dissection of the esophagus is performed bluntly. The plane of dissection is along the longitudinal muscle fibers of the esophagus. The pleura should not be violated. Blunt dissection can be performed to the thoracic outlet. During the blunt dissection of the esophagus, a second team (if available) may perform the neck dissection. Otherwise, the transhiatal dissection should proceed as far as possible before starting the neck dissection. Dissection of the esophagus is greatly facilitated if a bougie (38–48F) is placed and left in the lumen.

The approach to the cervical esophagus is similar to that of a pharyngoesophageal diverticulum. The longitudinal incision along the sternocleidomastoid muscle is extended to the suprasternal notch. The incision is developed through the avascular plane anterior to the sternocleidomastoid muscle. The carotid sheath is retracted laterally, the thyroid medially. Often, the middle thyroid vein is ligated and transected, as is the omohyoid muscle, to improve exposure. As the tracheoesophageal groove is approached, care must be taken to avoid injuring the recurrent laryngeal nerve. A bougie may be used to identify the extent of the esophageal diameter. Circumferential dissection of the esophagus is completed and a small Penrose drain is passed around the esophagus. The esophagus is then mobilized by a combination of blunt and sharp dissection toward the thoracic outlet. A sponge stick may be used to mobilize the inferior cervical esophagus. Simultaneous transhiatal and cervical dissection is done to facilitate esophageal mobilization. When the esophagus has been completely mobilized, a pyloroplasty is performed.

The stomach is then transected with an automatic stapling and cutting device so that a tube of stomach is created along the greater curvature. The stapler is placed at a point on the greater curvature 5 cm to the left of the GEJ and angled toward the incisura on the lesser curvature. Two loads of the automatic stapling and cutting device may be necessary. The portion of stomach attached to the esophagus is then sutured to a short segment of surgical tubing. The tubing is sutured to the tubular stomach. The esophagus is then delivered from the cervical incision, carrying the replacement conduit behind. The stomach should be guided into the chest to prevent torsion and undue pressure on the sutures.

Once the stomach is in the neck, the surgical tubing is removed. The stomach should reach the planned site of the anastomosis easily. Any tension increases the likelihood of an anastomotic leak postoperatively. If too much tension is present, the stomach must either be mobilized more, or an alternative conduit should be considered. A point on the cervical esophagus is chosen for the anastomosis. A double-layered hand-sewn or stapled anastomosis is performed. When the anastomosis is completed, the incisions are closed. The neck incision is drained with closed suction to allow egress of luminal contents in case a leak occurs. Patients are admitted to the intensive care unit for cardiopulmonary support and monitoring for postoperative bleeding. If the patient progresses well after the first day, they may be transferred out of the intensive care unit. A liquid diet is started on the third postoperative day. If an anastomotic leak is suspected, a barium contrast study is performed before the initiation of a diet. Patients are instructed to eat small meals in an upright position to limit gastric distention in the chest and facilitate transit to the abdominal portion of the stomach.

Outcome

Using the stomach as conduit, 78% of patients are able to swallow well and require no further intervention [135]. Although they will not have normal transit, they are able to maintain their weight and nutritional status. Fewer than 5% of patients have regurgitation that requires lifestyle modification consisting mostly of head elevation while supine. Overall, long-term follow-up 5 years after operative therapy shows good-to-excellent results in 68% of patients when all aspects of quality of life are considered [135]. Others have reported good results in 90% of patients undergoing esophageal resection for recurrent achalasia [84].

Complications

Perioperative mortality ranges from 1% to 8% [135–138]. Intraoperative death usually occurs from bleeding, which occurs during the blunt dissection in the mediastinum. Postoperative deaths occur as a result of nosocomial infections or an exacerbation of pre-existing conditions [137].

In a review of 23 papers reporting transhiatal esophagectomy in 1353 patients, the most common technical complications after surgery were found to be anastomotic leak (15%) and anastomotic stricture (14%) [139]. Most leaks may be treated without further operative intervention. Maintaining nutritional support and drainage of the wound via the closed suction catheter are all that is required. Anastomotic stricture is thought to occur as a result of a narrow anastomosis and the occurrence of a postoperative leak [140]. This is commonly and often successfully treated by serial dilations. Pulmonary complications are also quite common. Other complications include hoarseness resulting from recurrent laryngeal nerve injury, symptomatic gastroesophageal reflux, chylothorax, and infection. Perioperative cardiac dysrhythmia has been reported in nearly 50% of patients but can be controlled medically [141].

Controversies in treatment

The conduit used for esophageal replacement and the surgical approach to replacement are the main controversies in esophageal replacement. Of the conduits available, the stomach and the colon are the most common. The advantages of using the stomach are that only one anastomosis is performed as opposed to three, the blood supply to the stomach is better than that of the colon, and the plasticity of the stomach allows for easier lengthening [135–137]. Those who favor the colon as a conduit state that a longer segment may be replaced by the colon with less tension and long-term function is better [142, 143]. Furthermore, the likelihood of regurgitation and anastomotic stricture as a result of acid exposure is less with colonic interposition. Still, most gastrointestinal surgeons continue to use the stomach as the conduit of choice.

The surgical approach to a total esophagectomy for benign disease is accomplished efficiently through a transhiatal approach. The benefit is that the patient need not have a thoracotomy, with its inherent morbidity of the incision and single-lung ventilation. Although the procedure can be accomplished via a combined thoracoabdominal approach, this is generally not necessary for benign disease [137, 144]. A discussion of esophagectomy for malignancy is given in Chapter 35.

Conclusions

The esophagus can be safely resected and replaced with the stomach. The patient should fully understand the risks of the operation, especially if it is being considered for benign disease. Operative principles include preservation of the blood supply of the stomach, careful mediastinal dissection, and a tension-free anastomosis. Patients have a good functional outcome in 78–90% of cases. Benign stricture and anastomotic leak are the most common technical complications of the procedure.

References

1. Agur A. *Grant's Atlas of Anatomy*. Baltimore: Williams and Wilkins, 1991, p. 650.
2. Fremling C, Raivio M, Karppinen I. Endoscopic discision of Zenker's diverticulum. *Ann Chir Gynaecol* 1995;84:169–172.
3. van Overbeek JJ. Meditation on the pathogenesis of hypopharyngeal (Zenker's) diverticulum and a report of endoscopic treatment in 545 patients. *Ann Otolrhinolaryngol* 1994;103:178–185.
4. Westrin KM, Ergun S, Carlsoo B. Zenker's diverticulum—a historical review and trends in therapy. *Acta Otolaryngol* 1996;116:351–360.
5. Cote DN, Miller RH. The association of gastroesophageal reflux and otolaryngologic disorders. *Comprehens Ther* 1995; 21:80–84.
6. Ellis FH Jr. Pharyngoesophageal (Zenker's) diverticulum. *Adv Surg* 1995;28:171–189.
7. D'Ugo D, Cardillo G, Granone P, *et al.* Esophageal diverticula. Physiopathological basis for surgical management. *Eur J Cardiac Thorac Surg* 1992;6:330.
8. Migliore M, Payne H, Jeyasingham K. Pathophysiologic basis for operation on Zenker's diverticulum. *Ann Thorac Surg* 1994;57:1616–1620; discussion 1620–1621.
9. McConnel FM, Hood D, Jackson K, *et al.* Analysis of intrabolus forces in patients with Zenker's diverticulum. *Laryngoscope* 1994;104:571–581.
10. Lerut T, van Raemdonck D, Guelinckx P, *et al.* Zenker's diverticulum: is a myotomy of the cricopharyngeus useful? How long should it be? *Hepatogastroenterology* 1992;39:127–131.
11. Zaninotto G, Costantini M, Anselmino M, *et al.* Onset of oesophageal peristalsis after surgery for idiopathic achalasia. *Br J Surg* 1995;82:1532.
12. Venturi M, Bonavina L, Colombo L, *et al.* Biochemical markers of upper esophageal sphincter compliance in patients with Zenker's diverticulum. *J Surg Res* 1997;70:46–48.
13. Ghosh SK, Pandolfino JE, Zhang Q, *et al.* Deglutitive upper esophageal sphincter relaxation: a study of 75 volunteer subjects using solid-state high-resolution manometry. *Am J Physiol Gastrointest Liver Physiol* 2006;291:G525–531.
14. Rizzetto C, Zaninotto G, Costantini M, *et al.* Zenker's diverticula: feasibility of a tailored approach based on diverticulum size. *J Gastrointest Surg* 2008;12:2057–2064; discussion 2064–2065.
15. Barthlen W, Feussner H, Hannig C, *et al.* Surgical therapy of Zenker's diverticulum: low risk and high efficiency. *Dysphagia* 1990;5:13–19.
16. Laing MR, Murthy P, Ah-See KW, Cockburn JS. Surgery for pharyngeal pouch: audit of management with short- and long-term followup. *J R Coll Surg Edinb* 1995;40:315–318.
17. Zeitoun H, Widdowson D, Hammad Z, Osborne J. A video-fluoroscopic study of patients treated by diverticulectomy and cricopharyngeal myotomy. *Clin Otolaryngol* 1994;19:301–305.
18. Laccourreye O, Menard M, Cauchois R, *et al.* Esophageal diverticulum: diverticulopexy versus diverticulectomy. *Laryngoscope* 1994;104:889–892.
19. Mosher HP. Webs and pouches of the esophagus: their diagnosis and treatment. *Surg Gynecol Obstet* 1917;25:175–187.
20. Dohlman G, Mattsson O. The endoscopic operation for hypopharyngeal diverticula: a roentgencinematographic study. *AMA Arch Otolaryngol* 1960;71:744–752.
21. Collard JM, Otte JB, Kestens PJ. Endoscopic stapling technique of esophagodiverticulostomy for Zenker's diverticulum. *Ann Thorac Surg* 1993;56:573–576.
22. Bonavina L, Bona D, Abraham M, *et al.* Long-term results of endosurgical and open surgical approach for Zenker diverticulum. *World J Gastroenterol* 2007;13:2586–2589.
23. van Overbeek JJ, Hoeksema PE, Edens ET. Microendoscopic surgery of the hypopharyngeal diverticulum using electrocoagulation or carbon dioxide laser. *Ann Otol Rhinol Laryngol* 1984;93(1 Pt 1):34–36.
24. Benjamin B, Innocenti M. Laser treatment of pharyngeal pouch. *Aust NZ J Surg* 1991;61:909–913.
25. Wouters B, van Overbeek JJ. Endoscopic treatment of the hypopharyngeal (Zenker's) diverticulum. *Hepatogastroenterology* 1992;39:105–108.

26. van Overbeek JJ. Microendoscopic CO_2 laser surgery of the hypopharyngeal (Zenker's) diverticulum. *Adv Otorhinolaryngol* 1995;49:140–143.

27. Engel JJ, Panje WR. Endoscopic laser Zenker's diverticulotomy. *Gastrointest Endosc* 1995;42:368–370.

28. Chang CW, Burkey BB, Netterville JL, *et al*. Carbon dioxide laser endoscopic diverticulotomy versus open diverticulectomy for Zenker's diverticulum. *Laryngoscope* 2004;114:519–527.

29. Keck T, Rozsasi A, Grun PM. Surgical treatment of hypopharyngeal diverticulum (Zenker's diverticulum). *Eur Arch Otorhinolaryngol* 2010;267:587–592.

30. Counter PR, Hilton ML, Baldwin DL. Long-term follow-up of endoscopic stapled diverticulotomy. *Ann R Coll Surg Engl* 2002;84:89–92.

31. Narne S, Cutrone C, Bonavina L, *et al*. Endoscopic diverticulotomy for the treatment of Zenker's diverticulum: results in 102 patients with staple-assisted endoscopy. *Ann Otolrhinolaryngol* 1999:108:810–815.

32. Stoeckli SJ, Schmid S. Endoscopic stapler-assisted diverticuloesophagostomy for Zenker's diverticulum: patient satisfaction and subjective relief of symptoms. *Surgery* 2002;131:158–162.

33. Aly A, Devitt PG, Watson DI, *et al*. Endoscopic stapling for pharyngeal pouch: does it make the cut? *Aust NZ J Surg* 2004;74:116–121.

34. Visosky AM, Parke RB, Donovan DT. Endoscopic management of Zenker's diverticulum: factors predictive of success or failure. *Ann Otol Rhinol Laryngol* 2008;117:531–537.

35. Smith SR, Genden EM, Urken ML. Endoscopic stapling technique for the treatment of Zenker diverticulum vs standard open-neck technique. *Otolaryngol Head Neck Surg* 2002;128:141–144.

36. Gregoire J, Duranceau A. Surgical management of Zenker's diverticulum. *Hepatogastroenterology* 1992;39:132–138.

37. Lerut T, Van Raemdonck D, Guelinckx P, *et al*. Pharyngooesophageal diverticulum (Zenker's). Clinical, therapeutic and morphological aspects. *Acta Gastroenterol Belg* 1990;53:330–337.

38. Watemberg S, Landau O, Avrahami R. Zenker's diverticulum: reappraisal. *Am J Gastroenterol* 1996;91:1494–1498.

39. Dantas RO, Cook IJ, Dodds WJ, *et al*. Biomechanics of cricopharyngeal bars. *Gastroenterology* 1990;99:1269–1274.

40. Ekberg O. Cricopharyngeal bar: myth and reality. *Abdom Imaging* 1995;20:179–180.

41. Brady AP, Stevenson GW, Somers S, *et al*. Premature contraction of the cricopharyngeus: a new sign of gastroesophageal reflux disease. *Abdom Imaging* 1995;20:225–229.

42. Herberhold C, Walther EK. Endoscopic laser myotomy in cricopharyngeal achalasia. *Adv Otol Rhino Laryngol* 1995;49:144–147.

43. Wang AY, Kadkade R, Kahrilas PJ, Hirano I. Effectiveness of esophageal dilation for symptomatic cricopharyngeal bar. *Gastrointest Endosc* 2005;61:148–152.

44. Moerman MB. Cricopharyngeal Botox injection: indications and technique. *Curr Opin Otolaryngol Head Neck Surg* 2006; 14:431–436.

45. Monnig PJ. Familial achalasia in children. *Ann Thorac Surg* 1990;49:1019–1022.

46. Robertson CS, Martin BA, Atkinson M. Varicella-zoster virus DNA in the oesophageal myenteric plexus in achalasia. *Gut* 1993;34:299–302.

47. Facco M, Brun P, Baesso I, *et al*. T cells in the myenteric plexus of achalasia patients show a skewed TCR repertoire and react to HSV-1 antigens. *Am J Gastroenterol* 2008; 103:1598–1609.

48. Niwamoto H, Okamoto E, Fujimoto J, *et al*. Are human herpes viruses or measles virus associated with esophageal achalasia? *Dig Dis Sci* 1995;40:859–864.

49. Mearin F, Mourelle M, Guarner F, *et al*. Patients with achalasia lack nitric oxide synthase in the gastro-oesophageal junction. *Eur J Clin Invest* 1993;23:724–728.

50. Miyata M, Sakamoto T, Hashimoto T, *et al*. Effect of secretin on lower esophageal sphincter pressure in patients with esophageal achalasia. *Gastroenterol Jpn* 1991;26:712–715.

51. Pellegrini CA, Leichter R, Patti M, Somberg K, Ostroff JW, Way L. Thoracoscopic esophageal myotomy in the treatment of achalasia. *Ann Thorac Surg* 1993;56:680–682.

52. Ellingson TL, Kozarek RA, Gelfand MD, Botoman AV, Patterson DJ. Iatrogenic achalasia. A case series. *J Clin Gastroenterol* 1995;20:96–99.

53. Parrilla P, Aguayo JL, Martinez de Haro L, Ortiz A, Martinez DA, Morales G. Reversible achalasia-like motor pattern of esophageal body secondary to postoperative stricture of gastroesophageal junction. *Dig Dis Sci* 1992;37:1781–1784.

54. Myers NA, Jolley SG, Taylor R. Achalasia of the cardia in children: a worldwide survey. *J Pediatr Surg* 1994;29:1375.

55. Illi OE, Stauffer UG. Achalasia in childhood and adolescence. *Eur J Pediatr Surg* 1994;4:214–217.

56. Mattox HE, Albertson DA, Castell DO, Richter JE. Dysphagia following fundoplication: "slipped" fundoplication versus achalasia complicated by fundoplication. *Am J Gastroenterol* 1990;85:1468–1472.

57. Parrilla PP, Martinez DHLF, Ortiz EA, *et al*. Short myotomy for vigorous achalasia. *Br J Surg* 1993;80:1540.

58. Stuart RC, Byrne PJ, Lawlor P, O'Sullivan G, Hennessy TP. Meal area index: a new technique for quantitative assessment in achalasia by ambulatory manometry during eating. *Br J Surg* 1992;79:1162–1166.

59. Parrilla PP, Martinez DHL, Ortiz A, *et al*. Achalasia of the cardia: long-term results of oesophagomyotomy and posterior partial fundoplication. *Br J Surg* 1990;77:1371.

60. Crookes PF, Corkill S, DeMeester TR. Gastroesophageal reflux in achalasia. When is reflux really reflux? *Dig Dis Sci* 1997; 42:1354–1361.

61. Shoenut JP, Micflikier AB, Yaffe CS, Den Boer B, Teskey JM. Reflux in untreated achalasia patients. *J Clin Gastroenterol* 1995;20:6–11.

62. Stacher G, Schima W, Bergmann H, *et al*. Sensitivity of radionuclide bolus transport and videofluoroscopic studies compared with manometry in the detection of achalasia. *Am J Gastroenterol* 1994;89:1484–1488.

63. Mattioli S, Pilotti V, Felice V, Di Simone MP, D'Ovidio F, Gozzetti G. Intraoperative study on the relationship between the lower esophageal sphincter pressure and the muscular components of the gastro-esophageal junction in achalasic patients. *Ann Surg* 1993;218:635–639.

64. Oelschlager BK, Chang L, Pellegrini CA. Improved outcome after extended gastric myotomy for achalasia. *Arch Surg* 2003;138:490–495; discussion 495–497.

65. Delgado F, Bolufer JM, Martinez-Abad M, *et al*. Laparoscopic treatment of esophageal achalasia. *Surg Laparosc Endosc* 1996; 6:83–90.

66. Pellegrini C, Wetter LA, Patti M, *et al*. Thoracoscopic esophagomyotomy. Initial experience with a new approach for the treatment of achalasia. *Ann Surg* 1992;216:291–296; discussion 296–299.

67. Peracchia A, Rosati R, Bona S, Fumagalli U, Bonavina L, Chella B. Laparoscopic treatment of functional diseases of the esophagus. *Int Surg* 1995;80:336–340.

68. Shimi S, Nathanson LK, Cuschieri A. Laparoscopic cardiomyotomy for achalasia. *J R Coll Surg Edinb* 1991;36:152–154.

69. Patti MG, Pellegrini CA. Endoscopic surgical treatment of primary oesophageal motility disorders. *J R Coll Surg Edinb* 1996;41:137–142.

70. Horgan SHK, Eubanks TR, Pellegrini CA. Does Botox injection make esophagomyotomy a more difficult operation? Presented at SAGES Scientific Session, Seattle, WA, April 1–4, 1998.

71. Wright AS, Williams CW, Pellegrini CA, Oelschlager BK. Long-term outcomes confirm the superior efficacy of extended Heller myotomy with Toupet fundoplication for achalasia. *Surg Endosc* 2007;21:713–718.

72. Bonavina L, Nosadini A, Bardini R, Baesato M, Peracchia A. Primary treatment of esophageal achalasia. Long-term results of myotomy and Dor fundoplication. *Arch Surg* 1992;127:222–226; discussion 227.

73. Pandolfo N, Bortolotti M, Spigno L, Bozzano PL, Mattioli FP. Manometric assessment of Heller-Dor operation for esophageal achalasia. *Hepatogastroenterology* 1996;43:160–166.

74. Csendes A, Braghetto I, Mascaro J, Henriquez A. Late subjective and objective evaluation of the results of esophagomyotomy in 100 patients with achalasia of the esophagus. *Surgery* 1988;104:469–475.

75. Parrilla P, Martinez DHLF, Ortiz A, *et al*. Factors involved in the return of peristalsis in patients with achalasia of the cardia after Heller's myotomy. *Am J Gastroenterol* 1995;90:713.

76. Tatum RP, Wong JA, Figueredo EJ, *et al*. Return of esophageal function after treatment for achalasia as determined by impedance–manometry. *J Gastrointest Surg* 2007;11:1403–1409.

77. Martins P, Morais BB, Cunha MJR. Postoperative complications in the treatment of chagasic megaesophagus. *Int Surg* 1993;78:99–102.

78. Di Simone MP, Felice V, D'Errico A, *et al*. Onset timing of delayed complications and criteria of follow-up after operation for esophageal achalasia. *Ann Thorac Surg* 1996;61:1106–1110; discussion 1110–1111.

79. Richards WO, Torquati A, Holzman MD, *et al*. Heller myotomy versus Heller myotomy with Dor fundoplication for achalasia: a prospective randomized double-blind clinical trial. *Ann Surg* 2004;240:405–412; discussion 412–415.

80. Jaakkola A, Reinikainen P, Ovaska J, Isolauri J. Barrett's esophagus after cardiomyotomy for esophageal achalasia. *Am J Gastroenterol* 1994;89:165–169.

81. Parkman HE, Ogorek CE, Harris AD, *et al*. Nonoperative management of esophageal strictures following esophagomyotomy for achalasia. *Dig Dis Sci* 1994;39:2102.

82. Ellis FH. Esophagomyotomy by the thoracic approach for esophageal achalasia. *Hepatogastroenterology* 1991;38:498–501.

83. Johnson O. Achalasia of the cardia: experience of extramucosal cardiomyotomy during a ten-year period. *Ethiop Med J* 1994;32:89.

84. Miller DL, Allen MS, Trastek VF, Deschamps C, Pairolero PC. Esophageal resection for recurrent achalasia. *Ann Thorac Surg* 1995;60:922–925; discussion 925–926.

85. Csendes A, Braghetto I, Henriquez A, *et al*. Late results of a prospective randomised study comparing forceful dilatation and oesophagomyotomy in patients with achalasia. *Gut* 1989;30:299.

86. Gayet B, Fekete F. Surgical management of failed esophagomyotomy (Heller's operation). *Hepatogastroenterology* 1991; 38:488–492.

87. Gorecki PJ, Hinder RA, Libbey JS, *et al*. Redo laparoscopic surgery for achalasia. *Surg Endosc* 2002;16:772.

88. Ximenes MR. Esophageal resection for recurrent achalasia. *Ann Thorac Surg* 1996;62:322.

89. Schwartz HM, Cahow CE, Traube M. Outcome after perforation sustained during pneumatic dilatation for achalasia. *Dig Dis Sci* 1993;38:1409–1413.

90. Flynn AE, Verrier ED, Way LW, Thomas AN, Pelligrini CA. Esophageal perforation. *Arch Surg* 1989;124:1211–1214; discussion 1214–1215.

91. Pricolo VE, Park CS, Thompson WR. Surgical repair of esophageal perforation due to pneumatic dilatation for achalasia. Is myotomy really necessary? *Arch Surg* 1993;128:540–543; discussion 543–544.

92. Nathanson LK, Gotley D, Smithers M, Branicki F. Videothoracoscopic primary repair of early distal oesophageal perforation. *Aust NZ J Surg* 1993;63:399–403.

93. Ferguson MK, Reeder LB, Olak J. Results of myotomy and partial fundoplication after pneumatic dilation for achalasia. *Ann Thorac Surg* 1996;62:327–330.

94. Bourgeois N, Coffernils M, Sznajer Y, Panzer JM, Gelin M, Cremer M. Non-surgical management of achalasia. *Acta Gastroenterol Belg* 1992;55:260–263.

95. Efrati Y, Horne T, Livshitz G, Broide E, Klin B, Vinograd I. Radionuclide esophageal emptying and long-acting nitrates (Nitroderm) in childhood achalasia. *J Pediatr Gastroenterol Nutr* 1996;23:312–315.

96. Pasricha PJ, Kalloo AN. Recent advances in the treatment of achalasia. *Gastrointest Endosc Clin North Am* 1997;7:191–206.

97. Tack J, Janssens J, Vantrappen G. Non-surgical treatment of achalasia. *Hepatogastroenterology* 1991;38:493–497.

98. Abid S, Champion G, Richter JE, *et al*. Treatment of achalasia: the best of both worlds. *Am J Gastroenterol* 1994;89:979.

99. Anselmino M, Perdikis G, Hinder RA, *et al*. Heller myotomy is superior to dilatation for the treatment of early achalasia. *Arch Surg* 1997;132:233–240.

100. Makela J, Kiviniemi H, Laitinen S. Heller's cardiomyotomy compared with pneumatic dilatation for treatment of oesophageal achalasia. *Eur J Surg* 1991;157:411–414.

101. Csendes A, Velasco N, Braghetto I, Henriquez A. A prospective randomized study comparing forceful dilatation and esophagomyotomy in patients with achalasia of the esophagus. *Gastroenterology* 1981;80:789–795.

102. Kostic S, Kjellin A, Ruth M, *et al*. Pneumatic dilatation or laparoscopic cardiomyotomy in the management of newly

diagnosed idiopathic achalasia. Results of a randomized controlled trial. *World J Surg* 2007;31:470–478.

103. Vela MF, Richter JE, Khandwala F, *et al.* The long-term efficacy of pneumatic dilatation and Heller myotomy for the treatment of achalasia. *Clin Gastroenterol Hepatol* 2006;4:580–587.

104. Ancona E, Peracchia A, Zaninotto G, Rossi M, Bonavina L, Segalin A. Heller laparoscopic cardiomyotomy with antireflux anterior fundoplication (Dor) in the treatment of esophageal achalasia. *Surg Endosc* 1993;7:459–461.

105. Collard JM, Romagnoli R, Lengele B, *et al.* Heller-Dor procedure for achalasia: from conventional to video-endoscopic surgery. *Acta Chir Belg* 1996;96:62–65.

106. Graham AJ, Finley RJ, Worsley DF, *et al.* Laparoscopic esophageal myotomy and anterior partial fundoplication for the treatment of achalasia. *Ann Thorac Surg* 1997;64:785–789.

107. Morino M, Rebecchi F, Festa V, Garrone C. Laparoscopic Heller cardiomyotomy with intraoperative manometry in the management of oesophageal achalasia. *Int Surg* 1995;80:332–335.

108. Vara TC, Herrainz R. Esophageal achalasia: laparoscopic Heller cardiomyotomy. *Int Surg* 1995;80:376.

109. Ancona E, Anselmino M, Zaninotto G, *et al.* Esophageal achalasia: laparoscopic versus conventional open Heller-Dor operation. *Am J Surg* 1995;170:265–270.

110. Ellis FH Jr. Invited letter concerning: technique for prevention of gastroesophageal reflux after transthoracic Heller's operation. *J Thorac Cardiovasc Surg* 1993;105:555.

111. Gatzinsky P, Dernevik L, Bjork S, Sandberg N. Technique for prevention of gastroesophageal reflux after transthoracic Heller's operation. *J Thorac Cardiovasc Surg* 1993;105:553–555.

112. Holzman MD, Sharp KW, Ladipo JK, *et al.* Laparoscopic surgical treatment of achalasia. *Am J Surg* 1997;173:308–311.

113. Raiser F, Perdikis G, Hinder RA, *et al.* Heller myotomy via minimal-access surgery. An evaluation of antireflux procedures. *Arch Surg* 1996;131:593–597; discussion 597–598.

114. Hunter JG, Trus TL, Branum GD, Waring JP. Laparoscopic Heller myotomy and fundoplication for achalasia. *Ann Surg* 1997;225:655–664; discussion 664–665.

115. Patti MG, Arcerito M, Pellegrini CA. Thoracoscopic and laparoscopic Heller's myotomy in the treatment of esophageal achalasia. *Ann Chir Gynaecol* 1995;84:159–164.

116. Slim K, Pezet D, Chipponi J, Boulant J, Mathieu S. Laparoscopic myotomy for primary esophageal achalasia: prospective evaluation. *Hepatogastroenterology* 1997;44:11–15.

117. Shoenut JP, Duerksen D, Yaffe CS. A prospective assessment of gastroesophageal reflux before and after treatment of achalasia patients: pneumatic dilation versus transthoracic limited myotomy. *Am J Gastroenterol* 1997;92:1109–1112.

118. Rossetti G, Brusciano L, Amato G, *et al.* A total fundoplication is not an obstacle to esophageal emptying after heller myotomy for achalasia: results of a long-term follow up. *Ann Surg* 2005;241:614–621.

119. Katada N, Hinder RA, Hinder PR, *et al.* The hypertensive lower esophageal sphincter. *Am J Surg* 1996;172:439–442;discussion 442–443.

120. Benacci JC, Deschamps C, Trastek VF, *et al.* Epiphrenic diverticulum: results of surgical treatment. *Ann Thorac Surg* 1993;55:1109–1114; discussion 1114.

121. Barreca M, Oelschlager BK, Pellegrini CA. Outcomes of laparoscopic Nissen fundoplication in patients with the "hypercontractile esophagus." *Arch Surg* 2002;137:724–728.

122. Eypasch EP, Stein HJ, DeMeester TR, *et al.* A new technique to define and clarify esophageal motor disorders. *Am J Surg* 1990;159:144–151; discussion 151.

123. Stein HJ, DeMeester TR, Eypasch EP, *et al.* Ambulatory 24-hour esophageal manometry in the evaluation of esophageal motor disorders and noncardiac chest pain. *Surgery* 1991;110:753–761;discussion 761.

124. Mittal RK, Kassab G, Puckett JL, Liu J. Hypertrophy of the muscularis propria of the lower esophageal sphincter and the body of the esophagus in patients with primary motility disorders of the esophagus. *Am J Gastroenterol* 2003;98:1705–1712.

125. Jung HY, Puckett JL, Bhalla V, *et al.* Asynchrony between the circular and the longitudinal muscle contraction in patients with nutcracker esophagus. *Gastroenterology* 2005;128:1179–1186.

126. Filipi CJ, Hinder RA. Thoracoscopic esophageal myotomy-a surgical technique for achalasia diffuse esophageal spasm and "nutcracker esophagus." *Surg Endosc* 1994;8:921–925; discussion 925.

127. McBride PJ, Hinder RA, Filipi C, Raiser F, Katada N, Lund RJ. Surgical treatment of spastic conditions of the esophagus. *Int Surg* 1997;82:113–118.

128. Shimi SM, Nathanson LK, Cuschieri A. Thoracoscopic long oesophageal myotomy for nutcracker oesophagus: initial experience of a new surgical approach. *Br J Surg* 1992;79:533–536.

129. Patti MG, Gorodner MV, Galvani C, *et al.* Spectrum of esophageal motility disorders: implications for diagnosis and treatment. *Arch Surg* 2005;140:442–448; discussion 448–449.

130. Almansa C, Hinder RA, Smith CD, Achem SR. A comprehensive appraisal of the surgical treatment of diffuse esophageal spasm. *J Gastrointest Surg* 2008;12:1133–1145.

131. Patti MG, Pelligrini CA, Arcerito M, Tong J, Mulvihill SJ, Way LW. Comparison of medical and minimally invasive surgical therapy for primary esophageal motility disorders. *Arch Surg* 1995;130:609–615; discussion 615.

132. Del Genio A, Rossetti G, Maffetton V, *et al.* Laparoscopic approach in the treatment of epiphrenic diverticula: long-term results. *Surg Endosc* 2004;18:741–745.

133. Fernando HC, Luketich JD, Samphire J, *et al.* Minimally invasive operation for esophageal diverticula. *Ann Thorac Surg* 2005;80:2076–2080.

134. Melman L, Quinlan J, Robertson B, *et al.* Esophageal manometric characteristics and outcomes for laparoscopic esophageal diverticulectomy, myotomy, and partial fundoplication for epiphrenic diverticula. *Surg Endosc* 2009;23:1337–1341.

135. Orringer MB, Marshall B, Stirling MC. Transhiatal esophagectomy for benign and malignant disease. *J Thorac Cardiovasc Surg* 1993;105:265–276; discussion 276.

136. Daniel TM, Fleischer KJ, Flanagan TL, *et al.* Transhiatal esophagectomy: a safe alternative for selected patients. *Ann Thorac Surg* 1992;54:686–689; discussion 689.

137. Davis EA, Heitmiller RE Esophagectomy for benign disease: trends in surgical results and management. *Ann Thorac Surg* 1996;62:369–372.

138. Orringer MB, Marshall B, Chang AC, *et al*. Two thousand transhiatal esophagectomies: changing trends, lessons learned. *Ann Surg* 2007;246:363–372; discussion 372–374.

139. Katariya K, Harvey JC, Pina E, *et al*. Complications of transhiatal esophagectomy. *J Surg Oncol* 1994;57:157–161.

140. Honkoop P, Siersema PD, Tilanus HW, *et al*. Benign anastomotic strictures after transhiatal esophagectomy and cervical esophagogastrostomy: risk factors and management. *J Thorac Cardiovasc Surg* 1996;111:1141–1146; discussion 1147–1148.

141. Patti MG, Wiener KJP, Way LW, *et al*. Impact of transhiatal esophagectomy on cardiac and respiratory function. *Am J Surg* 1991;162:563–565; discussion 566.

142. Mansour KA, Bryan FC, Carlson GW. Bowel interposition for esophageal replacement: twenty-five-year experience. *Ann Thorac Surg* 1997;64:752–754.

143. Gupta NM, Goenka MK, Behera A, *et al*. Transhiatal oesophagectomy for benign obstructive conditions of the oesophagus. *Br J Surg* 1997;84:262–265.

144. Watson TJ, Peters JH, DeMeester TR. Esophageal replacement for end-stage benign esophageal disease. *Surg Clin North Am* 1997;77:1099–2103.

16 Esophageal Webs and Rings

Michael S. Smith
Temple University School of Medicine, Philadelphia, PA, USA

Introduction

Advances in our understanding of esophageal webs and rings have generated confusion as well as evolution in their identification and treatment. Other than Schatzki's rings, these are rare disorders. Their etiologies are, for the most part, poorly understood, and there is little agreement among experts as to what constitutes a web or ring. With better understanding of the "ringed esophagus" and its link to eosinophilic esophagitis (see Chapter 36), this chapter will focus on solitary lesions, their identification, possible etiologies for existence, and options for treatment.

Definitions

Webs and rings are membranous structures where a thin tissue fold creates at least partial obstruction of the esophageal lumen. Beyond this general definition, there is disagreement among esophagologists as to what constitutes each finding. Webs are thin mucosal folds covered with squamous epithelium. Previous editions of *The Esophagus* [1] have suggested that webs can occur anywhere in the esophageal lumen. Other textbooks, however, limit the definition of webs to include only proximal esophageal structures. Regardless, they are most commonly appreciated in the anterior portion of the proximal esophagus, leading to a narrowed esophageal lumen distal to the cricoid region. Webs are generally thought of as eccentric, though again some experts believe they have the potential to be concentric as well.

Compared to anatomic variations in esophageal webs, there is greater consensus that esophageal rings occur distally and are described as concentric. Schatzki [2] defined a ring as a thin mucosal structure at the gastroesophageal junction, covered by the normal esophageal squamous epithelium proximally and columnar epithelium on the distal side of the membrane. While some investigators have described rings as resulting from mucosal hypertrophy [3], others have shown normal wall layers on histologic evaluation [4]. For the purpose of clarity, this chapter will focus on anatomic position of the lesion, not nomenclature, as a means of organization.

Upper esophageal webs and rings

Prevalence and etiology

Without any significant prospective radiographic studies, it is difficult to estimate the prevalence of these proximal lesions. In several large series, 5–15% of patients undergoing either upper endoscopy or esophagrams for dysphagia demonstrate a cervical esophageal web. Detection of these often subtle lesions may be limited by suboptimal radiographic technique (see Symptoms and diagnosis below). However, it is important to remember that these subtle lesions may be incidental and have nothing to do with the source of the patient's complaint. A full dysphagia evaluation to exclude other etiologies such as a motility disorder or distal obstruction is appropriate in these cases.

The pathogenesis of proximal esophageal webs and rings is poorly understood, with most considered idiopathic. Cervical webs are not thought to be related to proximal stenoses, which can result from tracheobronchial remnants in esophageal atresia. As with Schatzki's rings, gastroesophageal reflux disease (GERD) may be a potential cause of proximal rings. Case reports and studies have identified multiple other associated diagnoses (Table 16.1) [5–25], including proximal lesions forming as extracutaneous sequelae of systemic skin disorders.

Symptoms and diagnosis

Proximal lesions typically present with dysphagia to pills or solid foods (see Chapter 3). Given their location, patients can present with a choking sensation resulting from tracheal

The Esophagus, Fifth Edition. Edited by Joel E. Richter, Donald O. Castell.
© 2012 Blackwell Publishing Ltd. Published 2012 by Blackwell Publishing Ltd.

Table 16.1 Conditions associated with upper esophageal webs.

Zenker's diverticulum [5]
Epidermolysis bullosa [6–10]
Pemphigus or pemphigoid vulgaris [11–14]
Psoriasis [15]
Celiac disease [16]
Heterotopic gastric mucosa [17–19]
Graft-versus-host disease [20]
Radiation therapy [1]
Bronchoesophageal fistula with an esophageal web [21]
Laryngeal carcinoma [22]
Esophageal duplication cyst [23]
Zinsser–Engman–Cole-Fanconi disease [24]
Pediatric growth failure [25]

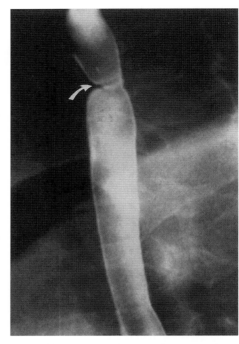

Figure 16.1 Double-contrast esophagram of upper esophageal web (arrow) (reproduced courtesy of Dr Marc Levine).

compression. Intolerance of liquids is rare, and other etiologies should be investigated in these patients. Weight loss, generated from an aversion to eating and the symptoms it creates, also can be seen [26].

The gold standard for diagnosing proximal lesions is a barium esophagram. The radiologist must be encouraged to focus on the upper esophagus if a lesion in this region is suspected. Full-column distention of the esophagus is essential [27], and is best accomplished with the patient in a prone position. Careful inspection of the esophagus just distal to the upper esophageal sphincter, using ciné technique with both anteroposterior and lateral views, is essential for complete visualization. Identification of a smaller web, as well as its clinical significance, may be aided by visualization of the passage of a barium pill (approximately 13 mm in diameter) or a solid food bolus. Esophageal webs are frequently best seen as a filling defect on a lateral view due to their often anterior location (Figure 16.1). While this technique will essentially identify all proximal lesions, standard upright double-contrast and mucosal relief techniques alone will identify fewer than half of all lesions [28], underscoring the importance of communicating with the radiologist prior to the study.

Upper endoscopy is a far inferior technique for diagnosing these lesions. Often, the lesion is not seen but only appreciated as resistance when the endoscope is passed through the upper esophageal sphincter and into the proximal esophagus. If the web or ring is seen, it will appear as a thin unilateral or circumferential band of tissue with normal overlying mucosa. The endoscopic detection rate is inversely proportional to the luminal diameter at the site of the lesion. Insertion of the endoscope may rupture the lesion, and all that may be visible to make the diagnosis is a small scar or spotting of blood due to mucosal trauma. Associated endoscopic findings, such as an "inlet patch" of gastric heterotopia, should be carefully assessed during visual inspection

[17–19]. As previously stated, a thorough endoscopy investigating other sources of dysphagia is crucial, as these findings are often incidental and can coexist with other lesions.

Treatment

Before embarking on treating a patient with a proximal web or ring, it is important to determine the likelihood that the lesion is actually the source of the patient's symptoms. The presence of concurrent esophageal findings, or other confounding variables, such as ineffective mastication due to dental problems or a stroke, or the need to consume large pills, can make this assessment difficult. If the benefits of treatment outweigh the risks, several options for endoscopic intervention are available (Table 16.2). If upper endoscopy itself does not rupture a web or ring, purposeful dilation should be attempted. Most frequently, Savary dilation over a guidewire is used [29, 30], although passage of Maloney bougies is an alternative approach [31]. Fluoroscopic guidance during the procedure is operator dependent. In both cases, a large (15 mm/45F or larger) dilator is preferred. More focal treatments to disrupt the mucosal integrity can be performed using a biopsy forceps [32] or electric or laser-based incision [33, 34]. As a last resort, surgical intervention with resection of the lesion and an end-to-end esophageal anastomosis can be considered [35].

Selection of the optimal therapy includes consideration of comorbidities. For example, in patients with Zenker's diverticulum, both diagnostic endoscopy and esophageal dilation

Table 16.2 Options for endoscopic treatment of esophageal webs and rings.

Upper esophageal webs and rings
Guidewire-directed Savary dilation [29, 30]
Maloney dilation [31]
Endoscopic balloon dilation
Endoscopic biopsy obliteration [32]
Electric or laser-based incision [33, 34]
Surgical resection [35]

Schatzki's rings
Large-bore guidewire-directed dilation [84]
Endoscopic biopsy [87]
Electrocautery [29, 88, 89]
Pneumatic dilation [92]
Injection with steroids
Surgical resection

carry a greater risk of perforation than in the standard population. Similarly, dilation in patients with bullous disease has a significant risk of generating further bullae or webs following dilation.

Plummer–Vinson syndrome

The controversial linkage between iron-deficiency anemia and upper esophageal webs, known most commonly as Plummer–Vinson syndrome, was first described by Plummer in 1912 [36]. Subsequent reports by two laryngologists, Paterson [37] and Brown Kelly [38], led to the name of Paterson–Brown Kelly syndrome. Vinson, a gastroenterologist, did not publish his observation until 1922 [39], and pleaded ignorance of the laryngologists' work [40].

The connection between iron-deficiency anemia and esophageal webs is based on a few key tenets. Iron deficiency is strongly associated with the presence of esophageal webs [41–43]. In fact, these webs have been reported to form after iron deficiency is documented [44]. Histologic examination has shown that iron deficiency leads to changes in the esophageal epithelium, increasing the likelihood of web formation [45]. Also, iron repletion can resolve these webs [44–46]. Both iron deficiency and Plummer–Vinson syndrome are decreasing in incidence [47, 48]. However, other studies have shown that patients with esophageal webs demonstrate the same prevalence of iron deficiency as controls from the general population, casting doubt on whether this disease state actually exists [49, 50].

Patients with Plummer–Vinson syndrome typically have webs, either single or multiple, in the hypopharynx or upper esophagus. It is most common in Caucasian women of middle or advanced age, although patients can be of other ethnicities, ages or sex [46, 51–53]. The webs may be associated with stricture formation, with biopsies showing fibrosis,

atrophic epithelium, hyperplasia and possibly chronic inflammation [48, 54]. Patients with Plummer–Vinson syndrome also have a higher likelihood of developing oral, hypopharyngeal or upper gastrointestinal malignancy [43, 48, 49], suggesting there is value to a screening program in these patients [55]. Other associated conditions include autoimmune diseases, such as thyroiditis, rheumatoid arthritis, and Sjögren's syndrome [56, 57]; celiac disease [58, 59]; glossitis and stomatitis [60]; and pernicious anemia [55].

Regardless of whether the syndrome actually exists, the patient must undergo evaluation to identify other potential sources of iron deficiency, particularly malignancy given the aforementioned association with proximal cancers. After completing the diagnostic evaluation, correction of the anemia is critical, particularly since it may lead to resolution of the web and also correction of possible esophageal motor abnormalities [61]. Some patients may require esophageal dilation along with iron supplementation [62].

Lower esophageal rings

Three distinct anatomic positions for lower esophageal rings can be identified on both barium esophagram and, to a lesser degree, on visual inspection. The most proximal, known as an "A" ring, is seen about 2 cm proximal to the gastroesophageal junction. It is believed to be the normal physiologic result of esophageal smooth muscle contractions. Clinically apparent symptoms are extremely rare. At the distal margin, "C" rings indicate extrinsic compression of the esophagus by the diaphragmatic crura. The intermediate or "B" ring, also known as Schatzki's ring, is the most commonly seen and studied ring.

Schatzki's ring

Lower esophageal rings were first described anatomically by Templeton in 1944 [63]. Nine years later, two teams of investigators each published articles regarding the clinical significance of these rings in causing dysphagia. The groups included Schatzki and Gary [64] and Ingelfinger and Kramer [65]. The continued study of this finding by Schatzki led to its eponym, although it commonly is referred to as a "lower esophageal ring."

Epidemiology, pathology and pathogenesis

Routine barium esophagram series demonstrate a broad prevalence of 0.2–14% of the general population having a Schatzki's ring [66–69] (Figure 16.2). As with upper esophageal webs and rings, variation in prevalence rates likely results from variations in radiographic technique and effort spent looking for these entities. Symptomatic rings most often include an internal ring diameter measuring less than 13 mm. They are found in 0.5% of all esophageal studies

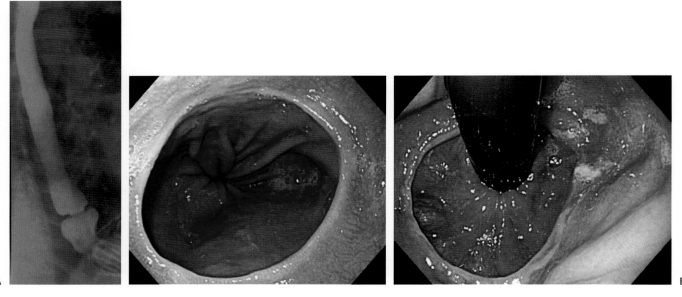

A ⋯ B,C

Figure 16.2 (A) Double-contrast esophagram, (B) antegrade endoscopic view (reproduced courtesy of Dr Benjamin Krevsky), and (C) retroflexed endoscopic view of a Schatzki's ring.

performed [68]. However, in studies performed for evaluation of dysphagia, much higher detection rates of 15–26% are seen [70]. There is a direct correlation between incidence and age; unlike proximal webs, Schatzki's rings are very uncommon in children [67].

Schatzki's rings are found at or near the gastroesophageal junction, and consist of annular membranes of mucosal and submucosal tissue [69]. As previously discussed, given their position at the squamocolumar junction, they are often composed of both squamous (proximal) and columnar (distal) epithelium. While chronic inflammation and fibrosis may be seen, this is not essential to make the diagnosis [71–73].

Initial theories regarding the origin of these distal esophageal rings included the possibility of both congenital formation and development following repeated pleating of the mucosa during muscular contractions [74]. Studies also have connected these rings with eosinophilic esophagitis [75], though solitary rings are an uncommon presentation of this disease. Current thinking most closely links Schatzki's rings with GERD for several reasons. In addition to the presence of chronic inflammation often seen on histologic examination, patients with these rings often present with reflux symptoms [73], and nearly two-thirds of patients have abnormal esophageal acid exposure on ambulatory pH monitoring [76]. Conditions predisposing to GERD, such as a hiatal hernia or scleroderma, frequently coexist in patients with Schatzki's rings [73, 77]. The high likelihood of ring recurrence suggests an underlying physiologic etiology, such as uncontrolled acid reflux disease.

Presentation and diagnosis

The classic presentation of a symptomatic Schatzki's ring is dysphagia to solid foods [78]. Food impaction, sometimes with an inability to manage secretions or chest pain leading to an emergency room visit, can be seen. Dysphagia may or may not be present in these cases. Very rarely, patients with Schatzki's rings can present with esophageal perforation [79]. However, most patients with these rings are asymptomatic. Schatzki himself demonstrated that the luminal diameter created within a ring correlates directly with the likelihood of developing symptoms [66]. Only when the diameter is less than 13 mm is the patient likely to be symptomatic, and only rarely will the subject have any symptoms if the lumen measures over 20 mm at the narrowest point. Patients with chronically symptomatic rings, through dietary modifications such as chewing food more thoroughly and eating slowly, may minimize the severity of their symptoms, even when a tight ring is present. However, poorly chewed food, such as a piece of steak, may cause food impaction, even if the ring has a diameter of over 20 mm. As a bolus of meat is the obstructing lesion in the majority of cases [80], these acute impactions have been termed "steakhouse syndrome" [81] or "backyard barbeque syndrome" [82].

Similar to upper esophageal webs and rings, the barium esophagram is the most sensitive test for diagnosing Schatzki's rings. Here again, technique is of great importance, and the radiologist should be alerted to the suspicion of a ring to utilize a large-volume, single-contrast examination with sufficient esophageal distention [83]. This method contrasts with the standard low-volume, double-contrast approach which is frequently used today. Pretest notification also permits use of a solid barium tablet or barium-soaked food bolus, which can provide insight into the clinical significance of a ring. Upper endoscopy, as long as sufficient insufflation is performed in the distal esophagus, can be diagnostic, but this is an invasive procedure that is less sensitive than a well-performed esophagram. Additional measures such as Valsalva during endoscopy may aid in detection, but this is difficult if the patient is well sedated for the procedure. If endoscopy follows the symptomatic ring diagnosis by barium esophagram, the endoscopist can proceed directly to treatment after obtaining informed consent.

Treatment and recurrence

Similar to upper esophageal webs, endoscopic treatment should be offered to those patients who are symptomatic from their Schatzki's rings. Large-bore dilation remains the mainstay of treatment once eosinophilic esophagitis has been ruled out as the etiology of dysphagia. Bougienage with a single dilator (at least 16 mm diameter) is preferred to serial dilations, the latter method chosen where the risk of perforation is increased by the presence of fibrotic tissue facilitating deeper mucosal tears. In a prospective study, Eckardt *et al.* showed that dilation provides symptom relief in all patients within 1 month [84].

After successfully dilating these patients, one study found that nearly half the patients had symptom recurrence significant enough to warrant repeat dilation within a mean follow-up of 2 years. Only 11% of patients were found to remain symptom free after 5 years. In another prospective study, 63% of patients developed recurrent dysphagia leading to repeat dilation [85]. In neither study did the initial luminal diameter of the ring predict the need for repeat bougienage. The first study considered the role of reflux in ring recurrence, but found that the need for repeat dilation did not correspond to either the presence or absence of reflux esophagitis on biopsy.

Sgouros *et al.*, however, demonstrated a clear benefit to acid suppressive therapy following ring dilation in a randomized prospective study [86]. Of the 44 patients enrolled, 14 had GERD diagnosed using objective measures such as endoscopy or ambulatory pH monitoring. These patients were placed on omeprazole 20 mg/day following successful ring dilation, and none developed recurrent dysphagia over the mean follow-up period of 43 months. The remaining 30 patients without demonstrated GERD were randomized to either omeprazole 20 mg/day or placebo treatment. Only one patient had a recurrence of a Schatzki's ring on proton pump inhibitor therapy, while seven patients on placebo relapsed during a mean follow-up period of nearly 20 months. This created a statistically significant increase in the actuarial probability to relapse (*P* = .008) (Figure 16.3). Use of omeprazole after successful Schatzki's ring dilation created an absolute risk reduction of recurrence of 40% and a rela-

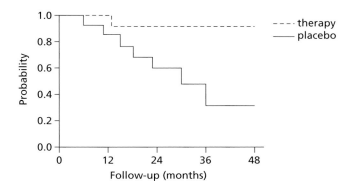

Patients at risk	0	12	24	36	48
Therapy	15	14	11	9	4
Placebo	15	11	7	3	1

Figure 16.3 Actuarial probability of remaining free from relapse of a Schatzki's ring following successful endoscopic dilation. This is significantly improved on prophylactic antisecretory therapy with daily proton pump inhibitor versus placebo (*P* = .008) (reproduced from Sgouros *et al.* [86]).

tive risk reduction of 85%, with a number needed to treat (NNT) of 3 to prevent a symptomatic recurrence. Given the results of another study suggesting radiographic evolution of classic Schatzki's rings into peptic strictures [87], acid suppression therapy should be considered in these patients, particularly those requiring dilation for recurrent symptoms.

Rings that are refractory to bougienage can be treated with alternative interventions similar to those used for proximal esophageal lesions (see Table 16.2). These include disrupting the ring with endoscopic biopsy and incision with electrocautery [88]. Multiple cases series have described the efficacy of electrocautery [29, 89]. Similarly, incision with a sphincterotome has been described [90]. One study showed that patients randomized to large-bore bougie dilation or four-quadrant biopsy interventions showed no difference in dysphagia scores after 3 and 12 months, and the biopsy procedure was better tolerated [91]. The biopsy method may be particularly useful in patients presenting with an acute food impaction. Concerns for perforation were allayed by a study which showed dilation at the time of presentation relieved symptoms without increasing perforation rates [92]. Deeper tissue injury may result from a prolonged impaction, significantly augmenting the risk of perforation. Biopsy-based therapy should also be considered for those patients whose coagulopathy or use of antiplatelet agents raise the complication rate of traditional bougienage. Pneumatic balloon dilation [93], injection of the ring with steroids, and surgery all have been described for these refractory patients.

References

1. Katzka DA. Esophageal rings and webs. In: Castell DO, Richter JE, eds. *The Esophagus*, 4th edn. Philadelphia: Lippincott, Williams and Wilkins, 2003, pp. 315–324.

2. Schatzki R. The lower esophageal ring. Long term follow-up of symptomatic and asymptomatic rings. *Am J Roentgenol Radium Ther Nucl Med* 1963;90:805.

3. Johnston JH, Griffin JC. Anatomic location of the lower esophageal ring. *Surgery* 1967;61:528–534.

4. MacMahon HE, Schatzki R, Gary JE. Pathology of the lower esophageal ring: report of a case, with autopsy, observed for nine years. *N Engl J Med* 1958;259:1–8.

5. Low DE, Hill LD. Cervical esophageal web associated with Zenker's diverticulum. *Am J Surg* 1988;156:34–37.

6. Orlando RC, Bozymksi EM, Briggaman RA, *et al.* Epidermolysis bullosa: gastrointestinal manifestations. *Ann Intern Med* 1974;81:203.

7. Marsden RA, Gowar FJS, MacDonald AF, *et al.* Epidermolysis bullosa of the esophagus with esophageal web formation. *Thorax* 1974;29:287–295.

8. Hillemeier C, Touloukian R, McCallum R, *et al.* Esophageal web: a previously unrecognized complication of epidermolysis bullosa. *Pediatrics* 1981;67:678.

9. Sehgal VN, Jain VK, Bhattadcharya SN, *et al.* Esophageal web in generalized epidermolysis bullosa. *Int J Dermatol* 1991;30:51–52.

10. Ergun GA, Lin AN, Dannenberg AJ, *et al.* Gastrointestinal manifestations of epidermolysis bullosa. A study of 101 patients. *Medicine* 1992;71:121.

11. Al-Kutoubi MA, Eliot A. Esophageal involvement in benign mucosa membrane pemphigoid. *Clin Radiol* 1984;35:131.

12. Foroozan P, Enta T, Winship DH, *et al.* Loss and regeneration of the esophageal mucosa in pemphigoid. *Gastroenterology* 1967;52:548.

13. Kaplan, RP, Touloukian, J, Ahmed, AR, Newcomer, VD. Esophagitis dissecans superficialis associated with pemphigus vulgaris. *J Am Acad Dermatol* 1981;4:682.

14. Naylor MF, MacCarty RL, Rogers RS. Barium studies in esophageal cicatricial pemphigoid. *Abdom Imaging* 1995;20:97.

15. Harty RF, Boharski MG, Harried RK. Psoriasis, dysphagia and esophageal webs or rings. *Dysphagia* 1988;2:136.

16. Sinha SK, Nain CK, Udawat HP, *et al.* Cervical esophageal web and celiac disease. *J Gastroenterol Hepatol* 2008;23:1149–1152.

17. Steadman C, Kerlin P, Teague C, *et al.* High esophageal stricture: a complication of "inlet patch" mucosa. *Gastroenterology* 1988;94:521–524.

18. Buse PE, Zuckerman GR, Balfe DM. Cervical esophageal web associated with a patch of heterotopic gastric mucosa. *Abdom Imaging* 1993;18:227–228.

19. Waring JP, Wo JM. Cervical esophageal web caused by an inlet patch of gastric mucosa. *South Med J* 1997;90:554–555.

20. McDonald GB, Sullivan KM, Plumley TE Radiographic features of esophageal involvement in chronic graft-vs.-host disease. *AJR Am J Roentgenol* 1984;142:501.

21. Turrentine MW, Kesler KA, Mahomed Y Bronchoesophageal fistula with an esophageal web. *Ann Thorac Surg* 1990;50:473–475.

22. Belafsky PC, Postma GN, Koufman JA. Laryngeal carcinoma and a lower esophageal web. *Ear Nose Throat J* 2001;80:788.

23. Snyder CL, Bickler SW, Gittes GK, *et al.* Esophageal duplication cyst with esophageal web and tracheoesophageal fistula. *J Pediatr Surg* 1996;31:968.

24. de Roux-Serratrice C, Serratrice J, Escoffier JM, *et al.* Esophageal web in Zinsser-Engman-Cole-Fanconi disease. *Gastrointest Endosc* 2000;52:561–562.

25. Kumuro H, Makino S, Tsuchiya I, *et al.* Cervical esophageal web in a 13-year old with growth failure. *Pediatr Int* 1999;41:568–570.

26. Lesser PB, Moyer P, Andrews PJ, *et al.* Upper esophageal ring. *Ann Intern Med* 1978;88:657–658.

27. Ott DJ, Gelfand DW, Lane TG, *et al.* Radiologic detection and spectrum of appearances of peptic esophageal strictures. *J Clin Gastroenterol* 1982;4:11–15.

28. Chen YM, Ott DJ, Gelfand DW, *et al.* Multiphasic examination of the esophagogastric region for strictures, rings, and hiatal hernia: evaluation of the individual techniques. *Gastrointest Radiol* 1985;10:311–316.

29. Lindgren S. Endoscopic dilatation and surgical myotomy of symptomatic cervical esophageal webs. *Dysphagia* 1991;6:235.

30. Webb WA, McDaniel L, Jones L. Endoscopic evaluation of dysphagia in two hundred and ninety-three patients with benign disease. *Surg Gynecol Obstet* 1984;158:152.

31. Huynh PT, de Lange EE, Shagger HA. Symptomatic webs of the upper esophagus: treatment with fluoroscopically guided balloon dilation. *Radiology* 1995;196:789.

32. Chotiprasidhi P, Minocha A. Effectiveness of single dilation with Maloney dilator versus endoscopic rupture of Schatzki's ring using biopsy forceps. *Dig Dis Sci* 2000;45:281–284.

33. Wills JC, Hilden K, Disario JA, *et al.* A randomized, prospective trial of electrosurgical incision followed by rabeprazole versus bougie dilation followed by rabeprazole of symptomatic esophageal (Schatzki's) rings. *Gastrointest Endosc* 2008;67:808–813.

34. Krevsky B, Pusateri JP. Laser lysis of an esophageal web. *Gastrointest Endosc* 1989;35:451–453.

35. Roy GT, Cohen RC, Williams SJ. Endoscopic laser division of an esophageal web in a child. *J Pediatr Surg* 1996;31:439–440.

36. Plummer HS. Diffuse dilation of the esophagus without anastomotic stenosis (cardiospasm), a report of ninety-nine cases. *PAM* 1912;34:285–288.

37. Paterson DR. A clinical type of dysphagia. *J Laryngol Rhinol Otol* 1919;34:289.

38. Kelly AB. Spasms at the entrance to the esophagus. *J Laryngol Rhinol Otol* 1919;34:285.

39. Vinson PP. Hysterical dysphagia. *Minn Med* 1922;5:107.

40. Baron JH. The Paterson–Brown Kelly syndrome of sideropenic dysphagia does not exist. *J R Coll Phys Lond* 1991;25:361.

41. Jacobs A, Kilpatrick GS. The Paterson–Kelly syndrome. *BMJ* 1964;2:79–82.

42. Chisolm M, Ardran GM, Gallender ST, *et al.* A follow-up study of patients with post-cricoid webs. *Q J Med* 1971;40:409–420.

43. Chisolm M. The association between webs, iron and postcricoid carcinoma. *Postgrad Med J* 1974;50:215–219.

44. Bredenkamp JK, Castro DJ, Mickel RA. Importance of iron repletion in the management of Plummer-Vinson syndrome. *Ann Otol Rhinol Laryngol* 1990;99:51–54.

45. Okamura H, Tsutsumi S, Inaki S, *et al.* Esophageal web in Plummer–Vinson syndrome. *Laryngoscope* 1988;98:994–998.

46. Malecki D, Cameron AJ. Plummer–Vinson syndrome associated with chronic blood loss anemia and large diaphragmatic hernia. *Am J Gastroenterol* 2002;97:190–193.

47. Chen TSN, Chen PSY. Rise and fall of the Plummer–Vinson syndrome. *J Gastroenterol Hepatol* 1994;9:654–658.

48. Larsson L-G, Sandstom A, Westling P. Relationship of Plummer-Vinson disease to cancer of the upper alimentary tract in Sweden. *Cancer Res* 1975;35:3308–3316.

49. Elwood PC, Jacobs A, Pitman RG, *et al*. Epidemiology of the Paterson–Kelly syndrome. *Lancet* 1964;2:716–720.

50. Nosher JL, Campbell WL, Seaman WB. The clinical significance of cervical esophageal and hypopharyngeal webs. *Diagn Radiol* 1975;117:45–47.

51. Mansell N, Jani P, Bailey CM. Plummer–Vinson syndrome-a rare presentation in a child. *J Laryngol Otol* 1999;113:475–476.

52. Crawford M, Jacobs A, Murphy B, *et al*. Paterson–Kelly syndrome in adolescence: a report of five cases. *Br Med J* 1965; 1:693–695.

53. Beyler AR, Yurdaydin C, Bahar K, *et al*. Dilation therapy of upper esophageal webs in two cases of Plummer-Vinson syndrome. *Endoscopy* 1996;28:260–267.

54. Entwhistle CC, Jacobs A. Histologic findings in the Paterson–Kelly syndrome. *J Clin Pathol* 1965;18:408–413.

55. Hoffman RM, Jaffe PE. Plummer-Vinson syndrome. A case report and literature review. *Arch Intern Med* 1995;155:2008–2011.

56. Chisolm M, Ardan GM, Callander ST, *et al*. Iron deficiency anemia and autoimmunity in post cricoid webs. *Q J Med* 1971;40:421–433.

57. Dejmkova H, Pavelka K. An unusual clinical manifestation of secondary Sjögren's syndrome and concomitant Paterson-Kelly syndrome. *Clin Rheumatol* 1994;13:305–308.

58. Rashid Z, Kumar A, Komar M. Plummer–Vinson syndrome and postcricoid carcinoma: late complications of unrecognized celiac disease. *Am J Gastroenterol* 1999;94:1991.

59. Dickey W, McConnell B. Celiac disease presenting as the Paterson–Brown Kelly (Plummer-Vinson) syndrome. *Am J Gastroenterol* 1999;94:527–529.

60. Geerlings SE, Statios van Eps LW. Pathogenesis and consequences of Plummer–Vinson syndrome. *Clin Invest* 1992;70:629–630.

61. Dantas RO, Villanova MG. Esophageal motility impairment in Plummer-Vinson syndrome. Correction by iron treatment. *Dig Dis Sci* 1993;38:968–971.

62. Beyler AR, Yurdaydin C, Bahar K, *et al*. Dilation therapy of upper esophageal webs in two cases of Plummer-Vinson syndrome. *Endoscopy* 1996;28:266–267.

63. Templeton FE. X-ray examination of the stomach. In: *A Description of the Roentgenologic Anatomy, Physiology and Pathology of the Esophagus, Stomach and Duodenum*. Chicago: University of Chicago Press, 1944, pp. 94–102.

64. Schatzki R, Gary JE. Dysphagia due to diaphragm-like narrowing in lower esophagus ("lower esophageal ring"). *Am J Roentgennol Radiat Ther Nucl Med* 1953;70:911–922.

65. Ingelfinger FJ, Kramer P. Dysphagia produced by contractile ring in lower esophagus. *Gastroenterology* 1953;23:419.

66. Kramer P. Frequency of the asymptomatic lower esophageal contractile ring. *N Engl J Med* 1956;254:692–694.

67. Keyting WJ, Baker G, McCarver RR, Daywitt AL. The lower esophagus. *AJR Am J Roentgenol* 1960;84:1070–1075.

68. Schatzki R. The lower esophageal ring. Long-term follow-up of symptomatic and asymptomatic rings. *AJR Am J Roentgenol* 1963;90:805–810.

69. Goyal RK, Glancy JJ, Spiro HM. Lower esophageal ring. *N Engl J Med* 1970;282:1298–1305.

70. Wilcox CM, Alexander LN, Clark WS. Localization of an obstructing esophageal lesion. Is the patient accurate? *Dig Dis Sci* 1995;40:2192–2196.

71. Postlewait RW, Musser AW. Pathology of the lower esophageal web. *Surg Gynecol Obstet* 1965;120:571.

72. Vansant JH. Surgical significance of the lower esophageal ring. *Ann Surg* 1972;175:733–739.

73. Eastridge CE, Pate JW, Mann JA. Lower esophageal ring: experiences in treatment of 88 patients. *Ann Thorac Surg* 1984; 37:103–107.

74. Steinnon OA. The anatomic basis for the lower esophageal contraction ring : plication theory and its application. *Am J Roentgenol Radiat Ther Nucl Med* 1963;90:811.

75. Nurko S, Teitelbaum JE, Husain K, *et al*. Association of Schatzki ring with eosinophilic esophagitis in children. *J Pediatr Gastroenterol Nutr* 2004;38:436–441.

76. Marshall JB, Kretschmar JM, Diaz-Arias AA. Gastroesophageal reflux as a pathogenic factor in the development of lower esophageal rings. *Arch Intern Med* 1990;150:1669–1672.

77. Lovy MR, Levine JS, Steigerwald JC. Lower esophageal rings as a cause of dysphagia in progressive systemic sclerosis – coincidence or consequence. *Dig Dis Sci* 1983;28:780–783.

78. Ott DJ, Gelfand DW Wu WC, *et al*. Esophagogastric region and its rings. *AJR Am J Roentgenol* 1984;142:281–287.

79. Miller S, Hines C, Ochsner JL. Spontaneous perforation of the esophagus associated with a lower esophageal ring. *Am J Gastroenterol* 1988;83:1405–1408.

80. Stadler J, Hölscher AH, Feussner H, Dittler J, Siewert JR. "The steakhouse syndrome". Primary and definitive diagnosis and therapy". *Surg Endosc* 1989;3:195–198.

81. Norton RA, King GD "Steakhouse syndrome": the symptomatic lower esophageal ring. *Lahey Clin Found Bull* 1963;13:55–59.

82. Palmer ED. Backyard barbecue syndrome. *JAMA* 1976; 235:2637–2638.

83. Ott DJ, Chen YM, Wu WC, *et al*. Radiographic and endoscopic sensitivity in detecting lower esophageal mucosal ring. *AJR Am J Roentgenol* 1986;147:261–265.

84. Eckardt VF, Kanzler G, Willems D. Single dilation of symptomatic Schatzki rings. A prospective evaluation of its effectiveness. *Dig Dis Sci* 1992;37:577–582.

85. Groskreutz JL, Kim CH. Schatzki's ring: long-term results following dilation. *Gastrointest Endosc* 1990;36:479–481.

86. Sgouros SN, Vlachogiannakos J, Karamanolis G, *et al*. Long-term acid suppressive therapy may prevent the relapse of lower esophageal (Schatzki's) rings: A prospective, randomized, placebo-controlled study. *Am J Gastroenterol* 2005;100:1929–1934.

87. Chen YM, Gelfand DW, Ott DJ, *et al*. Natural progression of the lower esophageal mucosal ring. *Gastrointest Radiol* 1987; 12:93–98.

88. Burdick JS, Venu RP, Hogan WJ. Cutting the defiant lower esophageal ring. *Gastrointest Endosc* 1993;39:616–619.

89. Raskin JB, Manten H, Harary A, *et al*. Transendoscopic electrosurgical incision of lower esophageal (Schatzki) rings: A new treatment modality. *Gastrointest Endosc* 1985;31:391.

90. Groskreutz JL, Kim CH. Late results in patients with Schatzki ring treated by endoscopic electrosurgical incision of the ring. *Gastrointest Endosc* 1987;33:96.

91. Chotiprasidhi P, Minocha A. Effectiveness of single dilation with Maloney dilator versus endoscopic rupture of Schatzki's ring using biopsy forceps. *Dig Dis Sci* 2000;45:281–284.

92. Vicari JJ, Johanson JF, Frakes JT Outcomes of acute esophageal food impaction: success of the push technique. *Gastrointest Endosc* 2001;53:178–181.

93. Arvanitakis C. Lower esophageal ring: endoscopic and therapeutic aspects. *Gastrointest Endosc* 1977;24:17–18.

17 Esophageal Diverticula

Francisco J. Marrero[1] and Edgar Achkar[2]
[1]Digestive Health Center, Lake Charles, LA, USA
[2]The Cleveland Clinic Foundation, Cleveland, OH, USA

Introduction

An esophageal diverticulum is a sac that protrudes from the esophageal wall. As in the rest of the gastrointestinal tract, a true diverticulum is one that contains all layers of the wall. A false diverticulum consists of mucosa, submucosa, and a few muscle fibers. Esophageal diverticula can be classified in many ways. They can be divided into congenital and acquired based on origin, into pulsion and traction based on etiology, or into false or true based on histology; but the simplest and most practical way is to classify them according to anatomy, into four categories: Zenker's (hypopharyngeal) diverticula, mid-esophageal diverticula; epiphrenic diverticula; and intramural pseudodiverticulosis.

Esophageal diverticula have been described in all age groups, but they are most commonly seen in adults. Esophageal diverticula are rare, occurring in fewer than 1% of upper gastrointestinal roentgenograms and accounting for fewer than 5% of dysphagia cases [1].

Esophageal diverticula are often associated with motor abnormalities of the esophagus, but the belief that all diverticula are due to a motor disorder of the esophagus is not established with certainty.

Zenker's diverticulum

Zenker's diverticulum, also called *pharyngoesophageal diverticulum*, is described as an esophageal pouch. In fact, this type of diverticulum occurs in a location proximal to the esophagus, above the upper esophageal sphincter (UES), and should be considered as a hypopharyngeal diverticulum.

The first report of hypopharyngeal pulsion diverticulum was published in 1764 by Abraham Ludlow. In 1867, Freidrich Albert Zenker published a monograph reviewing all previously documented cases of hypopharyngeal diverticula and this is how his name became attached to the lesion [2].

In Zenker's diverticulum, the pharyngeal constrictor muscles form a funnel, and the mouth of the esophagus is like a transverse slit at the bottom of this funnel. At endoscopy, the larynx with its moving vocal cords is in the center, the pyriform sinuses are lateral, and the esophageal opening appears as a posterior slit. The fibers of the cricopharyngeus muscle run transversely and form the UES at the esophageal inlet. Above the cricopharyngeus muscle, the walls of the hypopharynx contain oblique fibers of the inferior constrictor muscles. Between the transverse fibers of the cricopharyngeus muscle below and the oblique fibers of the inferior constrictors above, a triangular area containing fewer muscle fibers constitutes a region of relative weakness and is referred to as the triangle of Killian or Killian's dehiscence (Figure 17.1). The mucosa of the hypopharynx is allowed to bulge posteriorly at Killian's triangle, and with time, a pouch may develop, forming a Zenker's diverticulum.

Etiology and pathogenesis

Several mechanisms have been invoked to explain the pathogenesis of Zenker's diverticulum, but none of them has been definitely proven. Age may play a role in the development of Zenker's diverticulum. A decrease in tissue elasticity leading to an increased weakness of the triangle of Killian may explain why Zenker's diverticulum is rarely seen in individuals younger than 40 years. Additionally, the prevalence of Zenker's diverticulum increases in the elderly, reaching 50% in the seventh and eight decades of life, particularly in women [3].

The most widely accepted mechanism for Zenker's diverticulum is a functional disturbance of the hypopharynx, such as increased resting pressure of the sphincter, lack of complete sphincter relaxation or incoordination between the sphincter and the hypopharynx. The UES is formed mainly by the cricopharyngeus muscle, with participation from fibers from the inferior portion of the inferior pharyngeal constrictors and some fibers of the cervical esophagus. The sphincter is shaped like a slit, not a circle, leading to

The Esophagus, Fifth Edition. Edited by Joel E. Richter, Donald O. Castell.
© 2012 Blackwell Publishing Ltd. Published 2012 by Blackwell Publishing Ltd.

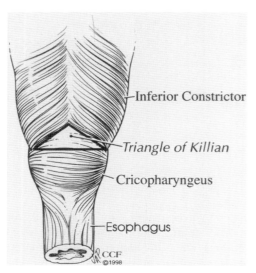

Figure 17.1 Triangle of Killian, an area of weakness that allows Zenker's diverticulum to develop.

marked radial asymmetry during tonic contractions. Normally, the UES is closed during tonic contraction and, immediately after a swallow, excitation of the muscle stops transiently and the UES relaxes, allowing passage of the bolus into the upper esophagus. UES function is under the influence of bolus volume as well as the nature of the upper esophageal contents [4, 5].

Traditionally, the most frequently proposed motility cause for a hypopharyngeal diverticulum is premature closure of the UES during swallowing, as shown by Ellis *et al.* [6]. The concept of *cricopharyngeal achalasia*, that is, failure of the sphincter to relax on time, was accepted for a long time as the reason for the development of Zenker's diverticula. Achalasia was demonstrated with the help of pharyngographs by Asherson in 1950 [7], and other authors, such as Sutherland [8], perpetuated this theory. Nilsson *et al.* studied 10 patients with symptomatic hypopharyngeal diverticulum using simultaneous radiography and manometry [8]. Pressures were measured using triple microtransducers, allowing the authors to measure pressures at three levels of the UES, including the level immediately below the neck of the diverticulum. Cineradiography used simultaneously provided a correlation between the pressures generated and the passage of contrast material. Results showed that below the entrance of the diverticulum the sphincter pressure exceeded UES resting pressure as the bolus entered the pharynx. The authors concluded that this phenomenon represented incoordination. They also found within the UES, during swallowing, double pressure peaks, which they called a "split UES." These results were not found in all patients, and no asymptomatic controls were used. Nevertheless, Nilsson *et al.* explained the pathogenesis of Zenker's diverticulum by pressures on the pharyngeal wall from the bolus

forced against a contracted UES [9]. Knuff *et al.* compared nine patients with Zenker's diverticulum, with a mean age of 60 years, to a control group of 15 patients matched for age [10]. Manometric measurements were obtained using a water-perfused system, which produces less reliable measurements than microtransducers. The tracings were analyzed into four time intervals, and the relationship of pharyngeal contractions to UES relaxation was studied and no difference between the two groups was found. However, the mean resting UES resting pressure was found to be significantly lower in patients with Zenker's diverticulum compared to those without. The authors had no explanation for the low resting pressure. Because of the absence of abnormal cricopharyngeal coordination, they questioned the concept that the diverticulum is the result of incomplete relaxation of the UES.

The notion of pharyngoesophageal incoordination or achalasia was contradicted further by Cook *et al.*, who studied 14 patients with diverticula and nine healthy, age-matched controls using simultaneous videoradiography and manometry [11]. Manometric studies were obtained with a sleeve catheter equipped with metallic markers, allowing exact localization of the recording sites during radiography. There was no difference between patients and controls in timing of pharyngeal contractions and sphincter relaxation. However, the authors found a significantly reduced sphincter opening associated with greater intrabolus pressure, suggesting an impairment of UES opening. The authors concluded that Zenker's diverticulum is a disorder of long-standing diminished UES opening with increased hypopharyngeal pressures, eventually causing formation of the diverticulum. They dispelled the notion that UES opening is impaired by pharyngoesophageal incoordination or lack of sphincter relaxation. A histologic study carried out by the same group [12] seems to support the concept of diminished UES opening. Muscle strips were obtained from 14 patients with Zenker's diverticulum during surgical myotomy. Tissue was also obtained from 10 control patients without history of dysphagia, nine from autopsy and one from a patient with laryngeal cancer. Of the 14 patients with Zenker's diverticulum, 10 showed greater than 50% replacement of cricopharyngeal muscle fibers by fibrous adipose tissue. None of the controls showed similar findings. The authors thought that degenerative changes may account for the abnormality observed in patients with Zenker's diverticulum. Muscle degeneration would prevent the sphincter from opening completely because of decreased elasticity, while normally the UES should relax during normal swallowing as a result of external traction and propulsive forces within the sphincter. Lerut *et al.* obtained biopsy specimens from 62 patients with Zenker's diverticulum and compared them to tissue obtained from 15 controls [13]. Histologic and immunochemical studies were carried out on most specimens and contractility studies on all specimens of cricopharyngeus

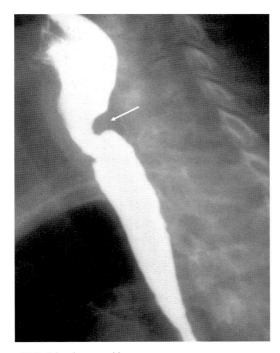

Figure 17.2 Cricopharyngeal bar.

muscles. Reduced amplitude and lower contractions were found in eight patients with Zenker's diverticulum and not in the controls. Neurogenic and myogenic abnormalities were also found on histologic examination. Some of the histologic changes may be due to local ischemia caused by traction and compression of the UES by the pouch [14].

A study of another condition thought to be due to cricopharyngeal spasm or achalasia may shed some light on the pathogenesis of Zenker's diverticulum. A cricopharyngeal bar (Figure 17.2), which is detected as a marked indentation on esophagram, was also thought to be due to incoordination.

Dantas *et al.* studied patients with cricopharyngeal bars who had a prominent indentation during radiography but in whom no diverticulum could be elicited [15]. Six patients with bars underwent concurrent fluoroscopic and manometric examination of the pharynx and UES, as did eight volunteers. Patients with bars were found to have smaller openings of the UES during swallowing and increased intrabolus pressure when compared to controls. These findings indicate reduced muscle compliance, preventing total relaxation of the cricopharyngeus. No evidence of spasm could be found and sphincter relaxation was complete during manometry. Studies such as this one and others performed on patients with Zenker's diverticulum indicate that there is little scientific data to support using the term *cricopharyngeal achalasia* to describe these disorders. Although no single pathogenic mechanism for the development of Zenker's diverticulum has been established, it appears that

reduced UES compliance rather than cricopharyngeal incoordination accounts for the genesis of the pouch. The consistent finding in recent studies is increased intrabolus pressure in patients with Zenker's diverticulum [16].

Gastroesophageal reflux has also been implicated in the genesis of Zenker's diverticulum. It was suggested that acid reflux leads to cricopharyngeal spasm and that eventually a pharyngoesophageal diverticulum will develop [17]. The UES is responsive to infusion of solutions in the esophagus and has been shown to react to the presence of acid. Gerhardt *et al.* studied nine normal subjects, infusing different solutions in the esophagus [4]. When 0.1 normal HCl was infused in the upper esophagus, high UES pressures were produced when compared to infusion of normal saline. Additionally, an increase in the rate of infusion resulted in further increases in pressure. These findings suggest that the UES acts as a barrier to acid reflux, possibly preventing aspiration. However, Vakil *et al.* found that esophageal acid exposure did not affect UES pressure in normal volunteers or in patients with esophagitis [18]. Although gastroesophageal reflux can result in throat symptoms, such as cough, hoarseness, and globus, as well as the lesion of posterior laryngitis, it is not known if anatomic abnormalities such as Zenker's diverticulum can result from chronic gastroesophageal reflux. Hunt *et al.* found a greater resting UES pressure in patients with reflux esophagitis than in controls. In five patients with Zenker's diverticulum, the UES pressure was also elevated, but there was no evidence of reflux esophagitis [17]. Others have tried using the presence of a hiatal hernia to establish a link between reflux and Zenker's diverticulum. Gage-White showed a 39% occurrence of hiatal hernia in patients with Zenker's diverticulum compared to 16% in controls, suggesting that the two disorders may be due to a common pathophysiologic phenomenon [19]. Resouly *et al.* reported an increased occurrence of reflux symptoms in patients with pharyngeal pouches, but did not show any objective results [20]. Some authors argue that there is no solid evidence that a direct relationship exists between Zenker's diverticulum and gastroesophageal reflux disease [3, 21]. Sasaki *et al.* theorized that acid-induced mucosal injury causes esophageal shortening thus weakening the space between pharyngeal constrictors which are anchored to the prevertebral fascia via a median raphe and the cricopharyngeus which has no anchoring raphe. This allows the cricopharyngeal muscle to be displaced inferiorly as the esophagus undergoes long axis shortening, eventually leading to a pouch [22]. This hypothesis has no supporting evidence. Nevertheless, should patients with Zenker's diverticulum exhibit symptoms of heartburn or chest pain, they should be studied for the presence of acid reflux. However, we cannot yet support aggressive medical or surgical treatment of reflux disease as a way to avoid the development of Zenker's diverticulum, or establish that the presence of a diverticulum is indicative of acid reflux.

Clinical features

Many pharyngoesophageal diverticula are asymptomatic and discovered by chance during radiologic evaluation. In general, symptoms of Zenker's diverticulum depend upon the stage of the disease. In the early phase, patients may complain only of a sensation of sticking in the throat or of vague irritation. They may also report intermittent cough, excessive salivation, and intermittent dysphagia, usually to solid foods. Some patients may present with such minor symptoms that they are dismissed as having "globus." Because of the vagueness of their symptoms, these patients are often labeled as *globus hystericus,* an unfortunate term since some patients with globus turn out to have a significant pathology such as reflux, diverticula, or other disorders of the voluntary phase of swallowing.

When the sac becomes large, more severe symptoms may develop. Dysphagia becomes more frequent. Regurgitation of food ingested several hours earlier is reported, and gurgling sounds may occur upon swallowing. Patients learn to use special maneuvers to empty the pouch by pressing on the neck or coughing and clearing the throat. In rare cases, the pouch is so large that it obstructs the esophagus, but more frequently a bulging in the left side of the neck takes place. Pulmonary aspiration leading to pneumonia or lung abscess may occur, but is rather infrequent [23].

Rare complications of Zenker's diverticulum have been described. Hendren *et al.* reported massive bleeding in a diverticulum [24]. Obstruction and tracheodiverticular fistula are rare. Isolated cases of squamous cell carcinoma associated with Zenker's diverticulum have been reported [25, 26]. In large series, the occurrence of carcinoma appears to be low; at the Mayo Clinic over a 53-year period, cancer was found in only 0.4% of 1249 patients [27]. The diagnosis of cancer is rarely made clinically and is suspected usually because of a defect on X-ray [25]. Most patients with carcinoma report additional symptoms, such as weight loss and increasingly worsening dysphagia. Cancer appears to be more frequent in men and in longstanding cases. Because of the long period of time between the discovery of a diverticulum and the occurrence of a carcinoma, it is speculated that cancer results from chronic irritation and inflammation of the diverticulum due to stasis. The frequency of carcinoma arising in Zenker's diverticulum has been less in recent years, perhaps because of earlier diagnosis and treatment. Bowdler and Stell reviewed this issue in 1987, finding only 38 cases in the English literature [26]. Most of the cancers in these reports were squamous cell carcinoma, with an occasional basal cell or spindle cell carcinoma. Bradley *et al.* reviewed 91 cases of Zenker's diverticulum seen over a period of 15 years and found two cases of squamous cell carcinoma and two of carcinoma *in situ* [28]. In three of the cases, the cancer was not found until histologic examination was performed post diverticulectomy. Since the authors believe that malignant transformation results from chronic irritation, they advocate excision of the pouch in patients younger than 65 in an attempt to avoid progression to cancer. Overall, the frequency of carcinoma arising in Zenker's diverticulum is not high enough by itself to justify surgery. From a practical standpoint, the decision to treat is based on the severity of symptoms.

Diagnosis

A barium esophagram with special attention to the oropharyngeal phase of swallowing is the best diagnostic test for Zenker's diverticulum. Small diverticula may be missed, but careful evaluation with lateral and oblique views will detect even small pouches. The diverticulum protrudes posteriorly, and barium tends to fall into the pouch before progressing into the esophagus (Figure 17.3). In the case of a very small diverticulum, the sac may be visible only during the phase of UES contraction and not during relaxation. Some authors have tried to classify Zenker's diverticula according to stage or categories based on the size and shape of the diverticulum, as well as the presence during contraction or relaxation of the UES. Ponette and Coolen reviewed 143 patients with diverticula and attempted to relate the morphology of the pouch to upper sphincter function [29]. These efforts to grade Zenker's diverticula based on shape and size result from the fact that barium studies will sometimes reveal a temporary posterior bulge at the level of or just above the UES. The bulge is not large enough and consistent enough through the study to be referred to as a diverticulum, and terms such as *transient diverticulum* and *early diverticulum* have been used [3]. Whether such changes represent a diverticulum or a manifestation of a cricopharyngeal bar, which can be seen in association with a diverticulum (Figure 17.4), or simply a trivial phenomenon is unknown. At any rate, such observations are of limited clinical importance and one must be guided by the patient's complaints. It is doubtful that a transient posterior bulge would cause significant throat symptoms, and if dysphagia is truly present, a more careful evaluation of the entire esophagus must be undertaken.

There is an area of weakness, distinct from Killian's triangle, located just below the cricopharyngeal muscle, called the Killian–Jamieson space [30]. Protrusions through this area of weakness are rare, but when they occur, they may be confused with a Zenker's diverticulum. However, a Killian–Jamieson diverticulum arises from the lateral wall, below the UES, and tends to be small (Figure 17.5). Patients with Killian–Jamieson pouches are usually asymptomatic. Rubisin and Levin found that three of 16 patients with Killian–Jamieson diverticula had symptoms; dysphagia in two and cough in one [31]. In contrast, 19 of 26 patients with Zenker's diverticula had symptoms.

Endoscopy adds very little to the evaluation of pharyngoesophageal pouches. If it has to be performed for other reasons, caution should be exercised to not enter the diverticulum and risk a perforation [32]. A large diverticulum

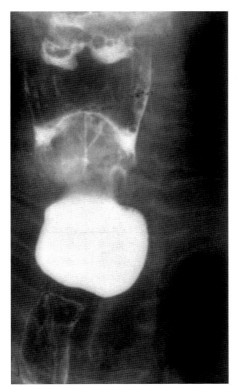 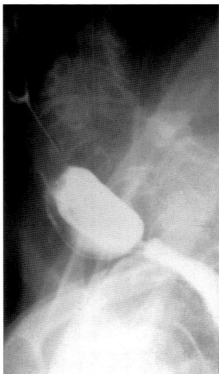

Figure 17.3 Zenker's diverticulum, anteroposterior and lateral views.

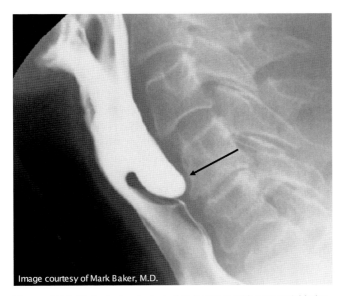

Image courtesy of Mark Baker, M.D.

Figure 17.4 Marked cricopharyngeal indentation with a posterial bulge (arrow), most likely representing a Zenker's diverticulum.

may make esophageal intubation difficult. Sometimes a guidewire may need to be passed into the stomach under fluoroscopy, with the endoscope then carefully passed over the guidewire.

Manometric testing of UES function has been recently refined, and accurate measurements with analysis of various phases of deglutition are possible [33]. However, the technique is of little value in the management of patients. Furthermore, manometry may be difficult to perform as the manometric catheter tends to coil in the diverticulum. There have been reports of low resting pressure of the sphincter [10, 34], as well as normal basal pressures [11] in patients with Zenker's diverticulum. The finding of cricopharyngeal incoordination is inconsistent, as discussed above in the section on pathogenesis. Manometric testing of the cricopharyngeal area should be reserved for clinical research and is not necessary in evaluating patients with pharyngeal pouches [35].

Treatment

Small Zenker's diverticula discovered by chance do not require any intervention and may be followed by periodic esophagrams. When needed, the only effective treatment of Zenker's diverticulum is surgical. Surgical techniques include, separately or in combination, diverticulopexy, diverticulectomy, and cricopharyngeal myotomy. Endoscopic treatment is emerging as an alternative to open surgery.

In the early 1900s, diverticulopexy became popular because attempts to excise the diverticulum in the 1800s were not encouraging. In diverticulopexy, the fundus of the

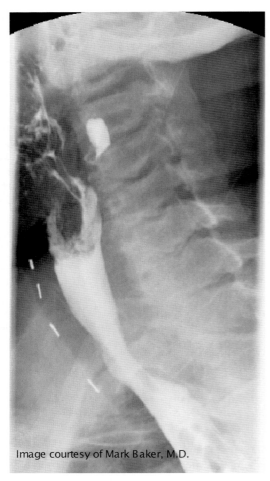

Image courtesy of Mark Baker, M.D.

Figure 17.5 Killian–Jamieson diverticulum. The pouch arises from the lateral esophageal wall below the upper esophageal sphincter.

diverticulum is attached high up in the neck to the prevertebral fascia after being dissected from surrounding tissues. By attaching the fundus of the diverticulum high in the neck, drainage is allowed to occur. A two-stage operation was also developed in which the diverticulum was ligated and an ostomy performed to allow drainage. In a second stage, the diverticulum was then resected. Various modifications to this operation were made to avoid infection and other complications. Today, diverticulopexy alone is rarely performed, while it is used sometimes in association with a myotomy. Diverticulectomy and myotomy, separately or together, constitute the most traditional approach to surgical treatment of Zenker's diverticulum [36]. At the Mayo Clinic, a one-stage pharyngoesophageal diverticulectomy with or without myotomy produced excellent results, with only a 3.6% recurrence rate [37]. In an updated report in 1992, Payne described his experience with over 900 patients treated for Zenker's diverticulum [38]. Mortality was low at 1.2%, morbidity was 8%, and the rate of recurrence was

still 3.6%. In the interval between the two reports, however, the surgical technique had varied from simple diverticulectomy to diverticulectomy associated with myotomy and, in some cases, myotomy alone without resection. Additionally, a mechanical stapling device was used in some cases. Therefore, it is difficult to conclude, based on this report, what is the single best technique to treat Zenker's diverticulum. When the diverticulum recurs, reoperation presents major technical difficulties, complications are more frequent, and mortality rises to 3.2% [39].

The open surgical technique involves usually a left cervical incision. The diverticulum once identified is retracted, dissected, and eventually resected, and the point of insertion either sutured or stapled. When a myotomy is performed, it is done either before [40] or after [41] the diverticulectomy. Myotomy is extramucosal, dissecting the fibers of the cricopharyngeal muscles away from the mucosa. The incision is extended 3–4 cm above the esophagus. Fegiz *et al.* reported 15 patients with Zenker's diverticulum [41]. Twelve were treated by resection only and three by resection and myotomy. The result was good in all three patients treated with a combined procedure. In the 12 treated by resection alone, results were good in eight and fair in three, with recurrence in one. Ellis and Crozier treated 10 patients, three of whom had undergone a diverticulotomy earlier [42]. Cricopharyngeal myotomy was performed in all patients, but diverticulectomy was performed in only two and diverticulopexy in one. There were no complications and follow-up showed good results in all patients. Lerut *et al.* justified the need to perform a cricopharyngeal myotomy by the pathophysiologic changes present in patients with Zenker's diverticulum [13]. They asked two questions: Is a myotomy of the cricopharyngeus useful? How long should it be? The finding of abnormal contractility and abnormal histology led them to advocate the use of myotomy, emphasizing that the incision should be no less than 4–5 cm long. These authors reported 100 consecutive patients treated by myotomy and in the majority of cases, diverticulopexy. The mean follow-up was 4 years and morbidity was minimal. Schmit and Zuckerbraun performed cricopharyngeal myotomy alone under local anesthesia [43]. Good results occurred in 70% of patients and fair results in 17%. Because of these favorable results, they concluded that the operation under local anesthesia without resecting the diverticulum was safe and effective even though the size of the diverticulum had a mean of 3.3 cm with a range of 1–8 cm. It should be noted that patient follow-up was conducted by telephone and direct contact was possible in only 63%. Diverticulectomy with cricopharyngeal myotomy achieves good results, but the physiologic consequences of this anatomic disruption have not been rigorously analyzed. A videofluoroscopic study of 15 patients treated surgically showed that the process of swallowing becomes abnormal following surgery [44]. Among the changes observed are pooling of contrast material, aspiration, and premature closure of the cricopharyngeus muscle. In this study, seven patients reported absence of symptoms after surgery, while six had mild residual dysphagia, one reported no difference, and one felt that the symptoms were worse than preoperatively. There was no significant difference in the number of abnormalities recorded postoperatively between asymptomatic and symptomatic patients. Shaw *et al.* studied eight patients pre- and post-operatively and showed that cricopharyngeal myotomy normalized UES opening by reducing hypopharyngeal intrabolus pressure [45]. Zaninotto *et al.* showed a significant decrease in UES resting pressure and pharyngeal intrabolus pressure after myotomy [46].

Open surgical treatment of Zenker's diverticulum may result in complications such as fistulae, infection, vocal cord paralysis, and aspiration [38, 39, 43]. A technique of inversion of the diverticulum resulting in invagination rather than excision has been advocated to avoid complications [47]. This technique is reserved for small diverticula and can be carried out in a short period of time. However, some authors disagree with its usefulness [48]. Other technical variations have also been suggested, such as the use of myotomy, diverticulectomy, and cervical esophagostomy with a feeding tube for the ostomy and removal of the feeding tube with closure of the esophagostomy in a second stage. This operation is advocated for severely debilitated patients [49].

Zenker's diverticulum may be treated endoscopically. Multiple reports have originated from non-US centers [50]. Endoscopic treatment of pharyngeal pouches was tried without success in the early 1900s. In 1960, a technique using a rigid esophagoscope with a double lip was established. The endoscope is positioned so it rides over the bridge between the diverticulum and the esophageal lumen. This wall and the cricopharyngeus muscle are then transected at the same time, creating a communication between the diverticulum and the esophagus. In other words, rather than resecting or draining the diverticulum, a common cavity is created and the diverticulum now drains openly into the esophagus. Van Overbeek and Hoeksema, from The Netherlands, reported 211 cases in whom a satisfactory rate of 91.5% was found with few complications [51]. The technique may be modified by using laser treatment for transection of the ridge rather than electrocoagulation [52, 53]. Benjamin and Innocenti treated 15 patients with a microsurgical laser procedure [54]. A minor leak occurred in two patients only, and they responded to conservative treatment. Long-term results in this series appeared favorable, although no details were given on follow-up. Wouters and van Overbeek compared their earlier experience with endoscopic electrocoagulation in 323 cases to the microendoscopic CO_2 laser treatment of 184 cases [55]. They found the results to be comparable, but thought that the laser technique produced less pain and allowed the patients to eat

earlier. Kos *et al.* reported good results in 229 patients treated with endoscopic diverticulotomy with electrocautery (EDE) or one of two forms of CO_2 laser [56].

Another modification to the endoscopic treatment of Zenker's diverticulum involves the use of staples [57]. An endoscopic stapler is used to divide the wall between the diverticulum and the esophagus, sealing the cut mucosal edges and preventing postoperative salivary leakage [58]. Results of this technique appear favorable with good symptom relief and patient satisfaction [58, 59]. Stapling is not possible in all cases because of inability to expose the esophagus and the diverticulum simultaneously [60]. Altman *et al.* reported on the use of a flexible fiberoptic endoscope and an overtube in five patients in whom a rigid laryngoscope could not be positioned in the diverticulum [61]. Treatment was successful in all patients. While the operative cost of endoscopic stapling diverticulectomy is comparable to that of the open technique, the overall cost is less and the hospital stay shorter [62].

It is extremely difficult to conclude from reviewing the literature which operation constitutes the best treatment for Zenker's diverticulum. The inclusion of patients with Zenker's diverticulum as well as cricopharyngeal achalasia, neurologic disorders, and other abnormalities; the variations in technique; the use of historic controls; and the lack of consistent and objectively structured follow-up are some of the reasons for the confusion. At this point, it appears that endoscopic treatment with or without laser or stapling is gaining popularity in the United States [58, 60, 63]. In spite of the debate over the need for myotomy, most surgeons continue to perform it while excising the diverticulum, unless it is very small. No causal relationship has been established between gastroesophageal reflux and Zenker's diverticulum. Antireflux surgery is therefore only appropriate when reflux is symptomatic [21, 64].

Mid-esophageal diverticula

Mid-esophageal diverticula are given this name to distinguish them from epiphrenic diverticula, which occur in the most distal part of the esophagus, and because most diverticula are found in the mid portion of the esophagus.

Etiology and pathogenesis

It is not known whether mid-esophageal diverticula are congenital. Most appear to develop in young and older adults. The development of esophageal diverticula in general has traditionally been explained by one of two mechanisms: traction or pulsion. This distinction was made in 1840 by Rokitansky [65]. A traction diverticulum is characteristically situated in the middle third of the esophagus and is thought to develop as a result of pulling of the esophageal wall by neighboring inflammatory or scar tissue. Therefore, a traction diverticulum is a true one as all layers of the esophagus are pulled out. A pulsion diverticulum, on the other hand, is thought to occur because of abnormal forces applied to a portion of the esophageal wall, resulting in an outpouching of mucosa through the muscle layer of the esophagus [66]. Zenker's diverticulum would be an example of pulsion diverticulum and so would the epiphrenic diverticulum, which will be discussed later. Mid-esophageal diverticula, based on this classification, could be of the traction or pulsion type.

Cross *et al.* showed that most esophageal diverticula occur because of an area of spasm or lack of sphincter relaxation; they found motor abnormalities even in cases of isolated mid-thoracic diverticulum [67]. Esophageal diverticula, which may be multiple, have been described in patients with achalasia, diffuse esophageal spasm, or other motor abnormalities [68]. Schima *et al.* studied 30 patients with mid-esophageal diverticula, some of which they considered to be of the pulsion type and some of the traction type [69]. Dysphagia was present in 22 patients. Esophageal manometry was performed in only 15 patients, but by associating cinefluoroscopy and manometry, the authors found a motor abnormality in 24 of 30 patients. Evander *et al.* reported 10 patients with motor abnormalities. Eight of these had epiphrenic diverticula [70]. The two patients with mid-esophageal diverticula had no abnormality in the lower esophageal sphincter (LES) function, but showed occasional simultaneous or repetitive contractions in the thoracic esophagus. An important study was carried out by Dodds *et al.* in 1975, who attempted to determine the importance of motor abnormalities in the genesis of mid-esophageal diverticula [71]. The authors purposely chose six patients who had no evidence of esophageal motor disorder by radiology and manometry. Pressures were measured by four recording ports positioned radially around the lumen. In five of six patients, the orifice facing the mouth of the diverticulum recorded a lower pressure than the other three ports. In two patients, bizarre wave forms were seen with abrupt onset or offset of the contraction, and in two others, high peristaltic pressure amplitude greater than 250 mmHg was found in the distal half of the esophagus. The radial asymmetry at the level of the diverticulum was attributed to the presence of the diverticulum, the bizarre forms were attributed to longitudinal motion of the diverticulum during recording, and the high peristaltic pressure was thought to be the reason the diverticulum forces pushed out the esophageal wall. However, this study does not prove that weakness at one point of the esophageal wall is the reason for the occurrence of diverticula as the pressure could be the result rather than the cause of the outpouching.

Clinical features

Most mid-esophageal diverticula are asymptomatic (Figure 17.6). Indeed, the diverticulum tends to be small and points upward, making food accumulation rare. In some patients,

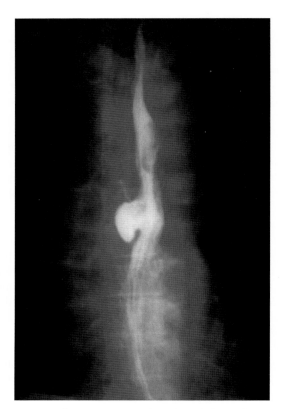

Figure 17.6 Small, asymptomatic mid-esophageal diverticulum.

chest pain and dysphagia are reported, but these are usually present in patients who have an esophageal motor disorder. Figure 17.7 illustrates a mid-esophageal diverticulum in a patient with diffuse esophageal spasm.

Gastroesophageal reflux is also noted in some patients with mid-esophageal diverticula [69]. Of the 30 patients studied by Schima *et al.* [69], five had gastroesophageal reflux [69].

Complications are unusual. Spontaneous rupture, exsanguination [72], aspiration [70, 73], fistula formation [74], and carcinoma [75] have been reported. These complications are usually seen in patients with motor disorders or when, in the distant past, traction diverticula were associated with pulmonary tuberculosis [66]. Inflammatory lymph nodes around the esophagus account for the outpouching of the tissue.

Atypical diverticula of the esophagus have been reported. Herman and McAlister found diverticula in two children who had developed strictures due to unsuspected foreign body ingestion [76]. Diverticula were present above the foreign body. Saccular dilatation was reported in a patient following excision of an asymptomatic congenital cyst [77] and may also be seen postoperatively after repair of an esophageal perforation or laceration. Intraluminal diverticula, which result in the appearance of a double esophageal lumen, are difficult to diagnose, may result in dysphagia or

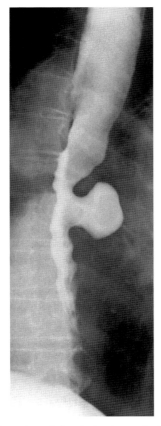

Figure 17.7 Mid-esophageal diverticulum in a patient with diffuse esophageal spasm.

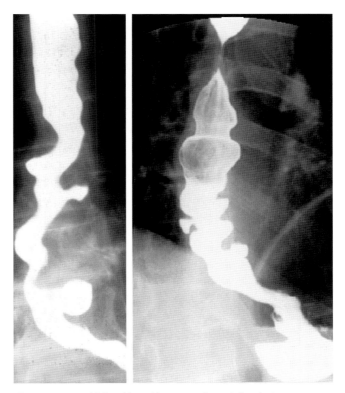

Figure 17.8 Multiple mid- and lower esophageal diverticula.

esophagitis, and are of unknown origin [78]. Finally, in progressive systemic sclerosis, pseudodiverticula of the esophagus may develop. Clements *et al.* reported five cases of unusual diverticula associated with progressive systemic sclerosis and other collagen vascular diseases [79]. Wide-mouthed saccular pouches were seen at various levels of the esophagus. Coggins *et al.* reported a similar case [80].

Diagnosis

Most mid-esophageal diverticula are discovered by chance during barium esophagram carried out for other reasons. Diverticula may be of various sizes and can be single or multiple [71, 81]. Figure 17.8 illustrates a case of multiple diverticula. In case of complication, radiology will determine the presence of a fistula. An intraluminal diverticulum may be missed on X-ray.

Endoscopy with today's flexible instruments is not contraindicated, but the procedure is not necessary for the diagnosis of diverticula.

Treatment

Since most mid-esophageal diverticula are uncomplicated and cause no symptoms, treatment is not required. If treat-

ment becomes necessary, the procedure of choice is diverticulectomy. It is imperative, however, to rule out an associated esophageal motility disorder before contemplating surgery. If a motor disorder is present, diverticulectomy alone may be followed by a recurrence of the diverticulum and symptoms would not be relieved [82]. Altorki *et al.* studied 20 patients with thoracic esophageal diverticula over a 20-year period and found that 45% had dysphagia, 55% regurgitation, and 25% pulmonary symptoms [73]. Seventeen patients agreed to the operation, with successful results. However, 18 of the 20 patients had an associated motor disorder, such as achalasia, diffuse esophageal spasm, Zenker's diverticulum, and other non-specific disorders.

Surgery is rarely necessary for mid-esophageal diverticula and, when indicated, is dictated by the presence of a motor abnormality or a complication [75]. Diverticulectomy with or without myotomy is the treatment of choice [65, 82]. Some surgeons add a fundoplication [70, 75].

Epiphrenic diverticula

As the name indicates, epiphrenic diverticula arise near the diaphragm (Figure 17.9). However, the epiphrenic segment of the esophagus has been defined by some as the distal 4 cm, by others as the distal 10 cm, and by others even as

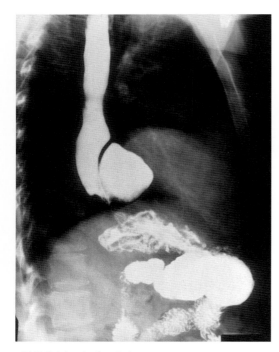

Figure 17.9 Epiphrenic diverticulum.

the distal one-third of the esophagus [83]. Most authors reserve the term *epiphrenic diverticulum* for those occurring in the distal 3–4 cm of the esophagus.

Etiology and pathogenesis

The issue of traction and pulsion diverticulum was discussed earlier. For a long time, epiphrenic diverticula were thought to be of the pulsion type and were therefore labeled as pseudodiverticula. Such considerations have little clinical relevance. The important issue is that epiphrenic diverticula are almost always the result of an esophageal motor abnormality, such as incoordination between the distal esophagus and the LES, or a more diffuse abnormality, such as achalasia or diffuse esophageal spasm.

The strong association between epiphrenic diverticula and motor abnormalities of the esophagus was noted even in early reports. Bruggeman and Seaman reported a motor abnormality in 48% of cases. It is probable that the proportion would have been higher had a method other than X-ray been used. In the same series, all patients with a diverticulum larger than 5 cm were found to have a significant abnormal motility disorder [83]. Debas *et al.* noted an abnormal motility disorder in 50 of 65 patients. This conclusion was reached based on manometry and roentgenology [84]. However, only 36 patients had complete motility studies. In the 15 patients who did not have an abnormal motility disorder, 13 had a hiatal hernia, five of whom had severe esophageal strictures. Tedesco *et al.* found an association

between epiphrenic diverticula and a motor disorder of the esophagus in 81% of 21 patients in a retrospective study [85]. D'Journo *et al.* found in a recent study that 20 of 23 patients had a spastic motor disorder of the esophagus and there was often evidence of LES abnormalities [86].

Clinical features

Epiphrenic diverticula occur at all ages. The series of Bruggeman and Seaman included 80 patients whose ages ranged from 18 to 88 years, with 75% being between 41 and 70 years old [83].

Although the exact incidence of epiphrenic diverticula is not known, the condition appears to be infrequent. In 20 years, 160 patients were reported from the Mayo Clinic [87], and 80 patients were seen over a period of 18 years at the Columbia Presbyterian Medical Center [83]. The frequency is estimated to be 20% that of Zenker's diverticula [88].

Patients with epiphrenic diverticula may be totally asymptomatic. Small diverticula may be discovered during an incidental roentgenographic examination. There appears to be no correlation between symptoms and size of the diverticulum. The presence and the severity of symptoms depend on the associated motor abnormality. It is imperative in patients with epiphrenic diverticula to obtain manometric studies to rule out a motility disorder. The most frequent abnormalities are achalasia and diffuse spasm [83, 84, 89], but other nonspecific abnormalities have been described as well [90]. Chest pain and regurgitation may also be presenting symptoms, particularly in giant diverticula [91]. Acute esophageal obstruction from food accumulating in the epiphrenic diverticulum has been reported [92]. Other complications are similar to those seen in mid-esophageal diverticula, such as perforation, fistula formation, and a rare case of carcinoma [93, 94].

Diagnosis

An epiphrenic diverticulum is easily diagnosed on a barium roentgenogram. Multiple views should be taken in different positions to evaluate the size of the diverticulum and the site of its mouth. A videoesophagram is helpful in subtle cases for identifying a motor abnormality. In patients with achalasia, the esophagus is tortuous and more than one diverticulum may be seen (Figure 17.10). On computed tomography (CT), a diverticulum will appear as a thin-walled or air–fluid-filled structure if an obstruction or motor disorder exists. The images may be confused with those of an abscess, tumor, or hiatal hernia [95].

Endoscopy, although not necessary, is helpful in diagnosing complications and esophageal inflammation. The procedure should be performed cautiously so that the endoscope does not inadvertently enter the cavity of the diverticulum.

Manometric studies are important to establish the presence of an associated motor abnormality. Usually, the area

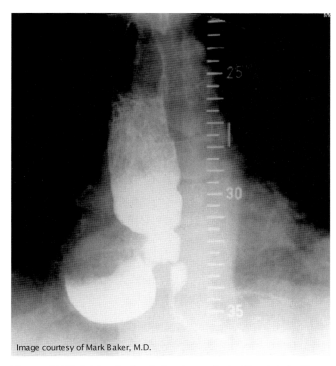

Image courtesy of Mark Baker, M.D.

Figure 17.10 Epiphrenic diverticulum in a patient with achalasia. The esophagus is dilated and tortuous, and other sacculations are seen.

of the diverticulum will reveal low, poorly transmitted, or simultaneous contractions. Whether these changes are the result or the cause of the diverticulum is not known. Attention therefore should be given to the pressures and relaxation of the LES and abnormalities in peristalsis throughout the entire esophagus.

Treatment

Small, asymptomatic epiphrenic diverticula probably do not require any treatment. However, the search for an associated motor abnormality should be carried out with the same intensity as in a symptomatic patient with a large diverticulum.

The goal of therapy should be to treat the motor disorder with the hope of avoiding further enlargement of the diverticulum. The traditional treatment of an epiphrenic diverticulum consists of diverticulectomy alone or with myotomy [87 –89, 96]. Surgical results are reported by most authors to be excellent, but little information is available about long-term follow-up. Hudspeth *et al.* treated nine patients surgically and reported a follow-up of 94%, ranging from 3 months to 12 years, with good-to-excellent results in all patients as measured by symptom relief, weight gain, and absence of clinical recurrence [96]. No details are given about radiographic appearance. On the other hand, Benacci *et al.* operated on 33 patients, half of whom at least had had an associated motor disorder, and follow-up in 29 patients

ranged from 4 months to 15 years [88]. The long-term results were good, but there were three operative deaths (9%) and an esophageal leak in 18%. All patients who showed an esophageal leak had had a diverticulectomy. In a related editorial, Orringer pointed out the risks associated with surgical treatment of epiphrenic diverticula and discussed the need to perform antireflux surgery in many patients [97]. Diverticulectomy with myotomy in all patients is advocated by Mulder *et al.* [98]. Chami *et al.* treated a patient successfully by the transhiatal laparoscopic approach [99].

It is quite difficult to assess the proper surgical technique for epiphrenic diverticula. Surgical series include a large proportion of patients with esophageal motor abnormalities. Some patients have been studied with manometry and many have not. It is not clear whether a diverticulectomy is necessary. Most authors agree that a diverticulectomy alone would result in a recurrence and advocate a long esophagomyotomy. The choice of operation should be based on the underlying disorder. For instance, in the case of a large, tortuous esophagus with esophageal sacculations due to achalasia, the addition of a diverticulectomy to myotomy would make no difference. If myotomy is not successful, esophagectomy should be considered. DeVault treated three elderly patients by injecting botulinum toxin in the area distal to the diverticulum in a manner and with a dose similar to those used in achalasia [100]. All patients reported improvement but follow-up information is given only for one with sustained benefit over 6 months.

Pneumatic dilation for achalasia has been considered dangerous when an epiphrenic diverticulum is present because of a possibly increased risk of perforation. This concern, however, is not based on any evidence. The presence of diverticula should not be a deterrent to pneumatic dilation if the procedure is carried out with the usual precautions and under fluoroscopic control. We have performed pneumatic dilation in a few patients with lower esophageal diverticular deformities without complications.

Esophageal intramural pseudodiverticulosis

Esophageal intramural pseudodiverticulosis is characterized by numerous minute, flask-like outpouchings along the esophageal wall.

Etiology and pathogenesis

Mendl *et al.* described the condition as intramural diverticulosis due to herniation of the mucosa through gaps in the muscularis as a result of increased pressure [101]. They likened the condition to the gallbladder sinuses of Rokitansky–Aschoff. Later studies using biopsy material and autopsy specimens revealed cystic dilatation of the esophageal gland ducts. The condition was thought to represent multiple mucous cysts of the submucosa, but since these pouches communicate with the lumen, the term *cyst* is not appropriate and the name *intramural pseudo-diverticulosis* would be more accurate [102]. Hammon *et al.* thought that the submucosal glands become impacted with inflammatory material secondary to stasis and suggested the term *esophageal adenitis* [103]. Others thought that the pseudocystic dilatations were an exaggeration of normal anatomy, i.e. dilated glandular ducts [104]. Umlas and Sakhuja, studying carefully an esophagus obtained at autopsy, found thickening of the esophageal wall due to submucosal fibrosis at the level of a stricture, and the diverticular structures represented the main excretory ducts of the submucosal glands rather than the glands themselves [105]. Mederios *et al.*, who described two similar cases, proceeded to study 100 esophageal specimens collected during past autopsies as well as 20 cases obtained prospectively, from whom sections were collected from various locations [106]. The results of this study showed that in the random specimens obtained retrospectively, dilated excretory ducts were found in 14% of cases and cysts in 7%. Comparatively, in the prospective study, 55% of specimens revealed dilated ducts and 15% cysts. In both groups, chronic inflammation was found in 65–67%. Additionally, cysts were found only in patients over the age of 40. From these findings, Mederios *et al.* concluded that the pathogenesis of intramural pseudodiverticulosis is extensive chronic inflammation leading to dilated ducts that in time develop small cysts and, when the cysts become large enough, possibly decreased inflammation [106]. They also pointed out that early changes of intramural pseudodiverticulosis were more common than described.

The frequent association of strictures in patients with pseudodiverticulosis and the frequent occurrence of pseudodiverticula above the stricture have been used as an argument to attribute the cause of the disorder to motor abnormalities. Various motor abnormalities have been described in these patients. Hammon *et al.* found non-peristaltic contractions in two of three patients [103], and others have described non-specific motility abnormalities [107]. One patient was reported with changes consistent with nutcracker esophagus [108], but esophageal motility may be normal in some cases [103, 104].

Clinical features

Intramural pseudodiverticulosis is a relatively rare condition. The exact prevalence is not known. In two large radiologic studies, it was present respectively in 0.09% [109] and 0.15% [110] of patients undergoing evaluation for a variety of conditions. Overall, fewer than 200 cases have been reported in the English literature [104].

The condition is found in both sexes. Most cases are discovered in the sixth and seventh decades [111], but a few cases have been reported in children and infants [112].

Patients with intramural pseudodiverticulosis almost always present with dysphagia [102, 103, 113]. Dysphagia usually occurs with solid foods and may be abrupt [114]. Bleeding from an associated web-like stricture has been reported in one case [115]. Spontaneous perforation after vomiting was the presenting manifestation of pseudodiverticulosis with stricture in another one [116].

When a stricture is associated with pseudodiverticulosis, it is most often proximal. In that case, pseudodiverticula occur above the stricture.

Other conditions have been described in association with intramural pseudodiverticulosis. Candidiasis is frequent and present in about 50% of cases. The presence of monilia may be attributed to stasis, which is quite frequent in cases of pseudodiverticulosis and does not seem to be the cause of the disease, even though chronic candidiasis may cause chronic esophageal inflammation [103, 107, 108].

Kochhar *et al.* studied 59 patients with sequelae of corrosive acid injury and found 14 with esophageal intramural pseudodiverticulosis [117]. The association with motor abnormalities has already been discussed. Pseudodiverticulosis was described in a case of achalasia [118]. Plavsic *et al.* reviewed the esophagrams of 245 patients with carcinoma of the esophagus and compared them to 6400 roentgenograms obtained for other reasons [109]. They found intramural pseudodiverticulosis in 4.5% of patients with cancer compared to 0.09% in the control group. They concluded that there may be an increased risk of carcinoma in pseudodiverticulosis and stated that periodic surveillance for carcinoma may be worthwhile in patients with intramural pseudodiverticulosis. The coexistence of carcinoma and pseudodiverticulosis does not indicate a cause-and-effect relationship. Indeed, it is possible that pseudodiverticulosis is simply the result of stasis caused by obstruction from the carcinoma just as it is observed in benign strictures. There is no evidence that intramural pseudodiverticulosis constitutes a risk for cancer, and surveillance should not be recommended.

Diagnosis

The diagnosis of esophageal intramural pseudodiverticulosis is usually made on a barium esophagram. The pouches are small, varying in length from 1 to 6 mm and usually less than 4 mm wide [117]. The neck of each diverticulum rarely measures more than 1 mm. The pouches are best seen when a double air contrast technique is performed [109]. Pseudodiverticulosis may be diffuse or segmental [105, 114, 119, 120] (Figures 17.11 and 17.12).

Pseudodiverticulosis is not always recognized during endoscopy, but visualization of pinpoint openings in the esophageal wall is easier since the advent of fiberoptic endoscopy [113, 121, 122].

Pearlberg *et al.* described the CT features of esophageal intramural pseudodiverticulosis in one patient [123].

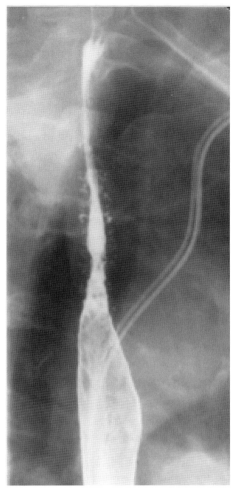

Figure 17.11 Segmental intramural pseudodiverticulosis. Image courtesy of David Einstein, M.D.

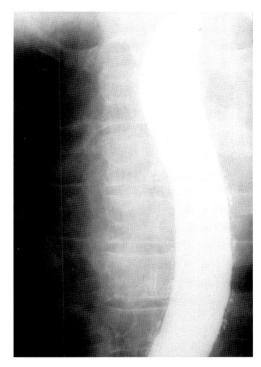

Figure 17.12 Diffuse intramural pseudodiverticulosis.

Treatment

Intramural pseudodiverticulosis responds to esophageal dilatation with relief of symptoms for a few years [1, 3 –5, 113]. Some patients may require periodic dilatations [113].

Medical treatment of candidiasis when present is appropriate and results in improvement [125], but is not always necessary [107]. In pseudodiverticulosis, treatment aims at relieving obstructive symptoms.

They found marked thickening of the esophageal wall and loss of normal soft tissue planes with small intramural gas collections. The loss of soft tissue planes raised the question of malignancy, leading to a repeat endoscopy and biopsies, which did not confirm the presence of a malignancy.

CT scanning does not seem to contribute to the diagnosis of pseudodiverticulosis and may create confusion in some cases. CT scans have been reported as normal [121] or showing thickening of the esophageal wall [122]. Devereaux and Savides recommend the use of endoscopic ultrasound to elucidate the nature of esophageal wall thickening based on experience with one case [124]. Ultrasound revealed thickening of the mucosal and submucosal layers with normal muscular propria and no adenopathy.

Esophageal manometry is indicated only in cases where a stricture is not present and when the radiographs suggest other abnormalities in the esophagus.

References

1. Ekberg O, Mylander G. Cineradiography of the pharyngeal phase of deglutition in 250 patients with dysphagia. *Br J Radiol* 1982;55:258.
2. Haubrich WS. Von Zenker of Zenker's diverticulum. *Gastrointest Endosc* 2004;126:1269.
3. Watemberg S, Landau O, Avrahami R. Zenker's diverticulum: Reappraisal. *Am J Gastroenterol* 1996;91:1494.
4. Gerhardt DC, Shuck TJ, Bordeaux RA, *et al.* Human upper esophageal sphincter. *Gastroenterology* 1978;75:268.
5. Kahrilas PJ, Dodds WJ, Dent J, *et al.* Upper esophageal sphincter function during deglutition. *Gastroenterology* 1988;95:52.
6. Ellis FH, Schlegel JF, Lynch VP, *et al.* Cricopharyngeal myotomy for pharyngoesophageal diverticulitis. *Ann Surg* 1969;170:340.
7. Asherson N. Achalasia of the cricopharyngeal sphincter: A record of cases, with profile pharyngograms. *J Laryngol Otol* 1950;64:747.

8. Sutherland HD. Cricopharyngeal achalasia. *J Thoracic Cardiovascular Surg* 1962;43:114.

9. Nilsson ME, Isberg A, Schiratzki H. The hypopharyngeal diverticulum. *Acta Otolaryngol* 1988;106:314.

10. Knuff TE, Benjamin SB, Castell DO. Pharyngoesophageal (Zenker's) diverticulum: A reappraisal. *Gastroenterology* 1982; 82:734.

11. Cook IJ, Gabb M, Panagopoulos V, *et al.* Pharyngeal (Zenker's) diverticulum is a disorder of upper esophageal sphincter opening. *Gastroenterology* 1992;103:1229.

12. Cook IJ, Blumbergs P, Cash K, *et al.* Structural abnormalities of the cricopharyngeus muscle in patients with pharyngeal (Zenker's) diverticulum. *J Gastroenterol Hepatol* 1992;7:556.

13. Lerut T, van Raemdonck D, Guelinckx P, *et al.* Zenker's diverticulum: is a myotomy of the cricopharyngeus useful? How long should it be? *Hepatogastroenterology* 1992;39:127.

14. Van Overbeek, JJM. Pathogenesis and methods of treatment of Zenker's diverticulum. *Ann Otol Rhinol Laryngol* 2003; 112:583.

15. Dantas RO, Cook IJ, Dodds WJ, *et al.* Biomechanics of cricopharyngeal bars. *Gastroenterology* 1990;99:1269.

16. McConnel FMS, Hood D, Jackson K, *et al.* Analysis of intrabolus forces in patients with Zenker's diverticulum. *Laryngoscope* 1994;104:1571.

17. Hunt PS, Connell AM, Smiley TB. The cricopharyngeal sphincter in gastric reflux. *Gut* 1970;11:303.

18. Vakil NB, Kahrilas PJ, Dodds WJ, *et al.* Absence of an upper esophageal sphincter response to acid reflux. *Am J Gastroenterol* 1989;84:606.

19. Gage-White L. Incidence of Zenker's diverticulum with hiatus hernia. *Laryngoscope* 1988;98:527.

20. Resouly A, Braat J, Jackson A, *et al.* Pharyngeal pouch: Link with reflux and oesophageal dysmotility. *Clin Otolaryngol* 1994;19:241.

21. Fuessner H, Siewert JR. Zenker's diverticulum and reflux. *Hepatogastroenterology* 1992;39:100.

22. Sasaki CT, Ross DA, Hundal J. Association between Zenker diverticulum and gastroesophageal reflux disease: development of a working hypothesis. *Am J Med* 2003;115:169S.

23. Welsh GF, Payne WS. The present status of one-stage pharyngoesophageal diverticulectomy. *Surg Clin North Am* 1973;53:953.

24. Hendren WG, Anderson T, Miller JI. Massive bleeding in a Zenker's diverticulum. *South Med J* 1990;83:362.

25. Johnson JT, Curtin HD. Carcinoma associated with Zenker's diverticulum. *Ann Otol Rhinol Laryngol* 1985;94:324.

26. Bowdler DA, Stell PM. Carcinoma arising in posterior pharyngeal pulsion diverticulum (Zenker's diverticulum). *Br J Surg* 1987;74:561.

27. Huang B, Unni KK, Payne WS. Long-term survival following diverticulectomy for cancer in pharyngoesophageal (Zenker's) diverticulum. *Ann Thorac Surg* 1984;38:207.

28. Bradley PJ, Kochaar A, Quraishi MS. Pharyngeal pouch carcinoma: real or imaginary risks? *Ann Otol Rhinol Laryngol* 1999; 108:1027.

29. Ponette E, Coolen J. Radiological aspects of Zenker's diverticulum. *Hepatogastroenterology* 1992;39:115.

30. Rubesin SE, Yousem DM. Structural abnormalities. In: Gore RM, Levine MS, Laufer I, eds. *Textbook of Gastrointestinal Radiology.* Philadelphia: WB Saunders, 1994, p. 244.

31. Rubesin SE, Levine MS. Killian-Jamieson diverticula: Radiographic findings in 16 patients. *AJR Am J Roentgenol* 2001;177:85.

32. Duranceau A. Oropharyngeal dysphagia and disorders of the upper esopharyngeal sphincter. *Ann Chirurgiae Gynaecologiae* 1995;84:225.

33. Castell JA, Dalton BC, Castell DO. Pharyngeal and upper esophageal sphincter manometry in humans. *Am J Physiol* 1990;258:G173.

34. Migliore M, Payne H, Jeyasingham K. Pathophysiologic basis for operation on Zenker's diverticulum. *Ann Thorac Surg* 1994;57:1616.

35. Fulp SR, Castell DO. Manometric aspects of Zenker's diverticulum. *Hepatogastroenterology* 1992;39:123.

36. Grégoire J, Duranceau A. Surgical management of Zenker's diverticulum. *Hepatogastroenterology* 1991;39:132.

37. Payne WS, Reynolds RR. Surgical treatment of pharyngoesophageal diverticulum (Zenker's diverticulum). *Surg Rounds* 1982;5:18.

38. Payne WS. The treatment of pharyngoesophageal diverticulum: The simple and complex. *Hepatogastroenterology* 1992; 39:109.

39. Huang B, Payne WS, Cameron AJ. Surgical management for recurrent pharyngoesophageal (Zenker's) diverticulum. *Ann Thorac Surg* 1984;37:189.

40. Brouillette D, Martel E, Chen LQ, *et al.* Pitfalls and complications of cricopharyngeal myotomy. *Chest Surg Clin North Am* 1997;7:457.

41. Fegiz G, Paolini A, DeMarchi C, *et al.* Surgical management of esophageal diverticula. *World J Surg* 1984;8:757.

42. Ellis FH, Crozier RE. Cervical esophageal dysphagia. Indications for and results of cricopharyngeal myotomy. *Ann Surg* 1981;194:279.

43. Schmit PJ, Zuckerbraun L. Treatment of Zenker's diverticula by cricopharyngeus myotomy under local anesthesia. *Am Surg* 1992;58:710.

44. Zeitoun H, Widdowson D, Hammad Z, *et al.* A videofluoroscopic study of patients treated by diverticulectomy and cricopharyngeal myotomy. *Clin Otolaryngol* 1994;19:301.

45. Shaw DW, Cook IJ, Jamieson GG, *et al.* Influence of surgery on deglutitive upper oesophageal sphincter mechanics in Zenker's diverticulum. *Gut* 1996;38:806.

46. Zaninotto M, Costantini M, Boccu C, *et al.* Functional and morphological study of the cricopharyngeal muscle in patients with Zenker's diverticulum. *Br J Surg* 1996;83:1263.

47. Morton RP, Bartley JRF. Inversion of Zenker's diverticulum: The preferred option. *Head Neck* 1993;15:253.

48. Banerjee AJ, Westmore GA. Letter to the Editor. Inversion of Zenker's diverticulum. *Head Neck* 1994;16:291.

49. Louie HW, Zuckerbraun L. Staged Zenker's diverticulectomy with cervical esophagostomy and secondary esophagostomy closure for treatment of massive diverticulum in severely debilitated patients. *Am Surg* 1993;12:842.

50. van Overbeek JJM. Meditation on the pathogenesis of hypopharyngeal (Zenker's) diverticulum and a report of endoscopic treatment in 545 patients. *Ann Otol Rhinol Laryngol* 1994;103:178.

51. Van Overbeek JJM, Hoeksema PE. Endoscopic treatment of the hypopharyngeal diverticulum: 211 cases. *Laryngoscope* 1982;92:88.

52. Mahieu HF, deBree R, Dagli SA, *et al*. The pharyngoesophageal segment: Endoscopic treatment of Zenker's diverticulum. *Dis Esophagus* 1996;9:12.

53. Nyrop M, Svendstrup F, Jorgensen KE. Endoscopic CO_2 laser therapy of Zenker's diverticulum—Experience from 61 patients. *Acta Otolaryngol* 2000;543 (Suppl):232.

54. Benjamin B, Innocenti M. Laser treatment of pharyngeal pouch. *Aust N Z J Surg* 1991;61:909.

55. Wouters B, van Overbeek JJM. Endoscopic treatment of the hypopharyngeal (Zenker's) diverticulum. *Hepatogastroenterology* 1992;39:105.

56. Kos MP, David EF, Mahieu HF. Endoscopie carbon dioxide laser Zenker's diverticulotomy revisited. *Ann Otol Rhinol Laryngol* 2009;118:512.

57. Collard JM, Otte JB, Kestens PJ. Endoscopic stapling technique of esophagodiverticulostomy for Zenker's diverticulum. *Ann Thorac Surg* 1993;56:573.

58. Scher RL, Richtsmeier WJ. Long-term experience with endoscopic staple-assisted esophagodiverticulostomy for Zenker's diverticulum. *Laryngoscope* 1998;108:200.

59. Stoeckli SJ, Schmid S. Endoscopic stapler-assisted diverticuloesophagostomy for Zenker's diverticulum: Patient satisfaction and subjective relief of symptoms. *Surgery* 2002;131:158.

60. Thaler ER, Weber RS, Goldberg AN, *et al*. Feasibility and outcome of endoscopic staple-assisted esophagodiverticulostomy for Zenker's diverticulum. *Laryngoscope* 2001;111:1506.

61. Altman JI, Genden EM, Moche J. Fiberoptic endoscopic-assisted diverticulotomy: a novel technique for the management of Zenker's diverticulum. *Ann Otol Rhinol Laryngol* 2005;114:347–351.

62. Smith SR, Genden EM, Urken ML. Endoscopic stapling technique for the treatment of Zenker diverticulum vs standard open-neck technique. *Arch Otolaryngol Head Neck Surg* 2002;128:141.

63. Adams J, Sheppard B, Andersen P, *et al*. Zenker's diverticulostomy with cricopharyngeal myotomy. *Surg Endosc* 2001; 15:34.

64. Duda M, Sery Z, Vojacek K, *et al*. Etiopathogenesis and classification of esophageal diverticula. *Int Surg* 1985;70:291.

65. Harrington SW. The surgical treatment of pulsion diverticula of the thoracic esophagus. *Ann Surg* 1949;129:606.

66. Case records of the Massachusetts General Hospital Weekly clinicopathological exercises Case 7-1977. *N Engl J Med* 1977; 296:384.

67. Cross FS, Johnson GF, Gerein AN. Esophageal diverticula. Associated neuromuscular changes in the esophagus. *Arch Surg* 1961;83:525.

68. Case records of the Massachusetts General Hospital. Weekly clinicopathological exercises. Case 32-1982. *N Engl J Med* 1982; 307:426.

69. Schima W, Schober E, Stacher G, *et al*. Association of midoesophageal diverticula with oesophageal motor disorders. *Acta Radiol* 1997;38:108.

70. Evander A, Little AG, Ferguson MK, *et al*. Diverticula of the mid- and lower esophagus: Pathogenesis and surgical management. *World J Surg* 1986;10:820.

71. Dodds WJ, Stef JJ, Hogan WJ, *et al*. Radial distribution of esophageal peristaltic pressure in normal subjects and patients with esophageal diverticulum. *Gastroenterology* 1975;69:584.

72. Schick A, Yesner R. Traction diverticulum of esophagus with exsanguination: Report of a case. *Ann Intern Med* 1953;39:345.

73. Altorki NK, Sunagawa M, Skinner DB. Thoracic esophageal diverticula. Why is operation necessary? *J Thorac Cardiovasc Surg* 1993;105:260.

74. Balthazar EJ. Esophagobronchial fistula secondary to ruptured traction diverticulum. *Gastrointest Radiol* 1977;2:119.

75. Fekete F, Vonns C. Surgical management of esophageal thoracic diverticula. *Hepatogastroenterology* 1992;39:97.

76. Herman TE, McAlister WH. Esophageal diverticula in childhood associated with strictures from unsuspected foreign bodies of the esophagus. *Pediatr Radiol* 1991;21:410.

77. Mahajan RJ, Marshall JB. Severe dysphagia, dysmotility, and unusual saccular dilation (diverticulum) of the esophagus following excision of an asymptomatic congenital cyst. *Am J Gastroenterol* 1996;91:1254.

78. Schreiber MH, Davis M. Intraluminal diverticulum of the esophagus. *AJR Am J Roentgenol* 1977;129:595.

79. Clements JL, Abernathy J, Weens HS. Atypical esophageal diverticula associated with progressive systemic sclerosis. *Gastrointest Radiol* 1978;3:383

80. Coggins CA, Levine MS, Kesack CD, et al. Wide-mouthed sacculations in the esophagus: A radiographic finding in scleroderma. *AJR Am J Roentgenol* 2001;176:953.

81. Jancu J, Marvan H. Multiple diverticula of the esophagus. *Am J Gastroenterol* 1973;60:408.

82. Ferraro P, Duranceau A. Esophageal diverticula. *Chest Surg Clin N Am* 1994;4:741.

83. Bruggeman LL, Seaman WB. Epiphrenic diverticula. An analysis of 80 cases. *AJR Am J Roentgenol* 1973;119:266.

84. Debas HT, Payne WS, Cameron AJ, *et al*. Physiopathology of lower esophageal diverticulum and its implications for treatment. *Surg Gynecol Obstet* 1980;151:593.

85. Tedesco P, Fisichella PM, Way LW, Patti MG. Cause and treatment of epiphrenic diverticula. *Am J Surg* 2005;190:891.

86. D'Journo XB, Ferraro P, Martin J, Chen LQ, Duranceau A. Lower oesophageal sphincter dysfunction is part of the functional abnormality in epiphrenic diverticulum. *Br J Surg* 2009:96:892.

87. Allen TH, Clagett OT. Changing concepts in the surgical treatment of pulsion diverticula of the lower esophagus. *J Thorac Cardiovasc Surg* 1965;50:455.

88. Benacci JC, Deschamps C, Trastek VF, *et al*. Epiphrenic diverticulum: Results of surgical treatment. *Ann Thorac Surg* 1993;55:1109.

89. Falk G. Regurgitation in a patient with an esophageal diverticulum. *Cleve Clin J Med* 1994;61:409.

90. Hurwitz AL, Way LW, Haddad JK. Epiphrenic diverticulum in association with an unusual motility disturbance: Report of surgical correction. *Gastroenterology* 1975;68:795.

91. Conrad C, Nissen F. Giant epiphrenic diverticula. *Eur J Radiol* 1982;2:48.

92. Niv Y, Fraser G, Krugliak P. Gastroesophagageal obstruction from food in an epiphrenic esophageal diverticulum. *J Clin Gastroenterol* 1993;16:314.

93. Schultz SC, Byrne DM, Cunzol DW, *et al*. Carcinoma arising within epiphrenic diverticula. A report of two cases and review of the literature. *J Cardiovasc Surg* 1996;37:649.

94. Guerra JM, Zuil M, Garcia I, *et al*. Epiphrenic diverticula, esophageal carcinoma and esophagopleural fistula. *Hepatogastroenterology* 2001;48:718.

95. Kim KW, Berkmen YM, Auh YH, Kazam E. Diagnosis of epiphrenic esophageal diverticulum by computed tomography. *J Comput Tomogr* 1988;12:25.

96. Hudspeth DA, Thorne MT, Conroy R, *et al*. Management of epiphrenic esophageal diverticula. A fifteen-year experience. *Am Surg* 1993;59:40.

97. Orringer MB. Epiphrenic diverticula: Fact and fable. *Ann Thorac Surg* 1993;55:1067.

98. Mulder DG, Rosenkranz E, DenBesten L. Management of huge epiphrenic esophageal diverticula. *Am J Surg* 1989;157:303.

99. Chami Z, Fabre JM, Navarro F, *et al*. Abdominal laparoscopic approach for thoracic epiphrenic diverticulum. *Surg Endosc* 1999;13:164.

100. DeVault KR. Dysphagia from esophageal diverticulosis respoonding to Botulinum toxin injection. *Am J Gastroenterol* 1997;92:895.

101. Mendl K, McKay JM, Tanner CH. Intramural diverticulosis of the esophagus and Rokitanski-Aschoff sinuses in the gallbladder. *Br J Radiol* 1960;33:496.

102. Boyd RM, Bogoch A, Greig JH, *et al*. Esophageal intramural pseudodiverticulosis. *Radiology* 1974;113:267.

103. Hammon JW Jr., Rice RP, Postlethwait RW, *et al*. Esophageal intramural diverticulosis. *Ann Thorac Surg* 1974;17:260.

104. Graham DY, Goyal RK, Sparkman J, *et al*. Diffuse intramural esophageal diverticulosis. *Gastroenterology* 1975;68:781.

105. Umlas J, Sakhuja R. The pathology of esophageal intramural pseudodiverticulosis. *Am J Clin Pathol* 1976;65:314.

106. Medeiros LJ, Doos WG, Balogh K. Esophageal intramural pseudodiverticulosis: A report of two cases with analysis of similar, less extensive changes in "normal" autopsy esophagi. *Hum Pathol* 1988;19:928.

107. Castillo S, Aburashed A, Kimmelman J, *et al*. Diffuse intramural esophageal pseudodiverticulosis. New cases and review. *Gastroenterology* 1977;72:541.

108. Murney RG, Linne JH, Curtis J. High-amplitude peristaltic contractions in a patient with esophageal intramural pseudodiverticulosis. *Dig Dis Sci* 1983;28:843.

109. Plavisc BM, Chen MYM, Gelfand DW, *et al*. Intramural pseudodiverticulosis of the esophagus detected on barium esophagograms: Increased prevalence in patients with esophageal carcinoma. *AJR Am J Roentgenol* 1995;165:1381.

110. Levine MS, Moolten DN, Herlinger H, *et al*. Esophageal intramural pseudodiverticulosis: A reevaluation. *AJR Am J Roentgenol* 1986;147:1165.

111. Herter B, Dittler HJ, Wuttge-Hannig A, *et al*. Intramural pseudodiverticulosis of the esophagus: A case series. *Endoscopy* 1997;29:109.

112. Daud AS, O'Connor F. Oesophageal intramural pseudodiverticulosis: a cause of dysphagia in a 10-year -old boy. *Eur J Pediatr* 1997;156:530.

113. Mahajan SK, Warshauer DM, Bozymski EM. Esophageal intramural pseudo-diverticulosis: endoscopic and radiologic correlation. *Gastrointest Endosc* 1993;39:565.

114. Montgomery RD, Mendl K, Stephenson SF. Intramural diverticulosis of the osophagus. *Thorax* 1975;30:278.

115. Hahne M, Schilling D, Arnold JC *et al*. Esophageal intramural pseudodiverticulosis. *J Clin Gastroenterol* 2001;33:378.

116. Murakami M, Tsuchiya K, Ichikawa H, *et al*. Esophageal intramural pseudodiverticulosis associated with esophageal perforation. *J Gastroenterol* 2000;35:702.

117. Kochhar R, Mehta SK, Nagi B, *et al*. Corrosive acid-induced esophageal intramural pseudodiverticulosis. *Gastroenterology* 1991;13:371.

118. Dua KS, Stewart E, Arndorfer R, *et al*. Esophageal intramural pseudodiverticulosis associated with achalasia. *Am J Gastroenterol* 1996;91:1859.

119. Flora KD, Gordon MD, Lieberman D, *et al*. Esophageal intramural pseudodiverticulosis. *Dig Dis* 1997;15:113.

120. Canon CL, Levine MS, Cherukuri R, *et al*. Intramural tracking: A feature of esophageal intramural pseudodiverticulosis. *AJR Am J Roentgenol* 2000;175:371.

121. Gillessen A, Konturek J, Roos N, *et al*. Esophageal intramural pseudodiverticulosis: A characteristically unusual path to diagnosis. *Endoscopy* 1996;28:640.

122. van der Putten ABMM, Loffeld RJLF. Esophageal intramural pseudodiverticulosis. *Dis Esophagus* 1997;10:61.

123. Pearlberg JL, Sandler MA, Madrazo BL. Computed tomographic features of esophageal intramural pseudodiverticulosis. *Radiology* 1983;147:189.

124. Devereaux CE, Savides TJ. EUS appearance of esophageal pseudodiverticulosis. *Gastrointest Endosc* 2000;51:228.

125. Cantor DS, Riley TL. Intramural Pseudodiverticulosis of the esophagus. *Am J Gastroenterol* 1982;77:454.

18 | Esophageal Involvement in Systemic Diseases

Siva Doma,[1] John M. Wo,[2] and Henry P. Parkman[1]

[1]Temple University School of Medicine, Philadelphia, PA, USA
[2]University of Louisville School of Medicine, Louisville, KY, USA

Introduction

Systemic diseases can affect the esophagus as well as other gastrointestinal organs. The clinical manifestations of systemic disorders affecting the esophagus can range from debilitating symptoms such as severe dysphagia to asymptomatic esophageal dysmotility. Occasionally, evaluation of the esophagus permits diagnosis of a systemic disorder, as seen in disorders such as scleroderma. This chapter reviews the esophageal manifestations of systemic diseases, including connective tissue diseases, endocrine and metabolic diseases, inflammatory diseases, and neuromuscular diseases.

Connective tissue diseases

Scleroderma and systemic sclerosis

Scleroderma is a rare, complex, fibrosing disease with insidious onset and unknown etiology. The characteristic attribute is skin thickening. Scleroderma comes from the Greek *"skleros"* for thickening and *"dermos"* for skin [1]. Scleroderma-related disorders can be broadly classified into: (1) localized limited cutaneous scleroderma without organ involvement; and (2) diffuse systemic sclerosis (SSc) with internal organ involvement. The localized forms of scleroderma, such as linea scleroderma and morphea, primarily affect children and, in contrast to systemic sclerosis, are not associated with Raynaud's phenomenon and do not affect the internal organs [2].

SSc is a generalized systemic disorder of the small arteries with the proliferation of fibrosis affecting the skin and multiple internal organs, including the pulmonary, peripheral vascular, renal, cardiac, and gastrointestinal systems. Gastrointestinal involvement can occur in nearly 90% of SSc patients [3]. The disorder is more common in women, particularly African-American women with initial symptoms presenting in the third decade.

Diagnosis of SSc is based on clinical findings, which have substantial heterogeneity and varying manifestations [2]. Patients with SSc can be classified into distinct clinical subsets with different patterns of skin and internal organ involvement, autoantibody production, and patient survival: a limited cutaneous form and a diffuse cutaneous form [2]. Patients with diffuse cutaneous disease tend to have more significant visceral organ involvement, particularly of the heart, lung, and kidney, than those with the limited cutaneous form. However, both subsets of patients commonly have gastrointestinal tract involvement.

The limited cutaneous subset is diagnosed when skin thickening is limited to areas distal to the elbows and knees. CREST (calcinosis cutis, Raynaud's phenomenon, esophageal dysfunction, sclerodactyly, telangiectaisa) syndrome is a variant of limited cutaneous SSc [4]. SSc sine scleroderma is a rare form of limited cutaneous scleroderma in which patients have the characteristic internal organ manifestations of the disease without skin thickening [2, 3]. Diagnosis of SSc sine scleroderma can be assessed with motility tests of the gastrointestinal tract, including esophageal manometry. These patients do not differ in their clinical or laboratory features and prognosis from classical SSc. In the absence of cutaneous signs/symptoms, its diagnosis is often delayed, leading to persistent gastrointestinal symptoms and morbidity. Patients with the diffuse cutaneous disease have skin thickening involving the torso, face and/or limbs proximal to the knees and elbows [2].

Pathology and pathogenesis

SSc appears to result from several pathologic processes: cellular, humoral autoimmunity, and specific vascular changes [5]. The disorder appears to start with microvascular changes and endothelial activation followed by immune cell activation with development of autoantibodies, and release of cytokines and growth factors. Subsequently, profibrotic fibroblastic cell proliferation occurs with resulting fibrosis [6].

The Esophagus, Fifth Edition. Edited by Joel E. Richter, Donald O. Castell.
© 2012 Blackwell Publishing Ltd. Published 2012 by Blackwell Publishing Ltd.

Histologic findings in the esophagus are dependent on the severity of SSc. In the early stages, there are arteriolar changes consisting of a disruption of the internal elastic lamina, a thickened capillary basement membrane, platelet aggregates, swollen endothelial cells, and arteriole sclerosis [7, 8]. Initially, muscle atrophy and fibrosis are scattered and patchy. In the later stages of the disease, extensive collagen infiltration and fibrosis of the smooth muscle occurs. The striated muscle remains unaffected in the proximal esophagus [7, 9]. Despite earlier reports of normal appearing myenteric plexus, electron microscopy studies have shown axonal degeneration in SSc.

Classically, SSc is thought to be associated with smooth muscle dysfunction from fibrosis of the smooth muscle. Physiologic and anatomic studies suggest that neural dysfunction precedes the smooth muscle dysfunction in the esophagus. As a result, impaired esophageal peristalsis is present despite normal smooth muscle histology [10]. Cohen et al. suggested that neural dysfunction occurs before smooth muscle fibrosis in the early stages of the disease [10]. Their studies showed that in patients with early disease, the response of the lower esophageal sphincter (LES) to gastrin, an agent acting through neural pathways, was diminished, while the response to methacholine, which acts directly on the smooth muscle, was not affected. Similar pattern of early neurologic involvement is also seen in the stomach. Gastric myoelectric activity was disorganized and hyperactive but the amplitude of the activity was preserved, suggesting neuropathic dysfunction in early SSc [11].

Autoantibodies have been postulated to play a role in the gastrointestinal manifestations of scleroderma. Acetylcholine is the principal excitatory neurotransmitter regulating gastrointestinal motility, acting predominantly via the muscarinic-3 receptor (M3R). There is recent evidence that patients with SSc and severe gastrointestinal involvement have anti-M3R antibodies at a strikingly high frequency [12]. In addition, autoantibodies linked to myositis (anti-U3-snRNP, antisignal recognition particle, anti-Ku and anti-U1 snRNP) have also been described in some patients with SSc and severe gastrointestinal involvement [13]. These myositis-antibodies may play a role in the smooth muscle atrophy and fibrosis seen in severe gastrointestinal tract involvement.

Clinical manifestations

More than 50% of SSc patients have esophageal disease [3, 14]. Patients' symptoms closely mirror the esophageal changes. Classically, in SSc, there is fibrosis of the smooth muscle in the distal two-thirds of the esophagus. This leads to low-amplitude peristaltic contractions in the mid and distal esophagus, which can progress to feeble simultaneous contractions. In addition, there is a marked reduction of the LES pressure.

The primary symptoms reported by patients are heartburn, regurgitation, and dysphagia. Heartburn is reported in 50–79% and dysphagia in 25–53% of scleroderma patients [4, 15–17]. Esophageal involvement in scleroderma appears to be associated with the presence of Raynaud's phenomenon [10], but not with the age at diagnosis, gender, and duration of disease [18]. The extent of skin involvement, either diffuse or limited, does not appear to correlate with the prevalence of esophageal manifestations [4, 17]. However, the degree of esophageal dysfunction and erosive esophagitis are generally more severe in patients with diffuse cutaneous SSc [4, 17].

Complications of gastroesophageal reflux disease (GERD) are common in SSc. The prevalence of erosive esophagitis varies in the literature from 36% to −63% of patients with SSc [15, 17, 19]. The main contributing factor appears to be decreased acid clearance from the distal esophagus due to impaired peristalsis. A study comparing patients with esophagitis with and without SSc found significantly longer acid reflux episodes in SSc patients [18]. LES pressure was similar in both groups in that study. Other studies reached similar conclusions where the presence of erosive esophagitis indicated impaired esophageal peristalsis [19]. The patients with normal peristalsis exhibited no signs of erosive esophagitis. Esophageal peptic stricture has been reported in 3–30% of the patients studied [15, 19].

The prevalence of Barrett's esophagus varies greatly from 6% to 37% in patients with SSc [20–22]. Barrett's esophagus appears to be prevalent in SSc patients, even in those on long-term proton pump inhibitor (PPI) therapy [22]. Although esophageal adenocarcinoma can occur, this complication appears to be rare. In a review of 2141 patients, Duncan and Winklemann reported that only one patient had esophageal adenocarcinoma [21]. In a review of 680 patients, Segel et al. also reported only one patient with undifferentiated esophageal carcinoma [23].

The contribution of acid reflux to pulmonary disease in SSc is unclear. Studies using esophageal impedance pH monitoring found higher frequency of acid and non-acid reflux episodes, and a higher frequency of reflux episodes reaching the proximal esophagus in patients with SSc and pulmonary fibrosis than in those without pulmonary fibrosis [24]. In another recent study, the decline in pulmonary function did not appear to be related to the degree of esophageal dysmotility [25].

Diagnostic features

Characteristic antibodies found in the diffuse SSc include a positive ANA (found in >90% of SSc patients). An ANA is not specific for this disease and can be seen with a number of autoimmune conditions, especially systemic lupus erythematosis (SLE). Anti-Scl-70 antibody is often present in diffuse SSc. Anticentromere antibody is often present in the limited cutaneous form.

Esophageal symptoms are not reliable in judging the presence or extent of esophageal dysfunction [26]. Radiographic findings are less sensitive than esophageal manometry [27]. Occasionally, an air-filled esophagus may be noted on a chest radiograph, but this finding is not sensitive or specific for SSc [28]. In the late stages of SSc, a dilated atonic esophagus and the absence of longitudinal mucosal folds may be present. Barium esophagography is useful to detect structural defects, such as an esophageal stricture, or hiatal hernia. Esophageal diameter of greater than 10 mm by high-resolution computed tomography (CT) correlated well with esophageal dysmotility as assessed by radionuclide scintigraphy [29].

Endoscopy should be performed in patients with dysphagia and odynophagia to detect erosive esophagitis, peptic stricture, and Barrett's esophagus. Impaired esophageal function may be appreciated during upper endoscopy. The LES tends not to close completely, and lumen-occluding contractions are mostly absent in the distal esophagus [30].

Characteristic findings on esophageal manometry (Figure 18.1) include decreased LES pressure, aperistalsis or hypomotility of the smooth muscle portion of the esophagus. Dysfunction of the esophageal body is reported to be more common than LES abnormalities in patients with SSc. In one study, esophageal body dysmotility was seen in 82% of patients, aperistalsis in 61%, and hypotonic LES in 39% [31]. Hypotonic LES was often associated with aperistalsis of the esophageal body. In the same study symptoms did not correlate with manometric abnormalities.

The presence of aperistalsis is more common in patients with diffuse cutaneous SSc compared to those with the limited variant [17]. Aperistalsis with very low LES pressure distinguishes SSc from primary achalasia. Peristalsis in the striated proximal esophagus and upper esophageal sphincter (UES) pressure are preserved in scleroderma [32]. The manometric findings in SSc are not specific, as they can be seen in mixed connective tissue disorder, Sjögren's syndrome, and rheumatoid arthritis [33].

Ambulatory pH monitoring is the most sensitive and specific test for detecting acid reflux [14]. In a study of 55 SSc patients by Stentoft et al., a positive pH test was reported in 67% of the patients with heartburn and in 25% of those without heartburn [34]. The severity of heartburn and regurgitation, however, does not correlate with the severity of GERD on pH monitoring [32].

Esophageal scintigraphy is a non-invasive test to quantify esophageal emptying. Classically, there is slow transit though the esophagus in the supine position, which requires esophageal peristalsis for emptying [35]. In contrast, esophageal transit is much improved in the upright position. An abnormal esophageal scintigraphy has been reported in approximately 85% of the patients [26]. The scintigraphy technique varies from liquid [36] to semisolid boluses [37]. In a study by Kaye et al., 301 patients were evaluated with scintigraphy using a semisolid ingested bolus to quantify the severity of esophageal dysfunction and to detect early dysfunction in

asymptomatic patients [27]. Esophageal scintigraphy is reported to be comparable to manometry in SSc [38, 39]. Scintigraphy can also provide information on gastric emptying and whole gut transit simultaneously [36, 37].

Treatment

Prognosis in SSc is determined by the degree of internal organ involvement. Although no disease-modifying therapy has been proven to be effective for SSc, the complications of SSc are treatable, and interventions for organ-specific manifestations have improved substantially [2]. Optimal patient care includes an integrated, multidisciplinary approach to promptly and effectively recognize, evaluate, and manage complications and limit end-organ dysfunction.

The medical treatment of acid reflux in SSc is similar to that of patients with typical GERD without SSc. In uncontrolled studies [10], symptoms improved in 59% of patients with SSc taking histamine-2-receptor antagonists (H2RAs) and in 94% taking with PPIs. Generally, twice daily PPI treatment is used. Nocturnal esophageal reflux is common in SSc patients on high-dose PPI and the addition of H_2 blockers may not reduce nocturnal acid exposure [40]. Patients treated with PPIs may be at a higher risk of developing esophageal candidiasis, but the clinical significance of this is uncertain [41]. If gastroparesis is present, prokinetic medications, such as metoclopramide, domperidone, and erythromycin, are appropriate. Oral doses of metoclopramide can increase the LES pressure, but have a minimal effect on esophageal function [42]. Dysphagia can be difficult to treat. High-dose PPIs, generally bid, are used to control acid reflux. Endoscopic dilation with Maloney, Savory, or TTS dilators may be needed for strictures. The treatment of skin manifestations in SSc with penicillamine does not improve esophageal manifestations [43].

Conventionally, it is taught not to perform antireflux surgery in SSc patients, as a fundoplication may worsen the dysphagia in those with significant esophageal peristaltic dysfunction. Fundoplication with a partial Nissen fundoplication (Toupet procedure) or Collis gastroplasty can reduce gastroesophageal reflux. Dysphagia can occur in 30–70% of patients and recurrence of reflux is high and can be seen in 10–100% of patients [44–47]. A modified short-limb Roux-en-Y gastric bypass has been reported to result in a lower incidence of dysphagia and recurrent reflux than fundoplication [48]. With the effectiveness of PPI therapy and the potential risks for post-fundoplication dysphagia and gastroparesis, antireflux surgery should be avoided in patients with SSc. Esophagectomy in these patients has a high complication rate [48].

Mixed connective tissue diseases

Mixed connective tissue disease (MCTD) is a syndrome characterized by overlapping clinical features of SSc, SLE, idiopathic inflammatory myopathy, and rheumatoid arthritis

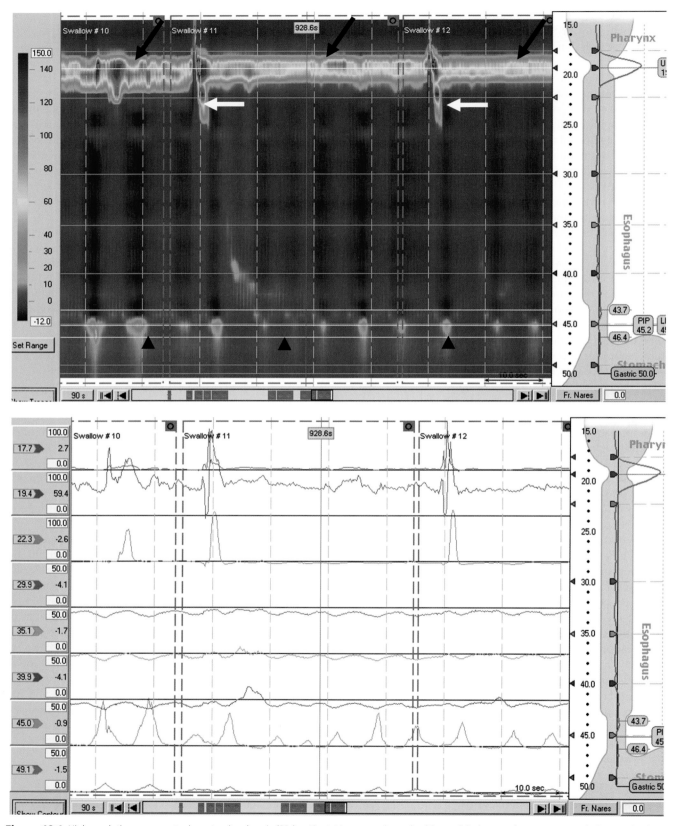

Figure 18.1 High-resolution manometry in systemic sclerosis (SSc) patient. Upper esophageal sphincter (black arrows) appears normal. Contraction in the proximal (skeletal muscle) part of the esophagus is present (white arrows). Characteristic features of SSc include aperistalsis in the smooth muscle part of the esophagus and low lower esophageal sphincter pressure (arrowheads).

[14, 49]. Often there is the presence of antibodies against the Ul-small nuclear ribonucleoprotein (snRNP) complex [50]. Patients with MCTD may be at a higher risk for gastrointestinal complications, as there is evidence that SSc patients with myositis have gastrointestinal involvement early in the course of the disease [13].

Similar to the overlapping clinical features of MCTD, histologic changes also seem to overlap. Histologic findings of the skin consist of vascular alterations and luminal thrombosis similar to SSc [51]. Biopsies of the skeletal muscle reveal inflammatory infiltration and focal interstitial myositis that are similar to polymyositis [52]. Abnormal autonomic testing suggesting parasympathetic dysfunction is frequently seen in MCTD [53]. One hypothesis suggests that the cause of esophageal manifestations is an overlap of the neural dysfunction and smooth muscle atrophy seen in SSc and striated muscle weakness seen in idiopathic inflammatory myopathy [49].

The clinical features of MCTD are Raynaud's phenomenon, polyarthritis, swelling of the hands, myalgia, and esophageal dysfunction. Unlike those with SSc, patients with MCTD may respond to corticosteroids. Gastrointestinal symptoms such as heartburn, regurgitation, dysphagia, dyspepsia, vomiting, diarrhea, and constipation are common in patients with MCTD [49]. Heartburn and regurgitation are common, occurring in 24–48% of the patients with MCTD [54, 55]. Dysphagia may be present [49, 55]. In a study by Doria et al., symptoms of oropharyngeal and esophageal dysphagia were both present [55]. In a study of 61 patients with MCTD by Marshall et al., one patient (2%) developed recurrent aspiration, and three (5%) developed esophageal stricture during a mean follow-up of 6.3 years [49].

Diagnostic findings

The barium esophagram findings in MCTD are similar to SSc, with diminished esophageal peristalsis and a dilated esophagus [53, 56]. Barium esophagography allows identification of esophageal strictures. Dilated small bowel and gastric bezoar have been reported, indicating a more diffuse gastrointestinal dysmotility [56]. Videofluoroscopic pharyngeal studies may detect oropharyngeal dysfunction similar to that of patients with polymyositis. The esophageal motility pattern in patients with MCTD is similar to that in patients with SSc. The LES pressure is diminished, but not as severely as in patients with SSc [55]. Distal esophageal peristaltic pressure is also reduced [55]. Aperistalsis has been reported in 17–64% of patients [55, 56]. The UES pressure was reduced in some studies but elevated in others [56, 57]. Up to 50% of patients could have abnormal acid reflux [54].

Treatment

Pharmacologic acid suppression with PPIs can be used when heartburn or complications of acid reflux are identified. Corticosteroids and alkylating agents have been used with some success for the skin and systemic manifestations of MCTD [51]. In a study of 10 patients by Marshall et al., the effect of corticosteroids on the esophagus was minimal, with the LES pressure improving, but the esophageal peristaltic pressures not changing [49].

Idiopathic inflammatory myopathies

Idiopathic inflammatory myopathies consist of a heterogeneous group of acquired disorders, including dermatomyositis (DM), polymyositis (PM), and inclusion-body myositis (IBM). DM and PM are more prevalent in women, whereas IBM is more prevalent in men [58, 59]. PM and DM are characterized by proximal muscle weakness with difficulty lifting the arms, climbing steps, and arising from chairs. PM affects mainly adults aged over 20 years, whereas DM may affect both children and adults [58, 59]. Dermatomyositis can be recognized by the characteristic heliotrope rash, periorbital edema, and papular scaly lesions over the knuckles (Gottren's signs). IBM causes a slowly progressive weakness of proximal and distal muscles in patients aged over 50 years [58, 59]. The diagnosis of inflammatory myopathy is based on elevated muscle enzymes, electromyography, and muscle biopsy. DM and PM can present as an isolated entity or may be associated with an overlapping connective tissue disorder [58]. DM and to a lesser extent with PM in adults can be associated with the paraneoplastic syndrome [58, 59]. It may be difficult to differentiate the histologic and clinical manifestations of various inflammatory myopathies because of their heterogeneous nature. Oropharyngeal dysphagia is the most prominent gastrointestinal complaint in inflammatory myopathies [60], with other intestinal manifestations including vasculitis, ulcerations, perforation, and intestinal bleeding [59].

Pathology and pathophysiology

The histologic changes of the striated cricopharyngeus and the upper esophagus in PM and DM consist of mononuclear inflammatory infiltration, a patchy area of necrosis, fiber degeneration, and prominent fibrosis [61, 62]. The inflammatory invasion of the muscle fibers is more characteristic of PM [59]. Involvement of the upper aerodigestive tract may cause weak pharyngeal muscles and uncoordinated oropharyngeal swallowing. Rare cases of smooth muscle fibrosis have been reported, but these patients may have an overlapping connective tissue disorder or a paraneoplastic syndrome [63]. Disturbances of the distal esophagus have also been reported [64, 65]. In a review of 18 patients, de Merieux et al. found radiographic dysfunction of the distal esophagus whereas smooth muscle fibrosis was mostly absent [66].

Clinical manifestations

Dysphagia has been reported in approximately one-third of patients with DM and PM [65–69] and in 40% of patients with IBM [70, 71]. In some cases, dysphagia can be the presenting complaint rather than the proximal weakness of skeletal muscles [69, 72, 73]. Dysphagia is mostly oropharyngeal with choking, coughing while eating, nasal regurgitation, dysphonia, and aspiration. Heartburn and regurgitation are uncommon [65].

Diagnostic features

A videofluoroscopic swallowing study is often used to detect oropharyngeal dysfunction, such as nasal regurgitation, laryngeal penetration, and residual barium in the pyriform sinuses. Assessment of the cricopharyngeus is particularly important to identify poor relaxation during swallowing, a prominent cricopharyngeal bar, and Zenker's diverticulum [61, 62]. Barium esophagram findings may be normal, but impaired peristalsis and aperistalsis have been reported [63, 64, 66]. Manometric abnormalities consist of weak pharyngeal pressures and poor relaxation of the cricopharyngeal muscle with swallowing [61, 66]. The proximal and distal esophageal peristaltic pressures may both be reduced [66]. The LES pressure is usually normal [66] unless the patient has an overlapping MCTD. Esophageal scintigraphy transit may be delayed [64].

The serum creatinine kinase (CPK) is a sensitive test to detect elevated muscle enzymes in DM and PM [58, 72].

Treatment

Corticosteroid therapy is the first line of treatment for patients with PM and DM [58–60]. Patients with IBM are usually refractory to corticosteroid therapy [59]. Oropharyngeal dysphagia in DM and PM may respond well with corticosteroid treatment [74]. Cricopharyngeal myotomy has been successful in selected patients with evidence of poor cricopharyngeal relaxation [61, 62]. Respiratory failure due to aspiration pneumonia is a common cause of death in these patients [75].

Sjögren's syndrome

Sjögren's syndrome is a chronic autoimmune inflammatory disorder associated with the destruction of salivary and lacrimal glands, causing xerostomia and keratoconjunctivitis sicca [14]. Other systemic manifestations include dysphagia, arthralgia, and pulmonary involvement. Sjögren's syndrome can present as a primary disorder or as a secondary disorder associated with other autoimmune diseases. The autoantibodies, anti-Ro and anti-La, are frequently present in Sjögren's syndrome. The histologic findings of the salivary and lacrimal glands in Sjögren's syndrome consist of lymphocytic infiltration, acinar atrophy, and hypertrophy of the ductal epithelial cells [76].

The precise mechanism causing dysphagia is unclear. Several hypotheses have been proposed, such as a lack of saliva, esophageal dysmotility, and a proximal esophageal web. The absence of saliva, which normally acts as a lubricant [77], may lead to impaired solid bolus transit through the esophagus [76]. Some investigators have found a significant correlation between esophageal and salivary gland dysfunction [78], but others have not [79, 80]. Dysphagia cannot be explained by esophageal dysmotility in most patients. Many case-controlled studies have failed to detect any differences in esophageal peristalsis when compared to normal volunteers [79–81]. A cervical esophageal web has been reported in approximately 10% of patients with Sjögren's syndrome [82].

The precise prevalence of dysphagia in Sjögren's syndrome is unclear. In the literature, dysphagia has been reported in 32–92% of patients [76, 78–83]. Dysphagia with solids is much more common than liquids [78–83]. Most patients localize the dysphagia sensation to the pharyngeal and upper esophageal region [78, 79, 82]. Patients can also present with odynophagia due to esophageal mucosal dissecans [84]. Heartburn, regurgitation and globus sensation occur in increased frequency in patients with Sjogren's syndrome when compared with controls [81].

Barium esophagram is normal in most patients. Close attention to the upper esophagus is needed to detect the subtle proximal esophageal web. Esophageal manometry, with dry and wet swallows, is usually normal in Sjögren's syndrome [78, 79, 83, 85]. Lower esophageal sphincter pressure varies, from low [78] to normal [82, 83] to elevated [79], while esophageal peristaltic pressures are usually normal, even when dysphagia is present [78, 79]. Rosztczy *et al.* reported in a study of 25 patients with primary Sjögren's syndrome that propagation velocity was slower than in normal controls [78]. Simultaneous esophageal contractions [80, 82, 83] and aperistalsis [83, 85] have been reported, but these occurrences are rare. In another study, non-specific esophageal dysmotility was the most common manometric abnormality in Sjögren's syndrome patients with dysphagia [86]. In the same study, these esophageal abnormalities did not correlate to clinical symptoms, disease duration, extraglandular manifestations, serological markers (RF, ANA, anti-Ro, and anti-La), or grade of minor salivary gland histopathology.

The treatment of Sjögren's syndrome is directed at correcting the lack of saliva. Patients are advised to increase intake of fluids with swallowing [76]. Other strategies include a change in diet, chewing sugarless gum, mucous-containing lozenges, and pharmacologic agents such as muscarinic cholinergic agonists [77].

Systemic lupus erythematosus

Anorexia, nausea, vomiting, and abdominal pain are common gastrointestinal symptoms associated with SLE. Esophageal involvement is less frequent. Approximately 16% of patients studied with SLE have an overlapping diagnosis of SSc, rheumatoid arthritis, polymyositis, or MCTD, which are all syndromes that can affect the esophagus [87]. Histologic findings of the esophagus are infrequent in patients with SLE. Harvey *et al.* reported that only four of 105 (4%) patients had arteritis in the esophagus [88].

Salivary gland dysfunction has been identified in SLE, which may contribute to symptoms of dysphagia or acid clearance [89]. Esophageal spasms have been suggested to be the cause of unexplained chest pain [90]. Reduced LES pressure and impaired peristalsis may contribute to heartburn and dysphagia. However, the correlation between esophageal symptoms and dysfunction has been poor with esophageal scintigraphy and manometry [89, 91]. Dysphagia is uncommon, occurring in 1.5–8% of patients with SLE [92]. The prevalence of heartburn and chest pain is unclear.

Physiologic esophageal dysfunction appears more common than the presence of esophageal symptoms. Esophageal scintigraphy may detect impaired esophageal transit in about 30% of the patients, including those with no esophageal complaints [87]. An abnormal esophageal manometry can be found in 32–72% of patients with SLE [87, 91]. Some patients have a manometric pattern similar to SSc with reduced LES and esophageal peristaltic pressures [87]. However, manometric abnormalities are less frequent in SLE than in SSc and MCTD [93]. The prevalence of esophageal aperistalsis is rare, only 4–7% [91].

Symptomatic patients should be evaluated for treatment. Therapy for acid suppression is reasonable when acid reflux is present.

Rheumatoid arthritis

Gastrointestinal manifestations of rheumatoid arthritis (RA) are rare, if complications of Aspirin and non-steroidal anti-inflammatory drugs are excluded, especially pill-induced esophagitis and stricture. Dysphagia has been reported in 10–38% of RA patients in a few small series studies, but usually does not require medical attention [94, 95]. There are many potential causes of dysphagia in RA. The prevalence of cricoarytenoid arthritis is estimated to be 26% [96]. The immobility of the cricoarytenoid joint can affect the coordination of oropharyngeal swallowing. RA may cause an inflammatory mass from chronic synovial inflammation that invades the adjacent laryngeal structures [97, 98]. This inflammatory mass consists of palisading histocytes, necrosis, confluent rheumatoid nodules, and destroyed cartilage [97, 98]. The anterior cervical spine spur may cause extrinsic compression on the upper esophagus, but in most cases it is an incidental finding rather than the cause of dysphagia. Geterud *et al.* reported that RA patients have reduced stimulated saliva production compared to normal controls, but this abnormality was not associated with dysphagia [94]. Bassotti *et al.* reported that esophageal motility disorders were common in RA, but the clinical significance was uncertain because the symptom correlation was poor [95]. The presence of dysphagia associated with hoarseness, nasal regurgitation, or stridor should alert clinicians to the possibility that oropharyngeal dysfunction may be present.

Radiating pain to the ears and pain with speech may indicate cricoarytenoid arthritis [96].

A videofluoroscopic study is helpful to identify functional abnormality. A laryngoscopic and physical examination may identify acute cricoarytenoid arthritis with erythema and edema over the arytenoids, immobile vocal processes, and tenderness on compressing the thyroid cartilage [96]. However, the examination in patients with chronic cricoarytenoid arthritis may be normal with minimal thickening over the arytenoids [96, 97]. An inflammatory rheumatoid mass may not be apparent on examination and usually requires a CT of the neck [97]. Esophageal manometry is likely to be normal in RA [99]. Some patients have non-specific triple-peaked waves, spasms, and spontaneous contractions [95], but distal peristaltic pressures are normal in most patients [94, 95].

The treatment of dysphagia in RA depends on the identifiable underlying etiology. Medical therapy of an inflammatory rheumatoid mass is usually ineffective, and surgical debridement is required in most patients [98].

Endocrine and metabolic diseases

Diabetes mellitus

Gastrointestinal symptoms are well recognized in patients with diabetes mellitus [14]. The most notable gastrointestinal symptoms in diabetic patients are often nausea and vomiting seen in diabetic gastroparesis. In addition, diarrhea and constipation can occur. Heartburn, dysphagia, and chest pain are infrequent symptoms among diabetic patients. The prevalence of heartburn is approximately 14% [100] and of dysphagia is 8–27% in diabetic outpatients [101, 102]. The presence of esophageal symptoms as a consequence of diabetes is not as clear: esophageal symptoms were reported to be more prevalent in diabetic than non-diabetic patients in an Australian study [103], whereas a US population study failed to find an increase in esophageal symptoms in diabetic patients compared to non-diabetic individuals [104].

Despite having relatively few symptoms, many patients have esophageal motility abnormalities. There is often a poor relationship with the presence of esophageal peristaltic dysfunction and esophageal symptoms. Approximately one-third of diabetic patients can have esophageal manometric abnormalities [105]. The most common esophageal motility abnormality in diabetic patients is ineffective peristalsis: non-transmitted esophageal contractions, simultaneous contractions, or low-amplitude esophageal contractions [106, 107]. A diminished LES pressure can also be seen. A close relationship has been reported between the level of peristaltic failure and the degree of bolus transit failure, as shown by esophageal scintigraphy [106].

The sensory function of the esophagus is also impaired in diabetes. Diabetics have a higher perception threshold for electrical stimuli and can produce erratic or absent cortical evoked potentials, suggesting vagal afferent sensory neuropathy [108].

The underlying causes for esophageal peristaltic dysfunction are primarily autonomic neuropathy (particularly vagal dysfunction) and hyperglycemia. The polyneuropathy seen in diabetes mellitus can affect the autonomic pathways of the esophagus, causing abnormalities in esophageal contractility. Hyperglycemia also has a significant effect on esophageal motor function. Acute hyperglycemia in normal subjects reduces LES pressure and prolongs peristaltic velocity of esophageal contractions [109]. Gastroesophageal reflux and esophageal motility abnormalities appear to worsen with longer duration of diabetes [110].

Treatment of esophageal dysmotility is aimed at the patient's symptoms and not the esophageal dysmotility *per se* [14]. Most diabetic patients who have esophageal dysmotility are asymptomatic. Patients with reflux symptoms should be treated with acid suppression. Prokinetic agents can be used if esophageal symptoms coexist with diabetic gastroparesis [14]. Control of hyperglycemia is advocated in any diabetic patient. Control of hyperglycemia can delay the onset and slow the progression of autonomic neuropathy [111]. However, the effectiveness of glycemic control for preventing the esophageal manifestations of diabetes is not yet known.

Obesity

See Chapter 33.

Thyroid disease

Thyroid disease is common, and its effects on the gastrointestinal system are widespread, affecting most hollow organs [112]. Hashimato's disease, the most common cause of hypothyroidism, may be associated with an esophageal motility disorder presenting as dysphagia or heartburn. The esophagus may be compressed by benign processes (thyroid enlargement) or even thyroid carcinomas. The gastrointestinal manifestations of thyroid disease are generally due to reduced motility in hypothyroidism, increased motility in hyperthyroidism, and esophageal compression by a thyroid process. Symptoms usually resolve with treatment of the thyroid process.

Hypothyroidism is a known cause of hypomotility of the gastrointestinal tract, particularly constipation from delayed colonic transit and early satiety and fullness from delayed gastric emptying. Reports of esophageal manifestations of hypothyroidism are rare and consist primarily of dysphagia [14]. The precise mechanism for the esophageal symptoms is unclear. Oropharyngeal dysphagia has been reported in some patients with myxedema. The cricopharyngeal muscle may not relax adequately with swallowing. Myxedema infiltration of the cricopharyngeus muscle has been suggested [113]. Other manometric abnormalities that have been reported include diminished LES pressure and low amplitude of peristaltic contractions [114, 115]. Dysphagia and the manometric abnormalities may improve with thyroid hormone replacement [113, 115, 116].

Hyperthyroidism can cause a variety of neurologic manifestations, including thyrotoxic myopathy and periodic paralysis [117]. Proximal muscle weakness and wasting of the striated muscles are common. Thyrotoxic myopathy involving the bulbar muscles can cause progressive oropharyngeal dysphagia [118–121]. Solid food dysphagia with esophageal dysfunction is rare [122, 123]. Dysphagia is usually progressive and associated with dysphonia, nasal regurgitation, and choking while swallowing [124]. The degree of hyperthyroidism in patients with dysphagia is usually very severe with marked weight loss and muscle wasting. Videofluoscopic studies can identify reduced pharyngeal movement, pooling of barium, and laryngeal penetration [120, 121]. Impaired esophageal peristalsis had been described with barium esophagram, and prolonged esophageal contraction velocity has been reported on esophageal manometry [123]. Dysphagia usually resolves completely after the patient is treated for hyperthyroidism, but improvement may take several months [124].

Electrolyte abnormalities

Hypercalcemia

Hypercalcemia can be seen in many disorders, including hyperparathyroidism and paraneoplastic syndrome. Gastrointestinal symptoms of hypercalcemia include constipation, anorexia, nausea, and vomiting. Esophageal manifestations are rare [14]. Chronic hypercalcemia can result in depression of the nervous system because the neuronal membrane is less likely to produce action potentials, resulting in reduced striated and smooth muscle contractility. Dysphagia to solids has been reported in patients with hypercalcemia associated with paraneoplastic syndrome [125, 126]. Heartburn has been reported to be seen by some investigators [127]. Esophageal manometry is generally normal, although a low LES pressure can be seen [127]. Dysphagia readily improves after correction of the hypercalcemia [125, 126]. Improvement of LES pressure has been reported during treatment of hypercalcemia [127].

Hypomagnesemia

Magnesium deficiency is a complication of nutritional deficiency states, such as starvation, short-bowel syndrome, diseases of malabsorption, and alcoholism [14, 128]. Magnesium deficiencies result in enhanced neuronal excitability. Dysphagia to solids and chest pain have been reported in patients with hypomagnesemia [129–131]. Interestingly, barium studies have shown rare cases of diffuse esophageal spasm and aperistalsis [129, 130]. Dysphagia and esophageal spasm may reverse after replenishing magnesium [129, 130].

Inflammatory diseases

Crohn's disease

Crohn's disease is a systemic inflammatory disorder affecting the entire gastrointestinal tract. Esophageal damage is an uncommon manifestation of Crohn's disease [132]. The prevalence of esophageal involvement is only 0.2–1.8% from two large retrospective series of patients with Crohn's disease [132, 133].

The diagnosis should be considered in patients who have other intestinal manifestations of Crohn's disease and present with esophageal symptoms. Dysphagia, odynophagia, retrosternal pain, and epigastric discomfort are symptomatic complaints associated with esophageal Crohn's disease [134]. Crohn's fistulae to the bronchopulmonary tree, mediastinum, pleura, and gastric cardia have been reported [135]. Ileitis or colitis is present in 95–100% of patients with esophageal involvement [133, 134, 136]. Isolated esophageal Crohn's disease is very rare [137, 138]. Diagnosis should be based on history, known extraesophageal Crohn's disease, endoscopic evaluation with biopsy, and exclusion of GERD.

A double-contrast barium esophagram is useful for evaluation of the esophagus. Aphthous ulcers appear as punctate, slit- or ring-like collections of barium [139]. Occasionally, thickened, irregular, and nodular mucosa folds may be seen. Strictures and fistulae can be identified with a barium esophagram. Endoscopy is very helpful to identify and biopsy the mucosal lesion. Esophageal erosions and ulcerations are the most common lesions found at endoscopy [133, 134]. The ulcers are usually superficial aphthous ulcers, but deep penetrating ulcers may occur [140].

The histologic findings in the esophagus consist of polymorphic inflammatory cells in the squamous epithelium and lamina propria [136]. The infiltrate consists of lymphocytes, eosinophils, mast cells, and neutrophils. A proliferation of histocytes and non-caseating granulomas may be present. The inflammation may be transmural, causing extensive fibrosis with anatomic obstruction of the esophageal lumen [137]. Fissures may penetrate deep into the muscularis, forming fistulae to adjacent organs [135].

Mild disease should be treated with acid suppression and a short course of steroids [14, 132]. 5-Aminosalicylates are unlikely to be effective due to drug release characteristics. Patients who have moderate to severe disease should be treated aggressively with acid suppression, a longer course of steroids, and consideration of immunosuppressive therapy with 6-mercaptopurine or azathioprine. Infliximab or other antitumor necrosis factor therapy also can be considered in refractory patients to try to prevent the complications of stricturing and fistula formation. In those patients who develop strictures of the esophagus, treatment with balloon dilatation of the stricture followed by injection of a long-acting steroid such as triamcinolone may help to alleviate symptoms. Surgery may be required for severe, refractory symptoms, but it has a high morbidity in this population.

Behçet's disease

Behçet's disease is a rare vasculitis with chronic relapsing symptoms diagnosed by the presence of recurrent oral ulcers and two of the following: genital ulcers, typical eye lesions, typical skin lesions, and a positive pathergy test [14]. It is most commonly seen in countries along the ancient silk road from Eastern Asia to the Mediterranean Basin [141], being highest in Turkey, with lower prevalence in Japan, Korea, China, Iran, and Saudi Arabia. Young adults between the second and fourth decades of life are mainly affected, with abdominal pain being the most common symptom. Gastrointestinal involvement in Behçet's disease mainly appears in mucosa and affects 5–40% of patients The ileocecal region is most commonly affected, with ulcerations that may penetrate or perforate. Rarely, the esophagus and stomach may have ulcerations. Bowel wall thickening is the most common finding on CT scan.

Esophageal involvement is uncommon, reported to occur in 2–11% of patients with Behçet's disease [142]. Esophageal symptoms of Behçet's disease consist of dysphagia, chest pain, and odynophagia [142, 143]. Importantly, esophageal lesions usually parallel oral ulcerations in Behçet's disease [142]. The most common lesions are recurrent esophageal erosions and ulcers [144, 145]. Deep penetrating ulcers can develop and dissect into the deep layers, and form a fistula to the adjacent organs [143, 146]. Luminal esophageal strictures can develop, causing persistent dysphagia [143, 145]. Pathology shows a vasculitis mainly involving the small veins or, alternatively, non-specific inflammation.

Diagnostic features in the esophagus are similar to esophageal Crohn's disease. Barium esophagram findings include mucosal ulcerations, irregular strictures, and fistula to the adjacent organs [143]. In one study using esophageal manometry in 25 patients with Behçet's disease [147], esophageal motor abnormalities were detected in 16% of patients (non-specific esophageal motor disorder in one, esophageal hypomotility in two, and LES hypotension in one patient). All cases with esophageal motor abnormalities were suffering from reflux, and endoscopy showed grade B esophagitis in two of these cases.

Esophageal symptoms are treated by treating the underlying Behçet's disease. Corticosteroids, with or without other immunosuppressive drugs, are used for severe eye disease. Their use in intestinal disease is largely empirical. Resolution of esophageal ulcers has been reported with corticosteroid therapy [144]. Long stenotic strictures and fistulae may require surgical interventions. Surgery may be required for perforation. Behçet's disease runs a chronic, unpredictable course with exacerbations and remissions that decrease in frequency and severity over time. Death is mainly due to major vessel disease and neurologic involvement.

Sarcoidosis

Sarcoidosis is a systemic disorder of unknown origin, characterized by accumulation of T lymphocytes, macrophages, and non-caseating epithelial granulomas. It affects the lungs in 90% of patients, and less frequently affects the lymph nodes, skin, and liver. Gastrointestinal tract sarcoidosis is an uncommon form of sarcoidosis [148]. The gastrointestinal tract can be involved as an isolated disease as a part of systemic sarcoidosis. The differential diagnosis of gastrointestinal sarcoidosis is extensive, including other granulomatous diseases of the gastrointestinal tract, such as tuberculosis, fungal infections, parasitic diseases, inflammatory bowel disease, and Whipple's disease.

Sporadic cases of esophageal sarcoidosis have been reported. Sarcoidosis can affect the esophagus in several different ways. The mid esophagus may be compressed extrinsically by mediastinal lymphadenopathy [149, 150]. Direct granulmatous infiltration of the esophagus has been reported, resulting in a markedly thickened esophagus. Development of strictures may also occur. The histologic findings consist of mononuclear inflammatory cells and non-caseating granuloma [151, 152]. Direct involvement of the myenteric plexus had been reported [154, 155], producing, in some cases, an achalasia-like picture.

Dysphagia is the most common presentation of esophageal sarcoidosis. Dysphagia can be mild with extrinsic compression of the esophagus or severe with marked weight loss in direct esophageal infiltration with sarcoidosis or secondary achalasia [151, 153].

The chest X-ray is abnormal in nearly all cases of esophageal sarcoidosis. A barium esophagram can identify areas of esophageal narrowing. Narrowing at the level of carina suggests extrinsic compression by subcarinal lymphadenopathy [149]. Mucosal irregularity and circumferential narrowing has been described in direct infiltration. Endoscopic biopsy may reveal the typical non-caseating, giant-cell granuloma and mononuclear infiltrates [154]. Special stains are needed to exclude tuberculosis and histoplasmosis. Manometric abnormalities vary.

Corticosteroid therapy is effective in the treatment of gastrointestinal sarcoidosis. Surgical intervention may be necessary in patients with bowel obstruction, perforation, or massive hemorrhage. Treatment with corticosteroids has been successful in relieving the dysphagia in esophageal sarcoidosis [150, 151, 153], and manometric abnormalities may return to normal. Among the rare cases of secondary achalasia, botulinum toxin injection [153] and Heller esophagomyotomy [153, 155] have improved dysphagia but residual symptoms may persist.

Systemic mastocytosis

Systemic mastocytosis is a rare heterogeneous disorder characterized by the accumulation of abnormal mast cells in various tissues [156]. The disease is usually divided into two categories. Localized cutaneous mastocytosis is the classical presentation. Systemic mastocytosis is more frequent in adults and is characterized by mast cell extracutaneous organ infiltration, including of the bone marrow, liver, spleen, and gastrointestinal tract. Esophageal lesions are rarely mentioned in the course of systemic mastocytosis. However, symptoms related to gastroesophageal reflux may occur and lesions can be found, including esophagitis and peptic esophageal stenosis. Rare esophageal motor disorders have been reported.

Neuromuscular diseases

Chagas disease (American trypanosomiasis)
See Chapter 13.

Amyloidosis

Amyloidosis is characterized by extracellular deposition of abnormal protein with a beta-sheet fibrillar structure and characteristic properties after staining with Congo Red dye [14, 157]. Primary amyloidosis (AL) is associated with monoclonal light chains in serum and/or urine, with 15% of patients having multiple myeloma. Secondary amyloidosis is associated with inflammatory, infections, and neoplastic diseases. The presentations are many, including macroglossia and a dilated and atonic esophagus. The most common oral manifestation of amyloidosis is macroglossia, which may cause sleep apnea, speech difficulties, oral dysphagia, difficulty in chewing, and eventually airway obstruction. The prevalence of esophageal disease in amyloidosis ranges from 13% to 22%. Symptoms include dysphagia, chest pain, heartburn, and hematemesis.

The most common radiographic feature is the dilated, atonic esophagus with decreased peristalsis, sometimes with distal narrowing and proximal dilatation. A variety of manometric abnormalities may be seen in the esophagus, with changes more common in AL than in AA amyloidosis. Generally, the LES pressure is normal or low, often with associated heartburn. The amplitude of esophageal contractions is decreased with the UES and pharynx operating normally.

Occasionally, the picture may mirror that seen in achalasia. Unlike idiopathic achalasia, patients experience a rapid onset of symptoms and significant, sometimes massive, weight loss. Neural involvement in esophageal amyloidosis is suggested by lack of the expected secondary peristalsis and LES relaxation caused by esophageal distention. Abnormal esophageal manometric findings can also be observed in some patients with familial Mediterranean fever regardless of amyloid status [158]. Amyloidosis should be considered in nondiabetic patients with nephrotic-range proteinuria, cardiomyopathy, hepatomegaly, and peripheral neuropathy.

Paraneoplastic syndromes

Paraneoplastic syndromes refer to the remote effects of neoplastic disorders on various organ systems. The underlying pathogenesis is believed to be that cancer cells express antigens mimicking the neuronal tissues, thus producing an autoimmune response [159]. Small cell lung cancer accounts for approximately 80% of the paraneoplastic syndromes, followed by breast, ovarian, and Hodgkin's lymphoma. Multiple paraneoplastic antineuronal antibodies have been identified. The most common antibody profile appears to be the anti-Hu antibody or antineuronal nuclear antibody 1 (ANNA-1) [159]. The paraneoplastic disorders affecting the esophagus are secondary achalasia and chronic intestinal pseudo-obstruction (CIP).

In secondary achalasia, typical symptoms and manometric findings to achalasia can be seen. The tumors can be at the gastroesophageal junction, in the lungs, or in remote areas away from the esophagus. Amyl nitrite has been suggested to differentiate secondary achalasia from idiopathic achalasia. Amyl nitrite produces a relaxation in idiopathic achalasia, but does not in secondary achalasia, especially from tumors at the gastroesophageal junction. In CIP, the findings on esophageal manometry are non-specific and include incomplete LES relaxation, simultaneous contractions, non-propagated contractions [160], and in some cases, secondary achalasia.

The gastrointestinal manifestations of paraneoplastic syndrome may occur before the primary cancer can be detected. Paraneoplastic syndrome should be considered in older individuals with weight loss and in patients at risk for lung and breast cancers. The treatment of the paraneoplastic esophageal symptoms depends on the severity of the esophageal disease compared of the stomach and the small bowel.

Dermatologic diseases affecting the esophagus

Many acquired and inherited cutaneous diseases may affect the oropharynx and proximal esophagus, since they share a similar stratified squamous epithelium. Cutaneous disease should be considered in patients with proximal esophageal ulcers and strictures. Underlying causes should be identified in the acquired syndromes.

Pemphigus and pemphigoid

Pemphigus and pemphigoid are autoimmune diseases characterized by bullous lesions on skin and mucous membranes. There are several variants of these diseases. Oropharyngeal and esophageal mucosal involvement commonly occurs in pemphigus vulgaris (PV) and cicatricial pemphigoid. Underlying pathogenic mechanisms include autoantibodies that induce disruption of the basement membrane zone. In PV, pathogenic antibodies are directed against desmoglein (Dsg), an adhesion molecule.

The frequency of esophageal involvement on PV is unclear. Earlier studies [161] suggested it is uncommon, whereas a later publication showed that the esophageal lesions can be seen in up to 70% of patients with PV [162]. Odynophagia and dysphagia are the usual symptoms of esophageal bullous disease. Endoscopy is the preferred diagnostic modality. Features on endoscopy include erosions, ulcers, bullous lesions, sheets of sloughed mucosa, and friability of the upper esophagus [163]. Esophageal mucosa can appear normal during initial passage of the endoscope and lesions can be seen during scope withdrawal [163]. There are case reports of severe esophageal mucosal desquamation (esophagitis dissecans superficialis) in bullous phemphigoid [164].

Histology provides the definitive diagnosis of esophageal involvement in PV: presence of basement membrane showing acantholysis deeply in the stratum spinosum with a suprabasal cleft [165]. The hallmark of PV is acantholysis (loss of cohesion among the keratinocytes of the stratum spinosum) with intact basement membrane and clumps of acantholytic cells floating in the blister fluid, the so-called Tzank cells [166]. Biopsies should be obtained both from the base of the lesions and surrounding normal appearing mucosa. Immunofluorescence of surrounding normal appearing mucosa will show deposits of IgG between epidermal cells. Enzyme-linked immunosorbent assay (ELISA) can be used to identify specific antibodies in PV, including Dsg 1 and Dsg3. Use of a special rocking-type biopsy forceps may allow for deep biopsy specimens to be obtained and better diagnosis. In one study, basement membrane was in 87% of biopsy specimens with rocking biopsy forceps compared to 16% with regular biopsy forceps [166]. On bullous phemphigoid, histopathologic examination shows a subepidermal blister with an underlying superficial inflammatory infiltrate containing lymphocytes, histiocytes, and eosinophils. Immunofluorescence shows linear deposits of C3 and IgG along the basement membrane zone.

Glucocorticoids are the mainstay of treatment for these diseases [167]. Long-term maintenance with prednisone may be required for the majority of patients [168]. Options for refractory cases include azathioprine, cyclophosphamide, mycophenolate mofetil, rituximab, methotrexate, and cyclosporine.

Epidermolysis bullosa

Epidermolysis bullosa acquisita is an acquired mucocutaneous syndrome characterized by skin fragility and by spontaneous and trauma-induced mucocutaneous blisters. It has been associated with amyloidosis, multiple myeloma, and inflammatory bowel disease. The underlying cause is the autoimmunity to type VII collagen, the anchoring protein for attaching the epidermis to the dermis layer. Tense blisters tend to occur on trauma-prone areas, such as the palms, soles, elbows, and knees. The clinical and endoscopic manifestations of epidermolysis bullosa are similar to pemphigus because they both cause blistering of the oral and upper esophageal mucosa. Esophageal mucosa may be damaged by the endoscope itself. Management is to identify and treat the underlying cause of epidermolysis bullosa. Endoscopic dilation may cause further blistering and scaring of the upper esophageal mucosa.

Lichen planus

Lichen planus (LP) is a chronic, relapsing, inflammatory disorder of the skin, nails and mucous membrane affecting 1% of the adult population. It causes mucocutaneous ulceration without blistering by a lymphocytic cell-mediated response against the basal epithelium. Esophageal involvement in LP is variable [169]. Patients usually present with odynophagia and dysphagia. Esophageal disease appears to be more common in the vulvoginal gingival subtype of LP. On endoscopy, esophageal strictures along with patchy white areas, superficial erosions, friability, and frequently linear ulceration are seen [170]. Histology may be non-specific or may show band-like inflammatory infiltrate and basal layer degeneration, including Civatte bodies (necrotic keratinocytes) [171]. Immunohistologic staining is not helpful in LP, except to exclude pemphigus and pemphigoid. Strictures can be treated with dilation with or without intralesional steroid injection [171]. Repeat injections may be needed. Strictures may not respond to systemic steroids [172, 173]. Oral and esophageal squamous carcinomas may develop in patients with mucosal lichen planus.

References

1. Domsic R, Fasanella K, Bielefeldt K. Gastrointestinal manifestations of systemic sclerosis. *Dig Dis Sci* 2008;53:1163–1174.
2. Hinchcliff M, Varga J. Systemic sclerosis/scleroderma: A treatable multisystem disease. *Am Family Physician* 2008; 78:961–968.
3. Sharma NL, Mahajan VK, Ranjan N, Sharma VC, Gupta M. Systemic scerlosis sine scleroderma and calcinosis cutis: report of a rare case. *Clin Rhuematol* 2010;29:215–219.
4. Akesson A, Wollheim FA. Organ manifestations in 100 patients with progressive systemic sclerosis: A comparison between the CREST syndrome and diffuse scleroderma. *Br J Rheumatol* 1989;28:281.
5. Bethards DM, Ouyang A. Scleroderma and collagen vascular disorders. In: Parkman HP, McCallum RW, Rao SC, eds. *A Handbook for the GI Motility Laboratory*. SLACK Inc, 2010.
6. Moore SC, DeSantis ER. Treatment of complications associated with systemic sclerosis. *Am J Health Syst Pharm* 2008; 65:315–322.
7. Treacy WL, Baggenstoss AH, Slocumb CH, *et al*. Scleroderma of the esophagus: a correlation of histologic and physiologic findings. *Ann Intern Med* 1963;59:351–356.
8. Russell ML, Friesen D, Henderson RD, et al. Ultrastructure of the esophagus in scleroderma. *Arthritis Rheumatol* 1982; 25:1117–1123.
9. Atkinson M, Summerling MD. Oesophageal changes in systemic sclerosis. *Gut* 1966;7:402–408.
10. Cohen S, Fisher R, Lipshutz W, *et al*. The pathogenesis of esophageal dysfunction in scleroderma and Raynaud's disease. *J Clin Invest* 1972;51:2663–2668.
11. Bortolotti M, Pinotti R, Sarti P, et al. Esophageal electromyography in scleroderma patients with functional dysphagia. *Am J Gastroenterol* 1989 ;84:1497–1502.
12. Kawaguchi Y, Nakamura Y, Matsumoto I, *et al*. Muscarinic-3 acetylcholine receptor autoantibody in patients with systemic sclerosis: contribution to severe gastrointestinal tract dysmotility. *Ann Rheum Dis* 2009;68:710–714.
13. Nishimagi E, Tochimoto A, Kawaguchi Y, *et al*. Characteristics of patients with early systemic sclerosis and severe gastrointestinal tract involvement. *J Rheumatol* 2007;34:2050–2055.
14. Wo JM. Esophageal involvement in systemic diseases. In: Castell DO, ed. *The Esophagus*. (3rd ed) Philadelphia: Lippincott, Williams and Wilkins, (2004) Chapter 37.
15. Abu-Shakra M, Guillemin F, Lee P. Gastrointestinal manifestations of systemic sclerosis. *Semin Arthritis Rheum* 1994; 24:29–39.
16. Weihrauch TR, Korting GW, Ewe K, *et al*. Esophageal dysfunction and its pathogenesis in progressive systemic sclerosis. *Klin Wochenschr* 1978,56:963–968.
17. Bassotti G, Battaglia E, Debernardi V, *et al*. Esophageal dysfunction in scleroderma: relationship with disease subsets. *Arthritis Rheumatol* 1997;40:2252–2259.
18. Murphy JR, McNally P, Peller P, *et al*. Prolonged clearance is the primary abnormal reflux parameter in patients with progressive systemic sclerosis and esophagitis. *Dig Dis Sci* 1992; 37:833–841.
19. Zamost BJ, Hirschberg J, Ippoliti AF, *et al*. Esophagitis in scleroderma. Prevalence and risk factors. *Gastroenterology* 1987; 92:421–428.
20. Katzka DA, Reynolds JC, Saul SH, *et al*. Barrett's metaplasia and adenocarcinoma of the esophagus in scleroderma. *Am J Med* 1987;82:46–52.
21. Duncan SC, Winklemann RK. Cancer and scleroderma. *Arch Dermatol* 1979;115:950–955.
22. Wipff J, Allanore Y, Soussi F, et al. Prevalence of Barrett's esophagus in systemic sclerosis. *Arthritis Rheumat* 2005; 52:2882–2888.
23. Segel MC, Campbell WL, Medsger TA Jr, *et al*. Systemic sclerosis (scleroderma) and esophageal adenocarcinoma: is increased patient screening necessary? *Gastroenterology* 1985; 89:485–488.
24. Savarino E, Bazzica M, Zentilin P, *et al.*. Gastroesophageal reflux and pulmonary fibrosis in scleroderma: a study using pH-impedance monitoring. *Am J Respir Crit Care Med* 2009; 179:408–413.
25. Gilson M, Zerkak D, Wipff J, *et al*. Prognostic factors for lung function in systemic sclerosis: prospective study of 105 cases. *Eur Respir J* 2010;35:112–117.
26. Kaye SA, Siraj QH, Agnew J, *et al*. Detection of early asymptomatic esophageal dysfunction in systemic sclerosis using a new scintigraphic grading method. *J Rheumatol* 1996; 23:297-301.
27. Weihrauch TR, Korting GW Manometric assessment of oesophageal involvement in progressive systemic sclerosis,

morphoea and Raynaud's disease. *Br J Dermatol* 1982; 107:325–332.

28. Olivé A, Juncosa S, Evison G, *et al.* Air in the oesophagus : a sign of oesophageal involvement in systemic sclerosis. *Clin Rheumatol* 1995;14:319–321.

29. Pitrez EH, Bredemeier M, Xavier RM, *et al.* Oesophageal dysmotility in systemic sclerosis: comparison of HRCT and scintigraphy. *Br J Radiol* 2006;79:719–724.

30. Cameron AJ, Malcolm A, Prather CM, *et al.* Videoendoscopic diagnosis of esophageal motility disorders. *Gastrointest Endosc* 1999;49:62–69.

31. Calderaro DC, de Carvalho MA. Moretzsohn LD, *et al.* Esophageal manometry in 28 systemic sclerosis Brazilian patients: findings and correlations. *Dis Esophagus* 2009;22:700–704.

32. Yarze JC, Varga J, Stampfl D, *et al.* Esophageal function in systemic sclerosis: a prospective evaluation of motility and acid reflux in 36 patients. *Am J Gastroenterol* 1993;88:870–876.

33. Schneider HA, Yonker RA, Longley S, *et al.* Scleroderma esophagus a nonspecific entity. *Ann Intern Med* 1984; 100:848–850.

34. Stentoft P, Hendel L, Aggestrup S. Esophageal manometry and pH-probe monitoring in the evaluation of gastroesophageal reflux in patients with progressive systemic sclerosis. *Scand J Gastroenterol* 1987;22:499–504.

35. Parkman HP, Miller DL, Maurer AH, Caroline DF, Krevsky B, Fisher RS. Optimal evaluation of esophageal dysphagia: Esophageal manometry, esophageal transit scintigraphy or videoesophagography? *Dig Dis Sci* 1996;41:1355–1368.

36. Wegener M, Adamek RJ, Wedmann B, *et al.* Gastrointestinal transit through esophagus, stomach, small and large intestine in patients with progressive systemic sclerosis. *Dig Dis Sci* 1994;39:2209–2215.

37. Geatti O, Shapiro B, Fig LM, *et al.* Radiolabelled semisolid test meal clearance in the evaluation of esophageal involvement in scleroderma and Sjogren's syndrome. *Am J Physiol Imaging* 1991;6:65–73.

38. Drane WE, Karvelis K, Johnson DA, *et al.* Progressive systemic sclerosis: radionuclide esophageal scintigraphy and manometry. *Radiology* 1986;160:73–76.

39. Klein HA, Wald A, Graham TO, *et al.* Comparative studies of esophageal function in systemic sclerosis. *Gastroenterology* 1992;102:1551–1556.

40. Janiak P, Thumshirn M, Menne D, *et al.* Clinical trial: the effects of adding ranitidine at night to twice daily omeprazole therapy on nocturnal acid breakthrough and acid reflux in patients with systemic sclerosis – a randomized controlled, cross-over trial. *Aliment Pharmacol Ther* 2007;26:1259–1265

41. Hendel L, Svejgaard E, Walsoe I, *et al.* Esophageal candidiasis in progressive systemic sclersosis. *Scand J Gastroenterol* 1988; 23:1182–1186.

42. Johnson DA, Drane WE, Curran J, *et al.* Metoclopramide response in patients with progressive systemic sclerosis. Effect on esophageal and gastric motility abnormalities. *Arch Intern Med* 1987;147:1597–1601.

43. Hendel L, Stentoft P, Aggestrup S. The progress of oesophageal involvement in progressive systemic sclerosis during D-penicillamine treatment. *Scand J Rheumatol* 1989;18:149–155.

44. Henderson R, Pearson F. Surgical management of esophageal scleroderma. *J Thorac Cardiovasc Surg* 1973;66:686.

45. Orringer M, Orringer J, Dabich L, Zarafonetis C. Combined Collis gastroplasty-fundoplication operations for scleroderma reflux esophagitis. *Surgery* 1981;90:624–630.

46. Poirer T, Taillefer R, Topart P, *et al.* Antireflux operations in patients with scleroderma. *Ann Thorac Surg* 1994;58:66.

47. Raftopoulos I, Awais O, Courcoulas A, Luketich J. Laparoscopic gastric bypass after antireflux surgery for the treatment of gastroesophageal reflux in morbidly obese patients: initial experience. *J Obes Surg* 2004;14:1373–1380.

48. Kent MS, Luketich JD, Irshad K, *et al.* Comparison of surgical approaches to recalcitrant gastroesophageal reflux disease in the patient with scleroderma. *Ann Thorac Surg* 2007; 84:1710–1715.

49. Marshall JB, Kretschmar JM, Gerhardt DC, *et al.* Gastrointestinal manifestations of mixed connective tissue disease. *Gastroenterology* 1990;98:1232–1238.

50. Hoffman RW, Greidinger EL. Mixed connective tissue disease. *Curr Opin Rheumatol* 2000;12:386–390.

51. Sharp GC, Irvine WS, Tan EM, *et al.* Mixed connective tissue disease-an apparently distinct rheumatic disease syndrome associated with a specific antibody to an extractable nuclear antigen (ENA). *Am J Med* 1972;52:148–115.

52. Oxenhandler R, Hart M, Corman L, *et al.* Pathology of skeletal muscle in mixed connective tissue disease. *Arthritis Rheumatol* 1977;20:985–988.

53. Stacher G, Merio R, Budka C, *et al.* Cardiovascular autonomic function, autoantibodies, and esophageal motor activity in patients with systemic sclerosis and mixed connective tissue disease. *J Rheumatol* 2000;27:692–697.

54. Fagundes MN, Caleiro MT, Navarro-Rodriguez T, *et al.* Esophageal involvement and interstitial lung disease in mixed connective tissue disease. *Respir Med* 2009;103:854–860.

55. Doria A, Bonavina L, Anselmino M, *et al.* Esophageal involvement in mixed connective tissue disease. *J Rheumatol* 1991; 18:685–690.

56. Prakash UB, Luthra HS, Divertie MB. Intrathoracic manifestations in mixed connective tissue disease. *Mayo Clin Proc* 1985;60:813–821.

57. Gutierrez F, Valenzuela JE, Ehresmann GR, *et al.* Esophageal dysfunction in patients with mixed connective tissue diseases and systemic lupus erythematosus. *Dig Dis Sci* 1982; 27:592–597.

58. Dalakas MC. Polymyositis, dermatomyositis, and inclusion body myositis. *N Engl J Med* 1991;325:1487–1498.

59. Amato AA, Barohn RJ. Idiopathic inflammatory myopathies. *Neurol Clin* 1997;15:615–648.

60. Plotz PH. NIH conference: current concepts in the idiopathic inflammatory myopathies: polymyositis, dermatomyositis, and related disorders. *Ann Intern Med* 1989;111:143–157.

61. Kagen LJ, Hochman RB, Strong EW. Cricopharyngeal obstruction in inflammatory myopathy (polymyositis/ dermatomyositis): report of three cases and review of the literature. *Arthritis Rheumatol* 1985;28:630–636.

62. Dietz F, Logeman JA, Sahgal V, *et al.* Cricopharyngeal muscle dysfunction in the differential diagnosis of dysphagia in polymyositis. *Arthritis Rheumatol* 1980;23:491–495.

63. O'Hara JM, Szemes G, Lowman RM. The esophageal lesions in dermatomyositis : a correlation of radiologic and pathologic findings. *Radiology* 1967;89:27–31.

64. de Merieux P, Verity MA, Clements PJ, *et al*. Esophageal abnormalities and dysphagia in polymyositis and dermatomyositis. *Arthritis Rheumatol* 1983;26:961–968.

65. Uthman I, Vazquez-Abad D, Senecal JL. Distinctive features of idiopathic inflammatory myopathies in French Canadians. *Semin Arthritis Rheum* 1996;26:447–458.

66. Jacob H, Berkowitz D, McDonald E, *et al*. The esophageal motility disorder of polymyositis: a prospective study. *Arch Intern Med* 1983;143:2262–2264.

67. Koh ET Seow A, Ong B, *et al*. Adult onset polymyositis/dermatomyositis: clinical and laboratory features and treatment response in 75 patients. *Ann Rheum Dis* 1993; 52:857–861.

68. Ramirez G, Asherson RA, Khamashta MA, *et al*. Adult-onset polymyositis-dermatomyositis : description of 25 patients with emphasis on treatment. *Semin Arthritis Rheum* 1990; 20:114–120.

69. Maugars YM, Berthelot JM, Abbas AA, *et al*. Long-term prognosis of 69 patients with dermatomyositis or polymyositis. *Clin Exp Rheumatol* 1996;14:263–274.

70. Horowitz M, McNeil JD, Maddern GJ, *et al*. Abnormalities of gastric and esophageal emptying in polymyositis and dermatomyositis. *Gastroenterology* 1986;90:434–439.

71. Lotz BE Engel AG, Nishino H, *et al*. Inclusion body myositis: observations in 40 patients. *Brain* 1989;112:727–747.

72. Tymms KE, Webb J. Dermatopolymyositis and other connective tissue diseases: a review of 105 cases. *J Rheumatol* 1985; 12:1140–1148.

73. Palace J, Losseff N, Clough C. Isolated dysphagia due to polymyositis. *Muscle Nerve* 1993;16:680–681.

74. Kornizky Y, Heller I, Isakov A, *et al*. Dysphagia with multiple autoimmune disease. *Clin Rheumatol* 2000;19:321–323.

75. Oh T, Brumfield KA, Hoskin KA, *et al*. Dysphagia in inflammatory myopathy: clinical characteristics, treatment strategies, and outcome in 62 patients. *Mayo Clinic Proc* 2007; 82:441–447.

76. Sheikh SH, Shaw-Stiffel TA. The gastrointestinal manifestations of Sjogren's syndrome. *Am J Gastroenterol* 1995; 90:9–14.

77. Sreebny LM. Saliva in health and disease: an appraisal and update. *Int Dental J* 2000;50:140–161.

78. Rosztczy A, Kovâcs L, Wittmann T, *et al*. Manometric assessment of impaired esophageal motor function in primary Sjogren's syndrome. *Clin Exp Rheumatol* 2001;19:147–152.

79. Grande L, Lacima G, Ros E, *et al*. Esophageal motor function in primary Sjogren's syndrome. *Am J Gastroenterol* 1993; 88:378–381.

80. Anselmino M, Zaninotto G, Costantini M, *et al*. Esophageal motor function in primary Sjogren's syndrome: correlation with dysphagia and xerostomia. *Dig Dis Sci* 1997;42:113–118.

81. Mandl T, Ekberg O, Wollmer P, *et al*. Dysphagia and dysmotility of the pharynx and oesophagus in patients with primary Sjogren's syndrome. *Scand J Rheumatol* 2007;36:394–401.

82. Kjellén G, Fransson SG, Lindström F, *et al*. Esophageal function, radiography, and dysphagia in Sjogren's syndrome. *Dig Dis Sci* 1986;31:225–229.

83. Palma R, Freire A, Freitas J, et al. Esophageal motility disorders in patients with Sjogren's syndrome. *Dig Dis Sci* 1994; 39:758–761.

84. Patel NK. Salathe C. Vu C. Anderson SH, *et al*. Esophagitis dissecans: a rare cause of odynophagia. *Endoscopy* 2007;39 (Suppl 1):E127.

85. Tsianos EB, Chiras CD, Drosos AA, *et al*. Oesophageal dysfunction in patients with primary Sjogren's syndrome. *Ann Rheum Dis* 1985;44:610–613.

86. Turk T, Pirildar T, Tunc E, *et al*. Manometric assessment of esophageal motility in patients with primary Sjogren's syndrome. *Rheumatol Int* 2005;25:246–249.

87. ter Borg EJ, Groen H, Horst G, *et al*. Clinical associations of antiribonucleoprotein antibodies in patients with systemic lupus erythematosus. *Semin Arthritis Rheum* 1990;20:164–173.

88. Harvey A, Shulman L, Tumulty P, *et al*. Systemic lupus erythematosus: review of the literature and clinical analysis of 138 cases. *Medicine* 1954;33:291–437.

89. Sultan SM, Ioannou Y, Isenberg DA. A review of gastrointestinal manifestations of systemic lupus erythematosus. *Rheumatology (Oxford)* 1999;38:917–932.

90. Peppercorn MA, Docken WP, Rosenberg S. Esophageal motor dysfunction in systemic lupus erythematosus. Two cases with unusual features. *JAMA* 1979;242:1895–1896.

91. Ramirez-Mata M, Reyes PA, Alarcon-Segovia D, *et al*. Esophageal motility in systemic lupus erythematosus. *Am J Dig Dis* 1974;19:132–136.

92. Dubois EL, Tuffanelli DL. Clinical manifestations of systemic lupus erythematosus. *JAMA* 1964;190:104–111.

93. Lapadula G, Muolo P, Semeraro F, *et al*. Esophageal motility disorders in the rheumatic diseases: a review of 150 patients. *Clin Exp Rheumatol* 1994;12:515–521.

94. Geterud A, Bake B, Bjelle A, *et al*. Swallowing problems in rheumatoid arthritis. *Acta Otolaryngol* 1991;111:1153–1161.

95. Bassotti G, Gaburri M, Biscarini L, *et al*. Oesophageal motor activity in rheumatoid arthritis : a clinical and manometric study. *Digest* 1988;39:144–150.

96. Lofgren RH, Montgomery WW. Incidence of laryngeal involvement in rheumatoid arthritis. *N Engl J Med* 1962;267:193–195.

97. Sorensen WT, Moller-Andersen K, Behrendt N. Rheumatoid nodules of the larynx. *J Laryngol Otol* 1998;112:573–574.

98. Erb N, Pace AV, Delamere JE, *et al*. Dysphagia and stridor caused by laryngeal rheumatoid arthritis. *Rheumatology (Oxford)* 2001;40:952–953.

99. Tsianos EB, Drosos AA, Chiras CD, *et al*. Esophageal manometric findings in autoimmune rheumatic diseases: is scleroderma esophagus a specific entity? *Rheumatol Int* 1987;7:23–27.

100. Talley NJ, Young L, Bytzer P, *et al*. Impact of chronic gastrointestinal symptoms in diabetes mellitus on health-related quality of life. *Am J Gastroenterol* 2001;96:71–76.

101. Keshavarzian A, Iber FL. Gastrointestinal involvement in insulin-requiring diabetes mellitus. *J Clin Gastroenterol* 1987; 9:685–692.

102. Feldman M, Schiller LR. Disorders of gastrointestinal motility associated with diabetes mellitus. *Ann Intern Med* 1983;98:378-384.

103. Bytzer E Talley NJ, Leemon M, *et al*. Prevalence of gastrointestinal symptoms associated with diabetes mellitus: a population-based survey of 15,000 adults. *Arch Intern Med* 2001;161:1989–1996.

104. Maleki D, Locke GR, III, Camilleri M, *et al*. Gastrointestinal tract symptoms among persons with diabetes mellitus in the community. *Arch Intern Med* 2000;160:2808–2816.

105. Pozzi M, Rivolta M, Gelosa M, *et al.* Upper gastrointestinal involvement in diabetes mellitus: study of esophagogastric function. *Acta Diabetologica Latina* 1988;25:333–341.

106. Holloway RH, Tippett MD, Horowitz M, *et al.* Relationship between esophageal motility and transit in patients with type I diabetes mellitus. *Am J Gastroenterol* 1999;94:3150–3157.

107. Stewart IM, Hosking DJ, Preston BJ, *et al.* Oesophageal motor changes in diabetes mellitus. *Thorax* 1976;31:278–283.

108. Kamath MV, Tougas G, Fitzpatrick D, *et al.* Assessment of the visceral afferent and autonomic pathways in response to esophageal stimulation in control subjects and in patients with diabetes. *Clin Invest Med* 1998;21:100–113.

109. De Boer SY, Masclee AA, Lam WF, *et al.* Effect of acute hyperglycemia on esophageal motility and lower esophageal sphincter pressure in humans. *Gastroenterology* 1992;103:775–780.

110. Kinekawa F, Kubo F, Matsuda K, *et al.* Esophageeal function worsens with long duration of diabetes. *J Gastroenterol* 2008;43:338–344.

111. The effect of intensive treatment of diabetes on the development and progression of long-term complications in insulin dependent diabetes mellitus. The Diabetes Control and Complications Research Group. *N Engl J Med* 1993; 329:977–986.

112. Ebert EC. The thyroid and the gut. *J Clin Gastroenterol* 2010;44:402–406.

113. Wright RA, Penner DB. Myxedema and upper esophageal dysmotility. *Dig Dis Sci* 1981;26:376–377.

114. Bassotti G, Pagliacci MC, Nicoletti I, *et al.* Intestinal pseudoobstruction secondary to hypothyroidism. Importance of small bowel manometry. *J Clin Gastroenterol* 1992;14:56–58.

115. Eastwood GL, Braverman LE, White EM, *et al.* Reversal of lower esophageal sphincter hypotension and esophageal aperistalsis after treatment for hypothyroidism. *J Clin Gastroenterol* 1982;4:307–310.

116. Urquhart AD, Rea IM, Lawson IT, *et al.* A new complication of hypothyroid coma: neurogenic dysphagia: presentation, diagnosis, and treatment. *Thyroid* 2001;11:595–598.

117. Engel AG. Neuromuscular manifestations of Grave's disease. *Mayo Clin Proc* 1972;47:919–925.

118. Kammer GM, Hamilton CR Jr. Acute bulbar muscle dysfunction and hyperthyroidism: a study of four cases and review of the literature. *Am J Med* 1974;56:464–470.

119. Ming RH, Dreosti LM, Tim LO, *et al.* Thyrotoxicosis presenting as dysphagia: a case report. *S Afr Med J* 1982;61:554.

120. Noto H, Mitsuhashi T, Ishibashi S, *et al.* Hyperthyroidism presenting as dysphagia. *Intern Med* 2000;39:472–473.

121. Marks P, Anderson J, Vincent R. Thyrotoxic myopathy presenting as dysphagia. *Postgrad Med J* 1980;56:669–670.

122. Sweatman MC, Chambers L. Disordered oesophageal motility in thyrotoxic myopathy. *Postgrad Med J* 1985;61:619–620.

123. Meshkinpour H, Afrasiabi MA, Valenta LJ. Esophageal motor function in Grave's disease. *Dig Dis Sci* 1979;24:159–161.

124. Joasoo A, Murray IP, Steinbeck AW. Involvement of bulbar muscles in thyrotoxic myopathy. *Aust Ann Med* 1970; 19:338–340.

125. Balcombe NR. Dysphagia and hypercalcemia. *Postgrad Med J* 1999;75:373–374.

126. Grieve RJ, Dixon PE. Dysphagia: a further symptom of hypercalcemia? *Br Med J* 1983;286:1935–1936.

127. Mowschenson PM, Rosenberg S, Pallotta J, *et al.* Effect of hyperparathyroidism and hypercalcemia on lower esophageal sphincter pressure. *Am J Surg* 1982;143:36–39.

128. Iannello S, Belfiore E. Hypomagnesemia: a review of pathophysiological, clinical and therapeutical aspects. *Panminerva Med* 2001;43:177–209.

129. Iannello S, Spina M, Leotta P, *et al.* Hypomagnesemia and smooth muscle contractility: diffuse esophageal spasm in an old female patient. *Mineral Electrol Metabol* 1998;24:348–356.

130. Harried IA, Lindeman RD. Dysphagia and vertical nystagmus in magnesium deficiency. *Ann Intern Med* 1978;89:222–223.

131. Flink EB. Dysphagia in magnesium deficiency. *Ann Intern Med* 1978;89:282.

132. Isaacs KL. Crohn's disease of the esophagus. *Curr Treat Options Gastroenterol* 2007;10:61–70.

133. Geboes K, Janssens J, Rutgeerts P, *et al.* Crohn's disease of the esophagus. *J Clin Gastroenterol* 1986;8:31–37.

134. Decker GA, Loftus EV Jr, Pasha TM, *et al.* Crohn's disease of the esophagus: clinical features and outcomes. *Inflamm Bowel Dis* 2001;7:113–119.

135. Clarke BW, Cassara JE, Morgan DR. Crohn's disease of the esophagus with esophagobronchial fistula formation: a case report and review of the literature. *Gastrointest Endosc* 2010; 71:207–209.

136. D'Haens G, Rutgeerts P, Geboes K, *et al.* The natural history of esophageal Crohn's disease: three patterns of evolution. *Gastrointest Endosc* 1994;40:296–300.

137. Gheorghe C, Aposteanu G, Popescu C, *et al.* Long esophageal stricture in Crohn's disease : a case report. *Hepatogastroenterology* 1998;45:738–741.

138. LiVolsi VA, Jaretzki A. Granulomatous esophagitis: a case of Crohn's disease limited to the esophoagus. *Gastroenterology* 1973;64:313–319.

139. Levine MS. Crohn's disease of the upper gastrointestinal tract. *Radiol Clin North Am* 1987;25:79–91.

140. Ghahremani GG, Gore RM, Breuer RI, *et al.* Esophageal manifestations of Crohn's disease. *Gastrointest Radiol* 1982;7:199–203.

141. Ebert EC. Gastrointestinal manifestations of Behçet's disease. *Dig Dis Sci* 2009;54:201–207.

142. Bayraktar Y, Özaslan E, Van Thiel DH. Gastrointestinal manifestations of Behcet's disease. *J Clin Gastroenterol* 2000;30:144–154.

143. Mori S, Yoshihira A, Kawamura H, *et al.* Esophageal involvement in Behcet's disease. *Am J Gastroenterol* 1983;78:548-553.

144. Ikezawa K, Kashimura H, Hassan M, *et al.* A case of Behcet's syndrome with esophageal involvement treated with salicylazosulfapyridine and prednisolone. *Endoscopy* 1998;30:552–553.

145. Bottomley WW, Dakkak M, Walton S, *et al.* Esophageal involvement in Behcet's disease. Is endoscopy necessary? *Dig Dis Sci* 1992;37:594–597.

146. Yashiro K, Nagasako K, Hasegawa K, *et al.* Esophageal lesions in intestinal Behcet's disease. *Endoscopy* 1986;18:57–60.

147. Bektas M, Altan M, Alkan M, Ormeci N, Soykan I. Manometric evaluation of the esophagus in patients with Behçet's disease. *Digestion* 2007;76:192–195.

148. Vahid B, Spodik M, Braun KN, Ghazi LJ, Esmaili A. Sarcoidosis of gastrointestinal tract: a rare disease. *Dig Dis Sci* 2007;52:3316–3320.

149. Cappell MS. Endoscopic, radiographic, and manometric findings in dysphagia associated with sarcoid due to extrinsic

esophageal compression from subcarinal lymphadenopathy. *Am J Gastroenterol* 1995;90:489–492.

150. Cook DM, Dines DE, Dycus DS. Sarcoidosis: report of a case presenting as dysphagia. *Chest* 1970;57:84–86.

151. Hardy WE, Tulgan H, Haidak G, *et al*. Sarcoidosis: a case presenting with dysphagia and dysphonia. *Ann Intern Med* 1967;66:353–357.

152. Polachek AA, Matre XJ. Gastrointestinal sarcoidosis: report of a case involving the esophagus. *Am J Dig Dis* 1964;9:429–433.

153. Lukens FJ, Machicao VI, Woodward TA, et al. Esophageal sarcoidosis: an unusual diagnosis. *J Clin Gastroenterol* 2002;34:54–56.

154. Boruchowicz A, Canva-Delcambre V, Guillemont F, *et al*. Sarcoidosis and achalasia: a fortuitous association? *Am J Gastroenterol* 1996;91:413–414.

155. Dufresne CR, Jeyasingham K, Baker RR. Achalasia of the cardia associated with pulmonary sarcoidosis. *Surgery* 1983;94:32–35.

156. Sokol H, Georgin-Lavialle S, Grandpeix-Guyodo C, *et al*. Gastrointestinal involvement and manifestations in systemic mastocytosis. *Inflamm Bowel Dis* 2010;16:1247–1253.

157. Ebert EC, Nagar M. Gastrointestinal manifestations of amyloidosis. *Am J Gastroenterol* 2008;103:776–787.

158. Doganay BM, Alkan M, Ustun Y, Soykan I. Esophageal motor function in Familial Mediterranean Fever: a prospective evaluation of motility in 31 patients. *Eur J Intern Med* 2009;20:548–550.

159. Lucchinetti CF, Kimmel DW, Lennon VA. Paraneoplastic and oncologic profiles of patients seropositive for type 1 antineuronal nuclear autoantibodies. *Neurology* 1998;50:652–657.

160. Lee HR, Lennon VA, Camilleri M, *et al*. Paraneoplastic gastrointestinal motor dysfunction: clinical and laboratory characteristics. *Am J Gastroenterol* 2001;96:373–379.

161. Gellis S, Glass FA. Pemphigus: a survey of 170 patients admitted to Bellevue Hospital from 1911 to 1941. *Arch Derm Syph* 1941;44:321–326.

162. Galloro G, Mignogna M, de Werra C, *et al*., The role of upper endoscopy in identifying oesophageal involvement in patients with oral pemphigus vulgaris. *Dig Liver Dis* 2005;37:195–199.

163. Faias S, Lage P, Sachse F, *et al*. Pemphigus vulgaris with exclusive involvement of the esophagus: case report and review. *Gastrointest Endosc* 2004;60:312–315.

164. Hwang JY, Park KS, Cho KB, Hwang JS, Ahn SH. Esophageal mucosal desquamation with hemorrhage in bullous pemphigoid: a case report. *Kor J Gastroenterol [Taehan Sohwagi Hakhoe Chi]* 2004;43:264–267.

165. Eversole LR. Immunopathology of oral mucosal ulcerative desquamative and bullous diseases: selective review of literature. *Oral Surg Oral Med Oral Pathol* 1994;77:555–571.

166. Galloro G, Diamantis G, Magno L, *et al*. Technical aspects in endoscopic biopsy of lesions in esophageal pemphigus vulgaris. *Dig Liver Dis* 2007;39:363–367.

167. Carson PJ, Hameed A, Ahmed AR. Influence of treatment on the clinical course of pemphigus vulgaris. *J Am Acad Dermatol* 1996;34:645.

168. Mourellou O, Chaidemenos GC, Koussidou T, Kapetis E. The treatment of pemphigus vulgaris. Experience with 48 patients seen over an 11-year period. *Br J Dermatol* 1995;133:83.

169. Quispel R, Van Boxel OS, Schipper ME, *et al*. High prevalence of lichen planus in esophagus: a study using magnification chromoendoscopy. *J Clin Gastroenterol*. 2006;40(8 Suppl 4):S189–S190.

170. Keate RF, Williams JW, Connolly SM. Lichen planus esophagitis: report of three patients treated with oral tacrolimus or intraesophageal corticosteroid injections or both. *Dis Esophagus* 2003;16:47–53.

171. Wedgeworth EK, Vlavianos P, Groves CJ, Neill S, Westaby D. Management of symptomatic esophageal involvement with lichen planus. *J Clin Gastroenterol* 2009;43:915–919.

172. Evans AV, Fletcher CL, Owen WJ, *et al*. Oesophageal lichen planus. *Clin Exp Dermatol* 2000;25:36–37.

173. Bobadillo J, Van der Hult R, Ften K, *et al*. Oesophageal lichen planus. *Gastrointest Endosc* 1999;50:268–271.

IV

Gastroesophageal Reflux

19 Clinical Spectrum and Diagnosis of Gastroesophageal Reflux Disease

Amit Agrawal and Donald O. Castell
Department of Medicine, Medical University of South Carolina, Charleston, SC, USA

Clinical spectrum

Thirty years ago, most patients who complained of heartburn, regurgitation, and water brash were given a diagnosis of "hiatal hernia" [1], despite evidence then emerging that a hernia is not found in all patients with these symptoms [2]. Twenty years ago, the diagnosis offered for the same symptoms would probably have been esophagitis, even though endoscopy sometimes showed a normal esophagus. Today, the acronym GERD has gained favor to denote the clinical manifestations of gastroesophageal reflux disease, being used as a diagnostic term that embraces the whole variety of symptoms and types of tissue damage that may be caused by reflux of gastric contents into the esophagus. GERD denotes abnormality and so should not be confused with the gastroesophageal reflux that occurs in healthy subjects (physiologic reflux), which does not cause symptoms or esophageal mucosal injury.

Clinical presentations of GERD vary considerably but can be logically grouped into three categories: typical symptoms, atypical symptoms, and complications. These comprise the spectrum of GERD (Figure 19.1).

Typical symptoms

Heartburn and regurgitation are the typical symptoms of GERD. When they are a patient's only symptoms, or predominant symptoms, they are specific but not sensitive as a basis for diagnosis [3]. Many patients with GERD have a less specific presentation, however, such as epigastric pain or other dyspepsia together with some retrosternal heartburn.

Reliable diagnosis on the basis of symptoms is not then possible. Fewer than 50% of patients with GERD have endoscopic evidence of esophagitis, and neither the pattern nor the severity of symptoms predict its presence or absence [1, 4–6].

Heartburn and regurgitation are characteristically worsened after eating, by bending or stooping, and by lying down in bed at night, especially by lying on the right side rather than the left. Heartburn and regurgitation may also be experienced during sexual intercourse (*reflux dyspareunia*)—a manifestation of reflux disease that is not commonly discussed. In one series of 100 women with chronic reflux symptoms, 77% complained of troubling heartburn during intercourse [7].

Atypical symptoms

Angina-like chest pain, sometimes including an exertional component, is one of the less typical symptoms of GERD. Ambulatory recordings of intraesophageal pH have been used to document directly the relationship of chest pain episodes to reflux. Findings of such studies indicate that previously unrecognized GERD is a major cause of non-cardiac chest pain [8–13].

Reflux also may be present as chronic hoarseness or other voice abnormalities associated with posterior inflammation of the larynx and vocal cords, a manifestation often referred to as *reflux laryngitis*. When studied with prolonged pH monitoring, more than 75% of such patients have been shown to have abnormal reflux, and acid exposure in the hypopharynx can be documented occasionally [14–16]. It has even been suggested that chronic reflux injury may promote malignant change. Ward and Hanson reported the occurrence of laryngeal cancer in 19 of 138 patients with moderate or severe reflux during a 10-year period [17]. None of these patients smoked or consumed alcohol, activities usually expected to be associated with laryngeal malignancies.

Various pulmonary symptoms may be associated with GERD. Nocturnal episodes of non-allergic asthma, particularly when preceded by a history of chronic reflux symptoms, are highly suggestive of reflux disease. Intraesophageal pH monitoring studies have demonstrated abnormal amounts of reflux in more than 20% of patients with chronic cough [18] and in more than 80% of unselected patients with chronic asthma [19]. Although pH monitoring may show that pulmonary symptoms occur after a reflux episode, often they may occur during reflux or even before it, making it hard to ascertain whether reflux is causing coughing or coughing is causing reflux [20].

Protracted hiccups also have been observed in reflux patients. In one such case, hiccups resolved in response to treatment with cimetidine and recurred on esophageal exposure to acid during a Bernstein test [21]. A specific causal relationship has been questioned, however, in that changes in esophageal pressures during hiccups are likely to cause reflux [22]. A variety of other atypical symptoms of GERD have been suggested. These include globus sensation, erosion of dental enamel, ear pain, night sweats, and intermittent torticollis or peculiar posturing in children (Sandifer's syndrome).

Complications

GERD can also present with the complications of reflux, such as erosive or ulcerative esophagitis, which may cause bleeding and anemia, or peptic stricture, which may cause dysphagia. However, intermittent dysphagia may be a feature of GERD even when no stricture is present [23]. Presumably it then occurs as a consequence of impaired bolus propulsion resulting from suboptimal esophageal body peristalsis [24]. Severe chronic reflux may also induce metaplastic change of the squamous epithelium of the lower

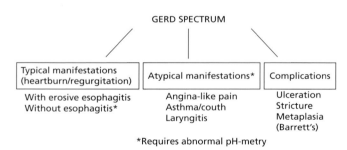

Figure 19.1 Demonstration of the various manifestations comprising the clinical spectrum of gastroesophageal reflux disease.

esophagus to a glandular (columnar) epithelium, referred to as Barrett's esophagus. This is of particular concern because it carries an increased risk of esophageal adenocarcinoma. In one study, 12% of unselected patients with chronic symptoms of heartburn and regurgitation had endoscopic and histologic changes in the esophageal epithelium consistent with Barrett's esophagus [6]. Recent epidemiologic evidence has given further strong support to the belief that longstanding reflux symptoms are associated with an enhanced risk of developing esophageal adenocarcinoma [25].

Prevalence

Quantitative estimates of the actual prevalence of GERD in the United States are difficult to obtain because of the sparsity of epidemiologic studies and because many individuals do not seek medical care for their symptoms. One often cited study provided information on the prevalence of heartburn from a questionnaire survey of 1004 individuals [26]. Included in the study population were 335 normal control subjects, 200 surgical inpatients, 246 medical inpatients, 121 patients attending a gastrointestinal clinic, and 102 pregnant patients attending an obstetrics clinic (Table 19.1). Overall, 11% of the entire study group reported daily heartburn, and an additional 12% and 15% described weekly and monthly heartburn, respectively, resulting in a total prevalence of 38% for heartburn in this sample of US adults. The substantially higher prevalence of daily heartburn (25%) described by pregnant women in the obstetrics clinic as compared with subjects in the other four groups reflects the well-known association between heartburn and pregnancy. The popular concepts that heartburn occurs daily in approximately 10% of US adults and that more than one-third of that population have occasional heartburn had their genesis in these data.

The concept of the GERD iceberg (Figure 19.2), was developed to demonstrate the clinical presentation of typical GERD symptoms. Most patients with heartburn and regurgitation have intermittent symptoms for which they do not consult their physicians and for which they frequently take

Table 19.1 Estimated heartburn prevalence in the United States (from Nebel *et al.*[26]).

Study group	Number of patients	Percentage experiencing heartburn			
		Daily	**Weekly**	**Monthly**	**Total**
Controls	335	7	14	15	36
Surgical inpatients	200	6	12	19	37
Medical inpatients	246	14	12	14	40
Gastrointestinal clinic patients	121	15	12	13	40
Obstetrics clinic patients	102	25	10	17	52
Total	1,004	11	12	15	38

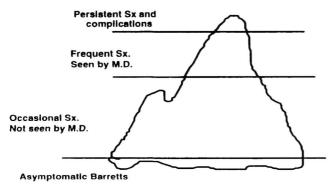

Figure 19.2 Gastroesophageal reflux disease iceberg displays the clinical presentations of typical manifestations. Details are provided in the text. Sx, symptoms.

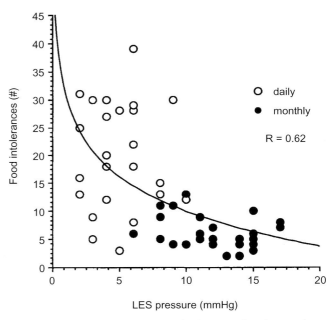

Figure 19.3 Relationship between 39 foods causing heartburn and resting lower esophageal sphincter (LES) pressure in 25 patients with daily and 25 patients with monthly reflux symptoms.

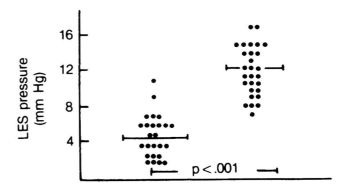

Figure 19.4 Resting lower esophageal sphincter pressures for 25 patients with daily heartburn (left) and 25 patients with monthly heartburn (right).

over-the-counter medications. Those with more persistent symptoms are more likely to see a physician for advice, with a small percentage of symptomatic individuals (probably 10% or less) represented by the group with complicated GERD seen by the gastroenterologist. Community-based studies suggest that the prevalence of reflux symptoms is much the same in adults of all ages, but that the proportion of individuals who seek medical help for the symptoms increases with age [27, 28]. One disturbing element in the clinical scenario is the group of patients who have Barrett's esophagus and who experience minimal reflux symptoms. They have little reason to consult a physician and consequently their increased risk of esophageal adenocarcinoma goes unrecognized. In one study, 28% of patients presenting with symptomatic adenocarcinoma in a Barrett's esophagus had no preceding history of reflux symptoms [29].

Influence of food on reflux symptoms

Although the pathophysiology of GERD is complex and the effects of eating on reflux are part of the complexity, there are some clear relationships between symptoms and certain foods. An early study of intolerance to 39 different types of food in 25 patients with daily heartburn and 25 patients with only monthly symptoms found an inverse correlation between the number of food intolerances and resting tonic lower esophageal sphincter (LES) pressure [30] (Figure 19.3). Individuals with a normal LES pressure reported heartburn only after eating certain foods, including fried foods, spicy foods, and hot dogs, whereas those with very low LES pressures experienced reflux symptoms after eating almost all types of food surveyed. Moreover, LES pressures were lower in the patients with daily heartburn than in the patients with less frequent symptoms. All the patients with daily symptoms had a resting LES pressure of less than 10mmHg (Figure 19.4), indicating that patients with poor

sphincter function tend to experience symptoms regardless of the type of food consumed.

Transient LES relaxations (TLESRs) are the dominant mechanism responsible for the occurrence of reflux episodes in normal subjects and in individuals with relatively mild reflux disease, whereas other mechanisms, notably sphincteric incompetence, make a progressively greater contribution as the severity of reflux disease increases (see Chapter 21). This difference explains, at least in part, some of the effects of meals in general and of specific foods in particular on reflux symptoms: the well-known relationship between fat ingestion and reflux can be examined against this background. Resting LES pressure in healthy volunteers is reduced by fat [30] and fat also increases the frequency of TLESRs

[31]. Thus, when TLESRs are the main mechanism of reflux, meals with a high fat content may be expected to have a relatively specific effect, predisposing to symptoms. However, in comparison with the fasting state, TLESR frequency is also increased by distention of the gastric fundus, so any meal that distends the stomach, regardless of its chemical composition, promotes reflux to some degree via this mechanism. In individuals with incompetence of the LES, the liability to post-prandial reflux occurs regardless of meal composition because the ineffectiveness of the LES barrier function has little to do with the nature of gastric contents. Patients with an incompetent sphincter are more likely to experience provocation of symptoms by bending down, by stooping, and by recumbency, however, because these maneuvers expose the incompetence of the sphincter.

One study illustrating these relationships compared the effect of high-fat (61% by calorie) and low-fat (16%) meals on esophageal acid exposure, determined by pH monitoring [32]. In normal subjects maintaining an upright posture post prandially, increased esophageal acid exposure occurred after the high-fat compared with the low-fat meal, particularly during the second and third hours after food ingestion. The fat content of the meal had little influence, however, on the acid exposure in reflux patients in the upright position, who experienced reflux after both the high-fat and the low-fat meals (Table 19.2). When normal subjects and reflux patients were studied in the recumbent position after eating, increased exposure of the esophagus to acid was observed in both groups after both high-fat and low-fat meals.

Many other observations illustrate the singular importance of dietary fat in predisposing to reflux. The effects of fat and of meals on tonic LES pressures, on TLESRs, and on gastric fundic distention and relaxation account for many of the observations, but an additional effect derives from the fact that gastric emptying takes longer with large meals than small meals, and with meals of high rather than low caloric density. When compared with a small meal of low nutrient

content, a large meal of high caloric density (such as one containing much fat) therefore causes the stomach to be in its post-prandial mode—when TLESRs occur at post-prandial frequency and facilitate reflux—for a longer period of time.

The risk of developing GERD may well be related in part to habits of the modern Western world. As discussed in subsequent chapters, these include a diet that is characterized by fatty and large meals, by obesity, smoking, and chocolate consumption, and, possibly, by long-term use of certain drugs.

Diagnostic evaluation

The diagnostic approach to the patient with possible GERD is multilayered, depending on the presentation. Because the symptoms are believed to be due to chronic reflux, the evaluation should attempt to document this abnormality. The patient who presents with typical heartburn and regurgitation with the usual positional and post-prandial relationships requires little, if any, additional information to establish a presumptive diagnosis and initiate therapy. The patient whose symptoms are less clear or include atypical manifestations usually needs additional diagnostic testing. The variety of tests and procedures available to evaluate the patient with possible GERD can cause diagnostic confusion if not used appropriately. It is preferable to begin the diagnostic approach by defining the question to be answered in the individual patient. In Table 19.3 the variety of diagnostic tests that has been advocated for the patient with possible reflux is categorized according to the question being asked.

Table 19.3 Diagnostic tests for gastroesophageal reflux disease categorized according to specific questions.

Is abnormal reflux present?
Barium upper gastrointestinal series
Gastroesophageal radionuclide scan
Standard acid reflux test
Ambulatory MII–pH monitoring

Is abnormal acid reflux present?
Ambulatory pH monitoring

Is there mucosal injury?
Endoscopy
Barium upper gastrointestinal (air contrast) study
Mucosal biopsy

Are symptoms due to acid reflux?
Ambulatory pH monitoring (with symptom index)
Bernstein test
Proton pump inhibitor (PPI) treatment response

Can prognostic or useful preoperative information be obtained?
Esophageal motility evaluation
Ambulatory pH monitoring

Table 19.2 Average upright esophageal acid exposure (% time) after high-fat versus low-fat meals in normals and reflux patients.[*]

	Low-fat meals	High-fat meals
Normals		
First hour	1.8	7.4
Second hour	2.1	8.1
Third hour	0.5	2.9
Reflux patients		
First hour	19.5	25.8
Second hour	22.3	27.2
Third hour	26.1	9.8

*The fat content, by calories, of the low-fat and high-fat meals was 16% and 61%, respectively.

Is abnormal reflux present?

The critical question often is whether the patient has abnormal reflux, particularly in the patient with an atypical symptom pattern. Simply confirming that abnormal reflux is present is often satisfactory to support the clinical impression.

Traditionally, the first test performed to evaluate possible reflux, particularly by the primary care physician, has been an upper gastrointestinal series. Despite being supplanted in recent years by upper gastrointestinal endoscopy, it is worth noting that endoscopy cannot answer the question "is abnormal reflux present?" Radiology can effectively rule out complications of GERD (ulcer, stricture) or other structural abnormalities of the esophagus, stomach, or duodenum, and can demonstrate reflux—the flow of barium from the stomach into the esophagus either spontaneously or induced by various maneuvers. However, radiographic reflux has limited diagnostic value. Reflux is dependent on the state of competence of the antireflux mechanism at a particular moment and has been demonstrated radiographically in as few as 60% of severely symptomatic patients or in as many as 25% of patients having no reflux symptoms. Thus, its reliability is questionable, with both poor specificity and sensitivity [33, 34]. Air contrast techniques provide more information (see Chapter 6). Because normal individuals have brief intermittent episodes of reflux (so-called physiologic reflux), particularly on those occasions when the LES spontaneously relaxes [35], observing the occurrence of reflux during a radiographic study does not itself imply abnormality.

Radionuclide scans have been advocated to document reflux and to provide quantitation of the amount of reflux. The gastroesophageal scan uses a radioisotope (technetium99m sulfur colloid) as a marker for reflux. Graded abdominal compression is used to unmask incompetence of the reflux barrier. Although originally proposed as a sensitive test of reflux [36], its reliability is doubtful [37] and it is no longer favored.

The use of an intraesophageal pH electrode to detect reflux was initially reported by Tuttle and Grossman in 1958 [38]. Subsequently, the standard acid reflux test was developed to stress the antireflux barrier in the laboratory while measuring reflux with a pH probe placed 5 cm above the LES. Following instillation of 300 mL of 0.1N hydrochloric acid into the stomach, the patient performs four maneuvers—deep breathing, Valsalva, Müller (inspiration against a closed glottis), and cough—repeated in the supine and right and left lateral decubitus positions and with the head down 20 degrees. Overall, 16 possibilities for acid reflux occur. A decrease in esophageal pH to less than 4 on at least three occasions is considered evidence of abnormal reflux. This test has relatively good overall sensitivity and specificity but is cumbersome and time-consuming in practice, so it is rarely used [34].

Prolonged ambulatory intraesophageal pH monitoring is considered the procedure of choice to demonstrate the occurrence of abnormal acid reflux (see Chapter 11). Patients record the time that they experience reflux symptoms during monitoring, thus allowing correlation of intraesophageal pH and subjective symptoms. A symptom index (SI) often helps clarify the association of specific symptoms with episodes of reflux, using the following equation [39]:

$$SI = \frac{\text{Number of symptoms occurring with pH} < 4.0 \times 100}{\text{Total number of symptoms}}$$

This test is of no value if the patient is incapable of gastric acid production. Clinical indications include difficult diagnostic problems or atypical reflux symptoms (chest pain, cough, hoarseness), non-response to therapy, and preoperative and postoperative evaluation of antireflux surgery.

Is there evidence of mucosal injury?

Esophagitis is the *sine qua non* of GERD. This can occasionally be documented by careful air–contrast barium esophagram showing mucosal lesions (erosions, ulcers) or stricture. Direct comparison of this technique with endoscopy has revealed that the finding of esophageal injury on air–contrast esophagram is highly specific, although not very sensitive [40].

Endoscopy is the diagnostic approach most frequently used to document esophageal injury. Erosions or ulcerations of the mucosa visualized through the endoscope are indications of reflex injury. The findings are definitive when unequivocally present but may be subtle or absent, and it is important that clinicians appreciate that many patients with GERD do not have esophagitis [4]. Only 34% of patients with chronic heartburn evaluated in one study had esophagitis apparent on endoscopy [6]. Moreover, many published studies of reflux and esophagitis have failed to address the problems of interpretation arising from interobserver variation in recognition of the milder degrees of esophagitis [41]. The Los Angeles system of grading esophagitis has been validated in this respect [42].

Potentially, esophageal mucosal biopsy should be a more sensitive test of the presence of reflux injury because histologic abnormalities may be present even when careful endoscopic examination indicates a normal-appearing esophagus. The most reliable criterion for esophagitis on endoscopic biopsy is the presence of acute inflammatory cells (polymorphonuclear leukocytes or eosinophils). These are present in esophageal biopsy specimens of only 20% of patients with reflux symptoms, however, and other epithelial changes have been proposed as providing better diagnostic criteria. Increased papillary extension and basal zone hyperplasia have been thought to be more sensitive findings occurring secondary to chronic gastroesophageal reflux [43]. However, there is no good evidence that these or other findings on biopsy are helpful in the context of ordinary clinical practice.

Indeed, there is persuasive evidence that conventional endoscopic pinch biopsies are of little value [44, 45]. Suction biopsies may be no better unless many samples are obtained [46]. Today, mucosal biopsies are more likely to be obtained to exclude eosinophilic esophagitis (see Chapter 36).

Are symptoms due to gastroesophageal reflux disease?

In many patients, a key question is whether their symptoms are clearly related to acid exposure and sensitivity of the esophageal mucosa to chronic reflux. The acid perfusion (Bernstein) test was used for many years as a test of acid sensitivity, with a reported specificity and sensitivity of approximately 80% in GERD [34]. If the patient's symptoms are reproduced during perfusion of the esophagus with dilute hydrochloric acid and resolve following saline perfusion, it is appropriate to conclude that chronic acid reflux is the cause of spontaneously occurring symptoms. This test is purely qualitative in character and provides no information on the magnitude of reflex.

If the SI is calculated as described earlier, 24-h pH monitoring can define the relationship between specific symptoms and reflux. This test is limited by the requirement that the patient's symptoms must occur during the test period. With this limitation, it is nonetheless considered by many investigators to represent an endogenous Bernstein test [16].

The opposite approach to acid reflux testing is the use of a proton pump inhibitor (PPI; omeprazole, 20 mg twice daily, or lansoprazole, 30 mg twice daily) as a diagnostic tool. The disappearance of symptoms by strong acid inhibition, given for at least 1 week, is a simple and inexpensive approach to the diagnosis of GERD and has the advantage of avoiding the day-to-day variation in magnitude of reflux that limits the reliability of 24-h pH monitoring [47]. However, systematic evaluation of this "PPI test" indicates it is perhaps less specific than might initially be supposed [48, 49].

Can prognostic information be obtained?

Measurement of tonic LES pressure was previously suggested as a possible means to diagnose reflux disease. The importance of the LES as a major barrier to reflux is well established. Although an LES pressure of less than 10 mmHg has been considered an indication of an incompetent gastroesophageal junction, there is much variation in this value. Many patients with well-documented esophagitis have an LES pressure greater than 10 mmHg, and some asymptomatic subjects have pressures less than this value. Consequently, LES pressure in a given patient is often too imprecise to identify a potential for reflux and its variability severely limits the sensitivity and specificity of LES pressure measurement as a diagnostic test. Nevertheless, a pressure of less than 6 mmHg correlates well with abnormal reflux on pH testing and very low LES pressures in this range are

predictive of a more severe degree of reflux and a worse prognosis [50]. The barrier function of the LES depends on the length of the sphincter as well as its pressure, and there is an inverse relationship between the length of the sphincter and the severity of GERD [51, 52].

In addition to LES pressure measurements, assessment of peristaltic activity in the esophageal body may be informative in evaluating reflux disease and assessing its prognosis [53, 54]. Until recently, these measurements have also been thought important in the preoperative assessment of GERD patients to inform the surgeon of potentially defective peristalsis that might constitute a risk for troublesome dysphagia after fundoplication. It seems that the occurrence of postoperative dysphagia correlates poorly with impaired peristalsis preoperatively [55].

Ambulatory pH monitoring can also provide important information about the severity of reflux disease and the reflux pattern present in a particular patient. That is, does the patient have reflux predominantly at night, or is upright, post-prandial reflex more prevalent?

What is the importance of a hiatal hernia?

Although once considered to be of major importance in the production of GERD, the finding of a hiatal hernia either radiographically or endoscopically has little value in predicting whether a patient's symptoms are secondary to reflux. When carefully sought, a sliding hiatal hernia can be found in a high percentage of persons, most of whom are asymptomatic. In a review of more than 1000 patients in 1968, Palmer estimated that only 9% of those with a radiographically demonstrated hiatal hernia had typical reflux symptoms [1]. Other careful studies have likewise indicated no consistent cause-and-effect relationship between the presence of symptomatic reflux and the finding of a hiatal hernia [56]. Nevertheless, it is clear that contraction of the crural diaphragm enhances pressure in the normally located LES [57]. Apart from any diminution of the LES barrier function resulting from hiatal hernia, there may also be a contribution to the severity of GERD by "trapping" acid in the hernial sac, which thus becomes more available to reflex during LES relaxation. This mechanism may prolong acid exposure and delay its clearance from the esophageal mucosa [5, 58]. Most patients undergoing endoscopy for upper gastrointestinal symptoms do not have esophagitis if they do not have a hiatal hernia, whereas a hiatal hernia is found in most patients with severe esophagitis [56].

Are symptoms with acid and non-acid reflux produced by different mechanisms?

It is well known that acid reflux can cause symptoms. Clinical testing at the Medical University of South Carolina of patients with persistent symptoms despite twice daily PPI has revealed that the patient's continuing symptoms are temporally related to non-acid reflux in about 35% of cases [59]. Obviously, the clinical approach to these different mechanisms of symptom production varies and is most reasonably pursued once the responsible mechanism has been better clarified.

The use of combined multichannel intraluminal impedance and pH (MII–pH) monitoring in our esophageal laboratory as described below has greatly expanded our ability to understand and manage this group of challenging patients. MII–pH is routinely performed on PPI therapy since the question being addressed is why symptoms are present despite acid suppression.

Many questions arise as to the mechanism of symptoms in patients with acid and non-acid reflux. Do patients with acid reflux perceive symptoms by a different mechanism from patients with non-acid reflux? Do patients with acid reflux and symptoms perceive symptoms earlier than patients with non-acid reflux?

Agrawal et al. showed that acid reflux is perceived sooner than non-acid episodes and that acid refluxate travels faster up the esophagus [60]. The main question raised by this study was whether there is evidence that different mechanisms may produce symptoms in patients with acid versus non-acid reflux? The relation between gastroesophageal reflux episodes and their conscious perception is complex. Despite many studies, the mechanisms responsible for the development of reflux symptoms are incompletely understood. The acid component of the refluxate plays a major role in the pathophysiology of GERD, especially in eliciting symptoms [61]. Ambulatory pH monitoring allows assessment of the temporal relationship between symptoms and acid reflux episodes. Although PPIs have a remarkable efficacy for mucosal healing and symptom relief [62], many patients continue to have symptoms despite adequate acid-suppressive therapy [63]. Many factors may be responsible for a poor response to PPI in patients with symptoms suggestive of GERD. When combined with pH monitoring, MII–pH identifies all types of reflux episodes and allows characterization of them as acid or non-acid [64].

There are many key reasons to understand mechanisms of symptoms since treatment may have a differential response depending on a particular symptom and whether it is related to acid or non-acid reflux. Other known variables important in reflux symptoms include age, volume of the meal, post-prandial timings, characteristics of food, and patient behavior.

Non-acid reflux has been shown to occur mainly post-prandially; perhaps suggesting that symptoms may be related to a larger volume and stimulate an intramural mechanoreceptor pathway. Esophageal mechanoreceptors can transduce painful sensations [65]. In contrast, patients with acid reflux may be more likely to perceive symptoms through a chemoreceptor-mediated pathway, perhaps explaining our results of earlier perception of symptoms in patients with acid reflux [60]. This was supported by a study showing that symptomatic reflux episodes were accompanied by a significantly larger pH drop compared with asymptomatic reflux

episodes. The results also suggested the concept that minute amounts of acid can induce a sensation of heartburn [66].

Another interesting finding in our study was the observation that patients were likely to perceive regurgitation sooner than heartburn and cough with both acid and non-acid reflux. Zerbib et al. found that high proximal extent of the refluxate was the only factor associated with greater likelihood of reflux perception in patients on double-dose PPI [67]. However, compared with regurgitation, composition of the refluxate, sensitization of the esophagus by preceding acid exposure, and delayed bolus clearance appeared to play a role in heartburn perception. Compared with regurgitation, they observed that reflux episodes eliciting heartburn were more frequently pure liquid and acidic, had a lower nadir pH, and were more frequently associated with preceding acid reflux episodes. These results suggest that the perception of heartburn is more sensitive to the chemical composition of the refluxate than regurgitation.

The findings in this study may have important clinical implications. Some centers currently use a 2-min window to define a positive or negative SI. Our study showed regurgitation, heartburn, and cough following non-acid reflux episodes occurring within the first 2 min were 79%, 54%, and 56%, respectively. Based on the data, a significant proportion of symptoms associated with non-acid reflux would be missed with the use of a 2-min window.

The study suggests that symptoms with acid and non-acid reflux are produced by different mechanisms. Further studies will be needed to better clarify the different mechanisms in the perception of symptoms in patients with acid versus non-acid reflux.

Do patients on proton pump inhibitors still experience gastroesophageal reflux disease symptoms?

Despite PPI therapy patients may have persistent symptoms of GERD. A study performed by Sharma et al. aimed to identify symptom types and frequency experienced by patients on PPI therapy, and to identify the type of reflux, if any, associated with these symptoms [68]. A retrospective review was performed of 200 patients on PPI with GERD symptoms during ambulatory MII–pH testing. The patients were divided into two groups: those with exclusively non-acid reflux episodes and those with mixed acid and non-acid reflux episodes. The symptom profiles were then compared between the groups. A total of 415 symptoms were reported by the 200 patients on twice-daily PPIs. Throat clearing was most common (24%). A total of 110 symptoms (27%) were typical symptoms and 305 (73%) were atypical. Typical symptoms were more likely to have a positive SI than atypical symptoms (48% vs 25%, $P < .01$). Eighty-four patients (42%) had a positive SI and 116 patients (58%) had a negative SI. One hundred patients (50%) had only non-acid reflux; the other 100 had mixed acid and non-acid reflux. Heartburn (21% vs 63%, $P < .01$) and nausea (8% vs 44%, $P < .01$) were more likely associated with reflux in the mixed acid and non-acid reflux group. The conclusion of the study was that patients on PPIs still experience GERD symptoms and that MII–pH monitoring identifies similar symptom associations with all types of reflux and also clarifies symptoms not related to any reflux.

References

1. Palmer ED. The hiatus hernia-esophagitis-esophageal stricture complex. Twenty year prospective study. *Am J Med* 1968;44:566.
2. Ellis FH. Esophageal hiatal hernia. *N Engl J Med* 1972;287:646.
3. Klauser AG, Schindlbeck NE, Muller-Lissner SA. Symptoms in gastro-esophageal reflux disease. *Lancet* 1990;335:205.
4. Johnston F, Joelsson B, Gudmundsson K, *et al*. Symptoms and endoscopic findings in the diagnosis of gastroesophageal efflux disease. *Scand J Gastroenterol* 1987;22:714.
5. Sloan S, Kahrilas PJ. Impairment of esophageal emptying with hiatal hernia. *Gastroenterology* 1991;100:596.
6. Winters C, Spurling TJ, Chobanian SJ. Barrett's esophagus. A prevalent, occult complication of gastroesophageal reflux disease. *Gastroenterology* 1987;92:118.
7. Kirk AJ. Reflex dyspareunia. *Thorax* 1986;41:215.
8. Breumelhof R, Nadorp JH, Akkermans LM, Smout AJ. Analysis of 24-hour esophageal pressure and pH data in unselected patients with noncardiac chest pain. *Gastroenterology* 1990;99:1257–1264.
9. Cherian P, *et al*. Esophageal tests in the evaluation of non-cardiac chest pain. *Dis Esophagus* 1995;8:129.
10. De Caestecker JS, Blackwell JN, Brown J, Heading RC.. The oesophagus as a cause of recurrent chest pain: which patients should be investigated and which tests should be used? *Lancet* 1985;2:1143–1146.
11. DeMeester TR, O'Sullivan GC, Bermudez G, Midell AI, Cimochowski GE, O'Drobinak J. Esophageal function in patients with angina-type chest pain and normal coronary angiograms. *Ann Surg* 1982;196:488–498.
12. Hewson EG, Sinclair JW, Dalton CB, Richter JE. Twenty-four hour esophageal pH monitoring: the most useful test for evaluating noncardiac chest pain. *Am J Med* 1991;90:576–583.
13. Schofield PM, Bennett DH, Whorwell PJ, *et al*. Exertional gastroesophageal reflux: a mechanism for symptoms in patients with angina pectoris and normal coronary angiograms. *Br Med J* 1987;294:1459–1461.
14. Katz PO. Ambulatory esophageal and hypopharyngeal pH monitoring in patients with hoarseness. *Am J Gastroenterol* 1989;85:38.
15. Shaker R, Milbrath M, Ren J, *et al*. Esophagopharyngeal distribution of refluxed gastric acid in patients with reflux laryngitis. *Gastroenterology* 1995;109:1575–1582.
16. Wiener GJ, Richter JE, Copper JB, Wu WC, Castell DO. The symptom index: a clinically important parameter of ambulatory 24-hour esophageal pH monitoring. *Am J Gastroenterol* 1988;83:358–361.

17. Ward PH, Hanson DG. Reflux as an etiological factor of carcinoma of the laryngopharynx. *Laryngoscope* 1988;98:1195.
18. Irwin RS, Curley FJ, French CL. Chronic cough. The spectrum and frequency of causes, key components of the diagnostic evaluation, and outcome of specific therapy. *Am Rev Respir Dis* 1990;141:640.
19. Sontag SJ, O'Connell S, Khandelwal S, *et al*. Most asthmatics have gastroesophageal reflux with or without bronchodilator therapy. *Gastroenterology* 1990;99:613–620.
20. Hetzel DJ, Heddle R. Gastroesophageal reflux disease, pH monitoring, and treatment. *Curr Opin Gastroenterol* 1993;9:629.
21. Gluck M, Pope CE. Chronic hiccups and gastroesophageal reflux disease. *Ann Intern Med* 1986;105:291.
22. Marshall JB, Landreneau RJ, Beyer KL. Hiccups: esophageal manometric features and relationship to gastroesophageal reflux. *Am J Gastroenterol* 1990;85:1172.
23. Dakkak M, Hoare RC, Maslin SC, Bennett JR. Oesophagitis is as important as oesophageal stricture diameter in determining dysphagia. *Gut* 1993;34:152–155.
24. Williams D, Thompson DG, Marples M, Heggie L, O'Hanrahan T, Bancewicz J. Diminished traction forces with swallowing in gastro-oesophageal reflux disease and in functional dysphagia. *Gut* 1994;35:165–171.
25. Lagergren J, Bergstrom R, Lindgren A, Nyren O.. Symptomatic gastroesophageal reflux as a risk factor for esophageal adenocarcinoma. *N Engl J Med* 1999;340:825–831.
26. Nebel OT, Fornes MF, Castell DO. Symptomatic gastroesophageal reflux: incidence and precipitating factors. *Am J Dig Dis* 1976;21:953.
27. Kennedy T, Jones R. Gastro-oesophageal reflux symptoms in the community. *Aliment Pharmacol Ther* 2000;14:1589.
28. Locke GR 3rd, Talley NJ, Fett SL, Zinsmeister AR, Melton LJ 3rd. Prevalence and clinical spectrum of gastroesophageal reflux: a population based study in Olmstead County, Minnesota. *Gastroenterology* 1997;112:1448–1456.
29. Cameron AJ, Ott BJ, Payne WS. The incidence of adenocarcinoma in columnar-lined (Barrett's) esophagus. *N Engl J Med* 1985;313:857.
30. Nebel OT, Castell DO. Lower esophageal sphincter pressure changes after food ingestion. *Gastroenterology* 1972;63:778.
31. Holloway RH, Lyrenas E, Ireland A, Dent J. Effect of intraduodenal fat on lower oesophageal sphincter function and gastro-oesophageal reflux. *Gut* 1997;40:449–453.
32. Becker DJ, Sinclair J, Castell DO, Wu WC. A comparison of high and low fat meals on postprandial esophageal acid exposure. *Am J Gastroenterol* 1989;84:782–786.
33. Johnston BT, Troshinsky MB, Castell JA, Castell DO. Comparison of barium radiography with esophageal pH monitoring in the diagnosis of gastroesophageal reflux disease. *Am J Gastroenterol* 1996;91:1181–1185.
34. Richter JE, Castell DO. Gastroesophageal reflux. Pathogenesis, diagnosis, and therapy. *Ann Intern Med* 1982;97:93.
35. Dodds WJ, Dent J, Hogan WJ, *et al*. Mechanisms of gastroesophageal reflux in patients with reflux esophagitis. *N Engl J Med* 1982;307:1547–1552.
36. Fisher RS, Malmud LS, Roberts GS, Lobis IF. Gastroesophageal (GE) scintiscanning to detect and quantitate GE reflux. *Gastroenterology* 1976;70:301–308.

37. Jenkins AF, Cowan RJ, Richter JE. Gastroesophageal scintigraphy: is it a sensitive test for gastroesophageal reflux disease? *J Clin Gastroenterol* 1985;7:127.

38. Tuttle SG, Grossman MI. Detection of gastroesophageal reflux by simultaneous measurements of intraluminal pressure and pH. *Proc Soc Exp Biol Med* 1958;93:225.

39. Wiener G, Koufman JA, Wu WC, Cooper JB, Richter JE, Castell DO. Chronic hoarseness secondary to gastroesophageal reflux disease. *Am J Gastroenterol* 1989;12:1503–1508.

40. Ott DJ, Gelfand DW, Wu WC. Reflux esophagitis: radiographic and endoscopic correlation. *Radiology* 1979;130:583.

41. Bytzer P, Havelund T, Hansen JM. Interobserver variation in the endoscopic diagnosis of reflux esophagitis. *Scand J Gastroenterol* 1993;28:119.

42. Lundell LR, Dent J, Bennett JR, *et al*. Endoscopic assessment of oesophagitis: clinical and functional correlates and further validation of the Los Angeles classification. *Gut* 1999;45:172–180.

43. Ismail-Beigi F, Horton PF, Pope CE. Histological consequences of gastroesophageal reflux in man. *Gastroenterology* 1970;58:163.

44. Knuff TE, Benjamin SB, Worsham GF, Hancock JE, Castell DO. Histological evaluation of chronic gastroesophageal reflux. *Dig Dis Sci* 1984;29:194–201.

45. Schindlbeck NE, Wiebecke B, Klauser AG, Voderholzer WA, Muller-Lissner SA. Diagnostic value of histology in non-erosive gastro-oesophageal reflux disease. *Gut* 1996;39:151–154.

46. Collins BJ, Elliott H, Sloan JM, McFarland RJ, Love AH. Oesophageal histology in reflux oesophagitis. *J Clin Pathol* 1985;38:1265–1272.

47. Schenk BE, Kuipers EJ, Klinkenberg-Knol EC, *et al*. Omeprazole as a diagnostic tool in gastroesophageal reflux disease. *Am J Gastroenterol* 1997;92:1997–2000.

48. Johnsson F, Weywadt L, Solhaug JH, Hernquist H, Bengtsson L. One-week omeprazole treatment in the diagnosis of gastro-oesophageal reflux disease. *Scand J Gastroenterol* 1998;33:15–20.

49. Juul-Hansen P, Rydning A, Jacobsen CD, Hansen T. High dose proton pump inhibitors as a diagnostic test of gastro-oesophageal reflux disease in endoscopic-negative patients. *Scand J Gastroenterol* 2001;36:806–810.

50. Lieberman DA. Medical therapy for chronic reflux esophagitis: long-term follow-up. *Arch Intern Med* 1987;147:1717.

51. DeMeester TR, Lafontaine E, Joelsson BE, *et al*. Relationship of a hiatal hernia to the function of the body of the esophagus and the gastroesophageal junction. *J Thorac Cardiovasc Surg* 1981;82:547–558.

52. Fein M, Ritter MP, DeMeester TR, *et al*. Role of the lower esophageal sphincter and hiatal hernia in the pathogenesis of gastroesophageal reflux disease. *J Gastrointest Surg* 1999;3:405–410.

53. Kahrilas PJ, Dodds WJ, Hogan WJ, Kern M, Arndorfer RC, Reece A. Esophageal peristaltic dysfunction in peptic esophagitis. *Gastroenterology* 1986;91:897–904.

54. Leite LP, Johnston BT, Barrett J, Castell JA, Castell DO. Ineffective esophageal motility (IEM): the primary finding in patients with non-specific esophageal motility disorder. *Dig Dis Sci* 1997;42:1853–1865.

55. Fibbe C, Layer P, Keller J, Strate U, Emmermann A, Zornig C. Esophageal motility in reflux disease before and after fundoplication: a prospective, randomized, clinical and manometric study. *Gastroenterology* 2001;121:5–14.

56. Kaul B, Petersen H, Myrvold HE, Grette K, Roysland P, Halvorsen T. Hiatus hernia in gastroesophageal reflux disease. *Scand J Gastroenterol* 1986;21:31–34.

57. Mittal RK. The crural diaphragm, an external lower esophageal sphincter: a definitive study. *Gastroenterology* 1993;105:1565.

58. Mittal RK, Lange RC, McCallum RW. Identification and mechanism of delayed esophageal acid clearance in subjects with hiatus hernia. *Gastroenterology* 1987;92:130.

59. Mainie I, Tutuian R, Shay S, *et al.*. Acid and non-acid reflux in patients with persistent symptoms despiteacid suppressive therapy. A Multicenter study using combined ambulatory impedance-pH monitoring. *Gut* 2006;55:1398–1402.

60. Agrawal A, Roberts J, Sharma N, *et al*. Symptoms with acid and non-acid reflux may be produced by different mechanisms. *Dis Esophagus* 2009;22:467–470.

61. Vaezi MF, Singh S, Richter JE. Role of acid and duodenogastric reflux in esophageal mucosal injury: a review of animal and human studies. *Gastroenterology* 1995;108:1897–1907.

62. Chiba N, De Gara CJ, Wilkinson JM, *et al*. Speed of healing and symptom relief in grade II to IV gastroesophageal reflux disease: a meta-analysis. *Gastroenterology* 1997;112:1798–1810.

63. Castell DO, Kahrilas PJ, Richter JE, *et al*. Esomeprazole (40 mg) compared with lansoprazole (30 mg) in the treatment of erosive esophagitis. *Am J Gastroenterol* 2002;97:575–583.

64. Sifrim D, Holloway R, Silny J, *et al*. Acid, nonacid, and gas reflux in patients with gastroesophageal reflux disease during ambulatory 24-hour pH–impedance recordings. *Gastroenterology* 2001;120:1588–1598.

65. Cervero F, Janig W. Visceral nociceptors: anew world order? *Trends Neurosci* 1992;15:374–378.

66. Bredenoord AJ, Weusten BL, Curvers WL, *et al*. Determinants of perception of heartburn and regurgitation. *Gut* 2006;55:313–318

67. Zerbib F, Duriez A, Roman S, Capdepont M, Mion F. Determinants of gastro-oesophageal reflux perception in patients with persistent symptoms despite proton pump inhibitors *Gut* 2008;57:156–160.

68. Sharma N, Agrawal A, Vela M, Castell DO. An analysis of persistent symptoms in acid suppressed patients undergoing impedance-pH monitoring. *Clin Gastroenterol Hepatol* 2008;6:482–483.

Hiatus Hernia and Gastroesophageal Reflux Disease

Albert J. Bredenoord and André J. P. M. Smout

Department of Gastroenterology and Hepatology, University Medical Center, Amsterdam, The Netherlands

Introduction

Over the past few decades, the views on the role of hiatus hernia in the pathophysiology of gastroesophageal reflux disease (GERD) have varied considerably. Once radiographic detection of hiatus hernia became possible, the high prevalence of hiatus hernia in patients with reflux disease became apparent, and at one point reflux disease was almost considered synonymous with hiatus hernia [1]. This changed with the arrival of esophageal manometry and the widespread acceptance of the notion that reflux disease was related to a low lower esophageal sphincter (LES) pressure [2]. Some time later, when prolonged LES pressure monitoring with a sleeve sensor made it clear that the majority of reflux episodes is caused by transient LES relaxations, interest in hiatus hernia was reduced even further [3, 4].

A renewed interest in hiatus hernia emerged after the discovery that the effectiveness of the antireflux barrier was dependent on the integrity of both the LES and diaphragm, and that the presence of a hiatus hernia interferes with this barrier function [5].

Anatomy of the diaphragm and gastroesophageal junction

The diaphragm is a musculotendinous plate consisting of a costal part connected to the ribs, and a crural part connected to the vertebra. The crural part of the diaphragm forms a canal, the esophageal hiatus , through which the esophagus, vagal nerve, and some lymph vessels, veins, and arteries cross and enter the abdominal cavity (Figure 20.1).

Under normal circumstances the gastroesophageal junction (GEJ) lies at or near the level of the diaphragm. At or near the GEJ, the esophageal squamous mucosa changes into gastric cylindric mucosa. This so-called squamocolumnar junction (SCJ) usually has a zigzag appearance at endoscopy and is therefore often called the z-line.

It is now clear that the antireflux barrier at the GEJ consists of an intrinsic and extrinsic sphincteric component. The intrinsic sphincter is called the LES, which is a combination of a thickening of the circular smooth musculature of the esophagus and oblique sling fibers of the proximal stomach [6]. The extrinsic sphincter is formed by striated muscular fibers of the diaphragm, which encircle the esophagus at the level of the LES. At the level of LES, the distal esophagus is attached to the diaphragm by the phrenoesophageal ligament [7].

The sphincteric complex is normally 2–4 cm long. Usually the most proximal one-third of the sphincter is located proximal to the diaphragm and the distal two-thirds of the sphincter is below the diaphragm and thus located intra-abdominally. The hiatus is formed primarily by the right crus of the diaphragm, and contraction of the crural diaphragm exerts a pinchcock-like action on the LES. The pressure exerted by the crural diaphragm is thus largest on the left lateral side of the GEJ, while the pressure exerted by the oblique gastric fibers is mainly on the right side of the GEJ. As a consequence the antireflux barrier is far from symmetrical [8].

Manometrically, the GEJ can be detected at the distal end of the esophagus as a high-pressure zone. Sphincter pressure is typically quantified with reference to the intragastric pressure [9]. Both the LES and crural diaphragm contribute to the high-pressure zone at the distal esophagus, although it is generally taken that the tonic component is mainly the result of the tonic contraction of the LES, and the superimposed increments in pressure during inspiration are caused by contractions of the crural diaphragm [10, 11]. However, the LES can also contract phasically, and the diaphragm also exerts a tonic pressure component, which was shown in esophagectomized patients [12]. The thickness of the LES varies considerably between subjects and correlates with

The Esophagus, Fifth Edition. Edited by Joel E. Richter, Donald O. Castell.

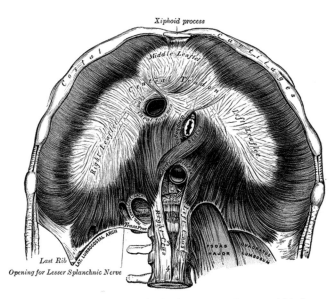

Figure 20.1 Inferior view on the diaphragm. Openings are visible for the vena cava, aorta, and esophagus. The esophageal hiatus is primarily formed by the right crus of the diaphragm (adapted from Gray H. *Henry Gray's Anatomy of the Human Body*. Philadelphia: Lea & Febiger, 1918, figure 391).

sphincter pressure. The magnitude of the increase in pressure during inspiration is directly proportional to the force of contraction of the crural diaphragm. During tidal inspiration, the increase in GEJ pressure is much smaller than during deep inspiration [13]. The crural diaphragm also contributes to the GEJ pressure increases during activities such as abdominal compression and straight leg raising [14, 15].

Physiology of the gastroesophageal junction

The main function of the high-pressure zone at the GEJ is to form a barrier against reflux of noxious gastric contents into the esophagus, while passage of a swallowed bolus is unaffected. Furthermore, reflux of gaseous gastric contents is needed for venting of gastric gas [16]. This requires a dedicated and complex one-way valve for liquids and solids, which does not affect reflux of gas.

The driving force behind the occurrence of gastroesophageal reflux is the positive pressure gradient from the stomach to the esophagus, resulting from the positive pressure gradient from the abdominal to the thoracic cavity [17, 18]. Normally, the pressure in the abdomen is higher than the pressure in the thoracic cavity and only the high-pressure zone at the GEJ prevents continuous influx of gastric contents into the esophagus. During increased abdominal pressure and inspiration, the pressure gradient between the stomach and esophagus increases as a result of a higher positive abdominal pressure combined with an unchanged or more negative esophageal body pressure. This would thus overcome the pressure at the GEJ and result in gastroesophageal reflux if not for the compensating physiologic mechanisms.

Prolonged manometry has shown that in the interdigestive state basal GEJ pressures fluctuate considerably during the day [19]. These variations are coupled with the interdigestive migrating motor complex of the stomach, the sphincter pressure typically peaking just before the onset of the gastric contractions of phase III. The participation of the LES in the interdigestive migrating motor complex serves to prevent reflux during periods with increased intragastric pressure.

As mentioned, the crural diaphragm rapidly contracts during events that increase intra-abdominal pressure, such as abdominal compression and straight leg raising. This rapid contraction results in an immediate sphincter pressure increase and thus protects against reflux that would otherwise have occurred with the increase in gastric pressure. In case of an intact GEJ, these mechanisms thus guarantee an effective antireflux barrier in all situations.

After swallowing, passage of the bolus across the GEJ is required; therefore the high-pressure zone has to be abolished temporarily. After the swallow reflex is initiated, relaxation of both the LES and crural diaphragm occurs and the LES is pulled upwards approximately 1–2 cm as a result of contraction of the longitudinal muscles of the esophagus [20–22]. The peristaltic wave pushes the bolus in a distal direction through the relaxed sphincter and simultaneously the LES moves distally again, pulled by the elastic fibers of the phrenoesophageal ligament. These mechanisms result in passage of the bolus over the GEJ into the stomach without the occurrence of reflux.

With each swallow, a variable volume of air is transported toward the stomach with the swallowed bolus. This air accumulates in the proximal stomach, together with gas that is released in the stomach, e.g. after drinking carbon dioxide-containing beverages. Distention of the proximal stomach results in activation of stretch receptors in the gastric wall and initiates a vagovagal reflex resulting in relaxation of the sphincteric complex. This reflex is called transient LES relaxation (TLESR), but the contractions of the crural diaphragm are also inhibited. TLESRs enable gaseous gastroesophageal reflux to occur and thus prevent the stomach from overdistention by gas. Therefore, TLESR is sometimes called the belch reflex [23]. TLESRs are also the most important mechanism through which gastroesophageal reflux of liquids can occur [24].

Hiatus hernia

A hiatus hernia is the extension of abdominal organs through the esophageal hiatus into the thoracic cavity. Usually hiatus hernias are divided into four types.

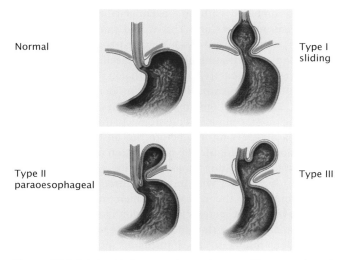

Normal

Type I
sliding

Type II
paraoesophageal

Type III

Figure 20.2 Relationship between the esophagus and lower esophageal sphincter and diaphragm in normal conditions and in various types of hiatus hernia.

Type I hiatus hernia

A type I hiatus hernia (Figure 20.2) refers to a herniation of the gastric cardia through the hiatus. This herniation can occur through widening of the hiatal opening and relaxation of the phrenoesophageal ligament. This type of hernia is referred to as a sliding hernia, as the herniated cardia can slide in and out of the thoracic cavity. This also implicates that the size of hernia is not constant but varies over time.

Estimates on the prevalence of sliding hiatus hernia vary enormously between 2.2% and 49% in the adult population, largely due to differences in definition and detection technique used [25–32]. Sliding hiatus hernias are more frequently observed in obese subjects and with increasing age [33]. The prevalence of hiatus hernia in Western populations seems higher than that in Asians [34, 35]. It is not known whether this is associated with differences in prevalence of obesity or demographic differences.

A genetic factor for the development of hiatus hernia has been suggested [36]. An autosomal dominant inheritance of hiatus hernia has been described in certain families [37]. Furthermore, a high concordance has been shown in identical twins [38]. Thus, both environmental and genetic factors seem to play a role in the development of hiatus hernia.

Most sliding hiatus hernias are asymptomatic; even the larger hernias do not necessarily evoke symptoms. Because a sliding hiatus hernia facilitates the occurrence of gastroesophageal reflux, the main implication of its presence is the development of GERD [39]. Larger hernias almost always lead to pathologic acid exposure of the esophagus, but this does not necessarily lead to symptoms or mucosal damage. Sometimes small ulcerative or erosive lesions are found at the herniated gastric mucosa at the level of the diaphragm. These lesions are called Cameron lesions and can be the

cause of occult or overt gastrointestinal hemorrhage [40]. Cameron lesions are thought to result from mild ischemia resulting from sliding of the gastric wall over the diaphragm in large hiatus hernias.

In case of a hiatus hernia, the diaphragmatic hiatus is no longer a small fissure in the diaphragmatic muscles but rather a rounded opening. The fixation of the distal esophagus to the diaphragm through the phrenoesophageal ligaments is more lax and these ligaments lose elasticity, resulting in a looser fixation of the distal esophagus. When during a TLESR or swallow, the distal esophagus is pulled upward through contraction of the longitudinal muscle layers, it is not immediately pulled back to its original position by the phrenoesophageal ligament. The LES and SCJ can thus remain proximal to the level of the diaphragm. In physiologic conditions, the LES can be pulled upward slightly during swallows and TLESRs, so that a small cavity is formed between the LES and the diaphragm; the phrenic ampulla [41]. By convention, when the longitudinal size of this cavity becomes more than 3 cm it is called a hiatus hernia rather than a phrenic ampulla. A small sliding hiatus hernia can thus be regarded as an exaggeration of a phrenic ampulla. Given the sliding character of this type of hernia, whether the hernia is encountered on endoscopic examination will depend on the moment of inspection. When a hernia becomes very large, complete reduction no longer occurs and the hernia is permanently present.

Sliding hiatus hernia is an acquired condition, and prevalence increases with age [27, 34, 42]. It is thought that age-related degeneration and factors that increase intra-abdominal pressure, such as pregnancy and obesity, result in the anatomic changes that lead to hiatus hernia [43]. Obesity seems to be an independent risk factor for the development of hiatus hernia [44, 45]. Furthermore, a high prevalence of hiatus hernia of up to 80% amongst power athletes supports a role for raised intra-abdominal pressure [46]. The increased abdominothoracic pressure gradient pushes the abdominal organs through the hiatus of the diaphragm, which becomes a challenge to the phrenoesophageal ligament [47]. It is no longer thought that shortening of the esophagus plays an important role in the pathogenesis of hiatus hernia [48].

Type II and III hiatus hernias

Type II and III hiatus hernias are different forms of paraesophageal hernias (Figure 20.2). These hernias constitute approximately 10% of all hernias. Although paraesophageal hernias can also lead to gastroesophageal reflux, their main clinical significance lies in their potential for mechanical complications.

A type II hernia results from a localized defect in the phrenoesophageal ligament, which leads to rolling of the gastric fundus into the thoracic cavity. As the largest part of the phrenoesophageal ligament is intact, the herniated fundus will be located left-lateral to the distal esophagus;

hence the description paraesophageal hernia. Usually more and more fundus will herniate until eventually the entire stomach can be located intrathoracically. For this to occur, the gastrosplenic and gastrocolic ligaments need to be abnormally lax. It is uncertain whether this is part of the cause or the effect of the herniation. As the hernia enlarges, the greater curvature of the stomach rolls up into the thorax. Because the stomach is fixed at the GEJ, the herniated stomach tends to rotate around its longitudinal axis, resulting in an organoaxial volvulus. Less frequently, rotation may alternatively occur around the transverse axis, resulting in a mesenteroaxial volvulus.

A type III hiatal hernia (Figure 20.2) has elements of both sliding hernias and paraesophageal hernias. This type of hernia starts as a type II paraesophageal hernia but after a large part of the stomach has herniated, the phrenoesophageal ligament stretches and a sliding component of the hernia is created.

Type IV hiatal hernia

A type IV hiatal hernia is associated with a large unilateral defect in the phrenoesophageal ligament through which, besides the stomach, other organs such as the colon, spleen, omentum, pancreas, and small intestine can herniate. The cause of the defect in the phrenoesophageal ligament that results in the paraesophageal hernia is usually unclear. However, sometimes the defect is a late complication of a surgical dissection of the hiatus, such as occurs during antireflux procedures and esophagectomy.

Many patients with paraesophageal hernias are asymptomatic. When symptoms occur, they are either related to mechanical obstruction or to ischemia. A paraesophageal hernia can present with non-specific symptoms such as epigastric pain, epigastric fullness, and nausea. Dyspnea can occur when the herniated organs fill a significant part of the thoracic cavity, while pressure on the esophagus can lead to dysphagia.

Congenital diaphragmatic hernias

Sliding hiatal hernias and paraesophageal hernias are believed to be acquired during life, but there are also congenital hernias. Symptomatic congenital diaphragmatic hernias appear in 1 in 2000 births, but asymptomatic defects are far from rare in adults. The anteromedial hernia of Morgagni is formed through herniation between the sternal and costal parts of the diaphragm, and the posterolateral hernia of Bochdalek is formed when there is a defect in the posterior growth of the diaphragm, resulting in a herniation between the diaphragm and lumbar muscles.

Hernias of Morgagni can contain stomach, colon or omentum. This type of hernia is usually small and can be asymptomatic. Hernias of Bochdalek are usually large and are associated with hypoplasia of the ipsilateral lung and mediastinal displacement to the contralateral side. The newborn with a large hernia of Bochdalek often presents with respiratory distress and this condition is generally not compatible with life. Smaller hernias can present with intestinal obstruction and are accompanied by symptoms of vomiting and respiratory symptoms, particularly after meals. Occasionally, herniation of the stomach and other abdominal organs through a Bochdalek or Morgagni defect is encountered in an adult patient. Usually the position of the hernia on chest X-ray or computed tomography (CT) scan makes it possible to differentiate it from hernia through the esophageal hiatus. Treatment of both types of congenital hernias of the diaphragm is surgical.

Sliding hiatus hernia and reflux disease

As previously described, the crural diaphragm functions as a second or external sphincter. In the normal situation, the pressures exerted by the LES and the crural diaphragm overlap and the two structures together form a strong antireflux barrier. Manometrically, one high-pressure zone is seen. Disruption of the spatial relationship between the LES and diaphragm will compromise the antireflux barrier. Indeed, a higher prevalence of GERD is found in patients with a hiatus hernia. As a group, patients with hiatus hernia have a higher esophageal acid exposure, a higher incidence of esophagitis, more severe esophagitis, and more frequent and more severe reflux symptoms [49–54].

Pull-through manometry reveals that in patients with a hiatus hernia two separate high-pressure zones exist [55]. Using radiography and clips placed at the SCJ and at the diaphragmatic impression, it was confirmed that the proximal high-pressure zone is located at the SCJ and the distal high-pressure zone at the level of the diaphragmatic impression [56]. Abdominal compression as well as inspiration were associated with augmentation of the pressure of the distal high-pressure zone in patients with a hiatal hernia to a degree that was equal to the pressure augmentation of the high-pressure zone during these events in healthy subjects. The pressure amplitude of the two separate high-pressure zones was lower than the pressure in healthy subjects in whom there is only one high-pressure zone. Mathematical summation of the pressure profiles of both high-pressure zones led to a pressure profile resembling that of a healthy subject.

Studies using simultaneous manometry and fluoroscopy showed that, regardless of the basal LES pressure, patients with a hiatus hernia more often had reflux provoked by the Valsalva procedure (expiration against a closed airway), Mueller maneuver (inspiration against closed airway), and increased abdominal pressure [57]. Other combined fluoroscopic and manometric LES recordings in patients with hiatus hernias showed that reflux of barium from the hernia sac into the esophagus occurs when the pressure of the sac exceeds the LES pressure [58, 59]. This may occur either during compartmentalization of the hiatal sac caused by inspiration-associated contractions of the diaphragm or by reduction of LES pressure during swallow-associated LES relaxation.

In one study ambulatory GERD patients with a hiatus hernia were compared to GERD patients without a hiatus hernia. The excess of reflux episodes found in the subjects with a hiatus hernia was due to reflux episodes that were not associated with a TLESR [60]. Much more reflux occurred in the patients with a hiatus hernia during periods of low LES pressure, swallow-associated LES relaxation, and straining during periods with a low LES pressure.

With high-resolution manometry, the two high-pressure zones that are caused by the LES and crural diaphragm can be distinguished in patients with a hiatus hernia and can be studied over time. A study in which high-resolution manometry of patients with a small hiatus hernia was performed for a prolonged period showed that sliding hernias do indeed slide. There was a frequent transition from a double high-pressure zone (non-reduced hernia) to a single high-pressure zone (reduced hiatus hernia), and back [61]. During the periods with a non-reduced hiatus hernia, the frequency of acidic and weakly acidic episodes was almost twice as high as in the periods with a reduced hernia. This increase in reflux frequency predominantly was the result of an increase in reflux episodes during swallowing and to a lesser extent to an increase in reflux episodes during periods with low LES pressure and straining. There was no difference in reflux episodes associated with TLESRs. This study thus showed that the increase in reflux episodes in case of a hiatus hernia can largely be explained as the result of the temporal spatial separation of the two components of the antireflux barrier.

The hypothesis that the crural diaphragm is of crucial importance in the prevention of gastroesophageal reflux during periods with low LES pressure is also supported by other studies, which have shown an absence of reflux during periods with low LES pressure in the presence of normal contractions of the diaphragm [57]. Thus, the frequency of TLESRs is similar in patients with and without a hiatal hernia, as is the frequency of TLESRs that are accompanied by reflux [62–64]. However, the excess of reflux episodes found in patients with a hiatal hernia is caused by reflux mechanisms other than TLESRs.

In addition to weakening of the barrier function caused by the spatial separation of LES and diaphragm, a large hiatus hernia may also impair the process of esophageal emptying. During swallowing the contents of the hernia sac may reflux into the esophagus [58, 65, 66]. Swallow-associated peristalsis will transport the refluxed fluids in a distal direction. However, with each swallow the LES will relax and the contents of the hernia sac will enter the esophagus again. This process will repeat with subsequent swallows.

Besides a lower maximum pressure at the GEJ, there is also evidence of an increased compliance of this region in patients with a hiatus hernia. Experiments with gradual

balloon distention showed that the GEJ opens more readily in patients with a hiatus hernia [67]. This can add to the impairment of the antireflux barrier in these patients.

Diagnosis

There are several techniques with which a hiatus hernia can be detected. Almost all tests used only offer a snapshot image of the GEJ, while a sliding hernia is a dynamic structure that varies over time. The gold standard for detection of a hiatus hernia and estimation of its size is still the barium esophagogram [50]. A well-performed barium study shows the narrowing of the lumen at the level of the LES, which is sometimes called the A ring [68, 69]. The hernia sac below the A ring is seen as a widening of the lumen which contains gastric folds. The hernia sac narrows distally by the impression of the diaphragm. In case of a weak LES, sometimes no A ring is observed. In case of a Schatzki's ring, a discrete circular narrowing at the level of the SCJ can be seen. A Schatzki's ring, which can be a cause of dysphagia, is called a B ring by radiologists. The barium esophagogram technique also allows detection of a paraesophageal hernia (Figure 20.3).

Probably, most sliding hiatus hernias are nowadays detected during upper endoscopy [70]. Endoscopically, the size of the hernia is usually measured as the distance from the diaphragmatic impression to the SCJ and it is assumed that the LES is located somewhere near the SCJ (Figure 20.4). Sometimes a Schatzki's ring is found (Figure 20.5). There are little data on the correlation between endoscopic and radiographic detection of hiatus hernia, although it

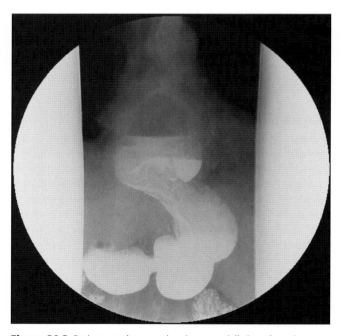

Figure 20.3 Barium esophagram showing a partially intrathoracic stomach with an air–fluid level, indicative of a paraesophageal hernia.

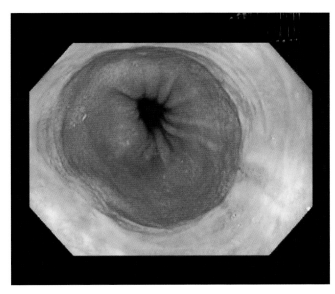

Figure 20.4 Endoscopic image of a sliding hiatus hernia. A small erosion is visible at 4 o'clock.

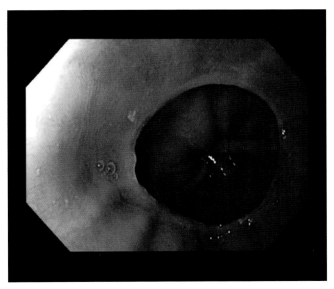

Figure 20.5 Endoscopic image of a sliding hiatus hernia with a Schatzki's ring.

seems that endoscopy underestimates the size of the hiatus hernia [71]. On the other hand, it has been suggested that many hiatus hernias detected with upper endoscopy would not have been detected with barium studies [72].

During pull-through manometry, the presence of a sliding hiatus hernia can be suspected when two distinct high-pressure zones are seen, the distal one being the diaphragm and the proximal one being the LES [55, 73–78]. High-resolution manometry allows detection of a sliding hiatus hernia as the high-pressure zones contributed by the LES and the diaphragm can be distinguished (Figure 20.6).

Studies using high-resolution manometry showed that the distance between the LES and diaphragm varies, and during a significant proportion of time a sliding hernia can be completely reduced [61, 79].

Sometimes a hiatus hernia can be seen on a plain radiograph of the thorax as an air pocket or an air–fluid level above the diaphragm (Figure 20.7). Sometimes the colon and other organs can be seen in the thoracic cavity (Figure 20.8). Hiatus hernias can also be recognized on CT (Figure 20.9).

Therapy

A sliding hiatus hernia usually is asymptomatic, but the subsequent increase in reflux episodes will predispose to the development of GERD. The decision on treatment of a sliding hiatus hernia should therefore be dependent on the presence of GERD symptoms and/or mucosal damage caused by reflux rather than on the presence of the hiatal hernia itself. Surgical reduction of a hernia brings the herniated gastric part intra-abdominally and overlaps the LES and diaphragm again, leading to a reduction of reflux episodes [80, 81]. Type II, III, and IV hernias carry a risk of incarceration and subsequent bleeding or perforation [82]. These complications are life-threatening. Furthermore, spontaneous regression does not occur and often the hernias grow larger with time. Therefore, in patients who are fit for surgery, an elective repair of a paraesophageal hernia is advised, even if no symptoms are present.

Surgical reduction of a paraesophageal hernia will include repositioning of the herniated stomach followed by closure of the hiatal defect and gastropexy, by attaching the stomach subdiaphragmatically to prevent recurrent herniation [83]. A mesh can be used to close a large hiatal defect. Controversy exists as to whether or not an antireflux procedure is required if no evidence of GERD is present. In the majority of cases, paraesophageal hernia repair is combined with a Nissen fundoplication. Gastropexy is performed only when the stomach is unusually mobile after repositioning in the abdomen. The operation was traditionally performed through either a laparotomy or thoracotomy. The transabdominal approach facilitates the reduction of gastric volvulus as well. In line with the success of laparoscopic antireflux surgery, laparoscopic paraesophageal hernia repair has been developed [84, 85]. This approach results in a reduction of hospital stay and reduced major and minor complications. However, perioperative mortality is still considerable and has been reported to be around 5%. The prognosis after successful surgical repair of a paraesophageal hernia is excellent, with a recurrence rate of less than 10% [86, 87].

As the majority of patients with paraesophageal hernias are of advanced age, many patients have significant comorbidities. In these patients the risks of surgery are substantial and less invasive techniques have been developed. A case series has been published in which patients with a paraesophageal hernia and severe comorbidity were treated

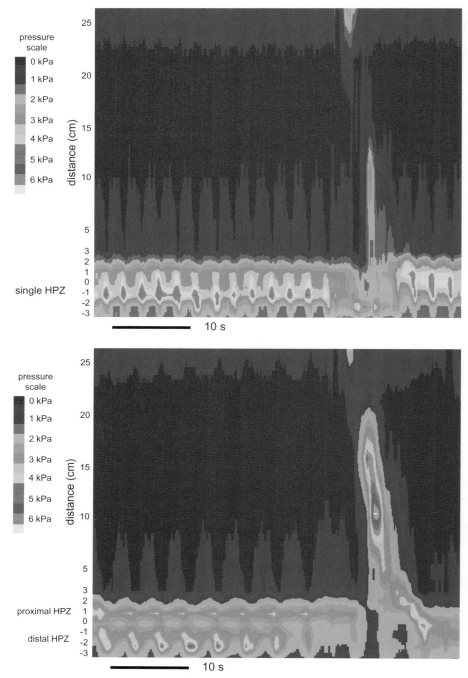

Figure 20.6 High-resolution manometry of a sliding hiatus hernia in reduced and unreduced state (adapted from Bredenoord *et al.* [61], with permission).

with endoscopic reduction of the hernia followed by percutaneous endoscopic gastrostomy (PEG) [88]. However, laparoscopic assistance for hernia reduction and gastropexy was required in nine patients and three major complications occurred. Although it remains questionable whether this can be regarded as a true alternative, selected patients with severe comorbidity might benefit from this approach.

Conclusions

Sliding hiatus hernia is a very common condition and the spatial separation of the LES and diaphragm associated with it leads to impaired functioning of the antireflux barrier. A sliding hiatus hernia is a dynamic condition in which the

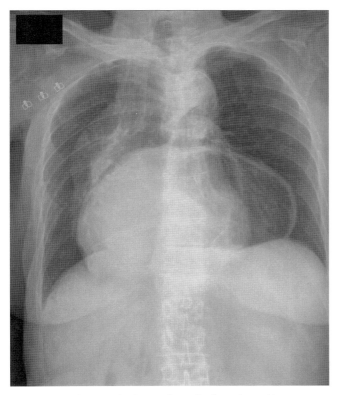

Figure 20.7 Plain upright chest radiograph of a patient with a very large sliding hiatus hernia.

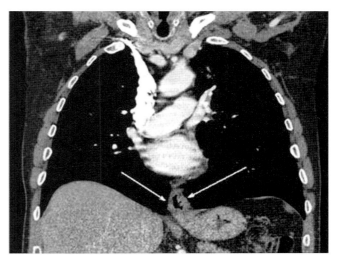

Figure 20.9 Coronal reconstruction of the gastroesophageal junction, scanned with computer tomography, showing a small hiatal hernia (arrows).

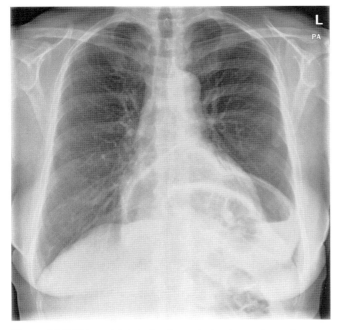

Figure 20.8 Plain upright chest radiograph showing a retrocardiac air–fluid level within a paraesophageal hernia and air-filled colon.

distance between the LES and diaphragm varies over time. Although a sliding hiatus hernia in itself usually does not lead to symptoms, the consequent increase in reflux episodes predisposes to the development of GERD. A paraesophageal hernia is encountered less frequently but represents a potentially dangerous condition that warrants careful management, usually including surgical correction.

References

1. Allison PR. Reflux esophagitis, sliding hiatal hernia, and the anatomy of repair. *Surg Gynecol Obstet* 1951;92:419–431.
2. Cohen S, Harris LD. Does hiatus hernia affect competence of the gastroesophageal sphincter? *N Engl J Med* 1971; 284:1053–1056.
3. Dent J. A new technique for continuous sphincter pressure measurement. *Gastroenterology* 1976;71:263–267.
4. Dodds WJ, Dent J, Hogan WJ, *et al.* Mechanisms of gastroesophageal reflux in patients with reflux esophagitis. *N Engl J Med* 1982;307:1547–1552.
5. Murray JA, Camilleri M. The fall and rise of the hiatal hernia. *Gastroenterology* 2000;19:1779–1781.
6. Liebermann-Meffert D, Allgower M, Schmid P, Blum AL. Muscular equivalent of the lower esophageal sphincter. *Gastroenterology* 1979;76:31–38.
7. Marchand P. The anatomy of esophageal hiatus of the diaphragm and the pathogenesis of hiatus herniation. *J Thorac Surg* 1959;37:81–92.
8. Stein HJ, Liebermann-Meffert D, DeMeester TR, Siewert JR. Three-dimensional pressure image and muscular structure of the human lower esophageal sphincter. *Surgery* 1995;117:692–698.

9. Fyke FE, Code CF, Schlegel JF. The gastroesophageal sphincter in healthy human beings. *Gastroenterologia* 1956;86:135–150.

10. Mittal RK, Rochester DF, McCallum RW. Sphincteric action of the diaphragm during a relaxed lower esophageal sphincter in humans. *Am J Physiol* 1989;256:G139–144.

11. Martin CJ, Dodds WJ, Liem HH, Dantas RO, Layman RD, Dent J. Diaphragmatic contribution to gastroesophageal competence and reflux in dogs. *Am J Physiol* 1992;263:G551–557.

12. Klein WA, Parkman HP, Dempsey DT, Fisher RS. Sphincterlike thoracoabdominal high pressure zone after esophagogastrectomy. *Gastroenterology* 1993;105:1362–1369.

13. Mittal RK, Rochester DF, McCallum RW. Electrical and mechanical activity in the human lower esophageal sphincter during diaphragmatic contraction. *J Clin Invest* 1988;81:1182–1189.

14. Boyle JT, Altschuler SM, Nixon TE, Tuchman DN, Pack AI, Cohen S. Role of the diaphragm in the genesis of lower esophageal sphincter pressure in the cat. *Gastroenterology* 1985;88:723–730.

15. Boyle JT, Altschuler SM, Nixon TE, Pack AI, Cohen S. Responses of feline gastroesophageal junction to changes in abdominal pressure. *Am J Physiol* 1987;253:G315–322.

16. Bredenoord AJ, Smout AJ. Physiologic and pathologic belching. *Clin Gastroenterol Hepatol* 2007;5:772–775.

17. Marchand P. A study of the forces productive of gastro-oesophageal regurgitation and herniation through the diaphragmatic hiatus. *Thorax* 1957;12:189–202.

18. Scheffer RC, Gooszen HG, Hebbard G, Samsom M. The role of transsphincteric pressure and proximal gastric volume in acid reflux before and after fundoplication. *Gastroenterology* 2005;129:1900–1909.

19. Dent J, Dodds WJ, Sekiguchi T, Hogan WJ, Arndorfer RC. Interdigestive phasic contractions of the human lower esophageal sphincter. *Gastroenterology* 1983;84:453–460.

20. Altschuler SM, Boyle JT, Nixon TE, Pack AI, Cohen S. Simultaneous reflex inhibition of lower esophageal sphincter and crural diaphragm in cats. *Am J Physiol* 1985;249:G586–591.

21. Mittal RK, Fisher MJ. Electrical and mechanical inhibition of the crural diaphragm during transient relaxation of the lower esophageal sphincter. *Gastroenterology* 1990;99:1265–1268.

22. Kahrilas PJ, Wu S, Lin S, Pouderoux P. Attenuation of esophageal shortening during peristalsis with hiatus hernia. *Gastroenterology* 1995;109:1818–1825.

23. Wyman JB, Dent J, Heddle R, Dodds WJ, Toouli J, Downton J. Control of belching by the lower oesophageal sphincter. *Gut* 1990;31:639–646.

24. Dent J, Dodds WJ, Friedman RH, *et al.* Mechanism of gastroesophageal reflux in recumbent asymptomatic human subjects. *J Clin Invest* 1980;65:256–267.

25. Wright RA, Hurwitz AL. Relationship of hiatal hernia to endoscopically proved reflux esophagitis. *Dig Dis Sci* 1979;24:311–313.

26. Kang JY, Ho KY. Different prevalences of reflux oesophagitis and hiatus hernia among dyspeptic patients in England and Singapore. *Eur J Gastroenterol Hepatol* 1999;11:845–850.

27. Loffeld RJ, van der Putten AB. Newly developing hiatus hernia: a survey in patients undergoing upper gastrointestinal endoscopy. *J Gastroenterol Hepatol* 2002;17:542–544.

28. Pridie RB. Incidence and coincidence of hiatus hernia. *Gut* 1966;7:188–189.

29. Chang CS, Poon SK, Lien HC, Chen GH. The incidence of reflux esophagitis among the Chinese. *Am J Gastroenterol* 1997;92:668–671.

30. Yeh C, Hsu CT, Ho AS, Sampliner RE, Fass R. Erosive esophagitis and Barrett's esophagus in Taiwan: a higher frequency than expected. *Dig Dis Sci* 1997;42:702–706.

31. Cronstedt J, Carling L, Vestergaard P, Berglund J. Oesophageal disease revealed by endoscopy in 1,000 patients referred primarily for gastroscopy. *Acta Med Scand* 1978;204:413–416.

32. Lee SJ, Song CW, Jeen YT, *et al.* Prevalence of endoscopic reflux esophagitis among Koreans. *J Gastroenterol Hepatol* 2001;16:373–376.

33. Dutta SK, Arora M, Kireet A, Bashandy H, Gandsas A. Upper gastrointestinal symptoms and associated disorders in morbidly obese patients: a prospective study. *Dig Dis Sci* 2009;54:1243–1246.

34. Furukawa N, Iwakiri R, Koyama T, *et al.* Proportion of reflux esophagitis in 6010 Japanese adults: prospective evaluation by endoscopy. *J Gastroenterol* 1999;34:441–444.

35. Sakaguchi M, Oka H, Hashimoto T, Asakuma Y, Takao M, Gon G et al. Obesity as a risk factor for GERD in Japan. *J Gastroenterol* 2008;43:57–62.

36. Goodman RM, Wooley CF, Ruppert RD, Freimanis AK. A possible genetic role in esophageal hiatus hernia. *J Hered* 1969;60:71–74.

37. Carre IJ, Johnston BT, Thomas PS, Morrison PJ. Familial hiatal hernia in a large five generation family confirming true autosomal dominant inheritance. *Gut* 1999;45:649–652.

38. Sidd JJ, Gilliam JI, Bushueff BP. Sliding hiatus hernias in identical twins. *Br J Radiol* 1966;39:703–704.

39. Ott DJ, Glauser SJ, Ledbetter MS, Chen MY, Koufman JA, Gelfand DW. Association of hiatal hernia and gastroesophageal reflux: correlation between presence and size of hiatal hernia and 24-hour pH monitoring of the esophagus. *AJR Am J Roentgenol* 1995;165:557–559.

40. Cameron AJ. Incidence of iron deficiency anemia in patients with large diaphragmatic hernia. A controlled study. *Mayo Clin Proc* 1976;51:767–769.

41. Lin S, Brasseur JG, Pouderoux P, Kahrilas PJ. The phrenic ampulla: distal esophagus or potential hiatal hernia? *Am J Physiol* 1995;268:G320–327.

42. Ho KY, Kang JY. Esophageal mucosal acid sensitivity can coexist with normal pH recording in healthy adult volunteers. *J Gastroenterol* 2000;35:261–264.

43. Wilson LJ, Ma W, Hirschowitz BI. Association of obesity with hiatal hernia and esophagitis. *Am J Gastroenterol* 1999;94:2840–2844.

44. Barak N, Ehrenpreis ED, Harrison JR, Sitrin MD. Gastrooesophageal reflux disease in obesity: pathophysiological and therapeutic considerations. *Obes Rev* 2002;3:9–15.

45. Stene-Larsen G, Weberg R, Froyshov LI, Bjortuft O, Hoel B, Berstad A. Relationship of overweight to hiatus hernia and reflux oesophagitis. *Scand J Gastroenterol* 1988;23:427–432.

46. Smith AB, Dickerman RD, McGuire CS, East JW, McConathy WJ, Pearson HF. Pressure-overload-induced sliding hiatal hernia in power athletes. *J Clin Gastroenterol* 1999;28:352–354.

47. de Vries DR, Van Herwaarden MA, Smout AJ, Samsom M. Gastroesophageal pressure gradients in gastroesophageal reflux disease: relations with hiatal hernia, body mass index, and esophageal acid exposure. *Am J Gastroenterol* 2008;103:1349–1354.

48. Paterson WG, Kolyn DM. Esophageal shortening induced by short-term intraluminal acid perfusion in opossum: a cause for hiatus hernia? *Gastroenterology* 1994;107:1736–1740.

49. Patti MG, Goldberg HI, Arcerito M, Bortolasi L, Tong J, Way LW. Hiatal hernia size affects lower esophageal sphincter function, esophageal acid exposure, and the degree of mucosal injury. *Am J Surg* 1996;171:182–186.

50. Kaul B, Petersen H, Myrvold HE, Grette K, Roysland P, Halvorsen T. Hiatus hernia in gastroesophageal reflux disease. *Scand J Gastroenterol* 1986;21:31–34.

51. Berstad A, Weberg R, Froyshov LI, Hoel B, Hauer-Jensen M. Relationship of hiatus hernia to reflux oesophagitis. A prospective study of coincidence, using endoscopy. *Scand J Gastroenterol* 1986;21:55–58.

52. Petersen H, Johannessen T, Sandvik AK, *et al.* Relationship between endoscopic hiatus hernia and gastroesophageal reflux symptoms. *Scand J Gastroenterol* 1991;26:921–926.

53. Jones MP, Sloan SS, Rabine JC, Ebert CC, Huang CF, Kahrilas PJ. Hiatal hernia size is the dominant determinant of esophagitis presence and severity in gastroesophageal reflux disease. *Am J Gastroenterol* 2001;96:1711–1717.

54. Sontag SJ, Schnell TG, Miller TQ, *et al.* The importance of hiatal hernia in reflux esophagitis compared with lower esophageal sphincter pressure or smoking. *J Clin Gastroenterol* 1991;13:628–643.

55. Code CF, Kelley ML, Schlegel JF, Olsen AM. Detection of hiatal hernia during esophageal motility tests. *Gastroenterology* 1962;43:521–531.

56. Kahrilas PJ, Lin S, Chen J, Manka M. The effect of hiatus hernia on gastro-oesophageal junction pressure. *Gut* 1999;44:476–482.

57. Sloan S, Rademaker AW, Kahrilas PJ. Determinants of gastroesophageal junction incompetence: hiatal hernia, lower esophageal sphincter, or both? *Ann Intern Med* 1992;117:977–982.

58. Sloan S, Kahrilas PJ. Impairment of esophageal emptying with hiatal hernia. *Gastroenterology* 1991;100:596–605.

59. Longhi EH, Jordan PH Jr. Pressure relationships responsible for reflux in patients with hiatal hernia. *Surg Gynecol Obstet* 1969;129:734–748.

60. Van Herwaarden MA, Samsom M, Smout AJ. Excess gastroesophageal reflux in patients with hiatus hernia is caused by mechanisms other than transient LES relaxations. *Gastroenterology* 2000;119:1439–1446.

61. Bredenoord AJ, Weusten BL, Timmer R, Smout AJ. Intermittent spatial separation of diaphragm and lower esophageal sphincter favors acidic and weakly acidic reflux. *Gastroenterology* 2006;130:334–340.

62. Dent J, Holloway RH, Toouli J, Dodds WJ. Mechanisms of lower oesophageal sphincter incompetence in patients with symptomatic gastrooesophageal reflux. *Gut* 1988;29:1020–1028.

63. Penagini R, Schoeman MN, Dent J, Tippett MD, Holloway RH. Motor events underlying gastro-oesophageal reflux in ambulant patients with reflux oesophagitis. *Neurogastroenterol Motil* 1996;8:131–141.

64. Bredenoord AJ, Weusten BL, Timmer R, Smout AJ. Air swallowing, belching, and reflux in patients with gastroesophageal reflux disease. *Am J Gastroenterol* 2006;101:1721–1726.

65. Mittal RK, Lange RC, McCallum RW. Identification and mechanism of delayed esophageal acid clearance in subjects with hiatus hernia. *Gastroenterology* 1987;92:130–135.

66. Emerenziani S, Habib FI, Ribolsi M, *et al.* Effect of hiatal hernia on proximal oesophageal acid clearance in gastro-oesophageal reflux disease patients. *Aliment Pharmacol Ther* 2006;23:751–757.

67. Pandolfino JE, Shi G, Trueworthy B, Kahrilas PJ. Esophagogastric junction opening during relaxation distinguishes nonhernia reflux patients, hernia patients, and normal subjects. *Gastroenterology* 2003;125:1018–1024.

68. Wolf BS. The definition of a sliding hiatal hernia. A radiologist's point of view. *Am J Dig Dis* 1960;5:168–173.

69. Heitmann P, Wolf BS, Sokol EM, Cohen BR. Simultaneous cineradiographic-manometric study of the distal esophagus: small hiatal hernias and rings. *Gastroenterology* 1966;50:737–753.

70. Trujillo NP. Endoscopic diagnosis of sliding-type diaphragmatic hiatal hernias. *Am J Dig Dis* 1968;13:855–867.

71. Gordon C, Kang JY, Neild PJ, Maxwell JD. The role of the hiatus hernia in gastro-oesophageal reflux disease. *Aliment Pharmacol Ther* 2004;20:719–732.

72. Panzuto F, Di Giulio E, Capurso G, *et al.* Large hiatal hernia in patients with iron deficiency anaemia: a prospective study on prevalence and treatment. *Aliment Pharmacol Ther* 2004;19:663–670.

73. Cuomo R, Sarnelli G, Grasso R, *et al.* Manometric study of hiatal hernia and its correlation with esophageal peristalsis. *Dig Dis Sci* 1999;44:1747–1753.

74. Clark MD, Rinaldo JA Jr, Eyler WR. Correlation of manometric and radiologic data from the esophagogastric area. *Radiology* 1970;94:261–270.

75. Klaus A, Raiser F, Swain JM, Hinder RA. Manometric components of the lower esophageal double hump. *Dig Dis* 2000;18:172–177.

76. Kasapidis P, Vassilakis JS, Tzovaras G, Chrysos E, Xynos E. Effect of hiatal hernia on esophageal manometry and pH-metry in gastroesophageal reflux disease. *Dig Dis Sci* 1995;40:2724–2730.

77. McCray WH, Jr., Chung C, Parkman HP, Miller LS. Use of simultaneous high-resolution endoluminal sonography (HRES) and manometry to characterize high pressure zone of distal esophagus. *Dig Dis Sci* 2000;45:1660–1666.

78. Agrawal A, Tutuian R, Hila A, Freeman J, Castell DO. Identification of hiatal hernia by esophageal manometry: is it reliable? *Dis Esophagus* 2005;18:316–319.

79. Bredenoord AJ, Weusten BL, Carmagnola S, Smout AJ. Double-peaked high-pressure zone at the esophagogastric junction in controls and in patients with a hiatal hernia. A study using high-resolution manometry. *Dig Dis Sci* 2004;49:1128–1135.

80. Bredenoord AJ, Draaisma WA, Weusten BL, Gooszen HG, Smout AJ. Mechanisms of acid, weakly acidic and gas reflux after anti-reflux surgery. *Gut* 2008;57:161–166.

81. Draaisma WA, Rijnhart-de Jong HG, Broeders IA, Smout AJ, Furnee EJ, Gooszen HG. Five-year subjective and objective

results of laparoscopic and conventional Nissen fundoplication: a randomized trial. *Ann Surg* 2006;244:34–41.

82. Hill LD. Incarcerated paraesophageal hernia. A surgical emergency. *Am J Surg* 1973;126:286–291.

83. Allen MS, Trastek VF, Deschamps C, Pairolero PC. Intrathoracic stomach. Presentation and results of operation. *J Thorac Cardiovasc Surg* 1993;105:253–258.

84. Schauer PR, Ikramuddin S, McLaughlin RH, *et al*. Comparison of laparoscopic versus open repair of paraesophageal hernia. *Am J Surg* 1998;176:659–665.

85. Livingston CD, Jones HLJ, Askew RE Jr, Victor BE, Askew RE Sr. Laparoscopic hiatal hernia repair in patients with poor esophageal motility or paraesophageal herniation. *Am Surg* 2001;67:987–991.

86. Yano F, Stadlhuber RJ, Tsuboi K, Gerhardt J, Filipi CJ, Mittal SK. Outcomes of surgical treatment of intrathoracic stomach. *Dis Esophagus* 2009;22:284–288.

87. Andujar JJ, Papasavas PK, Birdas T, *et al*. Laparoscopic repair of large paraesophageal hernia is associated with a low incidence of recurrence and reoperation. *Surg Endosc* 2004;18:444–447.

88. Kercher KW, Matthews BD, Ponsky JL, *et al*. Minimally invasive management of paraesophageal herniation in the high-risk surgical patient. *Am J Surg* 2001;182:510–514.

Pathophysiology of Gastroesophageal Reflux Disease: Motility Factors

Ravinder K. Mittal

Department of Medicine, University of California, San Diego and Gastroenterology Section San Diego Veterans Health Care Center, La Jolla, CA, USA

Introduction

Is gastroesophageal reflux disease (GERD) an acid or motility disorder of the esophagus? Indeed, gastric acid and pepsin are the major offenders and primarily responsible for the esophageal mucosal damage in reflux diseases. However, the gastric acid secretion in the majority of, if not all, patients with reflux disease is normal. The reason that gastric acid reaches the esophagus is due to motility abnormality of the lower esophageal sphincter (LES). Deranged esophageal peristalsis, when present, allows acid and possibly other noxious agents to remain in the esophagus for extended periods of time after reflux events and induce esophageal mucosal damage. Therefore, even though the major noxious agents in reflux disease are gastric acid and pepsin, the dysfunction of LES and esophageal peristalsis are primary etiologic factors and fundamental to the pathogenesis of reflux disease and esophagitis.

Lower esophageal sphincter

Historical perspective

A person can stand upside down after eating a large hearty meal, yet no food refluxes into the mouth or the esophagus. It is intuitively clear that there must be a valvular or sphincter mechanism at the lower end of the esophagus. In a 1958 review article, Ingelfinger stated that the pinchcock action of the diaphragm was important in the prevention of gastroesophageal reflux (GER) [1]. Code *et al.* were the first to record the intraluminal high-pressure zone between the esophagus and the stomach; they suggested that intrinsic muscles of the lower end of the esophagus were entirely responsible for maintaining this pressure [2]. It was not until 1985 that the diaphragmatic hiatus was convincingly proven to play a role in the valvular mechanism at the gastro-

esophageal junction (GEJ) [2, 3]. Studies conducted during the last 25 years convincingly show that there is not one, but two lower esophageal sphincters. The dual-sphincter mechanism at the GEJ is composed of intrinsic smooth muscles of the LES and extrinsic skeletal muscles of the diaphragmatic hiatus. In humans, under normal conditions, the LES is approximately 4 cm in length and is made up of clasp and sling fibers. On the other hand, crural diaphragm, which forms the esophageal hiatus, is about 2 cm in length. The crural diaphragm encircles the proximal 2 cm of the LES [4]. Therefore, a portion of the LES is intra-abdominal and a portion is located in the hiatus itself (Figure 21.1). The intra-abdominal portion of the LES is frequently termed the submerged segment of the esophagus [5]. The lower end of the esophagus has also been referred to as the phrenic ampulla by radiologists because it has a bulbar shape on barium swallow [6].

Morphology studies in cadavers [7, 8] and ultrasound imaging [8] in live humans demonstrate that the muscles of the LES are thicker than those of the adjacent esophagus. However, the muscle thickness in the LES region is not fixed; it increases with the increase in LES pressure. The smooth muscles of the LES are arranged in "C"-shaped clasp fibers on the right side of the esophagus and lesser curvature of stomach, and sling or oblique fibers of the stomach that are located on the left esophageal wall and greater curvature of the stomach [9]. Sling fibers are responsible for the flap–valve mechanism considered to be important in the prevention of GER [10].

The respiratory diaphragm, a major organ for the ventilatory function of the lung, also provides sphincter mechanism at the GEJ. The diaphragm is composed of a costal part arising from the ribs, and a crural part, which originates from the vertebral column. Embryologically, crural diaphragm develops in the dorsal mesentery of the esophagus, and the costal diaphragm from myoblasts originating in the lateral body wall [11]. The crural diaphragm, which forms the esophageal hiatus, can be considered as and is called the

The Esophagus, Fifth Edition. Edited by Joel E. Richter, Donald O. Castell.
© 2012 Blackwell Publishing Ltd. Published 2012 by Blackwell Publishing Ltd.

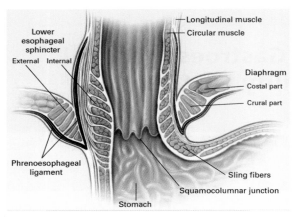

Figure 21.1 Anatomy of the gastroesophageal junction (GEJ). The smooth muscles of the lower end of the esophagus and the skeletal muscle of crural diaphragm are the two sphincter mechanisms at theGEJ. The two sphincters are anatomically superimposed and anchored to each other by the phrenoesophageal ligament (reproduced from Mittal RK, Balaban DH. The esophagogastric junction. *N Engl J Med* 1997;336:924–932, with permission).

"external lower esophageal sphincter;" it is actually shaped like a canal which is formed primarily by the right crus of the diaphragm [12].

The LES and crural diaphragm are anchored to each other by the phrenoesophageal ligament, a condensation of the loose areolar tissue. This ligament extends from the under surface of the diaphragm and attaches to the esophagus approximately at the upper border of the LES. Because of the firm anchoring of the LES and crural diaphragm by the phrenoesophageal ligament, the LES and crural diaphragm move together with inspiration and expiration. However, with longitudinal muscle contraction-related esophageal shortening during swallow and transient LES relaxation, the LES and crural diaphragm can be transiently separated from each other [13, 14]. Weakening of the phrenoesophageal ligament is the cause of sliding esophageal hiatus hernia. Prolonged LES pressure recordings using high-resolution manometry show that the LES and crural diaphragm separate from each other fairly frequently and reflux is more likely to occur when the two structure are anatomically apart rather than when they are together [15].

Gastroesophageal junction pressure under different physiologic conditions

The intraluminal pressure at the GEJ is a measure of the strength of the antireflux barrier. There are convincing data in both animals and humans that the two anatomic structures. i.e. the LES and crural diaphragm, contribute to the GEJ pressure. Electrical stimulation of the crural diaphragm increases the GEJ pressure in cats [16]. Furthermore, the crural diaphragm is capable of maintaining a high-pressure

zone at the abdominothoracic junction in patients who have undergone surgical resection of the smooth muscle LES [17].

To avoid confusion, the intraluminal pressure at the lower end of the esophagus will be referred to in this chapter as the GEJ pressure. The pressure generated from the contraction of LES smooth muscle is referred to as the LES pressure, and the pressure due to contraction of the crural diaphragm is termed the crural diaphragm pressure. Distinguishing these two pressures is important because it emphasizes the individual contributions of each structure to the GEJ pressure.

The LES or GEJ pressure is measured in reference to the intragastric pressure. Prolonged continuous pressure monitoring reveals that the GEJ pressure varies over time. These variations are either due to LES or crural diaphragm contractions. The LES pressure varies from minute to minute, and these pressure fluctuations are usually of small amplitude, ranging from 5 to 10 mmHg. However, large LES pressure fluctuations coupled with the migrating motor complex (MMC) activity of the stomach also occur. The frequency of these phasic pressure fluctuations is the same as that of the MMC, usually three per minute. The LES pressure may exceed 80 mmHg during phase III of the MMC, and typically peaks prior to the onset of gastric contraction [18].

The second type of variation in the GEJ pressure is related to the crural diaphragm contraction, which is linked with respiration. With each inspiration, as the crural diaphragm contracts, there is an increase in the GEJ pressure [19]. The amplitude of the inspiratory pressure increase is directly proportional to the force of crural diaphragmatic contraction. During tidal inspiration, the GEJ pressure increase is 10–20 mmHg, and with deep inspiration the pressure increase ranges from 100–150 mmHg or more. The crural diaphragm also contributes to the GEJ pressure during non-respiratory physical activities, such as straight leg raising and abdominal compression. These activities can induce sustained or tonic contractions of the crural diaphragm [20]. The crural diaphragm reflexively contracts during coughing, Valsalva maneuver, and any physical activity that increases intra-abdominal pressure.

Neural control of the lower esophageal sphincter and crural diaphragm

The tone in the LES muscle is the result of myogenic and neurogenic mechanisms. The relative contribution of these two mechanisms varies among different species. In humans, the LES tone is comprised of both neurogenic and myogenic components. A significant percentage of the LES tone in humans is due to cholinergic innervation [21]. Myogenic tone is due to shifts of intracellular calcium stores within the LES muscle [22].

There are large numbers of excitatory and inhibitory neurotransmitters and pharmacologic agents that act on the LES muscle; however, their physiologic significance remains unclear. The modulation of LES tone that occurs with MMC activity is largely mediated through the vagus nerve [23]. The swallow-associated LES relaxation is mediated through the central nervous system (dorsomotor nucleus of the vagus nerve). The efferent nerves travel to the LES via the vagus nerve and it is felt that they communicate with the excitatory and inhibitory motor neurons of the myenteric plexus, which in turn communicate with the smooth muscles of the LES. Interstitial cells of Cajal may play an intermediary role in the neuromuscular transmission even though several recent studies do not support such a role. The synapse between the vagal fibers and myenteric neurons employs a cholinergic mechanism, and the post-synaptic neurotransmitter is non-cholinergic and non-adrenergic [24]. Several studies confirm that nitric oxide is the non-cholinergic, nonadrenergic neurotransmitter [25], but vasoactive intestinal peptide, ATP, and other agents may also play minor roles.

LES muscles, as stated earlier, are made up of clasp and sling fibers; clasp fibers maintain stronger myogenic tone than the sling fibers [26]. On the other hand, sling fibers respond briskly to cholinergic agonist. Clasp fibers are predominantly innervated by the inhibitory neurons located in the body of the esophagus and sling fibers by the excitatory neurons located in the stomach [27, 28]. L-type calcium channels are predominantly seen in the clasp muscle fibers [29] and there are other differences as well in the mechanisms by which these sling and clasp muscles contract and relax [30]. Differences in the properties of sling and clasp muscle fibers may be responsible for the greater pressure and greater cholinergic responsiveness of the LES pressure on the left side. Sling fibers are likely to be responsible for the maintenance of the angle of His and flap–valve function, both of which are considered to be important in the prevention of reflux. LES relaxes with swallow, esophageal distention, and transient LES relaxation, and during all such times it moves in the oral direction because of contraction of the longitudinal muscles of the esophagus. Axial mechanical stretch exerted on the LES induces a neurologically-mediated LES relaxation that is mediated through mechanosensitive inhibitory motor neurons in the myenteric plexus [31]. Based on recent studies, it is possible that the vagus nerve actually innervates longitudinal muscles of the esophagus, which in turn activate inhibitory motor neurons to the LES through a stretch sensitive mechanism [32].

The crural diaphragm, like the remainder of the diaphragm, is controlled through the phrenic nerves. Although the diaphragmatic hiatus is composed of muscles, mainly from the right crus, it is innervated by the left and right phrenic nerves. Spontaneous inspiratory activity of the crural diaphragm is due to the activity of inspiratory neurons located in the syncitium of the brainstem [33]. This activity is transmitted to the phrenic nerve nucleus located in the cervical spinal cord. Voluntary control of the diaphragm originates within the cortical neurons. The crural diaphragm contracts a frac-

tion of a second earlier than the costal diaphragm, and this may have physiologic significance in relationship to its antireflux barrier function [34]. Crural diaphragm is also innervated by the vagus nerve (sensory as well as motor); however, its significance and role in neural control of crural diaphragm contraction and relaxation is unclear.

Esophageal sensory mechanisms can mediate reflex relaxation of the crural diaphragm. Esophageal distention and swallow induce selective inhibition of the crural diaphragm muscle [35]. Transient relaxation of the LES—a major mechanism of GER, belching, and vomiting—is also accompanied by simultaneous relaxation of the LES and crural diaphragm [36, 37].

Physiologic significance of two lower esophageal sphincters

Why do we need two lower esophageal sphincters, the LES and crural diaphragm? The answer to this question rests on the physical principle that the intraluminal GEJ pressure determines the strength of the antireflux barrier, and the pressure gradient between the esophagus and stomach (PGES) is the driving force for GER. Under normal situations, the GEJ pressure is constantly adapting to changes in the PGES that occur during various physiologic circumstances. The changes in PGES are related either to muscular contractions of the esophagus and stomach or to pressure changes within the intrathoracic and intra-abdominal cavities. Contraction of the esophagus is protective with respect to reflux. On the other hand, gastric contraction increases the pressure gradient in favor of reflux. Therefore, LES contraction is coupled with gastric contraction during MMC activity of the stomach, thus preventing reflux. Contraction of the inspiratory muscles of respiration produces negative intrathoracic and intraesophageal pressure, thus increasing the PGES. Similarly, contraction of the abdominal wall and diaphragm increases the stomach pressure and PGES. All of the maneuvers accompanied by contraction of the inspiratory and abdominal wall muscles that increase PGES are also accompanied by contraction of the crural diaphragm and a protective increase in GEJ pressure. The rapid changes in PGES caused by skeletal muscle contraction of the chest and abdomen are thus counteracted by the rapidly contracting skeletal sphincter muscle of the crural diaphragm.

Mechanisms of reflex

Based on an understanding of the two lower esophageal sphincters, one would intuitively think that weakness of either the LES or the crural diaphragm is the cause of GER. Indeed, some patients with reflux disease have a weak LES, some have a weak crural diaphragm, and some have both. However, in mild-to-moderate non-erosive reflux disease, the LES [38] and crural diaphragm pressures are normal. In fact, a number of patients with mild-to-moderate disease have a hypertensive LES [39]. The incidence of low LES pressure increases with the severity of esophagitis [38], and spontaneous inspiratory crural diaphragm pressure is low in patients with sliding hiatal hernias [40]. A large body of information indicates that transient relaxation of the LES and crural diaphragm (TLESR) is the major mechanism of reflux in normal subjects and patients with reflux disease [41].

Transient lower esophageal sphincter relaxation

McNally *et al.* were the first to observe non–swallow-related LES relaxation as a mechanism of belching in 1964 [42]. The TLESR and its relationship to GER were described in detail in 1980 by Dent *et al.* [43]. Overall, TLESR is the single most common mechanism underlying GER. In normal subjects, the majority of reflux episodes occur during TLESRs, with the remainder occurring during swallow-induced LES relaxation associated with failed or incomplete primary peristalsis, in both supine and ambulant positions [44]. TLESR is also the most common mechanism of reflux in patients with reflux disease and accounts for 63–74% of reflux episodes [41, 45]. Similar findings have also been reported in children with reflux disease [46, 47].

Mechanisms of reflux in patients with reflux disease are less homogeneous than in normal subjects. While more than 50% of patients, usually those without endoscopic evidence of esophagitis, reflux exclusively through TLESR, many patients have a mixed picture in which a significant number of reflux episodes occur during swallow-induced LES relaxation, persistently absent basal LES pressure, straining by deep inspiration, and increased intra-abdominal pressure. The proportion of reflux episodes that can be ascribed to TLESRs decreases inversely with the severity of reflux disease, presumably because of the increasing prevalence of defective basal LES pressure as the severity of esophagitis increases [38]. The presence or absence of esophagitis does not influence the rate of TLESRs. Presence of hiatus hernia introduces an additional mechanism of reflux as discussed in the following paragraphs.

Characteristics of transient lower esophageal sphincter relaxation

Transient LES relaxations are abrupt falls in LES pressure that are not triggered by swallowing, as manifested by pharyngeal or mylohyoid muscle contraction (Figure 21.2). Transient LES relaxations are typically of longer duration than swallow-induced LES relaxation, lasting from 10–45 s. The criteria that have proved optimal for the definition of TLESRs are (1) the absence of a pharyngeal swallow signal for 4 s before to 2 s after the onset of LES relaxation, or a mylohyoid EMG complex for 3 s before the onset of LES relaxation; (2) an LES pressure fall of greater than 1 mmHg/s; (3) time from the onset to complete relaxation of less than 10 s; and (4) a nadir pressure of less than 2 mmHg [48]. A number of events in

the esophagus, stomach, and crural diaphragm accompany TLESRs. Contractions in the pharynx and mylohyoid muscle occur at the onset of 20–45% of TLESRs, respectively [49], although these pharyngeal and mylohyoid complexes are much smaller (approximately 50%) than those associated with swallowing and can be interpreted as partial or incomplete swallows. Distal esophageal contractions often occur at the onset of TLESRs and when recorded at more than one site, usually have a synchronous onset. During the period of LES inhibition, there is also inhibition of the esophageal body. The gastric fundus also shows changes consistent with active inhibition during TLESRs. There is also selective and complete inhibition of the crural diaphragm, despite continued activity of the costal diaphragm during TLESRs [50]. Longitudinal muscle of the distal esophagus starts to contract before the onset of TLESR and remain contracted during the entire period of TLESR [51]. Longitudinal muscle contraction seems to traverse in a reverse peristaltic fashion. Thus, TLESR is a coordinated pattern of activity designed to facilitate the retrograde flow of gastric contents during reflux, belching and vomiting (Figure 21.3).

With relaxation of the LES and crural diaphragm during TLESR, the esophagus and stomach become one cavity (common cavity), resulting in equalization of pressure in the two cavities. Increase in esophageal pressure can occur a second or more sooner than the complete LES relaxation during TLESR [52]. Since reflux generally does not take place until LES is completely relaxed, it raises the possibility that the onset of esophageal pressure increase during TLESR is related to the longitudinal muscle contraction of the esophagus rather than the actual reflux event [52]. As discussed earlier, longitudinal muscle contraction of the esophagus is likely the key event that initiates relaxation of the LES and possibly the crural diaphragm.

Stimuli that trigger transient lower esophageal sphincter relaxations

Gastric distention
Gastric distention is a potent stimulus for TLESR. This is not surprising given the fact that TLESR is the mechanism by which gas is vented from the stomach during belching. Approximately 15 mL of air is delivered to the stomach with each swallow [53] and without a built-in venting mechanism, uncontrolled gastrointestinal bloating would occur. Subcardiac regions of the stomach appear to be primarily responsible for triggering the TLESR [54]. Reduction of the compliance of this region by buttressing it with mesh reinforcement substantially reduces TLESR in dogs. In humans, a gastric volume of 750–1000 mL causes a four-fold increase in the rate of TLESRs within the first 10 min; a similar effect has been reported after meals [55]. Meals are also associated with a significant increase in the proportion of TLESRs associated with reflux, and it is possible that this effect rather

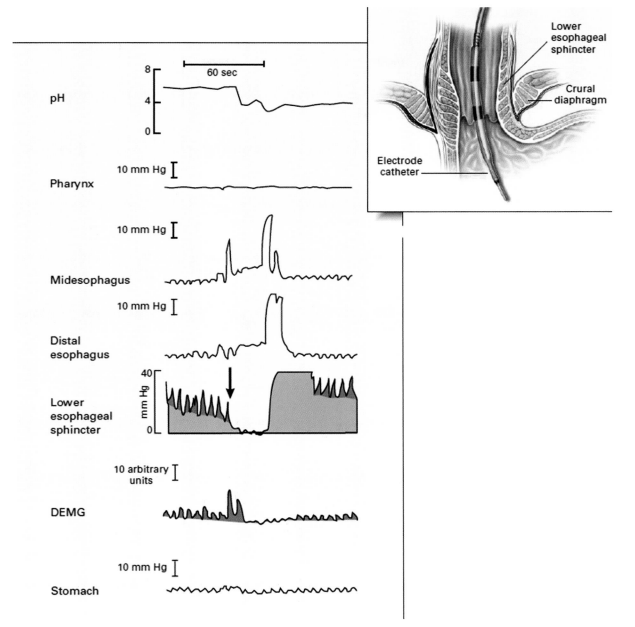

Figure 21.2 A spontaneous, transient lower esophageal sphincter relaxation (TLESR). The onset of TLESR is indicated by the vertical arrow. Relaxation occurs in the absence of a swallow as manifested by the absence of a pharyngeal pressure wave. The LES relaxation is complete to the level of the intragastric pressure (horizontal line at the bottom of the LES tracing) and is sustained for more than 20 s. TLESR is associated with the inhibition of crural diaphragm, as indicated by the loss of inspiratory LES pressure oscillations and inspiratory diaphragmatic electromyographic activity. Reflux (drop in esophageal pH) occurs following complete LES and crural diaphragm relaxation and is associated with an increase in intraesophageal pressure (reproduced Mittal RK, Balaban DH. The esophagogastric junction. *N Engl J Med* 1997;336: 924–932., with permission).

than an increase in the rate of TLESRs is responsible for the post-prandial increase in reflux.

Pharyngeal mechanisms

Pharyngeal intubation increases the rate of TLESRs. In fasted patients in whom LES pressure was monitored via a gastrostomy tube, pharyngeal intubation for 1 h increased the rate of TLESRs three-fold, from two to six per hour during the period of intubation [56]. Pharyngeal stimulation is usually associated with full expression of the oral, pharyngeal, and esophageal phases of deglutition; however LES relaxation without swallowing can be induced by instillation of minute

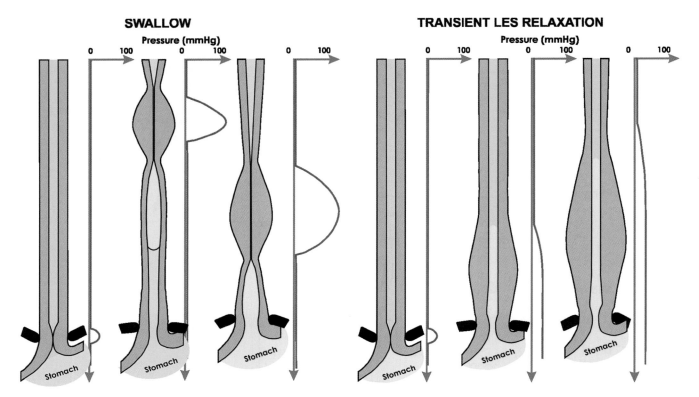

SWALLOW

Pressure (mmHg)

TRANSIENT LES RELAXATION

Pressure (mmHg)

Figure 21.3 Pattern of longitudinal muscle contraction of the esophagus during peristalsis and transient lower esophageal sphincter (LES) relaxation. Peristaltic contraction is associated with an aborally traversing simultaneous contraction of the circular and longitudinal muscles of the esophagus. On the other hand, transient LES relaxation is associated with contraction of the longitudinal muscle of the distal esophagus only that traverses in the oral directions (reverse peristalsis) (reproduced from Babaei *et al.* [51], with permission).

amounts of liquid into the hypopharynx in humans [45] and light stroking of the pharynx or low-frequency stimulation of the superior laryngeal nerve in the opossum [57]. This reflex depends on the afferent nerve fibers from the pharynx or larynx [58] travelling in the superior laryngeal branch of the vagus and the glossopharyngeal nerves; both nerves project to the nucleus tractus solitarius (NTS). The LES relaxation caused by stimulation of the pharynx with small amounts of water can last up to 60s or longer [45]. Interaction among stimuli is a real possibility; thus, pharyngeal stimulation may either trigger TLESRs directly or lower the threshold for triggering by gastric distension.

Factors modulating the rate of transient lower esophageal sphincter relaxations

In both healthy humans and dogs, the stimulation of TLESRs produced by gaseous gastric distension is almost totally suppressed in the supine posture [59]. In patients with reflux disease, TLESRs occur significantly less frequently in the supine [60] and lateral recumbent positions compared to the sitting position. TLESRs do not occur during stable sleep [61]; reflux episodes that do occur during the night-time sleep periods are totally confined to periods of arousal during sleep that may last for only 10s.

Spontaneous TLESRs are also completely suppressed in dogs by even light general anesthesia [62]. Cold stress has also been shown to reduce the frequency of TLESRs [63].

Neural pathways mediating transient lower esophageal sphincter relaxation: vagal control mechanisms

The vagus mediates swallow-induced LES relaxation [64, 65] and inhibition of gastric tone or receptive relaxation during swallowing (Figure 21.4). The efferent pathway for TLESRs is also presumably in the vagus nerve; in dogs, TLESRs are completely abolished by cooling of the cervical vagus [66], and eructation is substantially inhibited by truncal vagotomy, 5cm above the diaphragm [67]. The absence of TLESRs in patients with achalasia suggests that TLESRs share a final common pathway with swallow-induced LES relaxation [68]. Gastric distention probably triggers TLESRs through stimulation of tension receptors in the proximal stomach [69, 70]; particularly the gastric cardia. Afferent fibers, which signal gastric distension, are known to project to the NTS [71] and to the dorsal motor nucleus of the vagus (DMV), either directly or via interneurons [72]. The DMV contains the cell bodies of vagal efferent neurons that project to the LES. Gastric mechanoreceptors

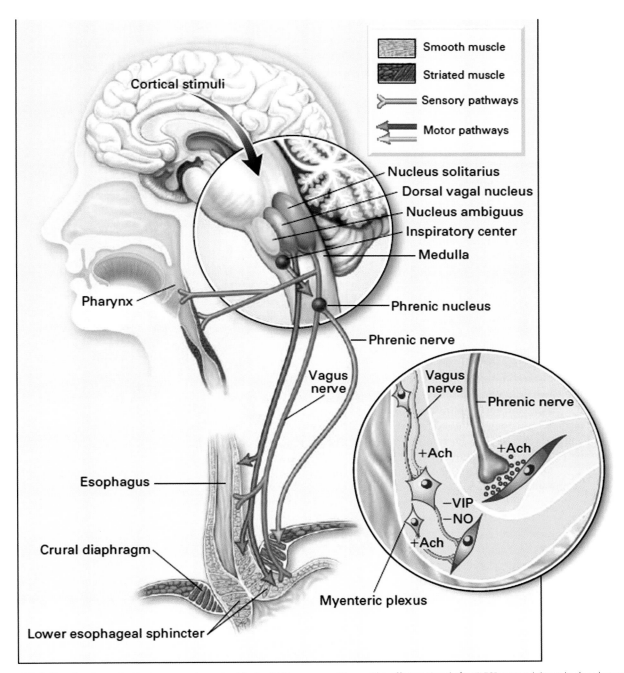

Figure 21.4 Neural pathway to the lower esophageal sphincter (LES) and crural diaphragm. Swallow-induced esophageal peristalsis and LES relaxation result from excitation of receptors located in the pharynx. The afferent stimulus travels to the sensory nucleus (nucleus tractus solitarius, NTS). A programmed set of events from the dorsomotor nucleus of the vagus and nucleus ambiguus mediate esophageal peristalsis and LES relaxation. The vagal fibers communicate with myenteric neurons, which in turn mediate LES relaxation. The post-ganglionic transmitter is nitric oxide (NO) and vasoactive intestinal peptide (VIP). Transient LES relaxation (TLESR, the major mechanism of reflux) appears to share the same neural pathway. The afferent signals for TLESR may originate in the pharynx, larynx, and stomach. The efferent pathway is in the vagus nerve, and NO is the post-ganglionic neurotransmitter. Crural diaphragm contraction is controlled by the inspiratory center in the brainstem, which communicates with the phrenic nerve nucleus. The crural diaphragm is innervated by right and left phrenic nerves through motor end plates and nicotinic cholinergic receptors. Ach, acetylcholine; +, excitatory; -, inhibitory (reproduced Mittal RK, Balaban DH. The esophagogastric junction. *N Engl J Med* 1997;336:924–932., with permission).

have been postulated to serve as the afferent pathway for a number of vagal reflexes, including reflex relaxation of the gastric corpus. Such a neural pathway could therefore potentially mediate TLESRs. In the opossum, LES relaxation can also be induced by intrinsic gastric nerves independently of extrinsic nerves [73]. Whether such a pathway mediates TLESRs is not known, but it cannot be involved in the associated inhibition of the crural diaphragm during TLESRs. The complete abolition of TLESRs by cervical vagal cooling [66] also argues against a dominant role for a local intramural pathway in mediating TLESRs.

The selective inhibition of the crural diaphragm that is characteristic of TLESRs also occurs during vomiting [37], esophageal distention [35], and, to a partial degree, during swallowing. Presumably, this inhibition is coordinated in the brainstem, although the precise site at which this occurs is unclear. Rhythmic respiration is controlled mainly by pre-motor neurons in the dorsal respiratory group within the NTS and the adjacent reticular formation [74], which in turn activate diaphragmatic motor neurons in the ventral horn of the cervical spinal cord. The NTS is also the destination for afferent input from the vagus and glossopharyngeal nerves and has been suggested as a potential site for the integrated neural control of inhibition of respiration during swallowing. However, inhibition of the crural diaphragm by esophageal distention and, by implication, during TLESRs does not appear to be through inhibition of the medullary premotor inspiratory neurons of the respiratory center, but via a separate, as yet unidentified, pathway [75].

The TLESR is a long period (10–60 s) of simultaneous LES and crural diaphragm relaxation. Relaxations of both the LES and crural diaphragm during TLESR are essential for the occurrence of reflux in normal subjects [76]. Based on the available information, it is possible to construct a hypothetical pathway for the triggering of TLESRs (Figure 21.5). The basic element is a vagal reflex pathway triggered by gastric distention or pharyngeal stimulation and integrated in the brainstem. The threshold for triggering is lowered by concurrent stimulation of the pharynx (and possibly larynx) and increased potentially by supine posture, sleep, and anesthesia. The efferent vagal output is controlled by a pattern generator in the brainstem and mediates the esophageal, LES, gastric, and diaphragmatic events during TLESR. Under usual circumstances, the pharyngeal components of deglutition are bypassed, but these can be partly activated on occasion, causing the small pharyngeal and mylohyoid complexes that occur with some TLESRs.

GERD is characterized by a higher frequency of reflux episodes. This has been attributed to both a higher frequency of TLESRs and a higher incidence of reflux during TLESRs [77]. However, several studies do not find higher frequency of TLESR in patients with reflux disease [78]. Some studies report that numbers of reflux episodes related to TLESR are no different between controls and patients but the total

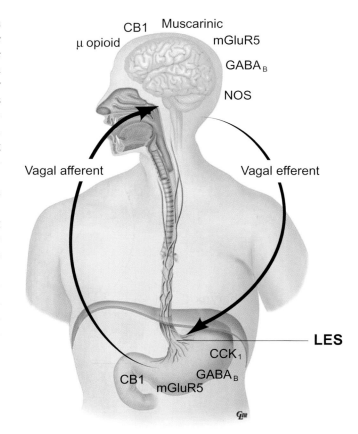

Figure 21.5 Proposed sites of action of pharmacologic agents targeting transient lower esophageal sphincter (LES) relaxation. CB1, cannabinoid 1, GABA$_B$, gamma amino butaric acid; CCK$_1$, cholecystokinin; NOS, nitric oxide synthase (reproduced from Lehmann A. *Esophageal Pain*. Plural Publihing, 2009, with permission).

number of reflux episodes is high in reflux patients because of the other mechanisms that are operative only in patients. The size of the meal, posture, and sleep status are some of the variables that influence the frequency of TLESRs and may vary among studies. The presence of a hiatal hernia also increases the frequency of TLESRs [79].

Earlier studies reported that 40–50% of TLESRs are accompanied by acid reflux compared with 60–70% of those in patients with reflux disease [41]. More recent studies that monitored air reflux, acid and non-acid reflux close to the LES, using impedance–pH monitoring, show that almost all TLESRs are accompanied by reflux of one kind or the other [80, 81].

Pharmacologic suppression of TLESRs is possible and a desirable form of therapy in reflux disease. TLESRs induced by gastric distention can be inhibited by cholecystokinin (CCK)-A receptor and nitric oxide (NO) antagonist [82]. The effect of CCK-A antagonist appears to be mediated through a peripheral rather than a central mechanism. Infusion of CCK-A increases the frequency of TLESRs and this increase can be abolished by administration of a NO antagonist. Even in the absence of CCK-A stimulation, NO antagonists can block TLESRs. However, NO is important in swallow-induced LES relaxation and its blockade can result in dysphagia and an "achalasia-like condition." Atropine also reduces the frequency of TLESRs and reflux after a meal, and the mechanism of its action appears to be at the level of the central nervous system [76, 83]. Morphine in small doses decreases TLESR frequency in normal subjects through an unknown mechanism [84]. Cannabinoid receptor stimulation also inhibits gastric distension-induced TLESR in the dog model [85]. The therapeutic potential, however, for most of pharmacologic agents that inhibit TLESRs is limited because of the anticipated side effects of these agents.

The GABA$_B$ agonist, baclofen, reduces induced gastric distention as well as spontaneous TLESR and GER in dogs, ferrets, and humans [86–89]. Baclofen inhibits relaxation of both the LES and crural diaphragm during TLESR. Esophageal distention-mediated relaxation of the LES and crural diaphragm, and esophageal shortening are significantly reduced by baclofen in cats [90, 91]. A single dose of baclofen, 40 mg by mouth, reduced GER as well as TLESR by 50% in normal subjects as well as in patients with GERD [88, 89]. It is possible that GABA agonist or related compounds could be useful in treating mild–to-moderate GERD, but the major limitation of this class of compounds is the central nervous system side effect profile. Metabotropic glutamate receptor subtype 5 (mGluR5) located on the afferent vagal nerve terminal is another possible target that blocks the triggering of TLESR in a dose-dependent fashion [92]. Preliminary studies in patients with symptomatic reflux disease with mGluR5 are encouraging, both for the reduction of reflux episodes as well as symptoms.

Effect of antireflux therapy on transient lower esophageal sphincter relaxation

The effect of medical therapy for reflux disease on TLESRs has been studied; omeprazole has been reported to have no effect [93], while H^2 antagonists decrease the rate of TLESRs [94]. Cisapride does not influence the rate of TLESRs up to 3 h after a meal [55]. The failure of therapy to influence the cause of reflux presumably explains why reflux disease relapses so promptly when medical therapy is terminated. Fundoplication has two major effects: a reduction in the rate of TLESRs and a reduction in the proportion of TLESRs that are accompanied by acid as well as non-acid reflux [95–97]. The mechanisms underlying these effects include (1) the creation of an artificial high-pressure zone around the LES by fundoplication that persists during transient and swallow-induced LES relaxation [95]; (2) prevention of axial stretch-induced LES relaxation; and (3) possibly a reduction in the degree of distension of the gastric cardia by the gastric wrap, which reduces the gastric distension-induced stimulation of TLESRs.

Lower esophageal sphincter hypotension and other factors in reflux disease

Even though TLESR is the major mechanism of reflex, low LES pressure is an important mechanism of reflex in patients with reflux disease [98, 99]. In the presence of a low LES pressure, reflux is thought to occur either freely from the stomach into the esophagus (free reflux) or during periods of abdominal strain (contraction of the abdominal wall, which increases intragastric pressure). Swallow-induced reflux and reflux episodes in which the mechanism cannot be clearly determined also occur in the setting of low LES pressure [100]. However, it is interesting that the low LES pressure induced by atropine in normal subjects does not cause reflux episodes [76]. All the straining maneuvers, i.e. coughing, abdominal straining, and straight leg raising, do not induce reflux during LES hypotension induced by atropine. The contraction of the crural diaphragm during these maneuvers is a protective antireflux barrier and is probably sufficient to guard against the occurrence of reflux during periods of increased intra-abdominal pressure. How low LES pressure causes reflux is not entirely clear. One possibility is that both low pressure and hiatal hernia are required for the occurrence of erosive esophagitis. A low LES pressure may allow movement of acid from the herniated pouch into the esophagus across a hypotensive LES. Alternatively, in the presence of a hernia, the diaphragmatic hiatus is incompetent and allows the stomach contents to move freely from the stomach below the diaphragm into the herniated sac and then into the esophagus. Along those lines, the severity of esophagitis appears to correlate directly with the size of the hiatal hernia and indirectly with the magnitude of the LES pressure [98, 101]. The larger the hernia, the wider the esophageal hiatus, and the more likely it is that the crural diaphragm component of the sphincter is incompetent. The hiatal hernia may play an important role in the pathophysiology of reflux from several other aspects [79, 102, 103] as well (see Chapter 20).

Patients with erosive esophagitis usually have low LES pressure. The degree of endoscopic esophagitis seems to correspond directly with LES pressure. Low LES pressure is the hallmark in patients with scleroderma of the esophagus and is considered to be the primary etiologic factor. Patients with scleroderma usually have the severe reflux esophagitis. Low LES pressure in scleroderma is due to the replacement of LES muscle by connective tissue [104]. The reason for low LES pressure in the more common variety of reflux disease is not entirely clear. Anatomic separation between the LES and crural diaphragm, as occurs in hiatal hernia, may contribute to low LES pressure [102]. It is possible that low LES pressure is due to primary myogenic or neurogenic failure of the LES muscle. Instillation of acid into the cat esophagus results in the reduction of LES pressure [105].

Studies in cats [106, 107] and human LES muscle strips show that products of inflammation induce excessive production of hydrogen peroxide, which in turn accelerates the production of platelet activating factor, prostaglandin E_2 (PGE_2), and F2-isoprostane to cause a decrease in the LES muscle tone. Catalase, a scavenger of hydrogen peroxide, increased LES tone in a patient with erosive esophagitis. Healing of esophagitis with omeprazole does not improve LES pressure in patients with erosive disease, the reason for which may be that acid-induced damage causes permanent and irreversible alterations in the contractile apparatus of the LES muscle.

Hiatal hernia is associated with an increased prevalence of reflux during swallow-induced LES relaxation presumably because of pooling of acid in the herniated gastric pouch [108]. Besides the increase in the frequency of reflux in patients, a higher volume of gastric contents may reflux into the esophagus with each reflux episode because of the higher compliance and larger opening of the GEJ in patients [103, 109]. Obesity is associated with higher intragastric pressure and a favorable pressure gradient for the reflux [110].

It is possible to propose a unifying hypothesis that incorporates TLESR, low LES pressure, and hiatal hernia in the pathogenesis of reflux disease. The initial pathologic event in reflux disease is most likely frequent TLESRs and acid reflux episodes. Acid in the esophagus causes esophagitis, which leads to low LES pressure and esophageal hypotension [105]. Furthermore, esophagitis induces esophageal shortening through acid-induced contraction of the longitudinal muscles [111]. Subsequently, fibrosis develops, which results in a hiatal hernia. The hiatal hernia, in turn, enlarges the esophageal hiatus, thus impairing the sphincter function of the crural diaphragm. The appearance of a hiatal hernia and a weak diaphragmatic sphincter introduces additional mechanisms of reflux, thus exacerbating the esophagitis.

Role of esophageal peristalsis in reflux disease

Esophageal peristalsis plays a key role in the clearance of refluxed material from the esophagus. Esophageal acid clearance is a two-step process, comprised of bolus clearance and acid neutralization [112, 113]. If a 15 mL or smaller bolus of acid is instilled into the esophagus, the majority of the acid can be cleared from the esophagus into the stomach by a single wave of peristaltic contraction of the esophagus. The remainder of the acid lining the esophageal mucosa is neutralized by saliva traversing the esophagus during subsequent swallow-induced peristaltic contractions. It takes seven to 10 swallows following esophageal acidification for the restoration of the normal esophageal pH of 5–7.

How strong must the esophageal peristaltic contraction be for an efficient bolus clearance? An esophageal contraction

of greater than 30 mmHg is usually sufficient in the supine position for bolus clearance [114]. However, depending upon the bolus viscosity, a contraction of even less than 30 mmHg may be able to clear the esophagus efficiently. A subgroup of patients, usually with severe reflux disease, have low esophageal contraction amplitude (termed "ineffective esophageal motility"; see Chapter 13), which could result in an impaired ability to clear acid bolus from the esophagus following a reflux episode [115]. The prevalence of peristaltic dysfunction increases with the increasing severity of esophagitis. The study by Kahrilas *et al*. reported that 25% of individuals with mild esophagitis and 50% of patients with severe esophagitis have severe peristaltic dysfunction [114]. The definition of abnormal peristalsis, based on studies in normal subjects, was that 50% of tested peristaltic sequences had to have a demonstrable abnormality. Whether esophageal peristaltic dysfunction is a primary defect or is secondary to acid-induced esophagitis is not clear. There is good experimental evidence to indicate that acid injury to the esophagus can impair esophageal contraction. However, healing of esophagitis in patients with low contraction amplitudes does not restore the contraction amplitude back to normal. Patients with scleroderma and mixed connective disorders have a similar defect in peristalsis due to the replacement of esophageal muscles with fibrous connective tissue [104].

Conclusions

The smooth muscle LES and crural diaphragm are two main components of the antireflux barrier. GER occurs primarily due to an incompetent LES. Transient relaxation of the lower esophageal sphincter and crural diaphragm is the single major mechanism of reflux in patients with reflux disease. Contraction of the longitudinal muscles of the distal esophagus is a key motor event in the induction of LES and crural diaphragm relaxation during TLESR. The nature of afferent dysfunction that causes frequent TLESRs is not known. Other reflux mechanisms are hypotensive LES and the presence of hiatal hernia. It appears that transient and intermittent separation of the LES and crural diaphragm (sliding hiatal hernia) is frequently associated with reflux episodes. The severity of esophagitis correlates directly with the hernia size and indirectly with the LES pressure. Ineffective esophageal motility found in patients with moderate-to-severe reflux disease impairs bolus clearance of the acid and thus increases acid contact time with the esophageal mucosa. Future studies need to address the nature of neural dysfunction that leads to TLESRs and the mechanism by which hiatus hernia develops and contributes to the pathogenesis of reflux disease. Novel pharmacologic therapies that inhibit TLESRs are definitely an important avenue that requires further investigation.

References

1. Ingelfinger FJ. Esophageal motility. *Physiol Rev* 1958; 38:533–584.

2. Code CF, Fyke FE Jr, Schlegel JF. The gastroesophageal sphincter in healthy human beings. *Gastroenterologia* 1956;86:135–150.

3. Boyle JT, Altschuler SM, Nixon TE, Tuchman DN, Pack AI, Cohen S. Role of the diaphragm in the genesis of lower esophageal sphincter pressure in the cat. *Gastroenterology* 1985;88:723–730.

4. Heine K, Dent J, *et al.* Anatomical relationship between the crural diaphragm and lower esophageal sphincter: an electrophysiological study. *J Gastrointest Motil* 1993;5:89–93.

5. Ott DJ, Gelfand DW, Wu WC, Castell DO. Esophagogastric region and its rings. *AJR Am J Roentgenol* 1984;142:281–287.

6. Lin S, Brasseur JG, Pouderoux P, Kahrilas PJ. The phrenic ampulla: distal esophagus or potential hiatal hernia? *Am J Physiol* 1995;268:G320–327.

7. Liu JB, Miller LS, Goldberg BB, Feld RI, Alexander AA, Needleman L, Castell DO, Klenn PJ, Millward CL. Transnasal US of the esophagus: preliminary morphologic and function studies. *Radiology* 1992;184:721–727.

8. Liu J, Parashar VK, Mittal RK. Asymmetry of lower esophageal sphincter pressure: is it related to the muscle thickness or its shape? *Am J Physiol* 1997;272:G1509–1517.

9. Liebermann-Meffert D, Allgower M, Schmid P, Blum AL. Muscular equivalent of the lower esophageal sphincter. *Gastroenterology* 1979;76:31–38.

10. Thor KB, Hill LD, Mercer DD, Kozarek RD. Reappraisal of the flap valve mechanism in the gastroesophageal junction. A study of a new valvuloplasty procedure in cadavers. *Acta Chir Scand* 1987;153:25–28.

11. Langman J. *Medical Embryology*. Philadelphia: William & Wilkins, 1975.

12. Delattre JF, Palot JP, Ducasse A, Flament JB, Hureau J. The crura of the diaphragm and diaphragmatic passage. Applications to gastroesophageal reflux, its investigation and treatment. *Anat Clin* 1985;7:271–283.

13. Dodds WJ. 1976 Walter B. Cannon Lecture: current concepts of esophageal motor function: clinical implications for radiology. *AJR Am J Roentgenol* 1977;128:549–561.

14. Pandolfino JE, Zhang QG, Ghosh SK, Han A, Boniquit C, Kahrilas PJ. Transient lower esophageal sphincter relaxations and reflux: mechanistic analysis using concurrent fluoroscopy and high-resolution manometry. *Gastroenterology* 2006;131:1725–1733.

15. Bredenoord AJ, Weusten BL, Timmer R, Smout AJ. Intermittent spatial separation of diaphragm and lower esophageal sphincter favors acidic and weakly acidic reflux. *Gastroenterology* 2006;130:334–340.

16. Liu J, Yamamoto Y, Schirmer BD, Ross RA, Mittal RK. Evidence for a peripheral mechanism of esophagocrural diaphragm inhibitory reflex in cats. *Am J Physiol Gastrointest Liver Physiol* 2000;278:G281–288.

17. Klein WA, Parkman HP, Dempsey DT, Fisher RS. Sphincterlike thoracoabdominal high pressure zone after esophagogastrectomy. *Gastroenterology* 1993;105:1362–1369.

18. Dent J, Dodds WJ, Sekiguchi T, Hogan WJ, Arndorfer RC. Interdigestive phasic contractions of the human lower esophageal sphincter. *Gastroenterology* 1983;84:453–460.

19. Mittal RK, Rochester DF, McCallum RW. Electrical and mechanical activity in the human lower esophageal sphincter during diaphragmatic contraction. *J Clin Invest* 1988;81:1182–1189.

20. Mittal RK, Fisher M, McCallum RW, Rochester DF, Dent J, Sluss J. Human lower esophageal sphincter pressure response to increased intra-abdominal pressure. *Am J Physiol* 1990;258:G624–630.

21. Dodds WJ, Dent J, Hogan WJ, Arndorfer RC. Effect of atropine on esophageal motor function in humans. *Am J Physiol* 1981;240:G290–296.

22. Biancani P, Hillemeier C, Bitar KN, Makhlouf GM. Contraction mediated by Ca2+ influx in esophageal muscle and by Ca^{2+} release in the LES. *Am J Physiol* 1987;253:G760–766.

23. Collman PI, Tremblay L, Diamant NE. The central vagal efferent supply to the esophagus and lower esophageal sphincter of the cat. *Gastroenterology* 1993;104:1430–1438.

24. Goyal RK, Rattan S. Nature of the vagal inhibitory innervation to the lower esophageal sphincter. *J Clin Invest* 1975;55:1119–1126.

25. Yamato S, Saha JK, Goyal RK. Role of nitric oxide in lower esophageal sphincter relaxation to swallowing. *Life Sci* 1992;50:1263–1272.

26. Preiksaitis HG, Tremblay L, Diamant NE. Cholinergic responses in the cat lower esophageal sphincter show regional variation. *Gastroenterology* 1994;106:381–388.

27. Brookes SJ, Chen BN, Hodgson WM, Costa M. Characterization of excitatory and inhibitory motor neurons to the guinea pig lower esophageal sphincter. *Gastroenterology* 1996;111:108–117.

28. Yuan S, Costa M, Brookes SJ. Neuronal pathways and transmission to the lower esophageal sphincter of the guinea Pig. *Gastroenterology* 1998;115:661–671.

29. Muinuddin A, Kang Y, Gaisano HY, Diamant NE. Regional differences in L-type Ca2+ channel expression in feline lower esophageal sphincter. *Am J Physiol Gastrointest Liver Physiol* 2004;287:G772–781.

30. L'Heureux MC, Muinuddin A, Gaisano HY, Diamant NE. Feline lower esophageal sphincter sling and circular muscles have different functional inhibitory neuronal responses. *Am J Physiol Gastrointest Liver Physiol* 2006;290:G23–29.

31. Dogan I, Bhargava V, Liu J, Mittal RK. Axial stretch: A novel mechanism of the lower esophageal sphincter relaxation. *Am J Physiol Gastrointest Liver Physiol* 2007;292:G329–334.

32. Jiang Y, Bhargava V, Mittal RK. Mechanism of stretch-activated excitatory and inhibitory responses in the lower esophageal sphincter. *Am J Physiol Gastrointest Liver Physiol* 2009;297:G397–405.

33. Roussos C, Macklem PT. The respiratory muscles. *N Engl J Med* 1982;307:786–797.

34. Darian GB, DiMarco AF, Kelsen SG, Supinski GS, Gottfried SB. Effects of progressive hypoxia on parasternal, costal, and crural diaphragm activation. *J Appl Physiol* 1989; 66:2579–2584.

35. Altschuler SM, Boyle JT, Nixon TE, Pack AI, Cohen S. Simultaneous reflex inhibition of lower esophageal sphincter and crural diaphragm in cats. *Am J Physiol* 1985;249:G586–591.

36. Martin CJ, Dodds WJ, Liem HH, Dantas RO, layman RD, Dent J. Diaphragmatic contribution to gastroesophageal competence and reflux in dogs. *Am J Physiol* 1992;263:G551–557.

37. Monges H, Salducci J, Naudy B. Dissociation between the electrical activity of the diaphragmatic dome and crura muscular fibers during esophageal distension, vomiting and eructation. An electromyographic study in the dog. *J Physiol (Paris)* 1978;74:541–554.

38. Dent J, Holloway RH, Toouli J, Dodds WJ. Mechanisms of lower oesophageal sphincter incompetence in patients with symptomatic gastrooesophageal reflux. *Gut* 1988;29:1020–1028.

39. Katzka DA, Sidhu M, Castell DO. Hypertensive lower esophageal sphincter pressures and gastroesophageal reflux: an apparent paradox that is not unusual. *Am J Gastroenterol* 1995;90:280–284.

40. Pandolfino JE, Kim H, Ghosh SK, Clarke JO, Zhang Q, Kahrilas PJ. High-resolution manometry of the EGJ: an analysis of crural diaphragm function in GERD. *Am J Gastroenterol* 2007;102:1056–1063.

41. Mittal RK, Holloway RH, Penagini R, Blackshaw LA, Dent J. Transient lower esophageal sphincter relaxation. *Gastroenterology* 1995;109:601–610.

42. McNally EF, Kelly JE Jr, Ingelfinger FJ. Mechanism of belching: effects of gastric distension with air. *Gastroenterology* 1964;46:254–259.

43. Dent J, Dodds WJ, Friedman RH, *et al.* Mechanism of gastroesophageal reflux in recumbent asymptomatic human subjects. *J Clin Invest* 1980;65:256–267.

44. Schoeman MN, Tippett MD, Akkermans LM, Dent J, Holloway RH. Mechanisms of gastroesophageal reflux in ambulant healthy human subjects. *Gastroenterology* 1995;108:83–91.

45. Mittal RK, Chiareli C, Liu J, Shaker R. Characteristics of lower esophageal sphincter relaxation induced by pharyngeal stimulation with minute amounts of water. *Gastroenterology* 1996;111:378–384.

46. Cucchiara S, Staiano A, Di Lorenzo C, De Luca G, della Rocca A, Auricchio S. Pathophysiology of gastroesophageal reflux and distal esophageal motility in children with gastroesophageal reflux disease. *J Pediatr Gastroenterol Nutr* 1988;7:830–836.

47. Werlin SL, Dodds WJ, Hogan WJ, Arndorfer RC. Mechanisms of gastroesophageal reflux in children. *J Pediatr* 1980;97:244–249.

48. Holloway RH, Penagini R, Ireland AC. Criteria for objective definition of transient lower esophageal sphincter relaxation. *Am J Physiol* 1995;268:G128–133.

49. Mittal RK, McCallum RW. Characteristics of transient lower esophageal sphincter relaxation in humans. *Am J Physiol* 1987;252:G636–641.

50. Mittal RK, Fisher MJ. Electrical and mechanical inhibition of the crural diaphragm during transient relaxation of the lower esophageal sphincter. *Gastroenterology* 1990;99:1265–1268.

51. Babaei A, Bhargava V, Korsapati H, Zheng WH, Mittal RK. A unique longitudinal muscle contraction pattern associated with transient lower esophageal sphincter relaxation. *Gastroenterology* 2008;134:1322–1331.

52. Tipnis NA, Liu J, Puckett JL, Mittal RK. Common cavity pressure during gastroesophageal reflux: reassessment using simultaneous pressure, impedance, and ultrasound imaging. *Am J Physiol Gastrointest Liver Physiol* 2006;290: G1149–1156.

53. Ergun GA, Kahrilas PJ, Lin S, Logemann JA, Harig JM. Shape, volume, and content of the deglutitive pharyngeal chamber imaged by ultrafast computerized tomography. *Gastroenterology* 1993;105:1396–1403.

54. Franzi SJ, Martin CJ, Cox MR, Dent J. Response of canine lower esophageal sphincter to gastric distension. *Am J Physiol* 1990;259:G380–385.

55. Holloway RH, Downton J, Mitchell B, Dent J. Effect of cisapride on postprandial gastro-oesophageal reflux. *Gut* 1989;30:1187–1193.

56. Mittal RK, Stewart WR, Schirmer BD. Effect of a catheter in the pharynx on the frequency of transient lower esophageal sphincter relaxations. *Gastroenterology* 1992;103:1236–1240.

57. Paterson WG, Rattan S, Goyal RK. Experimental induction of isolated lower esophageal sphincter relaxation in anesthetized opossums. *J Clin Invest* 1986;77:1187–1193.

58. Storey AT. Laryngeal initiation of swallowing. *Exp Neurol* 1968;20:359–365.

59. Little AF, Cox MR, Martin CJ, Dent J, Franzi SJ, Lavelle R. Influence of posture on transient lower oesophageal sphincter relaxation and gastro-oesophageal reflux in the dog. *J Gastroenterol Hepatol* 1989;4:49–54.

60. Freidin N, Mittal RK, McCallum RW. Does body posture affect the incidence and mechanism of gastro-oesophageal reflux? *Gut* 1991;32:133–136.

61. Freidin N, Fisher MJ, Taylor W, Boyd D, Surratt P, McCallum RW, Mittal RK. Sleep and nocturnal acid reflux in normal subjects and patients with reflux oesophagitis. *Gut* 1991;32:1275–1279.

62. Cox MR, Martin CJ, Dent J, Westmore M. Effect of general anaesthesia on transient lower oesophageal sphincter relaxations in the dog. *Aust N Z J Surg* 1988;58:825–830.

63. Penagini R, Bartesaghi B, Bianchi PA. Effect of cold stress on postprandial lower esophageal sphincter competence and gastroesophageal reflux in healthy subjects. *Dig Dis Sci* 1992;37:1200–1205.

64. Reynolds RP, El-Sharkawy TY, Diamant NE. Lower esophageal sphincter function in the cat: role of central innervation assessed by transient vagal blockade. *Am J Physiol* 1984;246:G666–674.

65. Ryan JP, Snape WJ Jr, Cohen S. Influence of vagal cooling on esophageal function. *Am J Physiol* 1977;232:E159–164.

66. Martin CJ, Patrikios J, Dent J. Abolition of gas reflux and transient lower esophageal sphincter relaxation by vagal blockade in the dog. *Gastroenterology* 1986;91:890–896.

67. Strombeck DR, Harrold D, Ferrier W. Eructation of gas through the gastroesophageal sphincter before and after truncal vagotomy in dogs. *Am J Vet Res* 1987;48:207–210.

68. Holloway RH, Wyman JB, Dent J. Failure of transient lower oesophageal sphincter relaxation in response to gastric distension in patients with achalasia: evidence for neural mediation of transient lower oesophageal sphincter relaxations. *Gut* 1989;30:762–767.

69. Andrews PL, Grundy D, Scratcherd T. Vagal afferent discharge from mechanoreceptors in different regions of the ferret stomach. *J Physiol* 1980;298:513–524.

70. Blackshaw LA, Grundy D, Scratcherd T. Vagal afferent discharge from gastric mechanoreceptors during contraction and relaxation of the ferret corpus. *J Auton Nerv Syst* 1987;18:19–24.

71. Rinaman L, Card JP, Schwaber JS, Miselis RR. Ultrastructural demonstration of a gastric monosynaptic vagal circuit in the nucleus of the solitary tract in rat. *J Neurosci* 1989;9:1985–1996.

72. Kalia M, Mesulam MM. Brain stem projections of sensory and motor components of the vagus complex in the cat: II. Laryngeal, tracheobronchial, pulmonary, cardiac, and gastrointestinal branches. *J Comp Neurol* 1980;193:467–508.

73. Schulze-Delrieu K, Percy WH, Ren J, Shirazi SS, Von Derau K. Evidence for inhibition of opossum LES through intrinsic gastric nerves. *Am J Physiol* 1989;256:G198–205.

74. Berger AJ, Mitchell RA, Severinghaus JW. Regulation of respiration (first of three parts). *N Engl J Med* 1977;297:92–97.

75. Altschuler SM, Davies RO, Pack AI. Role of medullary inspiratory neurones in the control of the diaphragm during oesophageal stimulation in cats. *J Physiol* 1987;391:289–298.

76. Mittal RK, Holloway R, Dent J. Effect of atropine on the frequency of reflux and transient lower esophageal sphincter relaxation in normal subjects. *Gastroenterology* 1995;109:1547–1554.

77. Dodds WJ, Dent J, Hogan WJ, *et al*. Mechanisms of gastroesophageal reflux in patients with reflux esophagitis. *N Engl J Med* 1982;307:1547–1552.

78. Sifrim D, Holloway R. Transient lower esophageal sphincter relaxations: how many or how harmful? *Am J Gastroenterol* 2001;96:2529–2532.

79. Kahrilas PJ, Shi G, Manka M, Joehl RJ. Increased frequency of transient lower esophageal sphincter relaxation induced by gastric distention in reflux patients with hiatal hernia. *Gastroenterology* 2000;118:688–695.

80. Sifrim D, Holloway R, Silny J, *et al*. Acid, nonacid, and gas reflux in patients with gastroesophageal reflux disease during ambulatory 24-hour pH-impedance recordings. *Gastroenterology* 2001;120:1588–1598.

81. Sifrim D, Silny J, Holloway RH, Janssens JJ. Patterns of gas and liquid reflux during transient lower oesophageal sphincter relaxation: a study using intraluminal electrical impedance. *Gut* 1999;44:47–54.

82. Boulant J, Fioramonti J, Dapoigny M, Bommelaer G, Bueno L. Cholecystokinin and nitric oxide in transient lower esophageal sphincter relaxation to gastric distention in dogs. *Gastroenterology* 1994;107:1059–1066.

83. Fang JC, Sarosiek I, Yamamoto Y, Liu J, Mittal RK. Cholinergic blockade inhibits gastro-oesophageal reflux and transient lower oesophageal sphincter relaxation through a central mechanism. *Gut* 1999;44:603–607.

84. Penagini R, Bianchi PA. Effect of morphine on gastroesophageal reflux and transient lower esophageal sphincter relaxation. *Gastroenterology* 1997;113:409–414.

85. Lehmann A, Blackshaw LA, Branden L, *et al*. Cannabinoid receptor agonism inhibits transient lower esophageal sphincter relaxations and reflux in dogs. *Gastroenterology* 2002;123:1129–1134.

86. Lehmann A, Antonsson M, Bremner-Danielsen M, Flardh M, Hansson-Branden L, Karrberg L. Activation of the GABA(B) receptor inhibits transient lower esophageal sphincter relaxations in dogs. *Gastroenterology* 1999;117:1147–1154.

87. Blackshaw LA, Staunton E, Lehmann A, Dent J. Inhibition of transient LES relaxations and reflux in ferrets by GABA receptor agonists. *Am J Physiol* 1999;277:G867–874.

88. Lidums I, Lehmann A, Checklin H, Dent J, Holloway RH. Control of transient lower esophageal sphincter relaxations and reflux by the GABA(B) agonist baclofen in normal subjects. *Gastroenterology* 2000;118:7–13.

89. Zhang Q, Lehmann A, Rigda R, Dent J, Holloway RH. Control of transient lower oesophageal sphincter relaxations and reflux by the GABA(B) agonist baclofen in patients with gastro-oesophageal reflux disease. *Gut* 2002;50:19–24.

90. Liu J, Pehlivanov N, Mittal RK. Baclofen blocks LES relaxation and crural diaphragm inhibition by esophageal and gastric distension in cats. *Am J Physiol Gastrointest Liver Physiol* 2002;283:G1276–1281.

91. Liu J, Puckett JL, Takeda T, Jung HY, Mittal RK. Crural diaphragm inhibition during esophageal distension correlates with contraction of the esophageal longitudinal muscle in cats. *Am J Physiol Gastrointest Liver Physiol* 2005;288:G927–932.

92. Frisby CL, Mattsson JP, Jensen JM, Lehmann A, Dent J, Blackshaw LA. Inhibition of transient lower esophageal sphincter relaxation and gastroesophageal reflux by metabotropic glutamate receptor ligands. *Gastroenterology* 2005;129:995–1004.

93. Downton J, Dent J, Heddle R, *et al*. Elevation of gastric pH heals peptic esophagitis-a role for omeprazole. *J Gastroenterology Hepatol* 1987;2:317.

94. Baldi F, Longanesi A, Frrarini F, *et al*. Oesophageal motor function and outcome of treatment with H2 blockers in erosive oesophagitis. *J Gastrointestinal Motil* 1992;4:165.

95. Ireland AC, Holloway RH, Toouli J, Dent J. Mechanisms underlying the antireflux action of fundoplication. *Gut* 1993;34:303–308.

96. Kiroff GK, Maddern GJ, Jamieson GG. A study of factors responsible for the efficacy of fundoplication in the treatment of gastro-oesophageal reflux. *Aust N Z J Surg* 1984; 54:109–12.

97. Bredenoord AJ, Draaisma WA, Weusten BL, Gooszen HG, Smout AJ. Mechanisms of acid, weakly acidic and gas reflux after anti-reflux surgery. *Gut* 2008;57:161–166.

98. Jones MP, Sloan SS, Rabine JC, Ebert CC, Huang CF, Kahrilas PJ. Hiatal hernia size is the dominant determinant of esophagitis presence and severity in gastroesophageal reflux disease. *Am J Gastroenterol* 2001;96:1711–1717.

99. van Herwaarden MA, Samsom M, Smout AJ. Excess gastroesophageal reflux in patients with hiatus hernia is caused by mechanisms other than transient LES relaxations. *Gastroenterology* 2000;119:1439–46.

100. Mittal RK, McCallum RW. Characteristics and frequency of transient relaxations of the lower esophageal sphincter in patients with reflux esophagitis. *Gastroenterology* 1988;95:593–599.

101. Sloan S, Rademaker AW, Kahrilas PJ. Determinants of gastroesophageal junction incompetence: hiatal hernia, lower esophageal sphincter, or both? *Ann Intern Med* 1992;117:977–982.

102. Kahrilas PJ, Lin S, Chen J, Manka M. The effect of hiatus hernia on gastro-oesophageal junction pressure. *Gut* 1999;44:476–482.

103. Pandolfino JE, Shi G, Curry J, Joehl RJ, Brasseur JG, Kahrilas PJ. Esophagogastric junction distensibility: a factor contributing to sphincter incompetence. *Am J Physiol Gastrointest Liver Physiol* 2002;282:G1052–1058.

104. Miller LS, Liu JB, Klenn PJ, et al. Endoluminal ultrasonography of the distal esophagus in systemic sclerosis. *Gastroenterology* 1993;105:31–39.

105. Eastwood GL, Castell DO, Higgs RH. Experimental esophagitis in cats impairs lower esophageal sphincter pressure. *Gastroenterology* 1975;69:146–153.

106. Cao W, Harnett KM, Cheng L, Kirber MT, Behar J, Biancani P. H(2)O(2): a mediator of esophagitis-induced damage to calcium-release mechanisms in cat lower esophageal sphincter. *Am J Physiol Gastrointest Liver Physiol* 2005; 288:G1170–1178.

107. Rieder F, Cheng L, Harnett KM, et al. Gastroesophageal reflux disease-associated esophagitis induces endogenous cytokine production leading to motor abnormalities. *Gastroenterology* 2007;132:154–165.

108. Mittal RK, Lange RC, McCallum RW. Identification and mechanism of delayed esophageal acid clearance in subjects with hiatus hernia. *Gastroenterology* 1987;92:130–135.

109. Pandolfino JE, Shi G, Trueworthy B, Kahrilas PJ. Esophagogastric junction opening during relaxation distinguishes nonhernia reflux patients, hernia patients, and normal subjects. *Gastroenterology* 2003;125:1018–1024.

110. Pandolfino JE, El-Serag HB, Zhang Q, Shah N, Ghosh SK, Kahrilas PJ. Obesity: a challenge to esophagogastric junction integrity. *Gastroenterology* 2006;130:639–649.

111. Paterson WG, Kolyn DM. Esophageal shortening induced by short-term intraluminal acid perfusion in opossum: a cause for hiatus hernia? *Gastroenterology* 1994;107:1736–1740.

112. Helm JF, Dodds WJ, Riedel DR, Teeter BC, Hogan WJ, Arndorfer RC. Determinants of esophageal acid clearance in normal subjects. *Gastroenterology* 1983;85:607–612.

113. Helm JF, Dodds WJ, Pelc LR, Palmer DW, Hogan WJ, Teeter BC. Effect of esophageal emptying and saliva on clearance of acid from the esophagus. *N Engl J Med* 1984;310:284–288.

114. Kahrilas PJ, Dodds WJ, Hogan WJ. Effect of peristaltic dysfunction on esophageal volume clearance. *Gastroenterology* 1988;94:73–80.

115. Kahrilas PJ, Dodds WJ, Hogan WJ, Kern M, Arndorfer RC, Reece A. Esophageal peristaltic dysfunction in peptic esophagitis. *Gastroenterology* 1986;91:897–904.

22 Esophageal Epithelial Resistance

Roy C. Orlando

University of North Carolina School of Medicine, Division of Gastroenterology and Hepatology, Chapel Hill, NC, USA

Introduction

Gastroesophageal reflux is for the most part a benign physiologic process that occurs in everyone every day, especially after meals [1]. This indicates that the antireflux barriers—as constituted by the lower esophageal sphincter (LES), diaphragm, acute angle of His, phrenoesophageal ligament, mucosal rosette, and other structures—are, by nature, functionally imperfect. This imperfection is necessitated by the regular need for reflexive gas venting (belching) from the stomach and occasional need for reflexive vomiting, which can remove all content from the stomach. Reflexive gas venting occurs by transient LES relaxation, a phenomenon that also permits liquids to spontaneously escape or "reflux" from the stomach into the esophagus [2]. Since gastric contents are predominantly acidic due to parietal cell secretion of hydrochloric acid (HCl), refluxates in healthy subjects typically have a pH of less than 4.0. Consequently, exposure of the human esophagus to gastric acid is almost universal, while acid-induced damage to the organ is not—perhaps, based on heartburn frequency, affecting around 25% of the adult population in the United States [3]. The reason for the obvious lack of correlation between prevalence of reflux and prevalence of damage is the presence of two additional defenses: (1) the luminal clearance mechanisms and (2) epithelial resistance [4]. The luminal clearance mechanisms, which include gravity, peristalsis, swallowed salivary secretions, and secretions of the esophageal submucosal glands, prevent damage by limiting the time of contact of the esophageal epithelia (EE) with the refluxate. Gravity and peristalsis do this by aiding bolus removal following reflux, while salivary and esophageal gland secretions do this by dilution and neutralization of the refluxate's acidic content. Nonetheless, acid clearance is neither immediate nor particularly effective during sleep when gravity is minimized by recumbency and primary peristalsis and salivary secretion

are infrequent [5–7]. This leaves epithelial resistance as a necessary defense for prevention of injury during the time of contact of acid with the EE [8]. Proof that epithelial resistance exists as a defensive phenomenon and is reasonably robust is evident during the Bernstein test—a test in which heartburn fails to occur despite the direct exposure of healthy human EE to HCl, pH 1.1, for 30 min [9, 10].

For purposes of discussion, the components of "epithelial resistance" can be divided into three compartments based on their relationship to the EE proper: pre-epithelial, epithelial, and postepithelial defenses (Table 22.1). This division is, however, artificial in that loss of one has consequences for the others that ultimately increase the risk of injury to the EE. At present, the cause of reflux esophagitis is unknown, and, in the final analysis, is likely to be multifactorial. There is little doubt, however, that contact of the EE with refluxed gastric acid plays a critical role. This is supported by the great success of proton pump inhibitors (PPIs) in relief of heartburn and healing of erosions [4]. Consequently, this chapter focuses on epithelial resistance as defense against luminal acid and the discussion based on the generally held, but recently challenged concept (see Rat model below), that the symptoms and signs of reflux esophagitis result from the direct attack and damage by luminal acid on the EE and on the subsequent diffusion of acid across the impaired apical junctional complex (AJC) into the intercellular space.

Pre-epithelial defense

The contributors to the pre-epithelial defense in gastrointestinal epithelia are listed in Table 22.1, and include mucus, bicarbonate ions (HCO_3^-), and the unstirred water layer [8]. They limit the contact between luminal acid and the EE proper. This is remarkably effective in the stomach and duodenum because they secrete mucoproteins that form a viscoelastic, adherent, surface layer. This layer entraps large molecules, e.g. pepsin, and HCO_3^-, the latter for dilution and

The Esophagus, Fifth Edition. Edited by Joel E. Richter, Donald O. Castell.
© 2012 Blackwell Publishing Ltd. Published 2012 by Blackwell Publishing Ltd.

neutralization of back-diffusing acid [11–14]. In the stomach the mucoproteins are MUC 5AC and MUC6 and in the duodenum, MUC2 and MUC3; and the HCO_3^- derived from surface cell secretion [13, 15, 16]. Consequently, the stomach and duodenum have a strong pre-epithelial defense in that they can maintain a surface pH of 5–7 even when the luminal pH is as low as 2.0. In contrast this defense is meagre in the esophagus, where the pH of the surface of the EE falls to 2–3 when luminal pH is 2.0 [15] (Figure 22.1). The reason for this is that the EE:

Table 22.1 Components of mucosal resistance against acid injury to esophageal epithelium.

Pre-epithelial:
Mucous layer
Unstirred water layer
Surface bicarbonate ion concentration

Epithelial:
Cell membranes
Intercellular apical junctional complex
Ion transporters
H+ buffers: intracellular and extracellular

Postepithelial:
Blood flow: nutrients, oxygen, CO_2, acid–base balance
Reparative mechanisms: cell restitution, cell replication

• Lacks a surface mucus coat [17]—mucoproteins secreted by esophageal glands, MUC5B, are soluble and used for lubrication but not barrier function [18];
• Does not secrete HCO_3^-;
• Being electrically "tight" does not permit free diffusion of HCO_3^- from blood to lumen [19, 20].

The result is that, unlike in the stomach and duodenum, luminal or refluxate acidity yields the same level of acidity at the surface of the EE. A likely consequence of this is that healing of the acid-damaged EE will require greater elevation of gastric, and therefore refluxate, pH to achieve the level of tissue neutrality for effective healing. Therefore, gastric and duodenal ulcers, with a surface barrier and buffer zone, heal well on H_2-receptor antagonists, while those with gastroesophageal reflux disease (GERD), especially erosive esophagitis, require treatment with PPIs [21].

Epithelial defense

This defense, whose components are listed in Table 22.1, comes into play when the pre-epithelial defense is inadequate to prevent acid contact with the EE [8]. It is formed by the EE proper which in humans is a non-keratinized stratified squamous epithelium. It has three layers: stratum corneum, stratum spinosum, and stratum germinativum; and at times is described as having a fourth layer, i.e. stratum granulosum. The stratum granulosum is identifiable by keratohyalin granules within the cytoplasm of its cells. The

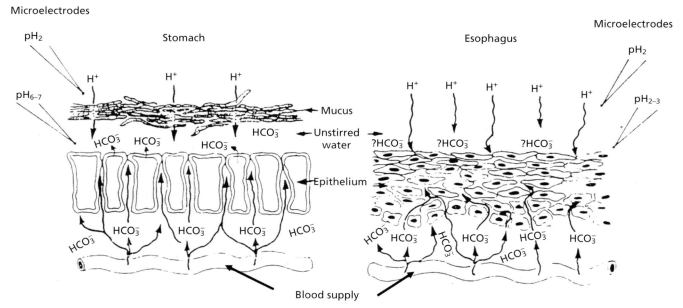

Figure 22.1 Pre-epithelial defense. In gastric and duodenal epithelia, H+ must cross the mucus–unstirred water layer–bicarbonate barrier before contact can be made with the surface of the epithelium. Diffusion of pepsin, but not H+, is blocked by mucus; however, H+ can be neutralized by HCO_3^- residing in the unstirred water layer. In contrast to gastric and duodenal epithelia, the pre-epithelial defense in the esophagus is poorly developed, having an ineffective mucus–HCO_3^- barrier to buffer back-diffusing H+ (reproduced from Orlando RC. Esophageal epithelial defense against acid injury. *J Clin Gastroenterol* 1991;13 (Suppl 2):51–S5, with permission).

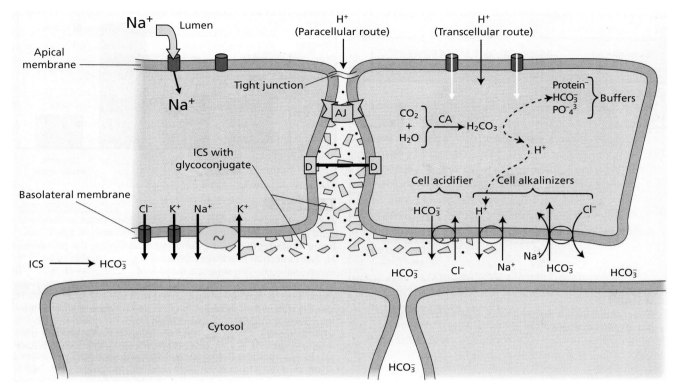

Figure 22.2 Epithelial defense. Some epithelial defenses against acid injury are illustrated. Structural barriers to H^+ diffusion include the cell membrane and apical junctional complex consisting of the tight junction, zonula adherens, and desmosomes. Functional components include the apical membrane epithelial sodium channel (ENaC), intracellular buffering by negatively charged proteins and HCO_3^- and H^+ extrusion processes (Na^+/H^+ exchanger and Na^+-dependent Cl^-/HCO_3^- exchanger) for regulation of intracellular pH. ICS, intercellular space (modified from Orlando RC. Esophageal epithelial defense. In: Castell DO, Wu WC, Ott DJ, eds. *Gastroesophageal Reflux Disease: Pathogenesis, Diagnosis, Therapy*. Mount Kisco, NY: Futura, 1985, p. 55, with permission).

stratum corneum is adjacent to the lumen and consists of multiple sheets of large, pancake-shaped, cells in varying stages of desquamation [22, 23]. This stratum provides protection by creation of a barrier that protects against the permeation of luminal ions and aqueous molecules from the lumen to the serosa [24, 25].

Structural components of the barrier in the stratum corneum include the lipid bilayer within the cell membrane and the protein bridges of the AJC that partially seal off the lumen from the aqueous intercellular space of neighboring cells. There are three components to the AJC, with the most luminal being the zonula occludens or tight junction (TJ), the subjacent zonula adherens or adherens junction (AJ), and the desmosome (Figure 22.2). The TJ and AJ, which are present in all layers of the stratum corneum and the upper layers of stratum spinosum, encircle the entire perimeter of the cells, thereby separating the luminal from the epithelial compartment [25–27]. Layers below this level lack this junctional barrier [25]. The desmosome, too, is part of the AJC; but its bridging proteins do not encircle the cell, thereby creating a "spot weld" that has no barrier function. Nonetheless, by tethering the lateral cell membranes (LCMs) of neighboring cells together, the desmosome indirectly contributes to barrier function by creating a long, narrow, serpiginous paracellular pathway that impedes diffusion of ions and molecules [28]. In effect, the low paracellular permeability created by the AJC and the low level of active sodium (Na^+) transport by squamous cells yield an EE of high electrical resistance, typically greater than $1000\,ohms/cm^2$ [29–31]. Further, circuit analysis has shown that the electrical resistance across the cells is greater than that across the paracellular route, and flux measurements have shown that the AJC are sufficiently porous to enable mannitol (MW 182), but not large dextrans (MW 4000), to diffuse through the paracellular route [28, 32].

Other important characteristics of the AJC include:
• The bridging proteins in the TJ are largely occludin and a family of claudins. In human EE, the most highly expressed of these are claudin-1 and claudin-4 [27]. These proteins, which bind heterotypically to family members in the adjacent cell membrane, are anchored to the membrane by interaction with the protein, zonula occludens. The zonula occludens protein in turn connects the bridging proteins to the cytoskeleton by binding to actin microfilaments [33].

• The bridging protein in the AJ is E-cadherin. This protein binds homotypically to other E-cadherin molecules from adjacent cells and does so in a calcium-dependent manner. E-cadherin binds intracellularly to catenins, which in turn connect E-cadherin to the cytoskeleton via actin microfilaments [34].

• The bridging proteins in the desmosome are desmoplakins and desmocollins. These proteins are anchored to the membrane by desmoplakins, and these in turn connect the bridging proteins to the cytoskeleton by binding to cytokeratins in the intermediate filaments [35].

Also noteworthy is that the intercellular space between the AJCs of the upper layers of the EE contain a ground substance secreted by membrane-coating granules in the cytoplasm of squamous cells (Figure 22.2). In human and rabbit EE this ground substance is composed of glycoproteins shown to be devoid of barrier properties, while that in mouse EE is composed of a lamellar lipid that contributes to barrier function [28, 36–38].

The EE has a number of properties that also serve a defensive function against acid. These are listed in Table 22.1 and include: (1) the epithelial Na^+ channel (ENaC); (2) buffering capacity; and (3) intracellular pH (pH_i) regulation. All of these properties relate to ion transport, and so a brief description of what is known about ion transport in EE follows. *In vivo* and *in vitro* the EE exhibits a lumen-negative potential difference (PD) [29, 30, 39, 40]. The PD, based on Ohm's Law, is a product of active transport and electrical resistance [29, 39]. The EE has a low current and this is a reflection of active Na^+ absorption [29, 30]. To achieve Na^+ absorption, luminal Na^+ diffuses down its concentration gradient through ENaC, a non-selective cation channel, in the apical membrane into the cell cytoplasm [41]. Cytoplasmic Na^+ is then actively transported by the sodium–potassium adenosine triphosphatase (sodium pump) across the basolateral membrane (Figure 22.2). For electroneutrality, the anion accompanying luminal Na^+, i.e. Cl^-, diffuses through the paracellular pathway. Since Na^+ is actively transported, this is relatively fast compared with the passive diffusion of Cl^-, yielding a net separation of charges in space that generates the PD.

ENaC, as noted, is a non-selective cation channel. It enables sodium, potassium, and lithium ions to diffuse across the apical membrane and into cells [41]. Yet, it has defensive properties at low pH that prevent excessive amounts of hydrogen ion (H^+) from entering the cell across the apical membrane. For instance, at a luminal pH of less than 4.0, cation transport via ENaC is inhibited, and at pH of around 2.0, cation transport is abolished [42]. Though H^+ entry via ENaC may occur at moderate luminal acidity, the rate of entry is known to be insufficient to lower luminal pH [43]. This is due to the presence of intracellular buffers, such as phosphates, proteins, and HCO_3^-. HCO_3^- ions are particularly important since their removal leads to cell necrosis in the acid-exposed EE [44]. There are two major

sources of HCO_3^- in the EE. One is its generation from carbonic acid via the action of carbonic anhydrases [45, 46]; and the other is its diffusion into the interstitium from blood. HCO_3^- in the interstitium enters cells in the EE by traversing the basolateral membrane on a Na^+-dependent, Cl^-/HCO_3^- exchanger (Figure 22.2). HCO_3^- in the interstitium also diffuses into the intercellular space where it buffers back-diffusing H^+ traversing the paracellular route.

Cell survival when attacked at low luminal pH is dependent upon preservation of a physiologic pHi.. Physiologic pHi is maintained in two ways: first, as noted above, is by buffering H^+ as they enter the cell; and second, by the action of membrane transporters that extrude H^+ from the cell. The latter include an amiloride-sensitive, Na^+/H^+ exchanger (NHE-1 isotype) and a disulfonic acid stilbene-sensitive, Na^+-*dependent*, Cl^-/HCO_3^- exchanger [47–51] (Figure 22.2). Both are present on the basolateral membrane and both are driven by the high to low, extracellular to intracellular, Na^+ gradient maintained by the sodium pump. The action of the acid extruders is counterbalanced by the presence on the basolateral membrane of a Na^+-*independent*, Cl^-/HCO_3^- exchanger that extrudes alkali. Thus, cells tightly regulate pHi and do so by taking their cue as to value by regulating it with respect to the pH of blood. This will have significance, as described below, to the pathogenesis cell death in the EE in GERD.

Postepithelial defense

This defense is almost exclusively a product of the blood supply (see Table 22.1). The blood supply protects by regulating tissue acid–base balance, by supporting cell metabolism, and by providing inflammatory cells for defensive and reparative processes (see below). Tissue acid–base balance is preserved under physiologic conditions by the delivery of HCO_3^- to buffer acidic by-products of cell metabolism, and under pathologic conditions by the delivery of HCO_3^- to neutralize back-diffusing luminal H^+ (see Figure 22.1). The blood supply also removes CO_2 from the tissue to the lungs after H^+ is neutralized by HCO_3^- and carbonic acid degraded by the action of tissue carbonic anhydrases. Further, the blood supply can rapidly adapt to changing conditions such as an increase in acid load; this by an increase in blood flow [46, 52–56]. The increase in blood flow, or hyperemic response, has been shown to be mediated both by capsaicin-sensitive afferent nerves carrying either transient receptor potential vanilloid-1 (TRPV-1) or acid-sensing ion channels (ASICs) [46] and by histamine, nitric oxide, calcitonin gene-related peptide (CGRP) or carbonic anhydrases [46, 52–56].

Models of reflux esophagitis

Rabbit model

The esophageal mucosa of the rabbit is structurally and functionally similar to that of human esophageal mucosa

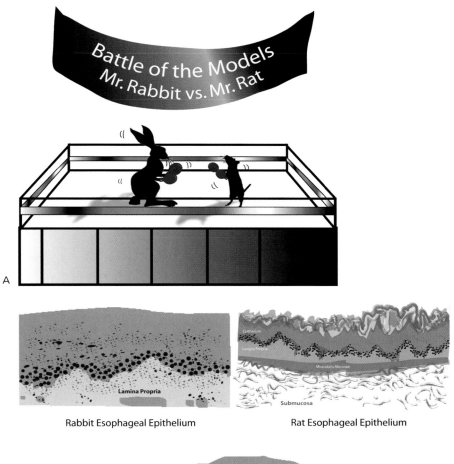

Rabbit Esophageal Epithelium

Rat Esophageal Epithelium

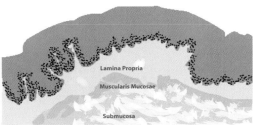

Human Esophageal Epithelium

B

Figure 22.3 Battle of the models. (A) The rabbit and the rat are two animal models that are being championed to represent the pathophysiology of human reflux disease. (B) Noteworthy, and fundamentally important to the debate, is that human EE is a *non-keratinized* stratified squamous epithelium, while rabbit is *partially-keratinized* and rat is *fully-keratinized* stratified squamous epithelium. These epithelia are diagrammatically depicted with the fully keratinized layers in the rat shown as a distinct surface covering.

with the exceptions that rabbit EE is a *partially keratinized* stratified squamous epithelium rather than a *non-keratinized* stratified squamous epithelium (Figure 22.3), and, unlike human mucosa, it lacks submucosal glands [57]. Absence of glands, however, is an advantage experimentally since it enables the pathobiology of EE to be monitored electrophysiologically in Ussing chambers without the observations being confounded by changes in glandular function. Rabbit, like human, EE has from 20 to 30 cell layers, a high electrical

resistance, and low rate of active Na^+ absorption. Rabbit, like human, EE also lacks a surface mucus coat, secretes neither Cl^- nor HCO_3^-, and contains a glycoprotein matrix within the intercellular spaces of the stratum corneum [25, 29, 30].

The pathobiology of acid injury to rabbit EE mirrors that observed in human EE and the changes to EE observed in patients with GERD [23, 31, 32, 58–61]. For instance, the lumen-negative PD in both exhibits a biphasic pattern when exposed to luminal acid [58, 60, 62]. PD initially increases

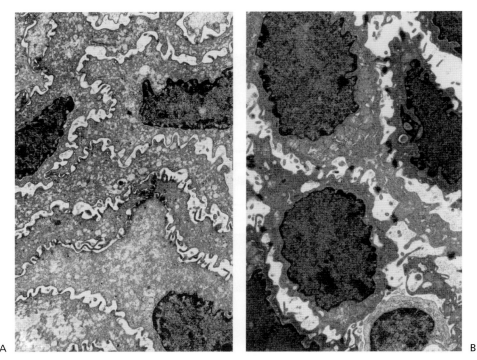

A   B

Figure 22.4 Dilated intercellular spaces in non-erosive reflux disease. Transmission electron micrographs showing the differences in size of the intercellular spaces for (A) normal and (B) non-erosive acid-damaged esophageal epithelia (original magnification 9000×) (adapted from Barlow and Orlando [75], with permission).

above baseline and then falls progressively to zero. The increase in PD is due to luminal H^+ diffusing across the EE [59] and the disappearance of H^+ from the lumen is utilized *in vivo* as a marker of increased permeability [63–65]. The path that H^+ takes as it passes through the EE is of fundamental importance to the pathogenesis of GERD. Its choices are to traverse the transcellular and/or paracellular routes. That H^+ does not traverse the apical cell membrane and so utilizes the transcellular route is evident by a lack of change in surface cell pHi until after it has induced a change in paracellular permeability. Moreover, despite an acid-induced increase in paracellular permeability, cell injury to the EE is preventable by the presence of a cell-impermeable buffer on the serosal side [43, 66]. That the initial decline in PD in acid-exposed rabbit EE is due to an increase in paracellular permeability is shown by observing a decline in electrical resistance, increase in mannitol flux, and dilated intercellular spaces (DISs) in EE in the absence of cell necrosis [58]. These experimental findings in the rabbit are mirrored in patients with non-erosive reflux disease (NERD) by observing: (1) a low PD in some [60]; (2) a fall in PD to low levels during acid perfusion in others [29]; (3) the presence of DISs in those with heartburn with or without pathologic acidity on pH monitoring; and (4) resolution of DISs along with heartburn on PPI therapy (Figure 22.4) [67–71]. As in the rabbit, DISs can also be readily produced by exposure of

healthy human EE to luminal acid *in vivo* [72]. Taken together, these data provide strong support for the concept that refluxed gastric acid initially attacks and damages the AJC to give rise to increased paracellular permeability. That this is the case has received recent support from the observation that the expression of claudin-4 is reduced and E-cadherin is cleaved in EE from patients with GERD [73]. It has also been shown experimentally in the rabbit model that DISs are the result of damage to the AJC by luminal H^+ and the subsequent diffusion of Cl^- into the intercellular space. The latter is necessary for the development of DISs because it generates an osmotic force for excess water to move into and to dilate the space [74].

Heartburn

Based on data largely obtained using the *rabbit model*, a hypothesis was generated as to the mechanism for heartburn in NERD [75] (Figure 22.5). Acid initially attacks and damages the AJC in the EE and by so doing increases paracellular permeability. The increase in paracellular permeability not only leads to DISs, but enables H^+ to back diffuse in quantities sufficient to overcome intercellular buffering and so to acidify the intercellular space. Sensory neurons in the EE, as shown in the macaque, reside within the intercellular space and come within three cell layers of the lumen [76, 77]. Consequently, acidification of the intercellular space

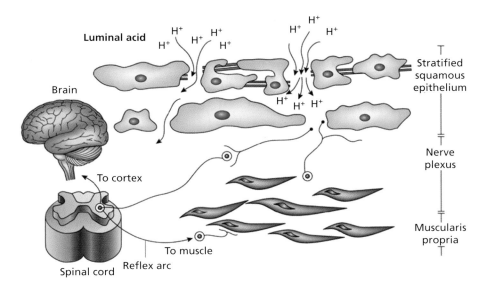

Figure 22.5 Mechanism for heartburn in non-erosive reflux disease. The presence of abnormal tissue resistance—demonstrated by defects within the intercellular junctional complex between the cells of the surface layers of esophageal (stratified squamous) epithelium—is shown to enable the ready diffusion of refluxed gastric acid (H^+) into the intercellular space. Within this space, it encounters and activates chemosensitive nociceptors whose signals are transmitted via the spinal cord to the brain for symptom (heartburn) perception. Activation of the same nociceptors are also capable of initiating a short reflex arc to esophageal (longitudinal) smooth muscle as a means of precipitating a sustained esophageal contraction (adapted from Barlow and Orlando [75], with permission).

can trigger the neuronal signal for heartburn, particularly because the neurons in the EE contain acid-sensitive nociceptors. The two types of nociceptors likely responsible for heartburn are TRPV1 and ASIC, type 3, which are capable of responding to pHs as high as 5.5–7.0 [78–84]. Given the small amounts of acid that it takes to trigger a sensory signal, it is easy to see how heartburn can be generated in NERD without producing cell necrosis. It should also not be surprising why such modest reductions in pH trigger the signal for heartburn. This is because heartburn is a device that warns the subject of an acidic pH on the wrong side of the epithelial barrier, and to be effective, this warning should occur before the onset of cell necrosis. Cell necrosis in the EE, as in other organs, can readily occur when pHs of less than 7.0 contact the basolateral cell membranes and this is apparent with the multiorgan failures observed with systemic acidosis, pHs of less than 7.0, in the critically ill.

Cell necrosis

When prolonged, intercellular acidification leads to cell edema and necrosis. This is heralded *in vivo* in the acid-perfused *rabbit model* and in human EE in GERD by the abolition of the esophageal PD [58, 60]. Abolition of esophageal PD is due to the decline in electrical resistance coupled with the inhibition of active Na^+ transport. The inhibition of active Na^+ transport in this setting is the result of acid-induced inhibition of the sodium pump [58, 59]. Although acid-induced inhibition of the sodium pump can abolish the

PD, it is insufficient to produce cell edema and necrosis since the latter do not occur with exposure to serosal ouabain [85, 86]. Cell edema and necrosis occur when *inter*cellular acidification is translated into *intra*cellular acidification, and *intra*cellular acidification readily occurs with *inter*cellular acidification because the basolateral membrane of squamous cells is highly permeable to acid. The acid permeability of the basolateral membrane is due to the presence of the Na^+-independent, Cl^-/HCO_3^- exchanger [66, 86–88]. The activity of this transporter is dependent on the electrochemical gradients for Cl^- and HCO_3^-. Consequently when intercellular pH is acidic, the exchanger enables the cell to absorb HCl by extruding HCO_3^- in exchange for Cl^- (Figure 22.6). As pHi falls toward intercellular pH, the basolateral Na^+/H^+ exchanger works to raise pHi to neutral levels. This means that the final pHi of the cell is determined by the relative activities of the two exchangers, the acid-unloading Na^+/H^+ exchanger and the acid-loading Na^+-independent, Cl^-/HCO_3^- exchanger [89–92]. That cell edema and necrosis occur in this way has been established in the rabbit model by blocking the acid-induced cell injury by pharmacologic inhibition of the Na^+-independent, Cl^-/HCO_3^- exchanger [66, 86–88].

The mechanisms by which low pHi in squamous cells are translated into cell edema and necrosis are unknown. However, one likely mediator is an acid-induced increased intracellular Ca^{2+}. This is because elevated Ca^{2+} activates a basolateral membrane NaK2Cl cotransporter; and activation of this transporter brings ions into the cell under a condition

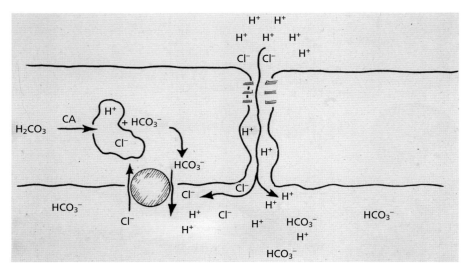

Figure 22.6 Mechanism of cell acidification in reflux disease. Acid diffusion via the paracellular pathway produces a low *inter*cellular pH. The low *inter*cellular pH is then translated into low *intra*cellular pH by the absorption of HCl across the basolateral membrane via the Na^+-independent, Cl^-/HCO_3^- exchanger. H^+ absorption is effected by loss of intracellular HCO_3^- along its concentration gradient in exchange for Cl^-, with intracellular HCO_3^- being derived from carbonic acid (CA; H_2CO_3). A low *intra*cellular pH is responsible for the sequence of events that leads to cell injury, swelling and death. (adapted from Orlando [8], with permission).

(low pH) where ion unloading is inactive due to inhibition of the sodium pump and potassium channels [93, 94]. Consequently, an osmotic force for water absorption is generated that can lead to cell edema. Since cell edema works to raise pHi by reducing H^+ concentration, one might speculate that volume regulation is being sacrificed for the regulation of pHi toward neutrality. Nonetheless, taken to extremes, osmotic water absorption could be severe and lead to cell death by membrane rupture. Alternatively, low pHi can lead to necrosis by other means, including calcium-mediated activation of endonucleases, proteases, and phospholipases [95], with endonucleases damaging nuclear chromatin, phospholipases and proteases damaging the cell membrane, and ATPases depleting energy stores. Further, low pHi and elevated calcium in hepatocytes are known to activate the mitochondrial permeability transition (MPT) [96]; the MPT causes opening of high-conductance pores in the inner mitochondrial membrane. Consequently, the MPT results in mitochondrial depolarization and uncoupling of oxidative phosphorylation. Cell death then ensues by either cell necrosis or apoptosis depending on whether cytosolic ATP is depleted (cell necrosis) or is retained (apoptosis) [96].

Inflammation

A consequence of cell injury is inflammation; and inflammation by design is a means of signaling a need of repair. The process is complex, but involves the release of signaling molecules by squamous and other cells in the area of damage to recruit to the area other cells from the environment and systemic circulation. The degree of inflammation is related to extent and severity of damage. For instance, there is minimal inflammation in the EE in NERD despite the presence of heartburn, DISs, and basal cell hyperplasia [68, 97–99]. In contrast, inflammation is prominent in the EE in erosive esophagitis where cell edema and necrosis are clearly evident. Among the mediators found in acid-damaged EE are: interleukin (IL)-1ß, IL-6, IL-8, interferon-γ, monocyte chemoattractant protein-1, RANTES, and platelet activating factor (PAF). At least three of these: IL-6, IL-8 and PAF, are produced and released from squamous cells [100–103], and serve to recruit lymphocytes, neutrophils, and eosinophils to the damaged area. In the damaged area, white cells release oxygen-derived free radicles, such as superoxide anion and hydrogen peroxide, and superoxide anion in turn reacts with nitric oxide to generate peroxynitrites [104–107]. These molecules, and others, aid repair by breaking down cellular debris and disabling invading organisms and antigens. Inflammation, however, is not always a finely tuned process as it can increase the apparent damage even as it aids repair. This is evident in the acid-pepsin exposed *rabbit model* where inflammation was found to convert microscopic esophagitis into macroscopic esophagitis. This was evident by the ability of the non-steroidal anti-inflammatory drug, ketotifen, white cell migration-inhibiting antibodies, CD-11, or the scavenger of superoxide anion, superoxide dismutase, to reduce the degree of damage when the EE was exposed to acidified pepsin [104–106].

Other unintended consequences of inflammation include affects on esophageal smooth muscle. For instance, LES pressure is often low or absent and peristalsis is often impaired in those with erosive esophagitis but not those with NERD. These abnormalities are likely a consequence and not the cause of inflammation due to the release of inflammatory mediators such as prostaglandin E_2, PAF, and IL-6. These products impair contractility of esophageal *circular* smooth muscle by inhibiting acetylcholine release or relaxing smooth muscle [101, 108, 109]. Other inflammatory products, however, increase contractility of the esophageal *longitudinal* smooth muscle and by so doing shorten the esophagus [110–112]. When shortened, the esophagus exerts upward tension on the gastric cardia, potentially creating a hiatal hernia or converting a sliding hiatal hernia into one that is fixed in the chest. That hernias are a consequence of inflammation rather than the cause is suggested by their high prevalence in erosive esophagitis and low prevalence in NERD [113–116]. These observations support the hypothesis that inflammation plays a key role in the pathogenesis of GERD. By impairing esophageal motor function, inflammation promotes more reflux and delays acid clearance, which both ensures chronicity and aids progression from NERD to erosive esophagitis. Progression is fostered by creation of a self-perpetuating cycle of reflux, cellular damage, inflammation, and muscle dysfunction, the latter leading to more reflux-induced cell damage and inflammation (Figure 22.7). Notably, if this sequence were always true, all NERD should eventually progress to erosive esophagitis, and this is clearly not the case with only around 25% of those with

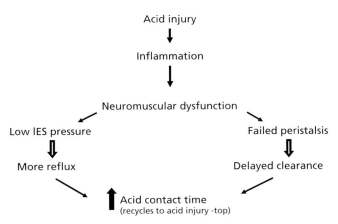

Figure 22.7 Mechanism of progression: non-erosive reflux disease (NERD) to erosive esophagitis. The process of inflammation is shown to promote the transition from NERD to erosive esophagitis by altering the neuromuscular function of esophageal smooth muscle. Impaired *circular* smooth muscle (illustrated) promotes more reflux by lowering lower esophageal sphincter (LES) pressure and delays luminal acid clearance by impairing esophageal peristalsis. Impaired *longitudinal* smooth muscle (not shown) produces a hiatal hernia that also increases reflux and impairs peristalsis. Since the smooth muscle defects result in an increase in acid contact with epithelium, injury and inflammation are increased and a vicious cycle is created that promotes more severe disease.

NERD reported to progress to erosive eosphagitis [117]. The reason for this likely relates to the host response to acid injury, with those having a robust inflammatory response progressing from NERD to erosive esophagitis and those with limited response remaining stable with NERD.

Squamous repair
Two mechanisms for the normal repair of EE are squamous replication and restitution. Only the cells within stratum germinativum are capable of replication, with these estimated to have a turnover rate of around 5–8 days [118, 119]. In GERD, the turnover rate in the EE is increased and this accounts for the morphologic feature of basal cell hyperplasia [98]. Although the stimulus for basal cell hyperplasia is contact of the EE with acid [120, 121], the mechanism by which the signal is transduced to replication is unclear. One hypothesis in the *rabbit model* is that the acid-induced increase in paracellular permeability enables swallowed salivary epidermal growth factor to diffuse across the EE to access its receptors on the basal cells [32]. An alternative hypothesis recently cited in reflux-exposed rat EE is that basal cell hyperplasia is a direct response to stimulation by released inflammatory cytokines [122]. Restitution also occurs in EE. This form of repair is very rapid—within 30–60 min—because, unlike replication, it occurs without the need for DNA and protein synthesis. In this instance, viable cells adjacent to areas denuded of dead and dying cells migrate over a scaffold or basement membrane to re-establish epithelial continuity. *In vitro* cells from rabbit EE exhibit restitution [94–96] and the rate of restitution is increased by exposure to epidermal and hepatocyte growth factors [123–125]. Restitution, like replication, however, is exquisitely acid sensitive, being inhibited at pH 6.5, and in a dose-dependent fashion is abolished at pH 3.0. This suggests that for replication or restitution to be effective in wound repair the acidity of the environment must be well controlled. Given an ineffective pre-epithelial defense, repairing a wound in the EE requires greater control over acidity than repair of a gastric or duodenal wound. This accounts, as noted previously, for the need for PPIs to heal erosive esophagitis, while H_2-receptor antagonists are usually sufficient for healing gastric and duodenal ulcers [21].

Erosions
As illustrated in the *rabbit model* exposure of the EE to luminal acid results in injury that progresses from non-erosive (DIS) to erosive disease (DIS, inflammation, cell necrosis) [23, 58]. Moreover, this sequence is ameliorated, but not abolished, by reducing the inflammatory response [104–106]. Thus, erosions are the macroscopic expression of accumulated microscopic (cell necrosis) disease and the culmination of an imbalance in which acid injury exceeds the rate of repair. That this sequence is relevant in GERD is supported by: (1) the presence of DISs in both NERD and erosive

eosphagitis; (2) the presence of inflammation and cell necrosis is erosive esophagitis; and (3) by resolution of all the markers of damage by controlling refluxate acidity with PPIs [72, 126–128].

Rat model

The concept that the symptom (heartburn) and signs of human reflux disease are the result of acid damage to the EE and subsequent back diffusion of H+ has recently been called into question, based on information obtained using the *rat model* (see Figure 22.3). A cornerstone of the counterview is that it is difficult to damage rat EE either by perfusion with acid or by exposure to refluxates containing acid and bile salts [56, 122, 128]. Perfusion with acid, however, does increase esophageal blood flow, and does so by stimulating sensory nerves without first acidifying the submucosa or basal layer of the EE [46, 56]. Since these findings were mimicked by perfusing the rat esophagus with a solution high in carbon dioxide (pCO$_2$ = 260 Torr), it was hypothesized that luminal CO$_2$ and *not* luminal H+ transduces the neural signal and, so by extension, is likely responsible for heartburn in NERD. How the high pCO$_2$ is produced in human esophagus is unclear, but it is postulated to be due to the neutralization reaction between refluxed H+ and HCO$_3^-$ secreted from esophageal submucosal glands or duodenum. Also, the hyperemic response to pCO$_2$ in the rat model was not only blocked by sensory nerve desensitization, but by pharmacologic inhibition of TRPV1, ASICs, and carbonic anhydrase; and these maneuvers were accompanied by submucosal acidification. Given the damaging action of serosal acidity on the EE, one or more defects in the chemosensing of CO$_2$ were hypothesized to cause the cell necrosis and inflammation in GERD [46].

In another investigation, high levels of luminal acidity for 3 h were unable to generate DISs in the EE of a *rat model*. Since this could be remedied by the addition of nitrites to the acid solution, it was concluded that DISs in the EE in GERD result from exposure to reactive nitrogen oxide species [128]. Among these species, nitric oxide was attractive since its generation under acidic luminal conditions could generate DISs through the formation of peroxinitrites when in contact with superoxide anion [129]. From this it was hypothesized that DISs in the EE in GERD result from the generation of reactive nitrogen oxide species when swallowed salivary nitrites come into contact with refluxed gastric acid.

In another *rat model* of reflux disease, it was noted that inflammation and basal cell hyperplasia preceded, not followed, the development of cell necrosis and erosions [122]. For instance, following esophagoduodenostomy, erosions developed at 28 days, while inflammatory cells appeared by day 3, basal cell hyperplasia by day 7, and papillary elongation by day 14. Inflammatory cells, principally T lymphocytes responding to IL-8, appeared initially in the submucosa (day 3), then in the lamina propria (day 7), and finally in the EE (day 21). Immunostaining showed IL-8 to be abundant by day 14, and while present in all layers, immunostaining was most intense within the intercellular spaces in the upper third of the EE. IL-8 was shown to be released from squamous cells and the secretion was found to be chemotactic for lymphocytes and neutrophils [122]. From these observations it was hypothesized that reflux esophagitis *in humans* is a cytokine-mediated immune response, rather than a response mediated by acid injury to the EE. The mechanisms of cytokine-mediated cell injury and death were not examined. However, basal cell hyperplasia before surface cell loss was ascribed to cytokine-stimulated basal cell replication, and this phenomenon was supported in human EE by the correlation of levels of IL-8 with basal cell hyperplasia in NERD [102].

Summary

In summary, models matter! Models using rat EE as surrogate for human EE present difficulties that are not present when rabbit EE serves as surrogate for human EE. This is because rat EE, unlike human and rabbit EE, is *fully keratinized* (see Figure 22.3B). Fully keratinized EE imbues the tissue with a more water-resistant (hydrophobic) surface, making it impermeable to small hydrophilic molecules like mannitol [36, 46, 128]. Consequently, it is difficult to damage rat EE with aqueous solutions even when highly acidic, while highly acidic solutions readily damage both human and rabbit EE. For example, DISs can be generated in human and rabbit EE within 30 min of acid exposure, while rat EE is impervious to such acidity even after 3 h [32, 56, 58, 67, 128]. To circumvent this difficulty, rat models mimic GERD by exposing the EE to noxious agents that are lipophilic. Examples of this include the exposure to: (1) high partial pressure of membrane-permeable CO$_2$ [46]; (2) high concentrations of nitrites to generate membrane-permeable nitrogen oxide species [128, 129]; and (3) high concentrations of membrane-permeable bile salts [122]. In the bile salt model, GERD was mimicked by creating an esophagoduodenostomy [122]. This hook-up ensures refluxates are high in bile salts (up to 20 mM) and low in acidity (gastric acid partially neutralized by duodenal content), which is the reverse of refluxates in GERD (~500 μM and pH <4) [1, 130–132]. In effect, the choice of the rat as a model of GERD is far from ideal, requiring an atypical offense (refluxate) to overcome an atypical defense (fully keratinized EE). The same is not the case for the rabbit model. The rabbit EE is structurally and functionally similar to human EE, and when exposed to acid recapitulates the findings observed in NERD and erosive esophagitis. Among the parallels between acid-exposed rabbit EE and GERD are changes in PD, electrical resistance, permeability and morphology—the latter including DIS as antecedent to cell necrosis and inflammation [23, 25, 29–32, 58–62].

Conclusions: lessons from the epithelium

Epithelial resistance is a phenomenon for esophageal defense against refluxed gastric acid. It is multidimensional, dynamic and complex, being comprised, as detailed above, of numerous structural and functional components. The sign of success when it prevents injury from acid contact with the EE is *silence*, i.e. freedom from symptoms. In contrast, the sign of failure in preventing injury when acid contacts the EE is *heartburn*! Heartburn, without endoscopic evidence of necrosis, is called NERD, and with endoscopic necrosis is called erosive esophagitis [4]. These conditions represent two ends of the spectrum of acid-induced damage [117], with the transition from NERD to erosive esophagitis, although challenged [133], not in question. This is because the EE in both have the same early lesion, i.e. DIS [67], the same early functional defect, i.e. increase in permeability [73], and the same pathogenetic pathway to these abnormalities, i.e. cleavage of E-cadherin [73]. Notably, the cleavage of E-cadherin also provides a means of ensuring the chronicity of NERD. How NERD transitions to erosive esophagitis is becoming clearer, and that is through inflammation. Inflammation creates a mucosal environment that alters smooth muscle function and it does so in ways that help explain why low LES pressure, impaired peristalsis, and hiatal hernias accompany severe (erosive) but not milder (non-erosive) disease [108–116]. These same motor abnormalities provide the means of ensuring the chronicity of erosive esophagitis. Finally, lessons from the epithelium also speak to the causation of GERD, suggesting that *GERD* is *not* a motor disease, but an *epithelial disease* (here there are shades of *Helicobacter pylori* and peptic ulcer disease). If a motor disease, the defects in antireflux barriers and luminal clearance mechanisms would lead to prolonged contact of acid with the EE. Based on 24-h esophageal pH monitoring, this is certainly the case in those with erosive esophagitis, but it is only one-half the story for those with NERD [4, 8]. The other story is that fully one-half of those with NERD have normal acid contact time on 24-h pH monitoring, and yet they have the same symptom, i.e. heartburn, the same pathologic lesion, i.e. DIS, and the same positive response to PPI therapy [67, 70, 71]. Since normal acid contact time excludes motor dysfunction, these individuals develop NERD through a defect in the only defense not factored into pH monitoring—epithelial resistance. Among the ways that a primary defect in epithelial resistance can be acquired are: (1) poor diet, e.g. too hypertonic due to salt, alcohol or pizza [134–136]; (2) physical stressors, e.g. restraint, heat [137, 138]; or possibly, (3) infection, e.g. colonization by Gram-negative bacteria [139, 140]. By impairment of barrier function, heartburn emerges from acid back diffusion during bouts of physiologic reflux. Over time, patients with NERD and physiologic reflux may progress to NERD with patho-logic reflux, and then, through inflammation, to erosive esophagitis. The proof of this awaits.

References

1. DeMeester TR, Johnson LF, Joseph GJ, Toscano MS, Hall AW, Skinner DB. Patterns of gastroesophageal reflux in health and disease. *Ann Surg* 1976;184:459–470.
2. Mittal RK, Holloway RH, Penagini R, *et al.* Transient lower esophageal relaxation. *Gastroenterology* 1995;109:601–610.
3. El Serag HB, Petersen NJ, Carter J, *et al.* Gastroesophageal reflux among different racial groups in the United States. *Gastroenterology* 2004;126:1692–1699.
4. Orlando RC. Reflux esophagitis. In: Yamada T, Alpers D, Owyang C, Powell DW, eds. *Textbook of Gastroenterology*, 3rd edn. Philadelphia: Lippincott Williams & Wilkins, 1999, pp. 1235–1263.
5. Dent J, Dodds WJ, Friedman RH, *et al.* Mechanism of gastroesophageal reflux in recumbent asymptomatic subjects. *J Clin Invest* 1980;65:256–267.
6. Lichter I, Muir RC. The pattern of swallowing during sleep. *Electroencephalogr Clin Neurophysiol* 1975;38:427–432.
7. Schneyer LH, Pigman W, Hanahan L, Gilmore RW. Rate of flow of human parotid, sublingual and submaxillary secretions during steep. *J Dent Res* 1956;35:109–114.
8. Orlando RC. Gastroesophageal reflux disease: Offensive factors and tissue resistance. In: Orlando RC, ed. *Gastroesophageal Reflux Disease*. New York: Marcel Dekker, Inc, 2000, pp. 165–192.
9. Bernstein LM, Baker LA. A clinical test for esophagitis. *Gastroenterology* 1958; 34:760–781.
10. Dent J. Review article: from 1906 to 2006 – a century of major evolution of understanding of gastro-oesophageal reflux disease. *Aliment Pharmacol Ther* 2006;24:1269–1281.
11. Allen A, Phil D. The structure and function of gastrointestinal mucus. In: Harmon JW, ed. *Basic Mechanisms of Gastrointestinal Mucosal Cell Injury and Protection*. Baltimore: Williams & Wilkins, 1981, pp. 351–367.
12. Pfeiffer CJ. Experimental analysis of hydrogen ion diffusion in gastrointestinal mucus glycoprotein. *Am J Physiol* 1981;240:G176–182.
13. Williams SE, Turnberg LA. Studies of the "protective" properties of gastric mucus: evidence for mucus bicarbonate barrier. *Gut* 1981;22:94–96.
14. Thomson ABR. Unstirred water layers: possible adaptive and cytoprotective function. In: Allen A, Flemström G, Garner A, Silen W, Turnberg LA, eds. *Mechanisms of Mucosal Protection in the Upper Gastrointestinal Tract*. New York: Raven Press, 1984, pp. 233–239.
15. Quigley EMM, Turnberg LA. pH of the microclimate lining the human gastric and duodenal mucosa in vivo-studies in control subjects and in duodenal ulcer patients. *Gastroenterology* 1987;92:1876–1884.
16. Williams SE, Turnberg LA. The demonstration of a pH gradient across mucus adherent to rabbit gastric mucosa: evidence for a mucus-bicarbonate barrier. *Gut* 1981;22:94–96.
17. Dixon J, Strugala V, Griffin SM, *et al.* Esophageal mucin: an adherent mucus gel barrier is absent in the normal esophagus

but present in Barrett's esophagus. *Am J Gastroenterol* 2001;96:2575–2583.

18. Guillem P, Billeret V, Buisine MP, *et al.* Mucin gene expression and cell differentiation in human normal, premalignant and malignant esophagus. *Int J Cancer* 2000;88:856–861.

19. Boyd DD, Carney CN, Powell DW. Neurohumoral control of esophageal epithelial electrolyte transport. *Am J Physiol* 1980;239:G5–11.

20. Hamilton BH, Orlando RC. In vivo alkaline secretion by mammalian esophagus. *Gastroenterology* 1989;97:640–648.

21. Orlando RC. Why is high grade inhibition of gastric acid secretion afforded by proton pump inhibitors often required for healing of reflux esophagitis? An epithelial perspective. *Am J Gastroenterol* 1996;91:1692–1696.

22. Powell DW. Barrier function of epithelia. *Am J Physiol* 1981;241:G275–288.

23. Carney CN, Orlando RC, Powell DW, Dotson MM. Morphologic alterations in early acid-induced epithelial injury of the rabbit esophagus. *Lab Invest* 1981;45:198–208.

24. Elias PM, McNutt NS, Friend DS. Membrane alterations during cornification of mammalian squamous epithelia: a freeze fracture, tracer and thin-section study. *Anat Rec* 1977;189:577–594.

25. Orlando RC, Lacy ER, Tobey NA, Cowart K. Barriers to paracellular permeability in rabbit esophageal epithelium. *Gastroenterology* 1992;102:910–923.

26. Tobey NA, Argote CM, Hosseini SS, Orlando RC. Calcium-switch technique and junctional permeability in native rabbit esophageal epithelium. *Am J Physiol Gastrointest Liver Physiol* 2004;286:G1042–1049.

27. Jovov B, Van Itallie CM, Shaheen NJ, Carson *et al.* Claudin-18: A dominant tight junction protein in Barrett's esophagus and likely contributor to its acid resistance. *Am J Physiol Gastrointest Liver Physiol* 2007;293:G1106–1113.

28. Tobey NA, Djukic Z, Brighton LE, Gambling TM, Carson JL, Orlando RC. Lateral cell membranes and shunt resistance in rabbit esophageal epithelium. *Dig Dis Sci* 2010;55:1856–1865.

29. Orlando RC, Powell DW Studies of esophageal epithelial electrolyte transport and potential difference in man. In: Allen A, Flemström G, Garner A, Silen W, Turnberg LA, eds. *Mechanisms of Mucosal Protection in the Upper Gastrointestinal Tract*. New York: Raven Press, 1984, pp. 75–79.

30. Powell DW, Morris SM, Boyd DD. Water and electrolyte transport by rabbit esophagus. *Am J Physiol* 1975;229:438–443.

31. Powell DW, Orlando RC, Carney CN. Acid injury of the EE. In: Harmon JW, ed. *Basic Mechanisms of Gastrointestinal Mucosal Cell Injury and Protection*. Baltimore: Williams & Wilkins, 1981, pp. 155–177.

32. Tobey NA, Hosseini SS, Argote CM, Dobrucali AM, Awayda MS, Orlando RC. Dilated intercellular spaces and shunt permeability in nonerosive acid-damaged esophageal epithelium. *Am J Gastroenterol* 2004;99:13–22.

33. Aijaz S, Balda MS, Matter K. Tight junctions: molecular architecture and function. *Int Rev Cytol* 2006;248:261–298.

34. Hartsock A, Nelson WJ. Adherens and tight junctions: structure, function and connections to the actin cytoskeleton. *Biochim Biophys Acta* 2008;1778:660–669.

35. Holthofer B, Windoffer R, Troyanovsky S, Leube RE. Structure and function of desmosomes. *Int Rev Cytol* 2007;264:65–163.

36. Elias PM, Friend DS. The permeability barrier in mammalian epidermis. *J Cell Biol* 1975;65:180–191.

37. Elias PM, Goerke J, Friend DS. Mammalian epidermal barrier layer lipids: composition and influence on structure. *J Invest Dermatol* 1977;69:535–546.

38. Hopwood D, Logan KR, Coghill G, *et al.* Histochemical studies of mucosubstances and lipids in normal human oesophageal epithelium. *Histochem J* 1977;9:153–161.

39. Tobey NA, Argote CM, Vanegas XC, Barlow W, Orlando RC. Electrical parameters and ion species for active transport in human esophageal stratified squamous epithelium and Barrett's specialized columnar epithelium. *Am J Physiol Gastrointest Liver Physiol* 2007;293:G264–270.

40. Turner KS, Powell DW Carney CN, Orlando RC, Bozymski EM. Transmural electrical potential difference in the mammalian esophagus in vivo. *Gastroenterology* 1978;75:286–291.

41. Awayda MS, Bengrine A, Tobey NA, Stockand JD, Orlando RC. Nonselective cation transport in native esophageal epithelia. *Am J Physiol Cell Physiol* 2004;287:C395–402.

42. Tobey NA, Argote CM, Awayda MS, Vanegas XC, Orlando RC. Effect of luminal acidity on the apical cation channel in rabbit esophageal epithelium. *Am J Physiol Gastrointest Liver Physiol* 2007;292:G796–805.

43. Khalbuss WE, Marousis CG, Subramanyam M, Orlando RC. Effect of HCl on transmembrane potentials and intracellular pH in rabbit EE. *Gastroenterology* 1995;108:662–672.

44. Tobey NA, Powell DW, Schreiner VJ, Orlando RC. Serosal bicarbonate protects against acid injury to rabbit esophagus. *Gastroenterology* 1989;96:1466–1477.

45. Christie KN, Thomson C, Xue L, Lucocq JM, Hopwood D. Carbonic anhydrase isoenzymes I, II, III, and IV are present in human EE. *J Histochem Cytochem* 1997;45:35–40.

46. Akiba Y, Mizumori M, Kuo M, *et al.* CO_2 chemosensing in rat esophagus. *Gut* 2008;57:1654–1664.

47. Layden TJ, Schmidt L, Agnone L, Lizitsa P, Brewer J, Goldstein JL. Rabbit esophageal cell cytoplasmic pH regulation: role of Na^+-H^+ antiport and Na^+-dependent HCO_3^- transport systems. *Am J Physiol* 1992;263:G407–G413.

48. Tobey NA, Reddy SP, Khalbuss WE, Silvers SM, Cragoe EJ Jr, Orlando RC. Na^+-dependent and -independent Cl^-/HCO_3^- exchangers in cultured rabbit esophageal epithelial cells. *Gastroenterology* 1993;104:185–195.

49. Tobey NA, Reddy SP, Keku TO, Cragoe EJ Jr, Orlando RC. Studies of pH_i in rabbit esophageal basal and squamous epithelial cells in culture. *Gastroenterology* 1992;103:830–839.

50. Tobey NA, Koves G, Orlando RC. Human esophageal epithelial cells possess an Na^+/H^+ exchanger for H^+ extrusion. *Am J Gastroenterol* 1998;93:2075–2081.

51. Lao-Sirieix P, Corovic A, Jankowski J, Lowe A, Triadafilopoulos G, Fitzgerald RC. Physiological and molecular acid loading mechanisms in squamous and columnar-lined esohagus. *Dis Esophagus* 2008;21:529–538.

52. Bass BL, Schweitzer EJ, Harmon JW, Kraimer J. H^+ back diffusion interferes with intrinsic reactive regulation of esophageal mucosal blood flow. *Surgery* 1984;96:404–413.

53. Hollwarth ME, Smith M, Kvietys PR, Granger DN. Esophageal blood flow in the cat. *Gastroenterology* 1986;90:622–627.

54. Feldman MJ, Morris GP, Paterson WG. Role of substance P and calcitonin gene-related peptide in acid-induced augmentation of opossum esophageal blood flow. *Dig Dis Sci* 2001;46:1194.

55. Feldman MJ, Morris GP, Dinda PK, Paterson WG. Mast cells mediate acid-induced augmentation of opossum esophageal blood flow via histamine and nitric oxide. *Gastroenterology* 1996;110:121–128.

56. Tanaka S, Chu S, Hirokawa M, Montrose MH, Kaunitz JD. Direct measurement of acid permeation into the rat oesophagus. *Gut* 2003;52:775–783.

57. Long J, Orlando RC. Esophageal submucosal glands: structure and function. *Am J Gastroenterol* 1999;94: 2818–2824.

58. Orlando RC, Powell DW Carney CN. Pathophysiology of acute acid injury in rabbit EE. *J Clin Invest* 1981;68:286–293.

59. Orlando RC, Bryson JC, Powell DW. Mechanisms of HCl injury in rabbit EE. *Am J Physiol* 1984;246:G718–724.

60. Orlando RC, Powell DW, Bryson JC, *et al.* Esophageal potential difference measurements in esophageal disease. *Gastroenterology* 1982;83:1026–1032.

61. Hopwood D, Milne G, Logan KR. Electron microscopic changes in human oesophageal epithelium in oesophagitis. *J Pathol* 1979;129:161–167.

62. Carlsson R, Fandriks L, Jonsson C, Lundell L, Orlando RC. Is the esophageal squamous epithelial barrier function impaired in patients with gastroesophageal reflux disease? *Scand J Gastroenterol* 1999;5:454–458.

63. Chung RSK, Magri J, DenBesten L. Hydrogen ion transport in the rabbit esophagus. *Am J Physiol* 1975;229:496–500.

64. Harmon JW, Johnson LF, Maydonovitch CL. Effects of acid and bile salts on the rabbit esophageal mucosa. *Dig Dis Sci* 1981;26:65–72.

65. Kivilaakso E, Fromm D, Silen W. Effect of bile salts and related compounds on isolated esophageal mucosa. *Surgery* 1980;87:280–285.

66. Tobey NA, Powell DW, Schreiner VJ, Orlando RC. Serosal bicarbonate protects against acid injury to rabbit esophagus. *Gastroenterology* 1989;96:1466–1477.

67. Tobey NA, Carson JL, Alkiek RA, Orlando RC. Dilated intercellular spaces: a morphological feature of acid reflux-damaged human EE. *Gastroenterology* 1996;111:1200–1205.

68. Solcia E, Villani L, Liunetti O, *et al.* Altered intercellular glycoconjugates and dilated intercellular spaces of EE in reflux disease. *Virchows Arch* 2000;436:207–216.

69. Villanacci V, Grigolato PG, Cestari R, *et al.* Dilated intercellular spaces as markers of reflux disease: histology, semiquantitative score and morphometry upon light microscopy. *Digestion* 2001;64:1–8.

70. Caviglia R, Ribolsi M, Maggiano N, *et al.* Dilated intercellular spaces of EE in nonerosive reflux disease patients with physiological esophageal acid exposure. *Am J Gastroenterol* 2005;100:543–548.

71. Calabrese C, Bortolotti M, Fabbri A, *et al.* Reversibility of GERD ultrastructural alterations and relief of symptoms after omeprazole treatment. *Am J Gastroenterol* 2005;100:537–542.

72. Bove M, Vieth M, Dombrowski F, Ny L, Ruth M, Lundell L. Acid challenge to the human esophageal mucosa: effects on epithelial architecture in health and disease. *Dig Dis Sci* 2005;50:1488–1496.

73. Jovov BJ, Djukic Z, Shaheen NJ, Orlando RC. E-cadherin cleavage in GERD. *Gastroenterology* 2009;136:M1834 (abstract).

74. Tobey NA, Gambling TM, Vanegas XC, Carson JL, Orlando RC. Physicochemical basis for dilated intercellular spaces in non-erosive acid-damaged rabbit EE. *Dis Esophagus* 2008;21:757–764.

75. Barlow WJ, Orlando RC. The pathogenesis of heartburn in non-erosive reflux disease: a unifying hypothesis. *Gastroenterology* 2005;128:771–778.

76. Robles-Chillida EM, Rodrigo J, Mayo I, Arnedo A, Gomez A. Ultrastructure of free-ending nerve fibers in oesophageal epithelium. *J Anat* 1981;133:227–233.

77. Rodrigo J, Hernandez DJ, Vidal MA, Pedrosa JA. Vegetative innervation of the esophagus 111. Intraepithelial endings. *Acta Anat* 1975;92:242–258.

78. Kollarik M UB. Mechanisms of acid-induced activation of airway afferent nerve fibres in guinea pig. *J Physiol* 2002;543:2591–2600.

79. Steen KH, Reeh PW. Sustained graded pain and hyperalgesia from harmless experimental tissue acidosis in humans. *Neurosci Lett* 1993;154:113–116.

80. Steen KH, Steen Ae, Reeh PW. A dominant role of acid pH in inflammatory excitation and sensitization of nociceptors in rat skin, in vitro. *J Neurosci* 1995;15:3982–3989.

81. Bhat YM, Bielefeldt K. Capsaicin receptor (TRPV1) and non-erosive reflux disease. *Eur J Gastroenterol Hepatol* 2006;18:263–270.

82. Carr MJ, Kollarik M, Meeker SN, Undem BJ. A role for TRPV1 in bradykinin-induced excitation of vagal airway afferent nerve terminals. *J Pharmacol Exp Ther* 2003;304:1275–1279.

83. Kollarik M, Ru F, Undem BJ. Acid-sensitive vagal sensory pathways and cough. *Pulm Pharmacol Ther* 2007;20:402–411.

84. Matthews PJ, Aziz Q, Facer P, Davis JB, Thompson DG, Anand P. Increased capsaicin receptor TRPV1 nerve fibres in the inflamed human oesophagus. *Eur J Gastroenterol Hepatol* 2004;16:897–902.

85. MacKnight ADC, Leaf A. Regulation of cellular volume. *Physiol Rev* 1977;57:510–573.

86. Tobey NA, Orlando RC. Mechanisms of acid injury to rabbit esophageal epithelium. Role of basolateral cell membrane acidification. *Gastroenterology* 1991;101:1220–1228.

87. Tobey NA, Reddy SP, Keku TO, Cragoe EJ Jr, Orlando RC. Mechanisms of HCl-induced lowering of intracellular pH in rabbit esophageal epithelial cells. *Gastroenterology* 1993;105:1035–1044.

88. Tobey NA, Orlando RC. Mechanisms of acid injury to rabbit esophageal epithelium. Role of basolateral cell membrane acidification. *Gastroenterology* 1991;101:1220–1228.

89. Layden TJ, Schmidt L, Agnone L, Lisitza P, Brewer J, Goldstein JL. Rabbit esophageal cell cytoplasmic pH regulation: role of Na^+-H^+ antiport and Na^+-dependent HCO_3^- transport systems. *Am J Physiol* 1992;263:G407–413.

90. Tobey NA, Reddy SP, Khalbuss WE, Silvers SM, Cargo EJ Jr, Orlando RC. Na^+-dependent and -independent Cl^-/HCO_3^- exchangers in cultured rabbit esophageal epithelial cells. *Gastroenterology* 1993;104:185–195.

91. Tobey NA, Reddy SP, Keku TO, Cragoe EJ Jr, Orlando RC. Studies of pH_i in rabbit esophageal basal and squamous epithelial cells in culture. *Gastroenterology* 1992;103:830–839.

92. Tobey NA, Koves G, Orlando RC. Human esophageal epithelial cells possess an Na$^+$/H$^+$ exchanger for H$^+$ extrusion. *Am J Gastroenterol* 1998;93:2075–2081.

93. Tobey NA, Cragoe EJ Jr, Orlando RC. HCl-induced cell edema in rabbit EE: a bumetanide-sensitive process. *Gastroenterology* 1995;109:414–421.

94. Tobey NA, Koves G, Orlando RC. HCl-induced cell edema in primary cultured rabbit EE. *Gastroenterology* 1997;112:847–854.

95. Cotran R, Vinay K, Robbins S, *et al. Pathologic Basis of Disease,* 5th edn. Philadelphia: WB Saunders, 1994, p. 1.

96. Lemasters JJ. Mechanisms of hepatic toxicity V. Necrapoptosis and the mitochondrial permeability transition: shared pathways to necrosis and apoptosis. *Am J Physiol Gastrointest Liver Physiol* 1999;276:G1–6.

97. Orlando RC. Pathology of reflux oesophagitis and its complications. In: Jamieson GG, ed. *Surgery of the Oesophagus.* New York: Churchill Livingstone, 1988, pp. 189–200.

98. Ismail-Beigi FHP, Pope CE. Histological consequences of gastroesophageal refluxes in man. *Gastroenterology* 1970;58:163–174.

99. Kanazawa Y, Isomoto H, Wen CY, *et al.* Impact of endoscopically minimal involvement on IL-8 mRNA expression in esophageal mucosa of patients with non-erosive reflux disease. *World J Gastroenterol* 2003;9:2801–2804.

100. Fitzgerald RC, Onwuegbusi BA, Bajaj-Elliott M, *et al.* Diversity in the oesophageal phenotype response to gastroesophageal reflux: immunological determinants. *Gut* 2002;50:451–459.

101. Rieder F, Cheng L, Harnett KM, *et al.* Gastroesophageal reflux disease–associated esophagitis induces endogenous cytokine production leading to motor abnormalities. *Gastroenterology* 2007;132:154–165.

102. Isomoto H, Wang A, Mizuta Y, *et al.* Elevated levels of chemokines n esophageal mucosa of patients with reflux esophagitis. *Am J Gastroenterol* 2003;98:551–556.

103. Oh DS, DeMeester SR, Valibohmer D, *et al.* Reduction of interleukin 8 gene expression in reflux esophagitis and Barrett's esophagus with antireflux surgery. *Arch Surg* 2007;142:554–559.

104. Naya MJ, Pereboom D, Ortego J, Alda JO, Lanas A. Superoxide anion produced by inflammatory cells play an important part in the pathogenesis of acid and pepsin induced esophagitis in rabbits. *Gut* 1997;40:175–181.

105. Lanas A, Soteras F, Jimenez P, *et al.* Superoxide anion and nitric oxide in high-grade esophagitis induced by acid and pepsin in rabbits. *Dig Dis Sci* 2001;46:2733–2743.

106. Soteras F, Lanas A, Fiteni I, *et al.* Nitric oxide and superoxide anion in low-grade esophagitis induced by acid and pepsin in rabbits. *Dig Dis Sci* 2000;45:1802–1809.

107. Uc A, Murray J, Kooy N, Conklin JL. Effect of peroxynitrite on motor function of the opossum esophagus. *Dig Dis Sci* 2001;46:30–37.

108. Cheng L, Cao W, Fiocchi C, Behar J, Biancani P, Harnett KM. HCl-induced inflammatory mediators on cat esophageal mucosa and inflammatory mediators in esophageal circular muscle in an in vivo model of acute esophagitis, *Am J Physiol* 2006;290:G1307–1317.

109. Cheng L, Cao W, Fiocchi C, Behar J, Biancani P, Harnett KM. Platelet-activating factor and prostaglandin E2 impair esopha-geal ACh release in experimental esophagitis. *Am J Physiol* 2005:289:G418–428.

110. White RJ, Zhang Y, Morris GP, Paterson WG. Esophagitis-related esophageal shortening in opossum is associated with longitudinal muscle hyperresponsiveness. *Am J Physiol* 2001;280:G463–469.

111. Paterson WG, Kolyn DM. Esophageal shortening induced by acute intraluminal acid perfusion: a cause for hiatus hernia? *Gastroenterology* 1994;107:1736–1740.

112. Dunne DP, Paterson WG. Acid-induced oesophageal shortening in humans: a cause for hiatus hernia? *Can J Gastroenterol* 2000;14:847–850.

113. Lord RV, DeMeester SR, Peters JH, *et al.* Hiatal hernia, lower esophageal sphincter incompetence, and effectiveness of Nissen fundoplication in the spectrum of gastroesophageal reflux disease. *J Gastrointest Surg* 2009;13:602–610.

114. Kawanishi M. Will symptomatic gastroesophageal reflux disease develop into reflux esophagitis? *J Gastroenterol* 2006;41:440–443.

115. Frazzoni M, DeMicheli E, Savarino V. Different patterns of oesophageal acid exposure distinguish complicated reflux disease from either erosive reflux oesophagitis or non-erosive reflux disease. *Aliment Pharmacol Ther* 2003;18:1091–1098.

116. Gordon C, Kang JY, Neild PJ, Maxwell JD. The role of the hiatus hernia in gastro-oesophageal reflux disease. *Aliment Pharmacol Ther* 2004;20:719–732.

117. Pace F, Bianchi Porro G. Gastroesophageal reflux disease: a typical spectrum disease (a new conceptual framework is not needed). *Am J Gastroenterol* 2004;99:946–949.

118. Bell B, Almy TP, Lipkin M. Cell proliferation kinetics in the gastrointestinal tract of man: III. Cell renewal in esophagus, stomach and jejunum of a patient with treated pernicious anemia. *J Natl Cancer Inst* 1967;38:615–628.

119. Eastwood GL. Gastrointestinal epithelial renewal. *Gastroenterology* 1977;72:962.

120. Livstone EM, Sheahan DG, Behar J. Studies of esophageal epithelial cell proliferation in patients with reflux esophagitis. *Gastroenterology* 1977;73:1315.

121. DeBacker A, Haentjens P, Willems G. Hydrochloric acid: a trigger of cell proliferation in the esophagus of dogs. *Dig Dis Sci* 1985;30:884–890.

122. Souza RF, Huo X, Mittal V, *et al.* Gastroesophageal reflux might cause esophagitis through a cytokine-mediated mechanism rather than caustic acid injury. *Gastroenterology* 2009;137:1776–1784.

123. Jimenez P, Lanas A, Piazuelo E, Esteva F. Effects of extracellular pH on restitution and proliferation of rabbit oesophageal epithelial cells. *Aliment Pharmacol Ther* 1999;13:545–52.

124. Jimenez P, Lanas A, Piazuelo E, Esteva F. Effect of growth factors and prostaglandin E2 on restitution and proliferation of rabbit esophageal epithelial cells. *Dig Dis Sci* 1998;43:2309–2316.

125. Takahashi M, Ota S, Ogura K, Nakamura T, Omata M. Hepatocyte growth factor stimulates wound repair of the rabbit esophageal epithelial cells in primary culture. *Biochem Biophys Res Commun* 1995;216:298–305.

126. Hetzel DI, Dent J, Reed WD, *et al.* Healing and relapse of severe peptic esophagitis after treatment with omeprazole. *Gastroenterology* 1988;95:903–912.

127. Schulman MI, Orlando RC. Treatment of gastroesophageal reflux: the role of proton pump inhibitors. In: Schrier RW Baxter JD, Abboud F, *et al.*, eds. *Advances in Internal Medicine*, vol 40. St. Louis: Mosby-Year Book, 1995, pp. 273–295.

128. Ito H, Iijima K, Ara N, *et al.* Reactive nitrogen oxide species induce dilatation of the intercellular space of rat esophagus. *Scand J Gastroenterol* 2010;45:282–291.

129. Ishiyama F, Iijima K, Asanuma K, *et al.* Exogenous luminal nitric oxide exacerbates esophagus tissue damage in a reflux esophagitis model of rats. *Scand J Gastroenterol* 2009;44:527–537.

130. Coleman R, Iqbal S, Godfrey PP, Billington D. Membranes and bile formation. Composition of several mammalian biles and their membrane-damaging properties. *Biochem J* 1979;178:201–208.

131. Takeuchi K, Furukawa O, Tanaka H, Okabe S. Determination of acid-neutralizing capacity in rat duodenum. Influences of 16,16-dimethyl prostaglandin E2 and nonsteroidal antiinflammatory drugs. *Dig Dis Sci* 1986;31:631–637.

132. Gotley DC, Morgan AP, Ball D, Owen RW, Cooper MJ. Composition of gastro-oesophageal refluxate. *Gut* 1991;32:1093–1099.

133. Navarro-Rodriguez T, Fass R. Functional heartburn, nonerosive reflux disease, and reflux esophagitis are all distinct conditions – a debate: pro. *Curr Treat Options Gastroenterol* 2007;10:294–304.

134. Long JD, Marten E, Tobey NA, Orlando RC. Effects of luminal hypertonicity on rabbit esophageal epithelium. *Am J Physiol* 1997;273:G647–654.

135. Bor S, Marten E, Tobey NA, Abdulnour-Nakhoul S, Orlando RC. The effect of ethanol on the structure and function of rabbit esophageal epithelium. *Am J Physiol* 1998;274:G819–826.

136. Lloyd DA, Borda IT. Food-induced heartburn: effect of osmolality. *Gastroenterology* 1981;80:740–741.

137. Farré R, De Vos R, Geboes K, *et al.* Critical role of stress in increased oesophageal mucosa permeability and dilated intercellular spaces. *Gut* 2007;56:1191–1197.

138. Tobey NA, Sikka D, Marten E, Caymaz-Bor C, Hosseini SS, Orlando RC. Effect of heat stress on rabbit esophageal epithelium. *Am J Physiol* 1999;276:G1322–1330.

139. Suerbaum S. Microbiome analysis in the esophagus. *Gastroenterology* 2009;137:419–421.

140. Yang L, Lu X, Nossa CW, Francois F, Peek RM, Pei Z. Inflammation and intestinal metaplasia of the distal esophagus are associated with alterations in the microbiome. *Gastroenterology* 2009;137:588–597.

23 Duodenogastroesophageal Reflux

Daniel Sifrim[1] and Roberto Penagini[2]
[1]Barts and The London School of Medicine and Dentistry, Queen Mary University of London, London, UK
[2]Università degli Studi and Fondazione IRCCS Cà Granda Ospedale Maggiore Policlinico, Milan, Italy

Introduction

A few reflux episodes of gastric contents into the esophagus occur after meals in most healthy individuals. These events, generally occurring during spontaneous relaxations of the lower esophageal sphincter (LES), called transient LES relaxations [1], are rapidly cleared and do not give rise to symptoms or esophageal lesions. However, when gastroesophageal reflux is excessive it may induce symptoms and/or erosive esophagitis, Barrett's esophagus or a stricture.

The gastric refluxate contains noxious agents, produced in the stomach, i.e. acid and pepsin, and a considerable body of evidence in animals and man has shown their importance in producing symptoms and inflammation. Gastric refluxate, however, may contain bile and pancreatic enzymes as well, which intermix with gastric juice, especially at night and after meals as a result of transpyloric reflux [2, 3]. It is suggested that, when duodenogastric reflux is excessive because of altered motility or partial gastrectomy, a chemically-induced gastritis and dyspeptic symptoms may occur [4].

Duodenogastroesophageal reflux (DGER) refers to the situation whereby duodenal contents reach the esophagus, a phenomenon which is increased when gastroesophageal reflux occurs frequently, as in patients with gastroesophageal reflux disease (GERD). DGER has been termed "bile reflux" or "alkaline reflux" but both terms are not correct on one side because not only bile refluxes into the esophagus and on the other because DGER is most often acid. Whereas it has long been demonstrated in animal studies that bile and pancreatic enzymes may injure esophageal mucosa independently of acid and pepsin, studies in humans have been more controversial, and the relative importance of acid and DGER to the development of symptoms and of injury of the esophageal, laryngeal and respiratory mucosa is still under debate. However, recent technologic advances have helped us greatly to progress knowledge in this field. This chapter reviews animal and human studies that clarify the role of gastric and duodenal contents in causing esophageal symptoms, and macroscopic and microscopic damage of the esophageal and respiratory mucosa. Furthermore, the available tests for identifying DGER are discussed and critically reviewed. Finally, medical and surgical treatments for DGER are discussed with a view to possible exciting developments in pharmacologic interventions.

Role of acid and pepsin

Animal studies

Experimental and clinical evidence supports the importance of acid and pepsin in causing esophageal mucosal injury. Experiments in dogs reported no esophageal damage with hydrochloric acid (HCl) infusion alone, while acid in combination with low concentrations of pepsin at pH of less than 2 caused the most severe esophagitis [5]. Experiments in cats demonstrated esophageal mucosal damage with either very high concentrations of acid (pH 1.0–1.3) or lower acid concentrations (pH 1.6–2.0) in the presence of pepsin [6].

More recently, Zhang *et al.* used acid–pepsin perfusions in a feline model to study the effect of repeated cycles of acute esophagitis and healing on esophageal motility. Acid perfusion induced severe esophagitis. At 24 h, distal peristaltic contractions disappeared, LES pressure was reduced by 60%, the esophagus length was 1–2 cm shorter, and esophageal compliance was reduced by 30%. Most parameters recovered in 4 weeks. Subsequent repeated acute injuries induced similar endoscopic esophagitis, but a different pattern of inflammatory infiltration and fibrosis in the mucosa and muscle layers, resulting in milder motor disturbances [7]. *Ex vivo* studies with rabbit esophagus confirmed that acid infusion alone did not produce mucosal damage or increase esophageal mucosal permeability. However, the addition of pepsin, in a dose-dependent manner, was associated with increased degrees of gross esophageal mucosal injury and changes in esophageal mucosal permeability [8]. These results were recently confirmed by Farre *et al.* studying changes in rabbit esophageal mucosal electrical resistance in Ussing chambers [9].

Thus, animal studies suggest that the esophageal mucosa is relatively resistant to reflux of acid alone unless it occurs at very high concentrations (pH 1.0–1.3). On the other hand, the combination of acid and even small concentrations of pepsin results in macroscopic as well as microscopic esophageal mucosal injury.

The mechanism of esophageal mucosal damage by pepsin is related to its proteolytic properties. Pepsin causes the most damage at its optimal pH activity range: pH 2–3. However, the activity of these enzymes depends on the substrate and pH with significant digestion occurring up to pH 4.5. It has also been shown that these enzymes can bind to substrates like collagen up to pH 5.5. Pepsin promotes detachment of the surface cells from the epithelium, presumably by digesting the intercellular substances and surface structures that contribute to the maintenance of cohesion between cells [10].

The mechanism for mucosal damage by HCl is more complicated and depends on a series of events. Based on experimental works by Orlando, Powell, and coworkers in the rabbit esophagus, H^+ impairs cell volume regulation, causing cell death by inactivation of the Na^+/K^+-ATPase pump located in the basolateral cell wall in the stratum spinosum of the mucosa. Inhibition of Na^+/K^+-ATPase occurs at the same time that an amiloride-sensitive Na^+ pump is activated, causing increased entry and accumulation of Na^+ and resulting in excess intracellular volume and subsequent cell death [11, 12].

Human studies

The importance of acid and pepsin in the development of heartburn and esophagitis was first observed many years ago. In 1953 Aylwin found that patients with esophagitis had aspirates of lower pH and higher pepsin concentration than those without esophagitis [13]. Later, Tuttle *et al.* performed short-term esophageal pH and motility studies in patients with esophagitis and documented the temporal relationship between falls in pH and onset of heartburn [14]. Subsequently, with the development of 24-h pH monitoring, several studies have shown increasing levels of esophageal acid exposure with increasing severity of esophageal lesions. DeMeester *et al.* found that 90% of patients with esophagitis had abnormal pH monitoring versus 55% of patients with normal endoscopy [15]. Robertson *et al.* observed that acid reflux was more severe in patients with complications (stricture, ulcer or Barrett's esophagus) compared to patients with uncomplicated esophagitis, and that the difference was more marked at night [16]. Percentage of total time at a pH below 4 was 26.2% and 35.6% (total and night time respectively) in the first group and 11.3% and 5.2% in the second group. Frazzoni *et al.* studied 88 patients with negative endoscopy,

76 with esophagitis, and 56 with complicated GERD, and found progressively higher % time at pH below 4; 11.8%, 14.9%, and 19.4%, respectively [17]. More recent studies performed with 48-h wireless pH monitoring confirmed these data. Pandolfino *et al.* found that 100% of esophagitis patients had an abnormal test (considering the worst day analysis) versus 55% of endoscopy-negative patients [18], whereas, with the same analysis, Wenner *et al.* showed that % time at pH below 4 was 8.4% in esophagitis and 4.0% in endoscopy negative-patients [19].

Other evidence for a role of acid in inducing esophageal lesions comes from Stein *et al.*, who reported that patients with Barrett's esophagus had greater exposure time to more caustic gastric acid concentrations (pH <3 or 2) [20], and from studies in patients with Zollinger–Ellison syndrome, a condition where acid output is high, which showed high prevalence of esophagitis [21].

The contribution of pepsin to esophageal injury is difficult to document in man since, as mentioned earlier, the optimum pH for the enzymatic activity of pepsin is below 3 [22]. A study by Gotley *et al.* showed that esophageal aspirates of patients with GERD collected over 2-h periods had progressively higher concentrations of pepsin as lesions became more severe, a finding which is probably related to the longer time during which refluxate was present in the esophagus of patients with more severe erosive disease [23].

In spite of the evidence presented in this section, it should be emphasized that acid reflux is not a strong predictor for severity of erosive esophagitis and Barrett's esophagus [24] as a substantial overlap in esophageal acid exposure has been observed in the various reports among patients with varying degrees of mucosal lesions. This may be partly due to the day-to-day variability of pH measurement, but it strongly suggests that other factors are important, such as DGER or resistance of the esophageal mucosa.

Several studies have demonstrated a marked correlation between symptom severity and the acidity of gastric refluxate. The relationship between the refluxate pH and the generation of heartburn was elegantly analyzed in an esophageal acid perfusion study by Smith *et al.* [25]. In this double-blind study, 25 patients with heartburn were randomly allocated to undergo esophageal perfusion with eight solutions of different pH (1.0, 1.5, 2, 2.5, 3, 4, 5, and 6). An overall positive correlation was demonstrated between the time to onset of pain and the pH of the solution infused. Reduced occurrence of heartburn and increased time between the start of acid perfusion and onset of heartburn were noted with increasing pH of the test solution. Solutions of pH 1 or 1.5 induced heartburn in all patients, but even the pH 6 solution induced heartburn in more than 40% of the patients (Figure 23.1).

In a study using impedance–pH monitoring, Bredenoord *et al.* demonstrated that heartburn and regurgitation are more likely to be evoked when the pH drop is large, the proximal extent of the refluxate is high, and the volume and

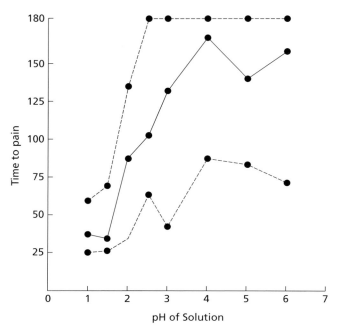

Figure 23.1 Time to onset of pain is related to the pH of the infused solution (reproduced from Smith *et al.* [25]).

acid clearance is delayed. Furthermore, sensitization of the esophagus occurs by preceding acid exposure [26].

Role of duodenal contents

The importance of DGER relates to findings in both animal and human studies that factors other than acid, namely bile and pancreatic enzymes, may play a significant role in mucosal injury and symptoms in patients with GERD.

The primary bile acids, cholate and chenodeoxycholate, are synthesized from cholesterol by hepatocytes. Secondary bile acids are formed as metabolic by-products of intestinal bacteria. In man, these include deoxycholic and lithocholic acid. Prior to secretion into bile, 98% of bile acids are conjugated with taurine or glycine. Conjugation, especially with taurine, increases the solubility of bile acids by lowering their pKa. Human bile consists of 54% cholic, 31% chenodeoxycholic, and 15% deoxycholic acid, of which about 80% is conjugated with taurin and 20% with glycine [27].

Since the reflux of gastroduodenal contents usually occurs intermixed with the acidic contents of the stomach, the synergistic and inhibitory interactions of HCl with pepsin, trypsin, and bile acids is critical to understand their effect on esophageal mucosa. For example, esophageal mucosal damage by bile acids is dependent on the conjugation state of the bile acids and the pH of the refluxate because of the different pKa of conjugated and unconjugated bile acids. Conjugated bile acids, which have a pKa of 1.9, are more injurious to the esophageal mucosa at acidic pH, while unconjugated bile acids (pKa 5.1) are more harmful at pH above 5. Injurious effect of trypsin on the esophageal mucosa occurs at pH 7.0. Lysolecithin is a normal constituent of duodenal juice formed by pancreatic phospholipase A hydrolysis of lecithin in bile. It causes histologic damage and alteration of the rabbit esophageal transmucosal potential difference only in the presence of HCl. Other studies have shown that acidification of bile to below pH 2 may result in a marked decrease of bile acid activity [28]. This was due to an irreversible bile acid precipitation. The clinical implications of this finding may be two-fold: (1) regurgitated bile acids may precipitate and become inactivated within a very acidic gastric environment; and (2) given an alkaline environment, such as after gastrectomy, bile acids may remain in solution and can reflux into the esophagus causing esophageal mucosal injury.

Figure 23.2 summarizes the proposed agents responsible for esophageal mucosal injury.

Bile acids in the pathogenesis of esophagitis, Barrett's esophagus and/or esophageal adenocarcinoma

Experimental exposure of esophageal mucosa to bile acids can provoke esophagitis and Barrett's epithelium. It has been suggested that undifferentiated multipotent stem cells in the basal layer of the esophagus can differentiate into columnar epithelium if exposed to components of the DGER [29]. The components thought to be most damaging are bile acids, either alone or in combination with acid [30]. Various animal models have been developed that, utilize different types of bypasses between the esophagus and parts of the stomach and/or duodenum to induce esophageal reflux. Using a dog model with biliary diversion and a jejunal conduit anastomozing directly to the esophagus, Moffat and Berkas showed that canine bile was capable of producing various degrees of erosive esophagitis [31]. In another dog model, columnar epithelial metaplasia in the distal esophagus could result from prolonged reflux of acid [32]. Under normal conditions, mucosal defects in the esophagus are regenerated by squamous epithelium. In the presence of gastroesophageal reflux of acid or a combination of acid and bile, regeneration is frequently by columnar epithelium [33].

Clark *et al.* performed an esophagoduodenostomy in rats with preservation of the stomach. The resulting DGER induced Barrett's esophagus in 27% of the rats and the development of esophageal adenocarcinoma in 35% [34]. Ireland *et al.*, too, performed an esophagoduodenostomy in rats, but with the removal of different parts of the stomach or diverting the stomach downstream. The prevalence of esophageal adenocarcinoma was 30% in rats with DGER, but 87% in rats with reflux of duodenal juice alone. These results show a progressive increase in the prevalence of Barrett's esophagus and esophageal adenocarcinoma as less

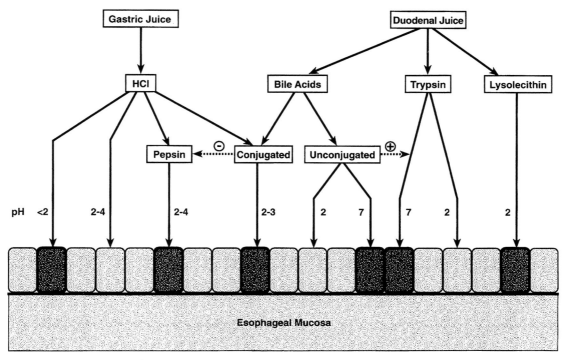

Figure 23.2 Proposed agents responsible for esophageal mucosal injury. Mucosal injury is illustrated by the heavy set boxes representing the epithelial surface.

gastric juice was permitted to reflux with duodenal juice into the esophagus. It was concluded from these results that the presence of gastric juice in refluxed duodenal juice protected against the development of Barrett's esophagus and/or esophageal adenocarcinoma. Likewise, the authors speculated that continuous acid suppression therapy in patients with GERD may be detrimental by encouraging esophageal metaplasia and tumorigenesis in patients with DGER [35]. Miwa *et al.* performed an esophagojejunostomy in rats with or without gastrectomy. In both groups, high incidences of Barrett's esophagus (92–100%) were found. In addition, 54–75% of rats developed esophageal adenocarcinoma. In this study, both DGER and duodenoesophageal reflux were able to induce Barrett's esophagus and/or esophageal adenocarcinoma [36].

These animal models show the importance of duodenal juice in inducing Barrett's esophagus and/or esophageal adenocarcinoma. However, it is not clear what the role of gastric acid is, as one study suggested a protective effect of gastric juice, whereas in another study gastric acid seemed to be an innocent bystander. Furthermore, these studies exposed animals to high concentrations of bile acids and extrapolation to the human setting should be made with caution.

The hypothesis that bile reflux could cause Barrett's esophagus and esophageal adenocarcinoma has also been evaluated in human cohort studies. Avidan *et al.* found no difference in the rate of gastric surgery (a surrogate marker of DGER), in 650 patients with short-segment or 366 patients with long-segment Barrett's esophagus compared to 3047 controls [37]. Similar conclusions were reached by Birgisson *et al.* in their retrospective review of 325 patients with esophageal adenocarcinoma and 117 patients with esophageal squamous cell carcinoma, finding a very low and similar rate of gastric surgery between the two groups [38]. Taha *et al.* compared prevalence of esophagitis and Barrett' esophagus in 140 patients with previous gastric surgery (a median of 27 years before) and 100 patients with an intact stomach, all referred for endoscopy, and found similar results in the two groups [39].

In vitro studies

Experiments using biopsies from Barrett's esophagus patients suggest an increase in cellular proliferation and decrease in cellular differentiation with exposure to pulses of either acid or bile.

In response to prolonged acid exposure, villin expression increased and correlated with the appearance of microvilli (differentiation) in Barrett's esophagus. In contrast, villin expression did not increase with pulsed exposure to acid. The opposite was found for proliferation, as determined by proliferating cell nuclear antigen (PCNA) expression. PCNA expression increased in Barrett's esophagus specimens exposed to pulses of acid, whereas continuous acid exposure reduced cell proliferation [40] (Figure 23.3). It was found that in Barrett's esophagus biopsies a brief exposure to a mixture of conjugated bile acids, but not unconjugated bile acids, in the

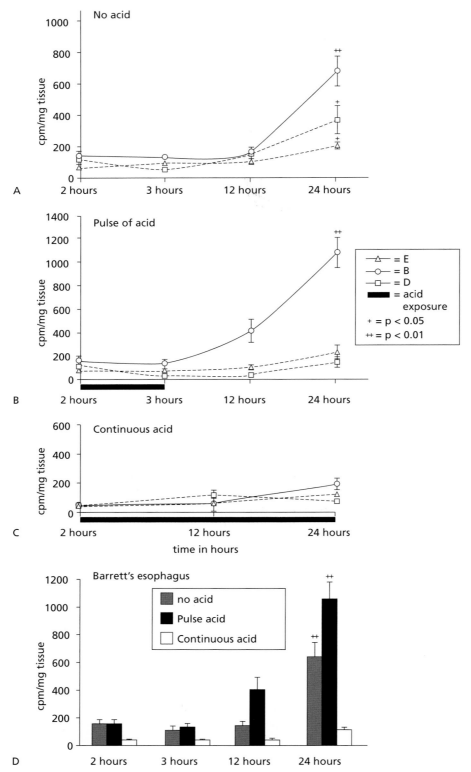

Figure 23.3 Cell proliferation under different pH conditions: (A) no acid; (B) pulse of acid; and (C) continuous acid. Endoscopic biopsies of normal esophagus (E), Barrett's esophagus (B), and duodenum (D) cultured in the presence of tritiated thymidine (1 mCi/mL) with either no acid (pH 7.4), for a 1-h acid pulse (pH 3.5) followed by pH 7.4, or with continuous acid (pH 3.5). At 2-, 3-, 12-, and 24-h time points, Barrett's esophagus proliferates more than normal esophagus and duodenum under all conditions, but particularly after an acid pulse. (D) Combines the data for Barrett's esophagus only, from (A), (B) and (C), to emphasize the augmented cell proliferation after an acid-pulse in this tissue (reproduced from Fitzgerald *et al.* [40]).

absence of acid increased proliferation, whereas exposure to a combination of bile acids *plus* acid resulted in an initial increased proliferation, which normalized after 24 h [41].

Shirvani *et al.* demonstrated a progressive increase in expression of cyclo-oxygenase (COX)-2 with disease progression from Barrett's metaplasia to dysplasia and adenocarcinoma in *ex vivo* human epithelial explants. COX-2 induction was increased significantly in the presence of acid and bile [42]. The highest induction could be found when the explants were exposed to a 1-h pulse of bile acids. Such induction could be related, in part, to protein C kinase activation by bile acids. This effect was attenuated by the selective COX-2 inhibitor NS-398, as was acid- and bile acid-induced proliferation. Combined exposure to acid and bile acids had no effect on COX-2 expression [43].

These *ex vivo* results suggest that pulsed exposure to acid or conjugated bile acids may contribute to the proliferative alterations and the molecular changes that are observed in Barrett's esophagus, and, in turn, play a key role in cancer development. Remarkably, the combination of acid and bile acids, which is most commonly found in the refluxate of patients with GERD and Barrett's esophagus, did not have these effects.

The mechanism by which bile acids cause mucosal damage is controversial. The most favored hypothesis suggests that bile acids gain entrance across the mucosa because of their lipophilic state, causing intramucosal damage primarily by disorganizing membrane structure or interfering with cellular function [44]. Once penetrating the mucosal barrier, bile acids are trapped inside the cells by intracellular ionization, explaining the several fold increase in intracellular concentrations of bile acids [45]. These findings explain the previous observations of increased mucosal injury by conjugated bile acids at pH 2, and unconjugated bile acids at pH 7 because of their different pKa (see above), which make them unionized at a different pH. The unionized forms of the bile acids are more lipophilic, allowing them to access through the esophageal mucosal barrier into the intracellular compartment where they are trapped by ionization and subsequently cause mucosal damage.

In conclusion, the predominant pathogenetic stimulus that causes Barrett's esophagus is still unclear. It has been suggested that undifferentiated multipotent stem cells in the basal layer of the esophagus can differentiate into columnar epithelium if exposed to components of the DGER [29]. In this regard, acid, pepsin, bile, pancreatic enzymes, the major constituents of the DGER, have all been proposed to be involved. However, the components of the refluxate thought to be most damaging are bile acids, either alone or in combination with acid. It is still an enigma as to why only a fraction of patients with GERD develop Barrett's esophagus and what factors in the refluxate (acid and/or bile) initiate metaplasia and/or promote carcinogenesis. The evidence thus far suggests that, for patients with Barrett's esophagus,

both acid and bile may be harmful. There is insufficient evidence to date suggesting that either acid or bile is less harmful than the other and can be left untreated. The ultimate goal is normalization of the esophageal milieu.

Bile acids in the pathogenesis of non-erosive reflux disease

Whereas previous studies have shown that bile acids are implicated in the pathogenesis of esophagitis and Barrett's esophagus, more recent studies have demonstrated the involvement of bile acids in the development of more subtle microscopic changes, such as dilated intercellular spaces (DISs), frequently observed in biopsies from patients with non-erosive reflux disease (NERD).

Experimental short exposure of the rabbit esophageal mucosa to solutions with a bile acid concentration and acidity similar to that observed in the gastric contents of patients with NERD may impair esophageal mucosal integrity and even induce DISs. Such a situation could, theoretically, underlie the occurrence and/or persistence of symptoms in these patients.

Incubation of rabbit esophageal mucosa with acidic solutions (pH 2.0) containing a range of bile acids (0.5–5 mmol/L) markedly decreased electrical resistance and increased mucosal permeability. Weakly acidic solutions (pH 5.0), and to some extent neutral solutions (pH 7.4), containing bile acids also decreased resistance and increased permeability, although the effects were much less marked. Exposure to bile acids provoked DISs in acid and weakly acidic conditions [9] (Figure 23.4).

Furthermore, perfusion of the distal esophagus in healthy humans subjects with acid and weakly acidic solutions containing bile acids provoked DISs not only in the "exposed" esophageal mucosa but also in the more proximal "non-exposed" mucosa, without producing visible erosions or significant inflammation [46]. It is suggested that these mucosal changes might be implicated in symptom perception in patients with NERD. Very interestingly, esophageal DISs induced by mucosal exposure to bile acids are associated with substance P release, a neurotransmitter implicated in the esophageal visceral perception [47].

Finally, it is known that exposure of esophageal epithelial cells to unconjugated bile acids increases intracellular reactive oxygen species, and this effect is blocked by antioxidants. Recent preliminary studies demonstrated that changes in esophageal mucosal integrity induced by weakly acidic solutions with unconjugated bile acids, similar to reflux in GERD patients "on" PPI, can be prevented with antioxidants [48].

Impact of duodenogastroesophageal reflux on laryngeal and respiratory mucosa

DGER has been implicated for producing laryngeal signs and symptoms. Adhami *et al.* studied the role of acid, pepsin, and duodenal ingredients (bile acids and trypsin) individually

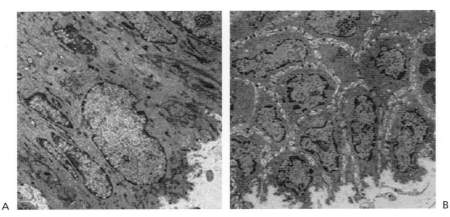

Figure 23.4 Transmission electron micrographs of rabbit esophageal mucosa. (A) Mucosa from control animals. (B) Mucosa exposed to weakly acidic solution that contains bile acids (2 mM taurodeoxycholic acid). Note the dilated intercellular spaces (reproduced from Farre *et al.* [9]).

and in combination on different laryngeal structures in an experimental canine model. They demonstrated that pepsin alone or combined with conjugated bile acids at pH 1–2 resulted in significant, severe histologic inflammation that was much greater than with other agents. Duodenal ingredients caused no or minimal histologic damage at all pH values. These authors concluded that in acidic refluxate, pepsin and conjugated bile acids are the most injurious agents affecting laryngeal tissue, but duodenal agents in a non-acidic refluxate do not play a significant role in causing laryngeal injury [49].

In preliminary studies, Mertens *et al.* evaluated the effect of non-acidic solutions with or without bile acids and bacterial subproducts (LPS) on the functional integrity of the rabbit tracheal mucosa. Studies used Ussing chambers for assessment of transepithelial mucosal resistance and measurements of substance P release (a neurotransmitter and marker of mucosal injury). Tracheal mucosa was exposed for 20 min to solutions containing deoxycholic acid, pepsin or endotoxin (LPS). As expected, exposure of the tracheal mucosa to acidic solutions induced a significant drop in electrical resistance. More interestingly, incubating the tissue with deoxycholic acid at a weakly acidic pH (pH 3–4) significantly reduced resistance. Furthermore, exposure to LPS significantly increased substance P release. These results show that not only acidic solutions but also weakly acidic solutions (pH 3–4) containing bile acids can harm the functional integrity of the tracheal mucosa *in vitro*. Local substance P release, induced by endotoxins present in gastroduodenal refluxate of patients "on" PPIs, may further promote an inflammatory reaction.

Finally, bile acids have been detected in bronchial secretions (bronchoalveaolar lavage and sputum) of patients with chronic cough, cystic fibrosis, and post lung transplant [50–52]. Interestingly, a recent study by Blondeau *et al.* showed that aspiration of bile acids in patients after lung transplant

seems to be associated with an increased number of nocturnal weakly acidic reflux events [53]. The presence of bile acids in the airways suggests aspiration following DGER. Whether bile acids *"per se"* are responsible for the inflammatory reaction in the airways or are only markers of aspiration of gastric contents is still controversial. A study by Vos *et al.* suggested that airway colonization is associated with bile acid aspiration after lung transplantation [54]. The presence of bile acids in bronchoalveolar lavage fluid is associated with significantly increased neutrophils, interleukins (IL-8, IL-1β, IL-10), monocyte chemotactic protein 1 and decreased levels of pulmonary collectins SP-A and SP-D [55]. Bile acid aspiration and reduced SP-A and SP-D levels might create a pulmonary environment with more aggressive T-cell-based alloimmune responses, leading to the development of chronic rejection (bronchiolitis obliterans syndrome).

Detection of duodenogastroesophageal reflux in humans

Various direct and indirect methodologies are employed for measuring DGER, including endoscopy, aspiration studies (both gastric and esophageal), scintigraphy, ambulatory pH monitoring, ambulatory bilirubin monitoring, and impedance–pH monitoring.

Endoscopy

Bile is frequently seen in the esophagus and especially in the stomach of patients during endoscopy, and many endoscopists report this finding, being convinced that it is pathophysiologically important for the symptoms and inflammatory lesions observed in the patient's stomach or esophagus. However, it should be borne in mind that endoscopy is an "unphysiologic" test during which the patient often retches, and it is quite likely that backward movements of contents across the stomach and esophagus during endoscopy bear little or no relationship to the real-life situation. This view is substantiated by the available evidence. Nasrallah *et al.* evaluated 25 patients who had bile in their stomach out of 110 patients undergoing endoscopy; increased gastric bile acid concentrations and evidence of duodenogastric reflux by scintigraphy were present in a minority of patients [56]. Stein *et al.* evaluated 135 patients undergoing endoscopy, 39 of whom had a bile lake in the stomach. Sensitivity, specificity, and positive predictive value of bile in the stomach were quite low for duodenogastric reflux as measured either with scintigraphy or with gastric pH monitoring [57].

It was also hypothesized that gastric biopsies could give a more reliable measure of duodenogastric reflux as it is known that duodenogastric reflux causes a typical form of gastritis, especially in the operated stomach, the so-called chemically induced/reactive gastritis according to the Sidney classification [4]. However, when hystopathologic findings suggestive for chemically-induced gastritis were correlated with evidence of duodenogastric reflux by the gold standard method used in the two previous studies, correlation was quite poor [56, 57]. This is not surprising because in the practical setting several issues complicate interpretation of biopsies, namely use of non-steroidal anti-inflammatory drugs which induce similar gastric damage and concomitant or previous infection with *Helicobacter pylori*.

It can be concluded therefore that both presence of bile in the stomach at endoscopy and hystopathologic features of gastric biopsies are not helpful in the assessment of DGER.

Gastric measurements

Gastric pH

Because of the alkaline nature of the duodenal contents, measurement of alkaline peaks in the acid's gastric environment seemed an attractive method for detecting duodenogastric reflux. The gastric pH environment is determined by a complex interplay of acid and mucous secretion, ingested food, swallowed saliva, regurgitated duodenal, pancreatic, and biliary secretions, and the effectiveness of the mixing evacuating the chyme. Simple measurement of alkaline episodes on gastric pH monitoring, therefore, proved inaccurate in the detection of duodenogastric reflux. Fuchs *et al.* consequently developed a scoring system based on 16 parameters of the 24-h gastric pH record, identified by regression analysis, to better estimate the presence and quantity of duodenogastric reflux on the basis of gastric pH monitoring [58]. Validation studies showed that this composite score can completely differentiate the gastric pH profile of normal volunteers from patients who have objectively proven excessive duodenogastric reflux.

Gastric aspiration

Detection of increased amounts of duodenal contents in the stomach might suggest a higher risk for DGER. However,

only half of duodenogastric reflux episodes into the antrum reach the fundus of the stomach and then all that is present in the fundus may not reflux into the esophagus. Measurements of bile acids in the stomach, in the context of DGER, should consider the above mentioned limitation. Aspiration of gastric contents with analysis for bile acids has been performed during fasting and post-prandial periods. In the fasting period, results were controversial with older studies showing no differences in bile acids concentrations between controls and GERD/Barrett's esophagus patients [59, 60] and more recent studies showing that fasting bile acid concentrations were higher in complicated (0.5 mM) compared to uncomplicated (0.24 mM) Barrett's patients, with concentrations in both groups being higher than controls (0.02 mM) [61]. In contrast, post-prandial measurements showed higher concentrations of bile acids in patients with complicated Barrett's esophagus [60].

Esophageal aspiration

Studies using esophageal aspiration techniques in humans have shown conflicting results regarding the role of DGER. On the one hand, a group of studies found no or very low concentrations of bile acids in esophageal aspirations in patients with GERD [62, 63]. On the other hand, several studies using prolonged aspiration techniques found increased esophageal bile acids in patients with GERD. Gotley *et al.* found increased amounts of conjugated bile acids in the majority (87%) of esophageal aspirates. Most bile acid reflux in that study occurred at night, with 7% of samples having bile acid concentrations above 1.0 mmol/L, the usual toxic concentration producing esophageal mucosal damage [64]. However, a later study by the same group found that esophageal aspirates of patients with esophagitis only rarely (2%) contained conjugated bile acid concentrations high enough (1.0 mmol/L) to cause esophageal mucosal damage [23].

Using prolonged ambulatory aspiration in the distal esophagus, Stein and Kauer showed that patients with GERD and Barrett's esophagus have greater and more concentrated bile acid exposure to the esophageal mucosa than normal subjects. This increased exposure occurs most commonly during the supine period while asleep and during the upright period after meals [65, 66]. These studies identified the glycine conjugates of cholic, deoxycholic, and chenodeoxycholic acids as the predominant bile acids aspirated from the esophagus of patients who have GERD.

Finally, Nehra *et al.* performed long-term (15 h) esophageal aspirations with simultaneous pH monitoring in 10 asymptomatic controls and 30 patients with GERD, including 10 with Barrett's esophagus [27]. They found significantly higher concentrations of conjugated primary bile acids, predominantly tauro and glycocholic acid, but also significantly greater proportions of the secondary conjugated bile acids, tauro- and glycol-deoxycholic acid, in patients with reflux esophagitis and Barrett's esophagus than in controls. Although bile acid reflux episodes occurred at variable pHs, a temporal relation existed between reflux of taurine conjugates and esophageal acid exposure [67].

Controversy among results is at least partly related both to methodologic differences, i.e. continuous versus intermittent aspiration and use of different methods for bile acid quantification, and to technical limitations of the aspiration technique, i.e. concentrations of bile acids refer to aspirates collected during periods of hours and not during single reflux episodes, meaning that they are a measure of the "mean concentration" and not of the "peak concentration" reached during individual reflux episodes. Nevertheless, data from the aspiration studies suggest a role for bile acids and acid in causing esophageal mucosal injury. Moreover, particularly taurine-conjugated primary (cholic acid) and secondary [deoxycholic acid (DCA)] bile acids seem important and responsible for esophageal damage.

Scintigraphy

Scintigraphic studies using ^{99m}Tc-HIDA found that DGER is a common phenomenon in normal individuals during the post-prandial period [3, 68]. However, patients with Barrett's esophagus, especially those with complicated Barrett's esophagus, have more frequent DGER detected by ^{99m}Tc-DISIDA scintigraphy than healthy volunteers [69]. Although less invasive than other methods for detecting DGER, the reliability and accuracy of scintigraphy have been challenged. Due to some technical problems, this technique can be considered a semiquantitative measure of bile reflux. The most common problem is the overlap of the small bowel and stomach, which is not correctable. Other problems include overlap of the left lobe of the liver and stomach, patient movement, and the intermittent nature of bile reflux [70].

Ambulatory pH monitoring

A few years ago it was thought that esophageal 24-h pH monitoring could be a reliable technique to study DGER, by measuring the % time at a pH of greater than 7.

Pellegrini et al. were the first to investigate both acid and alkaline reflux, defined as esophageal pH of less than 4 and greater than 7, respectively, in 100 patients with GER symptoms [71]. Normal values for both types of reflux were defined as the mean and two standard deviations of values obtained in 15 healthy volunteers. They found that 25 patients had both pathologic acid and alkaline reflux and six had pathologic alkaline reflux only. The latter group had a high incidence of severe regurgitation associated with mild symptoms of heartburn, and a higher rate of pulmonary diseases and of esophageal strictures. Attwood et al. performed 24-h esophageal pH monitoring in patients with uncomplicated and complicated (stricture, deep ulceration or dysplasia) Barrett's esophagus and compared them with esophagitis patients and normal volunteers [72]. They found

alkaline reflux (as % time pH >7) to be significantly greater in patients with complicated Barrett's esophagus. This result was confirmed in a later study [73]. In this report they measured gastric pH as well using a second electrode and documented increased gastric alkaline exposure in most of the patients who had increased esophageal alkaline exposure. From these data they suggested that prolonged exposure of the esophageal mucosa to duodenal contents may be an important factor promoting development of complications in Barrett's esophagus, including adenocarcinoma. A study by Vaezi and Richter, however, which enrolled 70 subjects—controls, and GERD patients with and without esophagitis, uncomplicated and complicated Barrett's esophagus, and found similar esophageal % time at pH greater than 7 in all groups [74].

Further studies showed that esophageal pH of greater than 7 is not a reliable marker of DGER and that other factors influence its occurrence. Penagini et al. studied patients with esophagitis, some of whom had undergone partial gastrectomy for peptic ulcer disease, using one pH electrode in the distal esophagus and a second one in the fundus of the stomach, and found similar alkaline esophageal exposure in the two groups and, above all, that elevations of esophageal pH of greater than 7 never occurred during episodes of alkalinization of gastric pH [75]. Other authors have confirmed these findings [76, 77]. In particular, Mattioli et al., using a triple-probe monitoring (probes placed in the distal esophagus, fundus, and antrum), found that alkaline reflux, defined as a rise in pH of greater than 7 from the antrum to the esophagus occurred in 0.75% of reflux episodes in 279 patients with an intact stomach [18]. Two other studies found no relationship between alkaline esophageal pH and esophageal bile acid concentration during aspiration studies in both controls and GERD patients [78, 79]. Furthermore, Champion et al. performed simultaneous 24-h esophageal pH and Bilitec monitoring in controls and patients with GERD both with and without Barrett's esophagus, including 10 after partial gastrectomy [80]. They found a poor relationship between DGER as measured with Bilitec (see next section for the technique) and % time at a pH of greater than 7 (Figure 23.5). Just et al. similarly found no relationship between overnight fasting intragastric pH and duodenogastric reflux measured with Bilitec [81]. Singh et al. performed saliva testing and pH monitoring in the proximal and distal esophagus, and in the fundus of the stomach of controls, and esophagitis and Barrett's esophagus patients [77]. They found that the three groups were similar regarding both salivary secretions, which were alkaline especially when stimulated by chewing, and alkaline proximal and distal esophageal pH, which occurred mainly during daytime when swallowing of saliva is frequent. Alkaline pH in the fundus at the time of alkaline esophageal pH was not observed. Similar results were reported by De Vault et al. [82].

Finally, a technical note needs to be mentioned. Antimony electrodes, contrary to glass electrodes which accurately evaluate pH in the alkaline range, are sensitive to oxygen, especially at low oxygen tension such as at the surface of the esophageal mucosa, and give false alkaline readings due to oxygen corrosion [83]. Some of the above mentioned studies used antimony electrodes [72, 73, 75, 78, 81, 82]

and the report of Pellegrini *et al.* did not mention the type of electrode used [71]. It is therefore conceivable that the time of alkaline pH in the esophagus was often overestimated.

From a review of the literature, it can therefore be concluded that an alkaline esophageal pH should not be used as a marker of DGER.

Ambulatory bilirubin monitoring (Bilitec)

In 1993 a fiberoptic sensor was developed (Bilitec 2000), which uses the optical properties of bilirubin, the most common bile pigment [84]. Bilirubin has a characteristic spectrophotometric absorption band at 450 nm. The working principle of this instrument is that absorption near this wavelength implies the presence of bilirubin and, therefore, represents DGER (Figure 23.6).

This system, resembling a standard ambulatory pH unit, consists of a miniaturized fiberoptic probe, which carries light signals into the tip and back to the optoelectronic system via a plastic bundle. The Teflon probe head is 9.5 mm in length and 4 mm in diameter. There is a 2-mm open groove in the probe across which two wavelengths of light are emitted and intraluminal material sampled. Two light-emitting diodes at 470 and 565 nm represent the source for the measurement of bilirubin and the reference signal, respectively. The portable photodiode system converts the light into an electrical signal. After amplification, the signals are processed by an integrated microcomputer, and the difference in absorption between the two diodes is calculated, representing absorption of the intraluminal liquid. Sampling frequency is 0.125 Hz; the software averages between the absorbance over two successive samples in order to decrease the noise of the measurements.

A good correlation has been shown between Bilitec readings and bile acid concentrations measured by gastric or esophageal aspiration studies [84–87]. However, it should be remembered that the Bilitec is only a semiquantitative

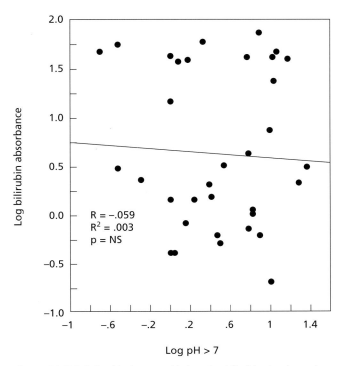

Figure 23.5 Relationship between % time that bilirubin absorbance is above 0.14 (a marker of bile reflux) and esophageal pH above 7 in a group of healthy controls, patients with gastroesophageal reflux disease, and those with Barrett's esophagus (reproduced from Champion *et al.* [80]).

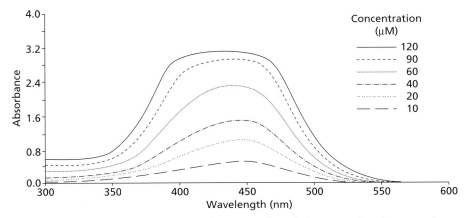

Figure 23.6 Laboratory spectrophotometric absorbance for bilirubin ditaurate in saline solution at pH 7.5 and concentrations ranging from 10 to 120 µm (reproduced from Vaezi *et al.* [87]).

method for detection of DGER and that it has several limitations (for interpretation of results). First, a variety of substances may result in false-positive readings which substantially alter the results of the test [87, 88]. They include heme (i.e. blood)-contaminated gastric contents, porphyrins, carotenoids, riboflavin, and many food products, such as tomatoes, bananas, carrots, beets, parmesan cheese, minestrone, beef, tea, and coffee. Additionally, solid food may clog the probe tip and markedly decrease accuracy of recordings [89]. Therefore studies have been performed with standardized liquid formulae. This implies two kinds of limitations with regards to the recorded pattern of gastroesophageal reflux compared to the one occurring in everyday life: one is that patients eat a diet different from their usual one and often of lower caloric content; the other one is that liquid meals empty from the stomach differently from the mixed solid–liquid meals of everyday life. Second, DGER is underestimated by at least 30% in an acidic medium (pH <3.5). In solution with a pH of less than 3.5 bilirubin undergoes monomer to dimer isomerization, which is reflected by the shift in the absorption wavelength from 453to 400nm. Since Bilitec readings are based on detection of absorption at 470nm, this shift results in underestimation of the degree of DGER [87]. Therefore, Bilitec measurement should always be accompanied by simultaneous measurement of esophageal acid exposure using 24-h pH monitoring.

Despite its limitations, Bilitec has been an important advance in the assessment of DGER and of its relevance in the clinical setting. DGER data are usually measured as % time at bilirubin absorbance greater than 0.14 (Figure 23.7),

although a cut-off of 0.2 has also been used [90, 91], and can be analyzed separately for total, upright, and supine periods. Normal values have been established [74, 89, 90].

Studies using combined esophageal pH and Bilitec monitoring have investigated the role of DGER in the development of esophageal lesions, i.e. esophagitis, and Barrett's esophagus and its complications, and in occurrence of reflux symptoms. Champion et al. studied four groups of subjects, i.e. healthy volunteers, reflux patients, Barrett's esophagus patients, and patients with esophageal symptoms after partial gastrectomy [80]. They reported two important findings: first that DGER increased significantly with the severity of reflux disease, being greatest in patients with Barrett's esophagus and comparable to that of patients with partial gastrectomy. Second, that there was a close association between total % time at pH of less than 4 and the amount of DGER (r = 0.78) (Figure 23.8). These findings were confirmed by studies from other groups. Kauer et al. found that patients with Barrett's esophagus had bilirubin exposures greater than those of the other GERD patients irrespective of esophagitis [90]. They also found that the majority of "bile reflux episodes" occurred when the pH of the esophagus was between 4 and 7. They remarked that at this pH range bile acids are more damaging because they are non-ionized, and they suggested that continuous PPI use may be detrimental by enhancing the effect of bile on cell proliferation and by promoting development of Barrett's esophagus and esophageal adenocarcinoma. This hypothesis is, however, not substantiated by epidemiologic studies showing on the one hand that long-term PPI use decreases incidence of dysplasia

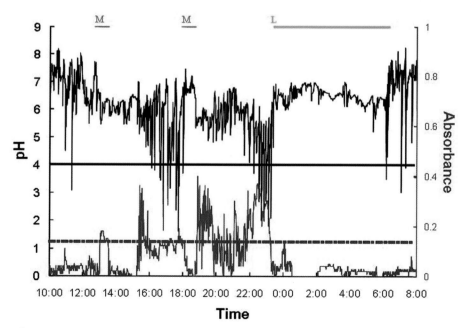

Figure 23.7 Typical pH–Bilitec recording. Upper tracing from pH-metry shows upright acid reflux episodes associated with increased bilirubin absorbance to greater than 0.14.

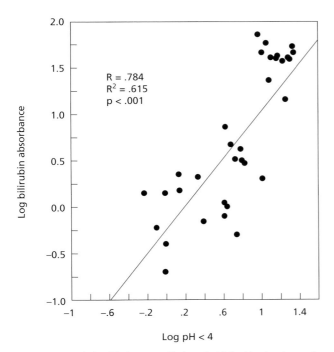

Figure 23.8 Relationship between % time that bilirubin absorbance is above 0.14 (a marker of bile reflux) and esophageal pH below 4 in a group of healthy controls, patients with gastroesophageal reflux disease, and those with Barrett's esophagus (reproduced from Champion *et al.* [80]).

in patients with Barrett's esophagus [92, 93] and on the other that prevalence of partial gastrectomy is not higher in patients with Barrett's esophagus or esophageal adenocarcinoma compared to controls (as mentioned above). Vaezi *et al.* studied both uncomplicated and complicated Barrett's esophagus and found that both bilirubin and acid exposure were significantly higher in complicated Barrett's esophagus compared to uncomplicated Barrett's esophagus [74] (Figure 23.9). Patients with complicated Barrett's esophagus had also higher fasting bile acid concentrations in the stomach. These authors did not confirm the weakly acidic nature of DGER episodes, reporting that the vast majority had a pH of less than 4. Similar findings were reported using simultaneous impedance–pH–Bilitec recordings [94]. Zaninotto *et al.* investigated patients with Barrett's esophagus of different lengths—long, short, and ultra-short—in comparison with GERD patients and healthy volunteers, and found bilirubin exposure to be particularly high in patients with long-segment Barrett's esophagus [91]. Stepwise logistic regression showed that increased bilirubin exposure, low LES pressure, advancing age, and male sex were the variables predicting long-segment Barrett's esophagus. Studies in patients with esophageal symptoms and partial gastrectomy for peptic ulcer disease gave further insight into the contribution of DGER in determining esophageal lesions. Sears *et al.* studied 13 patients and found that esophagitis was

present in those who had mixed acid and DGER, but not in those with DGER alone, suggesting that DGER by itself has low potential to induce lesions [95]. Vaezi and Richter confirmed these results in a larger series of patients (n = 32): 28% had mixed acid reflux and DGER, 50% had DGER only, and 22% had neither [96]. Esophagitis was present only in the group with mixed reflux.

Different results have been obtained in selected groups of patients. Tack *et al.*, studying PPI refractory patients, found that patients with persistent erosive esophagitis had significantly higher DGER episodes and a longer exposure to DGER, especially in the supine period, whereas the acid reflux parameters were similar those for endoscopy-negative patients [97] (Figure 23.10). Another study by Wilmer *et al.* looked at 25 mechanically ventilated patients in intensive care with a nasogastric tube and intravenous ranitidine therapy [98]. No patient had a previous history of GERD. After 5 days of mechanical ventilation, 12 had esophagitis, two pathologic acid reflux, and 12 pathologic DGER. The presence of esophagitis was significantly associated with pathologic DGER ($P = .017$) and the severity of esophagitis correlated with the gastric residual volume and with increasing DGER. These data strongly suggest that DGER alone can cause esophageal injury, at least in particular clinical settings.

Impedance–pH monitoring

This technique is based on measurement of electrical impedance between closely arranged electrodes mounted on an intraluminal probe. The measured impedance depends on the luminal contents surrounding the electrodes. When the esophagus is empty, the measured impedance reflects the conductivity of the esophageal mucosa. With multiple pairs of impedance rings along the length of the esophagus, temporal–spatial patterns of impedance changes allow the differentiation of swallowed and refluxed liquid or air. Liquid gastroesophageal reflux is detected as an orally progressing decrease in impedance, beginning at the LES [99]. A recent consensus report provided a detailed nomenclature for reflux patterns detected by impedance pH monitoring. An impedance-detected reflux is defined as acid when the esophageal pH falls to below 4, or when reflux occurs with the esophageal pH already below 4. When the esophageal pH falls by greater than 1 unit, but remains below 4, it is considered "weakly acidic reflux." The term "weakly alkaline reflux" is reserved for reflux episodes during which the esophageal pH increases to greater than 7 [100] (Figure 23.11). An alternative clinical classification prevalent in much of the literature considers acid (nadir pH <4) or non-acid (nadir pH >4) reflux, with non-acid reflux further separated into weakly acidic (nadir pH 4–7) or weakly alkaline (nadir pH >7).

Ambulatory impedance–pH studies suggest that patients with moderate and severe esophagitis have rates of weakly acidic reflux similar to or slightly greater than those in healthy

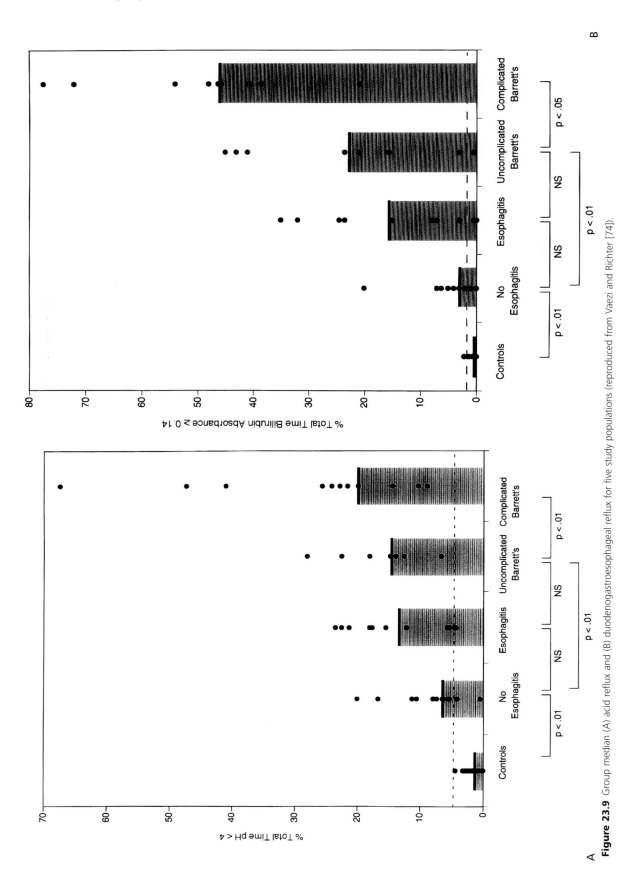

Figure 23.9 Group median (A) acid reflux and (B) duodenogastroesophageal reflux for five study populations (reproduced from Vaezi and Richter [74]).

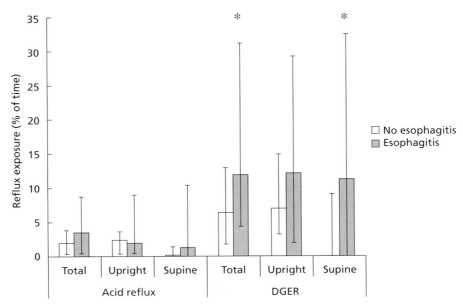

Figure 23.10 Acid exposure and duodenogastroesophageal reflux (DGER) in 65 patients with typical reflux symptoms poorly responsive to standard doses of proton pump inhibitor, according to the absence or presence of esophagitis. Compared to patients without esophagitis, patients with persistent esophagitis had significantly higher DGER exposure (reproduced from Tack *et al.* [97]).

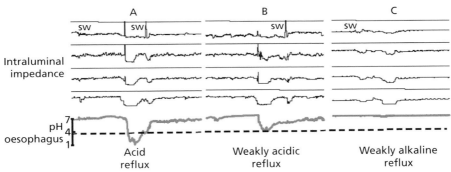

Figure 23.11 Gastroesophageal reflux is detected by impedance and defined by based on the pH of the refluxate. (A) Acid reflux is defined as reflux that reduces esophageal pH to below 4, or reflux that occurs when esophageal pH is already below 4. (B) Weakly acidic reflux is defined as a pH fall of at least one unit but the pH does not fall below 4. (C) Weakly alkaline reflux is defined as a reflux episode during which nadir esophageal pH does not drop below 7 (reproduced from Sifrim *et al.* [100]).

controls. Furthermore, distal esophageal exposure to weakly acidic refluxate is similar in esophagitis and NERD patients.

Does weakly acidic reflux contain duodenopancreatic material? Ambulatory esophageal aspiration studies have suggested that duodenogastric reflux is a physiologic phenomenon occurring mainly post prandially and at night [101]. Therefore, one should expect to detect bile in most post-prandial weakly acidic reflux events. However, studies using pH–Bilitec recordings have shown that most DGER events occur in an acid setting, with esophageal luminal pH below 4. Furthermore, in normal subjects, weakly acidic reflux is frequent, whereas DGER is rare [61, 74]. It should

be emphasized that weakly acidic reflux is not synonymous with bile reflux, which does provoke esophagitis in combination with acid. Bile reflux probably accounts for only 10–15% of weakly acidic and weakly alkaline reflux. A recent study using simultaneous Bilitec and impedance monitoring showed no correlation between the % time of bilirubin absorbance and weakly acidic or weakly alkaline reflux parameters [94]. To the contrary, the majority of bile reflux events occurred concomitantly with acid reflux [61, 67, 74] (Figure 23.12).

It is possible that differences in mixing and distribution of post-prandial gastric contents might explain the occurrence

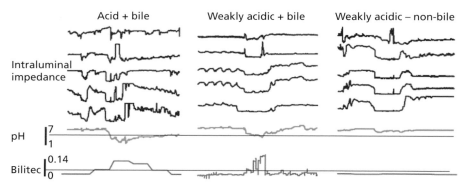

Figure 23.12 Simultaneous impedance–pH–Bilitec recordings: esophageal bilirubin concentration monitoring adds information about the chemical nature of acid and non-acid material that refluxes into the esophagus. Weakly acidic and weakly alkaline reflux may or may not include duodenal contents. The majority of bile reflux events occur concomitantly with acid reflux.

of either weakly acidic reflux with little or no bilio-pancreatic secretion or acid DGER containing a significant concentration of bile acids. Therefore, a clear distinction should be made between (1) weakly acidic reflux events occurring in the post-prandial period of healthy subjects or in patients with GERD, especially those on PPIs; and (2) acid DGER events detected with pH–Bilitec and occurring predominantly in patients with moderate and severe GERD.

Duodenogastroesophageal reflux and symptoms

A few studies have looked at the relevance of DGER in the perception of the symptoms complained of by GERD patients. Marshall *et al.* studied 59 patients with typical reflux symptoms, divided them into those with pathologic and those with normal acid exposure, and found that only 6% of symptomatic events in both groups were related to DGER versus 41% and 23% related to acid reflux in the pathologic and normal acid reflux groups, respectively [102]. Similar ambulatory monitoring studies by Koek *et al.* in patients with GERD "off" acid-suppressive therapy demonstrated that reflux symptoms are mainly related to acid reflux, or to mixed acid and bile acid reflux events; fewer than 10% of reflux episodes are related to bile reflux alone [103] (Figure 23.13). The role of DGER in the generation of persistent symptoms in patients "on" PPIs remains controversial. Initial studies by the Leuven group suggested a significant role for DGER in PPI refractoriness. When patients with persistent reflux symptoms despite PPI therapy were studied "on" PPI, there was a higher prevalence of DGER (64%) than of acid reflux (37%) [104, 105]. Tack *et al.* studied 65 patients with persistent typical symptoms and found DGER alone to be rather important, being related to 18% of symptomatic episodes versus 7% of acid and 10% of mixed reflux episodes [97]. Karamanolis *et al.* looked at a more heterogeneous group of patients (n = 184), only

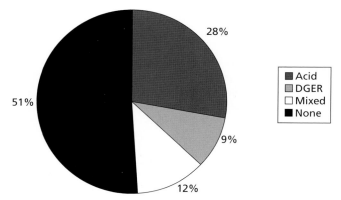

Figure 23.13 Reflux-associated symptom episodes in 72 patients: 165 symptom episodes occurred during acid reflux, 38 during bile reflux, 84 during combined reflux, and 257 in the absence of pathologic reflux. DGER, duodenogastroesophageal reflux (reproduced from Koek *et al.* [103]).

53% of whom had typical symptoms, and found DGER alone to be related to 4% of 415 symptomatic episodes versus 10% for acid reflux and 17% for mixed reflux episodes [106]. More recently, Gasiorowska *et al.* studied a similar group of patients (n = 24), but found DGER alone to be of lesser relevance, being related to 9% of symptom events versus 32% of acid and 32% of mixed reflux episodes [107].

DGER was more frequently responsible for symptoms when reflux patients with partial gastrectomy were studied: on 33% and 24% of the occasions, respectively, versus 65% and 69% for mixed reflux patients [95, 96].

To assess the causative role of bile acids in esophageal symptoms, Siddiqui *et al.* performed a modified Bernstein acid-infusion test (with 0.1 M HCl), and esophageal barostat balloon distentions, in healthy individuals and patients with NERD. The same procedure was repeated with infusions of chenodeoxycholic acid and ursodeoxycholic acid at doses of both 2 mM and 5 mM. These infusions were separated by at least 7 days. The volume of bile acid infused and length of time from onset of infusion to pain occurrence were compared for the three different substances. The pain thresholds (with regard to both volume and time) for ursodeoxycholic acid were significantly higher than for chenodeoxycholic acid, the pain thresholds of which were, in turn, higher than for acid infusion [108].

Findings from these studies provide evidence for a potential contribution of bile acids in the generation of esophageal symptoms, and the differing effects of bile salts in the generation of esophageal pain. It can be concluded that DGER alone may be responsible for symptoms, although its relevance appear less than that of acid.

Medical and surgical treatment

At present there are no drugs that specifically reduce DGER. It is, however, well established that inhibition of acid secretion with PPIs, besides decreasing acid reflux, decreases DGER as well, as measured by Bilitec. The first report came from Champion *et al.* in 1994 [80]. The authors studied nine patients with severe GERD (including six with Barrett's esophagus) and found that omeprazole 20 mg bid markedly decreased both acid and DGER (Figure 23.14). Further reports evaluating the effect of omeprazole or pantoprazole studied a total of 103 patients with either erosive esophagitis or Barrett's esophagus; all of them confirmed the first report, showing normalization of DGER in most patients [80, 109–113]. In one of these studies, however, performed in 25 patients with Barrett's esophagus on 40–60 mg of omeprazole/day, normalization of esophageal acid exposure did not guarantee control of pathologic DGER [113]; 20 of the patients had a normal 24-h pH profile and 11 still had pathologic DGER. Similarly, a report on 184 PPI refractory patients, most of whom were endoscopy negative and studied while on PPI once daily, found that ongoing pathologic acid exposure was present in only 27% of the patients, whereas pathologic DGER was found in 62% of them, of whom 40% had normal and 22% had pathologic acid reflux [106].

The likely mechanism whereby PPIs decrease DGER is a marked decrease in the volume of gastric secretions [114, 115], which means there is less gastric content available to reflux into the esophagus. These data have important implications, suggesting that PPIs are an effective treatment not only for acid, but also for bile reflux.

An advance in medical treatment which could potentially be particularly efficient in decreasing DGER is the development of drugs that decrease the rate of transient LES relaxation. Transient LES relaxation is a spontaneous and prolonged relaxation of the LES, stimulated by distention of the proximal stomach, through which most reflux episodes occur [1]. Inhibition of transient LES relaxation results in a decrease of both acid and weakly acidic reflux episodes [116]. This is an area of ongoing research with several drugs being developed [117]. Preliminary data are promising [118, 119]. A study has recently addressed control of DGER by this pharmacologic strategy [104]. Baclofen, a GABA$_B$ agonist currently used by neurologists to treat spasticity, has been evaluated in 16 patients with persistent heartburn or regurgitation and ongoing pathological DGER in spite of PPI therapy. Under PPI alone all patients had normal acid exposure, but pathologic duodenal reflux exposure as measured by Bilitec. After the addition of baclofen 20 mg tid, both duodenal reflux and severity of reflux symptoms

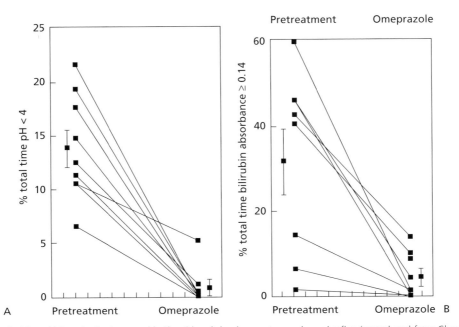

Figure 23.14 Omeprazole 20 mg bid markedly decreased both acid and duodenogastroesophageal reflux (reproduced from Champion *et al.* [80]).

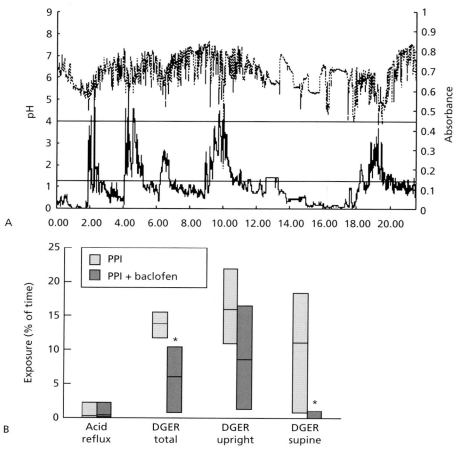

Figure 23.15 (A) Combined pH and Bilitec monitoring in a patient with typical reflux symptoms during omeprazole 20 mg twice daily treatment, showing normal acid exposure and pathologic duodenal reflux exposure. (B) Acid and duodenal reflux exposure during treatment with omeprazole 20 mg twice daily and during omeprazole 20 mg twice daily (PPI) plus baclofen 20 mg three times daily (reproduced from Koek *et al.* [104]).

significantly decreased (Figure 23.15). It should be stressed, however, that this study represents a proof of concept and not a current therapeutic option as baclofen crosses the blood–brain barrier and consequently has side effects (i.e. drowsiness, tiredness, nausea), preventing its use in routine clinical practice. More data are awaited with drugs devoid of central nervous system side effects.

Surgical treatment has been shown to be quite effective in decreasing DGER, at least in the short term. Stein *et al.* compared the effect of Nissen fundoplication 3–12 months after the operation to omeprazole 20 mg bid and found that duodenal reflux exposure was normalized in 15 of 16 GERD patients in the first group and nine of 15 patients in the second group, concluding that surgery is more effective than medical treatment [112].

Even considering the minority of patients with previous partial gastrectomy who suffer from reflux symptoms, it is important to be aware that gastric acid secretion is still present in some of these patients [120] and that acid reflux

is an important determinant of symptoms. Vaezi *et al.* have shown that in 32 patients with partial gastrectomy and upper gastrointestinal symptoms, 92% of heartburn and 89% of regurgitation episodes were associated with mixed acid and DGER reflux, suggesting that PPIs should be the first choice in these patients as well [96]. Theoretically, use of a prokinetic drug is also appealing. Vaezi *et al.* performed a placebo-controlled trial of cisapride in 10 patients with partial gastrectomy and found that it significantly decreased DGER and overall, improved symptoms in 70% of the patients compared to 10% of those given placebo [121]. Abdominal pain, regurgitation, and belching remained improved during a 4-month open-labeled treatment. Unfortunately, cisapride is no longer on the market; nevertheless these results suggest that a future prokinetic drug is a valid option or add-on therapy to PPIs. Before the advent of PPIs, Roux-en-Y gastrojejunostomy was often advocated in cases of severe enterogastric reflux (bile reflux gastritis) because there was no convincing evidence that antacids, H_2 antagonists, cytoprotective agents or bile salt absorbents were effective [122]. However, this surgical option should now be indicated with caution because it has been shown in the long term that 36% of patients were unsatisfied with the results of surgery, mainly because of Roux stasis syndrome [123].

Conclusions

Experimental and clinical evidence supports the importance of acid and pepsin in causing esophageal symptoms and mucosal injury, including Barrett's esophagus. However, it is clear that duodenal contents in the refluxate contribute to esophageal mucosal damage and symptoms. Experimental data have shown that pulsed exposure to acid or conjugated bile acids may contribute to the proliferative alterations and the molecular changes that are observed in Barrett's esophagus, and, in turn, play a key role in cancer development. Studies using aspiration and Bilitec measurements demonstrate that duodenal contents are often present in the esophageal refluxate. The degree of esophageal exposure to acid and DGER showed a graded increase from controls to esophagitis patients, with the highest value observed in patients with Barrett's esophagus. In conclusion, the predominant pathogenetic stimulus that causes Barrett's esophagus is still unclear. It is still an enigma as to why only a fraction of patients with GERD develop Barrett's esophagus and what factors of the refluxate (acid and/or bile) initiate metaplasia and/or promote carcinogenesis. The evidence thus far suggests that, for patients with Barrett's esophagus, both acid and bile may be harmful. There is insufficient evidence to date suggesting that either acid or bile is less harmful than the other and can be left untreated.

Added to their role in the pathogenesis of esophagitis and Barrett's esophagus, recent studies have demonstrated the involvement of bile acids in the development of subtle esophageal microscopic changes, such as DISs, which are frequently observed in biopsies from patients with NERD. Furthermore, DGER and bile acids can also be involved in the pathophysiology of extraesophageal GERD syndromes, particularly those associated with microaspiration of the airways.

Various direct and indirect methodologies are employed for measuring DGER, with ambulatory pH–bilirubin monitoring the most useful to identify increased esophageal exposure to duodenal contents.

Acid suppression with PPIs decreases both acid and DGER, perhaps by decreasing the volume of gastric contents available to reflux into the esophagus. Furthermore, the high intragastric and intraesophageal pH environment produced by PPIs inactivates conjugated bile acids, the main DGER ingredients implicated in causing esophagitis. Furthermore, baclofen-like drugs to reduce transient LES relaxations and new and more effective prokinetics to accelerate gastric emptying will probably become available to reduce or abolish DGER in patients with incomplete response to PPIs.

References

1. Mittal RK, Holloway RH, Penagini R, Blackshaw LA, Dent J. Transient lower esophageal sphincter relaxation. *Gastroenterology* 1995;109:601–610.
2. King PM, Pryde A, Heading RC. Transpyloric fluid movement and antroduodenal motility in patients with gastro-oesophageal reflux. *Gut* 1987;28:545–548.
3. Muller-Lissner SA, Fimmel CJ, Sonnenberg A, *et al.* Novel approach to quantify duodenogastric reflux in healthy volunteers and in patients with type I gastric ulcer. *Gut* 1983;24:510–518.
4. Dixon MF, Genta RM, Yardley JH, Correa P. Classification and grading of gastritis. The updated Sydney System. International Workshop on the Histopathology of Gastritis, Houston 1994. *Am J Surg Pathol* 1996;20:1161–1181.
5. Redo SF, Barnes WA, De La Sierra AO. Perfusion of the canine esophagus with secretions of the upper gastro-intestinal tract. *Ann Surg* 1959;149:556–564.
6. Goldberg HI, Dodds WJ, Gee S, Montgomery C, Zboralske FF. Role of acid and pepsin in acute experimental esophagitis. *Gastroenterology* 1969;56:223–230.
7. Zhang X, Geboes K, Depoortere I, Tack J, Janssens J, Sifrim D. Effect of repeated cycles of acute esophagitis and healing on esophageal peristalsis, tone, and length. *Am J Physiol Gastrointest Liver Physiol* 2005;288:G1339–1346.
8. Lillemoe KD, Johnson LF, Harmon JW. Role of the components of the gastroduodenal contents in experimental acid esophagitis. *Surgery* 1982;92:276–284.
9. Farre R, van MH, De VR, *et al.* Short exposure of oesophageal mucosa to bile acids, both in acidic and weakly acidic conditions, can impair mucosal integrity and provoke dilated intercellular spaces. *Gut* 2008;57:1366–1374.
10. Roberts NB. Review article: human pepsins—their multiplicity, function and role in reflux disease. *Aliment Pharmacol Ther* 2006;24 (Suppl 2):2–9.
11. Carney CN, Orlando RC, Powell DW, Dotson MM. Morphologic alterations in early acid-induced epithelial injury of the rabbit esophagus. *Lab Invest* 1981;45:198–208.
12. Orlando RC, Powell DW, Carney CN. Pathophysiology of acute acid injury in rabbit esophageal epithelium. *J Clin Invest* 1981;68:286–293.
13. Aylwin JA. The physiological basis of reflux oesophagitis in sliding hiatal diaphragmatic hernia. *Thorax* 1953;8:38–45.
14. Tuttle SG, Rufin F, Bettarello A. The physiology of heartburn. *Ann Intern Med* 1961;55:292–300.
15. Demeester TR, Wang CI, Wernly JA, *et al.* Technique, indications, and clinical use of 24 hour esophageal pH monitoring. *J Thorac Cardiovasc Surg* 1980;79:656–670.
16. Robertson D, Aldersley M, Shepherd H, Smith CL. Patterns of acid reflux in complicated oesophagitis. *Gut* 1987;28:1484–1488.
17. Frazzoni M, De ME, Savarino V. Different patterns of oesophageal acid exposure distinguish complicated reflux disease

from either erosive reflux oesophagitis or non-erosive reflux disease. *Aliment Pharmacol Ther* 2003;18:1091–1098.

18. Pandolfino JE, Richter JE, Ours T, Guardino JM, Chapman J, Kahrilas PJ. Ambulatory esophageal pH monitoring using a wireless system 1. *Am J Gastroenterol* 2003;98:740–749.

19. Wenner J, Johansson J, Johnsson F, Oberg S. Optimal thresholds and discriminatory power of 48-h wireless esophageal pH monitoring in the diagnosisof GERD. *Am J Gastroenterol* 2007;102:1862–1869.

20. Stein HJ, Hoeft S, Demeester TR. Functional foregut abnormalities in Barrett's esophagus. *J Thorac Cardiovasc Surg* 1993;105:107–111.

21. Miller LS, Vinayek R, Frucht H, Gardner JD, Jensen RT, Maton PN. Reflux esophagitis in patients with Zollinger-Ellison syndrome. *Gastroenterology* 1990;98:341–346.

22. Lillemoe KD, Johnson LF, Harmon JW. Alkaline esophagitis: a comparison of the ability of components of gastroduodenal contents to injure the rabbit esophagus. *Gastroenterology* 1983;85:621–628.

23. Gotley DC, Morgan AP, Ball D, Owen RW, Cooper MJ. Composition of gastro-oesophageal refluxate. *Gut* 1991;32:1093–1099.

24. Avidan B, Sonnenberg A, Schnell TG, Sontag SJ. Acid reflux is a poor predictor for severity of erosive reflux esophagitis. *Dig Dis Sci* 2002;47:2565–2573.

25. Smith JL, Opekun AR, Larkai E, Graham DY. Sensitivity of the esophageal mucosa to pH in gastroesophageal reflux disease. *Gastroenterology* 1989;96:683–689.

26. Bredenoord AJ, Weusten BL, Curvers WL, Timmer R, Smout AJ. Determinants of perception of heartburn and regurgitation. *Gut* 2006;55:313–318.

27. Miettinen TA, Peltokallio P. Bile salt, fat, water, and vitamin B 12 excretion after ileostomy. *Scand J Gastroenterol* 1971;6:543–552.

28. Barthlen WL. Influence of pH on bile acid concentration in human, pig and commercial bile: implications for alkaline gastro-esophageal reflux. *Dis Esophagus* 1994;7:127–130.

29. Jankowski JA, Harrison RF, Perry I, Balkwill F, Tselepis C. Barrett's metaplasia. *Lancet* 2000;356:2079–2085.

30. Theisen J, Peters JH, Stein HJ. Experimental evidence for mutagenic potential of duodenogastric juice on Barrett's esophagus. *World J Surg* 2003;27:1018–1020.

31. Moffat RC, Berkas EM. Bile esophagitis. *Arch Surg* 1965;91:963–966.

32. Bremner CG, Lynch VP, Ellis FH Jr. Barrett's esophagus: congenital or acquired? An experimental study of esophageal mucosal regeneration in the dog. *Surgery* 1970;68:209–216.

33. Gillen P, Keeling P, Byrne PJ, West AB, Hennessy TP. Experimental columnar metaplasia in the canine oesophagus. *Br J Surg* 1988;75:113–115.

34. Clark GW, Smyrk TC, Mirvish SS, *et al*. Effect of gastroduodenal juice and dietary fat on the development of Barrett's esophagus and esophageal neoplasia: an experimental rat model. *Ann Surg Oncol* 1994;1:252–261.

35. Ireland AP, Peters JH, Smyrk TC, *et al*. Gastric juice protects against the development of esophageal adenocarcinoma in the rat. *Ann Surg* 1996;224:358–370.

36. Miwa K, Sahara H, Segawa M, *et al*. Reflux of duodenal or gastro-duodenal contents induces esophageal carcinoma in rats. *Int J Cancer* 1996;67:269–274.

37. Avidan B, Sonnenberg A, Schnell TG, Sontag SJ. Gastric surgery is not a risk for Barrett's esophagus or esophageal adenocarcinoma. *Gastroenterology* 2001;121:1281–1285.

38. Birgisson S, Rice TW, Easley KA, Richter JE. The lack of association between adenocarcinoma of the esophagus and gastric surgery: a retrospective study. *Am J Gastroenterol* 1997;92:216–221.

39. Taha AS, Angerson WJ, Morran CG. Reflux and Barrett's oesophagitis after gastric surgery—long-term follow-up and implications for the roles of gastric acid and bile in oesophagitis. *Aliment Pharmacol Ther* 2003;17:547–552.

40. Fitzgerald RC, Omary MB, Triadafilopoulos G. Dynamic effects of acid on Barrett's esophagus. An ex vivo proliferation and differentiation model. *J Clin Invest* 1996;98:2120–2128.

41. Kaur BS, Ouatu-Lascar R, Omary MB, Triadafilopoulos G. Bile salts induce or blunt cell proliferation in Barrett's esophagus in an acid-dependent fashion. *Am J Physiol Gastrointest Liver Physiol* 2000;278:G1000–1009.

42. Shirvani VN, Ouatu-Lascar R, Kaur BS, Omary MB, Triadafilopoulos G. Cyclooxygenase 2 expression in Barrett's esophagus and adenocarcinoma: Ex vivo induction by bile salts and acid exposure. *Gastroenterology* 2000;118:487–496.

43. Kaur BS, Triadafilopoulos G. Acid- and bile-induced PGE(2) release and hyperproliferation in Barrett's esophagus are COX-2 and PKC-epsilon dependent. *Am J Physiol Gastrointest Liver Physiol* 2002;283:G327–334.

44. Batzri S, Harmon JW, Schweitzer EJ, Toles R. Bile acid accumulation in gastric mucosal cells. *Proc Soc Exp Biol Med* 1991;197:393–399.

45. Schweitzer EJ, Harmon JW, Bass BL, Batzri S. Bile acid efflux precedes mucosal barrier disruption in the rabbit esophagus. *Am J Physiol* 1984;247:G480–485.

46. Farre R, Fornari F, Blondeau K, *et al*. Acid and weakly acidic solutions impair mucosal integrity of distal exposed and proximal non-exposed human oesophagus. *Gut* 2010;59:164–169.

47. Farre R. Dilated intercellular spaces (DIS) are associated with released of Substance P after exposure of esophageal mucosa to bile acids. *Gastroenterology* 2010;134:A74.

48. Farre R, Cardozo L, Blondeau K. Esophageal mucosal damage induced by weakly acidic solutions containing unconjugated bile acids, similar to reflux in GERD patients "on" PPI, can be prevented with anti-oxidants. *Gastroenterology* 2009:136:5; A16.

49. Adhami TAdhami T, Goldblum JR, Richter JE, Vaezi MF. The role of gastric and duodenal agents in laryngeal injury: an experimental canine model. *Am J Gastroenterol* 2004; 99:2098–2106.

50. D'Ovidio F, Mura M, Tsang M, *et al*. Bile acid aspiration and the development of bronchiolitis obliterans after lung transplantation. *J Thorac Cardiovasc Surg* 2005;129:1144–1152.

51. Blondeau K, Mertens V, Vanaudenaerde BA, *et al*. Gastro-oesophageal reflux and gastric aspiration in lung transplant patients with or without chronic rejection. *Eur Respir J* 2008;31:707–713.

52. Blondeau K, Dupont LJ, Mertens V, *et al*. Gastro-oesophageal reflux and aspiration of gastric contents in adult patients with cystic fibrosis. *Gut* 2008;57:1049–1055.

53. Blondeau K, Mertens V, Vanaudenaerde BA, *et al.* Nocturnal weakly acidic reflux promotes aspiration of bile acids in lung transplant recipients. *J Heart Lung Transplant* 2009;28:141–148.

54. Vos R, Blondeau K, Vanaudenaerde BM, *et al.* Airway colonization and gastric aspiration after lung transplantation: do birds of a feather flock together? *J Heart Lung Transplant* 2008;27:843–849.

55. D'Ovidio F, Mura M, Ridsdale R, *et al.* The effect of reflux and bile acid aspiration on the lung allograft and its surfactant and innate immunity molecules SP-A and SP-D. *Am J Transplant* 2006;6:1930–1938.

56. Nasrallah SM, Johnston GS, Gadacz TR, Kim KM. The significance of gastric bile reflux seen at endoscopy. *J Clin Gastroenterol* 1987;9:514–517.

57. Stein HJ, Smyrk TC, Demeester TR, Rouse J, Hinder RA. Clinical value of endoscopy and histology in the diagnosis of duodenogastric reflux disease. *Surgery* 1992;112:796–803.

58. Fuchs KH, Fein M, Maroske J, Heimbucher J, Freys SM. The role of 24-hr gastric pH-monitoring in the interpretation of 24-hr gastric bile monitoring for duodenogastric reflux. *Hepatogastroenterology* 1999;46:60–65.

59. Kaye MD, Showalter JP. Pyloric incompetence in patients with symptomatic gastroesophageal reflux. *J Lab Clin Med* 1974;83:198–206.

60. Gillen P, Keeling P, Byrne PJ, Healy M, O'Moore RR, Hennessy TP. Implication of duodenogastric reflux in the pathogenesis of Barrett's oesophagus. *Br J Surg* 1988;75:540–543.

61. Vaezi MF, Richter JE. Synergism of acid and duodenogastro-esophageal reflux in complicated Barrett's esophagus. *Surgery* 1995;117:699–704.

62. Johnsson F, Joelsson B, Floren CH, Nilsson A. Bile salts in the esophagus of patients with esophagitis. *Scand J Gastroenterol* 1988;23:712–716.

63. Mittal RK, Reuben A, Whitney JO, McCallum RW. Do bile acids reflux into the esophagus? A study in normal subjects and patients with gastroesophageal reflux disease. *Gastroenterology* 1987;92:371–375.

64. Gotley DC, Morgan AP, Cooper MJ. Bile acid concentrations in the refluxate of patients with reflux oesophagitis. *Br J Surg* 1988;75:587–590.

65. Kauer WK, Peters JH, Demeester TR, *et al.* Composition and concentration of bile acid reflux into the esophagus of patients with gastroesophageal reflux disease. *Surgery* 1997;122:874–881.

66. Stein HJ, Feussner H, Kauer W, Demeester TR, Siewert JR. Alkaline gastroesophageal reflux: assessment by ambulatory esophageal aspiration and pH monitoring. *Am J Surg* 1994;167:163–168.

67. Nehra D, Howell P, Williams CP, Pye JK, Beynon J. Toxic bile acids in gastro-oesophageal reflux disease: influence of gastric acidity. *Gut* 1999;44:598–602.

68. Matikainen M, Taavitsainen M, Kalima TV. Duodenogastric reflux in patients with heartburn and oesophagitis. *Scand J Gastroenterol* 1981;16:253–255.

69. Liron R, Parrilla P, Martinez de Haro LF, *et al.* Quantification of duodenogastric reflux in Barrett's esophagus. *Am J Gastroenterol* 1997;92:32–36.

70. Drane WE, Karvelis K, Johnson DA, Silverman ED. Scintigraphic evaluation of duodenogastric reflux. Problems, pitfalls, and technical review. *Clin Nucl Med* 1987;12:377–384.

71. Pellegrini CA, Demeester TR, Wernly JA, Johnson LF, Skinner DB. Alkaline gastroesophageal reflux. *Am J Surg* 1978;135:177–184.

72. Attwood SE, Demeester TR, Bremner CG, Barlow AP, Hinder RA. Alkaline gastroesophageal reflux: implications in the development of complications in Barrett's columnar-lined lower esophagus. *Surgery* 1989;106:764–770.

73. Attwood SE, Ball CS, Barlow AP, Jenkinson L, Norris TL, Watson A. Role of intragastric and intraoesophageal alkalinisation in the genesis of complications in Barrett's columnar lined lower oesophagus. *Gut* 1993;34:11–15.

74. Vaezi MF, Richter JE. Role of acid and duodenogastroesophageal reflux in gastroesophageal reflux disease. *Gastroenterology* 1996;111:1192–1199.

75. Penagini R, Yuen H, Misiewicz JJ, Bianchi PA. Alkaline intraoesophageal pH and gastro-oesophageal reflux in patients with peptic oesophagitis. *Scand J Gastroenterol* 1988;23:675–678.

76. Mattioli S, Pilotti V, Felice V, *et al.* Ambulatory 24-hr pH monitoring of esophagus, fundus, and antrum. A new technique for simultaneous study of gastroesophageal and duodenogastric reflux. *Dig Dis Sci* 1990;35:929–938.

77. Singh S, Bradley LA, Richter JE. Determinants of oesophageal 'alkaline' pH environment in controls and patients with gastro-oesophageal reflux disease. *Gut* 1993;34:309–316.

78. Gotley DC, Appleton GV, Cooper MJ. Bile acids and trypsin are unimportant in alkaline esophageal reflux. *J Clin Gastroenterol* 1992;14:2–7.

79. Iftikhar SY, Ledingham S, Evans DF, *et al.* Alkaline gastro-oesophageal reflux: dual probe pH monitoring. *Gut* 1995;37:465–470.

80. Champion G, Richter JE, Vaezi MF, Singh S, Alexander R. Duodenogastroesophageal reflux: relationship to pH and importance in Barrett's esophagus. *Gastroenterology* 1994;107:747–754.

81. Just RJ, Leite LP, Castell DO. Changes in overnight fasting intragastric pH show poor correlation with duodenogastric bile reflux in normal subjects. *Am J Gastroenterol* 1996;91:1567–1570.

82. DeVault KR, Georgeson S, Castell DO. Salivary stimulation mimics esophageal exposure to refluxed duodenal contents. *Am J Gastroenterol* 1993;88:1040–1043.

83. Sjoberg F, Gustafsson U, Tibbling L. Alkaline oesophageal reflux—an artefact due to oxygen corrosion of antimony pH electrodes. *Scand J Gastroenterol* 1992;27:1084–1088.

84. Bechi P, Pucciani F, Baldini F, *et al.* Long-term ambulatory enterogastric reflux monitoring. Validation of a new fiberoptic technique. *Dig Dis Sci* 1993;38:1297–1306.

85. Barrett MW, Myers JC, Watson DI, Jamieson GG. Detection of bile reflux: in vivo validation of the Bilitec fibreoptic system. *Dis Esophagus* 2000;13:44–50.

86. Stipa F, Stein HJ, Feussner H, Kraemer S, Siewert JR. Assessment of non-acid esophageal reflux: comparison between long-term reflux aspiration test and fiberoptic bilirubin monitoring. *Dis Esophagus* 1997;10:24–28.

87. Vaezi MF, Lacamera RG, Richter JE. Validation studies of Bilitec 2000: an ambulatory duodenogastric reflux monitoring system. *Am J Physiol* 1994;267:G1050–1057.

88. Caldwell MT, Byrne PJ, Brazil N, *et al.* An ambulatory bile reflux monitoring system: an in vitro appraisal. *Physiol Meas* 1994;15:57–65.

89. Tack J, Bisschops R, Koek G, Sifrim D, Lerut T, Janssens J. Dietary restrictions during ambulatory monitoring of duodenogastroesophageal reflux. *Dig Dis Sci* 2003;48:1213–1220.

90. Kauer WK, Peters JH, Demeester TR, Ireland AP, Bremner CG, Hagen JA. Mixed reflux of gastric and duodenal juices is more harmful to the esophagus than gastric juice alone. The need for surgical therapy re-emphasized. *Ann Surg* 1995;222:525–531.

91. Zaninotto G, Portale G, Parenti A, *et al.* Role of acid and bile reflux in development of specialised intestinal metaplasia in distal oesophagus. *Dig Liver Dis* 2002;34:251–257.

92. El-Serag HB, Aguirre TV, Davis S, Kuebeler M, Bhattacharyya A, Sampliner RE. Proton pump inhibitors are associated with reduced incidence of dysplasia in Barrett's esophagus. *Am J Gastroenterol* 2004;99:1877–1883.

93. Hillman LC, Chiragakis L, Shadbolt B, Kaye GL, Clarke AC. Proton-pump inhibitor therapy and the development of dysplasia in patients with Barrett's oesophagus. *Med J Aust* 2004;180:387–391.

94. Pace F, Sangaletti O, Pallotta S, Molteni P, Porro GB. Biliary reflux and non-acid reflux are two distinct phenomena: a comparison between 24-hour multichannel intraesophageal impedance and bilirubin monitoring. *Scand J Gastroenterol* 2007;42:1031–1039.

95. Sears RJ, Champion GL, Richter JE. Characteristics of distal partial gastrectomy patients with esophageal symptoms of duodenogastric reflux. *Am J Gastroenterol* 1995;90:211–215.

96. Vaezi MF, Richter JE. Contribution of acid and duodenogastro-oesophageal reflux to oesophageal mucosal injury and symptoms in partial gastrectomy patients. *Gut* 1997;41:297–302.

97. Tack J, Koek G, Demedts I, Sifrim D, Janssens J. Gastroesophageal reflux disease poorly responsive to single-dose proton pump inhibitors in patients without Barrett's esophagus: acid reflux, bile reflux, or both? *Am J Gastroenterol* 2004;99:981–988.

98. Wilmer A, Tack J, Frans E, *et al.* Duodenogastroesophageal reflux and esophageal mucosal injury in mechanically ventilated patients. *Gastroenterology* 1999;116:1293–1299.

99. Sifrim D, Blondeau K, Mantilla L. Utility of non-endoscopic investigations in the practical management of oesophageal disorders. *Best Pract Res Clin Gastroenterol* 2009;23:369–386.

100. Sifrim D, Castell D, Dent J, Kahrilas PJ. Gastro-oesophageal reflux monitoring: review and consensus report on detection and definitions of acid, non-acid, and gas reflux. *Gut* 2004;53:1024–1031.

101. Kauer WK, Stein HJ. Emerging concepts of bile reflux in the constellation of gastroesophageal reflux disease. *J Gastrointest Surg* 2010;14 (Suppl 1):S9–16.

102. Marshall RE, Anggiansah A, Owen WA, Owen WJ. The relationship between acid and bile reflux and symptoms in gastro-oesophageal reflux disease. *Gut* 1997;40:182–187.

103. Koek GH, Tack J, Sifrim D, Lerut T, Janssens J. The role of acid and duodenal gastroesophageal reflux in symptomatic GERD. *Am J Gastroenterol* 2001;96:2033–2040.

104. Koek GH, Sifrim D, Lerut T, Janssens J, Tack J. Effect of the GABA(B) agonist baclofen in patients with symptoms and duodeno-gastro-oesophageal reflux refractory to proton pump inhibitors. *Gut* 2003;52:1397–1402.

105. Tack J. Review article: the role of bile and pepsin in the pathophysiology and treatment of gastro-oesophageal reflux disease. *Aliment Pharmacol Ther* 2006;24 (Suppl 2):10–16.

106. Karamanolis G, Vanuytsel T, Sifrim D, *et al.* Yield of 24-hour esophageal pH and bilitec monitoring in patients with persisting symptoms on PPI therapy. *Dig Dis Sci* 2008;53: 2387–2393.

107. Gasiorowska A, Navarro-Rodriguez T, Wendel C, *et al.* Comparison of the degree of duodenogastroesophageal reflux and acid reflux between patients who failed to respond and those who were successfully treated with a proton pump inhibitor once daily. *Am J Gastroenterol* 2009;104:2005–2013.

108. Siddiqui A, Rodriguez-Stanley S, Zubaidi S, Miner PB Jr. Esophageal visceral sensitivity to bile salts in patients with functional heartburn and in healthy control subjects. *Dig Dis Sci* 2005;50:81–85.

109. Marshall RE, Anggiansah A, Manifold DK, Owen WA, Owen WJ. Effect of omeprazole 20 mg twice daily on duodenogastric and gastro-oesophageal bile reflux in Barrett's oesophagus. *Gut* 1998;43:603–606.

110. Menges M, Muller M, Zeitz M. Increased acid and bile reflux in Barrett's esophagus compared to reflux esophagitis, and effect of proton pump inhibitor therapy. *Am J Gastroenterol* 2001;96:331–337.

111. Netzer P, Gut A, Brundler R, Gaia C, Halter F, Inauen W. Influence of pantoprazole on oesophageal motility, and bile and acid reflux in patients with oesophagitis. *Aliment Pharmacol Ther* 2001;15:1375–1384.

112. Stein HJ, Kauer WK, Feussner H, Siewert JR. Bile reflux in benign and malignant Barrett's esophagus: effect of medical acid suppression and nissen fundoplication. *J Gastrointest Surg* 1998;2:333–341.

113. Todd JA, Basu KK, de Caestecker JS. Normalization of oesophageal pH does not guarantee control of duodenogastro-oesophageal reflux in Barrett's oesophagus. *Aliment Pharmacol Ther* 2005;21:969–975.

114. Babaei A, Bhargava V, Aalam S, Scadeng M, Mittal RK. Effect of proton pump inhibition on the gastric volume: assessed by magnetic resonance imaging. *Aliment Pharmacol Ther* 2009;29:863–870.

115. Lind T, Cederberg C, Ekenved G, Haglund U, Olbe L. Effect of omeprazole – a gastric proton pump inhibitor—on pentagastrin stimulated acid secretion in man. *Gut* 1983;24:270–276.

116. Vela MF, Tutuian R, Katz PO, Castell DO. Baclofen decreases acid and non-acid post-prandial gastro-oesophageal reflux measured by combined multichannel intraluminal impedance and pH. *Aliment Pharmacol Ther* 2003;17:243–251.

117. Lehmann A. Novel treatments of GERD: focus on the lower esophageal sphincter. *Eur Rev Med Pharmacol Sci* 2008;12 (Suppl 1):103–110.

118. Beaumont H, Smout A, Aanen M, *et al.* The GABA(B) receptor agonist AZD9343 inhibits transient lower oesophageal sphincter relaxations and acid reflux in healthy volunteers: a phase I study. *Aliment Pharmacol Ther* 2009;30:937–946.

119. Keywood C, Wakefield M, Tack J. A proof-of-concept study evaluating the effect of ADX10059, a metabotropic glutamate receptor-5 negative allosteric modulator, on acid exposure and symptoms in gastro-oesophageal reflux disease. *Gut* 2009;58:1192–1199.

120. Mann O, Glaser J, Pausch J, Rosemeyer D, Tibroni T. [Prognostic value of long-term pH-metry in the B-II resected stomach]. *Gastroenterologia* 1993;31:392–394.

121. Vaezi MF, Sears R, Richter JE. Placebo-controlled trial of cisapride in postgastrectomy patients with duodenogastro-esophageal reflux. *Dig Dis Sci* 1996;41:754–763.

122. Nath BJ, Warshaw AL. Alkaline reflux gastritis and esophagitis. *Annu Rev Med* 1984;35:383–396.

123. McAlhany JC Jr, Hanover TM, Taylor SM, Sticca RP, Ashmore JD Jr. Long-term follow-up of patients with Roux-en-Y gastrojejunostomy for gastric disease. *Ann Surg* 1994; 219:451–455.

24 Role of *Helicobacter pylori* in Gastroesophageal Reflux Disease

Peter Malfertheiner and Arne Kandulski

Department of Gastroenterology, Hepatology and Infectious Diseases, Otto-von-Guericke University Magdeburg, Magdeburg, Germany

Introduction

The relationship between *Helicobacter pylori* infection and gastroesophageal reflux disease (GERD) continues to generate debate as to whether *H. pylori* is a protective, aggravating or neutral bystander of GERD. The overall prevalence of *H. pylori* and related diseases has been decreasing in developing countries during the last decades [1]. In patients with GERD, the prevalence of *H. pylori* has been reported to be lower than in healthy controls, but there is a considerable degree of variation [2, 3]. Several studies have described a negative association between *H. pylori* infection and GERD complications, Barrett's esophagus, and esophageal adenocarcinoma, again prompting the speculation that *H. pylori* is a protective factor, while others argue against this assumption [4–7].

This chapter will provide an overview of the complex relationship between *H. pylori* infection and GERD, including considerations of epidemiologic trends, pathophysiologic mechanisms, the impact of *H. pylori* eradication on GERD and related symptoms, and onset of *de novo* GERD after *H. pylori* eradication. A final section will be devoted to the interaction of *H. pylori* and GERD at the gastroesophageal junction (GEJ), resulting in intestinal metaplasia, Barrett's esophagus, and adenocarcinoma.

Epidemiologic trends

In epidemiologic studies, GERD is usually defined either based on typical symptoms (heartburn, regurgitation) as proposed by the Genval workshop and Montreal classification [8, 9] or on endoscopic findings, i.e. erosive esophagitis. The diagnosis of *H. pylori* is based either on blood serology or on biopsies assessed by the rapid urease test or histology.

In systematic reviews, the pooled odds ratio was 0.76 (0.61–0.96) in Europe and 0.70 (0.55–0.9) in North America, confirming the lower prevalence of *H. pylori* in patients with GERD. The data are limited by substantial heterogeneity between studies up to 2001 (Figure 24.1A) [3]. The latest published population-based study from Norway involving 65 363 individuals (HUNT study) reported that *H. pylori* infection—irrespective of the CagA status—was not associated with a decreased risk for GERD. However, when confounding factors were considered, gastric atrophy was found to be associated with an 80% reduction of GERD-related symptoms (OR 0.2, 95% CI 0.8–1.5) (Figure 24.1). The authors even demonstrated a dose dependence of reduced GERD-related symptoms and prostaglandin I (PGI) levels [10]. Based on current data, it is likely that the presence of *H. pylori*-induced corpus-predominant atrophic gastritis is the key to causing less gastric acid and, thereby, less esophageal acid reflux and GERD symptoms. This association is important for areas with high *H. pylori* prevalence and corpus-predominant colonization patterns.

Helicobacter pylori eradication and *de novo* gastroesophageal reflux disease

The first report of an increased incidence of esophagitis in patients with duodenal ulcers after *H. pylori* eradication [11] had a tremendous impact on the management of *H. pylori* infection for many years. The clinical observations were confirmed and extended by further studies in patients with corpus-predominant gastritis and associated hypochlorhydria [5, 12, 13]. The effect was attributed mainly to the recovery of acid secretion after *H. pylori* eradication in a condition of reversible atrophic gastritis. Other authors explained GERD after *H. pylori* eradication with the loss of the known production of ammonia by *H. pylori*, which aug-

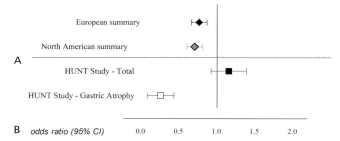

Figure 24.1 (A) Odds ratio (95% confidence interval) for the prevalence of *H. pylori* infection in patients with gastroesophageal reflux disease (GERD) from Europe and North America (according to Raghunath *et al.* [3]). (B) Risk of GERD-related symptoms in *H. pylori* infection (according to Nordenstedt *et al.* [10]).

ments the acid-suppressing effect of antacid medications [14]. A further explanation put forward was that successful eradication is associated with rebound acid secretion, which may cause GERD relapses [15]. The resolution of corpus gastritis after *H. pylori* eradication with the secondary recovery of gastric acid secretion was proposed as the plausible explanation for these physiologic changes. Following these early studies indicating an increased incidence of GERD after *H. pylori* eradication, a series of studies reported that *H. pylori* eradication in patients with gastric and duodenal ulcer disease did not induce GERD [7, 16, 17]. This was also the conclusion from a recent meta-analysis where no association was observed between *H. pylori* eradication and new cases of GERD in a large population of dyspeptic patients [18]. The risk for developing mild reflux esophagitis, however, was two-fold higher in a subset of patients with peptic ulcer, which likely indicates the frequent association of peptic ulcer and reflux esophagitis. While *H. pylori* eradication cures peptic ulcer disease with no further requirement for acid suppressant medications, the withdrawal of this medication may unmask GERD.

Helicobacter pylori eradication in patients with gastroesophageal reflux disease

A critical question to address is whether *H. pylori* eradication is beneficial in patients already suffering from GERD. A prospective randomized study of *H. pylori* eradication during long-term omeprazole therapy for GERD found no worsening of reflux disease, and no need for an increased omeprazole maintenance dose [19]. Another study reported a benefit even from *H. pylori* eradication during a 6-month follow-up among GERD patients [56]. In this study, GERD-associated symptoms relapsed even earlier in patients with persistent *H. pylori* infection than in patients in whom *H. pylori* had been successfully eradicated. The authors explained their result with the predominant pattern of antrum gastritis, which is linked to normal or increased acid

secretion, and concluded that there is lower acid output following eradication and healing of antrum-predominant gastritis.

Many GERD patients are dependent on the long-term use of acid suppressants. *H. pylori* infection increases the effect of PPIs, leading to a higher intragastric pH during acid suppressive treatment. Patients with *H. pylori* infection treated with pantoprazole had the best symptom relief and healing of severe forms of erosive esophagitis [20]. However, this benefit is marginal from a clinical perspective. In clinical reality, most patients with mild-to-moderate GERD will not notice a difference in the efficacy of PPI, regardless of their *H. pylori* status. The maintenance dose after healing of erosive esophagitis is not influenced by the patient's *H. pylori* status. The more important question to consider relates to the development of atrophic gastritis in patients on long-term PPI with persistent *H. pylori* infection [21, 22]. In a prospective, randomized trial of 231 patients on long-term treatment with omeprazole and in whom *H. pylori* had not been eradicated, Kuipers *et al.* described a progression of *H. pylori* colonization to a corpus-predominant gastritis [23]. PPI therapy induces changes in the gastric mucosa of *H. pylori*-positive patients, shifting the predominant pattern of gastritis from the antrum to the corpus. This cannot be overlooked as the strongest risk factor for developing gastric cancer is the presence of corpus-predominant gastritis [24]. *H. pylori* eradication before long-term PPI therapy is therefore recommended, at least in European guidelines, whereas in the United States clear recommendations are missing [25].

Impact of *Helicobacter pylori* infection on mechanisms related to gastroesophageal reflux disease

Helicobacter pylori, gastric acid secretion, esophageal acid exposure, gastric atrophy, and severity of gastroesophageal reflux disease

Analyzing esophageal pH-metry studies, endoscopy, and symptom severity in patients with GERD, no differences were seen between patients infected with *H. pylori* and those not infected [26, 27]. Although the gastric acid hypersecretion in cases of *H. pylori*-induced antrum-predominant gastritis is well known, the acid exposure in the distal esophagus does not differ between *H. pylori*-positive, *H. pylori*-negative, and *H. pylori*-eradicated patients, and only a delayed acid bolus clearance in the distal esophagus was described after *H. pylori* eradication therapy [28]. A second study of consecutive patients comparing *H. pylori* infected and non-infected patients with GERD demonstrated similar results in 24-h esophageal pH-metry, lower esophageal sphincter (LES) pressure, and motility, as well as the endoscopic severity of esophagitis [26].

The biologic mechanism explaining the negative association between *H. pylori* and GERD is the organism's ability to induce gastric atrophy, resulting in reduced gastric acid secretion. In the FINBAR case–control study, Anderson *et al.* described the relationship between *H. pylori* infection, gastric atrophy, and stages of esophageal inflammatory changes. Two hundred and thirty subjects with reflux esophagitis were included and *H. pylori* infection and CagA status were assessed, as well as gastric atrophy from the serum pepsinogen I:II ratio. The authors found a negative association between reflux esophagitis and *H. pylori* infection (OR 0.42; 95% CI 0.3–0.6) and further observed a strong negative association for severe gastric atrophy (pepsinogen I:II < 3) and esophagitis (OR 0.17), as well for mild-to-moderate atrophy (pepsinogen I:II < 7). The negative association for esophagitis was lost only when analyzing patients without atrophy. These results support the importance of gastric acid secretion in causing esophagitis, and the negative association between *H. pylori* infection and GERD is explained only in cases of atrophic body gastritis [29]. Similar results were found in the German ProGERD study, where no associations were found between gastrin-17 serum levels, pepsinogen I and II, and *H. pylori* status in patients with GERD, regardless of symptom or endoscopic severity [30]. Earlier studies investigated the effect of *H. pylori* infection on acid suppressive therapy. They described a more profound effect of acid suppressive medication in patients with *H. pylori* infection compared to in non-infected or eradicated patients [15, 31]. A likely mechanism explaining this effect is the colonization pattern of *H. pylori* with a corpus-predominant gastritis, thereby markedly decreasing the acid secreting region of the stomach.

For Barrett's esophagus and esophageal adenocarcinoma mechanisms other than gastric atrophy due to *H. pylori* are discussed and need further evaluation [32].

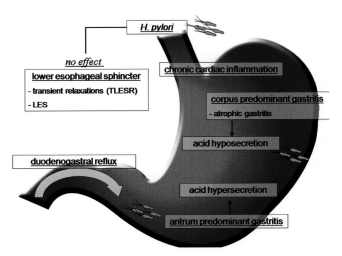

Figure 24.2 Pathophysiologic mechanisms involved in the pathogenesis of *H. pylori* infection and gastroesophageal reflux disease. LES, lower esophageal sphincter; TLESR, transient LES relaxations.

Helicobacter pylori and effects on lower esophageal sphincter, transient lower esophageal sphincter relaxations, and gastric motility

The LES constitutes an important component of the GEJ. The underlying pathologic mechanism of reflux events are transient LES relaxations (TLESR) (Figure 24.2). Although *H. pylori* colonization is known to induce higher amounts of nitric oxide and ammonium, it is unlikely that pharmacologic amounts reach the smooth muscle cells, lowering the resting LES pressure. On the other hand, the increase in serum gastrin noted with *H. pylori* infection may enhance LES pressure [33, 34]. No data exist about the interaction of different peptides and cytokines released during *H. pylori* infection and their influence on LES pressure. Wu *et al.* compared the LES resting pressure of *H. pylori*-positive and -negative patients with GERD. Besides a lower LES resting pressure, they described lower amplitude of the peristalsis in the distal esophagus of *H. pylori*-positive patients with GERD [35]. However, by investigating gastric compliance

and TLESR as underlying mechanisms in GERD, Zerbib *et al.* found no differences between *H. pylori*-infected and non-infected subjects [36]. Another debatable issue contributing to the genesis of reflux-related symptoms is the content of the small intestine and duodenum fluids moving retrograde into the stomach of *H. pylori*-infected patients. Artiko *et al.* described increased duodenogastric refluxate in *H. pylori*-positive compared to *H. pylori*-negative patients by scintigraphy, but the total reflux episodes did not differ between the groups [37]. Similar results were reported using the Bilitec method, demonstrating no differences between *H. pylori*-infected and non-infected subjects [38].

Helicobacter pylori and gastroesophageal reflux disease at the gastroesophageal junction

The GEJ has been attracting great attention from clinicians and pathologists since epidemiologic trends indicated an "overproportional" increase of malignancies in this location, paralleled by a decrease of gastric cancer in the distal part of the stomach [39, 40]. The speculation in the Western world has been that this results from the dramatic rise in the incidence of GERD and Barrett adenocarcinoma, and the decreasing incidence of *H. pylori* infection and related complications [41]. The pathophysiologic scenario is complex and gives room to various interpretations of an intriguing interplay of GERD and *H. pylori* at theGEJ. The current view favors that both conditions are independent rather than either mutually exclusive or synergistic at the GEJ [42, 43].

At the cardia region, both conditions—*H. pylori* infection and GERD—induce intestinal metaplasia in subsets of patients [44, 45] by distinct mechanisms. *H. pylori* leads to chronic inflammation involving the gastric mucosa from the most distal prepyloric region migrating up to the cardia. The pattern of chronic gastritis is variable, ranging from the phenotypic expression of an antrum-predominant gastritis to corpus-predominant gastritis or even pangastritis. The cardia presents with colonization and inflammation in all cases with *H. pylori* infection, but only around 20% of infected subjects in Western populations develop intestinal metaplasia at the cardia. The prevalence of intestinal metaplasia at the cardia is similar to that in the antrum and much higher than in the corpus region [46, 47]. In GERD, the development of intestinal metaplasia occurs within the columnar-lined epithelium (CLE) to constitute the condition of specialized "intestinalized" CLE (i.e. Barrett's esophagus). Barrett's esophagus is a preneoplastic lesion with an appropriately 4–10-fold increased risk for cancer development. Therefore the "meeting point" for *H. pylori* and GERD happens at the cardia, where both conditions may generate preneoplastic lesions that eventually might progress to cancer.

Helicobacter pylori and Barrett's esophagus and esophageal adenocarcinoma

H. pylori infection rates are inversely correlated with the presence of Barrett's esophagus. A recent systematic review reported a lower *H. pylori* prevalence in patients with Barrett's esophagus compared to normal controls at endoscopy (OR 0.50, 95% CI 0.27–0.93). Conflicting findings were reported if the diagnosis of *H. pylori* was based on serum-antibodies of patients with Barrett's esophagus compared to healthy blood donors as normal controls (OR 2.2, CI 1.07–4.55) [48]. Among the mechanisms involved in the pathogenesis of Barrett's esophagus and adenocarcinoma, the chronic exposure of the esophagus to acid and bile acids is considered to initiate and promote the development and neoplastic changes in Barrett's esophagus [49, 50]. In the large study of Anderson *et al.*, a negative association was reported between *H. pylori* infection in the presence of gastric atrophy and Barrett's esophagus and esophageal adenocarcinoma (OR 0.41–0.52). In the subgroup analysis for gastric atrophy (serum pepsinogen I:II ratio), even mild gastric atrophy (pepsinogen I:II < 7) was associated with a reduced risk for developing Barrett's esophagus [29]. Based on these observations, the claim was made that esophageal adenocarcinomas occur more commonly in subjects with non-atrophic gastric mucosa [51]. This protective role from Barrett's adenocarcinoma of *H. pylori* is supported by the findings of a recent meta-analysis showing an inverse relationship between the prevalence of *H. pylori* CagA-positive strains with Barrett's esophagus and adenocarcinoma [52]. However, individual studies reporting this inverse relationship between *H. pylori* infection and esophageal adenocarci-

noma are all characterized by a high degree of heterogeneity. The pattern of inflammation at the cardia is dependent on the consequences of reflux disease and the presence of *H. pylori* infection. Colonization of the gastric cardia by *H. pylori* is associated with an inflammatory infiltration of regulatory CD4$^+$CD25$^+$ T cells, which are absent in GERD-related inflammation [53, 54]. The pathophysiologic consequences of these distinct inflammatory reactions are poorly understood, especially in the relationship to the pathogenesis of Barrett's esophagus.

Conclusions

H. pylori infection interferes with gastric acid secretion depending on the pattern of gastritis. This is the key link to the hypothesis of the beneficial/protective effect of *H. pylori* in GERD. Hypothetically a benefit can occur only in the environment of less acid reflux due to the inhibition of gastric acid secretion by atrophic gastritis.

The never-ending debate about the relationship between *H. pylori* and GERD derives from many conflicting studies in which either the absence of *H. pylori* or its eradication indicated a higher prevalence and thus an increased risk for GERD and complications. By a careful summary of all the data, including recent meta-analyses, it is evident that most of the discrepancies in results are due to the heterogeneity of populations in these studies. In conclusion, *H. pylori* and acid reflux at the cardia are independent factors causing chronic inflammation at the cardia; increasing rather than reducing the risk of cancer.

In subsets of patients with reversible atrophic changes of the gastric mucosa and hypochlorhydria, *H. pylori* eradication may increase acid reflux in predisposed subjects (i.e. in the presence of a deficient reflux barrier). The clinical impact of this can be neglected, however, as overall eradication does not increase or decrease the incidence of GERD. European guidelines recommend eradication of *H. pylori* in patients with GERD who require long-term therapy with PPIs [55]; this recommendation is lacking in US guidelines.

References

1. Blaser MJ, Hypothesis: the changing relationships of *Helicobacter pylori* and humans: implications for health and disease. *J Infect Dis* 1999;179:1523–1530.
2. Metz DC, Kroser JA. *Helicobacter pylori* and gastroesophageal reflux disease. *Gastroenterol Clin North Am* 1999;28:971–985, viii.
3. Raghunath A, Hungin AP, Wooff D, Childs S. Prevalence of *Helicobacter pylori* in patients with gastro-oesophageal reflux disease: systematic review. *BMJ* 2003;326:737.
4. Graham DY. The changing epidemiology of GERD: geography and *Helicobacter pylori*. *Am J Gastroenterol* 2003;98:1462–1470.

5. El-Serag HB, Sonnenberg A, Jamal MM, Inadomi JM, Crooks LA, Feddersen RM. Corpus gastritis is protective against reflux oesophagitis. *Gut* 1999;45:181–185.

6. Sharma P, Vakil N. Review article: *Helicobacter pylori* and reflux disease. *Aliment Pharmacol Ther* 2003;17:297–305.

7. Malfertheiner P, Dent J, Zeijlon L, *et al.* Impact of *Helicobacter pylori* eradication on heartburn in patients with gastric or duodenal ulcer disease—results from a randomized trial programme. *Aliment Pharmacol Ther* 2002;16:1431–1442.

8. Vakil N, van Zanten SV, Kahrilas P, Dent J, Jones R. The Montreal definition and classification of gastroesophageal reflux disease: a global evidence-based consensus. *Am J Gastroenterol* 2006;101:1900–1920.

9. An evidence-based appraisal of reflux disease management—the Genval Workshop Report. *Gut* 1999;44 (Suppl 2):S1–16.

10. Nordenstedt H, Nilsson M, Johnsen R, Lagergren J, Hveem K. *Helicobacter pylori* infection and gastroesophageal reflux in a population-based study (The HUNT Study). *Helicobacter* 2007;12:16–22.

11. Labenz J, Tillenburg, Peitz U, *et al. Helicobacter pylori* augments the pH-increasing effect of omeprazole in patients with duodenal ulcer. *Gastroenterology* 1996;110:725–732.

12. Koike T, Ohara S, Sekine H, *et al. Helicobacter pylori* infection inhibits reflux esophagitis by inducing atrophic gastritis. *Am J Gastroenterol* 1999;94:3468–3472.

13. Yamaji Y, Mitsushima T, Ikuma H, *et al.* Inverse background of *Helicobacter pylori* antibody and pepsinogen in reflux oesophagitis compared with gastric cancer: analysis of 5732 Japanese subjects. *Gut* 2001;49:335–340.

14. Bercik P, Verdu EF, Armstrong D, *et al.* The effect of ammonia on omeprazole-induced reduction of gastric acidity in subjects with *Helicobacter pylori* infection. *Am J Gastroenterol* 2000;95:947–955.

15. Gillen D, Wirz AA, Neithercut WD, Ardill JE, McColl KE. *Helicobacter pylori* infection potentiates the inhibition of gastric acid secretion by omeprazole. *Gut* 1999;44:468–475.

16. Laine L, Sugg J. Effect of *Helicobacter pylori* eradication on development of erosive esophagitis and gastroesophageal reflux disease symptoms: a post hoc analysis of eight double blind prospective studies. *Am J Gastroenterol* 2002;97:2992–2997.

17. Vakil N, Hahn B, McSorley D. Recurrent symptoms and gastro-oesophageal reflux disease in patients with duodenal ulcer treated for *Helicobacter pylori* infection. *Aliment Pharmacol Ther* 2000;14:45–51.

18. Yaghoobi M, Farrokhyar F, Yuan Y, Hunt RH. Is there an increased risk of GERD after *Helicobacter pylori* eradication?: a meta-analysis. *Am J Gastroenterol* 2010;105:1007–1013.

19. Moayyedi P, Bardhan C, *et al. Helicobacter pylori* eradication does not exacerbate reflux symptoms in gastroesophageal reflux disease. *Gastroenterology* 2001;121:1120–1126.

20. Holtmann G, Cain C, Malfertheiner P. Gastric *Helicobacter pylori* infection accelerates healing of reflux esophagitis during treatment with the proton pump inhibitor pantoprazole. *Gastroenterology* 1999;117:11–16.

21. Kuipers EJ, Lundell L, Klinkenberg-Knol EC, *et al.* Atrophic gastritis and *Helicobacter pylori* infection in patients with reflux esophagitis treated with omeprazole or fundoplication. *N Engl J Med* 1996;334:1018–1022.

22. Lundell L, Miettinen P, Myrvold HE, *et al.* Lack of effect of acid suppression therapy on gastric atrophy. Nordic Gerd Study Group. *Gastroenterology* 1999;117:319–326.

23. Schenk BE, Kuipers EJ, Nelis GF, *et al.* Effect of *Helicobacter pylori* eradication on chronic gastritis during omeprazole therapy. *Gut* 2000;46:615–621.

24. Uemura N, Okamoto S, Yamamoto S, *et al. Helicobacter pylori* infection and the development of gastric cancer. *N Engl J Med* 2001;345:784–789.

25. Malfertheiner P, Megraud F, O'Morain C, *et al.* Current concepts in the management of *Helicobacter pylori* infection: the Maastricht III Consensus Report. *Gut* 2007;56:772–781.

26. Fallone CA, Barkun AN, Mayrand S, *et al.* There is no difference in the disease severity of gastro-oesophageal reflux disease between patients infected and not infected with *Helicobacter pylori*. *Aliment Pharmacol Ther* 2004;20:761V768.

27. Grande M, Cadeddu F, Villa M, *et al. Helicobacter pylori* and gastroesophageal reflux disease. *World J Surg Oncol* 2008;6:74.

28. Sarnelli G, Ierardi E, Grasso R, *et al.* Acid exposure and altered acid clearance in GERD patients treated for *Helicobacter pylori* infection. *Dig Liver Dis* 2003;35:151–156.

29. Anderson LA, Murphy SJ, Johnston BT, *et al.* Relationship between Helicobacter pylori infection and gastric atrophy and the stages of the oesophageal inflammation, metaplasia, adeno-carcinoma sequence: results from the FINBAR case-control study. *Gut* 2008;57:734–739.

30. Monkemuller K, Neumann H, Nocon M, *et al.* Serum gastrin and pepsinogens do not correlate with the different grades of severity of gastro-oesophageal reflux disease: a matched case-control study. *Aliment Pharmacol Ther* 2008;28:491–496.

31. Labenz J, Tillenburg B, Peitz U, *et al. Helicobacter pylori* augments the pH-increasing effect of omeprazole in patients with duodenal ulcer. *Gastroenterology* 1996;110:725–732.

32. McColl KE, Watabe H, Derakhshan MH. Role of gastric atrophy in mediating negative association between *Helicobacter pylori* infection and reflux oesophagitis, Barrett's oesophagus and oesophageal adenocarcinoma. *Gut* 2008;57:721–723.

33. Beales I, Blaser MJ, Srinivasan S, *et al.* Effect of *Helicobacter pylori* products and recombinant cytokines on gastrin release from cultured canine G cells. *Gastroenterology* 1997;113:465–471.

34. Calam J, Gibbons A, Healey ZV, Bliss P, Arebi N. How does *Helicobacter pylori* cause mucosal damage? Its effect on acid and gastrin physiology. *Gastroenterology* 1997;113:S43–S49.

35. Wu JC, Lai AC, Wong SK, Chan FK, Leung WK, Sung JJ. Dysfunction of oesophageal motility in *Helicobacter pylori*-infected patients with reflux oesophagitis. *Aliment Pharmacol Ther* 2001;15:1913–1919.

36. Zerbib F, Bicheler V, Leray V, Joubert M, Bruley D, Galmiche VJP. *H. pylori* and transient lower esophageal sphincter relaxations induced by gastric distension in healthy humans. *Am J Physiol Gastrointest Liver Physiol* 2001;281:G350–356.

37. Artiko VM, Chebib HY, Ugljesic MB, Petrovic MN, Obradovic VB. Relationship between enterogastric reflux estimated by scintigraphy and the presence of *Helicobacter pylori*. *Hepatogastroenterology* 1999;46:1234–1237.

38. Manifold DK, Anggiansah A, Rowe I, Sanderson JD, Chinyama CN, Owen WJ. Gastro-oesophageal reflux and duodenogastric

reflux before and after eradication in *Helicobacter pylori* gastritis. *Eur J Gastroenterol Hepatol* 2001;13:535–539.

39. Devesa SS, Fraumeni JF Jr. The rising incidence of gastric cardia cancer. *J Natl Cancer Inst* 1999;91:747–749.

40. Devesa SS, Blot WJ, Fraumeni JF Jr. Changing patterns in the incidence of esophageal and gastric carcinoma in the United States. *Cancer* 1998;83:2049–2053.

41. Labenz J, Malfertheiner P. *Helicobacter pylori* in gastro-oesophageal reflux disease: causal agent, independent or protective factor? *Gut* 1997;41:277–280.

42. Malfertheiner P, Peitz U. The interplay between *Helicobacter pylori*, gastro-oesophageal reflux disease, and intestinal metaplasia. *Gut* 2005;54 (Suppl 1):i13–i20.

43. Spechler SJ. The role of gastric carditis in metaplasia and neoplasia at the gastroesophageal junction. *Gastroenterology* 1999;117:218–228.

44. Peitz U, Vieth M, Malfertheiner P. Carditis at the interface between GERD and *Helicobacter pylori* infection. *Dig Dis* 2004;22:120–125.

45. Guenther T, Hackelsberger A, Kuester, Malfertheiner P, Roessner A. Reflux esophagitis or *Helicobacter* infection?—diagnostic value of the inflammatory pattern in metaplastic mucosa at the squamocolumnar junction. *Pathol Res Pract* 2007;203:831–837.

46. Hackelsberger A, Gunther T, Schultze V, Labenz J, Roessner A, Malfertheiner P. Prevalence and pattern of *Helicobacter pylori* gastritis in the gastric cardia. *Am J Gastroenterol* 1997;92:2220–2224.

47. Genta RM, Huberman RM, Graham DY. The gastric cardia in *Helicobacter pylori* infection. *Hum Pathol* 1994;25:915–919.

48. Wang C, Yuan Y, Hunt RH. *Helicobacter pylori* infection and Barrett's esophagus: a systematic review and meta-analysis. *Am J Gastroenterol* 2009;104492–500.

49. Fitzgerald RC. Molecular basis of Barrett's oesophagus and oesophageal adenocarcinoma. *Gut* 2006;55:1810–1820.

50. Shaheen NJ, Sharma P, Overholt BF, *et al.* Radiofrequency ablation in Barrett's esophagus with dysplasia. *N Engl J Med* 2009;360:2277–2288.

51. McColl KE, Going JJ, Aetiology and classification of adenocarcinoma of the gastro-oesophageal junction/cardia. *Gut* 2010; 59:282–284.

52. Rokkas T, Pistiolas D, Sechopoulos P, Robotis I, Margantinis G. Relationship between *Helicobacter pylori* infection and esophageal neoplasia: a meta-analysis. *Clin Gastroenterol Hepatol* 2007;5:1413–1417.

53. Kandulski A, Wex T, Kuester D, *et al.* Naturally occurring regulatory T cells (CD4+, CD25high, FOXP3+) in the antrum and cardia are associated with higher H. pylori colonization and increased gene expression of TGF-beta1. *Helicobacter* 2008;13:295–303.

54. Kandulski A, Wex T, Kuester D, *et al.* Chronic mucosal inflammation of the gastric cardia in gastroesophageal reflux disease is not regulated by FOXP3-expressing T cells. *Dig Dis Sci* 2009;54:1940–1946.

55. Malfertheiner P, Megraud F, O'Morain C, *et al.* Current concepts in the management of *Helicobacter pylori* infection: the Maastricht III Consensus Report. *Gut* 2007;56:772–781.

56. Moayyedi P, Wason C, Peacock R, Walan A, Bardhan K, Axon AT, Dixon MF; Changing patterns of Helicobacter pylori gastritis in long standing acid suppression. *Helicobacter*. 2000 Dec; 5(4): 206–14.

25 | Medical Management of Gastroesophageal Reflux Disease

Philip O. Katz and Ellen M. Stein
Department of Medicine, Division of Gastroenterology, Albert Einstein Medical Center, Philadelphia, PA, USA

Introduction

The medical therapy of gastroesophageal reflux disease (GERD) is based on knowledge of the pathophysiology of the disease and a defined set of goals based on symptom presentation and organ damage. Therapy must be individualized to obtain optimal results for the patient. The idealized medical therapy would augment lower esophageal sphincter (LES) pressure and/or reduce the number of transient LES relaxations (TLESRs), augment the ability of the esophagus to clear refluxed gastric contents, accelerate gastric emptying, augment mucosal resistance, and neutralize gastric acidity. While conceptually this is possible, we remain short of the ideal one-size-fits-all therapy. The clinician must utilize the available agents either alone or in combination in an attempt to achieve complete symptom relief and improvement of quality of life, to heal mucosal lesions should they exist, and to prevent complications. Hopefully, we are closer to delaying progression to malignancy in the patient with Barrett's esophagus.

Available interventions include lifestyle modifications, antacids, a mucosal protectant, a prokinetic (promotility) agent, H_2-receptor antagonists (H2RAs), and still the agents of choice at present, proton pump inhibitors (PPIs). In this chapter, we review each of these agents and modalities, discuss a general approach to acute and long-term therapy, and highlight specific clinical situations, including non-erosive GERD, unexplained chest pain, extraesophageal manifestations of GERD, pregnancy, and the medically refractory patient.

Lifestyle modifications

Throughout "history" many have felt that GERD is a lifestyle disease under a patient's control. As such, numerous dietary and lifestyle modifications continue to be advocated as important in the therapy of GERD and are sometimes aggressively "pushed" on patients (Table 25.1). Lifestyle and dietary modifications are for the most part based on physiologic data that certain foods, body positions, tobacco, alcohol, and body mass index (BMI) contribute to an increase in TLESRs, reflux or both. In addition, certain drugs have been documented to decrease LES pressure and have the potential to exacerbate reflux. Other medications may cause direct esophageal injury and may exacerbate reflux symptoms. These include Aspirin, non-steroidal anti-inflammatory drugs, some antibiotics, potassium chloride tablets, ferrous sulfate tablets, alendronate, and other bisphosphonates. Regardless of how sound the intent and solid the laboratory research, there are few outcomes data to support aggressively pushing lifestyles to reluctant patients (Table 25.2), with limited support for the effectiveness of any lifestyle intervention on symptom relief.

Physicians sometimes make different recommendations for lifestyle modifications in different patient populations. Physicians are more likely to recommend lifestyle changes in patients younger than 60 years of age than in older patients. Those with a BMI over $30\,kg/m^2$ also receive advice on eating habits more often than other patients. Heavy smokers are more likely to receive recommendations than light smokers. Despite this, lifestyle changes to counter GERD symptoms are often rather precise, involving specific foods, beverages, and sleeping positions. For many patients, changing their diet by giving up orange juice, coffee, carbonated beverages, and chocolate, for example, represents a serious impairment of their perceived quality of life. Many of these changes are a poor reflection of evidence-based medicine, because studies to prove benefits have produced contradictory results and have been conducted in small, often healthy populations. Some changes such as smoking cessation and weight reduction in patients who are obese carry well-accepted health benefits. Other changes may be less beneficial when measured against their cost in terms of quality of life. It is our experience that most patients have already attempted their own lifestyle changes based on their own evidence of which dietary indiscretions and lifestyle issues exacerbate their disease. Guidelines from the American College of Gastroenterology continue to recommend lifestyle changes as adjuncts to pharmacologic treatment [1].

Of all the recommendations, reminding and encouraging patients to avoid going to bed with a full stomach is the most logical. Proximal acid migration is greatest during sleep and sleep delays esophageal acid clearance. Since most reflux

occurs in the first 4 h of the sleeping period and patients eating within 1–2 h of sleep are much more likely to have abnormal nocturnal reflux [2], it is prudent to follow this dietary change. We see many who are helped with nocturnal symptoms if they can avoid a big meal late at night.

Sleep issues

It has been recommended that patients elevate the head of the bed 6–8 inches either on bed blocks or with a foam rubber wedge designed to elevate the shoulders and body angle in order to use gravity to aid in clearance of a reflux episode during the sleeping period. This is based on studies using prolonged pH monitoring that have shown an acceleration of esophageal clearance when the head of the bed is elevated compared to sleeping flat [3, 4]. Unfortunately, there are no clinical outcome studies to suggest that this individual recommendation will affect symptom relief or healing. Sleeping position might be of equal or greater importance than elevation of the head of the bed [5]. Reflux frequency as well as total time that esophageal pH was below 4 was decreased in the left-side down position, compared to the right-side down, prone, and supine positions. This study in adults augments a similar study in children, with similar findings [6]. This sleep study confirms other data showing an increase in esophageal acid exposure in the post-prandial period when right-side down compared to left-side down [7], likely due to a decrease in TLESRs in the left-side down position [8]. Unfortunately, there is no currently available commercial device that a patient can use to ensure they sleep left-side down, so this can only be suggested. In addition to these sleeping position recommendations, it is often recommended that the patient refrains from eating within 2–3 h of going to sleep. This suggestion is based on the premise that a full stomach produces gastric distention, an increase in TLESRs, and, therefore, an increase in

Table 25.1 Effects of foods and other substances on gastroesophageal reflux disease symptoms.

Decreases LES pressure	Mucosal irritant
Food	Food and drink
Fats	Citrus products
Chocolate	Tomato products
Onions	Spicy foods
Carminatives	Coffee, colas, tea, beer
Alcohol	Medications
Smoking	Aspirin
Medications	Non-steroidal anti-inflammatory
Progesterone	drugs
Theophylline	Tetracycline
Anticholinergic agents	Quinidine
Adrenergic agonists	Potassium tablets
Adrenergic antagonists	Iron salts
Diazepam	Alendronate
Meperidine	Zidovudine
Nitrates	
Calcium-channel blockers	

LES, lower esophageal sphincter.

Table 25.2 Recommendations based on results of a review of studies involving lifestyle modifications.

Lifestyle modification	Strength of scientific evidence	Pathophysiologically conclusive?	Recommendable?
Avoid fatty meals	Equivocal	Equivocal	Not generally
Avoid carbonated beverages	Moderate	Yes	Yes
Select decaffeinated beverages	Equivocal	Equivocal	Not generally
Avoid citrus products	Weak	Yes	Not generally
Eat smaller meals	Weak	Yes	Yes
Lose weight	Equivocal	Equivocal	Yes*
Avoid alcoholic beverages	Weak	Mechanisms not understood; different alcoholic beverages have different effects	Not generally
Stop smoking	Weak	Yes	Yes (in symptomatic persons)
Avoid excessive exercise	Weak	Yes	Yes*
Sleep with head elevated	Equivocal	Equivocal	Not generally
Sleep on left side	Unequivocal	Yes	Yes

*Obesity and smoking appear to be risk factors for cancer of the distal esophagus.

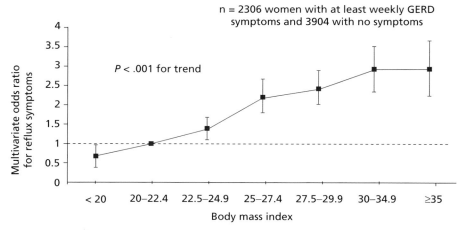

Figure 25.1 Study showing a clear relationship between increase in body mass index and gastroesophageal reflux disease (GERD) symptoms. Weight gain increases the odds of increasing frequency of GERD symptoms.

GER. As reflux is more frequent in the first half of the sleeping period, or even the first 2h, this makes sense [2, 9]. Insomnia (poor sleep) is common in the United States. Sleep aids may negatively affect the GERD patient. The sleep medication zolpidem increases night-time reflux and should be used with care in patients with GERD [10].

Food and weight

Acidic liquids, such as colas and teas, and citrus products, such as orange, grapefruit, and tomato juice, are direct esophageal irritants and will exacerbate symptoms in the GERD patient [11]. A variety of foods can decrease LES pressure [12–15]. Coffee can decrease LES pressure, and has been shown to augment acid production and to exacerbate reflux [16]. Some studies have shown that the effect of coffee on GER can be reduced if it is decaffeinated [16]. Studies have clearly shown that a high-fat meal will increase reflux frequency in both normals and patients with GERD [17, 18]; however, it is unclear whether this is based purely on the presence of fat or on meal size. Fat does delay gastric emptying, which may increase the risk of reflux. While there is reason to recommend a decrease in fat for other health reasons, good outcome studies in GERD patients are again lacking. Chocolate can also decrease LES due to its high xanthine content [19], and it increases esophageal acid exposure [20] and is on the list of foods to avoid.

There is a relationship between symptomatic GERD and body weight. In a cross-sectional study, a positive association between BMI and GERD symptoms was found in women. An increase in BMI of more than 3.5, as compared with no weight changes, was associated with an increased risk of frequency of GERD symptoms [21]. A BMI greater than $30 \, \text{kg/m}^2$ was associated with an almost three times higher risk of frequent reflux symptoms. Weight gain has been associated with an increased risk of symptoms of GERD and weight loss with a decrease in risk. A meta-analysis also

demonstrated a dose–response relationship between BMI and the risk of reporting symptoms of GERD among both men and women [22]. In the same meta-analysis both overweight (BMI 25–29) and obesity (BMI > 30) were associated with an increased risk for GERD symptoms with odds ratios of 1.43 and 1.94, respectively ($P < .001$). It has also been suggested that an increasing BMI is associated with an incremental increase in the risk of developing GERD symptoms [23] (Figure 25.1). An increase in BMI is a clear risk for the development of adenocarcinoma in patients with Barrett's esophagus [24] and a BMI of greater than 30 is a risk for failure of antireflux surgery [25], suggesting that there is some link between obesity and GERD. Ultimately, weight reduction is of clear value for a patient who needs it for other health reasons, and will likely reduce GERD symptoms.

Alcohol

Alcohol is a smooth muscle relaxant and reduces LES pressure. One study determined that 4 ounces of whiskey consumed 3h before the evening meal increased nocturnal acid reflux in healthy subjects. No participants experienced reflux on the night that they did not drink alcohol [26]. The effects of white and red wine on LES pressure and esophageal pH were assessed in a comparison study [27]. Although both types of wine increased the amount of time that esophageal pH was below 4, the effect of white wine was more pronounced than that of red wine, and in another study, the effect of beer was more pronounced than both types of wine. The results of this study suggest that patients with GERD should avoid white wine; however, some epidemiologic data suggest that drinking wine, as opposed to beer and other liquors, is associated with a reduced risk for esophageal adenocarcinoma [28].

Summary

Guidelines from the American College of Gastroenterology recommend lifestyle changes as adjuncts to treatment [1].

However, other experts have suggested that they play minimal to no role in the treatment of GERD today. Educating patients about the potential values of sleeping on their left side and going to bed on an empty stomach, and making them aware of the overall potential of these lifestyle modifications to reduce symptoms takes little time and ultimately might help. Unfortunately, in the absence of "hard data," it is difficult to push these interventions in patients who choose not to implement them.

Pharmacologic therapy

When one thinks of pharmacologic therapy, one immediately considers antisecretory therapy with H_2RAs or PPIs. Today, these antisecretory options are clearly the agents of choice for medical therapy for this disease. The clinician needs, however, to be familiar with the still widely used antacids, sucralfate, and prokinetic agents, despite limited data on their use in the patient with true GERD.

Antacids

Antacids should be used exclusively for symptom relief and rarely, if ever, are sufficient to adequately treat a patient with other than occasional heartburn. For all practical purposes all antacids should be considered equally efficacious at equivalent doses, whether tablet or liquid. Alginic acid combined with antacid has a slightly different mechanism of action but similar efficacy to other antacids. Clinicians often minimize the side effects of antacids, which is appropriate when they are used intermittently. However, with chronic use, magnesium-containing antacids may cause diarrhea, and should be avoided in the patient with heart failure or renal insufficiency, and in late trimester pregnancy. Aluminum-containing antacids may cause constipation [29–31].

Sucralfate

This mucosal protective agent binds to inflamed tissue, perhaps protecting the esophageal mucosa by blocking diffusion of gastric acid and pepsin across the mucosal barrier. Sucralfate may inhibit the erosive action of pepsin and bile [32]. Although rarely used in the GERD patient because of the need to administer the drug four times daily, there is value to this agent in special populations such as pregnant women (see below) [33]. Little systemic absorption of the agent has been demonstrated, so it is likely safe for this population. When compared to H_2RAs head to head, equivalent healing of erosive esophagitis is demonstrated, although overall healing rates are not as high [34, 35]. Constipation is seen in 2% of patients. This compound has little to no place in modern medical therapy for GERD, with the exception of pregnant patients.

Promotility therapy

Conceptually, a "promotility or motility-altering agent" might represent the ideal agent to treat GERD. The ideal therapy would address the underlying pathophysiologic defects, thus improving the strength and competence of the LES and augmenting esophageal clearance to shorten the time the esophageal mucosa is exposed to a pH below 4 and to improve gastric emptying. Unfortunately, the remaining agent available in the United States—metoclopramide—has limited therapeutic efficacy and a potentially unfavorable side effect profile. A brief review is presented, with the understanding that usefulness is currently limited in GERD patients.

Metoclopramide is a dopamine antagonist; the precise mechanism of action is unclear. Most commonly, it is reported to sensitize tissues to the action of acetylcholine and has been shown in some studies to increase the amplitude of gastric and esophageal contractions, increase LES pressure, and accelerate gastric emptying [35]. Because it crosses the blood–brain barrier and interacts with dopamine receptors, it produces clinically important central nervous system side effects, such as drowsiness and confusion [36], which preclude its widespread use. When studied head to head with H_2RAs, principally cimetidine, clinical trials have found equivalent efficacy of metoclopramide compared to H_2RAs in relieving heartburn and other GERD symptoms [37–39]. When compared to placebo, 10 mg of metoclopramide tid showed little symptom improvement. When the dose was increased to 10 mg qid, it was more effective than placebo in improving symptoms [40, 41]. No study has shown the agent to be more effective than placebo in promoting healing of erosive esophagitis. Because of its centrally acting effects, antidopaminergic side effects are observed in 20–30% of patients. Anxiety, agitation, confusion, motor restlessness, hallucinations, and drowsiness are the most common side effects; depression and tardive dyskinesia (potentially irreversible) are the most serious side effects. Side effects appear to be dose related and perhaps higher in children and the elderly. This agent has a black box warning for side effects. Some would get informed written consent if prescribed for long-term use. In a patient with clear evidence of gastroparesis and GERD symptoms refractory to antisecretory therapy, metoclopramide may be of additional benefit. The drug is not effective in treating patients with esophageal motility abnormalities.

Domperidone, a dopamine antagonist that stimulates esophageal peristalsis, increases LES pressure, and accelerates gastric emptying [42], is available outside the United States and in some US pharmacies that still compound the drug [42]. Unlike metoclopramide, it does not cross the blood–brain barrier, so has few of the central dopaminergic side effects of that drug. It should not be administered with antisecretory agents or antacids because reduced gastric acidity may impair its absorption. The few available studies are based on small samples and often lack controls. The efficacy studies suggest similarity to H₂RAs (ranitidine and famotidine) in symptom relief and in promotion of esophageal healing, and in one combination study with an H₂RA, the combination was not significantly better than each drug administered alone [42, 43]. Hyperprolactinemia, nipple tenderness, galactorrhea, and amenorrhea are the most common side effects of this agent, which is unlikely to be approved for distribution in the United States.

Combination therapy (H₂-receptor antagonists and promotility agents)

Prior to the availability of PPIs, the combination of an H₂RA and prokinetic was popularized as the management strategy to treat the difficult patient. This approach is presented here for historical information. While some studies have suggested that a combination of these two agents is more efficacious than either alone, the data are conflicting [39, 44]. The best study—a maintenance trial comparing ranitidine 150 mg tid, cisapride 10 mg tid, and a combination of ranitidine and cisapride, as part of a larger study including a PPI and combination of a PPI and cisapride—showed an advantage of combination therapy over H₂ blocker or cisapride alone [45]. This study showed a numeric, but not statistical, advantage for the combination of the prokinetic and PPI over a PPI alone. In general, the use of combination therapy with an antisecretory agent and a prokinetic should be discouraged as the therapeutic benefit, at best, is small and rarely results in improvement over an increase in the dose of antisecretory therapy. Combination therapy with an H₂RA and a PPI is discussed below.

Acid-suppressive therapy

Antisecretory agents are the medications of choice for pharmacologic therapy of GERD. Two classes of acid suppressive agents are still relevant today: H₂RAs and PPIs. Understanding of their active mechanisms and efficacy is crucial to optimal use of these agents alone or in combination. A brief review of acid production and active mechanism precedes the review of their overall efficacy.

Acid production

Parietal cells are located within the mucosa, predominantly in the body of the stomach. They produce an average of 2 L of gastric acid/day. There are three different types of receptors on the basal lateral membrane of the parietal cell, each of which when stimulated will affect the production of acid. Gastrin, present in the G cells in the gastric antrum, is stimulated by food in the stomach (gastric phase), reaching the parietal cells through the blood. Acetylcholine is released from the vagus nerve and is predominantly stimulated by the cephalic phase—the sight, sound, smell, and taste of food. Release of either of these two ligands stimulates the enterochromaffin-like (ECL) cell to release histamine, which

then binds to its receptor on the parietal cell. Activation of these receptors stimulates protein phosphokinases, principally cyclic adenosine 3′, 5′ monophosphate (cAMP), which then acts as a secondary messenger to stimulate the proton pump, which is in a resting state in the tubulovesicle of the parietal cell. Stimulation of the pump configures it into its active form at the secretory canaliculi where it will exchange an H⁺ for a K⁺ ion through the H⁺/K⁺-ATPase enzyme (the so-called proton pump), the final common path of acid secretion. Inhibition of any of the three receptors on the basal lateral membrane will inhibit acid production to some degree, while inhibition of the proton pump inhibits the final common pathway, thus creating the opportunity for superior acid suppression. There are no agents approved for use in GERD that inhibit the gastrin or acetylcholine receptor.

Both classes of agents, H₂RAs and PPIs, inhibit gastric secretion and raise intragastric pH. The number of hours of the day in which these agents raise intragastric pH to above 4 is an indirect measure of efficacy of symptom relief, correlates with healing of erosive esophagitis, and is important in understanding the overall efficacy data of these agents. When gastric pH is below 4, pepsinogen is activated to pepsin, which can exacerbate the esophageal mucosal damage caused by acid. An early meta-analysis linked healing of erosive esophagitis to the duration of time (> 24 h) that the intragastric pH is below 4 [46]. A recent proof of concept prospective study confirmed the relationship of control of intragastric pH and healing of grade C and D erosive esophagitis [47] (Figure 25.2), but suggests there may be a plateau effect, above which an increase in healing may not be obtained. In general, healing of erosive esophagitis by acid-suppressive agents is thus felt to be related to the duration of gastric acid suppression over a 24-h period. Unfortunately, a correlation between increase in intragastric pH control and symptom relief has not been conclusively documented.

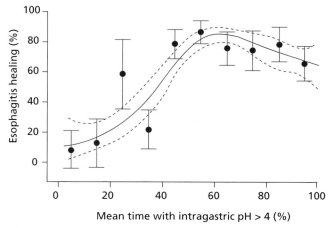

Figure 25.2 Prospective proof of concept study demonstrating an association between control of intragastric pH and healing of grade C and D erosive esophagitis [47].

H₂-receptor antagonists

Prior to the availability of PPIs, H₂RAs formed the mainstay of GERD therapy. The four available agents—cimetidine, ranitidine, famotidine, and nizatidine—derive their efficacy in GERD exclusively from inhibiting acid secretion. They do not affect LES pressure, TLESRs, esophageal clearance, or gastric emptying in humans. H₂RAs only block one receptor, and thus have limited effect on acid reduction, and are relatively weak inhibitors of meal-stimulated acid secretion, reducing acid secretion by almost 60–70% [48]. In general, the antisecretory capabilities of H₂RAs are best at night, with duration of acid inhibition longer when the drug is taken in the evening or before bedtime. Equally potent doses of H₂RAs equally inhibit acid secretion and as such provide reason for similar efficacy in GERD. H₂RAs were made available as over-the-counter agents in 1995, which is for the most part how they are used today. There are still however patients who do not tolerate PPIs and rare situations in which clinicians prefer to use an H₂RA, so understanding their efficacy is still important.

Symptom relief has been variable, ranging from 32% to 82% of patients, while endoscopic resolution ranges from 0% to 82% [49]. In a later meta-analysis, endoscopic improvement was demonstrated in 31–88% of patients, with healing in 27–45% of primarily grade 1 or 2 lesions [50]. The differences seen in these trials can be accounted for by various symptom endpoints, as well as the variability in erosive esophagitis baselines. This underscores the importance of carefully evaluating clinical trials in extrapolating clinical efficacy to specific patient populations.

Higher doses of H₂RAs given twice or four times a day may increase efficacy. Some comparative studies have produced 12-week healing rates as high as 70% with ranitidine at 150 mg two to four times daily [51–53] and 8-week healing rates of up 77% with 800 mg of cimetidine twice daily [52] and with famotidine 40 mg twice daily. These high healing rates are unusual in practice and when higher grades of erosive esophagitis are treated [53, 54]. The data above indicate that expectations for efficacy of higher doses may be overestimated in patients with severe disease who require greater acid suppression.

Maintenance of symptom relief and healing with H₂RAs are variable and parallel data from acute healing studies. One well-performed study examined symptom relapse over 4 weeks in 423 patients with GERD symptoms, randomized to either a placebo or 150 mg ranitidine twice or four times daily [55]. Approximately two-thirds had a normal-appearing esophagus endoscopically; 28%, grade-1 erosive esophagitis; and only 4.5%, grades 2–4 erosive esophagitis. Patients were randomized to receive 150 mg ranitidine twice daily or a placebo for 2 weeks. If patients were satisfied with their treatment (improved or complete relief), they continued with that therapy. If patients were not satisfied, they were re-randomized to receive 150 mg twice or four times

daily for another 2 weeks. If their symptoms did not respond after 4 weeks, they were removed from follow-up. After 4 weeks, all were taken off therapy, followed for an additional 20 weeks, and evaluated for overall symptom relapse. After 24 weeks, 52% who had non-erosive disease and 67% with erosive disease experienced relapse, giving an overall relapse rate of 59%. In general, dosage was unrelated to symptom relapse rate [34]. In a study comparing cisapride, ranitidine, and omeprazole, ranitidine 150 mg tid maintained remission in 49% at 1 year [56].

Overall, as a class, the H₂RAs are extremely safe with few overall side effects. Minor gastrointestinal side effects of clinical concern include nausea, abdominal pain, and bloating. There have been concerns about drug interactions with these agents, particularly interactions with agents affecting the cytochrome P450 system, and, in particular, with cimetidine. Serum concentrations of phenytoin, procainamide, theophylline, and warfarin have been altered after administration of cimetidine, and to a lesser degree ranitidine; these effects are not seen with famotidine and/or nizatidine [57, 58]. H2RAs do not appear to inhibit the effect of clopidogrel. The clinical consequences of these interactions are minimal and rarely result in a clinically important interaction. Nevertheless, these potential complications need to be considered if H₂RAs are prescribed.

Proton pump inhibitors

PPIs are clearly the most effective agents available for treatment of GERD at the present time. They provide superior control of intragastric pH over a 24-h period compared to H₂RAs and effect greater symptom relief and healing. By inhibiting the H⁺/K⁺-ATPase, the final common pathway of acid secretion, these agents suppress daytime, night-time, and meal-stimulated acid secretion to a significantly greater degree than H₂RAs [59]. There are seven PPIs available for use. The delayed-release PPIs are omeprazole, lansoprazole, rabeprazole, pantoprazole, and esomeprazole. Two newer formulations of PPIs have recently been added—omeprazole immediate release-sodium bicarbonate [a combination of non–enteric-coated omeprazole granules with sodium bicarbonate (OME-IR)] [60] and dexlansoprazole, the R-enantiomer of lansoprazole. The latter differs from traditional delayed-release PPIs by utilizing a dual delayed-release technology, with two types of enteric-coated granules soluble at different pHs. It is designed such that part will dissolve in the duodenum, like the traditional delayed-release PPI, and part in the distal small intestine [61].

PPIs are all weak bases that concentrate in the secretory canaliculi at pH below 4. They are highly selective and can concentrate up to 1000-fold in the acidic environment of the canaliculi. It is here that the inactive benzimidazole of the PPI is converted to a cationic sulfonamide, which binds to cysteines on the proton pump and therefore blocks acid-producing capabilities [62, 63]. The onset of inhibition may be delayed because PPIs need time to accumulate in the canaliculi and initiate activation of the acid production cycle. All available PPIs bind covalently and irreversibly to proton pumps; therefore, the degree of inhibition is related to area under the curve (AUC), not plasma concentration. PPIs block 70–80% of active pumps; therefore, for acid secretion to resume, new H^+/K^+-ATPase molecules must be synthesized, a process that takes 36–96 h. Although each of these agents has subtly different binding capabilities, delayed-release PPIs in general provide maximal efficacy in control of intragastric pH when taken immediately or longer before a meal, as the drugs bind to actively secreting pumps. It is for this reason that these drugs are administered before the first meal of the day, and when a second dose is needed, before the evening meal, rather than at bedtime. As not all pumps are active at any given time, a single dose of a PPI does not inhibit all pumps and, therefore, does not "completely" inhibit all acid secretion. Acid inhibition is never complete because of the continued synthesis of new pumps and a steady state is required in order to maintain continuous acid control [64]. When delayed-release PPIs are administered twice daily, more active pumps are exposed to the drug and the steady-state inhibition of gastric acid is more rapidly achieved and will be more complete. The sodium bicarbonate in OME-IR protects the PPI granules from acid degradation and may itself stimulate proton pumps. This may allow OME-IR to be effective when given at bedtime or perhaps when administered in the fasting state during the day. Limited data suggest the possibility that this drug may have a different absorption profile because of the bicarbonate and has a more rapid onset of action. Dexlansoprazole uses a dual delayed-release technology that results in a first peak in absorption at about 90 min after ingestion and a second 4–5 h after ingestion. Precise meal timing may not be required for optimal efficacy.

PPIs are metabolized in the liver by two enzymes in the cytochrome P450 system: CYP2C19, which forms an inactive 5-hydroxy and 5-O-desmethylmetabolite, and CYP3A4, which forms an inactive sulfone metabolite [63]. The subtle differences in how each PPI is metabolized within this system are responsible for the subtle differences in plasma concentration and drug interactions. While rarely a clinical problem, the absorption of other orally administered (acid-dependent) drugs may be affected (Table 25.3).

Clinical efficacy

pH control

The increase in pH control over a 24-h period accounts for the superiority of PPIs over the H_2RAs. Omeprazole, OME-IR, lansoprazole, pantoprazole, and rabeprazole are quite similar in their control of intragastric pH. Esomeprazole appears to provide a longer duration of pH control when the 40-mg dose is compared to the other delayed-release PPIs in doses

Table 25.3 Possible effects of increased intragastric pH on drug absorption.

Absorption increased	Absorption decreased
Aspirin	Ketoconazole
Benzylpenicillin	Itraconazole
Didanosine	Cefpodoxime proxetil
Nifedipine	Enoxacin
Midazolam	Indomethacin
Furosemide	Protein-bound cobalamin
Digoxin	

approved by the Food and Drug Administration (FDA) for healing of erosive esophagitis [65] (Figure 25.3). Direct comparisons between esomeprazole and OME-IR at similar dose timing have not been performed. With the newest PPI, dexlansoprazole, time at pH above 4 has been reported to be 17 h with once daily dosing, but again this drug has not been compared head to head with esomeprazole.

Symptom relief

To the patient the ultimate success of a drug is its ability to relieve symptoms. The PPIs are clearly superior to H_2RAs in this arena [66], though no PPI offers complete symptom relief in all patients when given once a day.

Although all PPIs provide a higher level of symptom improvement compared to H_2RAs, there are some variations and small difference in PPI performance when they are compared head to head [67–71]. The efficacy of OME-IR in symptom relief has been assumed, based on relative similarity in pH control to other delayed-release PPIs rather than clinical trials. There is speculation that the rapid onset of pH control seen with this agent should translate into faster symptom relief; however, no clinical trials are available to support this. Dexlansoprazole has demonstrated symptom relief that is superior to that with placebo in symptomatic GERD and has shown a similar percentage of symptom relief as other PPIs, although to date it has not been compared head to head with any other PPI. The overall clinical importance of the small differences seen among individual clinical trials is unknown. Because of the differences in endpoints, cross-study comparisons are extremely difficult. Consequently, a determination of whether any clinically important difference exists in symptom relief between PPIs is unknown based on available data. In clinical practice, there is likely no difference when the drugs are given as once a day doses.

Healing of erosive esophagitis

Ultimately, the most objective measure of drug efficacy is healing of erosive esophagitis. All PPIs provide excellent and likely clinically equivalent healing rates at 8 weeks. Esomeprazole 40 mg has a small statistical advantage in healing of erosive esophagitis after 8 weeks when compared

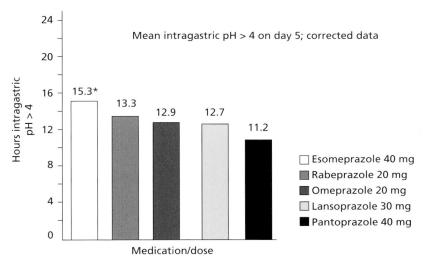

Figure 25.3 Percentage time intragastric pH above 4 for five delayed-release proton pump inhibitors given once daily before breakfast. Cross-over study in 34 patients. *P < .0004 (n = 34, all pairwise comparisons vs esomprazole).

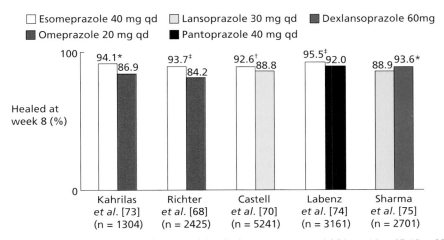

Figure 25.4 Healing of erosive esophagitis at 8 weeks with various delayed-release proton pump inhibitors. *P < .05; [+]P < .001; [‡]P = .0001.

separately head to head with omeprazole 20 mg, lansoprazole 30 mg, and pantoprazole 40 mg [68, 70, 72]. The superiority of esomeprazole 40 mg is predominantly seen with grades C and D, suggesting that the superior acid control seen with this agent compared to the others may augment healing. There are no healing studies available with OME-IR for comparison. Dexlansoprazole 60 mg demonstrated healing rates of 92–95% after 8 weeks, compared to 86–92% of those treated with lansoprazole 30 mg for a similar time frame. The overall pooled comparison showed no statistical difference. Los Angeles grade C and D erosive esophagitis seemed to be healed at a greater frequency with dexlansoprazole. A summary of healing rates for erosive esophagitis is given in Figure 25.4 [68, 70, 73–75]. It should be remembered that healing does not guarantee symptom relief and in clinical trials symptom relief does not reach the levels reported for the more objective healing data (Figure 25.5)

[68, 70, 73, 74, 76]. The reasons for this gap between healing and symptom relief are unclear, but it highlights the importance of individualizing therapy.

Maintenance therapy

Healing of mucosal injury or achievement of symptom control alone is not sufficient to alter the natural history of GERD, so relapse is almost universal if medication is stopped. Thus, almost all patients require some form of maintenance therapy. While numerous approaches have been advocated and studied, including on-demand, intermittent, and half-dose PPI, statistically patients with GERD will have better long-term symptom relief and maintenance of healing of erosive esophagitis with continuous PPI use. The optimal approach to maintenance therapy in clinical practice must be individualized, and depends on many factors. In general, patients who have non-erosive reflux disease (NERD) or Los Angeles grade

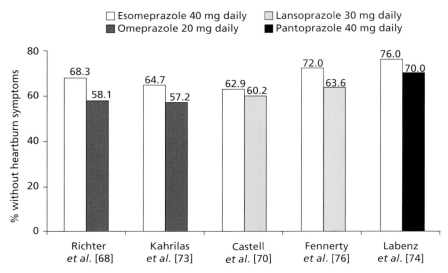

Figure 25.5 Symptom relief after 4 weeks of daily therapy on once-daily proton pump inhibitors.

A and B esophagitis are the best candidates for a regimen that does not involve daily continuous therapy [77]. Those with grades C and D erosive esophagitis, stricture, and Barrett's esophagus will in general need continuous therapy.

Dose response

Increasing the dose of PPIs if symptoms are not relieved is common in practice. Whether this will effectively increase healing of erosive esophagitis, i.e. whether a dose response is demonstrable with these agents, is difficult to prove. In a comparison study by Castell *et al.*, 15 mg of lansoprazole daily resulted in a healing rate that was lower than that for 30 mg of lansoprazole (79% vs 91%) [70]. A similar dose-dependent pattern was demonstrated in a study by Lundell *et al.*, who compared 10- and 20-mg doses of omeprazole in healing Los Angeles grades A–C of erosive esophagitis [78]. With the lower dose of omeprazole, efficacy in healing correlated with the grade of esophagitis (77% of grade A healed, 50% of B, and 20% of C). This correlation of efficacy with grade did not occur with the 20-mg dose, which healed 80% of grades A and B, and 40% of grade C erosive esophagitis. These are higher healing rates than seen with the lower dose and suggest that there is a dose response with antisecretory therapy with PPIs. However, Sontag *et al.* compared 20- and 40-mg daily doses of omeprazole to placebo in 230 patients with erosive esophagitis grades 2 to 4 [79]. At week 8, there was no difference in healing overall between the 20- and 40-mg groups (73.5% and 74.7%, respectively). The 40-mg dose resulted in faster symptom relief; however, no difference in overall symptom relief was observed at the end of 8 weeks. Esomeprazole 40 mg resulted in increased healing compared to esomeprazole 20 g. Clinical trials have failed to demonstrate improvement in healing (or symptom relief) when dosing strength is increased above that approved by the FDA. However, a long-term obser-vational study showed that by increasing omeprazole dose as needed, almost all patients refractory to ranitidine could be effectively healed, indicating that dose titration can be efficacious in individual patients [80].

Step therapy

As our understanding of the physiology of acid production, pathogenesis of heartburn, action mechanism of acid suppression, and drug safety profiles has changed over time, so has the therapy of choice. The once-dominant strategy involving lifestyle modifications and over-the-counter antacids followed by prescription H_2RAs, and then introduction of PPIs is no longer common practice. This strategy has been largely abandoned as we have become comfortable with the safety profile of PPIs, the cost of these agents has decreased, and clinical trials have been reported.

Step-down therapy for maintenance is still discussed and indeed advocated by some, due in the past (and now again) to concerns over long-term use (and cost) of PPIs. A study by Inadomi *et al.* examined the feasibility of step-down therapy in patients with non-erosive symptomatic GERD who were asymptomatic with PPIs [81]. After baseline demographic and quality-of-life information were obtained, the patients were withdrawn from PPIs in a stepwise fashion. Fifty-eight percent of patients were asymptomatic following discontinuation of treatment after 1 year of follow-up. Thirty-four percent required H_2RAs, 7% required prokinetic agents, 1% required both, and 15% remained asymptomatic without medication. Although quality of life was not significantly different, management costs decreased by 37%. Younger age and heartburn were the predominant factors predicting unsuccessful PPI step-down management, suggesting that individuals with "true GERD" will require full-dose maintenance therapy for optimal symptom relief.

Approach to the patient

Optimization of proton pump inhibitors

PPIs are generally approved for once-daily dosing and prescribed in the morning. Dexlansoprazole has been approved by the FDA for once-daily dosing without regard to food. Despite different food effects, the new data regarding pH control with dexlansoprazole and the potential for bicarbonate (OME-IR) to stimulate pumps in the absence of a meal in the vast majority of circumstances, we still recommend that all PPIs be given before a meal. In the majority, we suggest taking the PPI before the first meal of the day (usually breakfast). This is based on concepts previously discussed and results of an intragastric pH study addressing this issue [82]. This two-armed cross-over study treated normal subjects with 20 mg of omeprazole or 30 mg of lansoprazole at 7:30 am daily for 7 days, followed by intragastric pH monitoring performed with the dose given 15–30 min before breakfast and when given on an empty stomach with no food until lunchtime. A significant superiority in daytime pH control (time intragastric pH was above 4) was found when the PPI was taken before breakfast compared to an empty stomach [82] (Figure 25.6). Although the precise interval prior to a meal required to produce optimal pH control has not been determined, we suggest that PPIs should be given on an empty stomach and followed in 30 min by a meal, as done in the study described above. If dexlansoprazole is being used, we encourage similar dosing and remind patients that they should eat within 5 h of dosing. This type of once-daily dosing with any of the PPIs will result in good outcomes for the vast majority of patients.

Some patients require an increase in dosage due to incomplete symptom relief, the presence of extraesophageal symptoms (e.g. asthma, cough, laryngitis, and chest pain) and, perhaps, Barrett's esophagus. In this case, splitting the dose and giving a PPI twice daily before breakfast and dinner provides superior intragastric pH control, particularly at night, when compared to a double dose given once daily. At the time of writing, no data are available assessing intragastric pH control on dexlansoprazole given twice daily.

The difference in pH control relative to dose timing was first observed in a study in 19 normal subjects randomized to receive 40 mg of omeprazole before breakfast, 40 mg before dinner (pm), or 20 mg twice daily (before breakfast and dinner) [83]. Each was crossed over to all three regimens with a 1-week washout period between 24-h intragastric pH studies. The most important observation made from these data was the statistical superiority of the 20-mg twice-daily dose in control of 24-h intragastric pH compared to 40 mg in a single dose. A subsequent three-way cross-over study confirmed these observations by evaluating overnight pH control in subjects treated with 40 mg of omeprazole before breakfast, before dinner, or twice daily. Control in daytime pH was similar regardless of regimen; however, nocturnal pH control was significantly improved with the twice-daily regimen compared to a double-dose once daily [84] (Figure 25.7).

Another observation from intragastric pH studies is the finding of wide intersubject variability in intragastric pH control despite similar dosing regimens. This wide variability is illustrated by a study comparing 24-h intragastric pH control in normal subjects treated with omeprazole at 20 mg and lansoprazole at 30 mg twice daily for 7 days [85]. Both inter- and intra-subject variability in pH response were observed (Figure 25.8). This intra-subject variability in intragastric pH control is uncommon and not easy to explain, but it may account for the occasional patient who responds to a switch from one PPI to another after one seemingly fails.

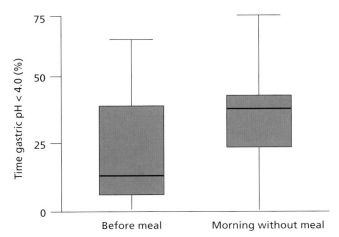

Figure 25.6 Cross-over study in healthy subjects demonstrating improvement in intragastric pH control when a delayed release proton pump inhibitor is taken prior to a meal as compared to in the morning with no food until lunch time. ——— median pH control.

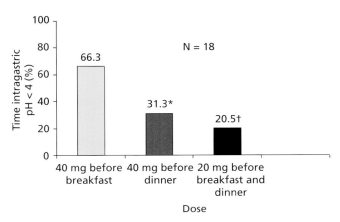

Figure 25.7 Cross-over study in healthy subjects assessing intragastric pH control in the sleeping period (10:00 pm–6:00 am) on 40 mg omeprazole. A split dose enhances overnight pH control. *$P = .01$; †$P < .02$.

Selected clinical situations

Nocturnal gastroesophageal reflux disease

Reflux that occurs while the patient is asleep (nocturnal reflux), whether or not it produces symptoms, has the potential to be more damaging to the esophageal mucosa, as esophageal clearance is delayed during sleep due to multiple factors. The approach to the patient with nocturnal reflux has evolved in part because of a series of careful studies using continuous intragastric pH monitoring that found that as many as 70% of patients continue to secrete acid and intragastric pH declines to below 4 for at least 1 continuous hour in the overnight period from 10 pm to 6 am even when taking a PPI twice daily [86]. This drop in pH, a pharmacologic phenomenon termed nocturnal gastric acid breakthrough (NAB), begins about 6–7 h after the evening dose of a PPI [86]. When PPIs are given as a once-daily dose before breakfast, this nocturnal gastric acid recovery occurs earlier in the evening, beginning around 11 pm [87]. This NAB appears to be a class effect, and can be demonstrated in normal subjects, and subjects with uncomplicated GERD, Barrett's esophagus, and scleroderma [86]. Large numbers of normal subjects and patients on all the once- and twice-daily dosages of all the PPIs (save dexlansoprazole) have been studied , documenting a consistent frequency of gastric acid recovery regardless of the PPI [88]. Overnight recovery of gastric acid is seen with dexlansoprazole once daily but it has not been studied twice daily.

The clinical importance of this common intragastric finding appears to have been overestimated, as esophageal reflux occurs during nocturnal breakthrough of intragastric pH in only 5% of normal subjects and about 15% of patients with uncomplicated GERD [89]. This is consistent with the observation from clinical trials that nocturnal heartburn is infrequent (10–15%) on once-daily PPIs. Symptoms during these nocturnal gastric pH drops have not been systematically studied but appear to be uncommon. Overnight gastric acid recovery may be of clinical importance in patients with severe GERD and those with Barrett's esophagus. Up to 50% of patients with Barrett's esophagus or scleroderma and GERD will have increased overnight esophageal acid exposure during NAB [90, 91]. NAB is not the result of PPI resistance, which is an extremely rare phenomenon [92].

When patients have acid reflux during the sleeping period it is often necessary to modify the dosing schedule of antisecretory therapy. In a patient with continued reflux on once-daily PPI there are several options. The single dose can be given before the evening meal, and consideration can be given to using OME-IR at bedtime, adding an H$_2$ blocker at bedtime (see below), increasing the PPI to twice daily (before breakfast and dinner or OME-IR before breakfast and bedtime), or in some cases twice daily PPI plus an H$_2$RA at bedtime. The use of OME-IR at bedtime is based on a study comparing overnight intragastric pH control in GERD patients with nocturnal symptoms treated with OME-IR 40 mg at bedtime or esomeprazole 40 mg and lansoprazole 30 mg given at a similar time [93] (Figure 25.9). The former showed more rapid onset of pH control, a decrease in NAB, and improved overnight pH control in the vulnerable period (first 4 h of sleep) compared to the other PPIs. It is important to be aware, however, that 24-h pH control with this dosing regimen of OME-IR was not as effective as esomeprazole 40 mg given at bedtime [93].

Another means of controlling NAB is to add an H$_2$RA given at bedtime to a PPI given once or twice daily. This was popularized in the early 2000s, based on a series of short-term studies prior to the release of OME-IR. Two papers reported longer-term use of nocturnal H$_2$RAs, evaluated the

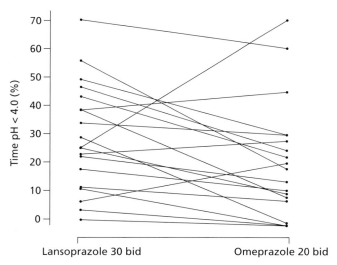

Figure 25.8 Study in 20 normal subjects demonstrating variability in intragastric pH control on twice-daily proton pump inhibitors. Note both inter- and intra-subject variability.

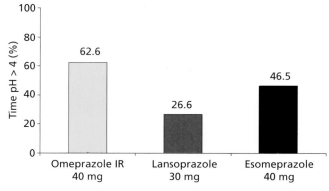

Figure 25.9 Study comparing overnight pH control in patients (n = 49) with night-time symptoms when proton pump inhibitors were given at bedtime. The study demonstrates the potential for immediate-release omeprazole (OME-IR) to be effective in this situation. OME-IR vs lanzoprazole, $P < .001$; OME-IR vs esomeprazole, $P < 0.02$.

control of intragastric pH in the subjects and patients, and raised important issues regarding long-term efficacy of this choice of regimen [94, 95].

One study prospectively evaluated 23 healthy volunteers and 20 patients with GERD initially treated with omeprazole 20 mg bid (before breakfast and dinner) followed by the addition of an H_2RA (ranitidine 300 mg qhs) at bedtime for 28 days [94]. Patients were studied with prolonged ambulatory pH monitoring after 2 weeks of omeprazole bid followed by pH testing after days 1, 7, and 28 of continuous H_2RAs at bedtime. The median time that pH was below 4 for the supine period was similar for GERD patients and normal volunteers. Four general patterns of gastric pH response were found. The first subgroup experienced a decreasing effect of H_2RA over time (tolerance). A second subgroup (21% of 43 subjects) exhibited a sustained response to H_2RA therapy (no tolerance). A third subgroup, consisting of three healthy subjects, had no NAB on the twice-daily PPI regimen, and NAB did not develop when H_2RA was added. All three in this group were *Helicobacter pylori* positive. The fourth subgroup was marked by an unpredictable response (26% of 43 subjects). This group showed variable outcomes at different time points in the study.

Another study reviewed prolonged ambulatory pH monitoring studies in GERD patients [95]. Group 1 (n = 60) took either 20 mg of omeprazole or 30 mg of lansoprazole bid. Group 2 (n = 45) received a PPI bid (omeprazole 20 mg or lansoprazole 30 mg) plus an H_2 blocker at bedtime (ranitidine 300 mg, famotidine 40 mg, or nizatidine 300 mg) for more than 28 days. Group 3 (n =11) patients were evaluated for response to both regimens. The authors evaluated percentage time that nocturnal and daytime intragastric pH was above 4 and percentage of patients with NAB for all groups. Overall, 27% of patients spent 100% of the recumbent period with intragastric pH above 4, and 32% spent greater than 90% of the recumbent period with pH above 4. Ten percent spent greater than 50% of the night with pH below 4. In contrast, 50% of patients on PPI bid experienced a pH below 4 over 50% of the recumbent period; 20% experienced a pH above 4 during more than 90% of the recumbent period (P < .001). For patients tested on both regimens (n = 11), the median percentage time overnight that intragastric pH was above 4 increased from 54.6% without an H_2RA to 96.5% with an H_2RA (P = .001).

These two studies [94, 95] come to different conclusions, but are in fact not dissimilar in their overall findings. Despite the finding of tolerance and the absence of statistical improvement in the randomized study (type 2 error?), both studies identify a substantial number of patients who do have a sustained effect and many who do not. The studies agree that total acid control (100% of the time that intragastric pH is above 4) is extremely difficult to achieve with modern pharmacology. Whether the newest PPI, dexlansoprazole twice daily, will make this control possible awaits

Table 25.4 Hierarchy of intragastric pH control.

PPI once a day
PPI plus H_2RA (OTC probably acceptable)*
PPI bid* (OME-IR at bedtime)
PPI bid plus H_2RA*

*These regimens have never been tested head to head in clinical trials. We use OME-IR at HS in selected patients but this has not been compared head to head with PPI bid plus H_2RA.
bid, twice daily; H_2RA, histamine 2-receptor antagonist; OME-IR, omeprazole immediate-release; OTC, over the counter; PPI, proton pump inhibitor.

further study. Fortunately, this high degree of pharmacologic control is rarely necessary and may raise safety issues if needed long term. Overall, it is fair to say that tolerance to H_2RAs at bedtime in addition to a PPI twice a day is real but relative, and that a sustained response may be seen in a large number of patients. Perhaps an on-demand H_2RA at bedtime should be considered in those situations in which night-time reflux is likely to occur. These studies underscore the importance of prolonged ambulatory reflux monitoring as a means of documenting the need for an aggressive acid control regimen, and the need to individualize antisecretory therapy in difficult-to-treat patients. A hierarchy of intragastric pH control is outlined in Table 25.4.

Non-erosive gastroesophageal reflux disease (symptomatic gastroesophageal reflux disease with normal upper endoscopy)

Patients with GERD and normal endoscopy have been considered to have less severe disease than patients with erosive esophagitis. However, clinical trials have suggested an interesting paradox: patients with GERD and a normal endoscopy may not respond as well to PPIs. Early studies highlight this paradox. Lind *et al.* compared 10- and 20-mg doses of omeprazole with a placebo in 509 patients with symptoms and normal endoscopy [96]. After 4 weeks of therapy, only 46% of patients on the 20-mg dose reported the complete absence of heartburn. Although superior to the placebo (13% with complete relief), this complete relief is inferior to that seen in erosive esophagitis trials. Bate *et al.* found similar results in a comparison of 20 mg of omeprazole to placebo in 209 patients [97]. After 4 weeks, 57% of the patients taking omeprazole were heartburn free and 43% completely asymptomatic (including no regurgitation), and thus omeprazole is superior to placebo; however, once again these results represent a decrease in efficacy compared to standard erosive esophagitis trials. A study by Carlsson *et al.* highlights this seeming paradox [98]. The authors conducted a 4-week comparison of the efficacy of omeprazole in 277 patients with and 261 patients without erosive esophagitis. A 20-mg dose of omeprazole achieved complete symptom relief. in 48% of those with erosions compared to only 29% of those without. While the outcome differences in these studies cannot be easily explained, the study by Lind *et al.* suggested that patients with an abnormal pH monitoring study were more likely to respond to omeprazole than those with a normal pH study [96]. Later studies with esomeprazole and dexlansoprazole do demonstrate improvement in symptom relief over these early studies. In clinical trials, increasing the dose of a PPI to twice daily does not improve symptom relief in patients with heartburn who have a normal endoscopy, though this strategy does work in individual patients. This group of patients is typically difficult to treat and this reflects a lack of clear understanding of the genesis of symptoms in these patients. We find it extremely helpful to study patients with NERD who do not respond well to PPIs with both prolonged reflux monitoring and esophageal function testing to carefully determine the association of GERD and symptoms.

Unexplained chest pain (non-cardiac chest pain)

It is very clear from a large body of research that many patients with unexplained chest pain in whom cardiac disease has been ruled out will have GERD as the proximate cause of their symptoms. When attempting to treat these and other patients with extraesophageal disease, the clinician should keep in mind that for the most part these patients require more aggressive antisecretory therapy for longer periods of time than the typical patient for heartburn. Unfortunately, there are few well-designed short-term studies in this patient population and no real maintenance trials. Therefore, long-term treatment of these patients, which is usually required, is based on extrapolation of data from maintenance trials of heartburn and erosive esophagitis.

A randomized, double-blind, placebo-controlled treatment trial compared omeprazole to placebo in 36 patients with non-cardiac chest pain and GERD documented by 24-h ambulatory pH testing [99]. Patients were treated with 20 mg of omeprazole twice daily or a placebo for 8 weeks and kept a daily diary of chest pain frequency and severity. Omeprazole produced a significant decrease in the fraction of chest pain days (39% ± 7.2% vs 10% ± 6.9%, $P = .006$) and pain severity (40.7 ± 8.1 vs 14.8 ± 8.2, $P = .03$). Fifteen of 18 (81%) patients receiving omeprazole reported symptomatic improvement, in contrast to only one of 18 (6%) in the placebo group.

A trial of antireflux therapy with a PPI is often recommended as initial therapy for suspected GERD. The most publicized trial addressing what is now called the PPI test was a randomized, double-blind, placebo-controlled trial that evaluated 1 week of high-dose omeprazole as a diagnostic test for GERD in 37 patients with non-cardiac chest pain [100]. All patients had chest pain at least three times a week. Endoscopy and 24-h ambulatory esophageal pH monitoring were performed in all, and a daily diary of the frequency and severity of chest pain was maintained. Patients were randomly assigned to receive either the placebo or omeprazole (40 mg in the morning and 20 mg in the evening) for 7 days with a cross-over to the other arm after a 2-week washout period and repeat baseline symptom assessment. Twenty-three patients (62.2%) were GERD positive and 14 GERD negative, based on the presence of erosive esophagitis or abnormal 24-h pH monitoring. The so-called "omeprazole test" was diagnostic for GERD if chest pain scores improved by greater than 50% after treatment. Eighteen GERD-positive patients (78%) and two GERD-negative patients (14%) had positive test results, yielding a sensitivity of 78.3% (95% CI 61.4–95.1) and specificity of 85.7% (95% CI 67.4–100), compared with endoscopy and ambulatory pH monitoring for the diagnosis of GERD. Subsequent economic analysis has estimated that this approach would save US$573 per patient with chest pain if a full work-up, including endoscopy, esophageal manometry, and 24-h ambulatory pH monitoring, is done in every patient. Subsequent studies of this type and a meta-analysis support PPI efficacy in GERD-related non-cardiac chest pain [101].

In the more typical patient with less-frequent pain (often less than once a week), a short pharmacologic trial may not be sufficient to evaluate improvement. Thus, this approach seems most useful for patients with frequent pain. In general, a 4–8-week trial of therapy seems more practical and most patients with chest pain related to GERD require long-term maintenance therapy.

Extraesophageal disease

Many patients present with a symptom other than heartburn or regurgitation but that is felt to be caused by GERD. Clinical trials of treatment involving patients with these so-called extraesophageal manifestations of GERD, specifically asthma, cough, and voice changes, are few, small, and in many instances uncontrolled. Early uncontrolled observations have led to the clinical impression that these patients require higher doses of PPIs (usually twice daily) for longer periods of time (up to 3–6 months) than patients with the typical symptoms of heartburn and regurgitation. Performing clinical trials in these patients is more difficult than in patients with erosive esophagitis as the "gold standard" for diagnosis of GERD with extraesophageal symptoms is not clear. As such, few randomized trials have been performed, many with negative results.

Only one study has examined the effect of lifestyle modifications, including raising the head of the bed by 6 inches, eliminating meals before bedtime, and using antacids in the treatment of patients with respiratory symptoms and GERD. Outcomes were compared to using no antireflux measures for 2-month periods. In this study, both esophageal and respiratory symptoms improved; however, there were no objective changes noted in pulmonary function [102]. This suggests that the addition of the conservative measures outlined in Table 25.1 may be useful in management, especially for patients with post-prandial reflux [103].

Early trials tested H_2RAs as treatment for patients with supraesophageal GERD and asthma or chronic cough. Larrain *et al.* performed a 6-month treatment trial that was the first to show that the clinical response was slower than that seen in patients with heartburn, with many patients achieving optimal response only after 4–6 months of therapy [104]. Several other short-term studies using H_2RAs have consistently demonstrated improvement in heartburn, but limited improvement in objective changes of pulmonary function and symptoms [105–107], an important finding even in PPI trials. A clear history of reflux-associated asthma appears to be the only predictive factor for improvement in respiratory symptoms. Clinical experience confirms these findings.

Improvement of cough believed to be associated with GERD has been reported in 70–100% of patients treated with H_2RAs [108–111], and again time to symptom improvement was quite prolonged, usually 161–179 days. Several clinical trials have been conducted using PPIs in patients with asthma, cough, and laryngitis. Patients taking omeprazole 20 mg once or twice a day for 4–6 weeks showed an improvement in pulmonary function tests, but little change in bronchodilator use or asthma scores [112, 113]. The patients who had control of their asthma also had healed esophagitis, reinforcing the fact that adequate acid control is required to decrease pulmonary symptoms. A randomized double-blind controlled trial by Boeree *et al.* in 36 patients, comparing omeprazole 40 mg twice daily to placebo for 3 months, showed a reduction in nocturnal cough during treatment with omeprazole [114]. Objective changes in forced expiratory volume in 1 s (FEV_1) and other pulmonary function tests could not be demonstrated, similar to the findings in asthma.

Important insights into medical treatment of patients with supraesophageal GERD can be gleaned from a well-designed study by Harding *et al.* in which 30 patients with documented asthma and GER proven by prolonged pH monitoring were treated with increasing doses of omeprazole [115]. Starting at 20 mg/day, the medication was increased by 20 mg after each 4-week treatment period for 3 months, or until esophageal acid exposure was reduced to "normal." Normalization of esophageal acid exposure resulted in improvement in pulmonary symptoms in 70% of patients. Several observations emerged from this trial: eight patients (28%) needed more than 20 mg/day of omeprazole to normalize esophageal acid exposure; many patients required the entire 3-month period of treatment to achieve optimal symptom relief, with improvement progressing continuously over the 3-month period, confirming the observations of Larrain *et al.* [104]; and a favorable response to omeprazole was seen in patients who presented with frequent regurgitation (more than once a week) and those with abnormal proximal acid exposure demonstrated by ambulatory pH monitoring. This study emphasized the importance of adequate esophageal acid control to achieve improvement

in patients with extraesophageal symptoms, and underscores that, despite the presence of an abnormal pH study, even optimal acid control may not completely relieve symptoms. The most recent trial, a large randomized study comparing esomeprazole 40 mg twice daily to placebo in patients with GERD-related asthma, found no difference between symptoms in the two groups [116].

Patients with voice disturbance suspected due to GERD present similar challenges to those in the respiratory group, and there is a similar lack of data on this group. Observational studies found variability in response of patients with this manifestation of GERD, the need to treat for longer periods before seeing a response when disease is severe, the need for higher doses of PPIs, and the rapid relapse of symptoms when therapy is discontinued, emphasizing that long-term treatment is often needed in these patients [117, 118].

A study by El-Serag *et al.* compared lansoprazole 30 mg twice daily with a placebo for 3 months in 20 patients with posterior laryngitis, abnormal laryngeal examination, and an abnormal pH monitoring study [119]. Complete relief of symptoms was seen in 50% of the PPI arm compared to 10% of the placebo arm ($P < .05$). Unfortunately, there were no predictive factors for improvement, either on laryngeal examination or pH monitoring. These data provide the "best" evidence for the efficacy of gastric acid suppression in the treatment of chronic laryngitis. A large, randomized controlled trial compared esomeprazole 40 mg twice daily to placebo for 24 weeks in patients with laryngeal findings consistent with GERD. No difference was found between the two groups [120]. A meta-analysis of all available trials also found no difference between PPIs and placebo in this difficult-to-treat group [121]. Nevertheless, some patients do extremely well with medical therapy.

Symptoms refractory to proton pump inhibitors and non-acid reflux

A substantial number of patients who are treated for symptoms of GERD have an incomplete response to PPIs. It is apparent from studies evaluating these patients with combined impedance pH testing [122] that a finite number will have symptoms that are related to weakly acidic or non-acid reflux. Treatment of these patients has not been systematically studied; however, small studies suggest that $GABA_B$ agonists like baclofen [123] decrease the number of reflux episodes, particularly after a meal, and may be useful in these patients, though are not FDA approved for this purpose (Figure 25.10). Multiple reflux inhibitors are in development.

Optimal treatment of extraesophageal manifestations of gastroesophageal reflux disease

The optimal treatment for patients with unexplained chest pain and other extraesophageal manifestations of GERD is

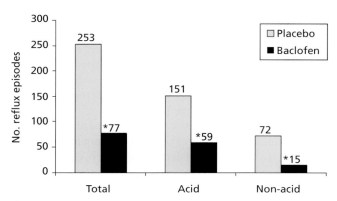

Figure 25.10 Study demonstrating a decrease in reflux episodes, both acid and non-acid in patients on baclofen 20 mg tid compared to placebo. The study assessed reflux episodes in the 2-h period after a refluxogenic meal. This is one of several studies to demonstrate that baclofen has potential to be helpful in the management of reflux.*P < .05.

not clear. Until better diagnostic tests are developed, the most efficient approach to is to begin empirical therapy with twice-daily PPI before breakfast and dinner for 2–3 months (note again that dexlansoprazole has not been studied twice daily). If patients do not respond to a trial of antireflux therapy, an evaluation with prolonged ambulatory reflux monitoring with impedance/pH testing while continuing therapy is the procedure of choice [122]. This allows assessment of pH control and symptom correlation. In the event that pH control is incomplete, and especially when overnight [86] esophageal acid exposure continues [89] and/or symptoms continue in association with continued reflux, antisecretory therapy should be adjusted or a reflux inhibitor added [86, 124]. Baclofen can be considered if non-acid reflux is present and associated with symptoms [124]. Patients successfully treated with acid suppression should be considered for long-term maintenance with PPI therapy, although no study has specifically addressed this issue.

Pregnancy

The frequency of GERD symptoms in pregnant women varies, with some estimating a prevalence of approximately 66% with others ranging from 45% to 80% [33]. Management of the pregnant patient with GERD presents a clinical challenge because of lack of data on the efficacy of traditional medical therapy and concerns about the risk of diagnostic studies. In general, endoscopy in the third trimester is safe, although it should rarely be needed. The treatment approach most often recommended is to begin with lifestyle and dietary modifications as the first step, using antacids alone or in combination with alginic acid for symptom relief. If this is not sufficient, sucralfate, a mucosal protectant with little or no systemic absorption, may be considered as a second-line agent. In fact, when this agent was given in doses of 1 g qid, greater relief of heartburn

(90% vs 30%) and regurgitation (83% vs 27%) compared to lifestyle and dietary modifications alone was demonstrated in one randomized study of 66 pregnant patients [33]. The clinician should be aware that sucralfate has been associated with the development of constipation, an important potential problem in pregnancy. The H$_2$RAs have been designated as FDA pregnancy class B (with the exception of nizatidine, which is classified as C because of animal studies demonstrating spontaneous abortions and low fetal birth weight) and can be considered in patients with severe, persistent symptoms despite the above interventions. Omeprazole, although designated as class C, has been administered to women immediately prior to labor and during elective cesarean section without complication, but it cannot be routinely recommended in pregnancy. The other PPIs—lansoprazole, rabeprazole, pantoprazole, esomeprazole, and dexlansoprazole—although designated as class B, have not been tested in clinical trials. A recent retrospective case–control study suggested that this class of agents is safe in pregnancy, maybe even in the first trimester [125]. Overall, the pharmacologic approach to the pregnant patient with GERD must be individualized and undertaken with extreme care. Fortunately, the condition is temporary and, despite uncomfortable symptoms, major complications are extremely unusual.

Side effects of proton pump inhibitors

As a class, PPIs have been amongst the safest. Initial concerns regarding development of gastric carcinoid tumors, B$_{12}$ deficiency, and colon cancer or polyps have not been substantiated in any credible long-term study. Recent concerns, however, have arisen regarding the potential for adverse events from long-term acid suppression [126–128] Emerging data illustrate the potential risks associated with both short- and long-term PPI therapy, including *Clostridium difficile*-associated diarrhea (CDAD), community-acquired pneumonia, osteoporotic fracture (Table 25.5), and inhibition of antiplatelet therapy [129–143]. These data are all from retrospective case–control studies, and demonstrate association not causality. No prospective, observational or randomized trial can substantiate the concerns discussed subsequently.

Clostridium difficile-associated diarrhea

C. difficile is the leading cause of diarrhea in hospitalized patients. Though the most common risk factors for acquiring CDAD is the use of antibiotics, there is evidence of a relationship between PPI therapy and CDAD based on the premise that the pathogenicity of *C. difficile* is related to the ability of its spores to resist destruction by the normal gastric acid environment, allowing for intestinal colonization. These data raise issues for clinicians caring for patients in the hospital

Table 25.5 Risks of proton pump inhibitor use.

Design *Clostridium difficile*-associated diarrhea	Outcomes	Adjusted OR (95% CI)
Case–control [130]	• Risk associated with PPI use within preceding 8 weeks	2.5 (1.5–4.2)
	• Risk associated with PPI use plus antibiotics	5.4 (2.2–13.2)
	• Risk associated with PPI use, antibiotics, and chemotherapy	43.2 (5.7–330.4)
Cohort [131]	• Risk associated with current PPI use	2.1 (1.2–3.5)
	• Risk associated with receipt of three or more antibiotics	2.1 (1.3–3.4)
	• Risk associated with being on a medical versus surgical ward	4.1 (2.3–7.3)
Case–control [131]	• Risk associated with current PPI use	2.6 (1.3–5.0)
	• Risk associated with prior renal failure	5.1 (1.7–15.2)
	• Risk associated with hospitalization within previous 3 months	2.9 (1.4–6.1)
	• Risk associated with female gender	2.5 (1.2–5.0)
	• Risk associated with MRSA colonization	7.8 (2.3–26.0)
Two population-based case–control studies [132]	• Risk associated with current PPI use	2.9 (2.4–3.4)
	• Risk associated with inflammatory bowel disease	3.6 (2.6–5.1)
	• Risk associated with renal failure	3.7 (2.4–5.6)
Prospective case–control study [133]	• Risk associated with antibiotic therapy	13.1 (6.6–26.1)
	• Risk associated with acid suppression therapy	1.90 (1.10–3.29)
Case–control [134]	• Risk associated with PPI use prior to or during admission	2.75 (1.68–4.52)
Case–control [135]	• Risk associated with PPI use	3.6 (1.7–8.3)
	• Risk associated with renal failure	5.7 (1.3–39.1)
Systematic review [136]	• Odds of taking antisecretory therapy among patients infected with *C. difficile*	1.94 (1.37–2.75)
		1.96 (1.28–3.00)
	• Risk associated with PPI use	1.40 (0.85–2.29)
	• Risk associated with H$_2$RA use	
Community-acquired pneumonia		
Nested case–control [137]	• Risk with any current acid-suppressive therapy	1.27 (1.06–1.54)
	• Risk among persons currently using PPIs	1.89 (1.36–2.62)
	• Risk among persons currently using H$_2$RAs	1.63 (1.07–2.48)
Case–control [138]	• Risk with current PPI use	1.5 (1.3–1.7)
	• Risk with initiation of PPIs 0–7 days prior to diagnosis	5.0 (2.1–11.7)
	• Risk when PPI was started >3 months prior to diagnosis	1.3 (1.2–1.4)
Nested case–control [139]	• Risk associated with current PPI use	1.02 (0.97–1.08)
	• Risk associated with current PPI therapy started:	6.53 (3.95–10.80)
	– within 2 days of diagnosis	3.79 (2.66–5.42)
	– within 7 days of diagnosis	3.21 (2.46–4.18)
	– within 14 days of diagnosis	
Bone fracture		
Nested case–control [140]	• Risk of hip fracture with PPI therapy >1 year	1.44 (1.30–1.59)
	• Risk of hip fracture with >1.75 average daily-dose PPI	2.65 (1.80–3.90)
Case–control [141]	• Risk of any fracture with PPI use within last year	1.18 (1.12–1.43)
	• Risk of hip fracture with PPI use within last year	1.45 (1.28–1.65)
	• Risk of spine fracture with PPI use within last year	1.60 (1.25–2.04)
Retrospective matched cohort [142]	• Risk of hip fracture after 5+ years of PPI use	1.62 (1.02–2.58)
	• Risk of hip fracture after 7+ years of PPI use	4.55 (1.68–12.29)
	• Risk of any osteoporosis-related fracture after 7+ years of PPI use	1.92 (1.16–3.18)

PPI, proton pump inhibitor; MRSA, methicillin-resistant *Staphylococcus aureus*.

setting, as many may already be on PPIs. Others may be inappropriately placed on a PPI for stress ulcer prophylaxis and then discharged on them. Should patients who are admitted on a PPI have it discontinued while hospitalized to minimize the risk of CDAD [139] or should we continue PPI therapy when indicated but at the lowest effective dose and practice protective barrier nursing and prudent hand washing [144]?

Community-acquired pneumonia

Few microorganisms survive the acidic environment in the stomach. PPIs may decrease this important defense mechanism, allowing gastric colonization with bacteria that are commonly found in the oral cavity and hypopharynx. Typically, the presence of pathogens in the stomach has been associated with nosocomial respiratory infections and ventilator-associated pneumonia [137, 143].

Bone fracture

There are conflicting data on the role of acid and absorption of calcium. PPIs inhibit intragastric secretion of acid, which mediates small intestinal calcium [145]. In those with normal gastric acid secretion, insoluble calcium is absorbed at the same rate as soluble calcium [146]. Osteoclasts possess proton pumps and are directly affected by PPIs, reducing bone resorption [147].

There are, however, no adequate long-term studies that have evaluated the effect of PPIs on calcium absorption. Short-term studies show a decrease in calcium absorption on PPIs; however, the patients studied were on hemodialysis [148, 149].

Yang *et al.* [150] drew similar conclusions to the study by Vestergaard *et al.* [140] with regard to the increased risk of hip fracture in patients taking PPIs. However, the study by Vestergaard *et al.* did not identify either a dose– or duration–response effect, in contrast to the Yang *et al.* study. Although neither study was designed to define underlying mechanisms to explain the potential association between fracture risk and PPI therapy, the authors postulated that there may be an alternative explanation for various effects with either standard- or high-dose PPIs. Clinically, it was suggested that elderly patients who require long-term and high-dose PPI therapy should consider increased dietary and/or supplementary calcium intake.

In contrast to the study by Yang *et al.*, the study by Targownik *et al.* found an increased overall risk for fracture in patients with 7 or more years of PPI therapy, as well as an increase in the risk of hip fracture when on PPI therapy for 5 years or more [141]. The short-term risk of fracture was not found to be significant. This study suggests that the duration of exposure to PPI therapy increases the risk of osteoporotic fracture, but not in a dose-dependent fashion.

Proton pump inhibitors and clopidogrel

In vitro studies have suggested that PPIs may decrease the antiplatelet effects of clopidogrel and this potential interaction has raised controversy as to whether patients on clopidogrel should remain on a PPI [142, 151–155]. This potential interaction underscores the importance of using PPIs only when needed and balancing benefit and risk of these excellent agents.

Conclusions

PPIs have revolutionized therapy for many upper gastrointestinal disorders and command a substantial percentage of the US pharmaceutical market share. Appropriate utilization of these drugs for diagnoses, periodic reassessment of patient symptoms to determine the lowest effective dosage and duration of therapy, as well as close surveillance for potential adverse risks, will not only minimize cost expenditure but will maximize favorable outcomes.

References

1. DeVault KR, Castell DO. Updated guidelines for the diagnosis and treatment of gastroesophageal reflux disease. *Am J Gastroenterol* 2005;100:190–200.
2. Hila A, Castell DO. Nighttime reflux is primarily an early event. *J Clin Gastroenterol* 2005;39:579–583.
3. Johnson LF, DeMeester TR. Evaluation of the head of the bed, bethanechol, and antacid foam tablets on gastroesophageal reflux. *Dig Dis Sci* 1981;26:673–680.
4. Stanciu C, Bennett JR. Effects of posture on gastro-oesophageal reflux. *Digestion* 1977;15:104–109.
5. Khoury RM, Camacho-Lobato LC, Katz PO, *et al.* Influence of spontaneous sleep positions on nighttime recumbent reflux in patients with gastroesophageal reflux disease. *Am J Gastroenterol* 1999;94:2069–2073.
6. Kapur KC, Trudgill NJ, Riley SA. Mechanism of gastroesophageal reflux in the lateral decubitus position. *Neurogastroenterol Motil* 1998;10:517–522.
7. Katz LC, Just R, Castell DO. Body position affects recumbent postprandial reflux. *J Clin Gastroenterol* 1994;18:280–283.
8. VanHerwaarden M, Katzka D, Smout AJPM, *et al.* Effect of different recumbent positions on postprandial reflex in normal subjects. *Am J Gastroenterol* 2000;95:2731–2736.
9. Dickman R, Parthasarathy S, Malagon IB, *et al.* Comparisons of the distribution of oesophageal acid exposure throughout the sleep period among the different gastro-oesophageal reflux disease groups. *Aliment Pharmacol Ther* 2007;26:41–48.
10. Gagliardi GS, Shah AP, Goldstein M, *et al.* Effect of zolpidem on the sleep arousal response to nocturnal esophageal acid exposure. *Clin Gastroenterol Hepatol* 2009;7:948–952.
11. McArthur K, Hogan D, Isenberg JI. Relative stimulatory effects of commonly ingested beverages on gastric acid secretion in humans. *Gastroenterology* 1982;83:199–203.
12. Babka JC, Castell DO. On the genesis of heartburn: the effects of specific foods on the lower esophagus sphincter. *Dig Dis* 1973;18:391–397.
13. Castell DO. Diet and the lower esophageal sphincter. *Am J Clin Nutr* 1975;28:1296–1298.

14. Vakily M, Lee RD, Wu J, *et al*. Drug interaction studies with dexlansoprazole modified release (TAK-390MR), a proton pump inhibitor with a dual delayed-release formulation: Results of four randomized, double-blind, crossover, placebo-controlled, single centre studies. *Clin Drug Investig* 2009;29:35–50.

15. Nebel OT, Castell DO. Lower esophageal sphincter pressure changes after food ingestion. *Gastroenterology* 1972;63:778.

16. Pehl C, Pfeiffer A, Wendl B, *et al*. The effect of decaffeination of coffee on gastro-esophageal reflux in patients with reflux disease. *Aliment Pharmacol Ther* 1997;11:483.

17. Becker DJ, Sinclair J, Castell DO, *et al*. A comparison of high and low fat meals on postprandial esophageal acid exposure. *Am J Gastroenterol* 1989;84:782.

18. Nebel OT, Castell DO. Lower esophageal sphincter pressure changes after food ingestion. *Gastroenterology* 1972;63:778–783.

19. Wright LE, Castell DO. Adverse effect of chocolate on lower esophageal sphincter pressure. *Dig Dis Sci* 1975;20:703–707.

20. Murphy DW, Castell DO. Chocolate and heartburn: evidence of increased esophageal acid exposure after chocolate ingestion. *Am J Gastroenterol* 1988;83:633–636.

21. Kjellin A, Ramel S, Rossner S, *et al*. Gastroesophageal reflux in obese patients is not reduced by weight reduction. *Scand J Gastroenterol* 1996;31:1047–1051.

22. Hampel H, Abraham NS, El-Serag HB. Meta-analysis: obesity and the risk for gastroesophageal reflux disease and its complications. *Ann Intern Med* 2005;143:199–211.

23. Jacobson BC, Somers SC, Fuchs CS, *et al*. Body-mass index and symptoms of gastroesophageal reflux in women. *N Engl J Med* 2006;354:2340–2348.

24. Chow WH, Blot WJ, Vaughan TL, *et al*. Body mass index and risk of adenocarcinoma of the esophagus and gastric, cardia. *J Natl Cancer Inst* 1998;90:150–155.

25. Perez AR, Moncure AC, Rattner DW. Obesity adversely affects the outcome of antireflux operations. *Surg Endosc* 2001;15:986–989.

26. Vitale GC, Cheadle WG, Patel B, *et al*. The effect of alcohol on nocturnal gastroesophageal reflux. *JAMA* 1987;258:2077–2079.

27. Pehl C, Pfeiffer A, Wendle B, *et al*. Different effects of white and red wine on lower esophageal sphincter pressure and gastroesophageal reflux disease. *Scand J Gastroenterol* 1998;33:118–122.

28. Meining A, Classen M. The role of diet and lifestyle measures in the pathogenesis and treatment of gastroesophageal reflux disease. *Am J Gastroenterol* 2000;95:2692–2697.

29. Tytgat GNJ, Nio CY. The medical therapy of reflux oesophagitis. *Bailleres Clin Gastroenterol* 1987;1:791–807.

30. Klinkenberg-Knol EC, Festen HPM, *et al*. Pharmacologic management of gastro-oesophageal reflux disease. *Drugs* 1995;49:695–710.

31. Furman D, Mensh R, Winan G, *et al*. A double-blind trial comparing high dose liquid antacid to placebo and cimetidine in improving symptoms and objective parameters in gastroesophageal reflux. *Gastroenterology* 1992;82:A1062.

32. Eslborg L, Beck B, Stubgaard M. Effect of sucralfate on gastroesophageal reflux in esophagitis. *Hepatogastroenterology* 1985;32:181–184.

33. Katz PO, Castell DO. Gastroesophageal reflux disease during pregnancy. *Gastroenterol Clin* 1998;27:153–167.

34. Simon B, Mueller P Comparison of the effect of sucralfate and ranitidine in reflux esophagitis. *Am J Med* 1987;83:43–47.

35. Hameeteman W, van de Boomgaard DM, Dekker W, *et al*. Sucralfate versus cimetidine in reflux esophagitis: single blind multicenter study. *J Clin Gastroenterol* 1987;9:390–394.

36. Barone JA, Jessen LM, Colaizzi JL, *et al*. Cisapride: a gastrointestinal prokinetic drug. *Ann Pharmacother* 1994;28:488–500.

37. McCallum RW, Ippoliti AF, Cooney C, *et al*. A controlled trial of metoclopramide in symptomatic gastroesophageal reflux. *N Engl J Med* 1977;296:354–357.

38. Bright-Asare P, El-Bassoussi M. Cimetidine, metoclopramide or placebo in the treatment of symptomatic gastroesophageal reflux. *J Clin Gastroenterol* 1980;2:149–156.

39. Temple JG, Bradby GVH, O'Connor F, *et al*. Cimetidine and metoclopramide in esophageal reflux disease. *Br Med J* 1983;286:1863–1865.

40. Paull A, Kerr A, Grant AK. A controlled trial of metoclopramide in reflux esophagitis. *Med J Aust* 1974;2:627–629.

41. Venables CW, Bell D, Eccleston D. A double-blind study of metoclopramide in symptomatic peptic esophagitis. *Postgrad Med J* 1973;49 (Suppl 4):73–77.

42. Ramirez B, Richter JE. Review article: promotility drugs in the treatment of gastro-oesophageal reflux disease. *Aliment Pharmacol Ther* 1993;7:5–20.

43. Blackwell JN, Heading RC, Fettes MR. Effects of domperidone on lower oesophageal sphincter pressure and gastro-oesophageal reflux in patients with peptic esophagitis. Progress with domperidone. *International Congress and Symposium Series*, vol 36. London: Royal Society of Medicine Press, 1981, p. 57.

44. Richter JE, Sabesin SM, Kogut DG, *et al*. Omeprazole versus ranitidine or ranitidine/metoclopramide in poorly responsive symptomatic gastroesophageal reflux disease. *Am J Gastroenterol* 1996;91:1766–1772.

45. Vignieri S, Termini R, Leandro G, *et al*. A comparison of five maintenance therapies for reflux esophagitis. *N Engl J Med* 1995;333:1106–1110.

46. Bell NJV, Burget DL, Howden CW, *et al*. Appropriate acid suppression for the management of gastro-esophageal reflux disease. *Digestion* 1992;51 (Suppl 1):59–67.

47. Katz PO, Ginsberg GG, Hoyle PE, *et al*. Relationship between intragastric acid control and healing status in the treatment of moderate to severe erosive esophagitis. *Aliment Pharmacol Ther* 2007;25:617–628.

48. Jones DB, Howden CW, Burget DW, *et al*. Acid suppression in duodenal ulcer: a meta-analysis to define optimal dosing with antisecretory drugs. *Gut* 1987;28:1120–1127.

49. DeVault KR, Castell DO. Guidelines for the diagnosis and treatment of gastroesophageal reflux disease. *Arch Intern Med* 1995;155:2165–73.

50. Bell NJV, Hunt RH. Role of gastric acid suppression in the treatment of gastro-oesophageal reflux disease. *Gut* 1992;33:118–124.

51. Cloud ML, Offen WW. Nizatidine versus placebo in gastroesophageal reflux disease: a six-week, multicenter, randomized, double-blind comparison. *Dig Dis Sci* 1992;37:865–874.

52. McCarty-Dawson D, Sue So, Morrill B, *et al*. Ranitidine versus cimetidine in the healing of erosive esophagitis. *Clin Ther* 1996;18:1150–1160.

53. Wesdorp ICE, Dekker W, Festen HPM. Efficacy of famotidine 20 mg twice a day versus 40 mg twice a day in the treatment

SECTION IV Gastroesophageal Reflux

of erosive or ulcerative reflux esophagitis. *Dig Dis Sci* 1993;38:2287–2293.

54. Euler AR, Murdock RH Jr, Wilson TH, *et al.* Ranitidine is effective therapy for erosive esophagitis. *Am J Gastroenterol* 1993;88:520–524.

55. Hallerback B, Glise H, Johansson B, *et al.* Gastroesophageal reflux symptoms: clinical findings and effect of ranitidine treatment. *Eur J Surg* 1998;583 (Suppl):6–13.

56. Vignieri S, Termini R, Leandor G, et al. A comparison of five maintenance therapies for reflux esophagitis. *N Engl J Med* 1995;333:1106–1110.

57. Feldman M, Burton ME. Histamine2-receptor antagonists: standard therapy for acid-peptic diseases. *N Engl J Med* 1990;323:1672–1680.

58. Lipsy RJ, Fennerty B, Fagan TC. Clinical review of histamine2 receptor antagonists. *Arch Intern Med* 1990;150:745–751.

59. Robinson M. Review article: current perspectives on hypergastrinemia and enterochromaffin-like-cell hyperplasia. *Aliment Pharmacol Ther* 1999;13 (Suppl 5):5–10.

60. Castell D. Review of immediate-release omeprazole for the treatment of gastric acid-related disorders. *Expert Opin Pharmacother* 2005;6:2501–2510.

61. Metz D, Vakily M, Dixit T, Mumford D. Review article: Dual delayed release formulation of dexlansoprazole MR, a novel approach to overcome the limitations of conventional single release proton pump inhibitor therapy. *Aliment Pharmacol Ther* 2009;29:928–937.

62. Massoomi F, Savage J, Destache CJ. Omeprazole: a comprehensive review. *Pharmacotherapy* 1993;13:46–59.

63. Lew EA. Review article: pharmacokinetic concerns in the selection of anti-ulcer therapy. *Aliment Pharmacol Ther* 1999;13 (Suppl 5):11–16.

64. Wolfe MM, Sachs G. Acid suppression: optimizing therapy for gastroduodenal ulcer healing, gastroesophageal reflux disease, and stress-related erosive syndrome. *Gastroenterology* 2000;118 (Suppl):9–31.

65. Miner P, Katz PO, Chen Y, Sostek M. Gastric acid control with esomeprazole, lansoprazole, omeprazole, pantoprazole, and rabeprazole: A five-way crossover study. *Am J Gastroenterol* 2003;98:2616–2620.

66. Chiba N, De Gara CJ, Wilkonson JM, *et al.* Speed of healing and symptom relief in grade II to IV gastroesophageal reflux disease: a meta-analysis. *Gastroenterology* 1997;112:1798–1810.

67. Castell DO, Richter JE, Robinson M, *et al.* Efficacy and safety of lansoprazole in the treatment of erosive esophagitis. *Am J Gastroenterol* 1996;91:1749–1758.

68. Richter JE, Kahrilas PJ, Johnston J, *et al.* Efficacy and safety of esomeprazole compared with omeprazole in GERD patients with erosive esophagitis: a randomized controlled study. *Am J Gastroenterol* 2001;96:656–665.

69. Dekkers CPM, Beker JA, Thjodleifsson B, *et al.* Double-blind, placebo-controlled comparison of rabeprazole 20 mg vs. omeprazole 20 mg in the treatment of erosive or ulcerative gastro-oesophageal reflux disease. *Aliment Pharmacol Ther* 1999;13: 49–57.

70. Castell DO, Kahrilas PJ, Richter JE, *et al.* Esomeprazole (40 mg) compared with lansoprazole (30 mg) in the treatment of erosive esophagitis. *Am J Gastroenterol* 2002;97:575–583.

71. Mossner J, Holscher Ah, Herz R, *et al.* A double-blind study of pantoprazole and omeprazole in the treatment of reflux oesophagitis: a multicentre trial. *Aliment Pharmacol Ther* 1995;9:321–326.

72. Kahrilas PJ, Fennerty MB, Joelsson B. High versus standard dose ranitidine for control of heartburn in poorly responsive acid reflux disease: a prospective, controlled trial. *Am J Gastroenterol* 1999;94:92–97.

73. Kahrilas PJ, Falk GW, Johnson DA, *et al.* Esomeprazole improves healing and symptom resolution as compared with omeprazole in reflux oesophagitis patients: a randomized controlled trial. The Esomeprazole Study Investigators. *Aliment Pharmacol Ther* 2000;14:1249–1259.

74. Labenz J, Armstrong D, Lauritsen K, *et al.* A randomized comparative study of esomeprazole 40 mg versus pantoprazole 40 mg for healing erosive oesophagitis: the EXPO study. *Aliment Pharmacol Ther* 2005;21:739–746.

75. Sharma P, Shaheen NJ, Perez MC, *et al.* Clinical trials: healing of erosive oesophagitis with dexlansoprazole MR, a proton pump inhibitor with a novel dual delayed-release formulation—results from two randomized controlled studies. *Aliment Pharmacol Ther* 2009;29:731–741.

76. Fennerty MB, Johanson JF, Hwang C, Sostek M. Efficacy of esomeprazole 40 mg vs lansoprazole 30 mg for healing moderate to severe erosive oesophagitis. *Aliment Pharmacol Ther* 2005;21:455–463.

77. Metz DC, Inadomi JM, Howden CW, *et al.* On-demand therapy for gastroesophageal reflux disease. *Am J Gastroenterol* 2007; 102:642–653.

78. Lundell LR, Dent J, Bennett JR, *et al.* Endoscopic assessment of oesophagitis: clinical and functional correlates and further validation of the Los Angeles classification. *Gut* 1999;45: 172–180.

79. Sontag SJ, Hirschowitz BJ, Holt S, *et al.* Two doses of omeprazole versus placebo in symptomatic erosive esophagitis: the US multicenter study. *Gastroenterology* 1992;102:109–118.

80. Klinkenberg-Knol EC, Nelis F, Dent J, *et al.* Long-term omeprazole treatment in resistant gastroesophageal reflux disease: efficacy, safety, and influence on gastric mucosa. *Gastroenterology* 2000;118:661–669.

81. Inadomi JM, Jamal R, Murata GH, *et al.* Step-down management of gastroesophageal reflux disease. *Gastroenterology* 2001;121:1095–1100.

82. Hatlebakk JG, Katz PO, Castell DO. Proton pump inhibitors: better acid suppression when taken before a meal than without a meal. *Aliment Pharmacol Ther* 2000;14:1267–1272.

83. Kuo B, Castell DO. Optimal dosing of omeprazole 40 mg daily: Effects on gastric and esophageal pH and serum gastrin in healthy controls. *Am J Gastroenterol* 1996;91:1532–1538.

84. Hatlebakk JG, Katz PO, Kuo B, *et al.* Nocturnal gastric acidity and acid breakthrough on different regimens of omeprazole 40 mg daily. *Aliment Pharmacol Ther* 1998;12: 1235–1240.

85. Katz PO, Hatlebakk JG, Castell DO. Gastric acidity and acid breakthrough with twice daily omeprazole or lansoprazole. *Aliment Pharmacol Ther* 2000;14:709–714.

86. Peghini PL, Katz PO, Bracy NA, *et al.* Nocturnal recovery of gastric acid secretion with twice-daily dosing of proton pump inhibitors. *Am J Gastroenterol* 1998;93:763–767.

87. Tutuian R, Katz PO, Castell DO. A PPI is a PPI is a PPI: Lessons from prolonged intragastric pH monitoring. *Gastroenterology* 2000;118:A17.

88. Katz P, Castell DO, Chen Y, *et al.* Esomeprazole 40 mg twice daily maintains intragastric pH > 4 more than 80% of a 24-hour time period. *Am J Gastroenterol* 2002;97:520.

89. Katz PO, Anderson C, Khoury R, *et al.* Gastro-oesophageal reflux associated with nocturnal gastric acid breakthrough on proton pump inhibitors. *Aliment Pharmacol Ther* 1998;12:1231–1234.

90. Hatlebakk J, Katz PO, Castell DO. Medical therapy: management of the refractory patient. *Gastroenterol Clin North Am* 1999;28:847–860.

91. Fass R, Sampliner RE, Malagon IB, *et al.* Failure of acid control in candidates for Barrett's oesophagus reversal on a very high dose of proton pump inhibitor. *Aliment Pharmacol Ther* 2000;14:597–602.

92. Leite LP, Johnston BT, Barrett J, *et al.* Persistent acid secretion during omeprazole therapy: A study of gastric acid profiles in patients demonstrating failure of omeprazole therapy. *Am J Gastroenterol* 1996;91:1527–1531.

93. Katz PO, Koch FK, Ballard ED, *et al.* Comparison of the effects of immediate-release omeprazole oral suspension, delayed-release lansoprazole capsules and delayed-release esomeprazole capsules on nocturnal gastric acidity after bedtime dosing in patients with night-time GERD symptoms. *Aliment Pharmacol Ther* 2007;25:197–205.

94. Fackler WK, Ours Tm, Vaezi MF, *et al.* Long-term effect of H₂RA therapy on nocturnal gastric acid breakthrough. *Gastroenterology* 2002;122:625–632.

95. Katz PO, Xue S, Castell DO. Control of intragastric pH with omeprazole 20 mg, omeprazole 40 mg and lansoprazole 30 mg. *Aliment Pharmacol Ther* 2001;15:647–652.

96. Lind T, Havelund T, Carlsson O, *et al.* Heartburn without oesophagitis: Efficacy of omeprazole therapy and features determining therapeutic response. *Scand J Gastroenterol* 1997;32:974–979.

97. Bate CM, Griffin SM, Keeling PWN, *et al.* Reflux symptom relief with omeprazole in patients without unequivocal oesophagitis. *Aliment Pharmacol Ther* 1996;10:547–555.

98. Carlsson R, Dent J, Watts R, *et al.* Gastro-oesophageal reflux disease in primary care: An international study of different treatment strategies with omeprazole. *Eur J Gastroenterol Hepatol* 1998;10:119–124.

99. Achem SR, Kolts BE, MacMath T, *et al.* Effects of omeprazole versus placebo in treatment of noncardiac chest pain and gastroesophageal reflux. *Am J Gastroenterol* 1997;42:2138–2145.

100. Fass R, Fennerty MB, Ofman JJ, *et al.* The clinical and economic value of a short course of omeprazole in patients with non-cardiac chest pain. *Gastroenterology* 1998;115:42–49.

101. Cremonini F, Wise J, Moayyedi P, Talley NJ: Diagnostic and therapeutic use of proton pump inhibitors in non-cardiac chest pain: A meta-analysis. *Am J Gastroenterol* 2005;100:1226–1232.

102. Kjellen G, Tibbling L, Wranne B. Effect of conservative treatment of oesophageal dysfunction in bronchial asthma. *Eur J Respir Dis* 1981;62:190–197.

103. Katz PO. Ambulatory esophageal and hypopharyngeal pH monitoring in patients with hoarseness. *Am J Gastroenterol* 1990;85:38–40.

104. Larrain A, Carrasco E, Galleguillos F, *et al.* Medical and surgical treatment of non-allergic asthma associated with gastro-esophageal reflux. *Chest* 1991;99:1330–1335.

105. Harper PC, Bergner A, Kaye MD. Antireflux treatment for asthma: improvement in patients with associated gastro-esophageal reflux. *Arch Intern Med* 1987;147:56–60.

106. Ekstrom T, Lindgren BR, Tibbling L. Effects of ranitidine treatment on patients with asthma and a history of gastro-oesophageal reflux: a double blind crossover study. *Thorax* 1989;44:19–23.

107. Gustafsson PM, Kjellman N-IM, Tibbling L. A trial of ranitidine in asthmatic children and adolescents with or without pathological gastro-oesophageal reflux. *Eur Respir J* 1992;5:201–206.

108. Irwin RS, Curley FJ, French CL. Chronic cough: the spectrum and frequency of causes, key components of the diagnostic evaluation, and outcome of specific therapy. *Am Rev Respir Dis* 1990;141:640–647.

109. Irwin RS, Azwacki JK, Curley FJ, *et al.* Chronic cough as the sole presenting manifestation of gastroesophageal reflux. *Am Rev Respir Dis* 1989;140:1294–1300.

110. Fitzgerald JM, Allen CJ, Craven MA, *et al.* Chronic cough and gastro-esophageal reflux. *CMAJ* 1989;140:520–524.

111. Waring JP, Lacayo L, Hunter J, *et al.* Chronic cough and hoarseness in patients with severe gastroesophageal reflux disease. Diagnosis and response to therapy. *Dig Dis Sci* 1995;40:1093–1097.

112. Ford GA, Oliver PS, Prior JS, *et al.* Omeprazole in the treatment of asthmatics with nocturnal symptoms and gastro-esophageal reflux: A placebo-controlled cross-over study. *Postgrad Med J* 1994;70:350–354.

113. Meier JH, McNally PR, Punja M, *et al.* Does omeprazole (Prilosec) improve respiratory function in asthmatics with gastroesophageal reflux? *Dig Dis Sci* 1994;39:2127–2133.

114. Boeree MJ, Peters FT, Postma, DS, Kleibeuker JH. No effects of high dose omeprazole in patients with severe airway hypersecretion and asymptomatic GER. *Eur Respir J* 1998;11:1070–1074.

115. Harding SM, Richter JE, Guzzo MR, *et al.* Asthma and gastro-esophageal reflux: acid suppression therapy improves asthma outcome. *Am J Med* 1996;100:395–405.

116. American Lung Association Asthma Clinical Research Centers, Mastronarde JG, Anthonisen NR, Castro M, *et al.* Efficacy of esomeprazole for treatment of poorly controlled asthma. *N Engl J Med* 2009;360:1487–1499.

117. Kamal PL, Hanson D, Kahrilas PJ. Omeprazole for the treatment of posterior laryngitis. *Am J Med* 1994;96:321–326.

118. Hanson DG, Karnel PL, Kahrilas PJ. Outcomes of antireflux therapy for the treatment of chronic laryngitis. *Ann Otol Rhinol Laryngol* 1995;104:550–555.

119. El-Serag HB, Lee P, Buchner A, *et al.* Lansoprazole treatment of patients with chronic idiopathic laryngitis: a placebo-controlled trial. *Am J Gastroenterol* 2001;96:979–983.

120. Park W, Hicks DM, Khandwala F, *et al.* Laryngopharyngeal reflux: Prospective cohort study evaluating optimal dose of proton-pump inhibitor therapy and pretherapy predictors of response. *Laryngoscope* 2005;115:1230–1238.

121. Leontiadis GI, Howden CW. The role of proton pump inhibitors in the management of upper gastrointestinal bleeding. *Gastroenterol Clin North Am* 2009;38:199–213.

122. Klinkenberg-Knol E, Meuwissen S. Combined gastric and oesophageal 24 hour monitoring in patients with reflux disease resistant to treatment with omeprazole. *Aliment Pharmacol Ther* 1990;4:485–495.

123. Vela MF, Tutuian R, Katz PO, Castell DO. Baclofen decreases acid and non-acid post-prandial gastro-oesophageal reflux measured by combined multichannel intraluminal impedance and pH. *Aliment Pharmacol Ther* 2003;17:243–251.

124. Peghini PL, Katz PO, Castell DO. Ranitidine controls nocturnal gastric acid breakthrough on omeprazole: a controlled study in normal subjects. *Gastroenterology* 1998;115:1335–1339.

125. Diav-Citrin O, Arnon J, Schechtman S, *et al.* The safety of proton pump inhibitors in pregnancy: A multicentre prospective controlled study. *Aliment Pharmacol Ther* 2005;21: 269–275.

126. Cote GA, Howden CW. Potential adverse effects of proton pump inhibitors. *Curr Gastroenterol Rep* 2008;10:208–214.

127. Inadomi JM, Fendrick AM. PPI use in the OTC era: Who to treat, with what, and for how long? *Clin Gastroenterol Hepatol* 2005;3:208–215.

128. Jacobsen BC, Ferris TG, Sheat TL, *et al.* Who is using chronic acid suppression and why? *Am J Gastroenterol* 2003;98:51–58.

129. Cunningham R, Dale B, Undy B, Gaunt N. Proton pump inhibitors as a risk factor for clostridium difficile diarrhoea. *J Hosp Infect* 2003;54:243–245.

130. Dial S, Delaney JAC, Barkun AN, Suissa S. Use of gastric acid-suppressive agents and the risk of community acquired clostridium difficile-associated disease. *JAMA* 2005;294: 2989–2995.

131. Dial S, Alrasadi K, Manoukian C, *et al.* Risk of clostridium difficile diarrhea among hospital inpatients prescribed proton pump inhibitors: Cohort and case-control studies. *CMAJ* 2004;171:33–38.

132. Yearsley KA, Gilby LJ, Ramadas AV, *et al.* Proton pump inhibitor therapy is a risk factor for clostridium difficile-associated diarrhea. *Aliment Pharmacol Ther* 2006;24:613–619.

133. Jayatilaka S, Shakov R, Eddi R, *et al.* Clostridium difficile infection in an urban medical center: Five-year analysis of infection rates among adult admissions and association with the use of proton pump inhibitors. *Ann Clin Lab Sci* 2007;37:241–247.

134. Aseeri M, Schroeder T, Kramer J, Zackula R. Gastric acid suppression by proton pump inhibitors as a risk factor for clostridium-difficile-associated diarrhea in hospitalized patients. *Am J Gastroenterol* 2008;103:2308–2313.

135. Leonard J, Marshall JK, Moayyedi P. Systematic review of the risk of enteric infection in patients taking acid suppression. *Am J Gastroenterol* 2007;102:2047–2056.

136. Gulmez SE, Holm A, Frederiksen H, *et al.* Use of proton pump inhibitors and the risk of community-acquired pneumonia: A population based case control study. *Arch Intern Med* 2007;167:950–955.

137. Inglis TJ, Sherrant MJ, Spoat LJ, *et al.* Gastroduodenal dysfunction and bacterial colonization of the ventilated lung. *Lancet* 1993;341:911–913.

138. Sarkar M, Hennessy S, Yang YX. Proton pump inhibitor use and the risk for community-acquired pneumonia. *Ann Intern Med* 2008;149:391–398.

139. Thachil J. Overprescribing PPIs: Time for a hospital antacid policy on *Clostridium difficile*. *BMJ* 2008;336:109.

140. Vestergaard P, Rejnmark L, Mosekilde L. Proton pump inhibitors, histamine H2 receptor antagonists, and other antacid medications and the risk of fracture. *Calcif Tissue Int* 2006;79:76–83.

141. Targownik LE, Lix LM, Merge CJ. Use of proton pump inhibitors and risk of osteoporosis-related fractures. *CMAJ* 2008;179:319–326.

142. Gilard M, Arnaud B, LeGal G, *et al.* Influence of omeprazole on the antiplatelet action of clopidogrel associated to aspirin. *J Thromb Haemost* 2006;4:2508–2509.

143. Laheij RJ, Van Ijzendoorn MC, Janssen MJ, *et al.* Gastric acid-suppressive therapy and community-acquired respiratory infections. *Aliment Pharmacol Ther* 2003;18:847–851.

144. Metz D. Clostridium difficile colitis: Wash your hands before stopping the proton pump inhibitor. *Am J Gastroenterol* 2008;103:2314–2316.

145. Bo-Linn GW, David GR, Buddrus DJ, *et al.* An evaluation of the importance of gastric acid secretion in the absorption of dietary calcium. *J Clin Invest* 1984;73:640–647.

146. Sheikh MS, Santa Ana CA, Nicar MJ, *et al.* Gastrointestinal absorption of calcium from milk and calcium salts. *N Engl J Med* 1987;317:532–536.

147. Farina C, Gagliardi S. Selective inhibition of osteoclast vacuolar H+-ATPase. *Curr Pharm Des* 2002;8:2033–2048.

148. Graziani G, Badalamenti S, Como G, *et al.* Calcium and phospate plasma levels in dialysis patients after dietary Ca-P overload. Role of gastric acid secretion. *Nephron* 2002;91: 474–479.

149. Hardy P, Secher A, Hottelart C, *et al.* Inhibition of gastric secretion by omeprazole and efficiency of calcium carbonate on the control of hyperphosphatemia in patients on chronic hemodialysis. *Artif Organs* 1998;22:569–573.

150. Yang YX, Lewis JD, Epstein S, Metz DC. Long-term proton pump inhibitor therapy and risk of hip fracture. *JAMA* 2006;296:2947–2953.

151. Gilard M, Arnaud B, Cornily JC, *et al.* Influence of omeprazole on the antiplatelet action of clopidogrel associated with aspirin: The randomized, double-blind OCLA (Omeprazole Clopidogrel Aspirin) study. *JACC* 2008;51:256–260.

152. Small DS, Farid NA, Payne CD, *et al.* Effects of the proton pump inhibitor lansoprazole on the pharmacokinetics and pharmacodynamics of prasugrel and clopidogrel. *J Clin Pharmacol* 2008;48:475–484.

153. Siller-Matula JM, Spiel AO, Lang IM, *et al.* Effects of pantoprazole and esomeprazole on platelet inhibition by clopidogrel. *Am Heart J* 2009;157:148e1–5.

154. Sibbing D, Morath T, Stegherr J, *et al.* Impact of proton pump inhibitors on the antiplatelet effects of clopidogrel. *Thromb Haemost* 2009;101:714–719.

155. O'Donoghue ML, Braunwald E, Antman EM, *et al.* Pharmacodynamic effect and clinical efficacy of clopidogrel and prasugel withor without a proton pump inhibitor: An analysis of two randomized trials. *Lancet* 2009;374:989–997.

26 | Endoscopic Therapies for Gastroesophageal Reflux Disease

Daniel von Renteln,[1] Melina C. Vassiliou[2] and Richard I. Rothstein[3]

[1]Department of Interdisciplinary Endoscopy, University Hospital Hamburg-Eppendorf, Hamburg, Germany
[2]Department of Surgery, Montreal General Hospital, McGill University, Montreal, Quebec, Canada
[3]Section of Gastroenterology and Hepatology, Dartmouth-Hitchcock Medical Center, Lebanon, NH, USA

Gastroesophageal reflux disease

The physiologic reflux barrier consists of the lower esophageal sphincter (LES) complex and the anatomy of the angle of His. Gastroesophageal reflux occurs when the LES pressure decreases and/or the anatomy of the angle of His is altered [1–3]. Esophageal erosions are the most commonly seen mucosal manifestations of esophageal exposure to excessive gastric acid. A minority of all symptomatic GERD patients has erosive esophagitis, and other complications, such as ulcers or stricture formation, are even less common. Barrett's esophagus can arise in the setting of long-standing gastroesophageal reflux and long-segment Barrett's esophagus, with intestinal type metaplasia is the most important risk factor for esophageal adenocarcinoma [4–7].

Therapy: perspectives on the role of medical, surgical, and endoscopic therapy

A meta-analysis of randomized controlled trials comparing different pharmacologic treatments for esophagitis was recently published. Five studies demonstrated that proton pump inhibitor (PPI) therapy was superior to placebo, and 26 demonstrated a statistically significant advantage of PPIs compared to H_2-receptor antagonists [8]. Based on these data, medical management with PPIs is considered to be the gold standard for the treatment of GERD. Effective in the majority of patients, these medications, however, are often required indefinitely, may require dose escalation over time, and can occasionally cause intolerable side effects. Furthermore, some patients on PPIs still suffer from persistent symptomatic non-acid regurgitation.

While surgical treatment offers a reasonable likelihood of symptom control (around 90%) and normalization of distal esophageal acid exposure (around 85%), it can have associated postoperative side effects and complications (3–8% develop dysphagia, inability to belch or vomit, gas bloat, diarrhea, and increased flatus) and the results of surgical intervention may not be durable for a sizeable minority. There is a need, therefore, for alternative treatment strategies in selected patients.

The less invasive endoscopic treatments can be repeated if needed, and one of the advantages of endoscopic treatment for GERD is that it does not preclude individuals going on to have surgical intervention if required in the future. In general, the ideal candidates for these treatments include patients who respond to acid suppressors but do not want to take chronic medications; individuals with incomplete or poor response to PPIs with documented GERD by pH-metry with reluctance to pursue surgical intervention; those with intolerance to the medications for GERD; and those with a failed surgical intervention as an alternative to re-do fundoplication. For all patients anticipating endoscopic treatment, preprocedural testing should include a thorough evaluation in similar fashion to that for surgical intervention: performance of pH study off antisecretory medications to establish baseline distal esophageal acid exposure, esophageal manometry, and upper endoscopy to stage the esophagus and identify individuals who have significant erosive esophagitis (> Los Angeles grade A or B) or Barrett's esophagus, which should preclude performing the endoscopic treatment. Procedures should be done on symptomatic individuals with documented reflux, and not to treat symptoms alone, especially given the high sham-response rate (>30%) for treatment of GERD symptoms. In general, for clinical situations like erosive esophagitis or Barrett's esophagus, the endoscopic treatments cannot be relied upon to provide effective acid control since they normalize acid exposure for only a minority (30–50%) of treated individuals.

Table 26.1 Endoscopic antireflux techniques and available levels of evidence.

Injection or implantation (level of evidence)	Thermal energy (level of Evidence)	Endoscopic suturing, plicating, or stapling (level of evidence)
Enteryx (2c)	Stretta (1b)	Endoscopic Suturing Device (2c)
Gatekeeper (2b)		EndoCinch (1b)
Durasphere (2c)		Plicator (1b)
Plexiglas PMMA (4)		EsophyX (2c)
		Syntheon (*)
		SafeStitch (*)
		Hiz-Wiz (*)
		Medigus (*)
		TOGA (*)

*No full-paper journal publication of clinical trials available to date.

Principles, techniques, and devices for endoscopic therapies

Endoscopic therapies have been designed to alter the anatomy of the gastroesophageal junction (GEJ) to prevent transient LES relaxations, increase baseline LES tone, or increase baseline LES length [1–3]. A number of endoscopic antireflux procedures have been evaluated for the treatment of GERD (Table 26.1. Over the past decade, these devices were developed and underwent initial evaluation with relatively small numbers of subjects in case series and some randomized sham-controlled trials. The desire was for a relatively easy and quick outpatient procedure which could be done with standard sedation as for routine or advanced endoscopies (not requiring general anesthesia). The majority of these devices was not commercially successful for a variety of reasons [not Food and Drug Administration (FDA) approved, not covered by third-party payers, not endorsed by clinicians] and have been removed from availability. These techniques include the application of radiofrequency energy, injection or implantation of biopolymers, and endolumenal suturing or stapling. A systematic review of the literature yielded 59 clinical studies including 3286 patients. Of those patients, 154 received sham treatment, 20 were in an observational control group, and 3132 received treatment with endoscopic reflux therapies [9–69]. Endoscopic treatment strategies typically targeted PPI-dependent GERD patients who had small (<3 cm) or no hiatal hernias, and who did not have severe esophagitis or Barrett's esophagus. This chapter reviews the devices, techniques and outcomes associated with endoscopic antireflux therapies that have been reported in peer-reviewed publications. Our focus is limited to clinical usage outcomes and we will not review the preclinical data that has been summarized in many topical reviews elsewhere.

Injection and implantation techniques

Enteryx

Enteryx (Boston Scientific, Natick, MA, USA) is a radio-opaque biocompatible polymer consisting of 8% ethylene vinyl alcohol mixed with tantalum powder (for radio-opacity) in a solution of dimethyl sulfoxide (DMSO). It is liquid before injection and becomes an inert spongy mass once in contact with tissue. The procedure requires a special 4-mm, 23G injector needle and the use of fluoroscopy. The standard procedure involves placement of 1 mL or more in each injection site circumferentially around the GEJ until about 6–8 mL of Enteryx have been implanted intramuscularly (Figure 26.1). Occasionally an arc or ring can be formed with a single injection and multiple milliliters of injectate can be placed through the same injection site. The LES length can be increased, although there has been no significant increased LES pressure after Enteryx treatment.

Gatekeeper

The Gatekeeper Reflux Repair System (Medtronic, Minneapolis, MN, USA) aims to restrict the luminal dimension of the distal esophagus by submucosal implantations of a polyacrylonitrile-based hydrogel prosthesis. The device consists of a 16-mm diameter overtube-type instrument through which a standard or pediatric-sized videogastroscope can be passed to monitor the procedure. Suction is used to draw mucosal tissue into multiple shallow holes in the distal part of the Gatekeeper instrument and to guide placement of the hydrogel prostheses submucosally. A 1-mm diameter flexible endoscopic injector needle and a 1-mm trocar needle catheter are employed through another channel in the overtube to prepare the submucosal region for implantation of the prosthesis. The technique creates a submucosal pillow into which the dry hydrogel implants are placed. Within 24–48 h the implants swell to full size and act as a mechanical barrier at the GEJ. Usually, four to six implants are placed in a radial fashion into the submucosa during one treatment session (Figure 26.2).

Durasphere

Durasphere (Carbon Medical Technologies, St Paul, MN, USA) is a sterile, biocompatible injectable bulking material composed of pyrolytic carbon-coated graphite beads suspended in a water-based carrier gel. It has been used clinically to treat urinary incontinence since 1999. The particles were specifically designed to prevent migration and are inert. The carrier gel is 2.8% beta-glucan, which is an absorbable polysaccharide used in several medical applications, including wound healing. Durasphere for injection is prepackaged in syringes containing 1.0 mL of Durasphere

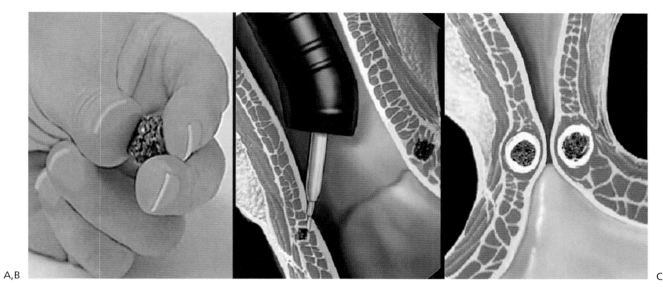

Figure 26.1 (A) Enteryx implant. (B) Endoscopic implant injection. (C) Implant after injection at the gastroesophageal junction.

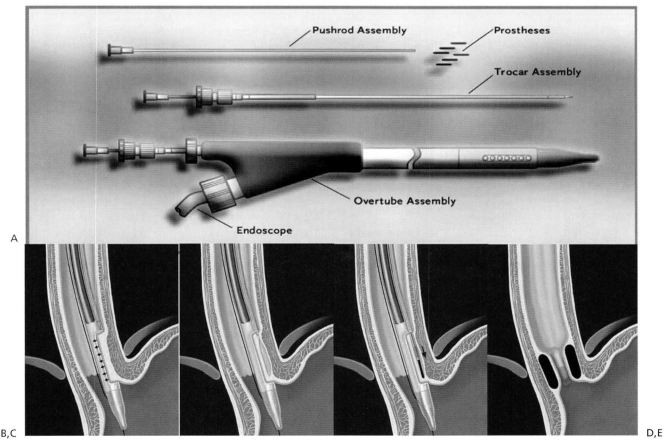

Figure 26.2 (A) Gatekeeper Device. (B) Tissue incorporation at the gastroesophageal junction into the applicator cap. (C) Pocket creation. (D) Injection of the implants. (E) Implants after injection.

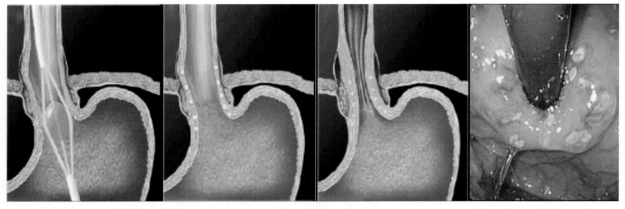

Figure 26.3 Stretta procedure. (A) Radiofrequency is delivered at the gastroesophageal junction (GEJ). (B, C) Scarring and remodeling of the GEJ. (D) Endoscopic image after Stretta therapy.

and is endoscopically delivered via a 20G sclerotherapy catheter. It is placed into the region of the LES to bulk and augment this area, and the treatment goal is to approximate the walls of the distal esophagus with narrowing of the GEJ.

Plexiglas (polymethylmethacrylate, PMMA)

Plexiglas implants consist of biocompatible 100 μm-PMMA microspheres, which have a smooth, round surface that permits injection through a needle and hinders phagocytosis and migration from the implantation site. The substance used as a carrier for PMMA is a heated 3.5% gelatin solution. The prepared implant is a 1:3 suspension of PMMA in gelatin. After implantation, the gelatin (75% of total volume) is phagocytozed by macrophages within 3 months and replaced by fibroblasts and collagen fibers, a reaction that is stimulated by the PMMA spheres (25% of total volume). The spheres are encapsulated by connective tissue, which replaces 50% of the gelatin volume, leaving at least two-thirds of the total volume of the implant remaining at the injection site.

Thermal energy

Stretta

The Stretta System (developed by Curon Medical, Sunnyvale, CA, USA; current manufacturer Mederi Therapeutics, Greenwich, CT, USA) delivers low-power, temperature-controlled radiofrequency (RF) energy to the GEJ. The system consists of a special 20F diameter balloon–basket single-use catheter with four radially-oriented nickel–titanium needles. Each needle has a dual thermocouple temperature sensor to maintain consistent energy delivery to the muscular layer of the LES. Ports in the catheters provide cold-water irrigation during the treatment to reduce mucosal heating and prevent surface injury. The RF generator is a computerized control module unit that delivers the RF energy to the needle electrodes. It provides pure sine-wave energy at 465 kHz and 2–5 W to four individually controlled channels. The system

has temperature feedback control designed to discontinue power to an individual needle electrode if the tissue temperature exceeds 100°C, if the mucosal surface temperature exceeds 50°C, or if recorded impedance exceeds 1000 Ω. The target temperature for the treatment is 85°C. The full Stretta procedure involves thermal RF treatment in four antegrade rings that straddle the GEJ from 1 cm above to just beneath the squamocolumnar junction in 0.5 cm increments (Figure 26.3). The Stretta procedure appears to provide mechanical alteration of the GEJ (increased esophageal wall thickness and modest increase in LES tone) and a significant reduction in transient LES relaxations.

Endoscopic suturing, plicating or stapling

Endoscopic suturing device

The Endoscopic Suturing Device (ESD; Wilson-Cook, Winston-Salem, NC, USA) consists of an external accessory channel, a flexible Sew-Right device, and a flexible Ti-Knot device. The external accessory channel is attached to a flexible endoscope and provides the channel for the Sew-Right and Ti-Knot devices. The Sew-Right device consists of a toggled dual-needle system that uses a single suture loop to create a tissue plication. The target tissue is aspirated into a suction chamber, and a needle with suture is then passed through the tissue. A continuous single-suture loop is used to stitch two adjacent areas in the proximal stomach to form a plication. The Ti-Knot device is passed through the external channel and guided to the tissue surface where a preloaded titanium crimp is placed to hold the sutures whose ends are cut. With the ESD, no repeated withdrawals of the endoscope are required to create the gastroplication. Typically two or three plications are placed during one treatment.

EndoCinch

The EndoCinch suturing device (CR Bard, Murray Hill, NJ, USA) is inserted via an overtube (Figure 26.4). A sewing capsule is attached to the distal tip of a standard videogastroscope and has a cavity into which tissue can be suctioned. A handle is attached to the biopsy port of the endoscope and controls a hollow-core suturing needle. A T-tag suture is back-loaded into the hollow-core needle, and is captured into the tip of the mounted capsule after being driven forward by a stiff wire pushed through the hollow needle. It can be reloaded and a second area of tissue can be captured about 1.5 cm from the initial suture site. The two areas are then drawn together to create a tissue placation, with a mean depth of placement of about 2.8 mm in the submucosal level. A catheter knotting device is guided down the sutures exiting the endoscope biopsy port and cuts the suture ends as it cinches together the submucosal sutures at

the luminal surface (Figure 26.5). Stitches to form plications can be placed in a linear, circumferential, or helical fashion. Typically two or three plications are placed during one treatment, and each plication can take 15–20 min. Preclinical studies suggested a post-procedural increase in LES tone and length, but this was not consistently found in human trials. Altered compliance and anatomy were also identified as possible mechanisms of action, and transient LES relaxations were demonstrated to be reduced.

Plicator

The NDO Plicator (developed by NDO Surgical, Mansfield, MA, USA, current IP holder Ethicon Endo-Surgery, Cincinnati, OH, USA) is designed to create a transmural full-thickness plication at the angle of His (Figure 26.6). The plication is formed with a pretied, suture-based implant (Figure 26.7). The Plicator can be advanced into the stomach over a Savary guidewire and is retroflexed for placement of the full-thickness sutures at the GEJ. Visualization is accomplished using a 5.9-mm flexible endoscope inserted through a dedicated channel in the device. This plicating device remodels the antireflux barrier at the angle of His by fashioning a pleat of full-thickness tissue and permitting serosa-to-serosa apposition. The components of the system include the plicator instrument, a tissue retracting helical catheter, and pretied pledgeted suture implants. The plicator has a

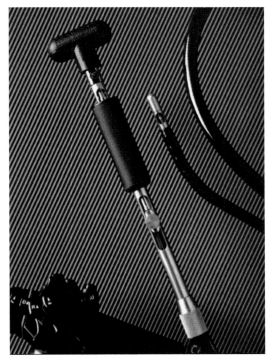

Figure 26.4 Bard EndoCinch device mounted on the endoscope working channel (reproduced courtesy of Bard/Davol).

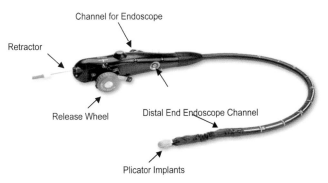

Figure 26.6 Endoscopic full-thickness Plicator.

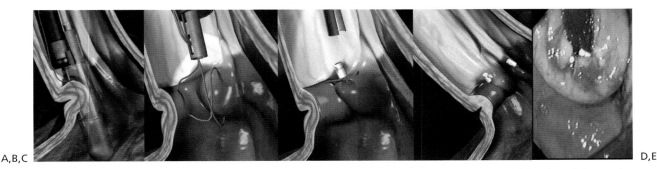

A,B,C · D,E

Figure 26.5 EndoCinch procedure. (A) Tissue is incorporated into the applicator cap. (B–D) Serial plications are placed. (E) Endoscopic image after implant placement. (reproduced courtesy of Bard/Davol).

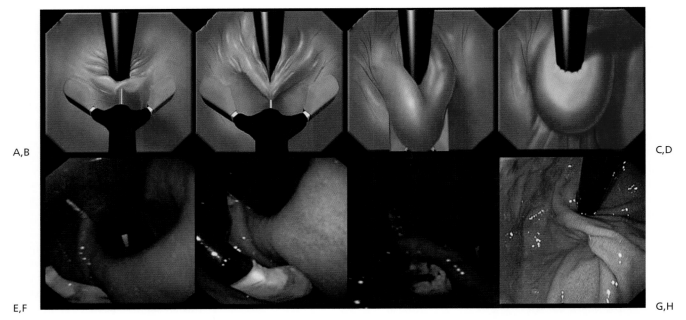

Figure 26.7 Endoscopic full-thickness plication. (A, B) Tissue is withdrawn into the Plicator jaws. (H) The implants are released creating a double layer full-thickness plication at the gastroesophageal junction. (E–G) Endoscopic images of the procedure.

handle with wheels for opening/closing the arms and sliding/locking the implant. The total procedure time is about 10–20 min to form a single plication. Recent studies have placed two to three implants for improved restructuring of the GEJ, the presumed major mechanism of action based on serosal-to-serosal apposition and fusing. The procedure required 10–20 min per plication implant.

EsophyX

The EsophyX (EndoGastric Solutions, Redmond, WA, USA) is a large overtube device with an insertion channel for a videogastroscope, and includes a bending section, which can articulate and retroflex to reach and manipulate tissue at the angle of His. The system is designed to create a circumferential endoscopic plication at the angle of His. The technique uses a helical retractor to engage and manipulate tissue in order to create the desired angle. After tissue grasping and fixation, preloaded double-sided T-tags (Treasury tags) can be passed through a double layer full-thickness plication. The method involves the placement of about 6–14 sutures, creating a near circumferential gastroplication of 180–260 degrees (Figure 26.8). It has been routinely done in operating room conditions and with general anesthesia, in contrast to all of the other endoscopic treatment methods.

Syntheon Anti-Reflux Device

The Syntheon Anti-Reflux Device (Syntheon LCC, Miami, FL, USA) delivers a titanium implant into the cardia to create a serosa-to-serosa apposition similar to the Plicator. The

Anti-Reflux Device differs from the Plicator in that it can be passed alongside the endoscope and controlled independently. A catheter-based tissue retractor through the biopsy channel of the endoscope is used to pull the gastric wall into the jaws of the Anti-Reflux Device. The titanium implant is deployed as the jaws close, to create a full-thickness pleat (Figure 26.9).

SafeStitch

The SafeStitch device is a system that utilizes two different instruments passed transorally and into which a videogastroscope can be placed to directly observe and assist in the procedure (Figure 26.10). One instrument captures and stabilizes tissue just below the GEJ, injects it with saline and performs a guillotine mucosectomy. Rotating the device allows several areas in the proximal stomach to be prepared for submucosal-to-submucosal tissue apposition. Using the second device, full thickness suturing can be performed with a circular needle and the denuded areas brought into apposition. This device can be used in the proximal stomach for therapy for GERD and can be extended into the stomach for a bariatric application fashioning a type of gastric sleeve.

His-Wiz Antireflux Procedure

The His-Wiz (Apollo Group/Olympus Optical, Tokyo, Japan) allows for full-thickness suturing and cutting in a single step. It is an overtube-based endoscopic suturing machine (Figure 26.11). Two tissue plications are performed, one on the anterior and the other on the posterior side of the GEJ, below the Z-line.

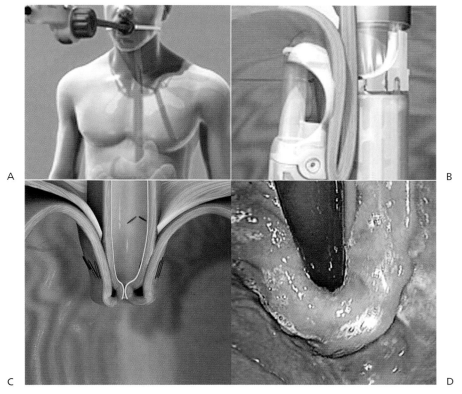

Figure 26.8 EsophyX procedure. (A) The EsophyX overtube is inserted transorally. (B) Tissue at the cardia is retracted and T-fasteners are placed, (C, D) creating a valve at the gastroesophageal junction (reproduced courtesy of Endosgastric Solutions).

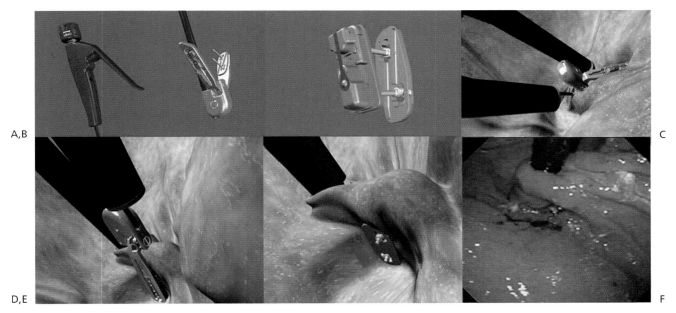

Figure 26.9 (A–E) Syntheon Anti-Reflux Device delivers a titanium implant into the cardia to create a serosa-to-serosa apposition. (F) Endoscopic image after the implant was deployed creating a full-thickness pleat.

Medigus Endoscopy System

The Medigus Endoscopy System (Medigus SRS, Tel Aviv, Israel) consists of an ultrasonic videoendoscope and an integrated surgical stapler. A stapler cartridge is mounted onto the shaft of the scope and the anvil is at the tip. B-shaped, 4.8-mm staples are fired under ultrasound guidance to create an anterior, full-thickness, 180-degree fundoplication. The fundus is caught and brought against the device where the stapler cartridge is located and the staples fired. Rotating 120 degrees, the procedure is repeated. This can create the remolding that results in tenting of the anterior stomach wall.

TOGA (Transoral Gastroplasty)

The TOGA (Transoral Gastroplasty) System (Satiety Inc, Palo Alto, CA, USA) was developed to create a transoral gastroplasty for treatment of obesity. The TOGA System is a transoral stapling device consisting of a dual-action handle, a long flexible braided shaft, and a short rigid capsule containing a stapler with a single vacuum pod for tissue acquisition. When fully opened, the largest width of the stapler is 17 mm and the width of opening between the stapler jaws is 4 mm.

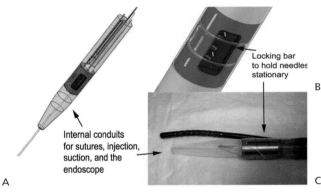

Figure 26.10 (A–C) SafeStitch device.

After acquiring a fold of tissue by vacuum, it fires two rows of six titanium staples over a 25-mm length without cutting the tissue. There has been interest in the use this bariatric device in a technique to treat GERD, and there has been preclinical study of this method.

Study outcomes of endoscopic therapies

Level of evidence and follow-up period

We employ the currently accepted standards of evidence in reporting the study outcomes of these therapies (Table 26.2). The majority of endoscopic reflux therapies have been studied in uncontrolled trials. Thus far, EndoCinch, Gatekeeper, Stretta, and the Plicator have been investigated in sham-controlled clinical trials (Tables 26.1 and 26.3). Sham-controlled studies overall have included 436 patients, of whom 262 received endoscopic reflux therapy at study

Table 26.2 Level of evidence according to Sackett *et al.* Evidence-based Medicine—How to Practice and Teach EBM, 2nd edn. London: Churchill Livingstone, 2000, pp. 173–175.

Level of evidence	Description
1a	Systematic review of randomized controlled trials (RCT)
1b	Individual randomized controlled trial (RCT)
2a	Systematic review of cohort studies
2b	Individual cohort study (including low-quality RCT)
2c	Outcomes research
3a	Systematic review of case–control studies
3b	Individual case–control study
4	Case series, poor quality case–control studies and reviews
5	Expert opinion

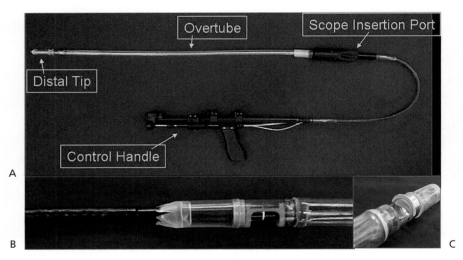

Figure 26.11 (A) Hiz-Wiz device. (B) Device loaded onto an endoscope and (C) close-up of the distal tip.

Table 26.3 Levels of evidence and follow-up intervals for endoscopic reflux therapy studies.

Author	Year	Treatment	Treatment principle	Patients (n)	Follow-up (months)[1]	Evidence level
Richards	2001	Stretta	Thermal energy	25	3	2c
Triadafilopoulos	2001	Stretta	Thermal energy	47	6	2c
Feretis	2001	Plexiglas	Injection or implantation	10	5–11 (7)	2c
Filipi	2001	EndoCinch	Endoscopic suturing	64	6	2b
Devière	2002	Enteryx	Injection or implantation	15	6	2c
DiBaise	2002	Stretta	Thermal energy	18	6	2c
Triadafilopoulos	2002	Stretta	Thermal energy	118	12	2c
Wolfsen	2002	Stretta	Thermal energy	558	1–33 (8)	2c
Chuttani	2003	Plicator	Endoscopic suturing	6	12	4
Houston	2003	Stretta	Thermal energy	41	6	2c
Johnson	2003	Enteryx	Injection or implantation	85	6	2c
Johnson	2003	Enteryx	Injection or implantation	85	12	2c
Mahmood	2003	EndoCinch	Endoscopic suturing	26	12	2c
Torquati	2004	Stretta	Thermal energy	36	27	2c
Pleskow	2004	Plicator	Endoscopic suturing	64	6	2c
Fockens	2004	Gatekeeper	Injection or implantation	68	6	2c
Schilling	2005	ESD	Endoscopic suturing	20	3	2c
Schiefke[2]	2005	ESD	Endoscopic suturing	20	6	2c
Liu[3]	2005	Stretta	Thermal energy	8	6–15	4
Cipolletta	2005	Stretta	Thermal energy	32	12	2c
Lutfi	2005	Stretta	Thermal energy	77	6–36 (26)	2c
Cicala	2005	Gatekeeper	Injection or implantation	9	6	4
Arts	2005	EndoCinch	Endoscopic suturing	20	12	2c
Schiefke	2005	EndoCinch	Endoscopic suturing	70	18	2c
Pleskow	2005	Plicator	Endoscopic suturing	64	12	2c
Schumacher	2005	Enteryx	Injection or implantation	93	12	2c
Abou-Rebyeh	2005	EndoCinch	Endoscopic suturing	38	12	2b
Mattar[4]	2006	Stretta	Thermal energy	7	20	4
Domagk	2006	EndoCinch	Endoscopic suturing	26	6	1b
		Enteryx	Injection or implantation	23	6	
Montgomery	2006	EndoCinch	Endoscopic suturing	22	12	1b
		Sham	Control group	24	12	
Rothstein	2006	Plicator	Endoscopic suturing	72	3	1b
		Sham	Control group	72	3	
Reymunde	2007	Stretta	Thermal energy	83	48	2c
Noar	2007	Stretta	Thermal energy	109	48	2c
McClusky[5]	2007	Stretta	Thermal energy	7	2–12 (8)	4
Arts	2007	Stretta	Thermal energy	13	6	2c
Meier	2007	Stretta	Thermal energy	60	12	2c
Pleskow	2007	Plicator	Endoscopic suturing	29	31–44 (36)	2c
Tierney	2007	EndoCinch	Endoscopic suturing	6	6	4
Higuchi	2007	Stretta	Thermal energy	9	6	4
Schwartz	2007	EndoCinch	Endoscopic suturing	20	3	1b
		Sham	Control group	20	3	
		Observation	Control group	20	3	
Dundon	2008	Stretta	Thermal energy	32	36–68 (53)	2c
Cadiere	2008	EsophyX	Endoscopic suturing	17	12	2c
Cadiere	2008	EsophyX	Endoscopic suturing	86	12	2c
Pleskow	2008	Plicator	Endoscopic suturing	33	50–65 (59)	2c
Thomson[6]	2008	EndoCinch	Endoscopic suturing	17	36	2c
von Renteln	2008	Plicator	Endoscopic suturing	41	6	2c
von Renteln	2008	Plicator	Endoscopic suturing	37	6	2c

(continued)

Table 26.3 (continued)

Author	Year	Treatment	Treatment principle	Patients (n)	Follow-up (months)[1]	Evidence level
Birk	2009	Plicator	Endoscopic suturing	81	12	2c
Cadiere	2009	EsophyX	Endoscopic suturing	17	24	2c
von Renteln	2009	Plicator	Endoscopic suturing	41	12	2c
Ganz	2009	Durasphere	Injection or implantation	10	12	2c
Jeansonne	2009	Stretta	Thermal energy	68	1–37 (5)	2b
		Plicator	Endoscopic suturing	58	1–29 (8)	
White	2009	Plicator	Endoscopic suturing	10	14	2b
		Stretta	Thermal energy	12	25	
Aziz	2010	Stretta[7]	Thermal energy	12	12	1b
		Stretta[8]	Thermal energy	12	12	
		Sham	Control group	12	12	
Demyttenaere	2010	EsophyX	Endoscopic suturing	26	10	2c
Testoni	2010	EsophyX	Endoscopic suturing	20	6	2c
von Renteln	2010	Plicator	Endoscopic suturing	12	6	4
Repici	2010	EsophyX	Endoscopic suturing	20	12	2c
Fockens[9]	2010	Gatekeeper	Injection or implantation	51	6	2b
		Sham	Control group	26	6	

[1]Numbers in brackets indicate median or average follow-up intervals.
[2]Study population are patients with retreatment after EndoCinch failure.
[3]Study population are children.
[4]Study population are patients post RYGB.
[5]Study population are patients after antireflux surgery failure.
[6]Study population are children.
[7]Single Stretta treatment.
[8]Double Stretta treatment.
[9]143 patients enrolled (25 lead in, 75 treatment, 43 sham, 6-month data available for 51 treatment and 26 sham patients [24 patients crossed over from sham to treatment]).

entry and 154 sham procedures, and 20 patients were included as observational controls in one study. GERD is a chronic condition, typically requiring lifelong therapy. Therefore, long-term follow-up is necessary to determine treatment efficacy. For 41 of the 59 studies (69%), follow-up data between 3 and 12 months is available (Table 26.3). Long-term follow-up data (>12 months) is available for nine of 59 studies (15%), including treatment with EndoCinch, EsophyX, Stretta, and the Plicator. Nine studies (15%) report data with inhomogeneous follow-up intervals ranging between less than 1 and up to 65 months after treatment. For the randomized sham-controlled trials, follow-up data are available for 3 and 12 months in two EndoCinch studies, for 6 months for Plicator and Gatekeeper studies, and for 12 months for one Stretta study (Table 26.3).

Symptom score outcomes

The majority of endoscopic antireflux therapies demonstrated significant improvements in health-related quality of life (HRQOL) and reflux scores (Table 26.4). This applies to the short-term follow-up for controlled and uncontrolled trials and for the available long-term follow-up in uncon-

trolled trials (Table 26.4). A sham-controlled Gatekeeper study terminated early due to lack of compelling efficacy data and for safety concerns. Uncontrolled studies suggest a sustained effect (≥24 months) for Plicator, EsophyX, and Stretta treatment (Table 26.4).

Proton pump inhibitor use outcomes

The majority of endoscopic reflux therapies demonstrated significant short-term improvements in PPI use (Table 26.5). Long-term follow-up data after endoscopic reflux therapy on PPI use is still limited. Interestingly, Stretta treatment demonstrated a sustained effect on PPI use in two long-term follow-up studies; however, it provided no difference in PPI usage compared to sham-treated patients in a randomized controlled trial. Unfortunately, the sustained effect of most endoscopic reflux therapies on PPI use remains unclear at present.

pH-metry outcomes

The majority of studies that reported pH-metry data demonstrated significantly improved esophageal acid exposure in the short-term follow-up compared to pretreatment values (Table 26.6). EndoCinch demonstrated significantly

Table 26.4 Symptom score outcomes.

Author	Year	Treatment	Patients (n)	Follow-up (months)	Symptom score	Score pre therapy	Score post therapy	P-value
Richards	2001	Stretta	25	3	QOLRD	3.5	5.5	<.001
Triadafilopoulos	2001	Stretta	47	6	HRQOL	26	7	≤.0001
Filipi	2001	EndoCinch	64	6	HBS	62.7	17	.0001
Feretis	2001	Plexiglas	10	7	HRQOL	12,2	6.2	<.005
Devière	2002	Enteryx	15	6	HRQOL	3.4	1.9	<.01
DiBaise	2002	Stretta	18	6	HRQOL	21.5	7	<.001
Triadafilopoulos	2002	Stretta	118	12	HRQOL	27	9	<.0001
Wolfsen	2002	Stretta	558	1–33	SC	23	87	<.0001
Chuttani	2003	Plicator	6	12	HRQOL	18.8	4.6	—
Houston	2003	Stretta	41	6	QOLRD	3.7	5.1	.002
Johnson	2003	Enteryx	85	6	HRQOL	24	4	<.001
Johnson	2003	Enteryx	85	12	HRQOL	24	5	<.001
Mahmood	2003	EndoCinch	26	12	HBS	19.2	7.5	<.0001
Torquati	2004	Stretta	36	27	HRQOL	6.1	4	<.0001
Pleskow	2004	Plicator	64	6	HRQOL	19	5	<0.001
Fockens	2004	Gatekeeper	68	6	HRQOL	24	5	<.01
Schilling	2005	ESD	20	3	HRQOL	28	4	≤.002
Schiefke[1]	2005	ESD	20	6	HBS	48	30	<.05
Liu[2]	2005	Stretta	8	6–15	—	—	—	—
Cipolletta	2005	Stretta	32	12	HRQOL	28	16	.003
Lutfi	2005	Stretta	77	6–36	QOLRD	3.6	5	<.001
Cicala	2005	Gatekeeper	9	6	HRQOL	35.5	9.4	<.01
Arts	2005	EndoCinch	20	12	HRQOL	—	6.4	—
Schiefke	2005	EndoCinch	70	18	HRQOL	58.2	36.8	≤.001
Pleskow	2005	Plicator	64	12	HRQOL	19	5	<.0001
Schumacher	2005	Enteryx	93	12	HRQOL	6	6	<.0001
Abou-Rebyeh	2005	EndoCinch	38	12	—	—	—	—
Mattar[3]	2006	Stretta	7	20	SC	0	83	—
Domagk	2006	EndoCinch	26	6	HBS	53.7	20.9	<.0001
		Enteryx	23	6	HBS	56.1	19.9	<.0001
Montgomery	2006	EndoCinch	22	12	GSRS	14	11	<.05
		Sham	24	12	GSRS	16	12	<.05
Rothstein	2006	Plicator	72	3	HRQOL	25.7	12.5	<.001
		Sham	72	3	HRQOL	26.3	20.1	<.001
Reymunde	2007	Stretta	83	48	HRQOL	2.7	0.6	<.001
Noar	2007	Stretta	109	48	HRQOL	27.8	7.1	<.001
McClusky[4]	2007	Stretta	7	2–12	HRQOL	1.6	0.3	<.03
Arts	2007	Stretta	13	6	HRQOL	12.5	7.5	<.05
Meier	2007	Stretta	60	12	HRQOL	19.2	6.6	<.0001
Pleskow	2007	Plicator	29	31–44	HRQOL	19	8	<.001
Tierney	2007	EndoCinch	6	6	HBS	2.6	2.4	—
Higuchi	2007	Stretta	9	6	HBS	5	0.7	.007
Schwartz	2007	EndoCinch	20	3	HBS	17.2	8.6	<.05
		Sham	20	3	HRQOL	15.6	14.7	—
		Observation	20	3	HRQOL	17.4	14.3	<.05
Dundon	2008	Stretta	32	36–68	HRQOL	2.4	1.8	—
Cadiere	2008	EsophyX	17	12	HRQOL	17	6	—
Cadiere	2008	EsophyX	86	12	HRQOL	24	7	<.0001
Pleskow	2008	Plicator	33	50–65	HRQOL	19	10	<.001
Thomson[5]	2008	EndoCinch	17	36	QOLRD	87	153.5	.002
von Renteln	2008	Plicator	41	6	HRQOL	25	6	<.001

(*continued*)

Table 26.4 (continued)

Author	Year	Treatment	Patients (n)	Follow-up (months)	Symptom score	Score pre therapy	Score post therapy	P-value
von Renteln	2008	Plicator	37	6	HRQOL	15	9	<.05
Birk	2009	Plicator	81	12	HRQOL	26.6	12	<.001
Cadiere	2009	EsophyX	17	24	HRQOL	17	7	.004
von Renteln	2009	Plicator	41	12	HRQOL	25.4	7.8	<.001
Ganz	2009	Durasphere	10	12	HRQOL	32.4	3.1	<.001
Jeansonne	2009	Stretta	68	1–37	HBS	55	22	<.01
		Plicator	58	1–29	HBS	53	43	.3
White	2009	Plicator	10	14	—	—	—	—
		Stretta	12	25	—	—	—	—
Aziz	2010	Stretta[6]	12	12	HRQOL	29.6	14.4	<.01
		Stretta[7]	12	12	HRQOL	31	10.7	<.001
		Sham	12	12	HRQOL	30.3	28.4	<.05
Demyttenaere	2010	EsophyX	26	10	HRQOL	22	10	.,0007
Testoni	2010	EsophyX	20	6	HRQOL	45	16	<.001
von Renteln	2010	Plicator	12	6	—	—	—	—
Repici	2010	EsophyX	20	12	HRQOL	40	10	<.05
Fockens[8]	2010	Gatekeeper	51	6	HRQOL	27.6	13.7	<.0001
		Sham	26	6	HRQOL	26	16.4	<.0001

[1]Study population are patients with retreatment after EndoCinch failure.

[2]Study population are children.

[3]Study population are patients post RYGB.

[4]Study population are patients after antireflux surgery failure.

[5]Study population are children.

[6]Single Stretta treatment.

[7]Double Stretta treatment.

[8]143 patients enrolled [25 lead in, 75 treatment, 43 sham, 6-month data available for 51 treatment and 26 sham patients (24 patients crossed over from sham to treatment)].

GSRS, gastrointestinal symptom rating scale. Disease-specific scale depicting reflux, abdominal pain, indigestion, diarrhea, and constipation, The GSRS has a seven-point graded Likert-scale where 1 represents absence of troublesome symptoms and 7 represents very troublesome symptoms.

HBS, heart burn score (0–5; lower numbers indicate better control).

HRQOL, health-related quality of life [gastroesophageal reflux disease (GERD) symptom index reflects the GERD–HRQOL; scale 0–50, a score <10 is considered normal].

SC, symptom control (percentage of patients with symptom control off drugs).

QOLRD, quality of life related to reflux disease (score 0–7; higher numbers indicate better control).

improved esophageal acid exposure in the short-term. This effect does not seem to be sustained in long-term follow-up due to suture loss in most studies. Only one study in children demonstrated significantly improved esophageal acid exposure ($P = .02$) at 36 months post treatment using EndoCinch. At 6-month follow-up, patients treated with the Plicator had significantly less esophageal acid exposure compared to the sham group. A randomized controlled study using Gatekeeper failed to demonstrate differences in acid exposure between the treatment and sham groups. Stretta demonstrated significantly reduced esophageal acid exposure in long-term follow-up in two uncontrolled studies. One of these studies had a follow-up of 27 months and one reported on a heterogeneous group with follow-up ranging between 6 and 36 months. The majority of studies with long-term follow-up report on symptom scores and do not provide pH-metry data (Table 26.6). The sustained effect of endoscopic reflux therapies on esophageal acid exposure remains unclear at present.

Serious adverse events

In the reviewed literature, minor transient adverse events related to the endoscopic therapy, like sore throat, chest pain, abdominal pain, mucosal injury with bleeding, and gas bloat syndrome, are quite common. Severe or potentially life-threatening complications, such as perforation, pneumothorax, dysphagia requiring dilatation, and severe bleeding, have been reported but are extremely rare. For the

Table 26.5 Proton pump inhibitor (PPI) use outcomes.

Author	Year	Treatment	Patients (n)	Follow-up (months)	PPI utilization (% pre therapy)	PPI utilization (% post therapy)	P-value
Richards	2001	Stretta	25	3	100	38	—
Triadafilopoulos	2001	Stretta	47	6	87.2	13	<.0001
Filipi	2001	EndoCinch	64	6	100	38	—
Feretis	2001	Plexiglas	10	5–11	100	10	—
Devière	2002	Enteryx	15	6	100	26.7	—
DiBaise	2002	Stretta	18	6	94.4	6	<.05
Triadafilopoulos	2002	Stretta	118	12	88.1	30	<.0001
Wolfsen	2002	Stretta	558	1–33	93.9	33.6	—
Chuttani	2003	Plicator	6	12	100	83.3	—
Houston	2003	Stretta	41	6	100	35	<.001
Johnson	2003	Enteryx	85	6	100	26	—
Johnson	2003	Enteryx	85	12	100	12.3	—
Mahmood	2003	EndoCinch	26	12	100	36	—
Torquati	2004	Stretta	36	27	100	44	—
Pleskow	2004	Plicator	64	6	92	26	—
Fockens	2004	Gatekeeper	68	6	100	47	—
Schilling	2005	ESD	20	3	100	80	≤.4
Schiefke[1]	2005	ESD	20	6	100	100	—
Liu[2]	2005	Stretta	8	6–15	—	—	—
Cipolletta	2005	Stretta	32	12	100	44	—
Lutfi	2005	Stretta	77	6–36	100	23	—
Cicala	2005	Gatekeeper	9	6	—	—	—
Arts	2005	EndoCinch	20	12	100	70	—
Schiefke	2005	EndoCinch	70	18	100	94.3	—
Pleskow	2005	Plicator	64	12	92	32	—
Schumacher	2005	Enteryx	93	12	100	35	—
Abou-Rebyeh	2005	EndoCinch	38	12	100	80	—
Mattar[3]	2006	Stretta	7	20	100	17	—
Domagk	2006	EndoCinch	26	6	100	77	<.0001
		Enteryx	23	6	100	87	<.0001
Montgomery	2006	EndoCinch	22	12	100	45.5	<.05
		Sham	24	12	100	20.8	<.05
Rothstein	2006	Plicator	72	3	100	43	—
		Sham	72	3	100	75	—
Reymunde	2007	Stretta	83	48	100	13.8	<.001
Noar	2007	Stretta	109	48	100	25	<.005
McClusky[4]	2007	Stretta	7	2–12	100	42.9	—
Arts	2007	Stretta	13	6	100	46	—
Meier	2007	Stretta	60	12	100	62	—
Pleskow	2007	Plicator	29	31–44	97	50	—
Tierney	2007	EndoCinch	6		83	67	—
Higuchi	2007	Stretta	9	6	100	78	—
Schwartz	2007	EndoCinch	20	3	100	—	—
		Sham	20	3	100	—	—
		Observation	20	3	100	—	—
Dundon	2008	Stretta	32	36–68	100	34	—
Cadiere	2008	EsophyX	17	12	100	18	—
Cadiere	2008	EsophyX	86	12	100	15	—
Pleskow	2008	Plicator	33	50–65	90,9	67	—
Thomson[5]	2008	EndoCinch	17	36	—	—	—
von Renteln	2008	Plicator	41	6	100	30	—

(continued)

Table 26.5 (continued)

Author	Year	Treatment	Patients (n)	Follow-up (months)	PPI utilization (% pre therapy)	PPI utilization (% post therapy)	P-value
von Renteln	2008	Plicator	37	6	100	41	—
Birk	2009	Plicator	81	12	94	42	—
Cadiere	2009	EsophyX	17	24	100	29	—
von Renteln	2009	Plicator	41	12	100	31	—
Ganz	2009	Durasphere	10	12	100	30	—
Jeansonne	2009	Stretta	68	1–37	84	50	.01
		Plicator	58	1–29	95	43	.01
White	2009	Plicator	10	14	91	50	.03
	2009	Stretta	12	25	64	40	NS
Aziz	2010	Stretta[6]	12	12	100	83.4	—
		Stretta[7]	12	12	100	50	—
		Sham	12	12	100	100	—
Demyttenaere	2010	EsophyX	26	10	100	68	—
Testoni	2010	EsophyX	20	6	100	44	—
von Renteln	2010	Plicator	12	6	—	—	—
Repici	2010	EsophyX	20	12	100	53	—
Fockens[8]	2010	Gatekeeper	51	6	100	45	—
		Sham	26	6	100	67	—

[1]Study population is patients with retreatment after EndoCinch failure.
[2]Study population is children.
[3]Study population is patients post RYGB.
[4]Study population is patients after antireflux surgery failure.
[5]Study population is children.
[6]Single Stretta treatment.
[7]Double Stretta treatment.
[8]143 patients enrolled [25 lead in, 75 treatment, 43 sham, 6-month data available for 51 treatment and 26 sham patients (24 patients crossed over from sham to treatment)].
NS, not significant.

Gatekeeper system, esophageal perforation was reported in the initial and the sham-controlled trial. One post-marketing death occurred outside of clinical trial and related to Enteryx injection into the aorta, after which the device was withdrawn from the market. For the Plicator treatment, two gastric perforations have been reported. Free intraperitoneal air occurs quite commonly after Plicator treatment, but this appears not to be clinically significant. It may be related to air translocating during placement of the transmural implants and does not have the consequences of a true perforation. Two esophageal perforations have been reported after treatment with the EsophyX device (Table 26.7). In general, mild adverse events are not unexpected due to the endoscopic treatments, and severe adverse events are either device or technique related, and fortunately rare. Some of the events that occurred were related to poor judgment or inadequate training of the clinician. It is imperative that for the introduction of any new endoscopic technology, the endoscopist needs to be adequately trained and has to follow the established protocols for safe use of the device.

Retreatment, reversibility, and issues of optimization of technique

All the endoscopic antireflux therapies allow for repeated use (Table 26.8). The initial assumption was that the effect on symptoms and pH control might be in the range of several years, allowing for retreatment when needed. Retreatment offers an ability to safely augment the initial treatment effect, and there is unfortunately extremely limited data on additive effects of additional endoscopic intervention following initial treatment. There is also no available experience with combining various treatment modalities, such as RF thermal treatment together with suture plication of the cardia. Unfortunately, all the initial trials were conducted for safety and not optimized for efficacy. The optimal number of thermal treatment sites, volume of injectate, or number of implants and pleats remains undetermined. Most implantation therapies are not reversible (Table 26.8), although it was possible to remove the Gatekeeper hydrogel prosthesis using a needle knife to incise over the implant and a suction cap to remove it from the

Table 26.6 pH-metry data outcomes.

Author	Year	Treatment	Patients (n)	Follow-up (months)	Esophageal acid exposure (pre therapy)	Esophageal acid exposure (post therapy)	P-value
Richards	2001	Stretta	25	3	31	—	—
Triadafilopoulos	2001	Stretta	47	6	11.7	4.8	<.001
Filipi	2001	EndoCinch	64	6	9.63	8.5	.011
Feretis	2001	Plexiglas	10	5–11	24.5	7.2	.007
Devière	2002	Enteryx	15	6	—	—	—
DiBaise	2002	Stretta	18	6	9.5	6.2	<.05
Triadafilopoulos	2002	Stretta	118	12	10.2	6.4	<.0001
Wolfsen	2002	Stretta	558	1–33	—	—	—
Chuttani	2003	Plicator	6	12	—	—	—
Houston	2003	Stretta	41	6	8.4	4.4	.03
Johnson	2003	Enteryx	85	6	9.5	7	<.001
Johnson	2003	Enteryx	85	12	9.5	7	<.001
Mahmood[1]	2003	EndoCinch	26	12	11.1	9.3	NS
Torquati	2004	Stretta	36	27	6.4	3.1	<.0001
Pleskow	2004	Plicator	64	6	10	8	<.008
Fockens	2004	Gatekeeper	68	6	9.1	6.1	<.05
Schilling	2005	ESD	20	3	8.5	7.8	0.74
Schiefke[2]	2005	ESD	20	6	9.9	12.3	0.6
Liu[3]	2005	Stretta	8	6–15	—	—	—
Cipolletta	2005	Stretta	32	12	11.7	8.4	.79
Lutfi	2005	Stretta	77	6–36	7.8	5.1	<.001
Cicala	2005	Gatekeeper	9	6	11.7	7.7	—
Arts	2005	EndoCinch	20	12	—	8.1	—
Schiefke	2005	EndoCinch	70	18	9,1	8.5	≤.82
Pleskow	2005	Plicator	64	12	10	—	—
Schumacher	2005	Enteryx	93	12	10.9	10.9	≤.55
Abou-Rebyeh	2005	EndoCinch	38	12	—	—	<.04
Mattar[4]	2006	Stretta	7	20	7	3	<.05
Domagk	2006	EndoCinch	26	6	14,5	9.6	≤.071
		Enteryx	23	6	15.5	13.9	≤.93
Montgomery	2006	EndoCinch	22	12	5.95	4.7	NS
		Sham	24	12	5.9	7.4	NS
Rothstein	2006	Plicator	72	3	10	7	<.001
		Sham	72	3	9	10	.686
Reymunde	2007	Stretta	83	48	—	—	—
Noar	2007	Stretta	109	48	—	—	—
McClusky[5]	2007	Stretta	7	2–12	—	—	—
Arts	2007	Stretta	13	6	11,6	8,5	<.05
Meier	2007	Stretta	60	12	16,7	8,8	.001
Pleskow	2007	Plicator	29	31–44	—	—	—
Tierney	2007	EndoCinch	6	6	25,6	23,5	—
Higuchi	2007	Stretta	9	6	—	—	—
Schwartz	2007	EndoCinch	20	3	10.2	7.5	.02
		Sham	20	3	9.5	7.6	—
		Observation	20	3	9.6	—	—
Dundon	2008	Stretta	32	36–68	—	—	—
Cadiere	2008	EsophyX	17	12	4,1	4.7	—
Cadiere	2008	EsophyX	86	12	10	7	,02
Pleskow	2008	Plicator	33	50–65	—	—	—
Thomson[6]	2008	EndoCinch	17	36	16.6	4.5	.02
von Renteln	2008	Plicator	41	6	11	9	<.02

(continued)

Table 26.6 (continued)

Author	Year	Treatment	Patients (n)	Follow-up (months)	Esophageal acid exposure (pre therapy)	Esophageal acid exposure (post therapy)	P-value
von Renteln	2008	Plicator	37	6	9.5	6.15	<.05
Birk	2009	Plicator	81	12	—	—	—
Cadiere	2009	EsophyX	17	24	—	—	—
von Renteln	2009	Plicator	41	12	—	—	—
Ganz	2009	Durasphere	10	12	13,2	7.4	.01
Jeansonne	2009	Stretta	68	1–37	10,8	9.1	NS
		Plicator	58	1–29	10	6.1	.05
White	2009	Plicator	10	14	—	—	—
		Stretta	12	25	—	—	—
Aziz	2010	Stretta[7]	12	12	9.4	6.7	<.01
		Stretta[8]	12	12	8.8	5.2	<.01
		Sham	12	12	9.9	8.2	NS
Demyttenaere	2010	EsophyX	26	10	—	—	—
Testoni[9]	2010	EsophyX	20	6	20	18	.57
von Renteln	2010	Plicator	12	6	6.8	3.4	.008
Repici	2010	EsophyX	20	12	3.8	3.3	NS
Fockens[10]	2010	Gatekeeper	51	6	12.7	11.4	.021
		Sham	26	6	12.3	10.7	.003

[1]pH-metry was performed at 3 months post treatment.
[2]Study population are patients with retreatment after EndoCinch failure.
[3]Study population are children.
[4]Study population are patients post RYGB.
[5]Study population are patients after antireflux surgery failure.
[6]pH metry was performed at 12 months post treatment; study population are children.
[7]Single Stretta treatment.
[8]Double Stretta treatment.
[9]DeMeester score.
[10]143 patients enrolled [25 lead in, 75 treatment, 43 sham, 6-month data available for 51 treatment and 26 sham patients (24 patients crossed over from sham to treatment)].
NS, not significant.

submucosal location. The suturing-based techniques allowed for implant removal since it was possible to cut the suture material with endoscopic scissors. The Syntheon implant had a removal process engineered into the device and a specific removal tool designed for this purpose. Removal of some of these devices and implants, or of sutures, was potentially difficult when scarring, tissue overgrowth or migration of the sutures or implants occurred. Thermal and stapler treatment, by design, is not reversible. The selection of various treatment options by clinicians and patients when these techniques were introduced could have been partly influenced by the safety margin of reversibility when needed.

Current availability (Table 26.8)

Gatekeeper was withdrawn from the market due to serious adverse events and lack of efficacy. Enteryx was withdrawn due to a procedure related death (see above). ESD outcomes demonstrated early loss of the sutures and inadequate acid contact control, and the device is therefore no longer mar-

keted by Wilson-Cook. The Plicator device and associated intellectual property were recently bought by Ethicon Endo-Surgery following the inability to successfully commercialize the device by the initial manufacturer (NDO Surgical); the technology is currently unavailable for clinical use. The Syntheon ARD and Olympus His-Wiz were not brought forward to commercialization. At present, only EndoCinch, EsophyX and Stretta are available for commercial use, and Medigus is undergoing study in a multicenter clinical trial. EndoCinch availability is specific to previously trained users and subject to approval by the company. EsophyX is commercially available in Europe, and has recently received FDA clearance for commercial sales in the United States.

Devices in development

Several devices were recently or currently under development. The outcomes of clinical study of the His-Wiz, Syntheon, and SafeStitch devices have not yet been published in peer-reviewed full manuscripts, and the experi-

Table 26.7 Procedure-related and possible procedure-related adverse events.

Author	Year	Treatment	Patients (n)	Follow-up (months)	Reported adverse events
Richards	2001	Stretta	25	3	1 ulcerative esophagitis, gastroparesis and hematemesis
Triadafilopoulos	2001	Stretta	47	6	1 linear mucosal injury during catheter positioning with fever for 24 h and odynophagia
Feretis	2001	Plexiglas	10	5–11	1 chest pain
					1 self-limited bleeding
					1 gas bloat syndrome
					1 transient dysphagia
Filipi	2001	EndoCinch	64	6	20 pharyngitis
					9 vomiting
					9 abdominal pain
					10 chest pain
					2 mucosal tear
					4 hypoxia
					2 gastric bleeding
					1 suture perforation
Devière	2002	Enteryx	15	6	8 mild retrosternal discomfort
DiBaise	2002	Stretta	18	6	1 mucosal injury during catheter positioning
Triadafilopoulos	2002	Stretta	118	12	2 fever
					3 superficial catheter injury
					2 chest pain
					1 transient dysphagia
					1 sedation-related hypotension
					1 submental swelling
Chuttani	2003	Plicator	6	12	2 mild epigastric pain
					1 gas bloat syndrome
Houston	2003	Stretta	41	6	1 gastroparesis
Johnson	2003	Enteryx	85	6	78 retrosternal chest pain
					17 dysphagia
					10 fever
					6 belching/burping
					5 bloating/flatulence
					4 body odor/bad taste
					1 rib pain
					9 sore throat
					7 nausea/vomiting
					5 nausea
					3 shoulder pain
					2 dry mouth
					2 anxiety
					1 breast pain
Mahmood	2003	EndoCinch	26	12	7 sore throat
					2 vomiting
					3 abdominal pain
					5 chest soreness
					2 dysphagia
					2 bloating
					2 bleeding necessitating transfusion
					1 gastric mucosal tear
Torquati	2004	Stretta	36	27	No adverse events

(*continued*)

Table 26.7 (*continued*)

Author	Year	Treatment	Patients (n)	Follow-up (months)	Reported adverse events
Pleskow	2004	Plicator	64	6	26 pharyngitis 13 abdominal pain 11 unspecified gastrointestinal disorder 11 gas bloating syndrome 9 dysphagia 4 nausea 1 gastric perforation 1 spontaneous pneumothorax 1 pneumoperitoneum 1 fundal mucosal injury 2 Intraprocedural dyspnea after overtube placement
Fockens	2004	Gatekeeper	68	6	15 erosion on the prosthesis 1 nausea and vomiting 1 retrosternal pain 1 stomach pain and skin rash 1 cough 1 hoarseness 1 ulcerations on the prosthesis 1 tiredness and poor sleep 1 pharyngeal perforation
Schilling	2005	ESD	20	3	13 transient abdominal or chest pain 2 acute bleeding 3 belching and burping 3 mild dysphagia 4 gas bloating syndrome
Schiefke	2005	ESD	20	6	2 bleeding episodes 17 transient chest pain, nausea, or abdominal pain
Liu	2005	Stretta	8	6–15	1 aspiration pneumonitis
Cipolletta	2005	Stretta	32	12	6 chest pain 4 mild fever 1 transient nausea/vomiting 1 Prolonged gastroparesis in patient with pre-existing gastric emptying disorder
Lutfi	2005	Stretta	77	6–36	1 transient gastroparesis
Arts	2005	EndoCinch	20	12	20 sore throat and mild epigastric pain 1 transient dysphagia
Schiefke	2005	EndoCinch	70	18	18 retrosternal and pharyngeal pain 12 nausea/vomiting 8 short intraprocedural bleeding episodes
Pleskow	2005	Plicator	64	12	26 pharyngitis 13 abdominal pain 11 unspecified gastrointestinal disorder 11 gas bloating syndrome 9 dysphagia 4 nausea 1 gastric perforation 1 spontaneous pneumothorax 1 pneumoperitoneum 1 fundal mucosal injury 2 intraprocedural dyspnea after overtube placement

Table 26.7 (*continued*)

Author	Year	Treatment	Patients (n)	Follow-up (months)	Reported adverse events
Schumacher	2005	Enteryx	93	12	1 pleural effusion 25 dysphagia/odynophagia 24 sensation of fever 3 belching 1 gas bloating syndrome 1 bradycardia 1 regurgitation
Cohen	2005	Enteryx	144	12	122 transient retrosternal chest pain 34 mild-to-moderate dysphagia 2 dysphagia requiring dilatation
		Enteryx	64	24	54 transient retrosternal chest pain 15 mild-to-moderate dysphagia 1 dysphagia requiring dilatation
Domagk	2006	EndoCinch	26	6	26 transient abdominal pain and pharyngitis
		Enteryx	23	6	1 Forrest IIa bleeding 1 painful singultus 3 fever
Montgomery	2006	EndoCinch	22	12	1 transient sore throat, mild dysphagia, and epigastric pain
		Sham	24	12	No adverse effects
Rothstein	2006	Plicator	72	3	2 gas bloat syndrome 2 leukocytosis 2 dysphagia 4 vomiting 6 nausea 7 abdominal pain or discomfort 9 radiating shoulder pain 9 epigastric pain or discomfort 7 pharyngolaryngeal pain 9 retrosternal/chest pain 2 pneumoperitoneum
		Sham	72	3	2 dysphagia 3 vomiting 1 nausea 3 epigastric pain or discomfort 8 pharyngolaryngeal pain 4 retrosternal/chest pain 1 intraprocedural oxygen desaturation
Reymunde	2007	Stretta	83	48	No adverse effects
Noar	2007	Stretta	109	48	11 dyspepsia 27 chest discomfort 2 minor gastric bleeding
McClusky	2007	Stretta	7	2–12	No adverse effects
Arts	2007	Stretta	13	6	13 sore throat and mild epigastric pain 1 dysphagia

(*continued*)

Table 26.7 (*continued*)

Author	Year	Treatment	Patients (n)	Follow-up (months)	Reported adverse events
Pleskow	2007	Plicator	29	31–44	13 sore throat 12 abdominal pain 7 chest pain 6 transient dysphagia 2 intraprocedural dyspnea 1 gastric mucosal injury
Tierney	2007	EndoCinch	6		2 transient dysphagia 1 dysphagia and gas bloat syndrome requiring dilatation
Higuchi	2007	Stretta	9	6	9 mucosal erosions 9 retrosternal or epigastric discomfort 1 fever
Schwartz	2007	EndoCinch	20	3	8 sore throat 6 chest soreness 10 transient dysphagia 1 belching 1 abdominal pain 2 gas bloating syndrome
		Sham	20	3	9 sore throat 1 transient dysphagia 1 abdominal pain 1 sedation-related complication
Cadiere	2008	Observation	20	3	—
		EsophyX	17	12	15 gas bloating syndrome 6 diarrhea 3 dysphagia 17 epigastric pain 2 fever 1 hematemesis 7 left shoulder pain 8 nausea 11 pharyngeal irritation 1 vomiting
Cadiere	2008	EsophyX	86	12	2 esophageal perforation 1 bleeding 8 musculoskeletal pain 8 abdominal pain 6 pharyngolaryngeal pain 6 nausea 4 epigastric pain 5 application site bleeding 3 fever 3 dysphagia 2 diarrhea 2 vomiting
Pleskow	2008	Plicator	33	50–65	2 intraprocedural dyspnea 1 gastric mucosal injury 13 sore throat 12 abdominal pain 7 chest pain 6 transient dysphagia
Thomson	2008	EndoCinch	17	36	17 sore throat and minor epigastric pain 2 retrosternal chest pain 3 nausea and vomiting 1 bleeding in a patient with platelet disorder

Table 26.7 (*continued*)

Author	Year	Treatment	Patients (n)	Follow-up (months)	Reported adverse events
von Renteln	2008	Plicator	41	6	17 abdominal pain 6 pharyngeal pain 8 shoulder pain 7 chest pain 2 pneumoperitoneum
von Renteln	2008	Plicator	37	6	24 mild abdominal pain 3 moderate or severe abdominal pain 21 retrosternal pain 11 shoulder pain 20 sore throat 9 bloating 4 nausea or vomiting 1 fever 3 hospitalizations for severe abdominal or chest pain
Birk	2009	Plicator	81	12	10 pharyngolaryngeal pain 10 chest pain 8 upper abdominal pain 1 shoulder pain and abdominal discomfort
Cadiere	2009	EsophyX	17	24	1 dysphagia 7 gas bloating syndrome
von Renteln	2009	Plicator	41	12	18 post-procedure abdominal pain 10 shoulder pain 7 chest pain
Ganz	2009	Durasphere	10	12	7 pain related to injection 4 sore throat 2 gas bloat syndrome 2 nausea 1 chest pain 1 difficulty belching 1 increased belching
White	2009	Plicator	10	14	No adverse events
		Stretta	12	25	No adverse events
Aziz	2010	Stretta	12	12	7 mild post-procedure chest pain 1 mild fever 2 transient nausea/vomiting 1 transient dysphagia 1 abdominal pain 1 pneumonia 1 pleural effusion 1 mucosal injury
		Stretta	12	12	6 mild post-procedure chest pain 1 mild fever 1 transient nausea/vomiting 1 transient dysphagia 2 abdominal pain 1 mucosal lacerations 2 prolonged gastroparesis
		Sham	12	12	2 mild post-procedure chest pain 1 mild fever 1 abdominal pain

(continued)

Table 26.7 (continued)

Author	Year	Treatment	Patients (n)	Follow-up (months)	Reported adverse events
Demyttenaere	2010	EsophyX	26	10	2 chest pain, Unspecified number ("many") with sore throat and left shoulder pain, 2 bleeding
Testoni	2010	EsophyX	20	6	1 nausea and vomiting 20 mild to moderate epigastric pain 15 pharyngeal irritation 18 leukocytosis
von Renteln	2010	Plicator	12	6	No adverse events
Repici	2010	EsophyX	20	12	2 hematemesis

Fockens[1]	2010	Gatekeeper	124	6	4 serious adverse events for Gatekeeper treatment:
					  2 perforation, one with emergency thoracotomy
					  1 pulmonary infiltrate and pleural effusion
					  1 severe chest pain
					Because of cross-over and lead-in, minor adverse events were not exactly determined but included :
					  odynophagia, epigastric pain, sore throat, dysphagia, cough, chest pain, nausea/vomiting, erosions over prostheses, hemorrhage, oxygen desaturation, mouth injury

		Sham	26	6	No serious adverse events

[1]Through lead in (n = 25) and cross-over from sham treatment to gatekeeper treatment (n = 124) patients with implanted prosthesis. Initially 143 patients enrolled [25 lead in, 75 treatment, 43 sham, treatment safety data available for 124 patients, 6-month follow-up available for 51 treatment and 26 sham patients (24 patients crossed over from sham to treatment)].

Table 26.8 Retreatment options, reversibility of the procedure, and current availability on the market.

Device	Retreatment	Reversibility	Current availability
Enteryx	+	−	−
Gatekeeper	+	+	−
Durasphere	+	−	−
Plexiglas	+	−	−
Stretta	+	−	+
Endoscopic Suturing Device	+	+	−
EndoCinch	+	+	+
Plicator	+	+	−
EsophyX	+	+	+
SafeStitch	+	+	−*
TOGA	−	−	−*
Syntheon	+	+	−
Hiz-Wiz	+	+	−
Medigus	+	−	+**

*Preclinical studies.
**Available only within early clinical trials.

ences reported in abstract form offer only limited details [70, 71]. TOGA is in use within clinical trials for obesity treatment. TOGA suggested improvement in pH-metry and manometry data in a porcine study [72]. For Medigus, a porcine study demonstrated procedural safety and feasibility of the device to create an anterior fundoplication [73]. The Medigus device is currently under investigation in clinical trials. All these devices are conceptually based on the same principles as the devices discussed above. Safety and efficacy of these new endoscopic GERD treatments will have to be determined in well-designed long-term clinical trials.

Issues related to understanding the role for endoscopic therapies for gastroesophageal reflux disease

The goals of any GERD therapy are to control symptoms, heal the esophageal mucosa, and prevent GERD-related complications. Pharmacologic therapy is effective for symptom relief and mucosal healing, as well as long-term maintenance of remission [8, 74]. However, the need for daily administration, occasional failure to provide complete symptom relief, and possible side effects may limit its use in some patients who may be candidates for alternative treatment strategies. Laparoscopic antireflux surgery is an alternative to long-term medical therapy for GERD. More than 90% of patients experience symptom control and maintenance of remission. The laparoscopic approach has been demonstrated to reduce perioperative and postoperative morbidity compared to the open surgical approach [75]. Nevertheless, the procedure is associated with considerable costs, and requires hospitalization and a prolonged recovery period. Moreover, the efficacy of Nissen fundoplication seems to decrease over time, with up to 50% of patients requiring medication to control recurrent reflux symptoms 10 years following surgery. After surgery 5–8% of patients experience new symptoms, such as dysphagia, gas bloating, increased flatus, and difficulty belching or vomiting [76, 77].

The idea of minimally invasive treatment has stimulated the development of several endoscopic techniques for GERD. Most available data on endoluminal GERD therapies suggest that, in short-term follow-up, endoscopic interventions produce significant improvements in GERD-related quality of life, reduction of antireflux medication intake, and esophageal acid exposure. The vast majority of the available data are still limited to follow-up periods of less than 24 months and uncontrolled trials. Since GERD is a chronic condition with a high placebo response rate, long-term follow-up in controlled trials is necessary to judge treatment efficacy.

RF treatment (Stretta) appears to be safe and, although relatively effective in the long-term in cohort studies, it failed to reduce medication usage in patients who underwent the treatment compared to those who received a sham procedure. Most implantation techniques have been abandoned due to lack of efficacy and serious side effects (Gatekeeper, Enteryx). First-generation endoluminal suturing techniques (EndoCinch, ESD) demonstrated a proof of principle, but the implants lacked durability. Second-generation endoscopic plication devices (Plicator, EsophyX) were developed with the intention to place more robust, transmural sutures. A randomized controlled trial has shown endoscopic full-thickness plication, employing the NDO Plicator device, to be significantly better compared to sham treatment for control of GERD symptoms, use of antisecretory medication, and distal esophageal acid exposure. The randomized controlled trial was limited to a 6-month follow-up. Three- and 5-year durability of the pledgeted sutures and the treatment effect (sustained symptom relief) has been demonstrated in uncontrolled trials. The use of multiple Plicator implants, as opposed to a single implant in the initial trials, demonstrated significant improvements in reflux symptoms, esophagitis, medication use, and esophageal acid exposure. The EsophyX technique allows for placement of transmural implants. Published data are limited to uncontrolled trials, with clinical data up to 24 months demonstrating improvement in GERD

symptoms and medication use, but the results from a randomized sham-controlled trial are necessary before conclusions about treatment efficacy can be made.

Endoscopic antireflux therapy is still in evolution. For all of the methods and devices, there continue to be challenges related to overall safety, long-term efficacy, ease of use, and cost-effectiveness. At present, no endoscopic antireflux procedure is widely utilized in the clinical setting. Insurance and third-party payment for these techniques has been lacking, due to the categorization of these techniques as "investigational" by reimbursers. Efficacy has been less than desired, but early studies were designed for safety outcomes and not for optimizing the technique for best clinical outcomes. In addition, the available published results were typically an amalgamated "learning curve" experience. Most investigators had performed few procedures before enrolling individuals into studies and the results were those from learning curve procedures and not necessarily reflective of later experience. We lack "dose-ranging" studies for most of the devices and techniques. None of the studies did a repetitive application of the treatment until pH normalization was achieved. Following subjects who had their symptoms improved after pH normalization would reveal the natural history and durability of these endoscopic interventions. For some of the most promising techniques, long-term data from randomized controlled trials is still lacking.

As for many new endoscopic technologies, a minority of the total experience has been reported in peer-reviewed publications. Beyond the safety issues reported in the clinical experiences in the literature are the device-related safety problems in the post-marketing experiences, including deaths associated with some of the techniques. In most of the studies to date, the subjects have had mild GERD and may not reflect the best usage of this technology. There are few experiences with situations such as post-Nissen endoscopic treatment rescue or treatment of extraesophageal manifestations of GERD. There are limited data using newer physiologic evaluations, such as impedance or functional lumen imaging probe (FLIP) technologies. [68, 69] Well-designed controlled trials comparing endoscopic reflux therapies with medical and/or surgical treatments are necessary to better understand the role of endoscopic treatments in the care of patients with GERD. The few comparative studies to surgical treatment have favored surgical intervention for long-term benefit, but better design and additional studies are needed. The typical choice for our patients with GERD is long-term use of antisecretory medications or surgical intervention. Some patients continue with regurgitation of poorly controlled acid or non-acid refluxes, and some patients do not want surgical intervention even when it is considered minimally invasive.

For many individuals, there remains a substantial need for an endoscopic approach to GERD therapy. The initial entrants into this arena have made an attempt to demonstrate efficacy and safety, but the many limitations have created an unsupportive climate for the current clinical use of endoscopic GERD treatments. Further development in this innovative area, with well-designed, prospective, multicenter, randomized, controlled trials, including optimized efficacy as an endpoint, may one day yield an ideal device and treatment.

References

1. Tack J. Recent developments in the pathophysiology and therapy of gastroesophageal reflux disease and nonerosive reflux disease. *Curr Opin Gastroenterol* 2005;21:454–460.

2. Massey BT. Potential control of gastroesophageal reflux by local modulation of transient lower esophageal sphincter relaxations. *Am J Med* 2001;111 (Suppl 8A):186S–189S.

3. Hirsch DP, Mathus-Vliegen EM, Dagli U, Tytgat GN, Boeckxstaens GE. Effect of prolonged gastric distention on lower esophageal sphincter function and gastroesophageal reflux. *Am J Gastroenterol* 2003;98:1696–1704.

4. Ye W, Chow WH, Lagergren J, Yin L, Nyren O. Risk of adenocarcinomas of the esophagus and gastric cardia in patients with gastroesophageal reflux diseases and after antireflux surgery. *Gastroenterology* 2001;121:1286–1293.

5. Lagergren J, Bergstrom R, Lindgren A, Nyren O. Symptomatic gastroesophageal reflux as a risk factor for esophageal adenocarcinoma. *N Engl J Med* 1999;340:825–831.

6. El-Serag HB. Epidemiology of non-erosive reflux disease. *Digestion* 2008;78 (Suppl 1):6–10.

7. el-Serag HB, Sonnenberg A. Associations between different forms of gastro-oesophageal reflux disease. *Gut* 1997;41:594–599.

8. Khan M, Santana J, Donnellan C, Preston C, Moayyedi P. Medical treatments in the short term management of reflux oesophagitis. *Cochrane Database Syst Rev* 2007:CD003244.

9. Feretis C, Benakis P, Dimopoulos C, *et al*. Endoscopic implantation of Plexiglas (PMMA) microspheres for the treatment of GERD. *Gastrointest Endosc* 2001;53:423–426.

10. Filipi CJ, Lehman GA, Rothstein RI, *et al*. Transoral, flexible endoscopic suturing for treatment of GERD: a multicenter trial. *Gastrointest Endosc* 2001;53:416–422.

11. Richards WO, Scholz S, Khaitan L, Sharp KW, Holzman MD. Initial experience with the stretta procedure for the treatment of gastroesophageal reflux disease. *J Laparoendosc Adv Surg Tech A* 2001;11:267–273.

12. Triadafilopoulos G, Dibaise JK, Nostrant TT, *et al*. Radiofrequency energy delivery to the gastroesophageal junction for the treatment of GERD. *Gastrointest Endosc* 2001;53:407–415.

13. Deviere J, Pastorelli A, Louis H, *et al*. Endoscopic implantation of a biopolymer in the lower esophageal sphincter for gastroesophageal reflux: a pilot study. *Gastrointest Endosc* 2002;55:335–341.

14. DiBaise JK, Brand RE, Quigley EM. Endoluminal delivery of radiofrequency energy to the gastroesophageal junction in uncomplicated GERD: efficacy and potential mechanism of action. *Am J Gastroenterol* 2002;97:833–842

15. Triadafilopoulos G, DiBaise JK, Nostrant TT, *et al*. The Stretta procedure for the treatment of GERD: 6 and 12 month follow-up of the U.S. open label trial. *Gastrointest Endosc* 2002;55:149–156.

16. Wolfsen HC, Richards WO. The Stretta procedure for the treatment of GERD: a registry of 558 patients. *J Laparoendosc Adv Surg Tech A* 2002;12:395–402.

17. Chuttani R, Sud R, Sachdev G, *et al*. A novel endoscopic full-thickness plicator for the treatment of GERD: A pilot study. *Gastrointest Endosc* 2003;58:770–776.

18. Houston H, Khaitan L, Holzman M, Richards WO. First year experience of patients undergoing the Stretta procedure. *Surg Endosc* 2003;17:401–404.

19. Johnson DA, Ganz R, Aisenberg J, *et al*. Endoscopic implantation of enteryx for treatment of GERD: 12-month results of a prospective, multicenter trial. *Am J Gastroenterol* 2003;98:1921–1930.

20. Johnson DA, Ganz R, Aisenberg J, *et al*. Endoscopic, deep mural implantation of Enteryx for the treatment of GERD: 6-month follow-up of a multicenter trial. *Am J Gastroenterol* 2003;98:250–258.

21. Mahmood Z, McMahon BP, Arfin Q, *et al*. Endocinch therapy for gastro-oesophageal reflux disease: a one year prospective follow up. *Gut* 2003;52:34–39.

22. Fockens P, Bruno MJ, Gabbrielli A, *et al*. Endoscopic augmentation of the lower esophageal sphincter for the treatment of gastroesophageal reflux disease: multicenter study of the Gatekeeper Reflux Repair System. *Endoscopy* 2004;36:682–689.

23. Pleskow D, Rothstein R, Lo S, *et al*. Endoscopic full-thickness plication for the treatment of GERD: a multicenter trial. *Gastrointest Endosc* 2004;59:163–171.

24. Torquati A, Houston HL, Kaiser J, Holzman MD, Richards WO. Long-term follow-up study of the Stretta procedure for the treatment of gastroesophageal reflux disease. *Surg Endosc* 2004;18:1475–1479.

25. Abou-Rebyeh H, Hoepffner N, Rosch T, *et al*. Long-term failure of endoscopic suturing in the treatment of gastroesophageal reflux: a prospective follow-up study. *Endoscopy* 2005;37:213–216.

26. Arts J, Lerut T, Rutgeerts P, *et al*. A one-year follow-up study of endoluminal gastroplication (Endocinch) in GERD patients refractory to proton pump inhibitor therapy. *Dig Dis Sci* 2005;50:351–356.

27. Cicala M, Gabbrielli A, Emerenziani S, *et al*. Effect of endoscopic augmentation of the lower oesophageal sphincter (Gatekeeper reflux repair system) on intraoesophageal dynamic characteristics of acid reflux. *Gut* 2005;54:183–186.

28. Cipolletta L, Rotondano G, Dughera L, *et al*. Delivery of radiofrequency energy to the gastroesophageal junction (Stretta procedure) for the treatment of gastroesophageal reflux disease. *Surg Endosc* 2005;19:849–853.

29. Cohen LB, Johnson DA, Ganz RA, *et al*. Enteryx implantation for GERD: expanded multicenter trial results and interim postapproval follow-up to 24 months. *Gastrointest Endosc* 2005;61:650–658.

30. Liu DC, Somme S, Mavrelis PG, *et al*. Stretta as the initial antireflux procedure in children. *J Pediatr Surg* 2005;40:148–151; discussion 151–142.

31. Lutfi RE, Torquati A, Kaiser J, Holzman M, Richards WO. Three year's experience with the Stretta procedure: did it really make a difference? *Surg Endosc* 2005;19:289–295.

32. Pleskow D, Rothstein R, Lo S, et al. Endoscopic full-thickness plication for the treatment of GERD: 12-month follow-up for the North American open-label trial. *Gastrointest Endosc* 2005;61:643–649.

33. Schiefke I, Neumann S, Zabel-Langhennig A, Moessner J, Caca K. Use of an endoscopic suturing device (the "ESD") to treat patients with gastroesophageal reflux disease, after unsuccessful EndoCinch endoluminal gastroplication: another failure. *Endoscopy* 2005;37:700–705.

34. Schiefke I, Zabel-Langhennig A, Neumann S, et al. Long term failure of endoscopic gastroplication (EndoCinch). *Gut* 2005;54:752–758.

35. Schilling D, Kiesslich R, Galle PR, Riemann JF. Endoluminal therapy of GERD with a new endoscopic suturing device. *Gastrointest Endosc* 2005;62:37–43.

36. Schumacher B, Neuhaus H, Ortner M, et al. Reduced medication dependency and improved symptoms and quality of life 12 months after enteryx implantation for gastroesophageal reflux. *J Clin Gastroenterol* 2005;39:212–219.

37. Domagk D, Menzel J, Seidel M, et al. Endoluminal gastroplasty (EndoCinch) versus endoscopic polymer implantation (Enteryx) for treatment of gastroesophageal reflux disease: 6-month results of a prospective, randomized trial. *Am J Gastroenterol* 2006;101:422–430.

38. Mattar SG, Qureshi F, Taylor D, Schauer PR. Treatment of refractory gastroesophageal reflux disease with radiofrequency energy (Stretta) in patients after Roux-en-Y gastric bypass. *Surg Endosc* 2006;20:850–854.

39. Montgomery M, Hakanson B, Ljungqvist O, Ahlman B, Thorell A. Twelve months' follow-up after treatment with the EndoCinch endoscopic technique for gastro-oesophageal reflux disease: a randomized, placebo-controlled study. *Scand J Gastroenterol* 2006;41:1382–1389.

40. Rothstein R, Filipi C, Caca K, et al. Endoscopic full-thickness plication for the treatment of gastroesophageal reflux disease: A randomized, sham-controlled trial. *Gastroenterology* 2006;131:704–712.

41. Arts J, Sifrim D, Rutgeerts P, et al. Influence of radiofrequency energy delivery at the gastroesophageal junction (the Stretta procedure) on symptoms, acid exposure, and esophageal sensitivity to acid perfusion in gastroesophagal reflux disease. *Dig Dis Sci* 2007;52:2170–2177.

42. Conchillo JM, Schwartz MP, Selimah M, et al. Role of intra-oesophageal impedance monitoring in the evaluation of endoscopic gastroplication for gastro-oesophageal reflux disease. *Aliment Pharmacol Ther* 2007;26:61–68.

43. Higuchi K, Fujiwara Y, Okazaki H, et al. Feasibility, safety, and efficacy of the Stretta procedure in Japanese patients with gastroesophageal reflux disease: first report from Asia. *J Gastroenterol* 2007;42:205–210.

44. McClusky DA, 3rd, Khaitan L, Swafford VA, Smith CD. Radiofrequency energy delivery to the lower esophageal sphincter (Stretta procedure) in patients with recurrent reflux after antireflux surgery: can surgery be avoided? *Surg Endosc* 2007;21:1207–1211.

45. Meier PN, Nietzschmann T, Akin I, Klose S, Manns MP. Improvement of objective GERD parameters after radiofrequency energy delivery: a European study. *Scand J Gastroenterol* 2007;42:911–916.

46. Noar MD, Lotfi-Emran S. Sustained improvement in symptoms of GERD and antisecretory drug use: 4-year follow-up of the Stretta procedure. *Gastrointest Endosc* 2007;65:367–372.

47. Pleskow D, Rothstein R, Kozarek R, et al. Endoscopic full-thickness plication for the treatment of GERD: long-term multicenter results. *Surg Endosc* 2007;21:439–444.

48. Reymunde A, Santiago N. Long-term results of radiofrequency energy delivery for the treatment of GERD: sustained improvements in symptoms, quality of life, and drug use at 4-year follow-up. *Gastrointest Endosc* 2007;65:361–366.

49. Schwartz MP, Wellink H, Gooszen HG, et al. Endoscopic gastroplication for the treatment of gastro-oesophageal reflux disease: a randomised, sham-controlled trial. *Gut* 2007;56:20–28.

50. Tierney B, Iqbal A, Haider M, Filipi C. Effects of prior endoluminal gastroplication on subsequent laparoscopic Nissen fundoplication. *Surg Endosc* 2007;21:321–323.

51. Cadiere GB, Buset M, Muls V, et al. Antireflux transoral incisionless fundoplication using EsophyX: 12-month results of a prospective multicenter study. *World J Surg* 2008;32:1676–1688.

52. Cadiere GB, Rajan A, Germay O, Himpens J. Endoluminal fundoplication by a transoral device for the treatment of GERD: A feasibility study. *Surg Endosc* 2008;22:333–342.

53. Dundon JM, Davis SS, Hazey JW, et al. Radiofrequency energy delivery to the lower esophageal sphincter (Stretta procedure) does not provide long-term symptom control. *Surg Innov* 2008;15:297–301.

54. Pleskow D, Rothstein R, Kozarek R, et al. Endoscopic full-thickness plication for the treatment of GERD: Five-year long-term multicenter results. *Surg Endosc* 2008;22:326–332.

55. Thomson M, Antao B, Hall S, et al. Medium-term outcome of endoluminal gastroplication with the EndoCinch device in children. *J Pediatr Gastroenterol Nutr* 2008;46:172–177.

56. von Renteln D, Brey U, Riecken B, Caca K. Endoscopic full-thickness plication (Plicator) with two serially placed implants improves esophagitis and reduces PPI use and esophageal acid exposure. *Endoscopy* 2008;40:173–178.

57. von Renteln D, Schiefke I, Fuchs KH, et al. Endoscopic full-thickness plication for the treatment of GERD by application of multiple Plicator implants: a multicenter study (with video). *Gastrointest Endosc* 2008;68:833–844.

58. Birk J, Pruitt R, Haber G, et al. The Plicator procedure for the treatment of gastroesophageal reflux disease: a registry study. *Surg Endosc* 2009;23:423–431.

59. Cadiere GB, Van Sante N, Graves JE, Gawlicka AK, Rajan A. Two-year results of a feasibility study on antireflux transoral incisionless fundoplication using EsophyX. *Surg Endosc* 2009;23:957–964.

60. Ganz RA, Fallon E, Wittchow T, Klein D. A new injectable agent for the treatment of GERD: results of the Durasphere pilot trial. *Gastrointest Endosc* 2009;69:318–323.

61. Jeansonne LOt, White BC, Nguyen V, et al. Endoluminal full-thickness plication and radiofrequency treatments for GERD: an outcomes comparison. *Arch Surg* 2009;144:19–24; discussion 24.

62. von Renteln D, Schiefke I, Fuchs KH, *et al.* Endoscopic full-thickness plication for the treatment of gastroesophageal reflux disease using multiple Plicator implants: 12-month multicenter study results. *Surg Endosc* 2009;23:1866–1875.

63. White B, Jeansonne LO, Cook M, *et al.* Use of endoluminal antireflux therapies for obese patients with GERD. *Obes Surg* 2009;19:783–787.

64. Aziz AM, El-Khayat HR, Sadek A, *et al.* A prospective randomized trial of sham, single-dose Stretta, and double-dose Stretta for the treatment of gastroesophageal reflux disease. *Surg Endosc* 2010;24:818–825.

65. Demyttenaere SV, Bergman S, Pham T, *et al.* Transoral incisionless fundoplication for gastroesophageal reflux disease in an unselected patient population. *Surg Endosc* 2010;24:854–858.

66. Fockens P, Cohen L, Edmundowicz SA, *et al.* Prospective randomized controlled trial of an injectable esophageal prosthesis versus a sham procedure for endoscopic treatment of gastroesophageal reflux disease. *Surg Endosc* 2010;24:1387–1397.

67. Repici A, Fumagalli U, Malesci A, *et al.* Endoluminal fundoplication (ELF) for GERD using EsophyX: a 12-month follow-up in a single-center experience. *J Gastrointest Surg* 2010;14:1–6.

68. Testoni PA, Corsetti M, Di Pietro S, *et al.* Effect of transoral incisionless fundoplication on symptoms, PPI use, and pH-impedance refluxes of GERD patients. *World J Surg* 2010;34:750–757.

69. von Renteln D, Schmidt A, Riecken B, Caca K. Evaluating outcomes of endoscopic full-thickness plication for gastroesophageal reflux disease (GERD) with impedance monitoring. *Surg Endosc* 2010;24:1040–1048.

70. Filipi CJ, Stadlhuber RJ. Initial experience with new intraluminal devices for GERD, Barrett's esophagus, and obesity. *J Gastrointest Surg* 2010;14 (Suppl 1):S121–126.

71. Ramage JI, Rothstein RI, Edmundowicz SA, *et al.* Endoscopically placed titanium plicator for GERD: Pivotal phase—preliminary 6-month results. *Gastrointest Endoscopy* 2006;63:AB126–AB126.

72. Sporn E, Miedema BW, Astudillo JA, *et al.* Evaluation of a novel endoluminal stapling procedure to restrict the lower esophageal sphincter and reduce reflux. *Endoscopy* 2008;40:752–758.

73. Kauer WK, Roy-Shapira A, Watson D, *et al.* Preclinical trial of a modified gastroscope that performs a true anterior fundoplication for the endoluminal treatment of gastroesophageal reflux disease. *Surg Endosc* 2009 Apr 9 [Epub ahead of print].

74. Vakil N, van Zanten SV, Kahrilas P, Dent J, Jones R. The Montreal definition and classification of gastroesophageal reflux disease: a global evidence-based consensus. *Am J Gastroenterol* 2006;101:1900–1920; quiz 1943.

75. Lundell L, Miettinen P, Myrvold HE, *et al.* Continued (5-year) followup of a randomized clinical study comparing antireflux surgery and omeprazole in gastroesophageal reflux disease. *J Am Coll Surg* 2001;192:172–179; discussion 179–181.

76. Peters JH, DeMeester TR, Crookes P, *et al.* The treatment of gastroesophageal reflux disease with laparoscopic Nissen fundoplication: prospective evaluation of 100 patients with "typical" symptoms. *Ann Surg* 1998;228:40–50.

77. Spechler SJ, Lee E, Ahnen D, *et al.* Long-term outcome of medical and surgical therapies for gastroesophageal reflux disease: follow-up of a randomized controlled trial. *JAMA* 2001;285:2331–2338.

27 Barrett's Esophagus

Gary W. Falk

Division of Gastroenterology, Hospital of the University of Pennsylvania, Philadelphia, PA, USA

Introduction

Barrett's esophagus is an acquired condition resulting from severe esophageal mucosal injury. It is unclear why some patients with gastroesophageal reflux disease (GERD) develop Barrett's esophagus whereas others do not. The diagnosis of Barrett's esophagus is established if the squamocolumnar junction (SCJ) is displaced proximal to the gastroesophageal junction (GEJ) and intestinal metaplasia is detected by biopsy, although controversy now exists regarding the need for intestinal metaplasia for the diagnosis. Diagnostic inconsistencies are a problem in Barrett's esophagus, especially in distinguishing short-segment Barrett's esophagus from intestinal metaplasia of the gastric cardia. Barrett's esophagus would be of little importance if not for its well-recognized association with adenocarcinoma of the esophagus. The incidence of esophageal adenocarcinoma continues to increase and the 5-year survival rate for this cancer remains dismal. However, the overall disease burden of esophageal cancer remains low and cancer risk for a given patient with Barrett's esophagus is also low. Current strategies for improved survival in patients with esophageal adenocarcinoma focus on cancer detection at an early and potentially curable stage. This can be accomplished either by screening more patients for Barrett's esophagus or with endoscopic surveillance of patients with known Barrett's esophagus. However, current screening and surveillance strategies are inherently expensive, inefficient, and of unproven benefit. New techniques to improve the efficiency of cancer surveillance continue to evolve and hold the promise to change clinical practice in the future. Treatment options include aggressive acid suppression, antireflux surgery, chemoprevention and ablation therapy, but there is still no clear consensus on the optimal treatment for these patients. This chapter will review our current understanding of this disorder.

Definition

Barrett's esophagus is defined as a metaplastic change in the lining of the tubular esophagus. Endoscopically, this is characterized by displacement of the SCJ proximal to the GEJ defined by the proximal margin of gastric folds. If the SCJ is above the level of the GEJ, biopsies should be obtained for confirmation of columnar metaplasia. There is ongoing debate regarding the presence of intestinal metaplasia for the diagnosis of Barrett's esophagus (see below) [1]. The professional societies of North America all require intestinal metaplasia for the diagnosis of Barrett's esophagus, whereas the British Society of Gastroenterology and a global consensus group do not [2–6].

Epidemiology

The incidence of Barrett's esophagus has increased markedly since the 1970s. This increase was once felt to be due the increased use of diagnostic upper endoscopy combined with the change in the definition of Barrett's esophagus to include shorter segments of columnar-lined epithelium [7]. However, data from the Netherlands suggest that the incidence of Barrett's esophagus has increased from 14.3 in 100 000 person years in 1997 to 23.1 in 100 000 person years in 2002 in the general population independent of the number of upper endoscopies (Figure 27.1) [8].

It is estimated that Barrett's esophagus is found in approximately 5–15% of patients undergoing endoscopy for symptoms of GERD [9]. A study of a high-risk patient population (chronic GERD, Caucasian, age >50 years) undergoing endoscopy for symptoms of GERD found Barrett's esophagus in 13.2% [9]. The prevalence of long-segment Barrett's esophagus (≥3 cm of intestinal metaplasia) is approximately 5%, whereas that of short-segment Barrett's esophagus

The Esophagus, Fifth Edition. Edited by Joel E. Richter, Donald O. Castell.
© 2012 Blackwell Publishing Ltd. Published 2012 by Blackwell Publishing Ltd.

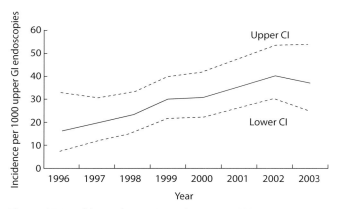

Figure 27.1 Incidence of Barrett's esophagus per 1000 upper gastrointestinal endoscopies over calendar time, with upper and lower confidence intervals (CI) in the Netherlands (reproduced from van Soest *et al.* [8], with permission).

(<3 cm of intestinal metaplasia) is approximately 6–12% in patients undergoing endoscopy in a variety of settings [10–12]. Population-based studies suggest that the prevalence of Barrett's esophagus is approximately 1.3–1.6% [13, 14]. Of note, most of these patients found in the general population have short segments of Barrett's esophagus and approximately 45% have no reflux symptoms.

Barrett's esophagus is predominantly a disease of middle-aged white males [15, 16]. However, it should be kept in mind that approximately 25% of Barrett's esophagus patients are women or younger than 50 years of age [17, 18]. The prevalence of Barrett's esophagus increases until a plateau is reached between the seventh and ninth decades [15, 19]. A variety of risk factors have been identified for the presence of Barrett's esophagus, including frequent and long-standing reflux episodes, smoking, male gender, older age, and central obesity [20–24]. Body mass index itself does not appear to be a risk factor for Barrett's esophagus, but rather the central obesity characteristic of male-pattern obesity [22, 23].

Pathophysiology

Barrett's esophagus is an acquired condition resulting from severe esophageal mucosal injury. However, it remains unclear why some patients with GERD develop Barrett's esophagus whereas others do not. Animal studies suggest that the development of Barrett's esophagus requires injury to the esophageal mucosa accompanied by an abnormal environment of epithelial repair [25]. Epidemiologic data suggest that once injury occurs, Barrett's esophagus develops to its full extent fairly rapidly with little subsequent change in length [15].

Barrett's esophagus is clearly associated with severe gastroesophageal reflux. Compared to patients with erosive and non-erosive GERD without Barrett's esophagus, patients with Barrett's esophagus typically have greater esophageal

acid exposure based on 24-h pH monitoring [26, 27]. Part of the increase in acid exposure in Barrett's patients may be related to the almost uniform presence of a hiatal hernia, which is typically longer and associated with larger defects in the hiatus than in controls or patients with esophagitis alone [28, 29]. In addition, patients with Barrett's esophagus have a lower basal lower esophageal sphincter (LES) pressure compared to GERD patients without Barrett's esophagus [27]. Reflux of duodenal contents is also increased in Barrett's esophagus patients compared to GERD patients without Barrett's esophagus [30]. Patients with short-segment Barrett's esophagus tend to have pathophysiologic abnormalities intermediate to those of long-segment Barrett's patients and normal controls [31, 32]. Esophageal pH monitoring studies suggest a correlation between the length of Barrett's mucosa and the duration of esophageal acid exposure [32]. Barrett's esophagus is also clearly associated with a distinct cytokine profile when compared to patients with reflux esophagitis, suggesting the possibility of different inflammatory responses to reflux disease as well [33].

Barrett's esophagus is characterized by columnar metaplasia, a process by which one adult cell type replaces another. This is thought to be a protective response to chronic inflammation as the metaplastic tissue is more resistant than the normal squamous lining of the esophagus to the noxious effects of refluxed acid and bile. The mechanism whereby injury triggers metaplasia and why this occurs in some but not all individuals remain unknown. Furthermore, the cell of origin of the columnar metaplasia remains unclear. One candidate pathway is the dedifferentiation of the normal squamous epithelium into columnar epithelium. The other candidate pathway is via stimulation of stem cells originating from either the basal layer of the esophageal epithelium or the ducts of the esophageal submucosal glands [34, 35]. Recent provocative animal studies suggest that multipotential stem cells originating from the bone marrow may be another potential source of columnar metaplasia in the esophagus [36].

The intestine-specific transcription factors CDX1 and CDX2, which promote the columnar cell differentiation pathway in intestinal epithelial cells, are ectopically expressed in Barrett's esophagus and are presently believed to be essential for the intestinal phenotype in Barrett's epithelium [37]. Moreover, both CDX1 and CDX2 can be induced in esophageal squamous cell lines by pulses of both acid and bile salts [38]. Another intestine-associated transcription factor potentially contributing to the intestinal metaplasia pathway is bone morphogenetic protein 4 (BMP-4), which is increased in inflamed esophageal tissue, Barrett's esophagus, and its underlying stroma [39]. Treatment of squamous esophageal cell lines with BMP-4 changes the cytokeratin expression profile from one characteristic of a squamous phenotype to a columnar phenotype. Putting these observations together, it appears that gastroduodenal refluxate first damages the

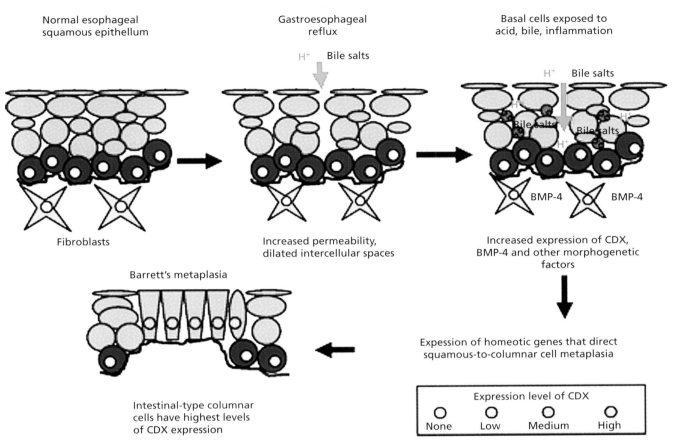

Figure 27.2 Schematic of how gastroesophageal reflux may lead to Barrett's esophagus. Refluxate damages the tight junction between squamous cells, which increases permeability. This exposes undifferentiated stem cells to acid, bile salts, and inflammatory mediators. This then causes these cells to express CDX and BMP-4, resulting in a squamous to columnar metaplasia (reproduced from Souza *et al.* [38], with permission).

superficial layer of the esophagus, thereby exposing stem cells in the basal layer and the submucosal ducts to the noxious effects of the refluxate, as well as the inflammatory response it engenders. This results in the expression of *Cdx* genes in the stem cells, perhaps activated by BMP4, which induces the progeny of those stem cells to differentiate along an intestinal rather than a squamous lineage [40]. A current conceptual model of the pathogenesis of Barrett's esophagus is shown in Figure 27.2 [38].

Clinical presentation

Patients with Barrett's esophagus are difficult to distinguish clinically from patients with GERD uncomplicated by a columnar-lined esophagus. However, some observational studies suggest that features such as the development of reflux symptoms at an earlier age, increased duration of reflux symptoms, increased severity of nocturnal reflux symptoms, and increased complications of GERD (e.g. esophagitis, ulceration, stricture, and bleeding) may distin-

guish Barrett's esophagus patients from GERD patients without Barrett's esophagus [21]. Interestingly, similar clinical risk factors have been identified for esophageal adenocarcinoma [41]. Identification of Barrett's esophagus patients may be hampered by the paradox that Barrett's esophagus patients have an impaired sensitivity to esophageal acid perfusion compared to patients with uncomplicated GERD [42]. However, many Barrett's esophagus patients are elderly, and this observation may be related to an age-related decrease in acid sensitivity [43]. A subset of Barrett's esophagus patients may have an inherited predisposition, as studies have reported on families with multiple affected relatives over successive generations [44–46]. These reports suggest an autosomal dominant pattern of inheritance in selected individuals with Barrett's esophagus.

Diagnosis

The diagnosis of Barrett's esophagus has clear implications for such individuals. Patients are subject to surveillance

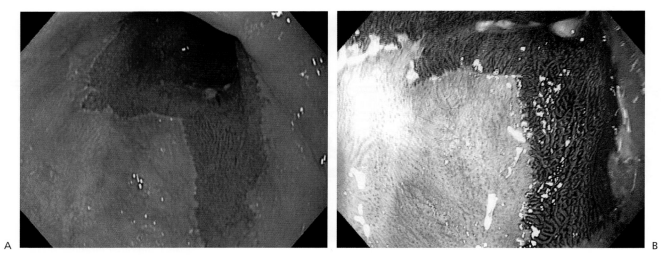

Figure 27.3 Endoscopic appearance of Barrett's esophagus with (A) high-definition white light and (B) narrow-band imaging.

endoscopy at regular intervals, worry about cancer risk, which they typically overestimate, face higher life insurance premiums, and are provided with conflicting information on how best to treat their condition [47, 48]. As such, it is essential to diagnose Barrett's esophagus as accurately as possible given the downstream effects of such a diagnosis.

Barrett's esophagus is defined as a metaplastic change in the lining of the tubular esophagus. Endoscopically, this is characterized by displacement of the SCJ proximal to the GEJ defined by the proximal margin of gastric folds (Figure 27.3). At the time of endoscopy, landmarks should be carefully identified, including the diaphragmatic pinch, the GEJ as best defined by the proximal margin of the gastric folds seen on partial insufflation of the esophagus, and level of the SCJ. It is commonly accepted that the proximal margin of the gastric folds is the most useful landmark for the junction of the stomach and the esophagus [49]. However, the precise junction of the stomach and the esophagus may be difficult to determine endoscopically due to the presence of a hiatal hernia, inflammation, and the dynamic nature of the GEJ, all of which may make targeting of biopsies problematic. Therefore, not surprisingly, endoscopists identify landmarks necessary for the diagnosis of the columnar-lined esophagus inconsistently [50]. The new Prague classification scheme should help improve our description of the columnar-lined esophagus [51]. This classification scheme describes the circumferential extent (C value) and maximum extent (M value) of columnar mucosa above the proximal margin of the gastric folds (Figure 27.4). The Prague classification does not include columnar islands. Reliability coefficients for both criteria are excellent for segments longer than 1 cm in length. However, recognition of columnar metaplasia shorter than 1 cm, even with this scoring system, is still problematic, pointing out the difficulties in measuring such short segments.

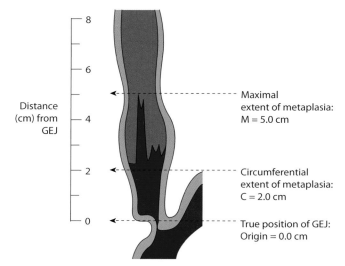

Figure 27.4 Schematic representation of the Prague classification for Barrett's esophagus classified as a C2M4. Note that C is the circumferential extent of metaplasia which extends up to 2 cm, whereas M is the maximal extent of metaplasia, which extends up to 4 cm from the gastroesophageal junction (GEJ) (reproduced from Sharma et al. [51], with permission).

If the SCJ is above the level of the GEJ, as defined by the proximal margin of the gastric folds, biopsies should be obtained for confirmation of columnar metaplasia. Biopsies of the SCJ, if appropriately located at the level of the GEJ, should not be routinely obtained in clinical practice. There is ongoing debate regarding the presence of intestinal metaplasia for the diagnosis of Barrett's esophagus. Recent evidence suggests that the non-goblet columnar metaplasia demonstrates DNA content abnormalities indicative of neoplastic risk similar to those encountered in intestinal metaplasia [52]. Additional supportive evidence for this concept comes from several pieces of evidence. The risk of developing esophageal adenocarcinoma is similar among patients with and without intestinal metaplasia [53]. Furthermore, more than 70% of early adenocarcinomas detected by endoscopic mucosal resection (EMR) have cardia and fundic-type mucosa adjacent to the cancer instead of intestinal metaplasia [54]. Currently, the issue of intestinal metaplasia versus columnar metaplasia as a diagnostic criterion remains unsettled.

There is also no agreement on the appropriate number of biopsies to obtain in order to detect intestinal metaplasia. Detection of intestinal metaplasia appears to be related to a number of factors, including location of biopsies, length of columnar-lined segment, number of biopsies obtained, male gender, and increasing age [55–57]. It would appear that if sufficient biopsies are obtained over time, intestinal metaplasia is eventually detected in the majority of patients. Intestinal metaplasia is more commonly found in biopsies obtained in the proximal portion of the columnar-lined esophagus where goblet cell density is also greater [58]. Detection of intestinal metaplasia increases with increasing number of biopsies per endoscopy: four biopsies had a yield of 34.7% whereas eight biopsies had a yield of 94% for intestinal metaplasia (Figure 27.5) [59]. Taking more than eight biopsies does not seem to enhance the yield of intestinal metaplasia.

Endoscopically it may be difficult to determine where the esophagus ends and the stomach begins for the reasons outlined above. Furthermore, it is not possible to reliably distinguish columnar metaplasia of the distal esophagus from that of the stomach. As such, it is recommended that a normal GEJ is not biopsied. Intestinal metaplasia may be seen in the cardia of normal individuals as well as in those with chronic reflux disease. The prevalence of intestinal metaplasia at a normal-appearing GEJ varies from 5% to 36% [60]. Unlike Barrett's esophagus, there is no clear gender predominance in patients with intestinal metaplasia of the GEJ and cardia, as this condition is more common in older patients who are often infected with *Helicobacter pylori* and have evidence of gastritis and/or intestinal metaplasia elsewhere in the stomach [12, 61]. However, a subset of these patients may have GERD and it is unclear if this condition is a sequella of aging, *H. pylori* infection, GERD or some combination of these factors.

Short-segment Barrett's esophagus is clearly associated with some risk of developing dysplasia and esophageal cancer, and this risk is not substantially lower than that in patients with long-segment Barrett's esophagus. Dysplasia and carcinoma have been reported in patients with intestinal metaplasia of the GEJ or cardia, but the magnitude of that risk appears to be less than that of short-segment Barrett's esophagus [62]. A reliable biomarker to distinguish between intestinal metaplasia of the cardia versus intestinal metaplasia of the esophagus would be beneficial. Techniques such as the Das-1 antibody and cytokeratin immunohistochemical staining patterns do not reliably distinguish between these two entities [63]. Some features, such as mucosal and submucosal esophageal glands, squamous epithelium overlying columnar crypts with intestinal metaplasia, and hybrid glands characterized by intestinal metaplasia confined to the superficial aspect of cardia-type mucus glands, are more often associated with the columnar-lined esophagus than intestinal metaplasia of the cardia [64]. As such, precise targeting of biopsies above the proximal margin of the gastric folds and communication of this information to pathologists is critical.

Pathology

The columnar-lined esophagus is characterized by a mosaic of three different types of columnar epithelium above the LES zone: fundic-type epithelium characterized by parietal and chief cells similar to the native gastric fundus (Figure 27.6); cardiac-type mucosa characterized by mucous glands and no parietal cells (Figure 27.7); and specialized columnar epithelium characterized by a villiform surface and Alcian-blue staining intestinal-type goblet cells (Figure 27.8) [65]. Currently, the diagnosis of Barrett's esophagus is established if the SCJ is displaced proximal to the GEJ and intestinal metaplasia, characterized by acid mucin-containing goblet cells detected by biopsy. However, the requirement of intestinal metaplasia for the diagnosis of Barrett's esophagus has

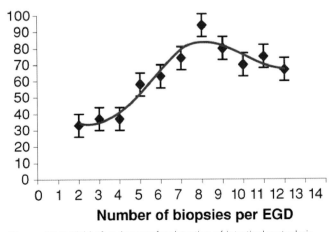

Figure 27.5 Yield of endoscopy for detection of intestinal metaplasia (IM) compared to the number of biopsies per endoscopy. The optimal number of biopsies to detect intestinal metaplasia is a minimum of eight. EGD, esophagogastroduodenoscopy (reproduced from Harrison *et al.* [59], with permission).

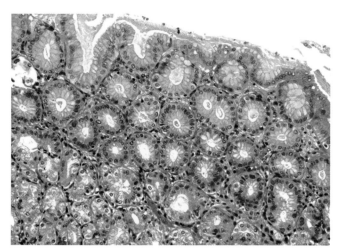

Figure 27.6 Fundic-type columnar cells. This biopsy from a columnar-lined esophagus reveals non-goblet cell-containing columnar epithelium with glands harboring pariental cells. These glands closely resemble those seen in the normal gastric fundus (20X) (reproduced courtesy of John Goldblum MD).

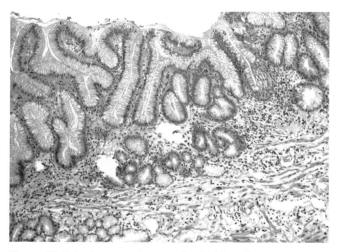

Figure 27.7 Cardiac-type columnar cells. This biopsy from a columnar-lined esophagus reveals non-goblet cell-containing columnar epithelium with mucin-containing glands that closely resemble those seen in the normal gastric cardia (10x) (reproduced courtesy of John Goldblum MD).

recently come under question as described above. In most cases, goblet cells are easily identified on routine hematoxylin and eosin preparations, and special stains such as Alcian blue/periodic acid-Schiff (PAS) are not necessary. Alcian blue/PAS stain can help avoid overinterpretation of pseudogoblet cells characterized by distended surface foveolar-type cells that stain for PAS but do not contain Alcian blue-positive acid mucins [66].

It is well recognized that pathologic interpretation of Barrett's esophagus specimens is problematic in the community as well as in academic centers. In a community study, only 35% of intestinal metaplasia were recognized

correctly and gastric metaplasia without intestinal metaplasia was identified as Barrett's esophagus in 38% of the cases [67]. Pathologic interpretation is also problematic for expert gastrointestinal pathologists, where interobserver reproducibility is substantial at the ends of the spectrum of Barrett's esophagus, namely negative for dysplasia and high-grade dysplasia/carcinoma, but not especially good for low-grade dysplasia or indefinite for dysplasia [68]. There are also problems with interobserver agreement among pathologists in distinguishing high-grade dysplasia from intramucosal cancer, even when evaluating esophagectomy specimens [69, 70]. Factors that contribute to some of the problems in pathologic interpretation include experience of the pathologist, quality of the slides, and size of the specimens [71]. In an effort to improve pathologic interpretation, current practice guidelines now recommend EMR of any nodularity in the Barrett's segment prior to making final treatment decisions [72, 73]. Recent data support just such an approach. Mino-Kenudson *et al.* found that the interobserver agreement for Barrett's esophagus-associated neoplasia on EMR specimens was higher than that for mucosal biopsies, especially in distinguishing intramucosal cancer from submucosal cancer [71].

Barrett's esophagus and esophageal adenocarcinoma

Barrett's esophagus is a clearly recognized risk factor for the development of esophageal adenocarcinoma compared to the general population [74]. Studies now show that the incidence of this cancer has increased by approximately six fold between 1975 and 2001, a rate greater than that of any other cancer in the United States during that time [75]. This increase has been accompanied by an increase in mortality rates from 2 to 15 deaths per million during that same time period [75]. Similar findings are occurring elsewhere in the Western world today. However, the overall burden of esophageal adenocarcinoma remains relatively low. It is estimated that there were 16 470 new cases of esophageal cancer (not all of which were adenocarcinoma) in the United States in 2009 [76].

Despite the alarming increase in the incidence of esophageal adenocarcinoma, the precise incidence of adenocarcinoma in patients with Barrett's esophagus is uncertain, with rates varying from approximately 1 in 52 to 1 in 694 years of follow-up [77]. However, the cancer risk for a given patient with non-dysplastic Barrett's esophagus is quite low. The most recent meta-analysis of cancer risk in Barrett's esophagus patient produced a pooled estimate of 0.6%/year [78]. The rate of progression to the combined endpoint of high-grade dysplasia or adenocarcinoma was 1%/year. The pooled incidence of fatal esophageal adenocarcinoma was 3%/year. Most importantly, this study again confirmed that

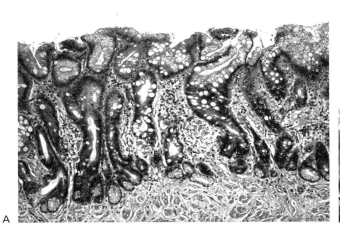

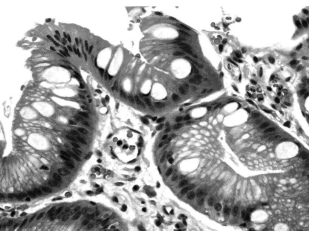

Figure 27.8 (A) Histologic appearance of specialized columnar epithelium. Goblet cells are characterized by a villiform appearance and distended barrel-shaped cytoplasm filled with acid mucins, resulting in a blue–gray tinge to the goblet cell cytoplasm, as seen on this hematoxylin and eosin stained section (10x) (reproduced courtesy of John Goldblum MD). (B) Histologic appearance of specialized columnar epithelium on high power. The goblet cells present in this biopsy from the Barrett's segment stand out from the surrounding non-goblet cell mucin-containing columnar cells (40x) (reproduced courtesy of John Goldblum MD).

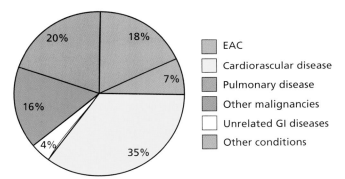

Figure 27.9 Causes of death in patients with Barrett's esophagus. EAC, esophageal adenocarcinoma (reproduced from Sikkema *et al.* [78], with permission).

adenocarcinoma was an uncommon cause of death in Barrett's esophagus patients: only 7% of deaths were due to adenocarcinoma, whereas 93% of the deaths were due to other causes, the most common being cardiovascular disease, which accounted for 35% of the deaths (Figure 27.9). Furthermore, the survival of patients with Barrett's esophagus is similar to that of the general population [79].

The reason for this increase in the incidence of esophageal adenocarcinoma is unknown. Barrett's esophagus is clearly a risk factor for adenocarcinoma of the esophagus. A variety of epidemiologic factors have been identified that either increase or decrease the risk for the development of esophageal adenocarcinoma. Among the well-accepted risk factors are increasing age, male gender, Caucasian ethnicity, obesity, especially male pattern central obesity, and smoking [80–83]. Protective factors include aspirin and non-steroidal anti-inflammatory drug (NSAID) ingestion, and a diet high in fruits and vegetables [84–86]. Factors of uncertain significance include family history, infection with *H. pylori*, alcohol consumption, antireflux therapy be it surgical or pharmacologic, and dietary supplements [83, 87].

Cancer biology

Compelling evidence exists for a dysplasia–carcinoma sequence in Barrett's esophagus whereby non-dysplastic columnar epithelium progresses to low-grade dysplasia, high-grade dysplasia, and finally carcinoma. Foci of carcinoma typically appear adjacent to dysplasia [88]. The time course for this progression is highly variable, and most patients never progress to dysplasia.

It is hypothesized that cancer develops in a subset of patients who have acquired genomic instability in Barrett's epithelium (Figure 27.10) [89]. This predisposes to the development of abnormal clones of cells that then accumulate progressively more genetic errors, which include numerical and structural chromosomal rearrangements, gene mutations, loss of normal cell cycle control, and increased cell proliferation rates [90, 91]. Among the most frequently described molecular changes that precede the development of adenocarcinoma in Barrett's esophagus are alterations in p53 [mutation, deletion or loss of heterozygosity (LOH)], and p16 (mutation, deletion, promoter hypermethylation, or LOH) [92–95]. However, there is no clearly predictable sequence of genetic abnormalities that leads to the development of cancer. Many of the genetic changes seen in esophageal adenocarcinoma do not directly contribute to carcinogenesis, but instead are "hitchhiker" mutations that are linked to other oncogenic mutations [96]. Upregulation of cyclo-oxygenase-2 (COX-2) expression also

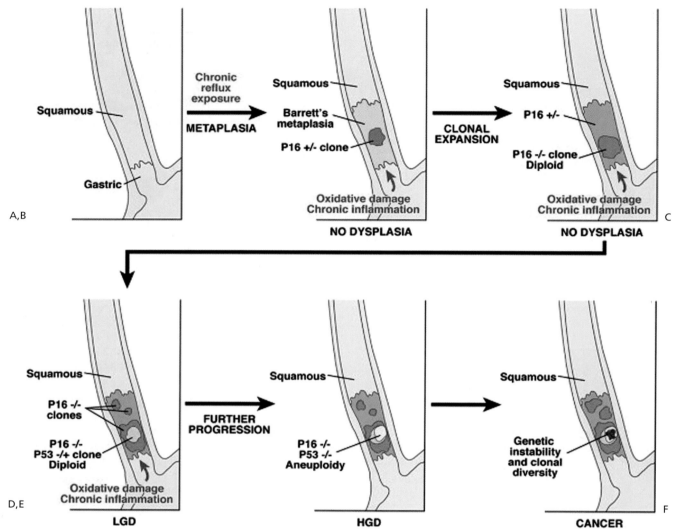

Figure 27.10 Schematic illustration of changes leading to adenocarcinoma in Barrett's esophagus. (A) Normal esophagus undergoes metaplastic change due to chronic exposure to refluxate. (B) Metaplastic change is followed by the loss of one p16 allele and this clone may expand (pink). (C) Loss of the second p16 allele results in an area that is p16 null. (D) Subsequent loss of p53 occurs within the p16 null clone. (E) Genetic instability develops leading to aneuploidy. (F) Numerous abnormal clones of cells develop, allowing for the development of adenocarcinoma. LGD, low-grade dysplasia; HGD, high-grade dysplasia (reproduced from Spechler *et al.* [40], with permission).

occurs in the metaplasia–dysplasia–carcinoma sequence [97, 98]. Increased COX-2 expression is associated with increased cellular proliferation and decreased apoptosis *in vitro*, and administration of selective COX-2 inhibitors can decrease cell growth and increase apoptosis in esophageal adenocarcinoma cell lines [99]. This finding may have implications for chemoprevention strategies currently under study.

Screening and surveillance strategies for Barrett's esophagus

Esophageal adenocarcinoma is a lethal disease with a 5-year survival of approximately 12–14% [100, 101]. Survival is stage dependent and early spread prior to the onset of symptoms is characteristic of this tumor. Early invasive cancer may be classified as intramucosal when neoplastic cells penetrate through the basement membrane to the lamina propria or muscularis mucosa, and submucosal when neoplastic cells infiltrate into the submucosa. The prognosis for these two lesions is very different because the risk of lymph node metastasis is approximately 0–7% for intramucosal cancer, but increases to 5–50% for submucosal cancer [102–105]. Lymph node metastases are a clear prognostic factor for decreased survival [106]. Thus, the best hope for improved survival of patients with esophageal adenocarcinoma is detection of cancer at an early and potentially curable stage.

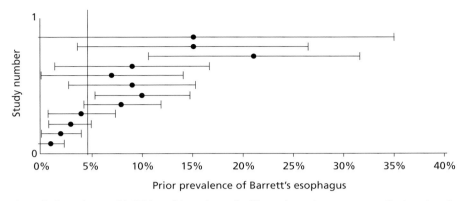

Figure 27.11 Prior prevalence (point estimate with 95% confidence interval) of Barrett's esophagus among patients undergoing resection for incident esophageal adenocarcinoma in 12 studies. The vertical line gives the summary estimate of 4.7% (reproduced from Dulai *et al.* [108], with permission).

Screening

One potential strategy to decrease the mortality rate of esophageal adenocarcinoma further is to identify more patients at risk, namely those with Barrett's esophagus. Population-based studies suggest that in patients with newly diagnosed esophageal adenocarcinoma, a prior endoscopy and diagnosis of Barrett's esophagus was associated with both early stage cancer and improved survival [107]. Unfortunately, only the minority of patients with esophageal adenocarcinoma has undergone prior endoscopy or has a prior diagnosis of Barrett's esophagus (Figure 27.11) [108, 109].

However, current professional society practice guidelines equivocate on screening patients with chronic GERD symptoms for Barrett's esophagus [2, 4, 5]. The 2009 American Cancer Society cancer screening guidelines do not include any recommendation for screening of either esophageal cancer or Barrett's esophagus [110].

Endoscopy with biopsy is still the only validated technique to diagnose Barrett's esophagus. However, it has clear limitations as a screening tool, including cost, risk, and complexity. If applied to the estimated 20% of the population with regular GERD symptoms, the cost implications would be staggering [111]. A recent study examined the yield of endoscopy in both symptomatic and asymptomatic individuals utilizing the Clinical Outcomes Research Initiative (CORI) database. Among white men with GERD symptoms, the yield of Barrett's esophagus increased from 3.3% in the fourth decade of life to 9.3% in the sixth decade prior to reaching a plateau (Figure 27.12) [112]. Interestingly, the yield in symptomatic middle-aged women was comparable to that in asymptomatic males. These findings suggest that screening should not be considered prior to age 50 years.

Unsedated upper endoscopy using small-caliber instruments still has the potential to change the economics of endoscopic screening, as this technique may decrease sedation-related complications and costs. Unsedated small-caliber endoscopy detects Barrett's esophagus and dysplasia with a sensitivity comparable to conventional endoscopy [113]. While both procedures are well tolerated by patients, a major hurdle for unsedated endoscopy is patient resistance to undergoing a test without sedation. Thus, it remains uncertain if endoscopy without sedation will meet with patient acceptance given the cultural preference for sedation in the United States. Otherwise, there are still no validated alternative techniques to screen for Barrett's esophagus that overcome the cost and risks associated with conventional upper endoscopy.

There has been considerable interest in esophageal capsule endoscopy as a screening alternative to conventional upper endoscopy. Unfortunately, studies to date demonstrate a sensitivity of 60–79% and a specificity of 75–100% when compared to conventional upper endoscopy [114–116]. Modeling studies suggest that capsule endoscopy is not a cost-effective alternative to conventional endoscopy either [117]. Thus, adoption of esophageal capsule endoscopy as a screening alternative to upper endoscopy is unlikely in the near future.

After a normal initial upper endoscopy, some wonder if a repeat screening upper endoscopy should be undertaken in symptomatic GERD patients at a later date. Several studies have addressed this point with consistent results. In patients with non-erosive reflux disease at the index endoscopy, Barrett's esophagus is rarely found if the repeat endoscopy is performed within 5 years [118, 119]. On the other hand, if erosive esophagitis is found at the time of index endoscopy, Barrett's esophagus may be present in 9–12% of these patients on repeat endoscopy, with higher grades of esophagitis associated with a higher case finding rate of Barrett's esophagus [120, 121]. As such, screening for Barrett's esophagus in GERD patients should only take place after initial proton pump inhibitor (PPI) therapy. A negative endoscopy at baseline makes it highly unlikely that Barrett's esophagus is found if endoscopy is repeated.

There are still no data from randomized controlled trials or observational studies to evaluate the strategy of

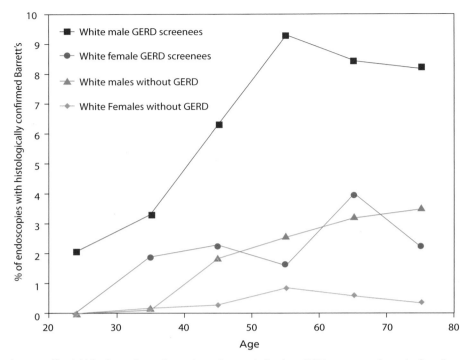

Figure 27.12 Age- and sex-specific yield for Barrett's esophagus by endoscopy indication. GERD, gastroesophageal reflux disease (reproduced from Rubenstein *et al.* [112], With permission).

screening. A decision-analysis model by Inadomi *et al.* examined screening of 50-year-old white men with chronic GERD symptoms for Barrett's esophagus, and found that one-time screening is probably cost-effective if subsequent surveillance is limited to patients with dysplasia on initial examination [122]. Other modeling studies support screening in patients with chronic GERD symptoms as well, but only if the following conditions are met: a group of patients at high risk for Barrett's esophagus, high-grade dysplasia or adenocarcinoma; high sensitivity and specificity of endoscopy with biopsy; and little or no reduction in quality of life with esophagectomy [123, 124]. Any variation of these ideal conditions quickly made this strategy cost-ineffective.

Thus, there is clearly a need to develop either a better profile of patients at high risk for Barrett's esophagus or a far less expensive tool to provide mass population screening. Problems inherent in demonstrating the utility of a screening program, such as healthy volunteer bias, lead time bias, and length time bias, will all need to be addressed as well.

Surveillance

Current practice guidelines recommend endoscopic surveillance of patients with Barrett's esophagus in an attempt to detect cancer at an early and potentially curable stage [2–5]. A number of observational studies suggest that patients with Barrett's esophagus in whom adenocarcinoma was detected in a surveillance program have their cancers detected at an earlier stage (Figure 27.13), with markedly improved 5-year

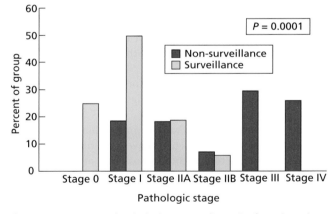

Figure 27.13 Improved pathologic stage at diagnosis of esophageal adenocarcinoma for patients diagnosed during endoscopic surveillance compared to patients diagnosed without prior surveillance (reproduced from Van Sandick *et al.* [127], with permission).

survival compared to similar patients not undergoing routine endoscopic surveillance (Figure 27.14) [109, 125–128]. Furthermore, nodal involvement is far less likely in surveyed patients compared to non-surveyed patients [127]. Since esophageal cancer survival is stage dependent, these studies suggest that survival may be enhanced by endoscopic surveillance. Several decision-analysis models support the concept of endoscopic surveillance [122, 129, 130]. The model of Provenzale *et al.* suggests that surveillance every 5

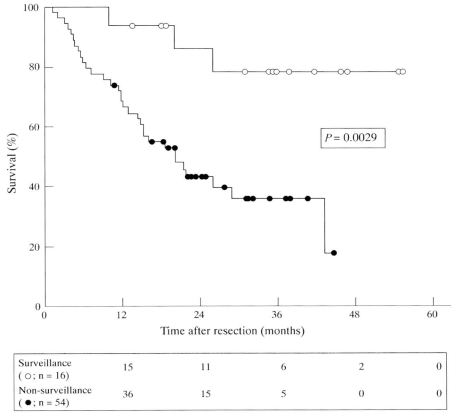

Surveillance (○; n = 16)	15	11	6	2	0
Non-surveillance (●; n = 54)	36	15	5	0	0

Figure 27.14 Improved postoperative survival in esophageal adenocarcinoma for patients diagnosed during endoscopic surveillance compared to patients diagnosed without prior surveillance (reproduced from Van Sandick *et al.* [127], with permission).

years is the most effective strategy to increase both length and quality of life, whereas the model of Inadomi *et al.* suggests that surveillance should be limited to individuals with dysplasia at the time of initial endoscopy [122, 129]. However, since most patients with Barrett's esophagus will not die from esophageal cancer, the entire concept of surveillance remains of uncertain benefit [131]. Design flaws, such as selection bias, healthy volunteer bias, lead time bias, and length time bias, are inherent in the observational studies that support endoscopic surveillance. Despite the concern regarding the esophageal cancer "epidemic," the overall burden of disease is rather limited in the Western world in comparison to other malignancies such as colon cancer.

Candidates for endoscopic surveillance

Patients with documented Barrett's esophagus are candidates for surveillance. Prior to entering into a surveillance program, patients should be advised about risks and benefits, including the limitations of surveillance endoscopy as well as the importance of adhering to appropriate surveillance intervals [132]. Other considerations include age, likelihood of survival over the next 5 years, and ability to tolerate

either endoscopic or surgical interventions for early esophageal adenocarcinoma.

Surveillance techniques

The aim of surveillance is the detection of dysplasia. The description of dysplasia should use a standard five-tier system: (1) negative for dysplasia; (2) indefinite for dysplasia; (3) low-grade dysplasia; (4) high-grade dysplasia; and (5) carcinoma [68]. Active inflammation makes it more difficult to distinguish dysplasia from reparative changes. As such, it is essential that surveillance endoscopy is only performed after any active inflammation related to GERD is controlled with antisecretory therapy. The presence of ongoing erosive esophagitis is a contraindication to performing surveillance biopsies.

Current guidelines suggest obtaining systematic four-quadrant biopsies at 2-cm intervals along the entire length of the Barrett's segment once inflammation related to GERD is controlled with antisecretory therapy [2–5]. A systematic biopsy protocol clearly detects more dysplasia and early cancer compared to *ad hoc* random biopsies [133, 134]. Subtle mucosal abnormalities, no matter how trivial, such as ulceration, erosion, plaque, nodule, stricture, or other luminal irregularity in the Barrett's segment, should also be extensively biopsied, as there is an association of such lesions with underlying cancer [135]. Current guidelines now recommend that mucosal abnormalities, especially in the setting of high-grade dysplasia, should undergo EMR [2]. Tumor staging with EMR is accurate when compared with surgical pathology following esophagectomy: negative margins on EMR specimens correlate well with absence of residual disease at the time of surgery, but submucosal involvement is associated with predictable rates of residual disease and/or lymph node metastases at the time of surgery [136]. Furthermore, EMR will change the diagnosis in approximately 50% of patients when compared to endoscopic biopsies, given the larger tissue sample available for review by the pathologist [137]. Interobserver agreement among pathologists is improved as well [138]. The safety of systematic endoscopic biopsy protocols has been demonstrated [139].

The rationale for such a comprehensive biopsy program comes from observations that high-grade dysplasia and early carcinoma in Barrett's esophagus often occur in the absence of endoscopic abnormalities, and from the focal nature of dysplasia. Systematic esophagectomy mapping studies demonstrate just how focal dysplasia and superficial cancer may be. In 30 esophagectomy specimens from patients undergoing surgery for either high-grade dysplasia or early invasive adenocarcinoma with no endoscopic evidence of cancer, the median surface area of total Barrett's esophagus was 32 cm²; of low-grade dysplasia 13 cm²; of high-grade dysplasia 1.3 cm²; and of adenocarcinoma 1.1 cm² (Figure 27.15) [140]. The three smallest cancers had surface areas of 0.02, 0.3, and 0.4 cm². There has been considerable debate over the years regarding the need for large particle (jumbo) forceps to obtain biopsies, but current guidelines suggest that evidence does not support the routine use of jumbo biopsy

forceps [4]. A new large capacity forceps that can be passed through standard diameter endoscopes provides larger samples than standard large capacity forceps and may increase the yield of dysplasia [141]. However, the extensive use of EMR has changed biopsy sampling considerably and makes much of this debate of historical interest only.

Surveillance intervals

Surveillance intervals, determined by the presence and grade of dysplasia, are based on our limited understanding of the biology of esophageal adenocarcinoma. The most recently published recommendations from the American College of Gastroenterology are shown in Table 27.1. However, these intervals are arbitrary, and have never been subject to a clinical trial and likely never will be. Guidelines from the various professional societies do not agree on surveillance intervals or techniques. Surveillance every 3 years is recommended as adequate in patients without dysplasia after two negative examinations by both the American College of Gastroenterology and the American Society for Gastrointestinal Endoscopy [2, 3]. However, the American Gastroenterological Association recommends extending the surveillance interval up to 5 years, whereas the British Society of Gastroenterology recommends continued surveillance at 2-year intervals in this setting [4, 5].

If low-grade dysplasia is found, the diagnosis should first be confirmed by an expert gastrointestinal pathologist due to the marked interobserver variability in interpretation of these biopsies. Data suggest that if there is a consensus diagnosis by two or three expert gastrointestinal pathologists, the risk of progression is greater than if there is no such agreement [142]. These patients should receive aggressive antisecretory

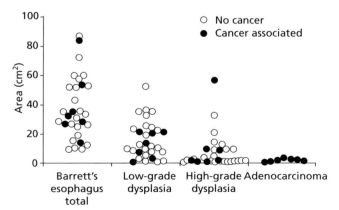

Figure 27.15 Surface area involved with Barrett's esophagus, low-grade dysplasia, high-grade dysplasia, and adenocarcinoma in 30 patients without obvious carcinoma undergoing resection for high-grade dysplasia or superficial adenocarcinoma (reproduced from Cameron and Carpenter [140], with permission).

Table 27.1 2008 American College of Gastroenterology practice guidelines for endoscopic surveillance of Barrett's esophagus (adapted from Wang and Sampliner [2], with permission).

Dysplasia grade	Interval
None	Every 3 years after two are negative within 1 year
Low grade	Expert gastrointestinal pathologist confirmation
	Repeat endoscopy within 6 months to insure no higher grade of dysplasia
	Every year until no dysplasia on two consecutive endoscopies
High grade	Expert gastrointestinal pathologist confirmation
	If Barrett's segment flat: redo endoscopy and biopsies within 3 months
	If mucosal abnormality: endoscopic mucosal resection
	Counsel patient with options:
	• Intensive surveillance
	• Endoscopic therapy
	• Esophagectomy

therapy for reflux disease with a PPI to decrease the changes of regeneration that make pathologic interpretation of this category so difficult. A repeat endoscopy should then be performed within 6 months of the initial diagnosis. If low-grade dysplasia is confirmed, annual surveillance is recommended when low-grade dysplasia is present until two consecutive examinations are negative [2]. There is no agreement on the biopsy protocol to use, although a protocol of four-quadrant biopsies at 1-cm intervals, as would be used for high-grade dysplasia, makes sense. EMR should be performed if any mucosal abnormality is present in these patients.

If high-grade dysplasia is found, the diagnosis should first be confirmed by an experienced gastrointestinal pathologist as well. If the segment is flat and without any mucosal abnormalities, the endoscopic biopsy protocol should then be repeated within 3 months to exclude an unsuspected carcinoma using careful inspection with high-quality white light endoscopy [2]. It is still unclear how much enhanced imaging techniques add to careful inspection with high-resolution or high-definition white light endoscopy (see below). The presence of any mucosal abnormality warrants EMR in an effort to maximize staging accuracy. If high-grade dysplasia is confirmed, there is no consensus on the appropriate management of these patients. Options include continued surveillance, endoscopic therapy or esophagectomy. While continued surveillance has been compared in randomized controlled trials to endoscopic approaches, esophagectomy has not been compared to endoscopic ablation therapy in any randomized controlled trials [143]. Observational studies, however, suggest that survival and cancer-free survival are comparable in patients treated either surgically or endoscopically for high-grade dysplasia [144]. If continued surveillance is chosen, one proposed option is surveillance at 3-month intervals for 1 year [145]. If there is no high-grade dysplasia on two consecutive endoscopies for the first year, endoscopy frequency is lengthened to every 6 months for the second year, then to annually thereafter as long as high-grade dysplasia is not encountered again. If high-grade dysplasia persists, then continued short-interval endoscopy is warranted.

Extent of high-grade dysplasia is thought by some to be a risk factor for the subsequent development of adenocarcinoma [146]. However, there are currently no uniform criteria for defining the extent of high-grade dysplasia and there are conflicting data on the clinical significance of extent of high-grade dysplasia in biopsy specimens and risk for unsuspected carcinoma [146, 147]. Mucosal abnormalities in patients with multifocal high-grade dysplasia may also be a risk factor for adenocarcinoma [148, 149]. Thus, high-grade dysplasia remains a worrisome lesion, although progression to carcinoma may take many years and is not inevitable.

The ultimate approach to the patient with high-grade dysplasia should consider factors such as available surgical and endoscopic expertise, age, length of Barrett's epithelium that would require biopsy to eliminate sampling error, compliance with endoscopic surveillance, future need for multiple surveillance endoscopies, and suspicious lesions such as plaques, nodules, and strictures.

Limitations of surveillance

Endoscopic surveillance of Barrett's esophagus, as currently practiced, has numerous shortcomings. Dysplasia and early adenocarcinoma are endoscopically indistinguishable from intestinal metaplasia without dysplasia. The distribution of dysplasia and cancer is highly variable, and even the most thorough biopsy surveillance program has the potential for sampling error. There are considerable interobserver variability and quality control problems in the interpretation of dysplasia in both the community and academic settings. Current surveillance programs are expensive and time consuming. Survey data indicate that while surveillance is widely practiced, there is marked variability in the technique and interval of surveillance as practice guidelines are not widely followed [150–153]. Recent work by Abrams *et al.* found that adherence to guidelines was seen in only 51% of cases and the longer the segment length, the worse the adherence encountered (Figure 27.16) [153]. However, education programs can enhance compliance with guidelines [152].

Currently, all Barrett's esophagus patients are handled in a similar fashion unless dysplasia is present. However, since most patients do not have dysplasia and will never develop cancer, it is necessary to make surveillance techniques more effective by either sampling larger areas of Barrett's mucosa, targeting biopsies to areas with a higher probability of harboring dysplasia, or developing risk stratification tools to allow efforts to be concentrated on individuals at greatest risk while decreasing the frequency and intensity of surveillance in individuals at lower risk.

Potential strategies to enhance surveillance

Chromoendoscopy

Methylene blue is a vital stain that selectively diffuses into the cytoplasm of absorptive epithelium of the small intestine and colon. The presence of staining in the esophagus indicates the presence of intestinal metaplasia [154]. Some studies suggest that methylene blue chromoendoscopy increases the efficiency of detecting dysplasia: fewer biopsies are required and more patients are identified with dysplasia compared to four-quadrant biopsies obtained at 2-cm intervals [155]. However, others have been unable to detect any differences in dysplasia detection between methylene blue-directed biopsies compared to a standard biopsy protocol [156]. Chromoendoscopy is appealing because it is simple, inexpensive, and safe. However, there is no agreement on application technique in terms of the concentration, volume,

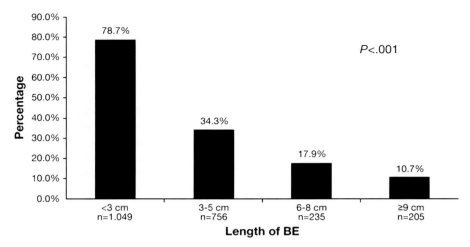

Figure 27.16 Adherence to the Seattle biopsy protocol in the community setting by length of Barrett's esophagus (BE) (reproduced from Abrams *et al.* [153], with permission).

and "dwell time" of various reagents, and interpretation of staining is subjective. Methylene blue chromoendoscopy also adds additional procedure time. A recent meta-analysis found that methylene blue chromoendoscopy resulted in no incremental yield when compared to random biopsies for the detection of intestinal metaplasia, high-grade dysplasia or early cancer [157].

Acetic acid has also been used as a chromoendoscopy technique. Application of 3% acetic acid in 100 Barrett's esophagus patients demonstrated a normal uniform pattern in 85 patients, none of whom had dysplasia, and an abnormal irregular pattern in 15, of whom 87% had dysplasia [158]. Others have shown that acetic acid-enhanced endoscopy improves image quality, but does not increase the detection rate of dysplasia or adenocarcinoma [159].

Optical contrast endoscopy

A variety of optical imaging enhancements have been developed to allow for detailed inspection of the mucosal and vascular surface patterns. Narrow-band imaging involves the placement of optical filters that narrow the bandwidth of white light to blue light. This allows for detailed imaging of the mucosal and vascular surface patterns in Barrett's esophagus without the need for chromoendoscopy. There are also two post-processing software-driven systems to accomplish similar visualization (I-scan and FICE). Most of the published literature to date has examined narrow-band imaging [160].

Studies of narrow-band imaging performed with optical zoom endoscopy found that an irregular mucosal and vascular appearance were highly predictive of early neoplasia [161, 162]. A tandem endoscopy study that compared standard resolution white light endoscopy to narrow-band imaging combined with high-definition white light endoscopy found the latter to be superior to conventional white

light endoscopy for the detection of early neoplasia, and required fewer biopsies to accomplish this [163]. However, other studies suggest that while narrow-band imaging improves overall image quality, it does not lead to enhanced detection of early neoplasia compared to high-resolution white light endoscopy [159, 164, 165].

A recent systematic review found that narrow-band imaging has a sensitivity of 77–100% and a specificity of 79–94% for the detection of intestinal metaplasia [166]. The sensitivity for the detection of high-grade dysplasia or cancer varies from 77% to 100%, with a specificity of 58–100%. There are a number of unresolved issues regarding narrow-band imaging, including the use of multiple classification schemes for mucosal and vascular patterns, image interpretation based on still images instead of real-time endoscopy, the use of optical versus electronic zoom, and the use of study populations enriched with early neoplasia in tertiary care centers.

Spectroscopy

Initial work with laser-induced fluorescence spectroscopy in a group of 36 patients had a sensitivity of 100% for high-grade dysplasia and a specificity of 70% for no dysplasia, but all six patients with low-grade dysplasia were classified as benign by laser-induced fluorescence spectroscopy [167]. A spectroscopic probe that combined the techniques of fluorescence, reflectance, and light scattering spectroscopy in 16 patients with Barrett's esophagus had a sensitivity and specificity of 100% for separating high-grade dysplasia from low-grade dysplasia and no dysplasia, and a sensitivity of 93% with a specificity of 100% for separating any dysplasia from no dysplasia [168]. Elastic scattering spectroscopy has also shown promise [169]. However, spectroscopic techniques, as currently configured, require a "point and shoot" method of touching the mucosa with the probe followed by biopsy. To be clinically helpful, these techniques will need to image a larger field by "spraying light," followed by targeted biopsies of abnormal optical regions.

Optical coherence tomography

Optical coherence tomography uses infrared light to produce high-resolution images of mucosal tissue *in vivo*. Current technology again is largely limited to a "touch and image" technique and is not yet able to sample large areas rapidly. Attempts at developing large-area image acquisition capabilities are still in their early stages [170]. Data to date suggest that the accuracy of current systems is insufficient for clinical application [170, 171].

Autofluorescence endoscopy

Autofluorescence endoscopy is a wide-area imaging technique, with the potential to rapidly examine a large surface area of gastrointestinal mucosa in order to detect small areas of dysplasia or cancer. Autofluorescence endoscopy is based on the principal that normal, metaplastic, and dysplastic tissues have different autofluorescence colors visible to the naked eye. It involves illumination of tissue of interest with short wavelength light, which leads to excitation of endogenous substances known as fluorophores and hence emission of fluorescence light of longer wavelengths [172].

Early work with autofluorescence endoscopy involved fiberoptic technology, but recent studies have examined video technology alone or combined with narrow-band imaging. Kara *et al.* found that video-based autofluorescence endoscopy increased the detection of high-grade dysplasia and early carcinoma lesions that were not seen with high-resolution white light videoendoscopy [173]. However, autofluorescence endoscopy, when used as a stand-alone technique was still associated with a high number of false-positive areas of abnormal fluorescence.

In an effort to decrease the high false-positive rates found with autofluorescence endoscopy as a stand-alone technique, autofluorescence endoscopy has been combined with high-resolution white light, narrow-band imaging and optical zoom technology in one endoscope. This "trimodal" technique involves the use of autofluorescence videoendoscopy as a "red flag technique" to identify suspicious areas of Barrett's mucosa, followed by narrow-band imaging combined with magnification endoscopy to examine the vascular and mucosal pattern of these suspicious lesions. In one study, the combination of the three techniques decreased the false-positive rate from 40% to 10%, whereas in a second study, the false-positive rate was decreased from 81% to 26%, while also increasing the detection rate of intramucosal carcinoma or high-grade dysplasia lesions compared to that achieved with high-resolution white light endoscopy alone [174, 175]. Unfortunately, despite the conceptual simplicity of autofluorescence endoscopy to provide enhanced endoscopic imaging, the technology in its current iteration is limited. In order for this technology to have future clinical applications, image quality still needs to be improved and the false-positive rate needs to be decreased further.

Confocal laser endomicroscopy

Confocal laser endomicroscopy is a new endoscopic imaging technique that allows for subsurface imaging and *in vivo* histologic assessment of the mucosal layer during standard white light endoscopy [176]. It is a potential ideal small field imaging technique that optimally should be used with a "red flag" method to target image acquisition. The goal of endomicroscopy is to distinguish neoplastic from non-neoplastic tissue in "real time" and thus provide the potential for a decreased number of biopsies. Two different platforms are available: a scope-based device that is integrated into the distal tip of the endoscope and a probe-based device that can be inserted through a standard endoscope. Both devices require administration of an intravenous fluorescence agent, fluorescein.

Several studies have examined confocal laser endomicroscopy in Barrett's esophagus. Using a scope-based device, a confocal Barrett's esophagus classification scheme involving cellular and vascular architecture was developed to predict histopathology in the columnar-lined segment. The sensitivity and specificity for the prediction of non-dysplastic Barrett's epithelium was 98% and 94%, respectively, and for Barrett's esophagus-associated neoplasia was 93% and 98%, respectively. The Kappa value for interobserver agreement was 0.843 [177]. Recent work also suggests that confocal endomicroscopy with the scope-based technique improves the diagnostic yield of endoscopically unapparent neoplasia compared to standard white light endoscopy and surveillance biopsies [178].

An initial pilot study of probe-based confocal laser microscopy yielded a sensitivity of 75–89% with a specificity of 75–91% for the detection of high-grade dysplasia of adenocarcinoma [179]. Preliminary studies examining the accuracy and interobserver agreement for intraepithelial neoplasia of probe-based confocal laser endomicroscopy using still images was encouraging with a sensitivity of 88%, specificity of 96%, and kappa value of 0.72 [180]. However, results were disappointing when the probe-based system was examined in real time in 68 patients [181]. When compared to conventional biopsies, "optical biopsies" obtained in real time had a sensitivity of 12% and a specificity of 97% for the detection of high-grade dysplasia or adenocarcinoma. Thus, while the conceptual paradigm is exciting, it is still premature to replace conventional surveillance biopsies with virtual optical biopsies.

Risk stratification

A number of clinical and biologic markers may define patients at increased risk for the development of adenocarcinoma. Clinical risk factors for the development of high-grade dysplasia or adenocarcinoma include gender, ethnicity, age, dysplasia, hiatal hernia size, length of the Barrett's segment, body mass index, and smoking [83]. While esophageal cancer develops in both short and long segments of Barrett's esophagus, segment length does not appear to be a strong risk factor for the development of cancer [77, 182].

Dysplasia is still the best available marker of cancer risk in clinical practice. Dysplasia is recognized adjacent to and distant from Barrett's esophagus-associated adenocarcinoma in resection specimens from patients with Barrett's esophagus. Barrett's esophagus patients progress through a phenotypic sequence of no dysplasia, low-grade dysplasia, high-grade dysplasia, and then on to adenocarcinoma, although the time course is highly variable and this stepwise sequence is not preordained [127, 183]. Furthermore, some patients may progress directly to cancer without prior detection of dysplasia of any grade [184].

The natural history of low-grade dysplasia is poorly understood. First, the diagnosis is often transient [185, 186]. In part, this may be due to the high degree of interobserver variability in establishing this diagnosis and the variable biopsy protocols by which these patients are followed, resulting in issues related to tissue sampling. While the majority of patients with low-grade dysplasia do not progress to adenocarcinoma or high-grade dysplasia, a subset of these patients do progress to a higher-grade lesion. Recent studies suggest an intermediate risk of progression to cancer with a weighted average incidence rate of 1.69%/year [187]. Factors associated with progression to cancer include consensus agreement among two or more pathologists as well as extent of low-grade dysplasia [142, 188].

High-grade dysplasia in Barrett's esophagus is a well-recognized risk factor for the development of adenocarcinoma [144, 145, 189]. Unsuspected carcinoma is detected at esophagectomy in approximately 40% of patients with high-grade dysplasia, with a range of 0–73% [190]. However, recent studies using EMR prior to esophagectomy suggest that finding unsuspected cancer is reduced considerably to approximately 13% [144]. Several studies have improved our understanding of the natural history of high-grade dysplasia. Buttar et al. followed 100 patients with high-grade dysplasia with continued endoscopic surveillance and found cancer at 1 and 3 years in 38% and 56% of individuals with diffuse high-grade dysplasia and 7% and 14% of individuals with focal high-grade dysplasia [146]. Reid et al. followed 76 patients for 5 years and encountered cancer in 59% [189]. On the other hand, Schnell et al., in a study of 79 patients, found cancer in 5% during the first year of surveillance and in 16% of the remaining patients followed for a mean of 7 years (20% of the total group developed cancer) [145]. Others have reported regression of high-grade dysplasia over time as well [145, 191]. A recent meta-analysis found that the incidence of adenocarcinoma in patients with high-grade dysplasia was approximately 6.58%/year [192].

Mucosal abnormalities in patients with multifocal high-grade dysplasia may also be a risk factor for adenocarcinoma [146, 193]. Thus, high-grade dysplasia remains a worrisome lesion, although progression to carcinoma may take many years and is not inevitable.

Unfortunately, dysplasia is an imperfect marker of increased cancer risk. It is typically not distinguishable endoscopically and is often focal in nature, thereby making targeting of biopsies problematic. Furthermore, there is considerable interobserver variability in the grading of dysplasia, and the ability of pathologists to distinguish between intramucosal carcinoma and high-grade dysplasia is problematic even in esophagectomy specimens as described above. Therefore, a less subjective marker for cancer risk that could supplement or replace the current dysplasia grading system is needed.

Biomarkers of increased risk

A number of molecular markers may define patients at increased risk for the development of esophageal adenocarcinoma. Among the most frequently described molecular changes that precede the development of adenocarcinoma in Barrett's esophagus are alterations in p53 (mutation, deletion or loss of heterozygosity [LOH]) [93, 194, 195] p16 (mutation, deletion, promoter hypermethylation, or LOH) [93, 94, 196], and aneuploidy by flow cytometry [197, 198]. Neoplastic progression in Barrett's esophagus is accompanied by flow cytometric abnormalities, such as aneuploidy or increased G2/tetraploid DNA contents, and these abnormalities may precede the development of high-grade dysplasia or adenocarcinoma. The potential of flow cytometry as a prognostic biomarker was illustrated in work by Reid et al., who found that for patients with no flow cytometric abnormalities at baseline and with histology that showed no dysplasia, indefinite or low-grade dysplasia, the 5-year incidence of cancer was 0% [199]. In contrast, aneuploidy, increased 4N fractions or high-grade dysplasia was detected in each of the 35 patients who went on to develop cancer within 5 years. Unfortunately, flow cytometry is not readily available for clinical practice and the technique typically requires fresh or frozen specimens. An alternative method for the detection of DNA ploidy abnormalities is image cytometry, which can analyze formalin-fixed tissue with automated analysis algorithms. Image cytometry may be comparable to flow cytometry for the detection of ploidy [200]. A recent study using image cytometry demonstrated that DNA ploidy abnormalities after successful photodynamic therapy (PDT) of high-grade dysplasia predicted subsequent relapse during follow-up [200]. Another technique with potential clinical applicability for the detection of abnormal DNA content is fluorescent in situ hybridization (FISH), which may also be simpler to apply in clinical practice [201].

Mutations of p53 and 17p LOH have been reported in up to 92% and 100%, respectively, of esophageal adencocarcinomas [202]. Furthermore, both abnormalities have been detected in Barrett's epithelium prior to the development of carcinoma. For example, Reid *et al.* found that the prevalence of 17p (p53) LOH at baseline increased from 6% in patients negative for dysplasia to 20% in patients with low-grade dysplasia, and to 57% in patients with high-grade dysplasia [93]. More importantly, the 3-year incidence of cancer was 38% for individuals with 17p (p53) LOH compared to 3.3% for individuals with two 17p alleles. However, techniques to detect p53 mutations and 17p LOH are also labor intensive and have not achieved widespread acceptance in clinical practice to date. Immunohistochemical staining for p53 suggests that p53 overexpression predicts progression regardless of histology [203]. However, immunostaining does not detect all forms of mutant p53 and thus has limitations as a biomarker technique as well. Similarly, p16 LOH and inactivation of the p16 gene by promoter region hypermethylation have been reported frequently in esophageal adenocarcinoma [95]. Furthermore, 9p LOH is commonly encountered in premalignant Barrett's epithelium and can be detected over large regions of the Barrett's mucosa [95]. It is hypothesized that clonal expansion occurs in conjunction with p16 abnormalities, creating a field in which other genetic lesions leading to esophageal adenocarcinoma can arise.

Epigenetic changes, in the form of hypo- and hypermethylation, and alteration to histone complexes have also been implicated in the progression of Barrett's esophagus to adenocarcinoma. Hypermethylation of p16, APC, RUNX3, and HPP1 are all independently associated with an increased risk of progression of Barrett's esophagus to high-grade dysplasia or esophageal adenocarcinoma [204, 205].

Given the complexity and diversity of alterations observed to date in the metaplasia–dysplasia–carcinoma sequence, it appears that a panel of biomarkers may be required for risk stratification. The combination of 17p LOH, 9p LOH, and DNA content abnormality has been shown to predict the 10-year adenocarcinoma risk better than any single biomarker alone [206]. Patients with a combination of these abnormalities had a markedly increased risk of developing cancer compared to those with no baseline abnormalities (relative risk 38.7; 95% CI 10.8–138.5). In those with no abnormalities of any of these biomarkers at baseline, 12% developed adenocarcinoma at 10 years. In contrast, those with the combination of 17p LOH, 9p LOH, and DNA content abnormality had a cumulative incidence of adenocarcinoma of 79% over the same time period. A risk stratification model utilizing a methylation index constructed from the methylation values for p16, HPP1, and RUNX3 also showed potential for prediction of progression to high-grade dysplasia or adenocarcinoma [207].

Thus, while all of these studies demonstrate the potential for biomarkers to predict risk of esophageal adenocarcinoma, none has been validated in large-scale clinical trials to date and as such are not yet useful for clinical decision-making. It is likely that in the future, the best predictor for the development of high-grade dysplasia or adenocarcinoma will be a combination of clinical, demographic, histologic, genetic, and epigenetic data.

Treatment

Medical therapy

Since Barrett's esophagus has the most severe pathophysiologic abnormalities of GERD, it should come as no surprise that PPIs are the cornerstone of medical therapy for Barrett's esophagus. PPIs consistently result in symptom relief and heal esophagitis in Barrett's esophagus patients [208–210]. However, PPIs, even at high doses, result in either no regression of the Barrett's segment or modest regression that is of uncertain clinical importance [211–213]. PPIs typically increase squamous islands in the Barrett's segment, but biopsies taken from such islands will often show underlying intestinal metaplasia [214].

Alleviation of reflux symptoms in Barrett's esophagus is not necessarily equivalent to normalization of esophageal acid exposure, despite the use of high-dose PPI therapy. Persistent abnormal acid exposure is encountered in approximately 25% of Barrett's esophagus patients despite twice-daily PPIs [215, 216]. The importance of complete control of esophageal acid exposure in Barrett's esophagus patients remains unknown. However, some studies provide conceptual support for the concept of aggressive acid suppression in these patients. Normalization of intraesophageal acid exposure in Barrett's patients decreases cellular proliferation rates and increases cellular differentiation rates over 6 months, whereas inability to normalize intraesophageal acid exposure results in no difference in proliferation or differentiation rates [217]. However, this change is not accompanied by any effect on apoptosis or COX-2 levels [218].

A recent Veteran's Association (VA) cohort study suggested that PPI therapy was associated with a decreased risk for the development of high-grade dysplasia and adenocarcinoma [219]. Similar observational data on reduction of dysplasia risk with administration of PPIs have been obtained in Australia [220]. However, no randomized controlled trials have examined the issue of PPIs and prevention of dysplasia or cancer.

Antireflux surgery

Antireflux surgery effectively alleviates GERD symptoms in Barrett's esophagus patients [221–223]. The outcome of laparoscopic antireflux surgery is comparable in Barrett's esophagus and GERD patients and similar to that with esomeprazole, although antireflux surgery may provide somewhat better intraesophageal acid control than PPI therapy [224]. As such, the indications for surgery in

Barrett's esophagus are the same as those for GERD patients without Barrett's esophagus.

Some have hypothesized that antireflux surgery provides protection from progression of Barrett's esophagus to adenocarcinoma [225]. However several lines of evidence suggest that antireflux surgery does not protect patients from developing esophageal adenocarcinoma. A large population-based cohort study of GERD patients from Sweden who underwent antireflux surgery found that surgery did not protect against the development of esophageal adenocarcinoma [226]. The standardized incidence ratio of esophageal adenocarcinoma in the surgically treated group was 14.1 (95% CI 8.0–22.8) compared to 6.3 (95% CI 4.5–8.7) in the medically treated group. A VA cohort study also found no attenuation of the risk for developing esophageal adenocarcinoma in GERD patients treated surgically compared to those treated medically (0.072%/year vs 0.04%/year) [227]. Similar findings are seen in Barrett's esophagus patients. A meta-analysis of surgical versus medical therapy of Barrett's esophagus found no difference in the risk of esophageal adenocarcinoma between the two groups [228]. A subsequent systematic review by Chang et al. found no difference in the incidence of esophageal adenocarcinoma in medically versus surgically treated patients, and that any evidence suggesting otherwise was driven by uncontrolled case series [229]. Thus, the best available evidence suggests that antireflux surgery does not decrease cancer risk in GERD or Barrett's esophagus patients.

Chemoprevention

Chemoprevention can be defined as pharmacologic intervention that leads either to the prevention of cancer or treatment of identifiable precancerous lesions [230]. A variety of chemoprevention agents have been proposed for Barrett's esophagus patients, including PPIs, aspirin, NSAIDs, celecoxib, lyophilized black raspberries, antioxidants, green tea, retinoids, ursodeoxycholic acid, statins, and curcumin [231–234].

Most attention currently is directed to the use of aspirin and NSAIDs. Observational studies suggest that NSAIDs, including aspirin, may play a protective role against esophageal adenocarcinoma by inhibiting the COX-1 and -2 enzymes, which regulate prostaglandin E2 (PGE2) production [84, 234–236]. Animal studies also suggest that administration of both selective and non-selective COX inhibitors decreases the development of esophageal adenocarcinoma in experimentally-induced Barrett's esophagus [237]. One possible mechanism that is involved in reflux-associated carcinogenesis in Barrett's esophagus is acid and bile salt-induced COX-2 activation and high levels of PGE2 production. A systematic review suggested that the protective effect of aspirin and NSAIDs was greater with more regular use, an observation supported by a recent cohort study as well [84, 85]. A single clinical trial examined the effect of celecoxib at a dose of 200 mg twice daily given for 48 weeks in patients with low- and high-grade dysplasia on change in proportion of biopsy samples with dysplasia between patients treated with celecoxib compared to those treated with a placebo [238]. No differences were found between the two groups. A small cross-over study demonstrated that high-dose PPI therapy in conjunction with aspirin at a dose of 325 mg daily can decrease mucosal PGE2 content in mucosal biopsies from Barrett's esophagus patients [239]. These findings have led to a large randomized clinical trial in the United Kingdom (ASPECT) and a smaller clinical trial in the United States in an effort to examine the potential for chemoprevention with aspirin in conjunction with PPIs as a clinical strategy in Barrett's esophagus patients. Given the overall low incidence of esophageal cancer in Barrett's esophagus, it is still premature to routinely administer aspirin or NSAIDs to these patients.

Endoscopic therapy

Given the limitations of conventional medical and surgical therapy as described above, a variety of mucosal ablation techniques have been studied, including thermal ablation, PDT, and EMR. The theory of mucosal ablation therapy is that reinjury of the metaplastic epithelium followed by the regeneration of normal squamous epithelium from a pluripotential stem cell in an environment of decreased acidity may decrease or eliminate the risk of developing esophageal adenocarcinoma.

Each of the available endoscopic techniques are able to eliminate much or all of the Barrett's epithelium, while the esophagus remains *in situ* and the risks of surgery for high-grade dysplasia or cancer are avoided. Recent data are encouraging, demonstrating low morbidity and mortality, and excellent 5-year survival with endoscopic therapy [240]. However, each of these techniques has disadvantages as well, including the need for continued meticulous surveillance, the potential for "at-risk" mucosa remaining behind after therapy, and diagnostic uncertainty. The decision to perform endoscopic therapy in patients with Barrett's esophagus is complex. Many factors enter into the decision-making process, including grade of dysplasia, characteristics of the lesion in question, patient characteristics, and institutional factors such as expertise in pathology, surgery, and interventional endoscopy.

Thermal ablation techniques

Thermal ablation of Barrett's esophagus can be accomplished by a variety of techniques, including laser, multipolar electrocoagulation, heater probe, argon plasma coagulation, radiofrequency ablation (RFA), and cryotherapy. Randomized controlled trials have compared a variety of thermal ablation techniques. These clinical trials have highlighted the difficulty in obtaining complete endoscopic and histologic ablation with argon plasma coagulation and multipolar electrocoagulation [241–243]. Studies of these techniques routinely found incomplete macroscopic regression of the Barrett's segment and buried intestinal metaplasia beneath the neosquamous epithelium, which not surprisingly, led to reports of subsquamous cancers developing in patients with previously non-dysplastic Barrett's epithelium [244–246]. As such, it appears that techniques such as multipolar electrocoagulation, heater probe, and argon plasma coagulation have all fallen by the wayside. The reasons that these techniques likely have no long-term future include difficulty in obtaining uniform ablation, cost, side effects, and persistent endoscopically evident or microscopic columnar epithelium after therapy. The only conceivable place at present for techniques such as multipolar electrocoagulation and argon plasma coagulation is when small islands and areas of residual Barrett's esophagus remain after treatment with another more effective modality. The most promising thermal techniques currently are RFA and cryotherapy. A key limitation of all thermal techniques is the inability to obtain complete pathologic confirmation of the index lesion, leaving some degree of uncertainty in the results of therapy for both the physician and patient.

Radiofrequency ablation

RFA involves the application of high-power radiofrequency energy using bipolar electrodes, thereby causing rapid heating of the tissue with ablation to a depth of approximately 0.5 mm. Studies on RFA have involved a step-wise progression from animal studies, to human studies prior to esophagectomy, to human dosimetry studies, single-center studies, multicenter non-randomized studies, and multicenter randomized controlled trials [247–249]. Buried intestinal metaplasia appears to be less common than with prior thermal techniques.

RFA has been studied for both non-dysplastic as well as dysplastic Barrett's esophagus. Sharma *et al.* described their 12-month results on the outcome of circumferential RFA of non-dysplastic Barrett's epithelium in 70 patients: complete elimination of intestinal metaplasia without any buried glands was achieved in 69% of subjects [249]. Buried intestinal metaplasia was not encountered in any of the biopsy specimens. Subsequently, longer-term follow-up for up to 30 months after additional focal RFA demonstrated complete elimination of metaplasia in 97% of patients at 30 months [250]. No buried intestinal metaplasia was encountered in any of the biopsy specimens at 12 and 30 months. The preliminary results of 5-year follow-up of 50 treated non-dysplastic patients report maintenance of remission of intestinal metaplasia in 92% of these patients [251]. Adverse events, most of which were minor, were encountered in 15.1% after the circumferential ablation phase of the study and 2.6% after the focal ablation phase of the study. Any postablation symptoms resolved within 4 days of the procedure.

A randomized sham-control study has evaluated RFA for low- and high-grade dysplasia [252]. This study demonstrated complete resolution of high-grade dysplasia in 81% of the treatment group compared to 19% of the sham group, and complete resolution of low-grade dysplasia in 91% of the treatment group compared to 23% of the sham group, using a combination of the circumferential and focal probes at 1-year follow-up (Figure 27.17). Among patients with high-grade dysplasia, progression to cancer occurred in 2.4% of the treatment group compared to 19% of the sham group. Complete elimination of intestinal metaplasia occurred in 77% of the treatment group compared to 2% of the sham group. Adverse events were encountered in three of 298 treatments, including bleeding and chest pain, whereas 6% developed strictures that were easily dilated.

Taken together with other data on RFA, we now know that a combination of circumferential and focal probes provide the optimal results, that this technique can be safely combined with EMR, that pre-existing genetic abnormalities resolve, and that buried intestinal metaplasia appears to be rare [253]. We also know that this method does not completely eliminate cancer risk or progression of low-grade dysplasia to high-grade dysplasia. As with other ablation techniques other than EMR, RFA does not allow tissue confirmation of efficacy, leaving a measure of uncertainty for each patient. Only a limited number of patients have been studied to date and we still do not know about the long-term durability of this technique.

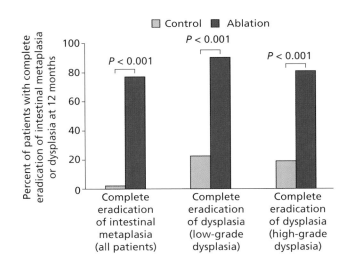

Figure 27.17 Complete histologic eradication of intestinal metaplasia and complete eradication of dysplasia in the subgroups with low-grade dysplasia and in the subgroup with high-grade dysplasia at 12 months after radiofrequency ablation (reproduced from Shaheen *et al.* [252], with permission).

Cryotherapy

Cryotherapy freezes the gut mucosa to induce cell death. There are two current techniques: carbon dioxide and liquid nitrogen. However, very limited data are available to date for either method and there are no randomized controlled trials. Johnston et al. treated 11 patients with liquid nitrogen with complete endoscopic and histologic reversal in seven at 6 months [254]. A case series reported on 26 patients with high-grade dysplasia treated with liquid nitrogen, of whom 32% were dysplasia free at 12-month follow-up [255]. The largest experience with liquid nitrogen cyrotherapy is a retrospective study of 60 patients with high-grade dysplasia who completed therapy of the Barrett's segment [256]. At a mean follow-up of 10.5 months, 97% had complete eradication of high-grade dysplasia, 87% had complete eradication of all dysplasia, and 57% had complete eradication of intestinal metaplasia. Buried subsquamous intestinal metaplasia was encountered in 3%. The side effect profile was excellent with no serious adverse events and strictures in 3%.

Thus, cryotherapy has potential as a simple, relatively inexpensive ablation option. However, a number of concerns remain, including uncertainty regarding optimal dosimetry, technique, limited number of patients studied, short-term follow-up, and lack of comparisons of carbon dioxide- versus liquid nitrogen-based techniques. Furthermore, the uneven application inherent in spraying of the cryogen rather than direct balloon-based application to isolated segments of the esophagus raises concerns regarding controlled depth of injury.

Photodynamic therapy

PDT is a process in which a light-sensitive drug concentrates in neoplastic tissue. The drug is activated by laser light of an appropriate wavelength directed at the abnormal tissue, producing a cytotoxic substance, singlet oxygen, which then selectively damages neoplastic tissue. PDT in Barrett's esophagus has involved a variety of different agents, including porfimer sodium, hematoporphyrin derivative, and 5-aminolevulinic acid (5-ALA). Each of these compounds is characterized by a different depth of tissue destruction and duration of cutaneous photosensitivity. Only sodium porfimer is available in the United States.

A randomized controlled study has evaluated PDT with porfimer sodium compared to a strategy of continued surveillance for patients with high-grade dysplasia [257]. At 2 years, complete ablation of high-grade dysplasia occurred in 77% of the PDT group compared to 39% of patients in the surveillance group, with progression to cancer in 13% and 28%, respectively. Importantly, complete elimination of all intestinal metaplasia and dysplasia occurred in only 52% of the PDT group and 7% of the surveillance group, and complications were common: strictures occurred in 36% and photosensitivity in 69%. At 5 years, the probability of complete ablation of high-grade dysplasia after PDT was only

48% and progression to cancer occurred in 15% [258]. However, work from the Mayo Clinic found that high-grade dysplasia patients treated with PDT, with or without concomitant EMR, had long-term survival comparable to that for patients treated with esophagectomy and low rates of cancer-associated death [259]. PDT has the advantages of leaving the esophagus in situ, evidence from randomized controlled trials that it is superior to continued surveillance, and evidence form cohort studies that survival is comparable to that for esophagectomy. Disadvantages include the considerable capital expense of the equipment required, high rate of strictures, prolonged photosensitivity, lack of tissue confirmation, and problems in attaining complete ablation of intestinal metaplasia. Persistent genetic abnormalities have been noted in residual dysplastic and non-dysplastic epithelium after PDT, with reports of subsequent redevelopment of high-grade dysplasia [260–263]. Important new biomarker work found that p16 loss, detected by FISH of cytology specimens obtained prior to PDT for high-grade dysplasia or intramucosal carcinoma, predicted a lesser response to PDT [264]. Given the advent of other techniques with a more favorable side effect profile, PDT appears to have a limited role today.

Endoscopic mucosal resection

EMR is a therapeutic option for patients with either high-grade dysplasia or intramucosal carcinoma in the setting of appropriate risk stratification. EMR permits accurate histologic staging of neoplasia arising in Barrett's epithelium when compared to esophageal resection specimens. Negative margins on EMR specimens correlate well with absence of residual disease at the time of surgery, but submucosal involvement is associated both with residual disease at the time of surgery and lymph node metastases [265]. As emphasized by the Wiesbaden group, EMR for superficial cancer with curative intent should only be attempted for lesions with the following criteria: lesion diameter less than 20 mm and macroscopically type I (polypoid), IIa (flat and slightly elevated), IIb (flat and level), or IIc (flat depressed <10 mm); well or moderately differentiated histologic grade; limited to the mucosa proven by histology of the resected specimens; and no invasion of lymph vessels or veins. The issue of submucosal cancer limited to the superficial layer is an evolving area of debate. Work by the Wiesbaden group suggests that EMR is a potential option for low-risk submucosal adenocarcinoma limited to the upper third of the submucosal layer with no tumor-related deaths at 5 years [266]. However, findings from the Mayo Clinic suggest that submucosal cancer at EMR has a prohibitive risk for both residual disease at esophagectomy (50%) and a high rate of lymph node metastases (31%) [136]. Comparable rates of lymph node metastases are found in patients with submucosal cancer undergoing esophagectomy for all depths of submucosal disease: 13% of patients with sm1 disease, 22%

with sm2 disease, and 19% with sm3 disease [267]. Thus, this area remains controversial and in evolution.

The pioneering work of the Wiesbaden group with EMR in 100 patients with intraepithelial neoplasia or intramucosal carcinoma with low-risk criteria as described above resulted in compete local remission in 99 after a mean of 1.47 EMRs, with no strictures and the only minor bleeding in 11 patients [268]. However, there were 11 metachronous lesions in 11 patients for a recurrence rate of 11%, characterized by local recurrence in six and disease at a different location in five. There were two deaths in the series unrelated to esophageal cancer. The 5-year life-table survival of these patients was 98%. It is important to emphasize some key methodologic aspects of the Wiesbaden group's work, including the meticulous multimodality staging, rigorous systemic biopsies of the Barrett's segment and all macroscopically visible lesions, and short-interval, long-term follow-up. Residual or metachronous disease, defined as high-grade epithelial neoplasia or early cancer after complete local remission was treated by repeat EMR. Overall, when EMR is used as a stand-alone therapy for early neoplasia in Barrett's esophagus, it is limited by the subsequent development of metachronous lesions in approximately 21% of patients [269]. A number of risk factors for recurrence have been identified with perhaps the most important being the lack of treatment of the residual at-risk mucosa [269].

Circumferential EMR has the goal of completely resecting the Barrett's segment with concomitant histologic confirmation of the underlying mucosal abnormalities. Studies to date suggest that circumferential EMR results in complete remission of intraepithelial neoplasia and Barrett's epithelium in 75–100% of patients [270–275]. Complication rates vary but early bleeding, the occasional perforation, and late strictures remain issues. A recent multicenter European cohort study provides the largest experience with this technique [276]. A total of 169 patients with high-grade dysplasia or early carcinoma in Barrett's esophagus with a segment length of 5 cm or shorter underwent complete EMR of their Barrett's segment with elimination of neoplasia in 97.6%, and all intestinal metaplasia in 85.2% at the end of the treatment phase. At the completion of follow-up (median 27 months), remission of neoplasia was maintained in 97.5%, and complete elimination of intestinal metaplasia was accomplished in 85%. The recurrence rate for metachronous disease was 1.8% and complications included perforation in 1%, delayed bleeding in 1%, and strictures requiring dilation in 50% of the study population. Importantly, the most advanced histologic findings were always encountered at the initial EMR session, where the most suspicious lesion was removed first.

Thus, EMR has the advantage of leaving the esophagus *in situ*, tissue confirmation of disease, as well as evidence from cohort studies regarding excellent long-term survival.

Disadvantages include need for continued and high frequency meticulous surveillance as well as at risk mucosa remaining behind. The role of circumferential EMR is evolving but it is clearly technically demanding and hampered by high stricture rates. Cancer risk is attenuated but not fully eliminated, and meticulous long-term follow up is still required.

Combination therapy

Studies now indicate that complete ablation of Barrett's esophagus with EMR in combination with RFA is feasible. A European multicenter experience of 23 patients who underwent EMR of visible lesions followed by RFA of the remaining Barrett's segment found eradication of neoplasia and intestinal metaplasia in 95% and 88% of patients, respectively [277]. Preliminary results of a randomized controlled clinical trial of circumferential EMR versus focal EMR plus RFA suggest that for the important endpoints of elimination of neoplasia and intestinal neoplasia, the two are comparable [278]. However, the complication rate is far lower for EMR plus RFA compared to circumferential EMR. Others have described excellent long-term results with a combination of EMR and PDT as well [259, 279].

Comparisons to surgical therapy

While there are no randomized controlled trials that have compared endoscopic to surgical approaches for the management of high-grade dysplasia and superficial carcinoma, a number of observational studies now suggest that long-term survival of the two techniques is comparable [259, 279, 280, 281]. Studies extending over 5 years are now available on EMR, PDT, and a combination of the two, and demonstrate comparable long-term survival to esophageal surgery for high-grade dysplasia or superficial carcinoma and low rates of cancer-associated death. A recent population-based study of patients with early esophageal cancer found comparable long-term survival for patients managed with endoscopic therapy compared to those treated with surgical resection [280]. However, while the 5-year survival is comparable between the two treatment modalities, cancer develops during follow-up of endoscopically-treated patients in approximately 6–12%.

Unresolved issues in endoscopic therapy

There are many unresolved issues in ablation therapy. Assuming equal endoscopic skills, it remains important to know which endoscopic therapy should be applied to a given patient. Should EMR be limited to focal lesions? What is the length threshold for circumferential EMR? Who should get thermal techniques and what parameters should be used to determine which patient should get which combination techniques? What factors predict if a patient will respond to a given therapy? Possible variables include segment length, hiatal hernia size, adequacy of acid suppression, and biomarkers. A recent multivariate analysis by Pech *et al.*, based on the long-term results of the Wiesbaden group's approach to patients with intraepithelial neoplasia with EMR with or without PDT, identified the following as risk factors for disease recurrence after ablation therapy: long-segment Barrett's esophagus, multifocal neoplasia, piecemeal resection, and no ablation therapy of the residual Barrett's segment after a complete response with EMR [269].

While early data are promising with RFA, it is difficult to conceive of any technique reliably eliminating all subsquamous intestinal metaplasia. Biomarker abnormalities persist in this subsquamous epithelium and we still do not know what degree of subsquamous columnar epithelium, if any, can be tolerated after ablation. Recent studies in a small number of patients with buried intestinal metaplasia after PDT found that buried Barrett's epithelium had reduced crypt proliferation and near normal DNA content compared to pretreatment Barrett's epithelium, raising the question of the neoplastic potential of the buried Barrett's epithelium [282]. Furthermore better techniques of detecting buried columnar epithelium are needed.

The neo-SCJ is an emerging concern for endoscopic eradication and is an area that warrants additional study. Several reports suggest that the cardia behaves in unexpected and potentially undesirable ways after ablation therapy. Nodules with high-grade dysplasia or cancer may develop months to years after therapy [283, 284]. The reason for this is unknown. While squamous epithelium may develop below the GEJ after ablation, it is unclear what the natural history of that metaplastic mucosa is [285]. Not only can problems develop at the cardia, but techniques such as RFA are difficult to apply to the cardia, even with the focal probe, due to positioning and the anatomic alterations in the setting of a large hiatal hernia.

As demonstrated by the studies cited above for EMR, PDT after EMR, and RFA, cancer may still develop in a small subset of these patients after endoscopic therapy. The emerging concept of EMR of visible lesions combined with either circumferential EMR or thermal injury treatment of the remaining at-risk mucosa is now taking hold.

Finally, despite the ready availability of a variety of different ablation techniques, it is difficult to justify a decision to embark on ablation for all Barrett's esophagus patients without dysplasia at this time for the following reasons: (1) cancer risk for a given patient is low; (2) need for surveillance is not changed; (3) all of the techniques involves considerable financial cost; and (4) adverse events still occur.

Surgery for high-grade dysplasia

Esophagectomy has long been viewed as the preferred approach to high-grade dysplasia, given the findings of unsuspected cancers in up to 73% of patients undergoing esophagectomy [286]. However, the prevalence of unsus-

pected carcinoma may be overestimated in these studies because of the lack of systematic preoperative biopsy protocols and failure to adequately sample mucosal abnormalities, which are known to be associated with the identification of carcinoma, at the time of preoperative endoscopy. Many of the studies on unsuspected cancer took place in the pre-EMR era as well. Surgery has a number of advantages as a treatment strategy for high-grade dysplasia: potential for cure of superficial adenocarcinoma, removal of remaining at-risk mucosa, elimination of the need for further surveillance, and removal of diagnostic uncertainty [287]. However, esophagectomy is a technically demanding operation and outcome is clearly related to surgical volumes, with a mortality rate of 18.8% for an annual surgical volume of fewer than two compared to 9.2% for a volume greater than six [288]. However, emerging data from selected tertiary care centers now suggest that surgery can be performed with a mortality of less than 1% in patients with high-grade dysplasia and consistently less than 5% for patients with intramucosal carcinoma [287, 289, 290, 291]. These excellent outcomes are most likely related to careful patient selection in high-volume centers with standardized clinical care pathways [292]. While there is considerable early morbidity associated with the operation, accompanied by a lengthy recovery time, quality of life in these patients is surprisingly good and approaches that of patients of similar age [293, 294]. Thus, when performed by skilled surgeons with adequate volume and careful patient selection, this operation can be done safely and remains an option for selected high-grade dysplasia patients.

References

1. Riddell RH, Odze RD. Definition of Barrett's esophagus: time for a rethink—is intestinal metaplasia dead? *Am J Gastroenterol* 2009;104:2588–2594.

2. Wang KK, Sampliner RE; Practice Parameters Committee of the American College of Gastroenterology. Updated guidelines 2008 for the diagnosis, surveillance and therapy of Barrett's esophagus. *Am J Gastroenterol* 2008;103:788–797.

3. Hirota WK, Zuckerman MJ, Adler DG, et al. ASGE guideline: the role of endoscopy in the surveillance of premalignant conditions of the upper GI tract. *Gastrointest Endosc* 2006;63:570–580.

4. Wang KK, Wongkeesong M, Buttar NS. American Gastroenterological Association technical review on the role of the gastroenterologist in the management of esophageal carcinoma. *Gastroenterology* 2005;128:1471–1505.

5. British Society of Gastroenterology. Guidelines for the diagnosis and management of Barrett's columnar-lined oesophagus. www.BSG.org.uk

6. Vakil N, van Zanten SV, Kahrilas P, Dent J, Jones R; Global Consensus Group. The Montreal definition and classification of gastroesophageal reflux disease: a global evidence-based consensus. *Am J Gastroenterol* 2006;101:1900–1920.

7. Conio M, Cameron AJ, Romero Y, *et al*. Secular trends in the epidemiology and outcome of Barrett's oesophagus in Olmsted County, Minnesota. *Gut* 2001;48:304–309.

8. van Soest EM, Dieleman JP, Siersema PD, Sturkenboom MC, Kuipers EJ. Increasing incidence of Barrett's oesophagus in the general population. *Gut* 2005;54:1062–1066.

9. Westhoff B, Brotze S, Weston A, *et al*. The frequency of Barrett's esophagus in high-risk patients with chronic GERD. *Gastrointest Endosc* 2005;61:226–231.

10. Spechler SJ, Zeroogian JM, Antonioli DA, Wang HH, Goyal RK. Prevalence of metaplasia at the gastro-oesophageal junction. *Lancet* 1994;344:1533–1536.

11. Nandurkar S, Talley NJ. Barrett's esophagus: the long and the short of it. *Am J Gastroenterol* 1999;94:30–40.

12. Hirota WK, Loughney TM, Lazas DJ, Maydonovitch CL, Rholl V, Wong RK. Specialized intestinal metaplasia, dysplasia, and cancer of the esophagus and esophagogastric junction: prevalence and clinical data. *Gastroenterology* 1999;116:277–285.

13. Ronkainen J, Aro P, Storskrubb T, *et al*. Prevalence of Barrett's esophagus in the general population: an endoscopic study. *Gastroenterology* 2005;129:1825–1831.

14. Zagari RM, Fuccio L, Wallander MA, *et al*. Gastro-oesophageal reflux symptoms, oesophagitis and Barrett's oesophagus in the general population: the Loiano-Monghidoro study. *Gut* 2008;57:1354–1359.

15. Cameron AJ, Lomboy CT. Barrett's esophagus: age, prevalence, and extent of columnar epithelium. *Gastroenterology* 1992;103:1241–1245.

16. Abrams JA, Fields S, Lightdale CJ, Neugut AI. Racial and ethnic disparities in the prevalence of Barrett's esophagus among patients who undergo upper endoscopy. *Clin Gastroenterol Hepatol* 2008;6:30–34.

17. Falk GW, Thota PN, Richter JE, Connor JT, Wachsberger DM. Barrett's esophagus in women: demographic features and progression to high-grade dysplasia and cancer. *Clin Gastroenterol Hepatol* 2005;3:1089–1094.

18. Guardino JM, Khandwala F, Lopez R, Wachsberger DM, Richter JE, Falk GW. Barrett's esophagus at a tertiary care center: association of age on incidence and prevalence of dysplasia and adenocarcinoma. *Am J Gastroenterol* 2006;101:2187–2193.

19. van Blankenstein M, Looman CW, Johnston BJ, Caygill CP. Age and sex distribution of the prevalence of Barrett's esophagus found in a primary referral endoscopy center. *Am J Gastroenterol* 2005;100:568–576.

20. Smith KJ, O'Brien SM, Smithers BM, *et al*. Interactions among smoking, obesity, and symptoms of acid reflux in Barrett's esophagus. *Cancer Epidemiol Biomarkers Prev* 2005;14:2481–2486.

21. Eisen GM, Sandler RS, Murray S, Gottfried M. The relationship between gastroesophageal reflux disease and its complications with Barrett's esophagus. *Am J Gastroenterol* 1997;92:27–31.

22. Corley DA, Kubo A, Levin TR, *et al*. Abdominal obesity and body mass index as risk factors for Barrett's esophagus. *Gastroenterology* 2007;133:34–41.

23. Edelstein ZR, Farrow DC, Bronner MP, Rosen SN, Vaughan TL. Central adiposity and risk of Barrett's esophagus. *Gastroenterology* 2007;133:403–411.

24. Smith KJ, O'Brien SM, Green AC, Webb PM, Whiteman DC. Current and past smoking significantly increase risk for Barrett's esophagus. *Clin Gastroenterol Hepatol* 2009;7:840–848.

25. Falk GW. Barrett's esophagus. *Gastroenterology* 2002;122:1569–1591.

26. Neumann CS, Cooper BT. 24 hour ambulatory oesophageal pH monitoring in uncomplicated Barrett's oesophagus. *Gut* 1994;35:1352–1355.

27. Singh P, Taylor RH, Colin-Jones DG. Esophageal motor dysfunction and acid exposure in reflux esophagitis are more severe if Barrett's metaplasia is present. *Am J Gastroenterol* 1994;89:349–356.

28. Cameron AJ. Barrett's esophagus: prevalence and size of hiatal hernia. *Am J Gastroenterol* 1999;94:2054–2059.

29. Wakelin DE, Al-Mutawa T, Wendel C, Green C, Garewal HS, Fass R. A predictive model for length of Barrett's esophagus with hiatal hernia length and duration of esophageal acid exposure. *Gastrointest Endosc* 2003;58:350–355.

30. Champion G, Richter JE, Vaezi MF, Singh S, Alexander R. Duodenogastroesophageal reflux: relationship to pH and importance in Barrett's esophagus. *Gastroenterology* 1994;107:747–754.

31. Loughney T, Maydonovitch CL, Wong RK. Esophageal manometry and ambulatory 24-hour pH monitoring in patients with short and long segment Barrett's esophagus. *Am J Gastroenterol* 1998;93:916–919.

32. Fass R, Hell RW, Garewal HS, *et al*. Correlation of oesophageal acid exposure with Barrett's oesophagus length. *Gut* 2001;48:310–313.

33. Fitzgerald RC, Onwuegbusi BA, Bajaj-Elliott M, Saeed IT, Burnham WR, Farthing MJ. Diversity in the oesophageal phenotypic response to gastro-oesophageal reflux: immunological determinants. *Gut* 2002;50:451–459.

34. Milano F, van Baal JW, Buttar NS, *et al*. Bone morphogenetic protein 4 expressed in esophagitis induces a columnar phenotype in esophageal squamous cells. *Gastroenterology* 2007;132:2412–2421.

35. Colleypriest BJ, Palmer RM, Ward SG, Tosh D. Cdx genes, inflammation and the pathogenesis of Barrett's metaplasia. *Trends Mol Med* 2009;15:313–322.

36. Sarosi G, Brown G, Jaiswal K, *et al*. Bone marrow progenitor cells contribute to esophageal regeneration and metaplasia in a rat model of Barrett's esophagus. *Dis Esophagus* 2008;21:43–50.

37. Peters JH, Avisar N. The molecular pathogenesis of Barrett's esophagus: common signaling pathways in embryogenesis metaplasia and neoplasia. *J Gastrointest Surg* 2010;14 (Suppl 1):S81–87.

38. Souza RF, Krishnan K, Spechler SJ. Acid, bile, and CDX: the ABCs of making Barrett's metaplasia. *Am J Physiol Gastrointest Liver Physiol* 2008;295:G211–218.

39. Milano F, van Baal JW, Buttar NS, *et al*. Bone morphogenetic protein 4 expressed in esophagitis induces a columnar phenotype in esophageal squamous cells. *Gastroenterology* 2007;132:2412–2421.

40. Spechler SJ, Fitzgerald RC, Prasad GA, Wang KK. History, molecular mechanisms, and endoscopic treatment of Barrett's esophagus. *Gastroenterology* 2010;138:854–869.

41. Lagergren J, Bergström R, Lindgren A, Nyrén O. Symptomatic gastroesophageal reflux as a risk factor for esophageal adenocarcinoma. *N Engl J Med* 1999;340:825–831.

42. Johnson DA, Winters C, Spurling TJ, Chobanian SJ, Cattau EL. Esophageal acid sensitivity in Barrett's esophagus. *J Clin Gastroenterol* 1987;9:23–27.

43. Grade A, Pulliam G, Johnson C, Garewal H, Sampliner RE, Fass R. Reduced chemoreceptor sensitivity in patients with Barrett's esophagus may be related to age and not to the presence of Barrett's epithelium. *Am J Gastroenterol* 1997;92:2040–2043.

44. Chak A, Lee T, Kinnard MF, *et al.* Familial aggregation of Barrett's oesophagus, oesophageal adenocarcinoma, and oesophagogastric junctional adenocarcinoma in Caucasian adults. *Gut* 2002;51:323–328.

45. Chak A, Ochs-Balcom H, Falk G, *et al.* Familiality in Barrett's esophagus, adenocarcinoma of the esophagus, and adenocarcinoma of the gastroesophageal junction. *Cancer Epidemiol Biomarkers Prev* 2006;15:1668–1673.

46. Drovdlic CM, Goddard KA, Chak A, *et al.* Demographic and phenotypic features of 70 families segregating Barrett's oesophagus and oesophageal adenocarcinoma. *J Med Genet* 2003;40:651–656.

47. Shaheen NJ, Green B, Medapalli RK, *et al.* The perception of cancer risk in patients with prevalent Barrett's esophagus enrolled in an endoscopic surveillance program. *Gastroenterology* 2005;129:429–436.

48. Shaheen NJ, Dulai GS, Ascher B, *et al.* Effect of a new diagnosis of Barrett's esophagus on insurance status. *Am J Gastroenterol* 2005;100:577–580.

49. McClave SA, Boyce HW, Gottfied MR. Early diagnosis of the columnar-lined esophagus: a new endoscopic criterion. *Gastrointest Endosc* 1987;33:413–416.

50. Ofman JJ, Shaheen NJ, Desai AA, Moody B, Bozymski EM, Weinstein WM. The quality of care in Barrett's esophagus: endoscopist and pathologist practices. *Am J Gastroenterol* 2001;96:876–881.

51. Sharma P, Dent J, Armstrong D, *et al.* The development and validation of an endoscopic grading system for Barrett's esophagus: the Prague C & M criteria. *Gastroenterology* 2006;131:1392–1399.

52. Liu W, Hahn H, Odze RD, Goyal RK. Metaplastic esophageal columnar epithelium without goblet cells shows DNA content abnormalities similar to goblet cell-containing epithelium. *Am J Gastroenterol* 2009;104:816–824.

53. Kelty CJ, Gough MD, Van Wyk Q, Stephenson TJ, Ackroyd R. Barrett's oesophagus: intestinal metaplasia is not essential for cancer risk. *Scand J Gastroenterol* 2007;42:1271–1274.

54. Takubo K, Aida J, Naomoto Y, *et al.* Cardiac rather than intestinal-type background in endoscopic resection specimens of minute Barrett adenocarcinoma. *Hum Pathol* 2009;4:65–74.

55. Wang A, Mattek NC, Corless CL, Lieberman DA, Eisen GM. The value of traditional upper endoscopy as a diagnostic test for Barrett's esophagus. *Gastrointest Endosc* 2008;68:859–866.

56. Csendes A, Smok G, Burdiles P, *et al.* Prevalence of intestinal metaplasia according to the length of the specialized columnar epithelium lining the distal esophagus in patients with gastroesophageal reflux. *Dis Esophagus* 2003;16:24–28.

57. Gatenby PA, Ramus JR, Caygill CP, Shepherd NA, Watson A. Relevance of the detection of intestinal metaplasia in non-dysplastic columnar-lined oesophagus. *Scand J Gastroenterol* 2008;43:524–530.

58. Chandrasoma PT, Der R, Dalton P, *et al.* Distribution and significance of epithelial types in columnar-lined esophagus. *Am J Surg Pathol* 2001;25:1188–1193.

59. Harrison R, Perry I, Haddadin W, *et al.* Detection of intestinal metaplasia in Barrett's esophagus: an observational comparator study suggests the need for a minimum of eight biopsies. *Am J Gastroenterol* 2007;102:1154–1161.

60. Sharma P, McElhinney C, Topalovski M, Mayo MS, McGregor DH, Weston A. Detection of cardia intestinal metaplasia: do the biopsy number and location matter? *Am J Gastroenterol* 2004;99:2424–2428.

61. Goldblum JR, Vicari JJ, Falk GW, *et al.* Inflammation and intestinal metaplasia of the gastric cardia: the role of gastroesophageal reflux and *H. pylori* infection. *Gastroenterology* 1998;114:633–639.

62. Sharma P, Weston AP, Morales T, Topalovski M, Mayo MS, Sampliner RE. Relative risk of dysplasia for patients with intestinal metaplasia in the distal esophagus and in the gastric cardia. *Gut* 2000;46:9–13.

63. Morales CP, Spechler SJ. Intestinal metaplasia at the gastroesophageal junction: Barrett's, bacteria, and biomarkers. *Am J Gastroenterol* 2003;98:759–762.

64. Srivastava A, Odze RD, Lauwers GY, Redston M, Antonioli DA, Glickman JN. Morphologic features are useful in distinguishing Barrett esophagus from carditis with intestinal metaplasia. *Am J Surg Pathol* 2007;31:1733–1741.

65. Paull A, Trier JS, Dalton MD, Camp RC, Loeb P, Goyal RK. The histologic spectrum of Barrett's esophagus. *N Engl J Med* 1976;295:476–480.

66. Weinstein WM, Ippoliti AF. The diagnosis of Barrett's esophagus: goblets, goblets, goblets. *Gastrointest Endosc* 1996;44:91–94.

67. Alikhan M, Rex D, Khan A, Rahmani E, Cummings O, Ulbright TM. Variable pathologic interpretation of columnar lined esophagus by general pathologists in community practice. *Gastrointest Endosc* 1999;50:23–26.

68. Montgomery E, Bronner MP, Goldblum JR, *et al.* Reproducibility of the diagnosis of dysplasia Barrett esophagus: a reaffirmation. *Hum Pathol* 2001;32:368–378.

69. Ormsby AH, Petras RE, Henricks WH, *et al.* Observer variation in the diagnosis of superficial oesophageal adenocarcinoma. *Gut* 2002;51:671–676.

70. Downs-Kelly E, Mendelin JE, Bennett AE, *et al.* Poor interobserver agreement in the distinction of high-grade dysplasia and adenocarcinoma in pretreatment Barrett's esophagus biopsies. *Am J Gastroenterol* 2008;103:2333–2340.

71. Mino-Kenudson M, Hull MJ, Brown I, *et al.* EMR for Barrett's esophagus-related superficial neoplasms offers better diagnostic reproducibility than mucosal biopsy. *Gastrointest Endosc* 2007;66:660–666.

72. Wang KK, Sampliner RE. Practice Parameters Committee of the American College of Gastroenterology Updated guidelines 2008 for the diagnosis, surveillance and therapy of Barrett's esophagus. *Am J Gastroenterol* 2008;103:788–797.

73. Wang KK, Wongkeesong M, Buttar NS. American Gastroenterological Association technical review on the role of the gastroenterologist in the management of esophageal carcinoma. *Gastroenterology* 2005;128:1471–1505.

74. Solaymani-Dodaran M, Logan RF, West J, Card T, Coupland C. Risk of oesophageal cancer in Barrett's oesophagus and gastro-oesophageal reflux. *Gut* 2004;53:1070–1074.

75. Pohl H, Welch HG. The role of overdiagnosis and reclassification in the marked increase of esophageal adenocarcinoma incidence. *J Natl Cancer Inst* 2005;97:142–146.

76. Jemal A, Siegel R, Ward E, Hao Y, Xu J, Thun MJ. Cancer statistics 2009. *CA Cancer J Clin* 2009;59:225–249.

77. Thomas T, Abrams KR, De Caestecker JS, Robinson RJ. Meta analysis: Cancer risk in Barrett's oesophagus. *Aliment Pharmacol Ther* 2007;26:1465–1477.

78. Sikkema M, de Jonge PJ, Steyerberg EW, Kuipers EJ. Risk of esophageal adenocarcinoma and mortality in patients with Barrett's esophagus: a systematic review and meta-analysis. *Clin Gastroenterol Hepatol* 2010;8:235–244.

79. Anderson LA, Murray LJ, Murphy SJ, *et al*. Mortality in Barrett's oesophagus: results from a population based study. *Gut* 2003;52:1081–1084.

80. van Blankenstein M, Looman CW, Hop WC, Bytzer P. The incidence of adenocarcinoma and squamous cell carcinoma of the esophagus: Barrett's esophagus makes a difference. *Am J Gastroenterol* 2005;100:766–774.

81. Kubo A, Corley DA. Marked multi-ethnic variation of esophageal and gastric cardia carcinomas within the United States. *Am J Gastroenterol* 2004;99:582–588.

82. Corley DA, Kubo A, Zhao W. Abdominal obesity and the risk of esophageal and gastric cardia carcinomas. *Cancer Epidemiol Biomarkers Prev* 2008;17:35235–35238.

83. Falk GW. Risk factors for esophageal cancer development. *Surg Oncol Clin North Am* 2009;18:469–485.

84. Corley DA, Kerlikowske K, Verma R, Buffler P. Protective association of aspirin/NSAIDs and esophageal cancer: a systematic review and meta-analysis. *Gastroenterology* 2003;124: 47–56.

85. Vaughan TL, Dong LM, Blount PL, *et al*. Non-steroidal anti-inflammatory drugs and risk of neoplastic progression in Barrett's oesophagus: a prospective study. *Lancet Oncol* 2005;6:945–952.

86. Engel LS, Chow WH, Vaughan TL, *et al*. Population attributable risks of esophageal and gastric cancers. *J Natl Cancer Inst* 2003;95:1404–1413.

87. Whiteman DC, Parmar P, Fahey P, *et al*. Australian Cancer Study. Association of *Helicobacter pylori* infection with reduced risk for esophageal cancer is independent of environmental and genetic modifiers. *Gastroenterology* 2010;139: 73–83.

88. McArdle JE, Lewin KJ, Randall G, Weinstein W. Distribution of dysplasias and early invasive carcinoma in Barrett's esophagus. *Human Pathol* 1992;23:479–482.

89. Reid BJ, Barrett MT, Galipeau PC, *et al*. Barrett's esophagus: ordering the events that lead to cancer. *Eur J Cancer Prev* 1996;5 (Suppl 2):57–65.

90. Maley CC. Multistage carcinogenesis in Barrett's esophagus. *Cancer Lett* 2007;245:22–32.

91. Paulson TG, Maley CC, Li X, *et al*. Chromosomal instability and copy number alterations in Barrett's esophagus and esophageal adenocarcinoma. *Clin Cancer Res* 2009;15:3305–3314.

92. Galipeau PC, Prevo LJ, Sanchez CA, Longton GM, Reid BJ. Clonal expansion and loss of heterozygosity at chromosomes 9p and 17p in premalignant esophageal (Barrett's) tissue. *J Natl Cancer Inst* 1999;91:2087–2095.

93. Reid BJ, Prevo LJ, Galipeau PC, *et al*. Predictors of progression in Barrett's esophagus II: baseline 17p (p53) loss of heterozygosity identifies a patient subset at increased risk for neoplastic progression. *Am J Gastroenterol* 2001;96:2839–2848.

94. Bian YS, Osterheld MC, Fontolliet C, Bosman FT, Benhattar J. P16 inactivation by methylation of the CDKN2A promoter occurs early during neoplastic progression in Barrett's esophagus. *Gastroenterology* 2002;122:1113–1121.

95. Wong DJ, Paulson TG, Prevo LJ, *et al*. p16INK4a lesions are common, early abnormalities that undergo clonal expansion in Barrett's metaplastic epithelium. *Cancer Res* 2001;61: 8284–8289.

96. Maley CC, Galipeau PC, Li X, Sanchez CA, Paulson TG, Reid BJ. Selectively advantageous mutations and hitchhikers in neoplasms: p16 lesions are selected in Barrett's esophagus. *Cancer Res* 2004;64:3414–3427.

97. Shirvani VN, Ouatu-Lascar R, Kaur BS, Omary MB, Triadafilopoulos G. Cyclooxygenase 2 expression in Barrett's esophagus and adenocarcinoma: ex vivo induction by bile salts and acid exposure. *Gastroenterology* 2000;118:487–496.

98. Morris CD, Armstrong GR, Bigley G, Green H, Attwood SE. Cyclooxygenase expression in the Barrett's metaplasia-dysplasia-adenocarcinoma sequence. *Am J Gastroenterol* 2001;96:990–996.

99. Souza RF, Shewmake K, Beer DG, Cryer B, Spechler SJ. Selective inhibition of cyclooxygenase-2 suppresses growth and induces apoptosis in human esophageal adenocarcinoma cells. *Cancer Res* 2000;60:5767–5772.

100. Sihvo EI, Luostarinen ME, Salo JA. Fate of patients with adenocarcinoma of the esophagus and the esophagogastric junction: a population-based analysis. *Am J Gastroenterol* 2004;99:419–424.

101. Enzinger PC, Mayer RJ. Esophageal cancer. *N Engl J Med* 2003;349:2241–2252.

102. Westerterp M, Koppert LB, Buskens CJ, *et al*. Outcome of surgical treatment for early adenocarcinoma of the esophagus or gastro-esophageal junction. *Virchows Arch* 2005;446:497–504.

103. Stein HJ, Feith M, Bruecher BL, Naehrig J, Sarbia M, Siewert JR. Early esophageal cancer: pattern of lymphatic spread and prognostic factors for long-term survival after surgical resection. *Ann Surg* 2005;242:566–573.

104. Nigro JJ, Hagen JA, DeMeester TR, *et al*. Prevalence and location of nodal metastases in distal esophageal adenocarcinoma confined to the wall: implications for therapy. *J Thorac Cardiovasc Surg* 1999;117:16–23.

105. Bollschweiler E, Baldus SE, Schröder W, *et al*. High rate of lymph-node metastasis in submucosal esophageal squamous-cell carcinomas and adenocarcinomas. *Endoscopy* 2006;38:149–156.

106. Rice TW, Blackstone EH, Goldblum JR, *et al*. Superficial adenocarcinoma of the esophagus. *J Thorac Cardiovasc Surg* 2001;122:1077–1090.

107. Cooper GS, Kou TD, Chak A. Receipt of previous diagnoses and endoscopy and outcome from esophageal adenocarcinoma: a population-based study with temporal trends. *Am J Gastroenterol* 2009;104:1356–1362.

108. Dulai GS, Guha S, Kahn KL, *et al.* Preoperative prevalence of Barrett's esophagus in esophageal adenocarcinoma: a systematic review. *Gastroenterology* 2002;122:26–33.

109. Corley DA, Levin TR, Habel LA, *et al.* Surveillance and survival in Barrett's adenocarcinomas: a population-based study. *Gastroenterology* 2002;122:633–640.

110. Smith RA, Cokkinides V, Brawley OW. Cancer screening in the United States, 2009: a review of current American Cancer Society guidelines and issues in cancer screening. *CA Cancer J Clin* 2009;59:27–41.

111. Shaheen NJ, Provenzale D, Sandler RS. Upper endoscopy as a screening and surveillance tool in esophageal adenocarcinoma: a review of the evidence. *Am J Gastroenterol* 2002;97:1319–1327.

112. Rubenstein JH, Mattek N, Eisen G. Age- and sex-specific yield of Barrett's esophagus by endoscopy indication. *Gastrointest Endosc* 2010;71:21–27.

113. Jobe BA, Hunter JG, Chang EY, *et al.* Office-based unsedated small-caliber endoscopy is equivalent to conventional sedated endoscopy in screening and surveillance for Barrett's esophagus: a randomized and blinded comparison. *Am J Gastroenterol* 2006;101:2693–2703.

114. Sharma P, Wani S, Rastogi A, *et al.* The diagnostic accuracy of esophageal capsule endoscopy in patients with gastroesophageal reflux disease and Barrett's esophagus: a blinded, prospective study. *Am J Gastroenterol* 2008;3:525–532.

115. Galmiche JP, Sacher-Huvelin S, Coron E, *et al.* Screening for esophagitis and Barrett's esophagus with wireless esophageal capsule endoscopy: a multicenter prospective trial in patients with reflux symptoms. *Am J Gastroenterol* 2008;103:538–545.

116. Lin OS, Schembre DB, Mergener K, *et al.* Blinded comparison of esophageal capsule endoscopy versus conventional endoscopy for a diagnosis of Barrett's esophagus in patients with chronic gastroesophageal reflux. *Gastrointest Endosc* 2007;65:577–583.

117. Gerson L, Lin OS. Cost-benefit analysis of capsule endoscopy compared with standard upper endoscopy for the detection of Barrett's esophagus. *Clin Gastroenterol Hepatol* 2007;5:319–325.

118. Stoltey J, Reeba H, Ullah N, *et al.* Does Barrett's oesophagus develop over time in patients with chronic gastro-oesophageal reflux disease? *Aliment Pharmacol Ther* 2007;25:83–91.

119. Rodriguez S, Mattek N, Lieberman D, *et al.* Barrett's esophagus on repeat endoscopy: should we look more than once? *Am J Gastroenterol* 2008;103:1892–1897.

120. Hanna S, Rastogi A, Weston AP, *et al.* Detection of Barrett's esophagus after endoscopic healing of erosive esophagitis. *Am J Gastroenterol* 2006;101:1416–1420.

121. Modiano N, Gerson LB. Risk factors for the detection of Barrett's esophagus in patients with erosive esophagitis. *Gastrointest Endosc* 2009;69:1014–1020.

122. Inadomi JM, Sampliner R, Lagergren J, *et al.* Screening and surveillance for Barrett esophagus in high risk groups: a cost-utility analysis. *Ann Intern Med* 2003;138:176–186.

123. Soni A, Sampliner RE, Sonnenberg A. Screening for high-grade dysplasia in gastroesophageal reflux disease: is it cost effective? *Am J Gastroenterol* 2000;95:2086–2093.

124. Gerson LB, Groeneveld PW, Triadafilopoulos G. Cost-effectiveness model of endoscopic screening and surveillance in patients with gastroesophageal reflux disease. *Clin Gastroenterol Hepatol* 2004;2:868–879.

125. Inacarbone R, Bonavina L, Saino G, *et al.* Outcome of esophageal adenocarcinoma detected during endoscopic biopsy surveillance for Barrett's esophagus. *Surg Endosc* 2002;16:263–266.

126. Ferguson MK, Durkin A. Long-term survival after esophagectomy for Barrett's adenocarcinoma in endoscopically surveyed and nonsurveyed patients. *J Gastrointest Surg* 2002;6:29–36.

127. Van Sandick JW, Lanschot JJ, Kuiken BW, *et al.* Impact of endoscopic biopsy surveillance of Barrett's esophagus on pathological stage and clinical outcome of Barrett's carcinoma. *Gut* 1998;43:216–222.

128. Peters JH, Clark GW, Ireland AP, *et al.* Outcome of adenocarcinoma arising in Barrett's esophagus in endoscopically surveyed and nonsurveyed patients. *Thorac Cardiovasc Surg* 1994;108:813–822.

129. Provenzale D, Schmitt C, Wong JB. Barrett's esophagus: a new look at surveillance based on emerging estimates of cancer risk. *Am J Gastroenterol* 1999;94:2043–2053.

130. Sonnenberg A, Soni A, Sampliner RE. Medical decision analysis of endoscopic surveillance of Barrett's oesophagus to prevent oesophageal adenocarcinoma. *Aliment Pharmacol Ther* 2002;16:41–50.

131. Conio M, Blanchi S, Lapertosa G, *et al.* Long-term endoscopic surveillance of patients with Barrett's esophagus: incidence of dysplasia and adenocarcinoma: a prospective study. *Am J Gastroenterol* 2003;98:1931–1939.

132. Wang KK, Wongkeesong M, Buttar NS. American Gastroenterological Association medical position statement: Role of the gastroenterologist in the management of esophageal carcinoma. *Gastroenterology* 2005;128:1468–1470.

133. Fitzgerald RC, Saeed I, Khoo D, *et al.* Rigorous surveillance protocol increases detection of curable cancers associated with Barrett's esophagus. *Dig Dis Sci* 2001;46:1892–1898.

134. Abela JE, Going JJ, Mackenzie JF, *et al.* Systematic four-quadrant biopsy detects Barrett's dysplasia in more patients than nonsystematic biopsy. *Am J Gastroenterol* 2008;103:850–855.

135. Reid BJ, Blount PL, Feng Z, *et al.* Optimizing endoscopic biopsy detection of early cancers in Barrett's high-grade dysplasia. *Am J Gastroenterol* 2000;95:3089–3096.

136. Prasad GA, Buttar NS, Wongkeesong LM, *et al.* Significance of neoplastic involvement of margins obtained by endoscopic mucosal resection in Barrett's esophagus. *Am J Gastroenterol* 2007;102:2380–2386.

137. Peters FP, Brakenhoff KP, Curvers WL, *et al.* Histologic evaluation of resection specimens obtained at 293 endoscopic resections in Barrett's esophagus. *Gastrointest Endosc* 2008;67:604–609.

138. Peters FP, Brakenhoff KP, Curvers WL, *et al.* Histologic evaluation of resection specimens obtained at 293 endoscopic resections in Barrett's esophagus. *Gastrointest Endosc* 2008;67:604–609.

139. Levine DS, Blount PL, Rudolph RE, *et al.* Safety of a systematic endoscopic biopsy protocol in patients with Barrett's esophagus. *Am J Gastroenterol* 2000;95:1152–1157.

140. Cameron AJ, Carpenter HA. Barrett's esophagus, high-grade dysplasia and early adenocarcinoma. *Am J Gastroenterol* 1997;92:586–591.

141. Komanduri S, Swanson G, Keefer L, Jakate S. Use of a new jumbo forceps improves tissue acquisition of Barrett's esophagus surveillance biopsies. *Gastrointest Endosc* 2009;70:1072–1078.

142. Skacel M, Petras RE, Gramlich TL, *et al.* The diagnosis of low-grade dysplasia in Barrett's esophagus and its implications for disease progression. *Am J Gastroenterol* 2000;95:3383–3387.

143. Green S, Tawil A, Barr H, *et al.* Surgery versus radical endo-therapies for early cancer and high grade dysplasia in Barrett's oesophagus. *Cochrane Database Syst Rev* 2009;(2):CD007334.

144. Prasad GA, Wang KK, Buttar NS, *et al.* Long-term survival following endoscopic and surgical treatment of high-grade dysplasia in Barrett's esophagus. *Gastroenterology* 2007;132:1226–1233.

145. Schnell TG, Sontag SJ, Chejfec G, *et al.* Long-term nonsurgical management of Barrett's esophagus with high-grade dysplasia. *Gastroenterology* 2001;120:1607–1619.

146. Buttar NS, Wang KK, Sebo TJ, *et al.* Extent of high-grade dysplasia in Barrett's esophagus correlates with risk of adeno-carcinoma. *Gastroenterology* 2001;120:1630–1639.

147. Dar M, Goldblum JR, Rice TW, *et al.* Can extent of high-grade dysplasia predict the presence of adenocarcinoma at esophagectomy? *Gut* 2003;52:486–489.

148. Tharavej C, Hagen JA, Peters JH, *et al.* Predictive factors of coexisting cancer in Barrett's high-grade dysplasia. *Surg Endosc* 2006;20:439–443.

149. Nigro JJ, Hagen JA, DeMeester TR, *et al.* Occult esophageal adenocarcinoma: extent of disease and implications for effective therapy. *Ann Surg* 1999;230:433–438.

150. Falk GW, Ours TM, Richter JE. Practice patterns for surveillance of Barrett's esophagus in the United States. *Gastrointest Endosc* 2000;52:197–203.

151. Gross CP, Canto MI, Hixson J, *et al.* Management of Barrett's esophagus: a national study of practice patterns and their cost implications. *Am J Gastroenterol* 1999;94:3440–3447.

152. Das D, Ishaq S, Harrison R, *et al.* Management of Barrett's esophagus in the UK: overtreated and underbiopsied but improved by the introduction of a national randomized trial. *Am J Gastroenterol* 2008;103:1079–1089.

153. Abrams JA, Kapel RC, Lindberg GM, *et al.* Adherence to biopsy guidelines for Barrett's esophagus surveillance in the community setting in the United States. *Clin Gastroenterol Hepatol* 2009;7:736–742.

154. Canto MI, Setrakian S, Petras RE, *et al.* Methylene blue selectively stains intestinal metaplasia in Barrett's esophagus. *Gastrointest Endosc* 1996;44:1–7.

155. Canto MI, Setrakian S, Willis J, *et al.* Methylene blue-directed biopsies improve detection of intestinal metaplasia and dysplasia in Barrett's esophagus. *Gastrointest Endosc* 2000;51:560–568.

156. Lim CH, Rotimi O, Dexter SP, *et al.* Randomized crossover study that used methylene blue or random 4-quadrant biopsy for the diagnosis of dysplasia in Barrett's esophagus. *Gastrointest Endosc* 2006;64:195–199.

157. Ngamruengphong S, Sharma VK, Das A. Diagnostic yield of methylene blue chromoendoscopy for detecting specialized intestinal metaplasia and dysplasia in Barrett's esophagus: a meta-analysis. *Gastrointest Endosc* 2009;69:1021–1028.

158. Vázquez-Iglesias JL, Alonso-Aguirre P, Diz-Lois MT, *et al.* Acetic acid allows effective selection of areas for obtaining biopsy samples in Barrett's esophagus. *Eur J Gastroenterol Hepatol* 2007;19:187–193.

159. Curvers W, Baak L, Kiesslich R, *et al.* Chromoendoscopy and narrow-band imaging compared with high-resolution magnification endoscopy in Barrett's esophagus. *Gastroenterology* 2008;134:670–679.

160. Song LM, Adler DG, Conway JD, *et al.* Narrow band imaging and multiband imaging. *Gastrointest Endosc* 2008;67:581–589.

161. Kara MA, Ennahachi M, Fockens P, *et al.* Detection and classification of the mucosal and vascular patterns (mucosal morphology) in Barrett's esophagus by using narrow band imaging. *Gastrointest Endosc* 2006;64:155–166.

162. Sharma P, Bansal A, Mathur S, *et al.* The utility of a novel narrow band imaging endoscopy system in patients with Barrett's esophagus. *Gastrointest Endosc* 2006;64:167–175.

163. Wolfsen HC, Crook JE, Krishna M, *et al.* Prospective, controlled tandem endoscopy study of narrow band imaging for dysplasia detection in Barrett's esophagus. *Gastroenterology* 2008;135:24–31.

164. Curvers WL, Bohmer CJ, Mallant-Hent RC, *et al.* Mucosal morphology in Barrett's esophagus: interobserver agreement and role of narrow band imaging. *Endoscopy* 2008;40:799–805.

165. Kara MA, Peters FP, Rosmolen WD, *et al.* High-resolution endoscopy plus chromoendoscopy or narrow-band imaging in Barrett's esophagus: a prospective randomized crossover study. *Endoscopy* 2005;37:929–936.

166. Curvers WL, van den Broek FJ, Reitsma JB, *et al.* Systematic review of narrow-band imaging for the detection and differentiation of abnormalities in the esophagus and stomach. *Gastrointest Endosc* 2009;69:307–317.

167. Panjehpour M, Overholt BF, Vo-Dinh T, *et al.* Endoscopic fluorescence detection of high-grade dysplasia in Barrett's esophagus. *Gastroenterology* 1996;111:93–101.

168. Georgakoudi I, Jacobson BC, Van Dam J, *et al.* Fluorescence, reflectance, and light- scattering spectroscopy for evaluating dysplasia in patients with Barrett's esophagus. *Gastroenterology* 2001;120:1620–1629.

169. Lovat LB, Johnson K, Mackenzie GD, *et al.* Elastic scattering spectroscopy accurately detects high grade dysplasia and cancer in Barrett's oesophagus. *Gut* 2006;55:1078–1083.

170. Peery AF, Shaheen NJ. Optical coherence tomography in Barrett's esophagus: the road to clinical utility. *Gastrointest Endosc* 2010;71:231–234.

171. Wallace MB. Detecting dysplasia with optical coherence tomography. *Clin Gastroenterol Hepatol* 2006;4:36–37.

172. Kara MA, DaCosta RS, Streutker CJ, *et al.* Characterization of tissue autofluorescence in Barrett's esophagus by confocal fluorescence microscopy. *Dis Esophagus* 2007;20:141–150.

173. Kara MA, Peters FP, Ten Kate FJ, *et al*. Endoscopic video autofluorescence imaging may improve the detection of early neoplasia in patients with Barrett's esophagus. *Gastrointest Endosc* 2005;61:679–685.

174. Kara MA, Peters FP, Fockens P, *et al*. Endoscopic video-autofluorescence imaging followed by narrow band imaging for detecting early neoplasia in Barrett's esophagus. *Gastrointest Endosc* 2006;64:176–185.

175. Curvers WL, Singh R, Song LM, *et al*. Endoscopic tri-modal imaging for detection of early neoplasia in Barrett's oesophagus: a multi-centre feasibility study using high-resolution endoscopy, autofluorescence imaging and narrow band imaging incorporated in one endoscopy system. *Gut* 2008;57:167–172.

176. Kantsevoy SV, Adler DG, Conway JD, *et al*. Confocal laser endomicroscopy. *Gastrointest Endosc* 2009;70:197–200.

177. Kiesslich R, Gossner L, Goetz M, *et al*. In vivo histology of Barrett's esophagus and associated neoplasia by confocal laser endomicroscopy. *Clin Gastroenterol Hepatol* 2006;4:979–987.

178. Dunbar KB, Okolo P 3rd, Montgomery E, *et al*. Confocal laser endomicroscopy in Barrett's esophagus and endoscopically inapparent Barrett's neoplasia: a prospective, randomized, double-blind, controlled, crossover trial. *Gastrointest Endosc* 2009;70:645–654.

179. Pohl H, Rösch T, Vieth M, *et al*. Miniprobe confocal laser microscopy for the detection of invisible neoplasia in patients with Barrett's oesophagus. *Gut* 2008;57:1648–1653.

180. Wallace MB, Sharma P, Lightdale C, *et al*. Preliminary accuracy and interobserver agreement for the detection of intraepithelial neoplasia in Barrett's esophagus with probe-based confocal laser endomicroscopy. *Gastrointest Endosc* 2010;72:19–24.

181. Bajbouj M, Vieth M, Rösch T,*et al*. Probe-based confocal laser endomicroscopy compared with standard four-quadrant biopsy for evaluation of neoplasia in Barrett's esophagus. *Endoscopy* 2010;42:435–440.

182. Rudolph RE, Vaughan TL, Storer BE, *et al*. Effect of segment length on risk for neoplastic progression in patients with Barrett esophagus. *Ann Intern Med* 2000;132:612–620.

183. Hameeteman W, Tytgat GN, Houthoff HJ, *et al*. Barrett's esophagus: development of dysplasia and adenocarcinoma. *Gastroenterology* 1989;96:1249–1256.

184. Sharma P, Falk GW, Weston AP, *et al*. Dysplasia and cancer in a large multicenter cohort of patients with Barrett's esophagus. *Clin Gastroenterol Hepatol* 2006;4:566–572.

185. Offman JJ, Lewin K, Ramers C, *et al*. The economic impact of the diagnosis of dysplasia in Barrett's esophagus. *Am J Gastroenterol* 2000;95:2946–2952.

186. Conio M, Blanchi S, Lapertosa G, *et al*. Long-term endoscopic surveillance of patients with Barrett's esophagus. Incidence of dysplasia and adenocarcinoma: a prospective study. *Am J Gastroenterol* 2003;98:1931–1939.

187. Wani S, Puli SR, Shaheen NJ, *et al*. Esophageal adenocarcinoma in Barrett's esophagus after endoscopic ablative therapy: a meta-analysis and systematic review. *Am J Gastroenterol* 2009;104:502–513.

188. Srivastava A, Hornick JL, Li X, *et al*. Extent of low-grade dysplasia is a risk factor for the development of esophageal adenocarcinoma in Barrett's esophagus. *Am J Gastroenterol* 2007;102:483–493.

189. Reid BJ, Levine DS, Longton G, *et al*. Predictors of progression to cancer in Barrett's esophagus: baseline histology and flow cytometry identify low- and high-risk patient subsets. *Am J Gastroenterol* 2000;95:1669–1676.

190. Pellegrini CA, Pohl D. High-grade dysplasia in Barrett's esophagus: surveillance or operation? *J Gastrointest Surg* 2000;4: 131–134.

191. Weston AP, Sharma P, Topalovski M, *et al*. Long-term follow-up of Barrett's high-grade dysplasia. *Am J Gastroenterol* 2000;95:1888–1893.

192. Rastogi A, Puli S, El-Serag HB, *et al*. Incidence of esophageal adenocarcinoma in patients with Barrett's esophagus and high-grade dysplasia: a meta-analysis. *Gastrointest Endosc* 2008;67:394–398.

193. Tharavej C, Hagen JA, Peters JH, *et al*. Predictive factors of coexisting cancer in Barrett's high-grade dysplasia. *Surg Endosc* 2006;20:439–443.

194. Reid BJ. P53 and neoplastic progression in Barrett's esophagus. *Am J Gastroenterol* 2001;96:1321–1323.

195. Prevo LJ, Sanchez CA, Galipeau PC, *et al*. Reid BJ P53-mutant clones and field effects in Barrett's esophagus. *Cancer Res* 1999;59:4784–4787.

196. Wong DJ, Barrett MT, Stoger R, *et al*. p16INK4*a* promoter is hypermethylated at a high frequency in esophageal adenocarcinomas. *Cancer Res* 1997 57:2619–2622.

197. Reid BJ, Haggitt RC, Rubin CE, *et al*. Barrett's esophagus. Correlation between flow cytometry and histology in detection of patients at risk for adenocarcinoma. *Gastroenterology* 1987;93:1–11.

198. Reid BJ, Blount PL, Rubin CE, *et al*. Flow-cytometric and histological progression to malignancy in Barrett's esophagus: prospective endoscopic surveillance of a cohort. *Gastroenterology* 1992;102:1212–1219.

199. Reid BJ, Levine DS, Longton G, *et al*. Predictors of progression to cancer in Barrett's esophagus: baseline histology and flow cytometry identify low- and high-risk patient subsets. *Am J Gastroenterol* 2000;95:1669–1676.

200. Dunn JM, Mackenzie GD, Oukrif D, *et al*. Image cytometry accurately detects DNA ploidy abnormalities and predicts late relapse to high-grade dysplasia and adenocarcinoma in Barrett's oesophagus following photodynamic therapy. *Br J Cancer* 2010;102:1608–1617.

201. Fritcher EG, Brankley SM, Kipp BR, *et al*. A comparison of conventional cytology, DNA ploidy analysis, and fluorescence in situ hybridization for the detection of dysplasia and adenocarcinoma in patients with Barrett's esophagus. *Hum Pathol* 2008;39:1128–1135.

202. Reid BJ. P53 and neoplastic progression in Barrett's esophagus. *Am J Gastroenterol* 2001;96:1321–1323.

203. Sikkema M, Kerkhof M, Steyerberg EW, *et al*. Aneuploidy and overexpression of Ki67 and p53 as markers for neoplastic progression in Barrett's esophagus: a case-control study. *Am J Gastroenterol* 2009;104:2673–2680.

204. Schulmann K, Sterian A, Berki A, *et al*. Inactivation of p16, RUNX3, and HPP1 occurs early in Barrett's-associated neoplastic progression and predicts progression risk. *Oncogene* 2005;24:4138–4148.

205. Wang JS, Guo M, Montgomery EA, *et al*. DNA promoter hypermethylation of p16 and APC predicts neoplastic progres-

sion in Barrett's esophagus. *Am J Gastroenterol* 2009;104: 2153–2160.

206. Galipeau PC, Li X, Blount PL, *et al*. NSAIDs modulate CDKN2A, TP53, and DNA content risk for progression to esophageal adenocarcinoma. *PLoS Med* 2007;4:e67.

207. Sato F, Jin Z, Schulmann K, *et al*. Three-tiered risk stratification model to predict progression in Barrett's esophagus using epigenetic and clinical features. *PLoS ONE* 2008;3:e1890.

208. Triadafilopoulos G. Proton pump inhibitors for Barrett's oesophagus. *Gut* 2000;46:144–146.

209. Sampliner RE. Effect of up to 3 years of high-dose lansoprazole on Barrett's esophagus. *Am J Gastroenterol* 1994;89: 1844–1848.

210. Neumann CS, Iqbal TH, Cooper BT. Long term continuous omeprazole treatment of patients with Barrett's oesophagus. *Aliment Pharmacol Ther* 1995;9:451–454.

211. Cooper BT, Chapman W, Neumann CS, Gearty JC. Continuous treatment of Barrett's oesophagus patients with proton pump inhibitors up to 13 years: observations on regression and cancer incidence. *Aliment Pharmacol Ther* 2006;23: 727–733.

212. Wilkinson SP, Biddlestone L, Gore S, *et al*. Regression of columnar-lined (Barrett's) oesophagus with omeprazole 40 mg daily: results of 5 years of continuous therapy. *Aliment Pharmacol Ther* 1999;13:1205–1209.

213. Sharma P, Sampliner RE, Camargo E. Normalization of esophageal pH with high-dose proton pump inhibitor therapy does not result in regression of Barrett's esophagus. *Am J Gastroenterol* 1997;92:582–585.

214. Sharma P, Morales TG, Bhattacharyya A, *et al*. Squamous islands in Barrett's esophagus: what lies underneath? *Am J Gastroenterol* 1998;93:332–335.

215. Spechler SJ, Sharma P, Traxler B, *et al*. Gastric and esophageal pH in patients with Barrett's esophagus treated with three esomeprazole dosages: a randomized, double-blind, crossover trial. *Am J Gastroenterol* 2006;101:1964–1671.

216. Wani S, Sampliner RE, Weston AP, *et al*. Lack of predictors of normalization of oesophageal acid exposure in Barrett's oesophagus. *Aliment Pharmacol Ther* 2005;22:627–633.

217. Ouatu-Lascar R, Triadafilopoulos G. Complete elimination of reflux symptoms does not guarantee normalization of intraesophageal acid reflux in patients with Barrett's esophagus. *Am J Gastroenterol* 1998;93:711–716.

218. Lao-Sirieix P, Roy A, Worrall C, *et al*. Effect of acid suppression on molecular predictors for esophageal cancer. *Cancer Epidemiol Biomarkers Prev* 2006;15:288–293.

219. Nguyen DM, El-Serag HB, Henderson L, Stein D, Bhattacharyya A, Sampliner RE. Medication usage and the risk of neoplasia in patients with Barrett's esophagus. *Clin Gastroenterol Hepatol* 2009;7:1299–1304.

220. Hillman LC, Chiragakis L, Shadbolt B, *et al*. Proton-pump inhibitor therapy and the development of dysplasia in patients with Barrett's oesophagus. *Med J Aust* 2004;180:387–391.

221. Abbas AE, Deschamps C, Cassivi SD, *et al*. Barrett's esophagus: the role of laparoscopic fundoplication. *Ann Thorac Surg* 2004;77:393–396.

222. O'Riordan JM, Byrne PJ, Ravi N, *et al*. Long-term clinical and pathologic response of Barrett's esophagus after antireflux surgery. *Am J Surg* 2004;188:27–33.

223. Hofstetter WL, Peters JH, DeMeester TR, *et al*. Long-term outcome of antireflux surgery in patients with Barrett's esophagus. *Ann Surg* 2001;234:532–528.

224. Attwood SE, Lundell L, Hatlebakk JG, *et al*. Medical or surgical management of GERD patients with Barrett's esophagus: the LOTUS trial 3-year experience. *J Gastrointest Surg* 2008;12: 1646–1654.

225. DeMeester S, DeMeester T. Columnar mucosa and intestinal metaplasia of the esophagus: fifty years of controversy. *Ann Surg* 2000;231:303–321.

226. Ye W, Chow WH, Lagergren J, *et al*. Risk of adenocarcinomas of the esophagus and gastric cardia in patients with gastroesophageal reflux diseases and after antireflux surgery. *Gastroenterology* 2001;121:1286–1293.

227. Tran T, Spechler SJ, Richardson P, *et al*. Fundoplication and the risk of esophageal cancer in gastroesophageal reflux disease: a Veterans affairs cohort study. *Am J Gastroenterol* 2005;100: 1002–1008.

228. Corey KE, Schmitz SM, Shaheen NJ. Does a surgical antireflux procedure decrease the incidence of esophageal adenocarcinoma in Barrett's esophagus? A meta-analysis. *Am J Gastroenterol* 2003;98:2390–2394.

229. Chang EY, Morris CD, Seltman AK, *et al*. The effect of antireflux surgery on esophageal carcinogenesis in patients with Barrett esophagus: a systematic review. *Ann Surg* 2007;246: 11–21.

230. Kelloff GJ, Lippman SM, Dannenberg AJ, *et al*. Progress in chemoprevention drug development: the promise of molecular biomarkers for prevention of intraepithelial neoplasia and cancer–a plan to move forward. *Clin Cancer Res* 2006;12: 3661–3697.

231. Ogunwobi OO, Beales IL. Statins inhibit proliferation and induce apoptosis in Barrett's esophageal adenocarcinoma cells. *Am J Gastroenterol* 2008;103:825–837.

232. Bozikas A, Marsman WA, Rosmolen WD, *et al*. The effect of oral administration of ursodeoxycholic acid and high-dose proton pump inhibitors on the histology of Barrett's esophagus. *Dis Esophagus* 2008;21:346–354.

233. Kubo A, Corley DA. Meta-analysis of antioxidant intake and the risk of esophageal and gastric cardia adenocarcinoma. *Am J Gastroenterol* 2007;102:2323–2330.

234. Nguyen DM, Richardson P, El-Serag HB. Medications (NSAIDs, statins, proton pump inhibitors) and the risk of esophageal adenocarcinoma in patients with Barrett's esophagus. *Gastroenterology* 2010;138:2260–2266.

235. Jayaprakash V, Menezes RJ, Javle MM, *et al*. Regular aspirin use and esophageal cancer risk. *Int J Cancer* 2006;119: 202–207.

236. Anderson LA, Johnston BT, Watson RG, *et al*. Nonsteroidal anti-inflammatory drugs and the esophageal inflammation-metaplasia-adenocarcinoma sequence. *Cancer Res* 2006;66: 4975–4982.

237. Buttar NS, Wang KK, Leontovich O, *et al*. Chemoprevention of esophageal adenocarcinoma by COX-2 inhibitors in an animal model of Barrett's esophagus. *Gastroenterology* 2002;122: 1101–1112.

238. Heath EI, Canto MI, Piantadosi S, *et al*. Chemoprevention for Barrett's Esophagus Trial Research Group. Secondary chemoprevention of Barrett's esophagus with celecoxib: results

of a randomized trial. *J Natl Cancer Inst* 2007;99: 545–557.

239. Triadafilopoulos G, Kaur B, Sood S, *et al*. The effects of esome-prazole combined with aspirin or rofecoxib on prostaglandin E2 production in patients with Barrett's oesophagus. *Aliment Pharmacol Ther* 2006;23:997–1005.

240. Falk GW. The future of endoscopic treatment of early Barrett neoplasia: the endoscopist's view. *Endoscopy* 2008;40: 1041–1047.

241. Kelty CJ, Ackroyd R, Brown NJ, *et al*. Endoscopic ablation of Barrett's oesophagus: a randomized-controlled trial of photo-dynamic therapy vs. argon plasma coagulation. *Aliment Pharmacol Ther* 2004;20:1289–1296.

242. Dulai GS, Jensen DM, Cortina G, *et al*. Randomized trial of argon plasma coagulation vs. multipolar electrocoagulation for ablation of Barrett's esophagus. *Gastrointest Endosc* 2005;61: 232–240.

243. Sharma P, Wani S, Weston AP, *et al*. A randomised controlled trial of ablation of Barrett's oesophagus with multipolar elec-trocoagulation versus argon plasma coagulation in combina-tion with acid suppression: long term results. *Gut* 2006;55: 1233–1239.

244. Van Laethem JL, Peny MO, Salmon I, *et al*. Intramucosal adenocarcinoma arising under squamous re-epithelialisation of Barrett's oesophagus. *Gut* 2000;46:574–577.

245. Shand A, Dallal H, Palmer K, *et al*. Adenocarcinoma arising in columnar lined oesophagus following treatment with argon plasma coagulation. *Gut* 2001;48:580–581.

246. Mino-Kenudson M, Ban S, Ohana M, *et al*. Buried dysplasia and early adenocarcinoma arising in Barrett esophagus after porfimer-photodynamic therapy. *Am J Surg Pathol* 2007;31: 403–409.

247. Ganz RA, Utley DS, Stern RA, *et al*. Complete ablation of esophageal epithelium with a balloon-based bipolar electrode: a phased evaluation in the porcine and in the human esopha-gus. *Gastrointest Endosc* 2004;60:1002–1010.

248. Dunkin BJ, Martinez J, Bejarano PA, *et al*. Thin-layer ablation of human esophageal epithelium using a bipolar radiofre-quency balloon device. *Surg Endosc* 2006;20:125–130.

249. Sharma VK, Wang KK, Overholt BF, *et al*. Balloon-based, cir-cumferential, endoscopic radiofrequency ablation of Barrett's esophagus: 1-year follow-up of 100 patients. *Gastrointest Endosc* 2007;65:185–195.

250. Fleischer DE, Overholt BF, Sharma VK, *et al*. Endoscopic abla-tion of Barrett's esophagus: a multicenter study with 2.5-year follow-up. *Gastrointest Endosc* 2008;68:867–876.

251. Fleischer DE, Overholt BF, Sharma VK, *et al*. Endoscopic radi-ofrequency ablation of Barrett's esophagus: five-year durabi-litry outcomes from a prospective multi-center study trial. *Gastrointest Endosc* 2010;71:AB117.

252. Shaheen NJ, Sharma P, Overholt BF, *et al*. Radiofrequency ablation in Barrett's esophagus with dysplasia. *N Engl J Med* 2009;360:2277–2288.

253. Pouw RE, Gondrie JJ, Rygiel AM, *et al*. Properties of the neos-quamous epithelium after radiofrequency ablation of Barrett's esophagus containing neoplasia. *Am J Gastroenterol* 2009;104: 1366–1373.

254. Johnston MH, Eastone JA, Horwhat JD, *et al*. Cryoablation of Barrett's esophagus: a pilot study. *Gastrointest Endosc* 2005;62: 842–848.

255. Dumot JA, Vargo JJ, Falk GW, *et al*. An open-label, prospective trial of cryospray ablation for Barrett's esophagus high-grade dysplasia and early esophageal cancer in high-risk patients. *Gastrointest Endosc* 2009;70:635–644.

256. Shaheen NJ, Greenwald BD, Peery AF, *et al*. Safety and efficacy of endoscopic spray cryotherapy for Barrett's esophagus with high-grade dysplasia. *Gastrointest Endosc* 2010;71:680–685.

257. Overholt BF, Lightdale CJ, Wang KK, *et al*. Photodynamic therapy with porfimer sodium for ablation of high-grade dys-plasia in Barrett's esophagus: international, partially blinded, ran-domized phase III trial. *Gastrointest Endosc* 2005;62:488–498.

258. Overholt BF, Wang KK, Burdick JS, *et al*. Five-year efficacy and safety of photodynamic therapy with Photofrin in Barrett's high-grade dysplasia. *Gastrointest Endosc* 2007;66:460–468.

259. Prasad GA, Wang KK, Buttar NS, *et al*. Long-term survival following endoscopic and surgical treatment of high-grade dysplasia in Barrett's esophagus. *Gastroenterology* 2007;132: 1226–1233.

260. Krishnadath KK, Wang KK, Taniguchi K, *et al*. Persistent genetic abnormalities in Barrett's esophagus after photody-namic therapy. *Gastroenterology* 2000;119:624–630.

261. Hage M, Siersema PD, Vissers KJ, *et al*. Molecular evaluation of ablative therapy of Barrett's oesophagus. *J Pathol* 2005;205: 57–64.

262. Hage M, Siersema PD, Vissers KJ, *et al*. Genomic analysis of Barrett's esophagus after ablative therapy: persistence of genetic alterations at tumor suppressor loci. *Int J Cancer* 2006;118:155–160.

263. Dvorak K, Ramsey L, Payne CM, *et al*. Abnormal expression of biomarkers in incompletely ablated Barrett's esophagus. *Ann Surg* 2006;244:1031–1036.

264. Prasad GA, Wang KK, Halling KC, *et al*. Utility of biomarkers in prediction of response to ablative therapy in Barrett's esophagus. *Gastroenterology* 2008;135:370–379.

265. Prasad GA, Buttar NS, Wongkeesong LM, *et al*. Significance of neoplastic involvement of margins obtained by endoscopic mucosal resection in Barrett's esophagus. *Am J Gastroenterol* 2007;102:2380–2386.

266. Manner H, May A, Pech O, *et al*. Early Barrett's carcinoma with "low-risk" submucosal invasion: long-term results of endo-scopic resection with a curative intent. *Am J Gastroenterol* 2008;103:2589–2597.

267. Badreddine RJ, Prasad GA, Lewis JT, *et al*. Depth of submu-cosal invasion does not predict lymph node metastasis and survival of patients with esophageal carcinoma. *Clin Gastroenterol Hepatol* 2010;8:248–253.

268. Ell C, May A, Pech O, *et al*. Curative endoscopic resection of early esophageal adenocarcinomas (Barrett's cancer). *Gastrointest Endosc* 2007;65:3–10.

269. Pech O, Behrens A, May A, *et al*. Long-term results and risk factor analysis for recurrence after curative endoscopic therapy in 349 patients with high-grade intraepithelial neo-plasia and mucosal adenocarcinoma in Barrett's oesophagus. *Gut* 2008;57:1200–1206.

270. Seewald S, Akaraviputh T, Seitz U, *et al*. Circumferential EMR and complete removal of Barrett's epithelium: a new approach to management of Barrett's esophagus containing high-grade intraepithelial neoplasia and intramucosal carcinoma. *Gastrointest Endosc* 2003;57:854–859.

271. Giovannini M, Bories E, Pesenti C, *et al*. Circumferential endoscopic mucosal resection in Barrett's esophagus with high-grade intraepithelial neoplasia or mucosal cancer. Preliminary results in 21 patients. *Endoscopy* 2004;36:782–787.

272. Peters FP, Kara MA, Rosmolen WD, *et al*. Stepwise radical endoscopic resection is effective for complete removal of Barrett's esophagus with early neoplasia: a prospective study. *Am J Gastroenterol* 2006;101:1449–1457.

273. Lopes CV, Hela M, Pesenti C, *et al*. Long-term follow-up of complete Barrett's eradication endoscopic mucosal resection (CBE-EMR) for the treatment of high grade dysplasia and intramucosal carcinoma. *Endoscopy* 2007;39:1086–1091.

274. Lopes CV, Hela M, Pesenti C, *et al*. Circumferential endoscopic resection of Barrett's esophagus with high-grade dysplasia or early adenocarcinoma. *Surg Endosc* 2007;21:820–824.

275. Chennat J, Konda VJ, Ross AS, *et al*. Complete Barrett's eradication endoscopic mucosal resection: an effective treatment modality for high-grade dysplasia and intramucosal carcinoma– an American single-center experience. *Am J Gastroenterol* 2009;104:2684–2692.

276. Pouw R, Seewald S, Gondrie JJ, *et al*. Stepwise radical enoscopic resection for eradication of Barrett's esophagus with early neoplasia in acohort of 169 patients. *Gut* 2010;59:1169–1177.

277. Pouw RE, Wirths K, Eisendrath P, *et al*. Efficacy of radiofrequency ablation combined with endoscopic resection for Barrett's esophagus with early neoplasia. *Clin Gastroenterol Hepatol* 2010;8:23–29.

278. van Vilsteren FG, Pouw RE, Seewald S, *et al*. A multi-center randomized trial comparing stepwise radical endoscopic resection versus radiofrequency ablation for Barrett esophagus containing high-grade dysplasia and/or early cancer. *Gastrointest Endosc* 2009;69:AB133.

279. Prasad GA, Wu TT, Wigle DA, *et al*. Endoscopic and surgical treatment of mucosal (T1a) esophageal adenocarcinoma in Barrett's esophagus. *Gastroenterology* 2009;137:815–823.

280. Das A, Singh V, Fleischer DE, Sharma VK. A comparison of endoscopic treatment and surgery in early esophageal cancer: an analysis of surveillance epidemiology and end results data. *Am J Gastroenterol* 2008;103:1340–1345.

281. Schembre DB, Huang JL, Lin OS, Cantone N, Low DE. Treatment of Barrett's esophagus with early neoplasia: a comparison of endoscopic therapy and esophagectomy. *Gastrointest Endosc* 2008;67:595–601.

282. Hornick JL, Mino-Kenudson M, Lauwers GY, *et al*. Buried Barrett's epithelium following photodynamic therapy shows reduced crypt proliferation and absence of DNA content abnormalities. *Am J Gastroenterol* 2008;103:38–47.

283. Weston AP, Sharma P, Banerjee S, Mitreva D, Mathur S. Visible endoscopic and histologic changes in the cardia, before and after complete Barrett's esophagus ablation. *Gastrointest Endosc* 2005;61:515–521.

284. Sampliner RE, Camargo E, Prasad AR. Association of ablation of Barrett's esophagus with high grade dysplasia and adenocarcinoma of the gastric cardia. *Dis Esophagus* 2006;19:277–279.

285. Fass R, Garewal HS, Hayden CW, Ramsey L, Sampliner RE. Preferential repair by squamous epithelium of thermal induced injury to the proximal stomach in patients undergoing ablation of Barrett's esophagus. *Gastrointest Endosc* 2001;53:711–716.

286. Kariv R, Plesec TP, Goldblum JR, *et al*. The Seattle protocol does not more reliably predict the detection of cancer at the time of esophagectomy than a less intensive surveillance protocol. *Clin Gastroenterol Hepatol* 2009;7:653–658.

287. Rice TW. Esophagectomy is the treatment of choice for high-grade dysplasia in Barrett's esophagus. *Am J Gastroenterol* 2006;101:2177–2179.

288. Birkmeyer JD, Stukel TA, Siewers AE, *et al*. Surgeon volume and operative mortality in the United States. *N Engl J Med* 2003;349:2117–2127.

289. Chang LC, Oelschlager BK, Quiroga E, *et al*. Long term outcome of esophagectomy for high-grade dysplasia or cancer found during surveillance for Barrett's esophagus. *J Gastrointest Surg* 2006;10:341–346.

290. Moraca RJ, Low DE. Outcomes and health-related quality of life after esophagectomy for high-grade dysplasia and intramucosal cancer. *Arch Surg* 2006;141:545–549.

291. Williams VA, Watson TJ, Herbella FA, *et al*. Esophagectomy for high grade dysplasia is safe, curative, and results in good alimentary outcome. *J Gastrointest Surg* 2007;11:1589–1597.

292. Low DE, Kunz S, Schembre D, *et al*. Esophagectomy–it's not just about mortality anymore: standardized perioperative clinical pathways improve outcomes in patients with esophageal cancer. *J Gastrointest Surg* 2007;11:1395–1402.

293. De Boer AG, Genovesi PI, Sprangers MA, *et al*. Quality of life in long-term survivors after curative transhiatal oesophagectomy for oesophageal carcinoma. *Br J Surg* 2000;87:1716–1721.

294. Headrick JR, Nichols FC, Miller DL, *et al*. High-grade esophageal dysplasia: long-term survival and quality of life after esophagectomy. *Ann Thorac Surg* 2002;73:1697–1702.

28 Esophageal Strictures

Jason M. Lake and Roy K. H. Wong

Walter Reed Army Medical Center, Department of Medicine, Gastroenterology Service, and Uniformed Services University of the Health Sciences, Washington, DC, USA

Introduction

Benign esophageal strictures are thought to arise from a variety of esophageal injuries. The injury induces collagen deposition and fibrous tissue formation, resulting in a narrowing of the esophageal lumen. Approximately 70% of all benign esophageal strictures are peptic in origin, arising as a result of gastroesophageal reflux disease (GERD). The incidence of peptic strictures appears to be stable or even decreasing in recent years despite an increase in the prevalence of GERD, likely as a result of the widespread use of proton pump inhibitors (PPIs) which minimize esophageal injury [1–3]. The differential diagnoses of the remaining benign esophageal strictures are listed in Table 28.1.

Etiology and pathogenesis

Peptic strictures are rare with an overall incidence of fewer than 1 per 10 000 patient years, but occur in 7–23% of patients with untreated reflux esophagitis [2, 4]. They occur more frequently in men than in women, and are ten-fold more common in whites than African Americans [5–7]. Most patients with peptic strictures are older, have had a longer duration of GERD symptoms, and have abnormal esophageal motility when compared to GERD patients without peptic strictures [2, 8]. The increased incidence in elderly patients is likely due to many factors, including an increased risk of severe esophagitis, increased incidence and size of hiatal hernias, and increased us of non-steroidal anti-inflammatory drugs (NSAIDs) [9].

The mechanisms predisposing to the development of peptic strictures are similar to those in other forms of GERD and include the breakdown of the three primary areas of defense: antireflux barriers, luminal clearance, and epithelial resistance. The major mechanisms that disrupt the reflux barriers include a hypotensive resting lower esophageal sphincter (LES), a hiatal hernia, or transient LES relaxations. Although transient LES relaxations occur more often and represent the majority of reflux episodes in GERD patients, they are unlikely to play the major role in those with peptic strictures [10]. More likely, hypotensive LES and hiatal hernias allow prolonged esophageal acid exposure, resulting in complicated GERD, including both peptic strictures and Barrett's esophagus [11]. Several studies have demonstrated decreased LES pressures in patients with peptic strictures compared with asymptomatic controls or patients with milder GERD [11–13]. Ahtaridis et al. compared 25 consecutive patients with heartburn and 25 patients with peptic strictures and noted that those with peptic strictures had a mean LES resting pressure of 4.9 mmHg compared with 7.5 mmHg in those with heartburn. Importantly, no patient in the peptic stricture group had an LES pressure greater than 8 mmHg [12]. Other data have confirmed the presence of a defective LES in approximately 90% of those with a peptic stricture [11, 13]. Hiatal hernias are found in approximately 90% of those with peptic strictures [14–16]. Hiatal hernias likely contribute to GERD and stricture formation through several mechanisms. First, since they displace the LES from the crural diaphragm, the basal LES pressure and the length of the high pressure zone are decreased [17]. Additionally, the hernia sac may trap a small amount of acid, which then refluxes into the esophagus during subsequent swallows when the LES relaxes [18]. This mechanism increases esophageal acid exposure and contributes to delayed acid clearance.

Impaired esophageal motility has been demonstrated in those with peptic structures and also contributes to the delayed acid clearance [11, 12, 19]. Typically, the dysmotility includes simultaneous or repetitive contractions, but occasionally includes aperistalsis [11, 12]. Despite the increased acid exposure in the esophagus, patients with peptic strictures have the same gastric acid and pepsin secretion rates as matched controls [20].

The Esophagus, Fifth Edition. Edited by Joel E. Richter, Donald O. Castell.

Table 28.1 Differential diagnoses of benign esophageal strictures.

Gastroesophageal reflux
Corrosive ingestion
Crohn's disease
Eosinophilic esophagitis
Schatzki's ring
Infectious esophagitis
Epidermolysis bullosa
Foreign body reaction
Pill esophagitis:
Alendronate
Non-steroidal anti-inflammatory drugs
Ferrous sulfate
Phenytoin
Potassium chloride
Tetracycline
Quinidine
Vitamin C
Iatrogenic
Post-surgical:
Anastomotic
Heller myotomy for achalasia
Postendoscopic therapy:
Sclerotherapy
Endoscopic mucosal resection
Photodynamic therapy
Cryotherapy
Radiofrequency ablation
External beam radiation

Factors contributing to the compromise of epithelial resistance are many and include the medications listed in Table 28.1, alkaline reflux, and lack of salivary bicarbonate, such as in the scleroderma patient. Alkaline reflux of trypsin, bile, and pancreatic enzymes has been implicated as a contributing factor to both GERD and esophageal strictures. Through prolonged ambulatory pH monitoring, Attwood et al. found that Barrett's patients with complications, including 92% with peptic strictures, had significant alkaline reflux defined as pH of over 7 [21]. Ultimately, this refluxate, whether acidic or alkaline, produces an inflammatory reaction and edema in the lamina propria. This may progress to destruction of the muscularis mucosae, with the formation of fibrosis down to and including the circular muscle layer, causing narrowing of the distal esophagus [22].

Iatrogenic esophageal strictures result as complications of both endoscopic and surgical interventions. Unlike peptic strictures which result from esophageal acid exposure, iatrogenic strictures result from local ischemia with the development of fibrosis. Strictures develop in approximately 6% of patients undergoing radiofrequency ablation of dysplastic Barrett's esophagus [23]. Photodynamic therapy (PDT) for treatment of Barrett's esophagus with high-grade dysplasia,

intramucosal carcinoma, or T1 esophageal cancers results in esophageal strictures in 23% of patients, with a noted increase from 16% in those undergoing a single PDT session to 43% following a second session [24]. Esophageal cryotherapy using low-pressure nitrogen spray for the treatment of Barrett's esophagus or focal esophageal carcinoma results in esophageal strictures in fewer than 4% of patients [25]. Treatment of esophageal varices results in strictures in 2–20% of those treated with sclerotherapy, but rarely results from treatment with band ligation [26]. The likelihood of developing an anastomotic stricture following a surgical esophagectomy ranges from as low as 5% to as high as 46%, and is related to several operative factors, including type of anastomosis, anastomotic leakage, and intraoperative blood loss [27–31].

Caustic injuries of the esophagus (discussed in detail in Chapter 40) often result in esophageal strictures. Solutions with a pH below 2 or above 12 are highly corrosive. Alkali ingestion induces liquefaction necrosis and rapid tissue injury, which results in tissue sloughing several days after the ingestion. The subsequent bacterial invasion and inflammatory response result in granulation tissue formation. Collagen deposition occurs after 2 weeks with scarring following shortly thereafter and lasting for several months [32]. The scar retraction results in shortening of the esophagus, diminishes esophageal motility, and alters LES pressure [33]. In effect, these alterations promote acid reflux which further accelerates stricture formation [34]. Acid ingestion induces coagulation necrosis and eschar formation [32]. The degree of injury determines the likelihood of stricture with a greater than 80% chance of developing a stricture if areas of necrosis are seen in the esophagus [35].

Eosinophilic esophagitis has become increasingly identified as a cause of dysphagia in adults (see Chapter 36). It is a chronic inflammatory disease which may lead to remodeling of the esophagus with the development of fibrosis in the subepithelial layers [36]. The prevalence of esophageal strictures in eosinophilic esophagitis varies in the literature and encompasses both short- and long-segment esophageal narrowing [36].

Epidermolysis bullosa encompasses many phenotypically distinct entities characterized by the presence of marked fragility of epithelial tissues. This results in the repeated development of blisters and non-healing wounds following minor trauma. Of the subtypes, dystrophic epidermolysis bullosa most commonly involves the esophagus. Acutely, esophageal blistering from minor food trauma may cause odynophagia and dysphagia. After repeating insults, fibrosis and scarring result in esophageal stricture formation [37].

Conditions predisposing to peptic strictures

In addition to those listed above, several other conditions may predispose to the development of esophageal strictures. These include scleroderma, the Zollinger–Ellison syndrome, prolonged placement of a nasogastric tube, esophageal inlet patches, and a history of NSAID use.

Systemic sclerosis, or scleroderma, involves the esophagus in up to 90% of patients [38]. It results in abnormal esophageal motility, typically distal esophageal aperistalsis (in the smooth muscle esophagus), and a hypotensive LES [39]. Delayed gastric emptying also occurs in about two-thirds of patients and contributes to the severity of GERD [40]. Peptic strictures develop in up to 41% of patients with scleroderma with erosive esophagitis [41].

The Zollinger-Ellison syndrome results in basal gastric acid secretion more than four times normal [42]. Hoffmann *et al.* studied 295 patients at the National Institutes of Health and demonstrated that 15% of those with Zollinger-Ellison syndrome associated with multiple endocrine neoplasia type 1 (MEN1) developed peptic strictures as compared with only 5% of those with sporadic Zollinger-Ellison syndrome. It is hypothesized that the hyperparathyroidism and hypercalcemia that results from the MEN1 makes acid secretion more difficult to control with PPIs and thus leads to a higher rate of peptic strictures [42].

Heterotopic gastric mucosa (inlet patch) located in the proximal esophagus has been associated with increased acid secretion and the development of peptic strictures [43–45]. The incidence of inlet patches has been reported to be 1–5% of patients with upper gastrointestinal complaints and may be associated with a higher rate of esophagitis and Barrett's esophagus, but its contribution to peptic strictures is based on isolated case reports [46–49].

Although the prolonged use of nasogastric tubes (NGTs) has been reported to be associated with the development of esophageal strictures, shorter term studies have not demonstrated an increase in reflux after NGT placement [50–52].

Aspirin and NSAID use, even low-dose Aspirin, are independently associated with esophageal strictures. Retrospective studies report from 31% to 64% of patients with benign esophageal strictures have taken NSAIDs [53–55]. The mechanism in which they contribute to stricture formation or aggravation is likely multifactorial and includes decreasing protective mucosal prostaglandins, as well as inducing direct effects when a pill lodges in the esophagus causing esophagitis [56].

Clinical presentation

The insidious onset of solid food dysphagia is the most common presentation in patients with benign esophageal strictures. Careful history alone can accurately diagnose the cause of dysphagia in 80% of cases [57]. A history of antecedent heartburn is present in at least two-thirds of cases of peptic strictures [2, 58]. In some patients, pyrosis may resolve over time and the diameter of the stricture decreases and impedes acid reflux. A history of intermittent solid food

dysphagia is most characteristic of a Schatzki's ring. A history of dysphagia to liquids suggests a motility disorder as opposed to an esophageal stricture. Weight loss is uncommon with peptic strictures and should increase the suspicion for a malignancy or achalasia. A careful history should include medications as they may complicate peptic strictures by causing pill-induced esophagitis. In other cases, strictures may be erroneously attributed to GERD when a medication was the true etiology [59, 60].

In certain cases, the patient's localization of the dysphagia may help to anticipate the location of the obstructing lesion. Generally, the lesion is located at the level of or distal to the point where the patient localizes the dysphagia. Symptoms in the lower sternal area reliably predict a distal esophageal stricture. On the other hand, proximal esophageal dysphagia does not reliably predict the location of the lesion as it may be caused by a stricture anywhere from that point to the distal esophagus [61].

Physical examination uncommonly delineates the cause of dysphagia. However, signs of joint abnormalities, calcinosis, sclerodactyly, or telangectasias are supportive of an esophageal abnormality secondary to scleroderma or other collagen vascular disease. A Virchow's node (palpable left supraclavicular lymph node) suggests an intra-abdominal neoplasm, such as adenocarcinoma of the gastroesophageal junction.

Diagnosis

Barium swallow is generally regarded as the initial diagnostic procedure of choice in patients experiencing solid food dysphagia. The barium esophagram is at least as sensitive as endoscopy for the detection of esophageal strictures of less than 1 cm in diameter and is likely more sensitive than endoscopy in strictures that are greater than 1 cm in diameter [62, 63]. It provides useful information, such as stricture location, diameter, and length, which may guide subsequent endoscopic evaluation and therapy. Additionally, barium swallow may more accurately identify alternate or coexistent conditions, such as Schatzki's ring, achalasia, Zenker's or epiphrenic diverticula, or paraesophageal hernias. When done by experienced radiologists, benign esophageal strictures can be confidently differentiated from malignant strictures by a smooth, symmetric, tapered appearance [16].

Endoscopy remains an essential component in the evaluation of esophageal strictures (Figure 28.1). Despite the high predictive value of benign features on a barium study in patients with peptic strictures, endoscopy offers evaluation for the presence of Barrett's esophagus or erosive esophagitis and allows for endoscopic therapy and dilation to relieve dysphagia [64, 65]. Interestingly, although initial studies reported a higher rate of Barrett's esophagus in those with peptic strictures, further data have suggested a similar rate

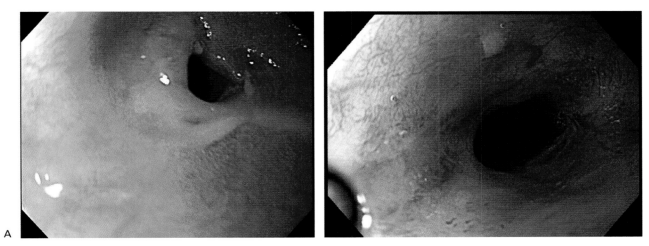

Figure 28.1 (A) Peptic stricture (reproduced courtesy of Milton Smith MD). (B) Radiation stricture.

of Barrett's esophagus in those with and without peptic strictures [66, 67]. Endoscopy also allows for the biopsy of indeterminate strictures that do not demonstrate classic benign features on barium swallow [16]. Typically, peptic strictures occur in the distal esophagus at the squamocolumnar junction and a location elsewhere should raise suspicion for other etiologies. Biopsy should not preclude dilation at the time of initial endoscopy in benign strictures as it has not been associated with an increase in complication rate.

Although other systems have been created to classify strictures, it is most clinically useful to designate them as either simple or complex [68, 69]. Simple strictures are those that are short, focal, not angulated, and easily traversed by an endoscope. Complex strictures are long (>2 cm), angulated or irregular, or have a diameter that does not allow passage of an endoscope [68]. The classification of these strictures aids in management decisions and may predict response to therapy.

Treatment

Acid-suppressive therapy

Dysphagia in patients with peptic stricture is due to both decreased luminal diameter and often coexistent esophagitis [70]. This is supported by multiple studies in which the use of PPIs, which are superior to H_2 blockers, has resulted in healed esophagitis, improved dysphagia, decreased need for esophageal dilation, and prolonged interval between esophageal dilations [71–77]. Prior to PPIs, the typical course of peptic strictures was one in which repeated dilations were required in the majority of patients regardless of whether or not they were taking H_2 blockers [58, 78–81]. Although the data are variable, it is likely that aggressive acid suppression decreases the need for repeated dilations in those with peptic

strictures to approximately 30% [72]. Ultimately, patients with peptic strictures should be maintained on long-term PPIs to maintain healing of esophagitis and reduce the need for stricture dilation.

Bougienage

Esophageal dilation has been practiced since at least the 16th century for the treatment of esophageal strictures. The use of tapered wax wands and whale bones to dislodge material stuck in the esophagus is well documented [82]. Whale bones and wax wands have been replaced by modern flexible bougies and balloon dilators passed through the scope. There are currently three types of dilators commonly used in the United States and the decision of which to use is based on several factors, including the characteristics of the stricture. Mercury- or tungsten-filled rubber bougies with blunt (Hurst) or tapered (Maloney) tips are passed blindly without the use of a guidewire, and are indicated in straight strictures with a diameter of greater than 10–12 mm. With narrower or irregular strictures, the tip may curl up and thus rubber bougie dilators should not be used [83]. Additionally, they should be avoided in those with a large hiatal hernia or esophageal diverticuli as the tip may lodge in the anatomic defect and increase the risk of perforation. Savary-Gilliard and American-type polyvinyl bougies are passed over a guidewire with or without fluoroscopy, and thus are indicated for irregular strictures or strictures with a diameter of less than 10–12 mm. Placement of the guidewire occurs through the endoscope after the stricture has been traversed. The tip of the guidewire should be placed distal to the stricture, ideally in the gastric antrum. Through-the-scope (TTS) balloon dilators are passed over a guidewire under direct endoscopic visualization (Figure 28.2). Used with fluoroscopy, they can be utilized to dilate strictures that cannot be traversed by the endoscope. Since TTS balloons generate a

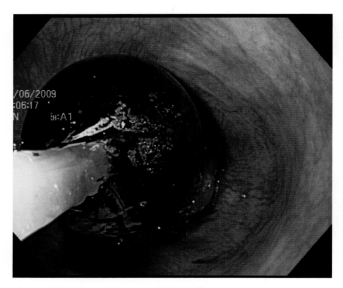

Figure 28.2 Through-the-scope balloon dilator.

radial dilating force, as opposed to bougies that depend on advancing a tapered dilator, they may provide an advantage when dilating epidermolysis bullosa-associated strictures by decreasing mucosal damage [84]. Unlike bougies, TTS balloons are not reusable and thus are more expensive to use. Fluoroscopy should be considered with guidewire-assisted bougies or TTS balloons if the stricture is complex and can aid in visualizing passage and location of guidewires, dilators, and balloons.

According to the American Society for Gastrointestinal Endoscopy (ASGE) guidelines for esophageal dilation released in 2006, patients should discontinue anticoagulants prior to dilation [85]. Based on updated American Heart Association recommendations for prevention of infective endocarditis, the ASGE guidelines for antibiotic prophylaxis for gastrointestinal endoscopy published in 2008 do not recommend the use of antibiotic prophylaxis in those undergoing esophageal dilation, regardless of pre-existing heart conditions [86]. Patients should be counseled about the risk of perforation prior to the procedure.

Although there is some retrospective data suggesting that more aggressive dilation can be safely performed, the "rule of threes" should generally be followed when dilating esophageal strictures [85, 87–89]. The initial dilator should approximate the estimated diameter of the stricture. Sequential dilation should then be performed with moderate resistance marking the first dilation. No more than three consecutive dilators in 1-mm increments should be passed in a single session. There have been numerous studies comparing the various types of dilators, but there is no clear evidence that one type is more effective than the others [90–98]. Regardless of the type of dilation performed, the goal is relief of dysphagia, which usually occurs when the

luminal diameter reaches at least 13–15 mm. In patients with peptic strictures a graded stepwise approach to between 13 and 20 mm improves symptoms in 85–93% of patients [87]. Caustic, post-radiation, and post-surgical strictures appear to be more refractory to dilation and may require several repeated dilation sessions, with difficultly achieving a diameter of greater than 15 mm [1]. Several factors have been suggested to predict the need for recurrent stricture dilation, including an initial presentation with weight loss and the absence of heartburn [99]. The need for repeated dilations increases as the stricture length increases and the luminal diameter decreases [100]. After dilation, the persistence of heartburn or inability to pass a 12-mm barium pill after dilation also predict the need for repeat dilation [101, 102]. For those patients with persistent or recurrent non-inflammatory strictures, a uniform classification has been proposed [103]. A refractory stricture is defined as one that is unable to be dilated to a diameter of 14 mm over five sessions at 2-week intervals. A recurrent stricture is defined as one that is dilated to the target diameter of 14 mm but does not maintain that diameter for 4 weeks.

The most serious complication of esophageal dilation is perforation. The rate of perforation after dilation of esophageal strictures has generally been reported to be 0.1–0.4%, but has been noted to be as high as 1.1% [83, 104, 105]. Factors that increase the perforation rate include the presence of a complex or post-radiation stricture as well as dilation performed by an inexperienced endoscopist [83, 105, 106].

Lastly, the technique of self-bougienage can be taught to motivated patients who require frequent dilation and are not candidates for other treatment modalities. Limited published data suggest that this may be both safe and effective in patients with benign esophageal strictures [107–109].

Intralesional injection of steroids

Studies evaluating the injection of corticosteroids into esophageal strictures date back over four decades. Corticosteroids are thought to reduce the inflammation and delay or prevent the fibrosis that are inherent in benign esophageal strictures. Until recently, data regarding the efficacy of intralesional steroid injection were limited to uncontrolled case series, which indicated that it may reduce stricture recurrence following dilation [110–115]. The limited randomized data support these case series and show that the combination of steroid injection and acid suppression significantly diminished the need for both repeat dilation and average time to repeat dilation compared to sham injection and acid suppression in those with recurrent peptic strictures [116, 117]. Endoscopic ultrasound may be useful in guiding the steroid injection into the thickest aspect of the stricture [118]. Typical injection regimens include four 1-mL aliquots of 10 mg/mL triamcinolone acetonide in a four-quadrant pattern in combination with stricture dilation. Although the role of intralesional steroid injection remains to be defined, it is reasonable to consider this therapy in those who have a short-lived response to dilation alone.

Esophageal stenting

Self-expanding metal stents (SEMSs) have long been used in the palliation of dysphagia from esophageal and gastric cardia malignancies. In 2009, Siersma collated the data from 12 studies including a total of 168 patients who underwent SEMS placement for benign esophageal strictures [119]. The earlier studies primarily used uncovered SEMS whereas the later studies primarily used partially or fully covered SEMS. Stent migration was noted in 14% of patients and hyperplastic tissue ingrowth or overgrowth was found to cause recurrent dysphagia in 17%. Although long-term data was only reported on 30 patients, 47% had no evidence of recurrent stricture. The type of stricture appears to influence long-term success with post-radiation strictures responding the best. Additionally, shorter strictures appeared to have a lower rate of recurrence than longer strictures [119].

Self-expanding plastic stents (SEPS) were developed in an attempt to decrease the risk of hyperplastic tissue ingrowth or overgrowth that occurs with the SEMS. In the 2009 systematic review, Siersma collated data from the nine published studies including 162 patients who underwent SEPS placement for benign esophageal strictures [119]. Hyperplastic overgrowth was rare and was seen in only one of the nine included series. Stent migration was higher than that seen with SEMS and occurred in 47–64%, with a greater likelihood when used in proximal and distal strictures as opposed to mid-esophageal strictures. In eight of the nine reviewed studies, long-term improvement in dysphagia after stent removal was seen in 50 of 129 (39%) of patients. In the other reviewed study, this proportion was even lower with only five of 83 (6%) interventions resulting in long-term success. Serious complications occurred in 6% of patients and included perforations (1%), fistulae (1%), bleeding (2%), and severe pain requiring stent removal (2%) [119]. Despite the inconsistent results, it has been proposed that placement of SEPS may be cost-effective if it results in two or more esophageal dilations being avoided [120].

Currently, given the overall success rate of less than 50% after stenting of benign esophageal strictures, it should cautiously be considered in those with refractory strictures that have not responded to other treatment modalities.

Endoscopic incision

Endoscopic incision has been proposed to treat patients with refractory, benign esophageal strictures. Reported methods for endoscopic incision include electrocautery with and without argon plasma coagulation (APC) as well as with endoscopic scissors [121–123]. In nearly all cases, these endoscopic therapies were applied to those with anastomotic strictures. In the largest of the retrospective studies, needle knife electrocautery in 20 patients with persistent anastomotic strictures resulted in complete relief of dysphagia in all 12 patients with strictures of less than 1 cm after a single session and in the remaining eight patients with longer strictures after a mean of three sessions [121]. A subsequent randomized study of 62 patients with refractory anastomotic strictures compared needle knife electrocautery to Savary bougienage, and found no differences in clinical outcomes or number of dilations required and there were no complications in either group [124]. Clearly, further data may help elucidate the role of endoscopic incisional therapy in those with refractory benign esophageal strictures.

Surgery

Surgical management for benign esophageal strictures is reserved for those who are not candidates or are not responsive to the above interventions, or those who have refractory esophagitis. There are several surgical approaches, ranging from minimally invasive techniques that are often used with less complex strictures to more invasive procedures for those who have complex strictures [125]. Typically, with peptic strictures, an antireflux surgery can be combined with intraoperative esophageal dilation. The ability to perform the antireflux procedure laparoscopically has decreased the morbidity of this option. In more complex strictures, or strictures of other etiologies, the strictured esophagus may need to be surgically resected. There are many surgical approaches for this, ranging from minimally invasive (e.g. transgastric stricture resection with endoscopic assistance) to complex [125, 126]. When more extensive resections are required, a gastric pull-up or intestinal (colon or jejunum) interposition is done to reconstruct the esophagus [125, 127].

References

1. Piotet E, Escher A, Monnier P. Esophageal and pharyngeal strictures: report on 1,862 endoscopic dilatations using the Savary-Gilliard technique. *Eur Arch Otorhinolaryngol* 2008;265: 357–364.

2. Ruigomez A, Garcia Rodriguez LA, Wallander MA, Johansson S, Eklund S. Esophageal stricture: incidence, treatment patterns, and recurrence rate. *Am J Gastroenterol* 2006;101:2685–2692.

3. Nayyar AK, Royston C, Bardhan KD. Oesophageal acid-peptic strictures in the histamine H2 receptor antagonist and proton pump inhibitor era. *Dig Liver Dis* 2003;35:143–150.

4. Richter JE. Peptic strictures of the esophagus. *Gastroenterol Clin North Am* 1999;28:875–891, vi.

5. Spechler SJ, Jain SK, Tendler DA, Parker RA. Racial differences in the frequency of symptoms and complications of gastro-oesophageal reflux disease. *Aliment Pharmacol Ther* 2002;16: 1795–1800.

6. Wang A, Mattek NC, Holub JL, Lieberman DA, Eisen GM. Prevalence of complicated gastroesophageal reflux disease and Barrett's esophagus among racial groups in a multi-center consortium. *Dig Dis Sci* 2009;54:964–971.

7. El-Serag HB, Sonnenberg A. Association of esophagitis and esophageal strictures with diseases treated with nonsteroidal anti-inflammatory drugs. *Am J Gastroenterol* 1997;92:52–56.

8. Marks RD, Shukla M. Diagnosis and management of peptic esophageal strictures. *Gastroenterologist* 1996;4:223–237.

9. Pilotto A, Franceschi M, Leandro G, et al. Clinical features of reflux esophagitis in older people: a study of 840 consecutive patients. *J Am Geriatr Soc* 2006;54:1537–1542.

10. Grossi L, Ciccaglione AF, Travaglini N, Marzio L. Transient lower esophageal sphincter relaxations and gastroesophageal reflux episodes in healthy subjects and GERD patients during 24 hours. *Dig Dis Sci* 2001;46:815–821.

11. Zaninotto G, DeMeester TR, Bremner CG, Smyrk TC, Cheng SC. Esophageal function in patients with reflux-induced strictures and its relevance to surgical treatment. *Ann Thorac Surg* 1989;47:362–370.

12. Ahtaridis G, Snape WJ Jr, Cohen S. Clinical and manometric findings in benign peptic strictures of the esophagus. *Dig Dis Sci* 1979;24:858–861.

13. Stein HJ, Barlow AP, DeMeester TR, Hinder RA. Complications of gastroesophageal reflux disease. Role of the lower esophageal sphincter, esophageal acid and acid/alkaline exposure, and duodenogastric reflux. *Ann Surg* 1992;216:35–43.

14. Berstad A, Weberg R, Froyshov Larsen I, Hoel B, Hauer-Jensen M. Relationship of hiatus hernia to reflux oesophagitis. A prospective study of coincidence, using endoscopy. *Scand J Gastroenterol* 1986;21:55–58.

15. Ho CS, Rodrigues PR. Lower esophageal strictures, benign or malignant? *J Can Assoc Radiol* 1980;31:110–113.

16. Gupta S, Levine MS, Rubesin SE, Katzka DA, Laufer I. Usefulness of barium studies for differentiating benign and malignant strictures of the esophagus. *AJR Am J Roentgenol* 2003;180:737–744.

17. Kahrilas PJ, Lin S, Chen J, Manka M. The effect of hiatus hernia on gastro-oesophageal junction pressure. *Gut* 1999;44: 476–482.

18. Mittal RK, Lange RC, McCallum RW. Identification and mechanism of delayed esophageal acid clearance in subjects with hiatus hernia. *Gastroenterology* 1987;92:130–135.

19. Barham CP, Gotley DC, Mills A, Alderson D. Oesophageal acid clearance in patients with severe reflux oesophagitis. *Br J Surg* 1995;82:333–337.

20. Hirschowitz BI. Gastric acid and pepsin secretion in patients with Barrett's esophagus and appropriate controls. *Dig Dis Sci* 1996;41:1384–1391.

21. Attwood SE, DeMeester TR, Bremner CG, Barlow AP, Hinder RA. Alkaline gastroesophageal reflux: implications in the development of complications in Barrett's columnar-lined lower esophagus. *Surgery* 1989;106:764–770.

22. Awad ZT, Filipi CJ. The short esophagus: pathogenesis, diagnosis, and current surgical options. *Arch Surg* 2001;136:113–114.

23. Shaheen NJ, Sharma P, Overholt BF, et al. Radiofrequency ablation in Barrett's esophagus with dysplasia. *N Engl J Med* 2009;360:2277–2288.

24. Yachimski P, Puricelli WP, Nishioka NS. Patient predictors of esophageal stricture development after photodynamic therapy. *Clin Gastroenterol Hepatol* 2008;6:302–308.

25. Greenwald BD, Dumot JA, Horwhat JD, Lightdale CJ, Abrams JA. Safety, tolerability, and efficacy of endoscopic low-pressure liquid nitrogen spray cryotherapy in the esophagus. *Dis Esophagus* 2010;23:13–19.

26. Eisen GM, Baron TH, Dominitz JA, et al. Complications of upper GI endoscopy. *Gastrointest Endosc* 2002;55:784–793.

27. Honkoop P, Siersema PD, Tilanus HW, Stassen LP, Hop WC, van Blankenstein M. Benign anastomotic strictures after transhiatal esophagectomy and cervical esophagogastrostomy: risk factors and management. *J Thorac Cardiovasc Surg* 1996;111:1141–1146; discussion 1147–1148.

28. McManus KG, Ritchie AJ, McGuigan J, Stevenson HM, Gibbons JR. Sutures, staplers, leaks and strictures. A review of anastomoses in oesophageal resection at Royal Victoria Hospital, Belfast 1977–1986. *Eur J Cardiothorac Surg* 1990;4: 97–100.

29. Griffin SM, Woods SD, Chan A, Chung SC, Li AK. Early and late surgical complications of subtotal oesophagectomy for squamous carcinoma of the oesophagus. *J R Coll Surg Edinb* 1991;36:170–173.

30. Fok M, Ah-Chong AK, Cheng SW, Wong J. Comparison of a single layer continuous hand-sewn method and circular stapling in 580 oesophageal anastomoses. *Br J Surg* 1991;78: 342–345.

31. Lam TC, Fok M, Cheng SW, Wong J. Anastomotic complications after esophagectomy for cancer. A comparison of neck and chest anastomoses. *J Thorac Cardiovasc Surg* 1992;104: 395–400.

32. Ramasamy K, Gumaste VV. Corrosive ingestion in adults. *J Clin Gastroenterol* 2003;37:119–124.

33. Bautista A, Varela R, Villanueva A, Estevez E, Tojo R, Cadranel S. Motor function of the esophagus after caustic burn. *Eur J Pediatr Surg* 1996;6:204–207.

34. Mutaf O, Genc A, Herek O, Demircan M, Ozcan C, Arikan A. Gastroesophageal reflux: a determinant in the outcome of caustic esophageal burns. *J Pediatr Surg* 1996;31:1494–1495.

35. Zargar SA, Kochhar R, Mehta S, Mehta SK. The role of fiberoptic endoscopy in the management of corrosive ingestion and modified endoscopic classification of burns. *Gastrointest Endosc* 1991;37:165–169.

36. Straumann A. The natural history and complications of eosinophilic esophagitis. *Gastrointest Endosc Clin North Am* 2008;18:99–118; ix.

37. Fine JD, Mellerio JE. Extracutaneous manifestations and complications of inherited epidermolysis bullosa: part I. Epithelial associated tissues. *J Am Acad Dermatol* 2009;61:367–384; quiz 385–386.

38. Ntoumazios SK, Voulgari PV, Potsis K, Koutis E, Tsifetaki N, Assimakopoulos DA. Esophageal involvement in scleroderma: gastroesophageal reflux, the common problem. *Semin Arthritis Rheum* 2006;36:173–181.

39. Yarze JC, Varga J, Stampfl D, Castell DO, Jimenez SA. Esophageal function in systemic sclerosis: a prospective evaluation of motility and acid reflux in 36 patients. *Am J Gastroenterol* 1993;88:870–876.

40. Sridhar KR, Lange RC, Magyar L, Soykan I, McCallum RW. Prevalence of impaired gastric emptying of solids in systemic sclerosis: diagnostic and therapeutic implications. *J Lab Clin Med* 1998;132:541–546.

41. Zamost BJ, Hirschberg J, Ippoliti AF, Furst DE, Clements PJ, Weinstein WM. Esophagitis in scleroderma. Prevalence and risk factors. *Gastroenterology* 1987;92:421–428.

42. Hoffmann KM, Gibril F, Entsuah LK, Serrano J, Jensen RT. Patients with multiple endocrine neoplasia type 1 with gastrinomas have an increased risk of severe esophageal disease including stricture and the premalignant condition, Barrett's esophagus. *J Clin Endocrinol Metab* 2006;91:204–212.

43. Yarborough CS, McLane RC. Stricture related to an inlet patch of the esophagus. *Am J Gastroenterol* 1993;88:275–276.

44. Steadman C, Kerlin P, Teague C, Stephenson P. High esophageal stricture: a complication of "inlet patch" mucosa. *Gastroenterology* 1988;94:521–524.

45. Galan AR, Katzka DA, Castell DO. Acid secretion from an esophageal inlet patch demonstrated by ambulatory pH monitoring. *Gastroenterology* 1998;115:1574–1576.

46. Jacobs E, Dehou MF. Heterotopic gastric mucosa in the upper esophagus: a prospective study of 33 cases and review of literature. *Endoscopy* 1997;29:710–715.

47. Tang P, McKinley MJ, Sporrer M, Kahn E. Inlet patch: prevalence, histologic type, and association with esophagitis, Barrett esophagus, and antritis. *Arch Pathol Lab Med* 2004;128:444–447.

48. Akbayir N, Alkim C, Erdem L, et al. Heterotopic gastric mucosa in the cervical esophagus (inlet patch): endoscopic prevalence, histological and clinical characteristics. *J Gastroenterol Hepatol* 2004;19:891–896.

49. Maconi G, Pace F, Vago L, Carsana L, Bargiggia S, Bianchi Porro G. Prevalence and clinical features of heterotopic gastric mucosa in the upper oesophagus (inlet patch). *Eur J Gastroenterol Hepatol* 2000;12:745–749.

50. Beg MH, Reyazuddin. Distal esophageal stricture due to indwelling nasogastric tube. *Indian J Chest Dis Allied Sci* 1988;30:64–66.

51. Zaninotto G, Bonavina L, Pianalto S, Fassina A, Ancona E. Esophageal strictures following nasogastric intubation. *Int Surg* 1986;71:100–103.

52. Kuo B, Castell DO. The effect of nasogastric intubation on gastroesophageal reflux: a comparison of different tube sizes. *Am J Gastroenterol* 1995;90:1804–1807.

53. Kim SL, Hunter JG, Wo JM, Davis LP, Waring JP. NSAIDs, aspirin, and esophageal strictures: are over-the-counter medications harmful to the esophagus? *J Clin Gastroenterol* 1999;29:32–34.

54. Wilkins WE, Ridley MG, Pozniak AL. Benign stricture of the oesophagus: role of non-steroidal anti-inflammatory drugs. *Gut* 1984;25:478–480.

55. Heller SR, Fellows IW, Ogilvie AL, Atkinson M. Non-steroidal anti-inflammatory drugs and benign oesophageal stricture. *Br Med J (Clin Res Ed)* 1982;285:167–168.

56. Marks RD, Richter JE. Peptic strictures of the esophagus. *Am J Gastroenterol* 1993;88:1160–1173.

57. Castell DO, Donner MW. Evaluation of dysphagia: a careful history is crucial. *Dysphagia* 1987;2:65–71.

58. Patterson DJ, Graham DY, Smith JL, et al. Natural history of benign esophageal stricture treated by dilatation. *Gastroenterology* 1983;85:346–350.

59. Bonavina L, DeMeester TR, McChesney L, Schwizer W, Albertucci M, Bailey RT. Drug-induced esophageal strictures. *Ann Surg* 1987;206:173–183.

60. Kikendall JW. Pill esophagitis. *J Clin Gastroenterol* 1999;28:298–305.

61. Wilcox CM, Alexander LN, Clark WS. Localization of an obstructing esophageal lesion. Is the patient accurate? *Dig Dis Sci* 1995;40:2192–2196.

62. Ott DJ, Chen YM, Wu WC, Gelfand DW. Endoscopic sensitivity in the detection of esophageal strictures. *J Clin Gastroenterol* 1985;7:121–125.

63. Ott DJ, Gelfand DW, Lane TG, Wu WC. Radiologic detection and spectrum of appearances of peptic esophageal strictures. *J Clin Gastroenterol* 1982;4:11–15.

64. Ott DJ. Radiographic techniques and efficacy in evaluating esophageal dysphagia. *Dysphagia* 1990;5:192–203.

65. Ott DJ. Barium evaluation of esophageal strictures: still useful or a bust? *Am J Gastroenterol* 2003;98:2563–2564.

66. Spechler SJ, Sperber H, Doos WG, Schimmel EM. The prevalence of Barrett's esophagus in patients with chronic peptic esophageal strictures. *Dig Dis Sci* 1983;28:769–774.

67. Kim SL, Wo JM, Hunter JG, Davis LP, Waring JP. The prevalence of intestinal metaplasia in patients with and without peptic strictures. *Am J Gastroenterol* 1998;93:53–55.

68. Lew RJ, Kochman ML. A review of endoscopic methods of esophageal dilation. *J Clin Gastroenterol* 2002;35:117–126.

69. Braghetto I, Csendes A, Burdiles P, Korn O, Compan A, Guerra JF. Barrett's esophagus complicated with stricture: correlation between classification and the results of the different therapeutic options. *World J Surg* 2002;26:1228–1233.

70. Dakkak M, Hoare RC, Maslin SC, Bennett JR. Oesophagitis is as important as oesophageal stricture diameter in determining dysphagia. *Gut* 1993;34:152–155.

71. Marks RD, Richter JE, Rizzo J, et al. Omeprazole versus H2-receptor antagonists in treating patients with peptic stricture and esophagitis. *Gastroenterology* 1994;106:907–915.

72. Smith PM, Kerr GD, Cockel R, et al. A comparison of omeprazole and ranitidine in the prevention of recurrence of benign esophageal stricture. Restore Investigator Group. *Gastroenterology* 1994;107:1312–1318.

73. Barbezat GO, Schlup M, Lubcke R. Omeprazole therapy decreases the need for dilatation of peptic oesophageal strictures. *Aliment Pharmacol Ther* 1999;13:1041–1045.

74. Swarbrick ET, Gough AL, Foster CS, Christian J, Garrett AD, Langworthy CH. Prevention of recurrence of oesophageal stricture, a comparison of lansoprazole and high-dose ranitidine. *Eur J Gastroenterol Hepatol* 1996;8:431–438.

75. Jaspersen D, Schwacha H, Schorr W, Brennenstuhl M, Raschka C, Hammar CH. Omeprazole in the treatment of patients with complicated gastro-oesophageal reflux disease. *J Gastroenterol Hepatol* 1996;11:900–902.

76. Silvis SE, Farahmand M, Johnson JA, Ansel HJ, Ho SB. A randomized blinded comparison of omeprazole and ranitidine in the treatment of chronic esophageal stricture secondary to acid peptic esophagitis. *Gastrointest Endosc* 1996;43:216–221.

77. Koop H, Arnold R. Long-term maintenance treatment of reflux esophagitis with omeprazole. Prospective study in patients with H2-blocker-resistant esophagitis. *Dig Dis Sci* 1991;36:552–557.

78. Ogilvie AL, Ferguson R, Atkinson M. Outlook with conservative treatment of peptic oesophageal stricture. *Gut* 1980;21:23–25.

79. Hands LJ, Papavramidis S, Bishop H, Dennison AR, McIntyre RL, Kettlewell MG. The natural history of peptic oesophageal strictures treated by dilatation and antireflux therapy alone. *Ann R Coll Surg Engl* 1989;71:306–309; discussion 309–310.

80. Ferguson R, Dronfield MW, Atkinson M. Cimetidine in treatment of reflux oesophagitis with peptic stricture. *Br Med J* 1979;2:472–474.

81. Farup PG, Modalsli B, Tholfsen JK. Long-term treatment with 300 mg ranitidine once daily after dilatation of peptic oesophageal strictures. *Scand J Gastroenterol* 1992;27:594–598.

82. Kelly HD. Origins of oesophagology. *Proc R Soc Med* 1969;62:781–786.

83. Hernandez LV, Jacobson JW, Harris MS. Comparison among the perforation rates of Maloney, balloon, and savary dilation of esophageal strictures. *Gastrointest Endosc* 2000;51:460–462.

84. McLean GK, LeVeen RF. Shear stress in the performance of esophageal dilation: comparison of balloon dilation and bougienage. *Radiology* 1989;172:983–986.

85. Egan JV, Baron TH, Adler DG, *et al.* Esophageal dilation. *Gastrointest Endosc* 2006;63:755–760.

86. Banerjee S, Shen B, Baron TH, *et al.* Antibiotic prophylaxis for GI endoscopy. *Gastrointest Endosc* 2008;67:791–798.

87. Riley SA, Attwood SE. Guidelines on the use of oesophageal dilatation in clinical practice. *Gut* 2004;53 (Suppl 1):i1–6.

88. Kozarek RA, Patterson DJ, Ball TJ, *et al.* Esophageal dilation can be done safely using selective fluoroscopy and single dilating sessions. *J Clin Gastroenterol* 1995;20:184–188.

89. Marshall JB, Afridi SA, King PD, Barthel JS, Butt JH. Esophageal dilation with polyvinyl (American) dilators over a marked guidewire: practice and safety at one center over a 5-yr period. *Am J Gastroenterol* 1996;91:1503–1506.

90. Yamamoto H, Hughes RW Jr, Schroeder KW, Viggiano TR, DiMagno EP. Treatment of benign esophageal stricture by Eder-Puestow or balloon dilators: a comparison between randomized and prospective nonrandomized trials. *Mayo Clin Proc* 1992;67:228–236.

91. Cox JG, Winter RK, Maslin SC, *et al.* Balloon or bougie for dilatation of benign esophageal stricture? *Dig Dis Sci* 1994;39:776–781.

92. Tytgat GN. Dilation therapy of benign esophageal stenoses. *World J Surg* 1989;13:142–148.

93. McBride MA, Ergun GA. The endoscopic management of esophageal strictures. *Gastrointest Endosc Clin North Am* 1994;4:595–621.

94. Tulman AB, Boyce HW, Jr. Complications of esophageal dilation and guidelines for their prevention. *Gastrointest Endosc* 1981;27:229–234.

95. Saeed ZA, Winchester CB, Ferro PS, Michaletz PA, Schwartz JT, Graham DY. Prospective randomized comparison of polyvinyl bougies and through-the-scope balloons for dilation of peptic strictures of the esophagus. *Gastrointest Endosc* 1995;41:189–195.

96. Cox JG, Winter RK, Maslin SC, *et al.* Balloon or bougie for dilatation of benign oesophageal stricture? An interim report of a randomised controlled trial. *Gut* 1988;29:1741–1747.

97. Scolapio JS, Pasha TM, Gostout CJ, *et al.* A randomized prospective study comparing rigid to balloon dilators for benign esophageal strictures and rings. *Gastrointest Endosc* 1999;50:13–17.

98. Shemesh E, Czerniak A. Comparison between Savary-Gilliard and balloon dilatation of benign esophageal strictures. *World J Surg* 1990;14:518–521; discussion 521–522.

99. Agnew SR, Pandya SP, Reynolds RP, Preiksaitis HG. Predictors for frequent esophageal dilations of benign peptic strictures. *Dig Dis Sci* 1996;41:931–936.

100. Chiu YC, Hsu CC, Chiu KW, *et al.* Factors influencing clinical applications of endoscopic balloon dilation for benign esophageal strictures. *Endoscopy* 2004;36:595–600.

101. Saeed ZA, Ramirez FC, Hepps KS, *et al.* An objective end point for dilation improves outcome of peptic esophageal strictures: a prospective randomized trial. *Gastrointest Endosc* 1997;45:354–359.

102. Said A, Brust DJ, Gaumnitz EA, Reichelderfer M. Predictors of early recurrence of benign esophageal strictures. *Am J Gastroenterol* 2003;98:1252–1256.

103. Kochman ML, McClave SA, Boyce HW. The refractory and the recurrent esophageal stricture: a definition. *Gastrointest Endosc* 2005;62:474–475.

104. Silvis SE, Nebel O, Rogers G, Sugawa C, Mandelstam P. Endoscopic complications. Results of the 1974 American Society for Gastrointestinal Endoscopy Survey. *JAMA* 1976;235:928–930.

105. Quine MA, Bell GD, McCloy RF, Matthews HR. Prospective audit of perforation rates following upper gastrointestinal endoscopy in two regions of England. *Br J Surg* 1995;82:530–533.

106. Clouse RE. Complications of endoscopic gastrointestinal dilation techniques. *Gastrointest Endosc Clin North Am* 1996;6:323–341.

107. Bapat RD, Bakhshi GD, Kantharia CV, Shirodkar SS, Iyer AP, Ranka S. Self-bougienage: long-term relief of corrosive esophageal strictures. *Indian J Gastroenterol* 2001;20:180–182.

108. Kim CH, Groskreutz JL, Gehrking SJ. Recurrent benign esophageal strictures treated with self-bougienage: report of seven cases. *Mayo Clin Proc* 1990;65:799–803.

109. Grobe JL, Kozarek RA, Sanowski RA. Self-bougienage in the treatment of benign esophageal stricture. *J Clin Gastroenterol* 1984;6:109–112.

110. Zein NN, Greseth JM, Perrault J. Endoscopic intralesional steroid injections in the management of refractory esophageal strictures. *Gastrointest Endosc* 1995;41:596–598.

111. Kochhar R, Makharia GK. Usefulness of intralesional triamcinolone in treatment of benign esophageal strictures. *Gastrointest Endosc* 2002;56:829–834.

112. Kochhar R, Ray JD, Sriram PV, Kumar S, Singh K. Intralesional steroids augment the effects of endoscopic dilation in corrosive esophageal strictures. *Gastrointest Endosc* 1999;49:509–513.

113. Miyashita M, Onda M, Okawa K, *et al.* Endoscopic dexamethasone injection following balloon dilatation of anastomotic stricture after esophagogastrostomy. *Am J Surg* 1997;174:442–444.

114. Holder TM, Ashcraft KW, Leape L. The treatment of patients with esophageal strictures by local steroid injections. *J Pediatr Surg* 1969;4:646–653.

115. Berenson GA, Wyllie R, Caulfield M, Steffen R. Intralesional steroids in the treatment of refractory esophageal strictures. *J Pediatr Gastroenterol Nutr* 1994;18:250–252.

116. Ramage JI, Jr., Rumalla A, Baron TH, *et al.* A prospective, randomized, double-blind, placebo-controlled trial of endoscopic steroid injection therapy for recalcitrant esophageal peptic strictures. *Am J Gastroenterol* 2005;100:2419–2425.

117. Altintas E, Kacar S, Tunc B, Sezgin O, Parlak E, Altiparmak E, et al. Intralesional steroid injection in benign esophageal strictures resistant to bougie dilation. *J Gastroenterol Hepatol* 2004;19:1388–1391.

118. Bhutani MS, Usman N, Shenoy V, *et al.* Endoscopic ultrasound miniprobe-guided steroid injection for treatment of refractory esophageal strictures. *Endoscopy* 1997;29:757–759.

119. Siersma PD. Stenting for benign esophageal strictures. *Endoscopy* 2009;41:363–373.

120. Martin RC, Woodall C, Duvall R, Scoggins CR. The use of self-expanding silicone stents in esophagectomy strictures: less cost and more efficiency. *Ann Thorac Surg* 2008;86:436–440.

121. Hordijk ML, Siersema PD, Tilanus HW, Kuipers EJ. Electrocautery therapy for refractory anastomotic strictures of the esophagus. *Gastrointest Endosc* 2006;63:157–163.

122. Schubert D, Kuhn R, Lippert H, Pross M. Endoscopic treatment of benign gastrointestinal anastomotic strictures using argon plasma coagulation in combination with diathermy. *Surg Endosc* 2003;17:1579–1582.

123. Beilstein MC, Kochman ML. Endoscopic incision of a refractory esophageal stricture: novel management with an endoscopic scissors. *Gastrointest Endosc* 2005;61:623–625.

124. Hordijk ML, van Hooft JE, Hansen BE, Fockens P, Kuipers EJ. A randomized comparison of electrocautery incision with Savary bougienage for relief of anastomotic gastroesophageal strictures. *Gastrointest Endosc* 2009;70:849–855.

125. Mamazza J, Schlachta CM, Poulin EC. Surgery for peptic strictures. *Gastrointest Endosc Clin North Am* 1998;8:399–413.

126. Lucktong TA, Morton JM, Shaheen NJ, Farrell TM. Resection of benign esophageal stricture through a minimally invasive endoscopic and transgastric approach. *Am Surg* 2002;68:720–723.

127. Keenan DJ, Hamilton JR, Gibbons J, Stevenson HM. Surgery for benign esophageal stricture. *J Thorac Cardiovasc Surg* 1984;88:182–188.

29 Gastroesophageal Reflux Laryngitis

Robert T. Kavitt and Michael F. Vaezi

Division of Gastroenterology, Hepatology, and Nutrition, Vanderbilt University Medical Center, Nashville, TN, USA

Introduction

Reflux of gastroduodenal contents into the laryngopharyngeal region is purported to be a significant cause of reflux-induced laryngitis often referred to as laryngopharyngeal reflux (LPR) [1]. Estimates range that from 4% to 10% of patients presenting to otolaryngologists present with symptoms related in part to gastroesophageal reflux disease (GERD) [2]. Such symptoms include hoarseness, sore or burning throat, chronic cough, globus, dysphagia, post-nasal drip, apnea, laryngospasm, and even laryngeal neoplasm, among other complaints (Table 29.1). Chronic laryngitis and sore throat symptoms are reportedly associated with GERD in up to 60% of patients [2–8]. Additionally, some studies suggest an association between laryngeal cancer and chronic laryngeal exposure with reflux of gastroduodenal contents [9–13].

The first association between GERD and laryngeal disease was suggested by Coffin in 1903. He wrote that symptoms of "post-nasal catarrh" may be due to "eructation of gases" from the stomach and hyperacidity [14]. In 1928, Jackson and Margulies described the "contact ulcer," and in 1937 Cherry and Margulies documented three patients with laryngeal contact ulcer refractory to vocal rehabilitation [15, 16]. On barium esophagram pharyngolaryngeal reflux of gastric contents into the larynx was noted, and the patients responded to antacids, dietary changes, and head of bed elevation. However, since these initial studies, the direct association between reflux of gastroduodenal contents and laryngeal signs and symptoms has been difficult to establish.

The 2006 Montreal consensus group distinguished GERD symptoms between esophageal and extraesophageal syndromes (Figure 29.1) [17]. Extraesophageal manifestations with established associations include chronic cough, laryngitis, and asthma, based on population-based studies, with odds ratios of 1.3–3.0 [18–21]. However, the causal relationship of GERD to these non-specific symptoms is not proven. The Montreal consensus group stated that present evidence indicates: "(1) The existence of an association between these syndromes and GERD, (2) the rarity of extraesophageal syndromes occurring in isolation without concomitant manifestations of the typical esophageal syndrome, (3) that those syndromes are usually multi-factorial with GERD as one of the several potential aggravating cofactors, and (4) that data substantiating a beneficial effect of reflux treatments on the extraesophageal syndromes are weak" [17]. More recently, the American Gastroenterological Association (AGA) guidelines for GERD recommended against treating laryngitis or asthma patients for acid reflux if they do not have concomitant typical reflux symptoms [18, 22]. Thus, the role of "silent" reflux, extraesophageal symptoms without concomitant heartburn or regurgitation, is controversial and divisive between the gastroenterology and otolaryngology communities.

Prevalence

GERD is a widely prevalent condition with significant impact on quality of life. In a Gallup poll of 1000 adults with heartburn at least weekly conducted for the AGA, 79% of respondents noted heartburn symptoms at night [23]. Of this subgroup, 75% reported that these symptoms affected their sleep, and 40% reported that night-time heartburn impacted their ability to function the next day. Twenty percent reported supraesophageal symptoms three to six times each week, and 43% reported these symptoms once or twice per week. In a population survey study, Locke et al. showed that heartburn and acid regurgitation are significantly associated with chest pain, dysphagia, dyspepsia, and globus sensation [19]. A subsequent VA-based case–control study by El-Serag et al. suggested that erosive esophagitis and esophageal stricture were associated with various extraesophageal symptoms, such as sinusitis (OR 1.60; 95% CI 1.51–1.70), pharyngitis (1.48; 1.15–1.89), aphonia (1.81; 1.18–2.80), and chronic laryngitis (2.01; 1.53–2.63), among

The Esophagus, Fifth Edition. Edited by Joel E. Richter, Donald O. Castell.
© 2012 Blackwell Publishing Ltd. Published 2012 by Blackwell Publishing Ltd.

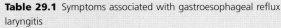

Table 29.1 Symptoms associated with gastroesophageal reflux laryngitis

Hoarseness
Dysphonia
Sore or burning throat
Excessive throat clearing
Chronic cough
Globus
Apnea
Laryngospasm
Dysphagia
Post-nasal drip
Neoplasm

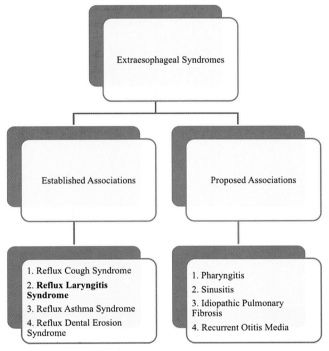

Figure 29.1 Montreal definition of constituent syndromes of GERD (adapted from Vakil *et al.* [17], with permission).

other symptoms [20]. The authors concluded that patients with reflux esophagitis are at an increased risk of harboring a large variety of sinus, pharyngeal, laryngeal, and pulmonary diseases. In an epidemiologic review of reflux disorders, it was estimated that the prevalence of esophagitis in the general population is approximately 1.4% [24]. Laryngeal disorders have been shown to be twice as likely in patients with esophagitis compared to those without [20]. Twenty-five percent of patients with LPR are found to have histologic evidence of esophagitis [25]. Thus, epidemiologic studies suggest an association between reflux disease and extraesophageal symptoms.

Mechanisms of gastroesophageal reflux laryngitis

The two predominant pathophysiologic mechanisms for LPR are direct and indirect exposure of the larynx to injurious gastric contents. The direct exposure is due to acid, pepsin, and bile acid exposure to laryngopharyngeal mucosa. The indirect mechanism is thought to be a result of refluxate interactions with structures distal to the larynx, evoking a vagally-mediated response of bronchoconstriction. This may cause the non-productive cough commonly associated with LPR [26]. The resting tone of the upper (UES) and lower esophageal sphincters (LES) as well as the magnitude of elevated intra-abdominal pressure all impact the bolus of refluxate involved.

The potential agents causing laryngitis may include gastric contents (acid and pepsin) and duodenal contents (bile acids and the pancreatic enzyme trypsin). Animal studies in the past have shown the potential of both acid and pepsin to cause laryngeal injury [27]. The role of conjugated and unconjugated bile and trypsin at pH values of 1–7 was investigated by Adhami *et al.*, who did not find histologic injury to the canine larynx by the above agents alone. However, they showed that the combination of the bile constituents with acid and pepsin in an acidic pH caused the greatest injury [28]. This is difficult to assess in humans, because refluxate into the esophagus is often a mix of gastric and duodenal contents [29]. However, these data indirectly suggest that reflux of duodenal contents into the larynx, although it may be associated with symptoms such as regurgitation, is less likely to cause mucosal damage unless it occurs in an acidic milieu.

A number of mechanisms exist in the supraesophageal region to prevent aspiration of gastric refluxate. The airway is protected during regurgitation of gastric fluid by complete adduction of the true vocal cords and arytenoids, as well as approximation of the adducted arytenoids at the base of the epiglottis, occluding entry to the closed vocal cords [30]. Furthermore, abrupt esophageal distention is shown to cause brief closure of the glottis [31]. This reflex may prevent aspiration of a larger refluxate. Fluid stimulation of the pharynx triggers a swallowing response to clear the pharynx, inducing a closure of the glottis [32]. The pharyngoglottal reflex, in addition to intrinsic defense mechanisms, which include the cough reflex and mucociliary actions of the bronchotracheal surface, work in tandem to minimize spread of any aspirated refluxate and to improve its clearance [33].

Defense mechanisms differ between the esophagus and the laryngopharynx. The esophagus has greater resistance to exposure to acid. One of the carbonic anhydrase isoenzymes, CA III, is noted to exhibit increased expression in esophageal mucosa in response to reflux, while the larynx has decreased CA III levels after exposure to chronic reflux.

The response of esophageal mucosa to acid and pepsin is often reversible, while laryngeal tissue can often exhibit irreversible damage [34, 35].

Clinical symptoms

Many patients with gastroesophageal reflux-induced chronic laryngitis present with symptoms such as sore throat, globus, chronic cough, hoarseness, dysphagia, apnea, or post-nasal drip, among others (Table 29.1). However, they may not present with classic GERD symptoms of heartburn and regurgitation. A 1991 study found that of 225 patients with otolaryngologic disorders and suspected GERD, only 43% reported symptoms of heartburn or acid regurgitation [6]. Additional symptoms that may be related to reflux-related laryngitis may include frequent throat clearing, dry mouth, prolonged voice warm-up time (>20–30 min), halitosis, excess phlegm, coated tongue, throat tickle, regurgitation of food, nocturnal cough, difficulty breathing especially at night, aspiration, laryngospasm, poorly controlled asthma, or pneumonia [33, 36].

The reflux symptom index (RSI) is a validated nine-item self-administered instrument published in 2002 to help assess the severity of LPR symptoms at the time of diagnosis and after therapy [37]. Symptoms assessed include throat clearing, difficulty swallowing, hoarseness, excess throat mucus or post-nasal drip, coughing after eating or lying down, breathing difficulties or choking episodes, troublesome or annoying cough, sensation of something sticking in the throat or a lump in the throat, and symptoms of heartburn, chest pain, or indigestion, on a scale from 0 to 5. An RSI score greater than 12 is defined as abnormal. The RSI was once believed to be significantly higher in untreated patients with LPR than controls; however, more recent studies suggest that it may be of lower clinical utility than previously believed [38]. Reliability of this instrument may vary based on patient population and clinical setting. Additionally, given the complexity of the symptoms and the scoring system, it is not widely used in clinical practice.

Evaluation of the larynx

Physical examination

Physical examination of patients with suspected gastroesophageal reflux laryngitis must be thorough, and include an examination of the head and neck, with assessment of ears and hearing, patency of the nares, oral cavity, temporomandibular joints, and larynx. One should also assess for signs of systemic disease (such as hypothyroidism) or neurologic impairment that may manifest with symptoms impacting the throat or voice, including Parkinson's disease, multiple sclerosis, or other conditions. When a patient reports symptoms of vocal difficulties, laryngeal examination by an otolaryngologist may include an assessment of the speaking and singing voice, and strobovideolaryngoscopy [33]. Objective voice analysis can quantify quality of voice, pulmonary function, harmonic spectral characteristics, valvular efficiency of vocal folds, and neuromuscular function on electromyography [39]. Use of flexible transnasal laryngoscopy plays a vital role in excluding more ominous causes for patients' laryngeal symptoms. Hoarseness is a symptom that can be present in patients with LPR; however it also may be a symptom of vocal fold paresis, polyps, post-viral inflammatory reactions, allergies, vocal abuse, dysplasia, and cancer [40]. If hoarseness persists for longer than 2 weeks, laryngoscopy is indicated [41]. Some patients with severe LPR may experience reflux that impacts the oral cavity, leading to a loss of dental enamel.

Physical examination by a gastroenterologist is in general not useful since in nearly all cases normal findings are the rule. Gastroenterologists may observe laryngeal abnormalities during upper endoscopy, in which case we recommend referral to an experienced otolaryngologist for further evaluation and therapy. Interpretation of endoscopic views between gastroenterologists and otolaryngologists can vary. Gastroenterologists' abilities to detect abnormalities of the larynx have been questioned in the literature [42]. However, the role of the gastroenterologist in this area is not to make a specific diagnosis of laryngeal pathology, but to determine globally that a more thorough evaluation may be in order.

Laryngeal signs

Normal laryngeal tissue has sharply demarcated landmarks with glistening mucosa and minimal or no laryngeal edema (Figure 29.2), unlike abnormal laryngeal findings (Figure 29.3). The epithelium of the larynx is thin and is not adapted

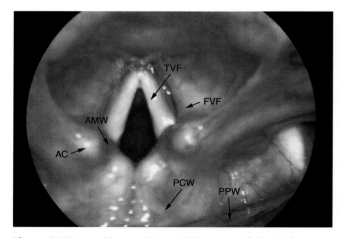

Figure 29.2 Normal laryngeal tissue. TVF, true vocal fold; FVF, false vocal fold; AMW, arytenoid medial wall; AC, arytenoid complex; PCW, posterior cricoid wall; PPW, posterior pharyngeal wall (adapted from Vaezi *et al.* [1], with permission).

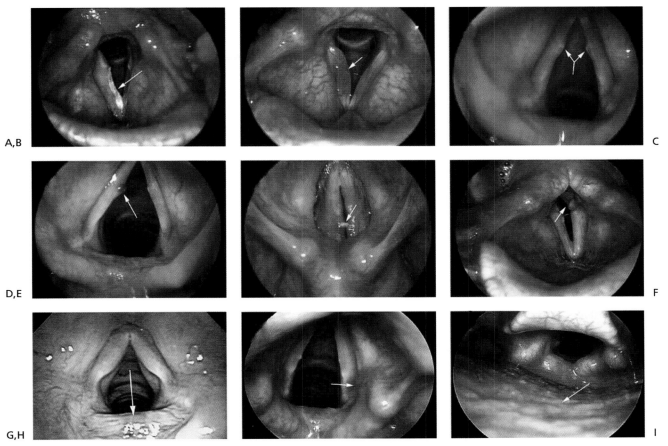

Figure 29.3 Abnormal larynx. (A) Leukoplakia; (B) Reinke's edema; (C) bilateral true vocal cord nodules; (D) true vocal fold hemorrhagic polyp; (E) true vocal fold erythema; (F) vocal fold granuloma; (G) interarytenoid bar; (H) arytenoid medial wall erythema; and (I) posterior pharyngeal wall cobble stoning (adapted from Vaezi *et al.* [1], with permission).

Table 29.2 Potential laryngopharyngeal signs associated with gastroesophageal reflux laryngitis

Edema and hyperemia of larynx
Hyperemia and lymphoid hyperplasia of posterior pharynx (cobblestoning)
Contact ulcers
Laryngeal polyps
Granuloma
Interarytenoid changes
Subglottic stenosis
Posterior glottic stenosis
Reinke's edema
Tumors

to accommodating injury from acid and pepsin [34]. Several laryngeal signs are attributed to GERD, including edema, erythema, pseudosulcus, ventricular obliteration, and postcricoid hyperplasia (Table 29.2) [1].

In a study reporting survey results of otolaryngologists regarding the signs likely used to diagnose LPR, subjective signs of laryngeal erythema and edema were the most commonly employed findings to diagnose GERD [43, 44]. However, these signs are criticized for their lack of specificity for GERD. Several signs of posterior laryngitis thought to be markers for LPR are actually present in a high percentage of asymptomatic healthy volunteers, raising questions about the specificity of such findings [45]. Forty-three of 50 healthy subjects (86%) may exhibit one or more findings considered pathognomonic of laryngeal complaints due to GERD. This finding suggests that GERD may be over-diagnosed, as the laryngeal signs used in clinical practice are non-specific [46]. The advantages and disadvantages of laryngoscopy and other diagnostic tests in detecting reflux are shown in Table 29.3.

First described in 2001, the reflux finding score (RFS) received considerable attention initially as a validated sign for reflux-induced laryngeal pathology. This instrument is an eight-item clinical severity scale based on laryngoscopic findings, including subglottic edema, vocal fold edema, diffuse laryngeal edema, ventricular obliteration, erythema/hyperemia, posterior commissure hypertrophy, granuloma/granulation tissue, and thick endolaryngeal mucus, ranging

Table 29.3 Advantages and disadvantages of methods for detecting esophageal reflux

Method	Advantages	Disadvantages
Endoscopy	• Easy visualization of mucosal damage/erosions	• Poor sensitivity/specificity/positive predictive value • Requires sedation • High cost
Laryngoscopy	• No sedation required • Direct visualization of the larynx and laryngeal pathology	• No specific laryngeal signs for reflux • Over-diagnoses gastroesophageal reflux disease (GERD)
pH monitoring	• Easy to perform • Relatively non-invasive • Prolonged monitoring • Ambulatory	• Catheter-based, may have up to a 30% false-negative rate • No pH predictors of treatment response in laryngopharyngeal reflux (LPR)
Impedance monitoring	• Easy to perform • Relatively non-invasive • Prolonged monitoring • Ambulatory • Measures acidic and non-acidic gas and liquid reflux (combined with pH)	• Catheter-based • False-negative rate unknown but most likely similar to catheter-based pH monitoring • Unknown clinical relevance when abnormal on proton pump inhibitor (PPI) therapy • Unknown importance in LPR
ResTech Dx-pH	• Faster detection rate and faster time to equilibrium pH than traditional pH catheters	• Unknown if clinically useful in patients with LPR

from 0 to 26 [47, 48]. However, similar to RSI, RFS is not commonly employed in clinical practice. A recent study found that both the RSI and RFS have poor specificity, with no significant difference between patients and control groups [38].

The variability of detecting laryngeal signs may also be impacted by the quality and sensitivity of the detection instrument. Abnormal laryngeal signs are more likely to be suspected with flexible laryngoscopy as opposed to rigid laryngoscopy in the same individual, indicating that flexible laryngoscopy may be more sensitive and less specific for

detecting laryngeal irritation [49]. Laryngeal signs appear to be poorly specific for identifying gastroesophageal reflux. One study showed that lesions of the vocal fold may represent more specific signs for LPR, exhibiting 91% specificity and 88% response to treatment with proton pump inhibitors (PPIs) [50]. The non-specific nature of laryngoscopy may also be due to poor inter- and intra-observer variability. A randomized prospective analysis by five otolaryngologists blinded to patient information of 120 video segments of rigid fiberoptic laryngoscopy found poor inter-rater reliabilities of the laryngoscopic findings associated with LPR (intra-class correlation coefficient of 0.265), and intra-rater reliability was extremely variable for the various physical findings (Kendall correlation coefficients ranging from -0.121 to 0.837). Taken together, these studies suggest that accurate assessment of laryngeal involvement with LPR is quite difficult as interpretation of physical findings is subjective and varies among physicians.

Ambulatory pH studies

Ambulatory pH monitoring allows for detection of esophageal or hypopharyngeal acid exposure. Since even healthy individuals have some reflux, the normal values have a range with an accepted upper limit, based on studies in healthy subjects. Up to 50 acid reflux events into the esophagus each day may occur normally and the upper limit for gastroesophageal reflux episodes is four [25]. When compared to physical examination findings, dual pH probe monitoring is reported to have superior sensitivity and specificity [6]. A meta-analysis of 16 studies involving a total of 793 subjects who underwent 24-h pH monitoring (529 patients with LPR, 264 controls) showed that the number of pharyngeal reflux events for the control group and for LPR patients differed significantly ($P < .0001$). The authors concluded that the "upper probe gives accurate and consistent information in normal subjects and patients with LPR," and that the acid exposure time and number of reflux events are most important in distinguishing normal subjects from patients with LPR [51]. However, there is a great degree of variability in the reported prevalence of pH abnormalities in the literature for patients with LPR (Table 29.4). This heterogeneity may be due to different patient populations and non-standard pH probe placement [52]. Some investigators utilized direct laryngoscopy for probe placement, while others utilized esophageal manometry to identify the UES and LES [1]. Current recommendations suggest that the hypopharyngeal probe be placed 1–2 cm above the UES as determined by manometry, while the distal and proximal pH probes be placed 5 and 15 cm above the manometric LES [1].

Initial studies of patients with suspected gastroesophageal reflux laryngitis investigated the role of proximal esophageal

Table 29.4 Prevalence of abnormal pH monitoring in the distal and proximal esophagus and the hypopharynx

Study	Proportion of patients with LPR	Number of patients with reflux identified during proximal pH monitoring	Number of patients with reflux identified during distal pH monitoring	Number of patients with reflux identified during hypopharyngeal pH monitoring	Prevalence (%)
Ossakow et al. (1987) [102]	43/63	NR	43	NR	68
Koufman et al. (1988) [2]	24/32	NR	24	7	75
Wiener et al. (1989) [103]	12/15	NR	12	3	80
Wilson et al. (1989) [104]	17/97	17	NR	NR	18
Katz (1990) [105]	7/10	NR	7	7	70
Woo et al. (1996) [106]	20/31	20	20	NR	65
Metz et al. (1997) [107]	6/10	?	6	NR	60
Vaezi et al. (1997) [108]	21/21	11	21	NR	100
Chen et al. (1998) [109]	365/735	NR	229	255	50
Havas et al. (1999) [80]	10/15	NR	6	4	67
Ulualp et al. (1999) [110]	15/20	15	15	15	75
Smit et al. (2001) [111]	7/15	7	3	NR	47
Ulualp et al. (2001) [58]	28/39	28	28	28	72
Noordzij et al. (2002) [57]	29/42	NR	29	29	69
Park et al. (2005) [50]	33/78	20	28	NR	42
Cumulative	**637/1223**	**46%**	**42%**	**38%**	**52**

NR, not reported; LPR, laryngopharyngeal reflux; ?, unclear how many patients tested.

pH probes. A 1991 study assessed the prevalence of abnormal acid exposure on the proximal esophagus in 15 patients with typical GERD (group 1), 15 patients with laryngeal symptoms without abnormal findings on laryngoscopy (group 2), and 10 patients with both laryngeal symptoms and findings on laryngoscopy (group 3) [53]. Increased proximal esophageal acid exposure was observed in patients in groups 1 and 2, indicating that proximal esophageal acid exposure may differentiate patients with laryngitis from patients with typical GERD. Measurement of hypopharyngeal pH exposure was initially used to objectively measure laryngeal extension of reflux. An earlier study suggested that hypopharyngeal pH assessment may be useful when used in conjunction with findings on laryngoscopy to identify patients whose symptoms may be related to GERD [54]. In this study, 76 patients with respiratory complaints thought to be related to GERD were divided into three groups based on reflux finding score and pharyngeal reflux events. The patients were classified as RFS+ if the RFS was greater than 7, and pharyngeal reflux positive if they had more than one episode of reflux noted during pH assessment. Controls were found to have a significantly lower RFS and fewer episodes of pharyngeal reflux. None of the controls had more than one episode of pharyngeal reflux during a 24-h period. Twenty-one patients had both an abnormal RFS and pharyngeal reflux, and these patients also had significantly higher heartburn scores and acid exposure in the distal esophagus. The authors conclude that agreement between detection of pharyngeal reflux by pH monitoring and an increased RFS greater than 7 help establish or refute the diagnosis of GERD as an etiology of laryngeal symptoms. When both are normal, GERD is most like not playing a role in a patient's extraesophageal symptoms.

However, the initial enthusiasm about the diagnostic ability of hypopharyngeal reflux monitoring has now been replaced by skepticism. The positioning of the hypopharyngeal pH probe is operator dependent and varies with regard to placement via direct visualization with laryngoscopy as compared to measurement by manometry [55]. Artifacts commonly occur and computer-driven interpretations must be manually reviewed [56]. Several studies have found that positive results of pharyngeal testing do not predict a favorable response to antireflux therapy [57, 58]. One study showed that the degree of improvement in symptoms among 19 of 27 patients with pharyngeal reflux was similar to that for the eight patients not exhibiting pharyngeal reflux [58]. Additionally, there are no universally accepted diagnostic criteria for pH monitoring of the hypopharynx. The range of normal pH values is not uniformly defined, and can vary from none to 4 pH drops less than 4 [57, 59, 60]. Less restrictive pH values, including a drop in pH of 1.0 or 1.5 units instead of 2.0 units, does not differentiate healthy volunteers from patients with suspected ear, nose, and throat (ENT) complaints [61].

The 2008 AGA Technical Review on the Management of GERD suggested that the role of pH or impedance–pH monitoring in diagnosing extraesophageal reflux is controversial and unproven (Table 29.5) [18]. This evidence-based technical review concludes that the value of a negative pH or impedance–pH study is of greater clinical utility, and states "In the absence of troublesome esophageal symptoms or endoscopic findings, with a failed 8-week therapeutic trial of twice-daily PPI therapy, and with normal esophageal acid exposure (PPI therapy withheld) on 24-h monitoring, one has gone as far as currently possible to rule out GERD as a significant contributor to these nonspecific syndromes. Such patients should have etiologies other than GERD explored" [18].

This conclusion is in direct contrast to guidelines published by the American Academy of Otolaryngology–Head and Neck Surgery (AAOHNS) Committee on Speech, Voice, and Swallowing Disorders. These guidelines state that LPR can be diagnosed based on symptoms or laryngeal findings, but ambulatory 24-h double-probe (simultaneous esophageal and pharyngeal) pH assessment is considered the gold standard diagnostic tool (Table 29.5) [25]. They also suggest that barium esophagraphy or esophagoscopy provide far less sensitive assessments of LPR, but these may be advisable for screening of the esophagus for related pathology [6, 25, 62]. However, in line with the AGA guidelines, the American College of Gastroenterology (ACG) practice guidelines suggest that pH testing may not be the gold standard diagnostic test in this group of patients [55] (Table 29.5). These guidelines refer to data indicating that the overall pretherapy prevalence of an abnormal pH test in a population with chronic laryngeal symptoms is 53%, with the prevalence of excessive distal, proximal, and hypopharyngeal acid exposure being 42%, 44%, and 38%, respectively [52], suggesting that this population may have abnormal reflux symptoms, but not proving causality. In support of the ACG and AGA guidelines, a placebo-controlled study of 145 patients with

suspected GERD-related ENT symptoms treated with high-dose esomeprazole or placebo for 16 weeks, found that the degree of symptomatic or laryngeal involvement was independent of pretherapy pH findings and that neither esophageal nor hypopharyngeal acid reflux predicted a response to PPI use [63].

In patients who remain symptomatic despite aggressive acid suppressive therapy, recent studies suggest that non-acid reflux may play a role in their symptoms [64–67]. The combination of impedance and pH monitoring allows for distinction between acid, weakly acidic, and weakly alkaline reflux [65]. A multicenter trial using impedance–pH-metry in healthy adults developed normal values to be utilized for comparison with reflux patients [68]. Studies assessing patients with heartburn and regurgitation in addition to patients with extraesophageal symptoms suggest that 10–40% of patients on twice-daily PPI therapy may have persistent non-acid reflux [66, 69]. However, causation between these non-acid reflux events and persistent symptoms is difficult to establish [29]. A recent study found that abnormal impedance in patients on therapy predicts acid reflux in patients off therapy [70]. The study also concluded that in patients with refractory reflux, combined impedance–pH monitoring might provide the single best strategy for evaluating reflux symptoms. However, the clinical significance of abnormal impedance findings in this group of patients awaits further study.

Two indices are utilized to establish a relationship between symptoms and GERD observed on pH testing. The symptom index (SI) refers to the number of symptoms associated with reflux divided by the total number of symptoms. A symptom is determined to be associated with reflux if a reflux episode is detected by pH monitoring 5 minutes in advance of symptom onset. Symptom association probability (SAP) is determined by dividing 24-h pH data into 2-minute segments, each of which is assessed to determine if reflux occurred and if symptoms occurred. The probability of the distribution of symptoms and episodes of reflux is then calculated to assess if it could have occurred by chance. An overall positive SI or SAP is concluded if at least one symptom is positive. These indices are of greater utility when used for patients with intermittent symptoms, as opposed to those patients with constant symptoms of sore throat, hoarseness, cough, or globus, among other complaints [66, 71–74].

The Restech Dx-pH Measurement System™ (Respiratory Technology Corp, San Diego, CA, USA) is a new device developed to detect acid reflux in the posterior oropharynx [75] (Figure 29.4). A nasopharyngeal catheter is utilized to assess pH in liquid or aerosolized droplets. A comparison of this device to the traditional pH catheters has shown a faster detection rate and a faster time to equilibrium pH. A typical tracing of distal esophageal and oropharyngeal pH monitoring in a healthy volunteer is shown in Figure 29.5. A recent prospective observational study in healthy volunteers

Table 29.5 Summary of AGA, AAOHNS, and ACG guidelines regarding pH testing and treatment modalities for patients with suspected laryngopharyngeal reflux (LPR)

	AGA	AAOHNS	ACG
	American Gastroenterological Association Institute Technical Review on the Management of Gastroesophageal Reflux Disease, 2008 [18]	Laryngopharyngeal Reflux: Position Statement of the Committee on Speech, Voice, and Swallowing Disorders of the American Academy of Otolaryngology-Head and Neck Surgery, 2002 [25]	American College of Gastroenterology Practice Guidelines: Esophageal Reflux Testing, 2007 [55]
pH Testing	Role of pH or impedance–pH monitoring in diagnosing extraesophageal reflux is controversial and unproven. "In the absence of troublesome esophageal symptoms or endoscopic findings, with a failed 8-week therapeutic trial of twice-daily PPI therapy, and with normal esophageal acid exposure (PPI therapy withheld) on 24-hour monitoring, one has gone as far as currently possible to rule out GERD as a significant contributor to these nonspecific syndromes. Such patients should have etiologies other than GERD explored."	Diagnosis of LPR can be made based on symptoms and laryngeal findings, but ambulatory 24-h double-probe pH assessment is considered the gold standard diagnostic tool. Barium esophagraphy or esophagoscopy provide far less sensitive assessments of LPR, but may be advisable for screening of the esophagus for related pathology.	"The accumulating data seriously question the clinical usefulness of esophageal or hypopharyngeal pH monitoring in the initial evaluation of patients with suspected acid-related ENT complaints." "Studies using impedance pH monitoring in patients with extraesophageal symptoms unresponsive to PPI therapy show little evidence of nonacid reflux, except in the chronic cough patient."
Treatment	Empiric therapy with twice-daily PPI for 2 months for patients with concomitant esophageal GERD syndrome and laryngitis remains a pragmatic clinical strategy (USPSTF grade B, quality fair). Do not support use of once- or twice-daily PPIs (or H_2-receptor antagonistss) for acute treatment of potential extraesophageal GERD syndromes, including laryngitis and asthma, in absence of esophageal GERD (USPSTF grade D, quality fair). "Step-down therapy should be attempted in all patients with extraesophageal reflux syndromes after empirical twice-daily PPI therapy. Continuing maintenance PPI therapy should be predicated on either the requirements of therapy for concomitant esophageal GERD syndromes or extraesophageal syndrome symptom response. In both cases, maintenance therapy should be with the lowest PPI dose necessary for adequate symptom relief."	Treatment for LPR needs to be more aggressive and prolonged than that for GERD, and depends on symptoms and severity of LPR and on response to therapy. Mild or intermittent LPR symptoms can be treated with dietary and lifestyle changes and H_2 antagonists, while the majority of patients require at least twice-daily PPI (minimum of 6 months). Fundoplication has been shown to be effective.	"The practical and popular approach is an empiric trial with a BID PPI regimen for several months, reserving pH testing for patients with persistent symptoms. However, here again, the results of acid pH testing have limited clinical utility."

GERD, gastroesophageal reflux disease; ENT, ear, nose, and throat; PPI, proton pump inhibitor.

developed normative data for this device at pH cut-offs of 4, 5, and 6 for the distal esophagus and oropharynx [75] (Figure 29.6). Although the initial studies with this device in patients with LPR are encouraging [76], controlled studies are needed to assess its future role in patients with LPR.

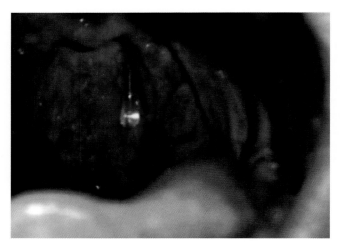

Figure 29.4 Dx-pH probe and light-emitting diode positioned in the oropharynx (adapted from Sun *et al.* [75], with permission).

Managing laryngeal complications of reflux disease

Medical management

Given the poor sensitivity and specificity of diagnostic tests, empiric treatment of suspected gastroesophageal reflux laryngitis using PPIs is common [1]. A recent study assessed response to PPIs based on change in 24-h pH studies in 27 patients with LPR with abnormal pH studies at baseline. Of five patients who did not have a measurable pH response to PPI, four reported improvements in their symptoms, highlighting poor prediction of treatment response based on pH results [77]. Most trials have utilized twice-daily PPIs for 3–4 months [1, 78]. The primary reason for this unapproved high-dose acid suppression is based on pH monitoring data indicating that the chances of normalizing exposure of the esophagus to acid in patients with chronic cough, laryngeal symptoms, or asthma is 99% with a twice-daily PPI [79]. A prospective cohort study (uncontrolled and open-label) assessed optimal PPI dose in patients with LPR, and indicated that twice-daily PPI is more effective than daily PPI in achieving clinical symptom response in patients with suspected LPR [50].

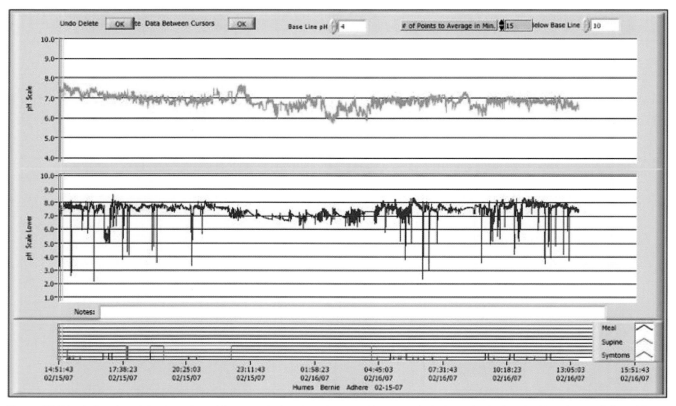

Figure 29.5 Typical tracing of distal esophageal (lower tracing) and oropharyngeal (upper tracing) pH monitoring in a healthy volunteer (adapted from Sun *et al.* [75], with permission).

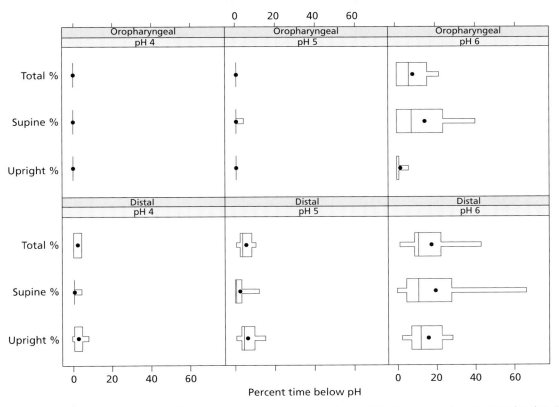

Figure 29.6 Extended box plot (25th, 75th percentile) of percentage of time below pH 4, 5, or 6 for the distal and oropharyngeal probes. The large, solid dots indicate the mean, and the line within the box plot represents the median values. The horizontal whiskers represent 5th and 95th percentile values (adapted from Sun *et al.* [75], with permission).

Although PPIs are widely used in patients with suspected LPR, high-quality supporting evidence for this remains minimal at this time as most trials have utilized small sample sizes and are uncontrolled [1, 17, 18, 78]. Placebo-controlled studies assessing lansoprazole, esomeprazole, pantoprazole, and rabeprazole for 2–4 months have observed no significant difference in symptoms experienced by LPR patients on placebo as compared to PPIs (Table 29.6) [63, 80–82]. Similarly, a meta-analysis of randomized controlled trials assessing PPIs for suspected GERD-related chronic laryngitis noted no benefit of PPIs over placebo (Figure 29.7) [83]. On the other hand, in support of the role of acid suppression in LPR, a more recent double-blind, placebo-controlled trial noted a significant improvement in LPR symptoms with 3 months of esomeprazole therapy [84]. One reason for the positive nature of this study is that the RSI was used as one of the outcome measures assessed. Of all symptoms queried, patients experienced the greatest improvement in heartburn symptoms after 3 months (and less marked improvements in hoarseness, throat clearing, coughing after meals, breathing difficulties, and other symptoms addressed). The improvement in heartburn symptoms had the most significant effect on the overall RSI score. Similarly, an earlier study comparing lansoprazole with placebo in 22 patients

with idiopathic chronic laryngitis noted that after 3 months 50% of patients in the lansoprazole group had noted resolution of symptoms, compared to 10% of patients in the placebo group [85]. Furthermore, another study reported that LPR patients who tested positive for *Helicobacter pylori* antibody were more likely to respond to PPI than those seronegative for *H. pylori* [86]. However, the clinical relevance of the latter study is still uncertain.

The AGA guidelines advise empiric therapy with twice-daily PPI for 2 months for patients with a concomitant esophageal GERD syndrome and laryngitis (USPSTF grade B recommendation) [18]. These recommendations do not support the use of PPIs for acute treatment of laryngitis in the absence of esophageal GERD (USPSTF grade D) [18]. However, the AAOHNS position statement indicates that treatment for LPR needs to be more aggressive and prolonged than that for GERD, and depends on the symptoms and severity of LPR and on the response to therapy [25]. The authors advise that patients with mild or intermittent symptoms of LPR can be treated with dietary and lifestyle changes and with H₂ antagonists, while the majority of patients require at least twice-daily PPI therapy [5, 6, 26, 47, 87–92]. Some patients require therapy with both a PPI and an H₂ antagonist, and the AAOHNS recommends the use of

Table 29.6 Placebo-controlled trials assessing use of proton-pump inhibitors (PPIs) in laryngopharyngeal reflux (LPR)

Study	PPI studied	Duration (weeks) Number of subjects	Inclusion criteria	Important exclusion criteria	pH monitoring	Gastrointestinal endoscopy	Outcome measured	Response to therapy
Havas et al. (1999) [80] (Australia)	Lansoprazole 30 mg twice daily	12 15	Posterior pharyngolaryngitis	CNS disorder, COPD, pre-existing acid suppression, severe esophagitis	Yes	Yes	50% reduction in global symptom score	35% reduction in symptoms
Noordzij et al. (2001) [112] (USA)	Omeprazole 40 mg twice daily	8 30	LSx for 3 months LPR four episodes	Infection Cancer Allergies	Yes	Optional	50% reduction in global symptom score	Comparable symptom score improvement in both groups
El-Serag et al. (2001) [85] (USA)	Lansoprazole 30 mg twice daily	12 20	LSx for >3 weeks LPR on laryngoscopy	Infection, cancer, previous gastrointestinal surgery	Yes	Yes	Complete symptom resolution	50% with complete resolution vs 10% in placebo group
Eherer et al. (2003) [113] (Austria)	Pantoprazole 40 mg twice daily	12 14	Hoarseness for 2 months (+) pH test		Yes	Optional	50% reduction in global symptom score	Significant improvement in symptoms in both groups
Steward et al. (2004) [82] (USA)	Rabeprazole 20 mg twice daily	8 42s	LSx for >4 weeks LPR on laryngoscopy	Gastrointestinal surgery PPI in 1 month	Optional	Optional	50% reduction in global symptom score	53% resolution in treatment group, 50% resolution in placebo group
Wo et al. (2006) [81] (USA)	Pantoprazole 40 mg daily	12 39	LSx for 3 days a week (+) pH test		Yes	Optional	50% reduction in global symptom score	40% with resolution in both groups
Vaezi et al. (2006) [63] (USA)	Esomeprazole 40 mg twice daily	16 145	LSx for 3 months LPR on laryngoscopy	Heartburn >3 episodes/week PPI in 2 weeks	Optional	Optional	50% reduction in symptoms	~15% resolution of symptoms in both groups, with 45% of both groups experiencing improvement in symptoms
Reichel et al. (2008) [84] (Germany)	Esomeprazole 20 mg twice daily	12 62	RFS > 7 and RSI > 13	PPI in 3 months, GI surgery, laryngeal malignancy	No	No	Reduction of total RSI and RFS	Significantly greater improvement in laryngeal appearance and LPR symptoms

LSx, laryngeal symptoms; RFS, reflux finding score; RSI, reflux symptom index; COPD, chronic obstructive pulmonary disease; CNS, central nervous system.

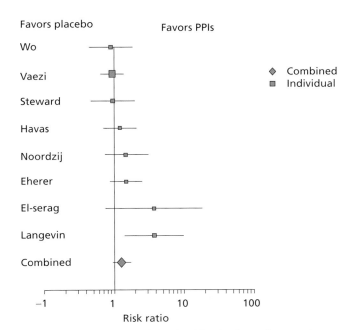

Figure 29.7 Forest plot depicting the risk ratios for studies assessing efficacy of proton pump inhibitor (PPI) in reflux laryngitis and pooled risk ratio by random effects method (adapted from Qadeer *et al.* [83], with permission).

twice-daily PPI for a minimum of 6 months [25, 89]. The authors of the AAOHNS statement suggest that fundoplication has been shown to be an effective treatment for LPR [93, 94]. However, this point is controversial, as discussed in the next section.

The need for chronic therapy in patients suspected of GERD-related laryngitis comes from uncontrolled observational studies with small sample sizes. For example, patients with LPR with concomitant GERD symptoms may have esophagitis (12%) and Barrett's esophagus (7%) [95, 96]. Studies suggest a possible association between chronic reflux-induced inflammation of the larynx and laryngeal cancer [13, 18, 40]. However, the main purpose of maintenance use of PPIs in patients with LPR is for control of symptoms, and stepdown therapy should always follow the initial empiric trial [18]. Long-term PPI is the current practice in many patients, as evidenced by a double-blind placebo-controlled trial finding only 21–48% likelihood of remaining PPI free at 1 year [97]. However, evidence supporting the use of long-term PPI therapy for patients with LPR is primarily anecdotal and future studies are needed to assess appropriate duration and use of PPI in patients with suspected LPR.

Surgical therapy

A number of uncontrolled observational studies have suggested efficacy of antireflux surgery in patients with gastro-esophageal reflux laryngitis. An earlier study assessed the effect of laparoscopic Hill repair in 145 patients. The Hill repair involves securing the gastroesophageal junction in the abdomen, recalibrating the LES, and recreating the acute angle of His, thus surgically recalibrating the antireflux barrier. The authors found that after a mean follow-up of 20 months, reports of sore throat decreased from 43% to 8% of patients. Symptoms of cough decreased from 41% to 8%, and voice loss decreased from 25% to 11% [98]. Similarly, another study evaluated 40 patients who underwent laparoscopic Nissen fundoplication for complaints of reflux laryngitis. After 3 months, 79.3% of patients had decreased inflammation noted on otorhinolaryngeal examination, and 41.4% of patients described improvement in voice quality. After 12 months, these figures were 92.3% and 38.5%, respectively. After a median follow-up of 42 months, 62.5% of patients reported either no cough or mild cough or hoarseness [99].

A more recent prospective concurrent controlled study in patients with LPR symptoms refractory to PPI therapy did not find Nissen fundoplication to be of benefit. One year after surgery only 10% of patients noted improvement in laryngeal symptoms, while signs of LPR on laryngoscopy improved in 80% of patients [100]. Recent controversy surrounds the role of surgical fundoplication in patients with PPI-refractory symptoms who have abnormal non-acid reflux by impedance monitoring. A retrospective review assessed patients with chronic cough referred for fundoplication after documentation of an association between their symptoms and reflux disease using multichannel intraluminal impedance and pH testing. In all six patients who underwent surgery, fundoplication was found to eliminate chronic cough due to non-acid reflux [101]. In this subgroup of patients, an uncontrolled telephone survey study suggested symptom improvement in most patients with laparoscopic Nissen fundoplication [67]. However, controlled studies are needed before this practice can be advocated. Based on published data, the role of fundoplication is best delineated in those who have a positive symptom response to PPI therapy and caution should be exercised in referring patients who do not respond to aggressive acid suppression, especially those with extraesophageal complaints.

Conclusions

GERD is associated with laryngeal signs and symptoms; however, the frequency of the association between these two entities is not firmly established. Improvement in the specificity of laryngeal examination would be an important goal in improving the accuracy of diagnosis of gastroesophageal reflux laryngitis. pH or impedance–pH studies can serve as diagnostic tools in patients whose symptoms are refractory to an empiric trial of PPIs. If these tests are normal on

PPI therapy despite persistence of symptoms, other etiologies for abnormal laryngeal signs and symptoms should be investigated [1]. Table 29.5 summarizes and contrasts the most recent national society guidelines regarding pH testing and treatment modalities for patients with suspected LPR. These guidelines are at times opposing and result in further confusion in the care of this group of patients.

It is prudent to remember that patients with suspected extraesophageal GERD syndromes, including those with LPR, may have GERD as a contributing etiology but rarely as the sole cause of their complaints [18]. Based on our experiences in treating patients with reflux-suspected chronic laryngitis, we suggest the treatment algorithm illustrated in Figure 29.8. Initial empiric therapy with twice-daily PPI for 2 months is a reasonable starting point for patients with suspected GERD-related laryngitis and no ominous symptoms or signs. If symptoms improve, then acid suppression should be tapered to the minimum dose for symptom control. If symptoms persist despite twice-daily PPI therapy, diagnostic testing with pH monitoring "off or on" PPIs or impedance–pH monitoring on therapy is recommended. In patients with normal test results, a search for an alternative explanation for symptoms should be pursued. In the infrequent cases of abnormal test results on therapy, clinical judgment should be exercised regarding the role of surgical fundoplication given lack of controlled studies in this area.

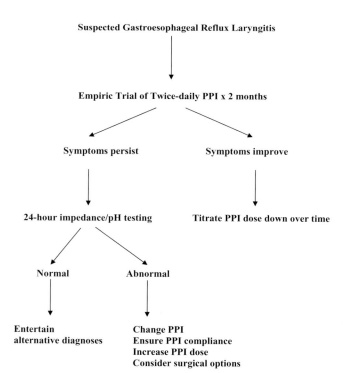

Figure 29.8 Suggested algorithm for evaluation and treatment of suspected gastroesophageal reflux laryngitis. PPI, proton pump inhibitor.

References

1. Vaezi MF, Hicks DM, Abelson TI, Richter JE. Laryngeal signs and symptoms and gastroesophageal reflux disease (GERD): a critical assessment of cause and effect association. *Clin Gastroenterol Hepatol* 2003;1:333–344.
2. Koufman JA, Wallace CW, *et al.* Reflux laryngitis and its sequela. *J Voice* 1988;2:78–79.
3. Gaynor EB. Otolaryngologic manifestations of gastroesophageal reflux. *Am J Gastroenterol* 1991;86:801–808.
4. Graser A. Gastroesophageal reflux and laryngeal symptoms. *Aliment Pharmacol Ther* 1994;8:265–272.
5. Koufman J, Sataloff RT, Toohill R. Laryngopharyngeal reflux: consensus conference report. *J Voice* 1996;10:215–216.
6. Koufman JA. The otolaryngologic manifestations of gastroesophageal reflux disease (GERD): a clinical investigation of 225 patients using ambulatory 24-hour pH monitoring and an experimental investigation of the role of acid and pepsin in the development of laryngeal injury. *Laryngoscope* 1991;101 (Suppl 53):1–78.
7. Richter JE. Typical and atypical presentations of gastroesophageal reflux disease. The role of esophageal testing in diagnosis and management. *Gastroenterol Clin North Am* 1996;25: 75–102.
8. Toohill RJ, Kuhn JC. Role of refluxed acid in pathogenesis of laryngeal disorders. *Am J Med* 1997;103:100S–106S.
9. Ward PH, Hanson DG. Reflux as an etiological factor of carcinoma of the laryngopharynx. *Laryngoscope* 1998;98: 1195–1199.
10. Freije JE, Beatty TW, Campbell BH, Woodson BT, Schultz CJ, Toohill RJ. Carcinoma of the larynx in patients with gastroesophageal reflux. *Am J Otolaryngol* 1996;17:386–390.
11. Morrison MD. Is chronic gastroesophageal reflux a causative factor in glottic carcinoma? *Otolaryngol Head Neck Surg* 1988;99:370–373.
12. Vaezi MF, Qadeer MA, Lopez R, Colabianchi N. Laryngeal cancer and gastroesophageal reflux disease: a case-control study. *Am J Med* 2006;119:768–776.
13. Qadeer MA, Colabianchi N, Strome M, Vaezi MF. Gastroesophageal reflux and laryngeal cancer: causation or association? A critical review. *Am J Otolaryngol* 2006;27: 119–128.
14. Coffin L. The relationship of upper airway passages to diseases of gastrointestinal tract. *Ann Otol Rhinol Laryngol* 1903;12: 521–526.
15. Jackson CMS. Contact ulcer of larynx. *Ann Otol Rhinol Laryngol* 1928;37:227–230.
16. Cherry J, Margulies SI. Contact ulcer of the larynx. *Laryngoscope* 1968;78:1937–1940.
17. Vakil N, van Zanten SV, Kahrilas P, Dent J, Jones R. The Montreal definition and classification of gastroesophageal reflux disease: a global evidence-based consensus. *Am J Gastroenterol* 2006;101:1900–1920; quiz 1943.
18. Kahrilas PJ, Shaheen NJ, Vaezi MF. American Gastroenterological Association Institute technical review on the management of gastroesophageal reflux disease. *Gastroenterology* 2008;135: 1392–1413,1413 e1–5.

19. Locke GR 3rd, Talley NJ, Fett SL, Zinsmeister AR, Melton LJ 3rd. Prevalence and clinical spectrum of gastroesophageal reflux: a population-based study in Olmsted County, Minnesota. *Gastroenterology* 1997;112:1448–1456.

20. el-Serag HB, Sonnenberg A. Comorbid occurrence of laryngeal or pulmonary disease with esophagitis in United States military veterans. *Gastroenterology* 1997;113:755–760.

21. Sontag SJ, O'Connell S, Khandelwal S, et al. Asthmatics with gastroesophageal reflux: long term results of a randomized trial of medical and surgical antireflux therapies. *Am J Gastroenterol* 2003;98:987–999.

22. Kahrilas PJ, Shaheen NJ, Vaezi MF, et al. American Gastroenterological Association Medical Position Statement on the management of gastroesophageal reflux disease. *Gastroenterology* 2008;135:1383–1391, 1391 e1–5.

23. Shaker R, Castell DO, Schoenfeld PS, Spechler SJ. Nighttime heartburn is an under-appreciated clinical problem that impacts sleep and daytime function: the results of a Gallup survey conducted on behalf of the American Gastroenterological Association. *Am J Gastroenterol* 2003;98:1487–1493.

24. Johanson JF. Epidemiology of esophageal and supraesophageal reflux injuries. *Am J Med* 2000;108 (Suppl 4a):99S–103S.

25. Koufman JA, Aviv JE, Casiano RR, Shaw GY. Laryngopharyngeal reflux: position statement of the committee on speech, voice, and swallowing disorders of the American Academy of Otolaryngology-Head and Neck Surgery. *Otolaryngol Head Neck Surg* 2002;127:32–35.

26. Hanson DG, Jiang JJ. Diagnosis and management of chronic laryngitis associated with reflux. *Am J Med* 2000;108 (Suppl 4a):112S–119S.

27. Loughlin CJ, Koufman JA, Averill DB, et al. Acid-induced laryngospasm in a canine model. *Laryngoscope* 1996;106:1506–1509.

28. Adhami T, Goldblum JR, Richter JE, Vaezi MF. The role of gastric and duodenal agents in laryngeal injury: an experimental canine model. *Am J Gastroenterol* 2004;99:2098–2106.

29. Vaezi MF. Laryngitis: from the gastroenterologist's point of view. In: Vaezi MF, ed. *Extraesophageal Reflux*. San Diego, CA: Plural Publishing Inc, 2009, pp. 37–47.

30. Shaker R, Ren J, Kern M, Dodds WJ, Hogan WJ, Li Q. Mechanisms of airway protection and upper esophageal sphincter opening during belching. *Am J Physiol* 1992;262: G621–628.

31. Shaker R, Dodds WJ, Ren J, Hogan WJ, Arndorfer RC. Esophagoglottal closure reflex: a mechanism of airway protection. *Gastroenterology* 1992;102:857–861.

32. Kelly JH. Management of upper esophageal sphincter disorders: indications and complications of myotomy. *Am J Med* 2000;108 (Suppl 4a):43S–46S.

33. Sidhu H, Shaker R, Hogan WJ. Gastroesophageal reflux laryngitis. In: Castell DO, Richter JE, eds. *The Esophagus*, 4th edn. Philadelphia: Lippincott, Williams and Wilkins, 2003, pp. 518–529.

34. Axford SE, Sharp N, Ross PE, et al. Cell biology of laryngeal epithelial defenses in health and disease: preliminary studies. *Ann Otol Rhinol Laryngol* 2001;110:1099–1108.

35. Johnston N, Bulmer D, Gill GA, et al. Cell biology of laryngeal epithelial defenses in health and disease: further studies. *Ann Otol Rhinol Laryngol* 2003;112:481–491.

36. Hogan WJ, Shaker R. Supraesophageal complications of gastroesophageal reflux. *Dis Mon* 2000;46:193–232.

37. Belafsky PC, Postma GN, Koufman JA. Validity and reliability of the reflux symptom index (RSI). *J Voice* 2002;16:274–277.

38. Park KH, Choi SM, Kwon SU, Yoon SW, Kim SU. Diagnosis of laryngopharyngeal reflux among globus patients. *Otolaryngol Head Neck Surg* 2006;134:81–85.

39. Sataloff RT. *Professional Voice: The Science and Art of Clinical Care*, 2nd edn. San Diego: Singular Publishing Group, 1997.

40. Ford CN. Evaluation and management of laryngopharyngeal reflux. *JAMA* 2005;294:1534–1540.

41. Weinberger PM, Postma GN. Laryngopharyngeal reflux from the otolaryngologist's perspective. In: Vaezi MF, ed. *Extraesophageal Reflux*. San Diego: Plural Publishing Inc, 2009, pp. 49–66.

42. Young JL, Shaw GY, Searl JP, Miner PB Jr. Laryngeal manifestations of gastroesophageal reflux disease: endoscopic appearance and management. *Gastrointest Endosc* 1996;43:225–230.

43. Ahmed TF, Khandwala F, Abelson TI, et al. Chronic laryngitis associated with gastroesophageal reflux: prospective assessment of differences in practice patterns between gastroenterologists and ENT physicians. *Am J Gastroenterol* 2006;101: 470–478.

44. Book DT, Rhee JS, Toohill RJ, Smith TL. Perspectives in laryngopharyngeal reflux: an international survey. *Laryngoscope* 2002;112:1399–1406.

45. Hicks DM, Ours TM, Abelson TI, Vaezi MF, Richter JE. The prevalence of hypopharynx findings associated with gastroesophageal reflux in normal volunteers. *J Voice* 2002;16: 564–579.

46. Vaezi MF, Ours TM, Hicks DM, et al. Laryngoscopic signs of gastroesophageal reflux disease: science or fiction? *Am J Gastroenterol* 1999;94:2601.

47. Belafsky PC, Postma GN, Koufman JA. The validity and reliability of the reflux finding score (RFS). *Laryngoscope* 2001;111: 1313–1317.

48. Mesallam TA, Stemple JC, Sobeih TM, Elluru RG. Reflux symptom index versus reflux finding score. *Ann Otol Rhinol Laryngol* 2007;116:436–440.

49. Milstein CF, Charbel S, Hicks DM, Abelson TI, Richter JE, Vaezi MF. Prevalence of laryngeal irritation signs associated with reflux in asymptomatic volunteers: impact of endoscopic technique (rigid vs. flexible laryngoscope). *Laryngoscope* 2005;115: 2256–2261.

50. Park W, Hicks DM, Khandwala F, et al. Laryngopharyngeal reflux: prospective cohort study evaluating optimal dose of proton-pump inhibitor therapy and pretherapy predictors of response. *Laryngoscope* 2005;115:1230–1238.

51. Merati AL, Lim HJ, Ulualp SO, Toohill RJ. Meta-analysis of upper probe measurements in normal subjects and patients with laryngopharyngeal reflux. *Ann Otol Rhinol Laryngol* 2005;114:177–182.

52. Ahmed T, Vaezi MF. The role of pH monitoring in extraesophageal gastroesophageal reflux disease. *Gastrointest Endosc Clin North Am* 2005;15:319–331.

53. Jacob P, Kahrilas PJ, Herzon G. Proximal esophageal pH-metry in patients with 'reflux laryngitis'. *Gastroenterology* 1991;100: 305–310.

54. Oelschlager BK, Eubanks TR, Maronian N, *et al.* Laryngoscopy and pharyngeal pH are complementary in the diagnosis of gastroesophageal-laryngeal reflux. *J Gastrointest Surg* 2002;6: 189–194.

55. Hirano I, Richter JE. ACG practice guidelines: esophageal reflux testing. *Am J Gastroenterol* 2007;102:668–685.

56. Wo JM, Jabbar A, Winstead W, Goudy S, Cacchione R, Allen JW. Hypopharyngeal pH monitoring artifact in detection of laryngopharyngeal reflux. *Dig Dis Sci* 2002;47:2579–2585.

57. Noordzij JP, Khidr A, Desper E, Meek RB, Reibel JF, Levine PA. Correlation of pH probe-measured laryngopharyngeal reflux with symptoms and signs of reflux laryngitis. *Laryngoscope* 2002;112:2192–2195.

58. Ulualp SO, Toohill RJ, Shaker R. Outcomes of acid suppressive therapy in patients with posterior laryngitis. *Otolaryngol Head Neck Surg* 2001;124:16–22.

59. Eubanks TR, Omelanczuk PE, Maronian N, Hillel A, Pope CE 2nd, Pellegrini CA. Pharyngeal pH monitoring in 222 patients with suspected laryngeal reflux. *J Gastrointest Surg* 2001;5: 183–190; discussion 190–191.

60. Maldonado A, Diederich L, Castell DO, Gideon RM, Katz PO. Laryngopharyngeal reflux identified using a new catheter design: defining normal values and excluding artifacts. *Laryngoscope* 2003;113:349–355.

61. Shaker R, Bardan E, Gu C, Kern M, Torrico L, Toohill R. Intrapharyngeal distribution of gastric acid refluxate. *Laryngoscope* 2003;113:1182–1191.

62. Belafsky PC, Postma GN, Daniel E, Koufman JA. Transnasal esophagoscopy. *Otolaryngol Head Neck Surg* 2001;125: 588–589.

63. Vaezi MF, Richter JE, Stasney CR, Spiegel JR, Iannuzzi RA, Crawley JA, et al. Treatment of chronic posterior laryngitis with esomeprazole. *Laryngoscope* 2006;116:254–260.

64. Vaezi MF. Reflux-induced laryngitis (laryngopharyngeal reflux). *Curr Treat Options Gastroenterol* 2006;9:69–74.

65. Sifrim D, Blondeau K. Technology insight: The role of impedance testing for esophageal disorders. *Nat Clin Pract Gastroenterol Hepatol* 2006;3:210–219.

66. Mainie I, Tutuian R, Shay S, *et al.* Acid and non-acid reflux in patients with persistent symptoms despite acid suppressive therapy: a multicentre study using combined ambulatory impedance-pH monitoring. *Gut* 2006;55:1398–1402.

67. Mainie I, Tutuian R, Agrawal A, Adams D, Castell DO. Combined multichannel intraluminal impedance-pH monitoring to select patients with persistent gastro-oesophageal reflux for laparoscopic Nissen fundoplication. *Br J Surg* 2006;93: 1483–1487.

68. Shay S, Tutuian R, Sifrim D, *et al.* Twenty-four hour ambulatory simultaneous impedance and pH monitoring: a multicenter report of normal values from 60 healthy volunteers. *Am J Gastroenterol* 2004;99:1037–1043.

69. Vaezi MF, Hicks DM, Ours TM, Richter JE. ENT manifestation of GERD: a large prospective study assessing treatment outcome and predictors of response. *Gastroenterology* 2001;120: A636.

70. Pritchett JM, Aslam M, Slaughter JC, Ness RM, Garrett CG, Vaezi MF. Efficacy of esophageal impedance/pH monitoring in patients with refractory gastroesophageal reflux disease, on and off therapy. *Clin Gastroenterol Hepatol* 2009;7:743–748.

71. Bogte A, Bredenoord AJ, Smout AJ. Diagnostic yield of oesophageal pH monitoring in patients with chronic unexplained cough. *Scand J Gastroenterol* 2008;43:13–19.

72. Wunderlich AW, Murray JA. Temporal correlation between chronic cough and gastroesophageal reflux disease. *Dig Dis Sci* 2003;48:1050–1056.

73. Patterson N, Mainie I, Rafferty G, *et al.* Nonacid reflux episodes reaching the pharynx are important factors associated with cough. *J Clin Gastroenterol* 2009;43:414–419.

74. Taghavi SA, Ghasedi M, Saberi-Firoozi M, Alizadeh-Naeeni M, Bagheri-Lankarani K, Kaviani MJ, et al. Symptom association probability and symptom sensitivity index: preferable but still suboptimal predictors of response to high dose omeprazole. *Gut* 2005;54:1067–1071.

75. Sun G, Muddana S, Slaughter JC, *et al.* A new pH catheter for laryngopharyngeal reflux: Normal values. *Laryngoscope* 2009;119:1639–1643.

76. Wiener GJ, Tsukashima R, Kelly C, *et al.* Oropharyngeal pH monitoring for the detection of liquid and aerosolized supraesophageal gastric reflux. *J Voice* 2009;23:498–504.

77. Reichel O, Keller J, Rasp G, Hagedorn H, Berghaus A. Efficacy of once-daily esomeprazole treatment in patients with laryngopharyngeal reflux evaluated by 24-hour pH monitoring. *Otolaryngol Head Neck Surg* 2007;136:205–210.

78. Field SK, Sutherland LR. Does medical antireflux therapy improve asthma in asthmatics with gastroesophageal reflux?: a critical review of the literature. *Chest* 1998;114:275–283.

79. Charbel S, Khandwala F, Vaezi MF. The role of esophageal pH monitoring in symptomatic patients on PPI therapy. *Am J Gastroenterol* 2005;100:283–289.

80. Havas T, Huang S, Levy M, *et al.* Posterior pharyngolaryngitis: double-blind randomised placebo-controlled trial of proton pump inhibitor therapy. *Aust J Otolaryngol* 1999;3:243.

81. Wo JM, Koopman J, Harrell SP, Parker K, Winstead W, Lentsch E. Double-blind, placebo-controlled trial with single-dose pantoprazole for laryngopharyngeal reflux. *Am J Gastroenterol* 2006;101:1972–1978; quiz 2169.

82. Steward DL, Wilson KM, Kelly DH, *et al.* Proton pump inhibitor therapy for chronic laryngo-pharyngitis: a randomized placebo-control trial. *Otolaryngol Head Neck Surg* 2004;131:342–350.

83. Qadeer MA, Phillips CO, Lopez AR, *et al.* Proton pump inhibitor therapy for suspected GERD-related chronic laryngitis: a meta-analysis of randomized controlled trials. *Am J Gastroenterol* 2006;101:2646–2654.

84. Reichel O, Dressel H, Wiederanders K, Issing WJ. Double-blind, placebo-controlled trial with esomeprazole for symptoms and signs associated with laryngopharyngeal reflux. *Otolaryngol Head Neck Surg* 2008;139:414–420.

85. El-Serag HB, Lee P, Buchner A, Inadomi JM, Gavin M, McCarthy DM. Lansoprazole treatment of patients with chronic idiopathic laryngitis: a placebo-controlled trial. *Am J Gastroenterol* 2001;96:979–983.

86. Oridate N, Takeda H, Yamamoto J, *et al. Helicobacter pylori* seropositivity predicts outcomes of acid suppression therapy for laryngopharyngeal reflux symptoms. *Laryngoscope* 2006;116:547–553.

87. Ulualp SO, Toohill RJ. Laryngopharyngeal reflux: state of the art diagnosis and treatment. *Otolaryngol Clin North Am* 2000;33:785–802.

88. Belafsky PC, Postma GN, Koufman JA. Laryngopharyngeal reflux symptoms improve before changes in physical findings. *Laryngoscope* 2001;111:979–981.

89. Bough ID Jr, Sataloff RT, Castell DO, Hills JR, Gideon RM, Spiegel JR. Gastroesophageal reflux laryngitis resistant to omeprazole therapy. *J Voice* 1995;9:205–211.

90. Chiverton SG, Howden CW, Burget DW, Hunt RH. Omeprazole (20 mg) daily given in the morning or evening: a comparison of effects on gastric acidity, and plasma gastrin and omeprazole concentration. *Aliment Pharmacol Ther* 1992;6:103–111.

91. Kahrilas PJ, Falk GW, Johnson DA, *et al*. Esomeprazole improves healing and symptom resolution as compared with omeprazole in reflux oesophagitis patients: a randomized controlled trial. The Esomeprazole Study Investigators. *Aliment Pharmacol Ther* 2000;14:1249–1258.

92. Shaw GY, Searl JP. Laryngeal manifestations of gastroesophageal reflux before and after treatment with omeprazole. *South Med J* 1997;90:1115–1122.

93. Hunter JG, Trus TL, Branum GD, Waring JP, Wood WC. A physiologic approach to laparoscopic fundoplication for gastroesophageal reflux disease. *Ann Surg* 1996;223:673–685; discussion 685–687.

94. Dallemagne B, Weerts JM, Jeahes C, Markiewicz S. Results of laparoscopic Nissen fundoplication. *Hepatogastroenterology* 1998;45:1338–1343.

95. Koufman JA, Belafsky PC, Bach KK, Daniel E, Postma GN. Prevalence of esophagitis in patients with pH-documented laryngopharyngeal reflux. *Laryngoscope* 2002;112:1606–1609.

96. Halum SL, Postma GN, Bates DD, Koufman JA. Incongruence between histologic and endoscopic diagnoses of Barrett's esophagus using transnasal esophagoscopy. *Laryngoscope* 2006;116:303–306.

97. Bjornsson E, Abrahamsson H, Simren M, *et al*. Discontinuation of proton pump inhibitors in patients on long-term therapy: a double-blind, placebo-controlled trial. *Aliment Pharmacol Ther* 2006;24:945–954.

98. Wright RC, Rhodes KP. Improvement of laryngopharyngeal reflux symptoms after laparoscopic Hill repair. *Am J Surg* 2003;185:455–461.

99. Salminen P, Sala E, Koskenvuo J, Karvonen J, Ovaska J. Reflux laryngitis: a feasible indication for laparoscopic antireflux surgery? *Surg Laparosc Endosc Percutan Tech* 2007;17: 73–78.

100. Swoger J, Ponsky J, Hicks DM, *et al*. Surgical fundoplication in laryngopharyngeal reflux unresponsive to aggressive acid suppression: a controlled study. *Clin Gastroenterol Hepatol* 2006;4:433–441.

101. Tutuian R, Mainie I, Agrawal A, Adams D, Castell DO. Nonacid reflux in patients with chronic cough on acid-suppressive therapy. *Chest* 2006;130:386–391.

102. Ossakow SJ, Elta G, Colturi T, Bogdasarian R, Nostrant TT. Esophageal reflux and dysmotility as the basis for persistent cervical symptoms. *Ann Otol Rhinol Laryngol* 1987;96: 387–392.

103. Wiener GJ, Koufman JA, Wu WC, Cooper JB, Richter JE, Castell DO. Chronic hoarseness secondary to gastroesophageal reflux disease: documentation with 24-h ambulatory pH monitoring. *Am J Gastroenterol* 1989;84:1503–1508.

104. Wilson JA, White A, von Haacke NP, *et al*. Gastroesophageal reflux and posterior laryngitis. *Ann Otol Rhinol Laryngol* 1989;98:405–410.

105. Katz PO. Ambulatory esophageal and hypopharyngeal pH monitoring in patients with hoarseness. *Am J Gastroenterol* 1990;85:38–40.

106. Woo P, Noordzij P, Ross JA. Association of esophageal reflux and globus symptom: comparison of laryngoscopy and 24-hour pH manometry. *Otolaryngol Head Neck Surg* 1996;115: 502–507.

107. Metz DC, Childs ML, Ruiz C, Weinstein GS. Pilot study of the oral omeprazole test for reflux laryngitis. *Otolaryngol Head Neck Surg* 1997;116:41–46.

108. Vaezi MF, Schroeder PL, Richter JE. Reproducibility of proximal probe pH parameters in 24-hour ambulatory esophageal pH monitoring. *Am J Gastroenterol* 1997;92:825–829.

109. Chen MY, Ott DJ, Casolo BJ, Moghazy KM, Koufman JA. Correlation of laryngeal and pharyngeal carcinomas and 24-hour pH monitoring of the esophagus and pharynx. *Otolaryngol Head Neck Surg* 1998;119:460–462.

110. Ulualp SO, Toohill RJ, Hoffmann R, Shaker R. Pharyngeal pH monitoring in patients with posterior laryngitis. *Otolaryngol Head Neck Surg* 1999;120:672–677.

111. Smit CF, Copper MP, van Leeuwen JA, Schoots IG, Stanojcic LD. Effect of cigarette smoking on gastropharyngeal and gastroesophageal reflux. *Ann Otol Rhinol Laryngol* 2001;110: 190–193.

112. Noordzij JP, Khidr A, Evans BA, *et al*. Evaluation of omeprazole in the treatment of reflux laryngitis: a prospective, placebo-controlled, randomized, double-blind study. *Laryngoscope* 2001;111:2147–2151.

113. Eherer AJ, Habermann W, Hammer HF, Kiesler K, Friedrich G, Krejs GJ. Effect of pantoprazole on the course of reflux-associated laryngitis: a placebo-controlled double-blind crossover study. *Scand J Gastroenterol* 2003;38:462–467.

30 Pulmonary Complications of Gastroesophageal Reflux

Radu Tutuian[1] and Donald O. Castell[2]

[1]Division of Gastroenterology, University Clinics of Visceral Surgery and Medicine, Bern University Hospital, Switzerland
[2]Division of Gastroenterology, Department of Internal Medicine, Medical University of South Carolina, Charleston, SC, USA

Introduction

Gastroesophageal reflux disease (GERD) is a prevalent condition with 40% of the adult US population experiencing reflux symptoms at least weekly [1]. According to the Montreal classification GERD is ". . . a condition that develops when the reflux of stomach contents causes troublesome symptoms and/or complications" [2]. Clinical manifestations of GERD include typical reflux symptoms (heartburn, regurgitation) and findings (erosive esophagitis, Barrett's esophagus), and atypical symptoms (cough, chest pain, throat burning, etc.) and manifestations (asthma, dental erosions, laryngitis, etc.). In the group of extraesophageal syndromes, the Montreal classification differentiates between established associations (reflux cough syndrome, reflux laryngitis syndrome, reflux asthma syndrome, reflux dental erosion syndrome) and proposed associations (pharyngitis, sinusitis, idiopathic pulmonary fibrosis, recurrent otitis media) between gastroesophageal reflux (GER) and extraesophageal symptoms.

The association between pulmonary diseases and GERD has been documented in a large case–control study by El Serag and Sonnenberg, including 101 366 patients with asthma, chronic bronchitis, chronic obstructive pulmonary disease (COPD), pulmonary fibrosis, chronic bronchitis, pulmonary collapse, and pneumonia with esophageal erosions of stricture as evidence of GERD, and matched subjects with the above-mentioned problems and no endoscopic findings suggestive of GERD [3]. Patients with endoscopic visible esophageal lesions had a higher incidence of pulmonary findings compared to the control patients without esophageal erosions (Table 30.1).

Recognizing pulmonary manifestations of GERD is important for both pulmonologists and gastroenterologists as pulmonary symptoms may be the only clinical manifestations of GERD. On the other hand, it is important to recognize that pulmonary disorders and GERD are highly prevalent and can coexist without causal relationship. The aim of the present chapter is to discuss the prevalence of pulmonary manifestations of GERD, pathophysiologic mechanisms leading to reflux causing pulmonary symptoms, and diagnostic tools and treatment options for pulmonary manifestations of GERD.

Epidemiology

The difficulty in establishing the prevalence of GERD as the cause of chronic cough is the multifactorial etiology of cough. Investigating 102 patients complaining of cough for an average of 53 ± 97 month, Irwin et al. identified GERD as the cause of cough in 21%, GERD being the third most common cause of chronic cough after post-nasal drip (41%) and asthma (24%) [4]. The authors noted that cough was due to only one condition in 73% of patients, 23% of patients had two conditions causing chronic cough, and 3% of patients had three conditions causing chronic cough. Conversely, in this patient group, cough was the only manifestation of GERD in 43% of patients. This observation is supported by another study by Irwin et al. in 12 patients whose chronic cough was likely due to reflux based on the results of chest radiographs, barium esophagogram, 24-h esophageal pH monitoring, esophagoscopy, and bronchoscopy, and the fact that cough disappeared with antireflux therapy. In nine of 12 (75%) of these patients GERD was, with the exception of chronic cough, clinically "silent" [5].

Asthma affects almost 9% of the US population [6], GERD symptoms occur daily in approximately 7–20% of the US adult population [7], and the coexistence of asthma and GERD is more frequent than chance association. The prevalence of GERD in patients with asthma is estimated to be between 34% and 89% [8, 9], and depends on the methods used to diagnose GERD. According to Field *et al.*, 77% of asthmatics experience heartburn, 55% report regurgitation, and 24% dysphagia [10]. More recently, Kiljander and Laitinen found typical reflux (heartburn and/or regurgitation at least once a week) in 52% of patients with asthma, while 25% of asthmatics diagnosed with GERD (based on endoscopy, 24-h pH monitoring) were free of typical reflux symptoms [11]. On the other hand, presence of typical reflux symptoms in asthmatics did not guarantee the presence of abnormal acidic reflux.

Pathophysiology

The classical mechanisms of reflux inducing pulmonary symptoms and manifestations include: (1) macroaspiration:

Table 30.1 Pulmonary conditions associated with erosive esophagitis and/or esophageal strictures.

Pulmonary condition	Cases (n = 101366)	Controls (n = 101366)	Odds ratio	P-value
Asthma	4314	2604	1.51	<.01
Pulmonary fibrosis	1511	952	1.36	<.01
Pulmonary collapse	2463	1595	1.31	<.01
Chronic bronchitis	8659	4931	1.28	<.01
Bronchiectasis	522	280	1.26	<.01
Chronic obstructive lung disease	8557	4920	1.22	<.01
Pneumonia	17283	12794	1.15	<.01

fairly large amounts of gastric content moving up the esophagus, past the upper esophageal sphincter (UES) and then penetrating into the lungs; (2) microaspiration: small amounts of gastric content moving through the esophagus, past the UES and then "dribbling" into the trachea and large bronchi; and (3) vago-vagal esophageal–bronchial reflex: gastric content reaching the distal esophagus stimulates either chemical or mechanical receptors leading to reflex bronchial constriction mediated through vagal nerves (Figure 30.1).

Macroaspiration is probably the least frequently occurring mechanism, as it implies increased abdominal pressure, filled stomach, penetration of the UES (with average resting pressure of approx. 100 mmHg), and failure of the laryngeal/epiglottic closing reflex, it is probably the most aggressive mechanisms due to the large amount of gastric content entering the pulmonary tree. Clinical scenarios in which this occurs include aspiration in alcoholic or neurologically impaired patients (stroke, Parkinson's disease, amyotrophic lateral sclerosis, etc.).

Microaspiration implies GER episodes, regardless of their volume, traveling all the way up the esophagus, an inappropriate opening of the UES, accumulation in the hypopharynx, and then small amounts penetrating the larynx into the trachea and bronchi. This mechanism is supported by studies by Tuchman *et al.* in a cat model, which documented a five-fold increase in airflow resistance when 0.5 mL of acid were instilled into the trachea compared to an 1.5-fold increase in airflow resistance when 1.5 mL of acid were instilled into the esophagus [12]. In addition, this response occurred in all (100%) animals when acid was infused directly into the trachea, whereas only 60% of animals had a bronchial response to esophageal acid infusion. Data to support the existence of microaspiration in humans were provided by Jack *et al.* who examined four asthmatics and three non-asthmatic GERD patients with 24-h esophageal

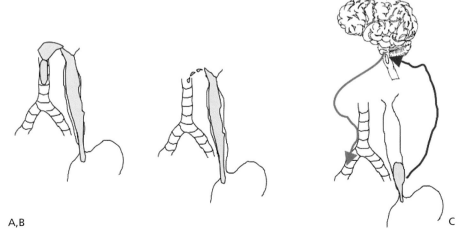

A,B   C

Figure 30.1 Major mechanisms by which gastroesophageal reflux can induce pulmonary symptoms and manifestations: (A) macroaspiration, (B) microaspiration, and (C) vagovagal reflex bronchoconstriction.

and tracheal pH monitoring placed under general anesthesia [13]. The authors noted 37 reflux episodes with prolonged (i.e. >5 min) distal esophageal acid exposure, five of which were associated with a drop in tracheal pH from 7.1 ± 0.2 to 4.1 ± 0.4. Peak expiratory flow rate (PEFR) dropped by 84 ± 16 L/min at times of tracheal acidification compared to a PEFR drop of 8 ± 4 L/min during esophageal pH drops as part of GER episodes.

Vago-vagal esophageal–bronchial reflex is considered a protective mechanism by which airways are protected from noxious intragastric agents. Mansfield and Stein investigated pulmonary response to intraesophageal acid in 15 asthmatics [14]. They documented increased airflow resistance following intraesophageal acid infusion, which was promptly restored by antacids, and postulated that a nervous, vagal mechanism is involved in this response. A few years later the same group performed animal studies in a dog model, documenting an increased airflow resistance following intraesophageal acidification that was ablated by bilateral vagotomy [15]. Schan *et al.* further clarified the distal esophageal location of this reflex by using dual pH monitoring in order to document no proximal extension (and hence no microaspiration) of intraesophageally infused acid [16]. In a study including 20 asthmatics with GERD, seven asthmatics without GERD, 10 patients with GERD but no asthma, and 10 normal controls, they infused acid in the distal esophagus. While a decrease in PEFR was noted in all patient groups, the PEFR did not return to normal in patients with asthma and GERD, suggesting that this group of patients is more sensitive to distal esophageal acid exposure and longer acid suppression might be required for the normalization of their pulmonary function tests. The vago-vagal esophageal–bronchial reflex contributes to a heightened bronchial reactivity to stimuli other than GERD. This hypothesis was proposed by Herve *et al.*, following observations that the total dose of methacholine required to reduce forced expiratory volume in 1 s (FEV_1) by 20% was lower following esophageal acid versus normal saline infusion [17].

In addition to this mechanism linking GER to asthma, there are factors promoting GER in patients with asthma. Pressure swings during acute asthma exacerbation can cause a more negative intrathoracic pressure and increased intra-abdominal pressure that might overcome more easily the normal (10–35 mmHg) LES resting pressure, this finally leading to an increased frequency of GER episodes [18]. In addition, chronic hyperinflation with subsequent flattening and stretching of the diaphragmatic crura [19] can lead to more frequent transient lower esophageal sphincter relaxations (TLESRs), the main mechanisms of GER episodes [20]. Furthermore, medications used to treat asthma can promote GER. Investigating 25 patients with asthma using 24-h esophageal pH monitoring, Ekström and Tibbling found that asthmatics with therapeutic levels of theophyline had a 24% increase in total esophageal acid exposure and 170% increase

in reflux symptoms [21]. In contrast beta2-adrenergic agents do not alter distal esophageal acid exposure [22], although repeated doses of albuterol have been shown to decrease LES pressure and distal contractile amplitude [23]. Oral corticoids may also affect GER as shown by Lazenby *et al.* in a prospective, placebo-controlled, cross-over trial in 20 moderately severe, stable asthmatics [24]. Esophageal acid exposure was increased in both the distal and proximal esophagus after 1-week therapy with prednisone 60 mg daily. Despite evaluation of various parameters (esophageal peristalsis, acid secretion, LES pressure, etc.), the mechanisms by which steroids worsen esophageal acid exposure remain unclear. Of note, medications to treat asthma have not been shown to increase the incidence of esophageal erosions [25] or increase the frequency of typical GERD symptoms such as heartburn and/or regurgitation [10].

Clinical evaluation

Pulmonary manifestations due to GERD include chronic cough, wheezing (i.e. asthma attacks), and recurrent pulmonary infections such as pneumonias or chronic bronchitis. Clinicians should be aware that these symptoms could be caused by GERD since they may be the only manifestation of GER. On the other hand, careful pulmonary evaluation and exclusion of other causes is equally important as establishing the association between pulmonary symptoms and GERD. For example, chronic cough might be secondary to asthma, chronic bronchitis, pneumonia, etc., but also due to smoking and medications [i.e. angiotensin-converting enzyme (ACE) inhibitors]. Similarly, asthma could be allergic, due to medication [i.e. Aspirin, non-steroidal anti-inflammatory drugs (NSAIDs), etc.] or exercise induced. Thus, GERD should be considered a cause for pulmonary symptoms not responding to conventional pulmonary treatments, but one should also be prepared to reject this consideration when there is no supporting evidence for GERD or patients continue to have symptoms despite adequate antireflux therapies. Last but not least, it is worthwhile mentioning that pulmonary symptoms and GERD might coexist without causal effect on each other ("true–true but unrelated").

Diagnostic tools

The armamentarium for diagnosing GERD in patients with pulmonary symptoms includes endoscopy, reflux monitoring, scintigraphy ,and bronchoalveolar lavage fluid (BALF) analysis.

Endoscopy

Upper gastrointestinal endoscopy (EGD) is the gold standard in diagnosing erosive esophagitis, the hallmark finding of GERD. Sontag *et al.* reported a prevalence of GERD of 43%

in asthmatics (79 of 186 consecutive patients with asthma) [25]. A study by Nakase *et al.* in 72 asthmatics undergoing upper gastrointestinal endoscopy found erosive esophagitis in 20 (27%) patients, 15 (21%) having a mild form (Los Angeles class A–B), while the remaining five (6%) had a more severe erosive esophagitis (class C–D) [26]. Severe asthma attacks and post-prandial exacerbation of asthma attacks were more frequent in the group of patients with severe GERD (class C–D) compared to the non-erosive reflux disease (NERD) and mild GERD group. Still, while EGD provides information on the coexistence of erosive esophagitis and pulmonary symptoms, its clinical value is limited in patients with reflux disease in the absence of esophageal erosions (i.e. NERD) and it does not provide information on the association between symptoms and reflux episodes.

Reflux monitoring (including impedance-pH-pressure)

Esophageal pH monitoring is the most widely used clinical tool to quantify GER. Spencer *et al.* were among the first to describe prolonged intraesophageal pH measurements in the late 1960s [27]. The technique became widely used both in clinical and research settings after Johnson and DeMeester published normal values in the mid 1970s [28]. Esophageal pH monitoring provides information on distal esophageal acid exposure and on the association between symptoms and acid reflux episodes. Technical details on esophageal pH monitoring are provided in Chapter 11. The clinical utility of esophageal pH monitoring in patients with pulmonary symptoms has been intensively investigated over the past 30 years. In a retrospective study, Harding *et al.* compared the results of esophageal pH monitoring in asthmatics with reflux symptoms and GERD and asthmatics without reflux symptoms and endoscopic evidence of GERD [29]. Of 199 asthmatics who qualified for analysis, 164 (82%) had reflux symptoms. The results of 24-h esophageal pH tests were abnormal in 72% (118 of 164) of asthmatics with reflux symptoms compared with 29% (10 of 35) of asthmatics without reflux symptoms. Among asthmatics with GERD, 79% (119 of 151) were found to have respiratory symptoms associated with esophageal acid and 91% (76 of 84) of patients reporting cough had a positive association of their symptoms with esophageal acid.

Following these results, the same authors performed a prospective cohort study comparing demographics, esophageal manometry, and 24-h esophageal pH testing in 26 patients with stable asthma without reflux symptoms and 30 age-matched asthmatics with symptomatic GER [30]. The study revealed that the prevalence of abnormal 24-h esophageal pH tests in asthmatics without reflux symptoms was 62% (16 of 26), and that asthmatics with asymptomatic GER had higher amounts of proximal esophageal acid exposure ($P < .05$) compared with asthmatics with symptomatic GER. Because demographic variables do not predict abnormal

24-h esophageal pH tests in asthmatics without reflux symptoms, the authors concluded that 24-h esophageal pH testing in asthmatics is required since GER is present in asthma patients, even in the absence of esophageal symptoms.

The most recent report comes from a multicenter study including 304 patients who underwent 24-h esophageal pH probe monitoring and lung function testing, and were assessed for methacholine responsiveness, asthma symptoms, and quality-of-life scores [31]. Abnormal GER in the distal esophagus was identified in 53% of patients, and among the 242 patients with proximal pH monitoring, 38% had an abnormal proximal esophageal acid exposure. Although there was no difference in need for short-acting bronchodilators, nocturnal awakenings, dose of inhaled corticosteroid, use of long-acting beta-agonists, lung function, or methacholine reactivity between individuals with and without proximal or distal GER, patients with GER reported more use of oral corticosteroids and had worse asthma quality of life, and subjects with proximal GER had significantly worse asthma quality of life and health-related quality of life compared with participants without GER. While esophageal pH monitoring provides information on esophageal acid exposure and relationship between pulmonary symptoms and acid GER, it provides insufficient information on the relationship between symptoms and reflux with pH above 4 (i.e. non-acid reflux).

In the early 1990s, Silny introduced multichannel intraluminal impedance (MII) for detection of esophageal bolus movement though the esophagus [32]. Details on the methodology of MII monitoring to detect and differentiate swallowing and reflux episodes of liquids and gas in the esophagus are discussed in Chapter 10. Combined impedance–pH monitoring expands the abilities of conventional pH monitoring to identify GER, providing information on bolus presence in the esophagus and height of reflux episodes, and, since it detects reflux episodes independent of the pH of the refluxate, it allows evaluation GER in patients on acid suppressive therapy.

To date, probably the most comprehensive evaluation on the relationship between GER and cough was performed by Sifrim *et al.* in 22 patients off acid suppressive therapy [33]. They found that the majority (70%) of cough episodes occurred "independent" of reflux, but 30% of cough episodes were temporally associated with reflux. In half (51%) of these cases, cough preceded reflux, while in the other half cough was preceded by acid (32%) or non-acid (17%) reflux (Figure 30.2). Using the information from the pressure transduces as "objective cough detector," the authors were able to evaluate not only the temporal association between reflux and cough, but also the causality between reflux and cough.

The same group followed up on these findings and performed a cross-sectional study in 100 patients with chronic cough [77 "off" and 23 "on" a proton pump inhibitor (PPI)] investigated with impedance–pH monitoring for reflux detection and manometry for objective cough monitoring

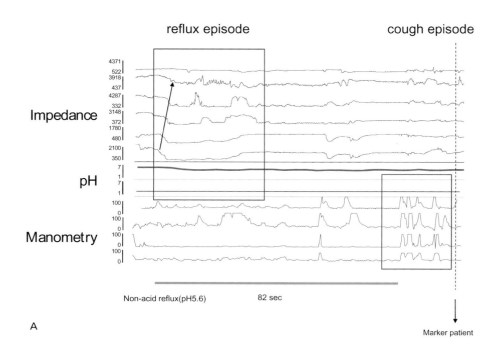

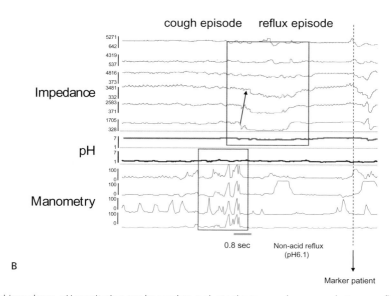

Figure 30.2 Combined impedance–pH monitoring can be used to evaluate the temporal sequence between reflux episodes and cough. (A) Example of a reflux episode followed by cough (i.e. reflux-induced cough). (B) Example of a cough episode followed by reflux (i.e. cough-induced reflux).

[34]. Symptom association probability (SAP) analysis was used to characterize the reflux–cough association. The authors found that acid reflux was a potential mechanism for cough in 45 patients (with either heartburn, high acid exposure or positive SAP for acid reflux), and non-acid reflux in 24 patients (with either increased esophageal volume exposure, increased number of weakly acidic reflux or positive SAP for weakly acidic reflux), and that reflux made no contribution to the mechanism for cough in 31 patients. The authors summarized their findings as a positive association between cough and weakly acidic reflux found in a significant subgroup of patients with unexplained chronic cough, and concluded that impedance–pH-manometry identified patients in whom cough can be related to reflux that would have been disregarded using the standard diagnostic criteria for acid reflux. Further, inter-ventional studies are warranted to investigate if this sus-pected causality is truly a predictor of treatment response.

We performed a study evaluating the relationship between cough and GER episodes in 50 patients on acid-suppressive therapy [PPI bid ± histamine 2 receptor antagonists (H$_2$RA) qhs] [35]. The association of cough and reflux was evaluated by calculating the symptom index (SI) (positive if ≥50%). Of 50 patients (38 female; mean age 43 years; age range 6 months to 84 years) who were monitored while receiving therapy, 13 (26%) had a positive SI for cough. The SI-positive group had a lower percentage of female patients and patients of younger age compared to the SI-negative group. Laparoscopic Nissen fundoplication was performed in six SI-positive patients who became asymptomatic and stopped taking acid-suppressive therapy during follow-up evaluations (median time 17 months; range 12–27 months). We concluded that, in patients with persistent pulmonary symptoms who are receiving PPI therapy, impedance–pH monitoring should be performed "on therapy," since a positive SI for non-acid reflux may be helpful in selecting patients who will benefit from antireflux surgery.

Rosen and Nurko reported similar results in 28 children (mean age 6.5 ± 5.6 years) with persistent respiratory symptoms on antacid medications who underwent 24-h impedance–pH monitoring [36]. The authors calculated the SI for each patient, followed by logistic regression to determine which reflux characteristics were associated with a high degree of symptom correlation present during the occurrence of symptoms. Overall, impedance–pH monitoring identified a total of 1822 reflux episodes, 45% of which were non-acidic (pH > 4). The mean SI increased using impedance–pH monitoring (35.7 ± 28.5) compared to pH-only monitoring (14.6 ± 18.9; $P = .002$), and significantly ($P = .035$) more patients had a positive SI with impedance–pH monitoring compared to pH-only monitoring. Multivariate analysis revealed that symptoms occurred more frequently when the reflux was non-acidic, mixed (liquid–air), and reaching the proximal esophagus. The authors concluded that non-acid reflux may be an important predictor of respiratory symptoms and that impedance–pH monitoring provides important information in the evaluation of children with intractable respiratory symptoms.

In summary, reflux monitoring provides important information on the relationship between GER and cough. Conventional pH monitoring allows distal esophageal acid exposure and the association between cough and acid reflux to be quantified. Combined impedance–manometry adds the capability of correlating reflux episodes, both acid and non-acid, with cough, while combined impedance–pH–pressure monitoring allows the time sequence between reflux and cough episodes to be determined (i.e. distinguishes between reflux-induced cough and cough-induced reflux).

Gastroesophageal ^{99}Tc scintigraphy

Delayed pulmonary scintigraphy after oral ingestion of radiolabeled ^{99}Tc colloid sulfur has been used to document pulmonary aspiration as a consequence of GER since the late 1970s. Chernow et al. were among the first to document abnormal scintigraphic activity in the lungs of three of six asthmatics suspected of having nocturnal aspirations from GER [37]. While this method is not designed to identify individual reflux episodes, it does document abnormal pulmonary depositions of orally ingested radiolabeled substances. Still, its routine use in clinical practice is limited by the need for radioactive markers and the availability of other diagnostic tools such as endoscopy and esophageal pH monitoring. Of note is a recent study by Ravelli et al. comparing 24-h intraesophageal pH monitoring and gastroesophageal ^{99}Tc scintigraphy with lung scan 18–20 h after the test meal in 51 patients with refractory respiratory symptoms (18 with cough, 14 with pneumonia, eight with apnea, seven with asthma, and four with laryngitis) [38]. Abnormal intraesophageal acid exposure was documented in 13 of 51 patients (25.5%) and overnight scintigraphy showed pulmonary aspiration in 25 of 51 patients (49%). Nineteen of these 25 patients had entirely normal pH study results, whereas six of 13 patients with abnormal pH study results had aspiration, highlighting the differences between the two methods in identifying pulmonary complications of GER.

Bronchoalveolar lavage fluid analysis

Corwin and Irwin were among the first to propose evaluating lipid-laden macrophages in the BALF as a marker for aspiration [39]. Staining BALFs from nine aspirators, 40 non-aspirators, and nine normal subjects with Oil-Red-O, the authors graded the amount of intracellular Oil-Red-O per 100 alveolar macrophages and computed a semiquantitative, lipid-laden alveolar macrophage index (LLMI). The authors found a mean index for aspirators of 207 ± 80 that was significantly greater than the mean indexes of non-aspirators (121 ± 97, $P < .02$) and normal subjects (0.6 ± 1.7, $P < .001$). An index of 100 or greater had a sensitivity and negative predictive value of 100% each, a false-negative rate of 0%, and a specificity of 57% in identifying patients with aspiration. Over the years the clinical utility of the LLMI to diagnose aspiration has been challenged, mainly due to its poor specificity [40, 41].

A more recent concept for BALF analysis to diagnose pulmonary complications of GERD relies on documenting the presence of pepsin, a highly specific gastric fluid marker in the bronchial secretions. Since pepsin is a large protein, the only way for it to reach the pulmonary tree is by aspiration of gastric fluid. In the late 1990s, Badellino et al. demonstrated in an animal model that peptic activity in BALF, due to the presence of the gastric proteolytic enzyme pepsin, could serve as a biochemical marker for pulmonary aspiration of gastric contents [42]. Its applicability to clinical practice was recently proposed by Farrell et al. [43] based on the results in 33 children with GERD, 13 asymptomatic negative controls, and five positive controls with observed aspirations. While none of the controls had pepsin activity in the BALF and the positive controls has higher median pepsin levels in the BALF, patients with proximal reflux episodes and chronic cough had also significantly elevated pepsin levels. The extent to which BALF analysis will establish itself as diagnostic test for pulmonary complications of GERD for clinical use outside study protocols will be clarified in the years to come.

Therapy

Medical therapy: acid suppressive therapy

Therapy for pulmonary complications of GERD follows the general principles of GERD therapy with some specific adaptations. Medical therapy for GERD-induced asthma and chronic cough includes H_2RAs and PPIs. Many studies have design limitations, including cross-over design (allowing for carry-over effect), small or selected populations, inconsistent outcome parameters, and/or lack of objective evidence of acid suppression. Nevertheless, placebo-controlled trials have shown symptom improvement and reduction in the use of asthma medication in 60–70% of patients. An improvement in PEF was seen in only 26% of patients [44].

Harding *et al.* evaluated the effects of acid suppressive therapy in 30 non-smoking adult asthmatics found to have GERD based on structured questionnaires, esophageal manometry, and dual-pH probe 24-h esophageal pH monitoring [45]. Acid suppressive therapy was started at omeprazole 20 mg daily and the dose was titrated until acid suppression was documented by 24-h pH monitoring. Patients then remained on this acid suppressive dose for 3 months and responders were identified by *a priori* definitions: asthma symptom reduction by greater than 20% and/or PEF increase by greater than 20%. At 3 months, 22 patients (73%) were asthma symptom and/or PEF responders: 20 (67%) were asthma symptom responders and six (20%) were PEF responders. In responders, asthma symptoms were reduced by 57% ($P < .001$), morning and night PEFs improved by 8% and 9%, respectively (both $P < .005$), and FEV_1 ($P < .02$), mean forced expiratory flow during the middle half of the forced vital capacity ($P < .04$), and PEF ($P < .01$) also improved. The authors concluded that acid suppressive therapy improves asthma symptoms and/or PFTs in up to 73% of asthmatics with GERD, and that many asthmatics require high doses (i.e. higher doses than omeprazole 20 mg daily) for a longer duration (i.e. at least 3 months).

A cross-over study in 107 asthmatics with GERD diagnosed by ambulatory esophageal pH monitoring [46]. Following 8 weeks of omeprazole 40 mg qid versus placebo, patients who received active therapy reported a reduction in nocturnal asthma symptoms ($P = .04$) and had improved corrected FEV_1 values ($P = .049$). When assessing symptom scores, 35% of patients were classified as responders.

A systematic review by Chang *et al.* of randomized controlled studies published up to 2006 in the Cochrane, Medline, and Embase databases identified five studies comparing PPIs with placebo [47]. All outcomes favored PPIs: the odds ratio for clinical failure (primary outcome) was 0.24 (95% CI 0.04–1.27); number needed to treat (NNT) was 5 (harm 50 to ∞ to benefit 2.5). The authors concluded that PPIs used to treat cough associated with GERD have some effect, even though the effect is less universal than suggested in consensus guidelines on chronic cough.

On the other hand, Littner *et al.* investigated in a double-blind placebo-controlled study the effects of 24 weeks of lansoprazole therapy on asthma symptoms, exacerbations, quality of life, and pulmonary function in adult asthmatics with acid reflux symptoms [48]. In this study 207 patients with moderate-to-severe asthma and acid reflux symptoms were followed with daily asthma symptom scores (diaries) while receiving either lansoprazole 30 mg or placebo bid for 24 weeks. Secondary outcomes included albuterol use, daily morning and evening PEF, FEV_1, forced vital capacity (FVC), asthma quality of life with standardized activities questionnaire score, investigator-assessed symptoms, exacerbations, and oral corticosteroid-treated exacerbations. At the end of 6 months, daily asthma symptoms, albuterol use, PEF, FEV_1, FVC, and investigator-assessed asthma symptoms had not improved significantly with lansoprazole treatment compared to placebo. Yet, fewer patients receiving lansoprazole (8.1% vs 20.4%, respectively; $P = .017$) had exacerbations and oral corticosteroid-treated (i.e. moderate-to-severe) exacerbations (4% vs 13.9%, respectively; $P = .016$) of asthma. The authors concluded that in adult patients with moderate-to-severe persistent asthma and symptoms of acid reflux, treatment with 30 mg of lansoprazole bid for 24 weeks did not improve asthma symptoms or pulmonary function, or reduce albuterol use. However, this dose significantly reduced asthma exacerbations and improved asthma quality of life, particularly in those patients receiving more than one asthma-control medication.

Mastronarde *et al.* reported on the results of a parallel-group, double-blind, controlled study evaluating the effects of 24-week treatment of esomeprazole 40 mg versus placebo bid in 412 participants with inadequately controlled asthma without typical GER symptoms [49]. The authors found that episodes of poor asthma control occurred with similar frequency in the placebo and esomeprazole groups (2.3 and 2.5 events per person-year, respectively; $P = 0.66$) and that there was no treatment effect with respect to individual components of the episodes of poor asthma control or with respect to secondary outcomes (pulmonary function, airway reactivity, asthma control, symptom scores, nocturnal awakening, quality of life, etc.). The presence of GER, documented by 24-h distal esophageal pH monitoring in 40% of participants, did not identify a subgroup of patients who benefited from PPI treatment. The authors concluded that despite a high prevalence of asymptomatic GER among patients with poorly controlled asthma, treatment with PPIs does not improve asthma control.

Most recently, Kiljander et al. reported the results of a 26-week, randomized, double-blind, placebo-controlled study including 961 adult patients (18–70 years) with moderate-to-severe asthma and symptomatic GERD [50]. The study collected data on the change in morning PEF (primary variable), evening PEF, FEV$_1$, asthma symptoms, Asthma Quality of Life Questionnaire, Reflux Disease Questionnaire, and tolerability. Relative to baseline, improvement in morning PEF was observed for both esomeprazole 40 mg once daily (+3.5 L/min; 95% CI, −3.2–10.2) and 40 mg twice daily (+5.5 L/min; 95% CI, −1.2–12.2), although no statistically significant between-treatment differences were apparent. At treatment end, both doses of esomeprazole significantly improved FEV$_1$ versus placebo (+0.09 L and +0.12 L; $P = .0039$ and $P < .0001$, respectively). The authors concluded that esomeprazole may improve pulmonary function and asthma-related quality of life, even though improvements were minor and of small clinical significance.

In summary, while initial studies have suggested a benefit in patients with pulmonary symptoms receiving acid suppressive therapy, recently published large, randomized studies provide less enthusiastic data. The challenge remains to define criteria by which to identify patients with pulmonary symptoms who would benefit from GERD therapy.

Surgical therapy: antireflux surgery

The idea of antireflux surgery to treat pulmonary manifestations of GERD is based on the concept that gastric components other than acidity contribute to the pathogenesis of cough and asthma. This concept is supported by Irwin et al.'s study in eight patients whose chronic coughs were due to GERD resistant to intensive medical therapy and who responded well to antireflux surgery [51].

Sontag et al. reported on the long-term results of a randomized trial of medical and surgical antireflux therapies in 62 asthmatics with GERD [52]. In this study, 62 patients with both GER and asthma were randomized to either antacids as needed (24 controls), ranitidine 150 mg tid (22 in the medical arm) or Nissen fundoplication (16 in the surgical arm). Asthma was defined as a previous diagnosis of asthma with discrete attacks of wheezing and 20% reversibility in airway disease. GER was defined as an abnormal ambulatory 24-h esophageal pH test and macroscopic or microscopic evidence of GER disease. Over at least 2 years general clinical status, asthma symptom scores, and pulmonary medication requirements were recorded monthly. By the end of 2 years, improvement, marked improvement, or cure in the overall asthma status occurred in 74.9% of the surgical group, 9.1% of the medical group, and 4.2% of the control group, whereas the overall status worsened in 47.8% of the control group, 36.4% of the medical group, and 12.5% of

the surgical group ($P < .001$, surgical vs medical and control). The authors concluded that in asthmatics with GERD, antireflux surgery (but not medical therapy with ranitidine 150 mg tid) has minimal effect on pulmonary function, pulmonary medication requirements, or survival, but significantly improves asthma symptoms and overall clinical status.

Kaufman et al. reported on the long-term results (median follow-up 53 month) of laparoscopic antireflux surgery in 128 patients with airway symptoms and GERD [53]. Following antireflux surgery, cough, hoarseness, wheezing, sore throat, and dyspnea improved in 65–75% of patients. Heartburn improved in 91% (105 of 116) of patients and regurgitation in 92% (90 of 98). The response rate for airway symptoms was the same in patients with and without heartburn. The only factor that predicted a successful surgical outcome was the presence of abnormal reflux in the pharynx as determined by 24-h pharyngeal pH monitoring. The authors summarized their findings as indicative for antireflux surgery providing an effective and durable barrier to reflux, and in so doing improved GERD-related airway symptoms in approximately 70% of patients, and pharyngeal pH monitoring as a useful tool to identify those patients more likely to benefit from antireflux surgery.

Gastroesophageal reflux and pulmonary fibrosis

Tobin et al. were among the first to investigate the prevalence of GER in patients with idiopathic pulmonary fibrosis (IPF) [54]. Seventeen patients with biopsy-proven IPF and eight control patients with interstitial lung disease other than IPF underwent dual-channel pH measurements. Patients with IPF had more severe distal and proximal esophageal acid exposure both upright and supine compared to those without pulmonary fibrosis. Sixteen of 17 (94%) patients with IPF had abnormal distal esophageal acid exposure, whereas only four of eight (50%) patients with non-IPF lung disease had an elevated percentage of time the pH was less than 4 in the distal esophagus. In summary, this study documented that patients with IPF have a high prevalence of increased esophageal acid exposure, usually without typical GER symptoms, and GER episodes in these patients tended to occur at night and extend into the proximal esophagus. The authors concluded that acid reflux may be a contributing factor in the pathogenesis of IPF.

A few year later the same group compared reflux monitoring results in 65 patients with IPF versus 133 patients with intractable asthma [55]. Esophageal pH monitoring was abnormal in 87% of IPF patients compared to abnormal esophageal acid exposure in 68% of patients with intractable asthma ($P = .014$). In the group of IPF patients, 12 (63%) of the 19 patients who were on acid suppressive therapy still had abnormal esophageal acid exposure, suggesting that these patients require higher doses of PPI or alternative approaches.

In 2009 Savarino *et al.* investigated the relationship between GER and pulmonary fibrosis in patients with systemic sclerosis (SSc) [56]. Forty patients with limited or diffuse SSc diagnosed according to the American Rheumatism Association (ARA) criteria underwent high-resolution computed tomography (HRCT) scan and 24-h impedance–pH monitoring off acid suppressive therapy. Patients with SSc and pulmonary fibrosis (i.e. HRCT fibrosis score ≥7) had higher distal esophageal acid exposure, higher number of acid and non-acid reflux episodes, and increased number of reflux episodes reaching the proximal esophagus. In addition, the HRCT score correlated well with the total number of reflux episodes in the distal ($r^2 = 0.637$) and proximal ($r^2 = 0.644$) esophagus (Figure 30.3). While this study nicely

documents the association between pulmonary fibrosis and reflux episodes, it does not answer the causality question, i.e. whether patients had more severe pulmonary findings due to an increased number of reflux episodes or if an increased number of reflux episodes is due to more severe lung fibrosis and symptoms. Thus the question whether or not development or progression of pulmonary fibrosis in SSc patients can be prevented/reduced by GERD therapy remains to be answered.

Gastroesophageal reflux and lung transplant

In 1990 Reid *et al.* reported on the importance of chronic aspiration in a series of 11 heart–lung transplant patients [57]. Five of the 11 (45%) patients had chronic cough, delayed gastric emptying, and/or esophageal dysmotility. While three patients improved once antireflux therapy was introduced, the authors concluded that GER could represent a potential cause of pulmonary complications after lung transplant. Almost one decade later, Palmer *et al.* reported a 23-year-old patient who underwent lung transplant for cystic fibrosis and who developed bronchiolitis obliterans syndrome (BOS) 15 months after lung transplant that required a second lung transplant [58]. Although the patient did not complain of typical reflux symptoms following the first lung transplant, approximately 4 months after retransplantation he reported typical reflux symptoms, the upper gastrointestinal endoscopy documenting severe reflux esophagitis. Since reflux symptoms persisted while on acid suppressive therapy, the patient underwent fundoplication. Following antireflux surgery the patient's pulmonary function tests improved and he maintained excellent pulmonary function for more than 2 years after fundoplication. The authors interpreted this first report of improved pulmonary function test following fundoplication as indicative of GER being a potentially reversible cause of BOS in lung transplant recipients. The same group reported a few years later a 73% prevalence of abnormal esophageal pH studies in patients undergoing lung transplant [59]. Among 43 patients who underwent fundoplication, 26 (60%) met criteria for BOS at the time of fundoplication; in 13 (50%) of these patients BOS was reversed by the surgical antireflux procedure. The authors concluded that GERD is very common in lung transplant patients and fundoplication should be recommended in the early stages of BOS as the surgical intervention improves lung functions.

Recently, Blondeau *et al.* reported one of the most detailed characterizations of GER and gastric aspiration in lung transplant recipients who underwent impedance–pH monitoring and BALF analysis [60]. Pepsin was found in BAL fluid of all patients and bile acids in BALF of 50% of the patients. Patients with BOS had neither increased GER nor elevated

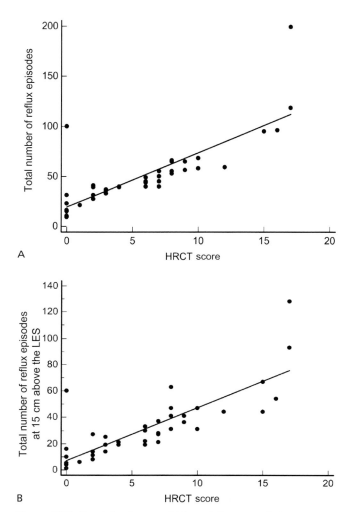

Figure 30.3 Correlation between high-resolution computed tomography (HRCT) scores and number of reflux episodes in the (A) distal ($r^2 = 0.637$; $P < .001$) and (B) proximal esophagus in patients with scleroderma and interstitial lung disease ($r^2 = 0.644$; $P < .001$). LES, lower esophageal sphincter (adapted from *Savarino et al.* [56]).

pepsin in BALF. However, 70% of the patients with BOS had bile in BALF compared with 31% of stable patients. PPI treatment reduced acid reflux but did not affect non-acid reflux nor prevent gastric aspiration. The same group reported on the effects of azithromycin to reduce GER and gastric aspiration in patients who underwent lung transplant [61]. Measuring acid and non-acid reflux using 24-h impedance–pH monitoring and gastric aspiration by quantifying pepsin and bile acid in the BALF in 47 lung transplant recipients before and after treatment with azithromycin, the authors found a significantly lower total number of reflux events [41 (30–61) vs 22.5 (7–37.5)], number of acid reflux events [24 (16–41) vs 8 (4–18)], esophageal acid exposure [2.9% (0.7–7.3) vs 0.2% (0.1–2.0)], bolus exposure [0.73% (0.5–1.4) vs 0.21% (0.12–0.92)], and proximal extent of reflux [14 (9–24) vs 5 (2–7)]) in patients treated with azithromycin. The authors interpreted these findings as supportive for the indication to recommend reflux reducing therapies rather than acid suppressive therapy in patients undergoing lung transplant.

Regarding the role of GER in lung transplant patients, current data indicate an elevated prevalence of GERD in patients considered for lung transplant and in patients who have undergone lung transplant. In addition, data from the surgical literature document improved outcome in lung transplant patients undergoing fundoplication. Accordingly, many centers recommend fundoplication at the time of lung transplant. Thus, the role of preoperative reflux monitoring is minimal since on the one hand, finding abnormal amounts of reflux supports the indication for fundoplication, and on the other hand, documenting normal GER cannot be used as a good argument against fundoplication in this set of patients.

Conclusions

Pulmonary manifestations of GERD include chronic cough, asthma, wheezing, chronic bronchitis, pneumonia, and pulmonary fibrosis. Mechanisms by which GER triggers pulmonary manifestations include macro- and micro-aspirations as well as esophageal–bronchial reflex loops. Pulmonary symptoms are often independent of typical reflux symptoms and can be the only manifestation of GERD. Lung scintigraphy and BALF analysis complement upper gastrointestinal endoscopy and esophageal reflux monitoring (pH or impedance–pH monitoring) in the diagnostic armamentarium in patients with extraesophageal reflux symptoms and findings. With regards to therapy, acid suppressive therapy may be successfully employed in patients with asthma and/or cough associated with GERD, while careful diagnostics may help identify patients benefiting from antireflux surgery as treatment for extraesophageal symptoms.

References

1. Shaheen NJ, Hansen RA, Morgan DR, *et al*. The burden of gastrointestinal and liver diseases, 2006. *Am J Gastroenterol* 2006;101:2128–2138.
2. Vakil N, van Zanten SV, Kahrilas P, Dent J, Jones R; Global Consensus Group. The Montreal definition and classification of gastroesophageal reflux disease: a global evidence-based consensus. *Am J Gastroenterol* 2006;101:1900–1920.
3. El-Serag H, Sonnenberg A. Comorbid occurrence of laryngeal or pulmonary disease with esophagitis in United States military veterans. *Gastroenterology* 1997;113:755–760.
4. Irwin RS, Curley FJ, French CL. Chronic cough. The spectrum and frequency of causes, key components of the diagnostic evaluation, and outcome of specific therapy. *Am Rev Respir Dis* 1990;141:640–647.
5. Irwin RS, French CL, Curley FJ, Zawacki JK, Bennett FM. Chronic cough due to gastroesophageal reflux. Clinical, diagnostic, and pathogenetic aspects. *Chest* 1993;104:1511–1517.
6. Eaton DK, Kann L, Kinchen S, *et al*. Youth risk behavior surveillance—United States, 2009. *MMWR Surveill Summ* 2010;59:1–142.
7. Locke GR 3rd, Talley NJ, Fett SL, *et al*. Prevalence and clinical spectrum of gastroesophageal reflux: a population-based study in Olmsted County, Minnesota. *Gastroenterology* 1997;112:1448–1456.
8. Irwin RS, Curley FJ, French CL. Difficult-to-control asthma. Contributing factors and outcome of a systematic management protocol. *Chest* 1993;103:1662–1669.
9. Cheung TK, Lam B, Lam KF, *et al*. Gastroesophageal reflux disease is associated with poor asthma control, quality of life, and psychological status in Chinese asthma patients. *Chest* 2009;135:1181–1185.
10. Field SK, Underwood M, Brant R, Cowie RL. Prevalence of gastroesophageal reflux symptoms in asthma. *Chest* 1996;109:316–322.
11. Kiljander TO, Laitinen JO. The prevalence of gastroesophageal reflux disease in adult asthmatics. *Chest* 2004;126:1490–1494.
12. Tuchman DN, Boyle JT, Pack AI, *et al*. Comparison of airway responses following tracheal or esophageal acidification in the cat. *Gastroenterology* 1984;87:872–881.
13. Jack CI, Calverley PM, Donnelly RJ, *et al*. Simultaneous tracheal and oesophageal pH measurements in asthmatic patients with gastro-oesophageal reflux. *Thorax* 1995;50:201–204.
14. Mansfield LE, Stein MR. Gastroesophageal reflux and asthma: a possible reflex mechanism. *Ann Allergy* 1978;41:224–226.
15. Mansfield LE, Hameister HH, Spaulding HS, Smith NJ, Glab N. The role of the vague nerve in airway narrowing caused by intraesophageal hydrochloric acid provocation and esophageal distention. *Ann Allergy* 1981;47:431–434.
16. Schan CA, Harding SM, Haile JM, Bradley LA, Richter JE. Gastroesophageal reflux-induced bronchoconstriction. An intraesophageal acid infusion study using state-of-the-art technology. *Chest* 1994;106:731–737.
17. Herve P, Denjean A, Jian R, Simonneau G, Duroux P. Intraesophageal perfusion of acid increases the bronchomotor

response to methacholine and to isocapnic hyperventilation in asthmatic subjects. *Am Rev Respir Dis* 1986;134:986–989.

18. Holmes PW, Campbell AH, Barter CE. Acute changes of lung volumes and lung mechanics in asthma and in normal subjects. *Thorax* 1978;33:394–400.

19. Roussos C, Macklem PT. The respiratory muscles. *N Engl J Med* 1982;307:786–797.

20. Mittal RK, Rochester DF, McCallum RW. Effect of the diaphragmatic contraction on lower oesophageal sphincter pressure in man. *Gut* 1987;28:1564–1568.

21. Ekström T, Tibbling L. Influence of theophylline on gastro-oesophageal reflux and asthma. *Eur J Clin Pharmacol* 1988;35:353–356.

22. Schindlbeck NE, Heinrich C, Huber RM, Müller-Lissner SA. Effects of albuterol (salbutamol) on esophageal motility and gastroesophageal reflux in healthy volunteers. *JAMA* 1988;260:3156–3158.

23. Crowell MD, Zayat EN, Lacy BE, Schettler-Duncan A, Liu MC. The effects of an inhaled beta(2)-adrenergic agonist on lower esophageal function: a dose-response study. *Chest* 2001;120:1184–1189.

24. Lazenby JP, Guzzo MR, Harding SM, Patterson PE, Johnson LF, Bradley LA. Oral corticosteroids increase esophageal acid contact times in patients with stable asthma. *Chest* 2002;121:625–634.

25. Sontag SJ, Schnell TG, Miller TQ, *et al*. Prevalence of oesophagitis in asthmatics. *Gut* 1992;33:872–876.

26. Nakase H, Itani T, Mimura J, *et al*. Relationship between asthma and gastro-oesophageal reflux: significance of endoscopic grade of reflux oesophagitis in adult asthmatics. *J Gastroenterol Hepatol* 1999;14:715–722.

27. Spencer J. Prolonged pH recording in the study of gastro-oesophageal reflux. *Br J Surg* 1969;56:912–914.

28. Johnson LF, DeMeester TR. Twenty-four-hour pH monitoring of the distal esophagus. A quantitative measure of gastroesophageal reflux. *Am J Gastroenterol* 1974;62:325–332.

29. Harding SM, Guzzo MR, Richter JE. 24-h esophageal pH testing in asthmatics: respiratory symptom correlation with esophageal acid events. *Chest* 1999;115:654–659.

30. Harding SM, Guzzo MR, Richter JE. The prevalence of gastroesophageal reflux in asthma patients without reflux symptoms. *Am J Respir Crit Care Med* 2000;162:34–39.

31. DiMango E, Holbrook JT, Simpson E, *et al*. Effects of asymptomatic proximal and distal gastroesophageal reflux on asthma severity. *Am J Respir Crit Care Med* 2009;180:809–816.

32. Silny J. Intraluminal multiple electric impedance procedure for measurement of gastrointestinal motility. *J Gastrointest Motil* 1991;3:151–162.

33. Sifrim D, Dupont L, Blondeau K, Zhang X, Tack J, Janssens J. Weakly acidic reflux in patients with chronic unexplained cough during 24 hour pressure, pH, and impedance monitoring. *Gut* 2005;54:449–454.

34. Blondeau K, Dupont LJ, Mertens V, Tack J, Sifrim D. Improved diagnosis of gastro-oesophageal reflux in patients with unexplained chronic cough. *Aliment Pharmacol Ther* 2007;25:723–732.

35. Tutuian R, Mainie I, Agrawal A, Adams D, Castell DO. Nonacid reflux in patients with chronic cough on acid-suppressive therapy. *Chest* 2006;130:386–391.

36. Rosen R, Nurko S. The importance of multichannel intraluminal impedance in the evaluation of children with persistent respiratory symptoms. *Am J Gastroenterol* 2004;99:2452–2458.

37. Chernow B, Johnson LF, Janowitz WR, Castell DO. Pulmonary aspiration as a consequence of gastroesophageal reflux: a diagnostic approach. *Dig Dis Sci* 1979;24:839–844.

38. Ravelli AM, Panarotto MB, Verdoni L, Consolati V, Bolognini S. Pulmonary aspiration shown by scintigraphy in gastroesophageal reflux-related respiratory disease. *Chest* 2006;130:1520–1526.

39. Corwin RW, Irwin RS. The lipid-laden alveolar macrophage as a marker of aspiration in parenchymal lung disease. *Am Rev Respir Dis* 1985;132:576–581.

40. Knauer-Fischer S, Ratjen F. Lipid-laden macrophages in bronchoalveolar lavage fluid as a marker for pulmonary aspiration. *Pediatr Pulmonol* 1999;27:419–422.

41. Kazachkov MY, Muhlebach MS, Livasy CA, Noah TL. Lipid-laden macrophage index and inflammation in bronchoalveolar lavage fluids in children. *Eur Respir J* 2001;18:790–795.

42. Badellino MM, Buckman RF Jr, Malaspina PJ, Eynon CA, O'Brien GM, Kueppers F. Detection of pulmonary aspiration of gastric contents in an animal model by assay of peptic activity in bronchoalveolar fluid. *Crit Care Med* 1996;24:1881–1885.

43. Farrell S, McMaster C, Gibson D, Shields MD, McCallion WA. Pepsin in bronchoalveolar lavage fluid: a specific and sensitive method of diagnosing gastro-oesophageal reflux-related pulmonary aspiration. *J Pediatr Surg* 2006;41:289–293.

44. Field SK, Sutherland LR. Does medical antireflux therapy improve asthma in asthmatics with gastroesophageal reflux?: a critical review of the literature. *Chest* 1998;114:275–283.

45. Harding SM, Richter JE, Guzzo MR, Schan CA, Alexander RW, Bradley LA. Asthma and gastroesophageal reflux: acid suppressive therapy improves asthma outcome. *Am J Med* 1996;100:395–405.

46. Kiljander TO, Salomaa ER, Hietanen EK, Terho EO. Gastroesophageal reflux in asthmatics: A double-blind, placebo-controlled crossover study with omeprazole. *Chest* 1999;116:1257–1264.

47. Chang AB, Lasserson TJ, Kiljander TO, Connor FL, Gaffney JT, Garske LA. Systematic review and meta-analysis of randomised controlled trials of gastro-oesophageal reflux interventions for chronic cough associated with gastro-oesophageal reflux. *BMJ* 2006;332:11–17.

48. Littner MR, Leung FW, Ballard ED 2nd, Huang B, Samra NK; Lansoprazole Asthma Study Group. Effects of 24 weeks of lansoprazole therapy on asthma symptoms, exacerbations, quality of life, and pulmonary function in adult asthmatic patients with acid reflux symptoms. *Chest* 2005;128:1128–1135.

49. American Lung Association Asthma Clinical Research Centers, Mastronarde JG, Anthonisen NR, Castro M, *et al*. Efficacy of esomeprazole for treatment of poorly controlled asthma. *N Engl J Med*. 2009;360:1487–1499.

50. Kiljander TO, Junghard O, Beckman O, Lind T. Effect of esomeprazole 40mg once or twice daily on asthma: a randomized, placebo-controlled study. *Am J Respir Crit Care Med* 2010;181:1042–1048.

51. Irwin RS, Zawacki JK, Wilson MM, French CT, Callery MP. Chronic cough due to gastroesophageal reflux disease: failure

to resolve despite total/near-total elimination of esophageal acid. *Chest* 2002;121:1132–1140.

52. Sontag SJ, O'Connell S, Khandelwal S, *et al*. Asthmatics with gastroesophageal reflux: long term results of a randomized trial of medical and surgical antireflux therapies. *Am J Gastroenterol* 2003;98:987–999.

53. Kaufman JA, Houghland JE, Quiroga E, Cahill M, Pellegrini CA, Oelschlager BK. Long-term outcomes of laparoscopic antireflux surgery for gastroesophageal reflux disease (GERD)-related airway disorder. *Surg Endosc* 2006;20:1824–1830.

54. Tobin RW, Pope CE 2nd, Pellegrini CA, Emond MJ, Sillery J, Raghu G. Increased prevalence of gastroesophageal reflux in patients with idiopathic pulmonary fibrosis. *Am J Respir Crit Care Med* 1998;158:1804–1808.

55. Raghu G, Freudenberger TD, Yang S, *et al*. High prevalence of abnormal acid gastro-oesophageal reflux in idiopathic pulmonary fibrosis. *Eur Respir J* 2006;27:136–142.

56. Savarino E, Bazzica M, Zentilin P, *et al*. Gastroesophageal reflux and pulmonary fibrosis in scleroderma: a study using pH-impedance monitoring. *Am J Respir Crit Care Med* 2009;179: 408–413.

57. Reid KR, McKenzie FN, Menkis AH, *et al*. Importance of chronic aspiration in recipients of heart-lung transplants. *Lancet* 1990;336:206–208.

58. Palmer SM, Miralles AP, Howell DN, Brazer SR, Tapson VF, Davis RD. Gastroesophageal reflux as a reversible cause of allograft dysfunction after lung transplantation. *Chest* 2000;118:1214–1217.

59. Davis RD Jr, Lau CL, Eubanks S, *et al*. Improved lung allograft function after fundoplication in patients with gastroesophageal reflux disease undergoing lung transplantation. *J Thorac Cardiovasc Surg* 2003;125:533–542.

60. Blondeau K, Mertens V, Vanaudenaerde BA, *et al*. Gastro-oesophageal reflux and gastric aspiration in lung transplant patients with or without chronic rejection. *Eur Respir J* 2008;31:707–713.

61. Mertens V, Blondeau K, Pauwels A, *et al*. Azithromycin reduces gastroesophageal reflux and aspiration in lung transplant recipients. *Dig Dis Sci* 2009;54:972–979.

31 Gastroesophageal Reflux Disease in Infants and Children

Carlo Di Lorenzo[1] and Yvan Vandenplas-[2]

[1]Nationwide Children's Hospital, Columbus, OH, USA,
[2]Universitair Ziekenhuis Brussels, Vrije Universiteit, Brussels, Belgium

Introduction

There are many reasons justifying the need for a chapter on pediatric gastroesophageal reflux disease (GERD) in a book dedicated to the esophagus: GERD is very common in infants and children [1], it is associated with high societal cost [2], and there are very few other gastrointestinal diseases in which children and adults differ so much as in GERD. One could make the case that in peptic ulcer disease, inflammatory bowel disease, irritable bowel syndrome, just to name a few other common gastrointestinal conditions, the pathophysiology, symptoms, diagnostic work-up, and treatment are similar in a toddler and in a fully grown adult. This is certainly not the case for GERD. What makes such a chapter even timelier is the publication in 2009 of two consensus documents: a practice guideline [3], endorsed by both the European and North American pediatric gastrointestinal societies; and a consensus paper [4] on the definitions of GERD in the pediatric population. Finally, in the past few years, new technologies have allowed the study of GERD in children of all ages including preterm infants, pharmacologic agents have been evaluated in well-designed, controlled studies in children with GERD, and much more is now known about the long-term outcome of children with esophagitis and reflux disease. This is an exciting time for clinicians and researchers with an interest in children with GERD!

Epidemiology

Healthy and sick individuals do not differ in whether they experience daily reflux, but in the frequency and/or characteristics of reflux episodes, and/or in the symptoms associated with such reflux episodes [5]. In young infants, regurgitation is the most common symptom associated with

reflux, but daily regurgitation is also within the range of expected behaviors and the great majority of regurgitating infants are happy, healthy, and thriving. More than half of 3–6-month-old infants regurgitate at least once a day, with a peak of regurgitation at 4 months [1] and a decrease in frequency during the second semester of the first year of life (Figure 31.1) [6]. Almost 25% of the parents of these infants consider the frequency and/or volume of regurgitation concerning enough to consult a physician [1]. Only one study has looked at the prevalence of symptoms in older children and adolescents: symptoms of reflux (heartburn, epigastric pain, and sour taste in the mouth) were present in 2–8% of children. Interestingly, the parents reported that the symptoms were less frequent than reported by the adolescents [7]. Treatment in the previous week with antacids was reported by 0.5% of parents of children aged 3–9 years, and by 1.9% and 2.3% of parents of children aged 10–17 years and children aged 10–17 years, respectively [7].

Few longitudinal follow-up studies have been performed to evaluate whether or not infants with significant GER are more likely to have persistent symptoms through childhood and/or adulthood. Although scientifically convincing evidence is missing, most studies indicate an association between reflux symptoms early and later in life. Nelson et al. followed 6–12-month-old infants with frequent regurgitation and compared them to a control group [8]. One year later, regurgitation had stopped in all, but eating and meals were still considered unpleasant experiences, suggesting that infant regurgitation may result in a "negative eating experience" that may persist for a longer period than the regurgitation itself. In a group of 69 children with a median age of 16 months referred to a tertiary care referral center, "standard medical therapy" was stopped successfully in 63% 1 year later [9]. A less favorable outcome was reported in older children (age 2–17 years) who had a mean follow-up of 28 months; symptoms persisted in 76%. Johnston et al. reported on the long-term follow-up of 118 children who had been found to have a hiatal hernia more than 20 years before

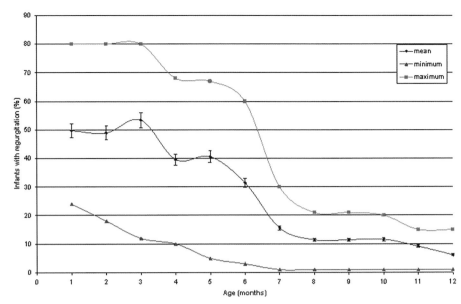

Figure 31.1 Natural evolution of regurgitation in infants (data from Hegar *et al.* [6]).

[10]. The hiatal hernia persisted in 53% of the non-surgically treated patients, but only a few individuals were symptomatic (46% had monthly heartburn, judged to be "severe" in only 2%). In another study, adults classified as "refluxers" were far more likely than "non-refluxers" to recall having experienced GER symptoms during childhood [11]. Adults with GER were also more likely to have taken antireflux medications as children and their symptoms as adults were more significant if they had exhibited symptoms of GERD by 11 years of age.

The mode of inheritance of GERD is not completely understood. The genetic influence on GERD is supported by increased GER symptoms in relatives of GERD patients [12]. Moreover, the concordance for GER is higher in monozygotic than dizygotic twins [13]. Genes in question have been localized to chromosomes 9 and 13. A locus on chromosome 13q, between microsatellite D13S171 and D13S263, has been linked with severe GERD in five multiple affected families [14]. This could not be confirmed in another five families, probably due to the genetic heterogeneity of GERD and the different clinical presentation of patients [15]. Carre *et al.* described autosomal dominant inheritance of hiatal hernia by discovering familial hiatal hernia in five generations of a large family, but without demonstrating the link to GERD [16]. Barrett's esophagus seems to be at least partially genetically determined [17].

Pathophysiology

It has been demonstrated that transient lower esophageal sphincter relaxations (TLESRs) not associated with swallows account for most episodes of GER in individuals of all ages, from prematurity into adulthood [18, 19]. Much like in adults, low resting LES pressure and increased intragastric pressure also play a role in the pathophysiology of pediatric GERD. In this section, we will highlight the pathogenic factors that differentiate children (especially infants) from adults.

The LES in infants measures only a few millimeters in length, compared to 2–3 cm in adults. The antireflux barrier provided by the LES is reinforced by the diaphragmatic crura and the acute angle of His. This angle is less acute in infants than in adults, acting almost like an inverted funnel directing gastric contents toward the esophagus when intragastric pressure increases. Intragastric pressure is more often raised in infants compared to adults. Healthy infants cry for an average of 2 h daily [20] and are routinely placed in infant chairs or car seats where they frequently lean forward due to their poor trunk control, situations that lead to increase in intragastric pressure. Children with chronic respiratory problems, such as bronchopulmonary dysplasia or cystic fibrosis, who frequently cough and wheeze, are at even a higher risk for GERD [3].

The intra-abdominal esophagus is a segment that collapses with increases in intra-abdominal pressure. This collapse contributes to the barrier to GER. The shorter length of the infant intra-abdominal esophagus limits its barrier function. The stomach of newborn infants has also been noted to have poor accommodation, a factor that may contribute to regurgitation early on in life [21] Prolonged supine positioning and a relatively large feeding volume in relation to gastric and esophageal size further contribute to regurgitation. Lying prone would be ideal in order to decrease episodes of

GER in infants, but prone positioning has been associated with an increased risk for sudden infant death syndrome (SIDS), leading to the "Back to Sleep" educational campaign. Another reason explaining why regurgitation is very common in healthy infants is the enormous volume of nutrients ingested over a short period of time during the first year of life, when birth weight triples. A typical 180-mL feeding for a 5-kg infant would be equivalent to a 3 L meal in an 80-kg adult, swallowed in 5 min. Feeding frequency is also higher in infants than in adults, resulting in more post-prandial periods during which TLESRs are more common.

A variety of motility disturbances have been described in children with GERD. Delayed gastric emptying has been reported in approximately half of children with GERD referred to pediatric gastroenterologists [22]. Prolonged stasis of ingested material in the stomach favors post-prandial reflux, possibly by increasing the rate of TLESRs and the likelihood of reflux occurring during the TLESRs. Motility dysfunction (low amplitude, simultaneous, broad-based peristaltic waves) is seen often in the distal esophagus of children with esophagitis, and resolves after successful treatment of inflammation [23]. Clearance of refluxate is further impaired by the prolonged time infants spend recumbent, a position which does not allow gravity to contribute to the esophageal emptying. Children with hiatal hernia have less effective esophageal clearance and are at higher risk for failure of non-surgical treatment compared to children without hiatal hernia [24]. Salivary production and rate of swallowing are reduced during sleep. Children sleep more than adults, thus further reducing the buffering of acid reflux episodes.

The relation between *Helicobacter pylori* infection and GER seems multifactorial and is still open for debate. Eradication of *H. pylori* does not seem to be associated with increased symptoms of GER in children and adolescents. In a population of 119 children, improvement of epigastric pain was significantly correlated with the improvement in GER symptoms, but not with eradication of *H. pylori* [25].

Clinical presentation

Tables 31.1–31.3 summarize the clinical manifestations of pediatric GER.

Esophageal manifestations

Regurgitation with occasional projectile vomiting is the most common presentation of infantile GER (Figure 31.1) [6]. Although most studies report a comparable incidence of regurgitation in unselected populations of formula- versus breast-fed infants, Hegar *et al.* reported a higher incidence in formula-fed infants [6]. This observation fits with the knowledge that GER and symptoms of GERD may be indis-

Table 31.1 Symptoms and signs that may be associated with gastroesophageal reflux.

Symptoms
Recurrent regurgitation with/without vomiting
Weight loss or poor weight gain
Feeding refusal
Irritability
Heartburn or chest pain
Hematemesis
Dysphagia, odynophagia
Wheezing
Stridor
Cough
Hoarseness

Signs
Esophagitis
Esophageal stricture
Barrett's esophagus
Laryngeal/pharyngeal inflammation
Aspiration pneumonia
Bronchospasm
Iron-deficiency anemia
Dental erosion
Dystonic neck and trunk posturing (Sandifer syndrome)
Apnea
Bradycardia
Apparent life-threatening events (ALTE)

Table 31.2 Symptoms and signs requiring investigation in infants with regurgitation or vomiting.

Consistently forceful vomiting
Bilious vomiting
Gastrointestinal bleeding
Onset of vomiting after 6 months of life
Failure to thrive
Diarrhea
Constipation
Fever
Lethargy
Bulging fontanelle
Macro/microcephaly
Seizures
Hepatosplenomegaly
Abdominal distention
Developmental delay
Other congenital abnormalities

tinguishable from those of food allergy [3, 4]. The incidence of cow's milk protein allergy is 3–5%, and is 5–10 times higher in formula-fed than in breastfed infants [26].

Poor weight gain is a critical warning sign that requires a thorough diagnostic work-up. Failure to thrive in an infant with GERD may be due to excessive regurgitation or to reduced

Table 31.3 Symptoms according to age.

Manifestations	Infants	Children	Adults
Regurgitation/vomiting	+++	+	+
Excessive crying/irritability	+++	+	−
Food refusal/feeding disturbancies/anorexia	++	+	+
Persisting hiccups	++	+	+
Failure to thrive	++	(+)	−
Abnormal posturing/Sandifer syndrome	++	+	?
Esophagitis	+	++	+++
Persistent cough	+	++	+
Aspiration pneumonia	++	+	+
Wheezing/laryngitis	+	++	+
Laryngomalacia/stridor/croup	+	++	−
Sleeping disturbancies	+	+	++
Anemia/hematemesis	+	(+)	+
Apnea/ALTE/desaturation	+	−	−
Bradycardia	+	?	?
Heartburn	?	++	+++
Epigastric pain	?	+	++
Chest pain	?	+	++
Dysphagia	?	+	++
Dental erosions/water brush	?	+	+
Chronic asthma/sinusitis	−	++	+
Laryngostenosis/vocal nodules problems	−	+	+
Esophageal stricture	−	(+)	+
Barrett's/esophageal adenocarcinoma	−	(+)	+

+++ very common; ++ common; + possible; (+) rare; − absent; ? unknown.
ALTE, acute life-threatening event.

oral intake. Food refusal may be related to the discomfort felt when food travels through the inflamed esophagus. GERD is only one of the many etiologies of "feeding problems" in infancy. Primary GER without associated anatomic malformations is only seldom a cause of failure to thrive.

Children who present with "distressed behavior" (excessive crying, back arching, lack of interest in eating, poor sleep) constitute a particularly challenging group of patients. Parents are often convinced that all the child's problems are due to reflux and demand diagnostic and therapeutic interventions. The same amount of distress and crying may be perceived by some parents as acceptable, while it may be unbearable for other parents. Many factors, some of them infant related (e.g. cow's milk protein allergy) and others not infant related (e.g. exposure to tobacco smoke), may cause infant irritability. Parents need to be educated that there is substantial interindividual variability and healthy infants may cry for up to 5 h a day [20]. In the absence of other alarm signs, medical providers need to provide education and reassurance, and resist the urge to prescribe medications that have no proven benefit in this scenario. Two controlled studies with proton pump inhibitors (PPIs) in distressed infants have shown an equal decrease in dis-

tressed behavior in the active treatment and the placebo groups [27, 28].

Descriptions of intensity, location, and severity of pain (caused by reflux) may be unreliable until the age of 8–12 years [3, 4, 8]. In adolescents, heartburn is the most characteristic symptom of GERD. Diagnosis and management of GERD in older children (>12 years) and adolescents follow the recommendations for adults [3 −5].

Esophagitis is defined as visible breaks of the esophageal mucosa [4]. Esophagitis is present in 15–62% of children with GER symptoms. Incidence of erosive esophagitis in 0–17-year-old children with GER symptoms was 12.4%, and increased with age [29]. Erosive esophagitis is rare in infants and premature babies. This finding is in sharp contrast with the extremely high incidence (24.8%) of antireflux medication prescribed in extremely low birth weight infants at the moment of discharge [30]. Hiatal hernia is more frequent in children with erosive esophagitis than in those without (7.7% vs 2.5%) [29]. Esophagitis typically presents with pain, but it can also be asymptomatic. Children with severe neurologic impairment may have a limited ability to localize the source of their distress and constitute the most difficult group to diagnose and treat appropriately.

One the most common current challenges for the clinician is differentiating reflux esophagitis from eosinophilic esophagitis (EoE). In children with EoE, the mucosa may appear pale, granular, and furrowed, and occasionally rings may be seen during endoscopy [4, 31]. In reflux esophagitis, the distal and lower eosinophilic infiltrate is mostly limited to fewer than 5/high power field (HPF). In primary eosinophilic esophagitis, there are more than 20 eosinophils/HPF. Recently, failure of PPI treatment as a condition to diagnose EoE has increased the attention on GER as a coexistent or even predisposing factor for the development of EoE [31]. It has been suggested that excessive use of PPIs may be associated with the development of EoE [32].

Although GERD is frequently mentioned as a cause of dysphagia or odynophagia, there are no convincing pediatric data demonstrating this association. Feeding difficulty and/or refusal are terms often used to describe uncoordinated sucking and swallowing, gagging, and irritability during feeding. A relation between GER, GERD, and feeding refusal has not been established.

Extraesophageal manifestations

Reactive airway disease and recurrent pneumonia may be caused by direct aspiration, by vagally-mediated bronchial and laryngeal spasm, or by neurally-mediated inflammation. Esophageal acidification in patients with asthma can produce airway hyperresponsiveness and airflow obstruction [33]. An association between wheezing, especially if nocturnal, and reflux measured by pH or impedance probe has been frequently reported. However, a correlation between pH-metry results and pulmonary function tests was not found [34]. There is no uniformity in the criteria to use in order to identify patients in whom reflux treatment may result in improvement of asthma. It is not clear if recording in the upper esophagus or pharynx helps in making therapeutic decisions in children with chronic respiratory problems [35, 36]. A new technique to record pharyngeal reflux has been developed (Restech®), with promising results needing confirmation [36]. The measurement of pepsin in bronchoalveolar lavage seems to be a promising technique for the identification of children with reflux-related pulmonary symptoms, although substantial overlap seems to exist between patients and controls [37]. A study evaluating nuclear scintigraphy with late imaging reported that 50% of patients with a variety of respiratory symptoms had pulmonary aspiration after 24 h [38]. However, aspiration also occurs in healthy subjects, especially during sleep [39], and later studies failed to reproduce these findings [40]. The majority of children with cystic fibrosis (CF) have pathologic acid reflux [3]. A high prevalence of acid GER was reported in very young CF infants, before respiratory symptoms developed. Early reflux treatment seems to slow down the respiratory deterioration. In children with CF, a better weight gain was reported during PPI treatment [41], but whether this is due a reduction of acid reflux or better buffering of acid gastric content in the intestine is unclear.

The relationship between apnea and apparent life-threatening events (ALTE) and GER has been debated for decades. The literature can best be summarized as follows: most series fail to show a temporal association between pathologic apnea and GER, and GER and bradycardia and GER and ALTE [3, 5]. However, impedance in combination with polysomnographic recording has shown a relation between GER and short, physiologic apnea [42]. There are also well-described case reports or small case series that demonstrate that pathologic apnea can occur as a consequence of GER. However, reflux as a cause of pathologic apnea and/or ALTE remains rare.

Sandifer syndrome involves abnormal posturing with torsional dystonia mainly involving the neck and back in children with GERD, probably due to a vagally-mediated reflex triggered by esophageal acid exposure. A multichannel physiologic study demonstrated association of rectus abdominis contraction with onset of reflux episodes, and association of reflux episodes with Sandifer syndrome posturing in a child with resolution of symptoms after fundoplication [43]. Awareness of the relationship between GERD and Sandifer syndrome may spare affected children from persistent symptoms and inappropriate neurologic testing and treatment.

GER has been suggested as a potential contributing factor in children with recurrent sinusitis, rhinopharyngitis, and otitis media. In a small case series of children with chronic sinusitis, reflux treatment dramatically reduced the number of children requiring sinus surgery [44]. The amount of time with pH below 6 in the pharynx was higher in children with chronic rhinopharyngitis compared to controls [45]. However, in another study, the frequencies of ear, sinus, and upper respiratory infections and of episodes of wheezing were comparable in infants with or without GER [8]. No convincing data demonstrate an association of otitis media and GER in children. However, otalgia has been associated with GER in a small group of children and was reported to improve with treatment of GER [46].

Diagnosis

Many of the symptoms and signs that may be associated with GER in infants and children are non-specific. GERD is diagnosed when tests show excessive frequency or duration of reflux events, esophagitis, or a clear association between symptoms and signs and reflux events in the absence of an alternative diagnosis. Diagnostic tests can be subdivided into those measuring only post-prandial reflux (barium meal, nuclear scintigraphy, ultrasonography), those measuring reflux over prolonged periods (pH monitoring for acid reflux, impedance–pH measurement for acid, weakly acid and non-acid reflux, and bilirubin measurement for bile reflux), and endoscopy evaluating mainly the histologic consequence of reflux. In general, the severity of symptoms does not correlate to the degree of abnormality on reflux investigations [3, 47].

The main role of history and physical examination is to exclude other disorders that present with symptoms similar to GERD and to identify complications of GERD [4]. In adults, GERD is often diagnosed based on a history of heartburn defined as substernal, burning chest pain, with or without regurgitation. Recent adult and pediatric consensus guidelines have applied the terms "typical reflux syndrome" or "reflux chest pain syndrome" to this presentation [4]. Based on expert opinion, the diagnosis of GERD can be made in adolescents presenting with typical heartburn symptoms. However, a clinical diagnosis based on a history of heartburn cannot be used in infants, children or non-verbal adolescents (e.g. those with neurologic impairment) as these individuals cannot reliably communicate the quality and quantity of their symptoms. The verbal child can communicate pain, but descriptions of quality, intensity, location, and severity generally are unreliable until at least 8 and possibly 12 years of age [48]. Parent or patient-reported questionnaires based on clusters of symptoms have been developed because symptoms do not consistently correlate with objective findings or response to medical treatment. Orenstein *et al.* developed a diagnostic questionnaire for infants, with a score of greater than 7 (of 25 possible) having a sensitivity of 0.74 and specificity of 0.94 during primary validation [49]. The questionnaire has undergone several revisions [50]. However, when applied to another population, it had a sensitivity and specificity of only 43% and 79%, respectively. According to Salvatore *et al.*, the questionnaire had a sensitivity and specificity of 47% and 81%, respectively, for a reflux index of greater than 10%, and 65% and 63%, respectively, for a reflux index of greater than 5%, and failed to identify 26% of infants with GERD [47]. In infants and young children, no symptom or cluster of symptoms has been shown to reliably predict complications of reflux or to predict those infants likely to respond to therapy [4].

Radiographic tests

Upper gastrointestinal series is neither sensitive nor specific for diagnosing GERD. The brief duration of the upper gastrointestinal series produces false-negative results, while the frequent occurrence of non-pathologic reflux during the examination produces false-positive results. The upper gastrointestinal series is useful to detect anatomic abnormalities and its routine performance to diagnose reflux or GERD is not justified [3].

The technetium-99m nuclear scan evaluates post-prandial reflux independent of the gastric pH, and may demonstrate aspiration of gastric contents. Scintigraphy can also measure gastric emptying, which may be delayed in children with GERD [22]. A lack of standardized techniques and the absence of age-specific norms limit the value of this test. A negative test does not exclude aspiration, as it may occur intermittently. Nuclear scintigraphy is not recommended in the routine diagnosis and management of GERD in infants and children [3].

Ultrasound is not recommended as a routine test to measure GER, but the technique may provide some useful information as it measures fluid movements over short periods of time. It can also detect hiatus hernia, length and position of the LES relative to the diaphragm, and magnitude of the gastroesophageal angle of His. A barium upper gastrointestinal series can provide the same information, but it is associated with radiation exposure. Compared to esophageal pH-metry, the sensitivity of color Doppler ultrasound performed for 15 min post-prandially is about 95% with a specificity of only 11%, and there is no correlation between reflux frequency detected by ultrasound and pH monitoring [51]. At present, there is no role for ultrasound as a routine diagnostic tool for GERD in children [3].

Endoscopy and biopsy

Esophagogastroduodenoscopy with biopsies is the only method to reliably diagnose esophageal manifestations of GERD, such as erosive esophagitis or Barrett's esophagus. Mucosal biopsies are always obtained during endoscopy in children and enable evaluation of the microscopic anatomy. Recent Global Consensus guidelines define reflux esophagitis as the presence of endoscopically visible breaks in the esophageal mucosa at or immediately above the gastroesophageal junction [4]. Evidence from adult studies indicates that visible breaks in the esophageal mucosa are the endoscopic sign of greatest interobserver reliability [52]. However, it is not clear if the experience in adults can be extrapolated to children. Mucosal erythema and an irregular Z-line are not reliable signs of reflux esophagitis. Grading the severity of esophagitis, using a recognized endoscopic classification system is useful for evaluation of the severity of esophagitis and response to treatment. The Hetzel–Dent classification has been used in several pediatric studies, while the Los Angeles classification is generally used for adults, but is suitable also for children [4]. Eosinophilia, elongation of papillae (rete pegs), basal hyperplasia, and dilated intercellular spaces (spongiosis) are non-specific reactive changes that may be found in esophagitis of other causes, or in healthy volunteers [4]. The presence of endoscopically normal esophageal mucosa does not exclude a diagnosis of non-erosive reflux disease or esophagitis of other etiologies. Recent studies have shown considerable overlap between the histology of reflux esophagitis and EoE [31, 53]. When EoE is considered as part of the differential diagnosis, it is advisable to take esophageal biopsies from the proximal and distal esophagus. Mucosal eosinophilia may be

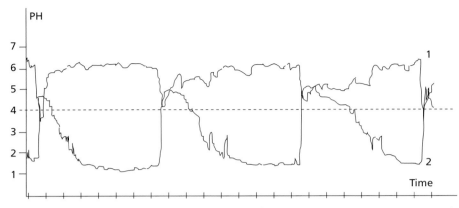

Figure 31.2 Esophageal (tracing 1) and gastric (tracing 2) pH monitoring in an infant presenting with regurgitation. Automatic computer analysis of the tracing is normal because esophageal pH does not drop below 4.0. This is the consequence of gastric acid buffering caused by the milk feeding. Yet, the regurgitation episodes are visible on the esophageal pH tracing.

present in the esophageal mucosa in asymptomatic infants under 1 year of age [54], and in symptomatic infants eosinophilic infiltrate may be due to milk protein allergy [55].

Esophageal luminal monitoring

Esophageal pH monitoring measures the frequency and duration of acid reflux episodes. Wireless capsule sensors that can be clipped to the esophageal mucosa during endoscopy allow pH monitoring without a nasal probe. By convention, a drop in pH below 4.0 is considered an acid reflux episode. This cut-off was initially chosen because heartburn induced by acid perfusion of the esophagus in adults generally occurs at pH below 4.0 [56]. Although pH monitoring data analysis is performed automatically by computer programs, visual inspection of the tracing is required to detect artifacts and for correct interpretation (Figure 31.2). The reflux index (percentage of the entire record with esophageal pH < 4.0) is the most commonly used summary score in children. Other commonly measured parameters include total number of reflux episodes, number of reflux episodes lasting longer than 5 min, and duration of the longest reflux episode. The area under the pH 4.0 curve has been associated with erosive esophagitis in children [57]. However, this parameter has not entered routine use. Most of the data above pertain to infants, in whom frequency, volume, and type of feeding may have different buffering effects. "Cut-off" values that discriminate between physiologic GER and pathologic GERD are misleading because there is a continuum between both. Normal ranges should be regarded as guidelines rather than absolutes. Esophageal pH monitoring is insensitive to weakly acid and non-acid reflux events. The degree of abnormality of pH monitoring has not been shown to correlate with symptom severity [47]. Esophageal pH monitoring is also useful for evaluating the efficacy of acid suppression therapy. Esophageal pH monitoring results may

help correlate symptoms with acid reflux by applying various analytic methods, including the symptom index, symptom sensitivity index, and symptom association probability. The optimal cut-offs of these parameters and thus the clinical utility of pH studies to determine a causal relationship between specific symptoms (pain, cough, etc) and reflux have been insufficiently studied in pediatric patients.

Multiple intraluminal impedance (MII) is a pH-independent procedure for measuring the movement of fluids, solids, and air in the esophagus (Figure 31.3). Esophageal impedance tracings are analyzed for changes in impedance caused by the passage of liquid or gas (or mixed) boluses. Although MII can detect very small bolus volumes, pH-only reflux (acid reflux without bolus movement) exists as well [58]. Therefore, impedance measurement should always be combined with pH detection in a single catheter. The combined measurement of pH and impedance (MII–pH) provides additional information as to whether refluxed material is acid, weakly acidic, or non-acidic. Variable reproducibility of this technique has been reported [59, 60]. Evaluation of MII recordings is aided by automated analysis tools, but the automatic analysis software stills needs validation in children. Although normal values for all age groups have not yet been established, these are unlikely to be detrimental because the main advantage and indication of the technique is demonstration of a symptom–reflux association in time.

The combination of pH and MII with simultaneous monitoring of symptoms using video-polysomnography has proven useful for the evaluation of symptom correlations between reflux episodes and apnea, cough, other respiratory symptoms, and behavioral symptoms [42]. However, the nasal presence of a probe alters the quality of sleep.

Continuous monitoring of biluribin in the esophagus has been suggested as a means of detecting esophageal reflux of duodenal juice or duodenogastroesophageal reflux (DGER).

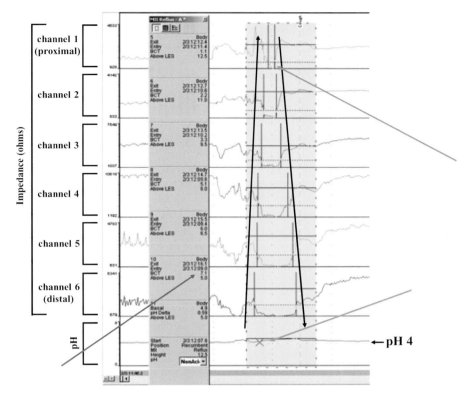

Figure 31.3 Example impedance tracing showing a weakly acid reflux episode in an infant with respiratory symptoms. The black arrows indicate the direction of bolus movement. The absence of "spikes" within the drops of impedance waveforms indicates a purely "liquid" reflux episode. The red arrow demarcates the duration (7.1s) of bolus exposure in the distal esophagus. The green arrow points to the pH which, because it is above 4 but below 7, indicates that it is a weakly acidic reflux event. The fact that the bolus is detectable even in the most proximal channel near the oropharynx (black arrow) suggests increased likelihood/possibility of aspiration.

One study indicated that therapy with PPI decreased the esophageal damage caused by DGER [61]. The role of bile reflux in children resistant to PPI treatment has not been established.

Other investigations

Recent studies reported the finding of pepsin, a gastric enzyme, in middle ear effusions of children with chronic otitis media [62]. This relation has not been validated in controlled treatment trials. Also, many infants with acute otitis media do vomit. As a consequence, the finding of pepsin can be a consequence and not causal. The presence of lactose, glucose, pepsin, or lipid-filled macrophages in bronchoalveolar lavage fluid has been proposed to implicate aspiration secondary to reflux as a cause of chronic pulmonary conditions [37].

GERD cannot be diagnosed by esophageal manometry. Esophageal manometry measures esophageal peristalsis, upper and lower esophageal sphincter pressures, and the coordinated function of these structures during swallowing. Manometry is critical to diagnosing achalasia or other motor disorders of the esophagus which may mimic GERD, but is not useful for the diagnosis of GERD. Recent studies indicate there is no role for manometry in predicting outcome of fundoplication [63].

Empiric treatment with acid suppression as a diagnostic test has been studied in adults in many clinical situations. However, empiric therapy has only modest sensitivity and specificity as a diagnostic test for GERD, depending upon the comparative reference standard used (endoscopy, pH monitoring, symptom questionnaires) [64], and the appropriate duration of a "diagnostic trial" of acid suppression has not been determined. There are no data in infants, children, and adolescents on the utility of a therapeutic trial as a diagnostic test.

Treatment

Conservative therapy and lifestyle modifications in infants

Parental education, guidance, and support are always required, and are usually sufficient to manage healthy, thriving infants presenting with regurgitation or other signs and symptoms likely due to physiologic GER. Whether regurgitation is considered "troublesome" or not depends largely on the coping capacity of the parents. Therefore, reassurance is essential in the management of regurgitation. However, frequently parents will expect some therapeutic intervention. In these circumstances, it is important that therapeutic advice be without risk and use of medications is not recommended.

Although about 50% of normal 1–4-month-old infants regurgitate at least once a day, up to 20% of caregivers in the United States seek medical help for this reason [1]. A subset of infants with allergy to cow's milk protein experience regurgitation and vomiting indistinguishable from that associated with GER [3, 4, 26]. Elimination of cow's milk protein from the diet is followed by a rapid decrease (usually within 2 weeks) of episodes of vomiting and regurgitation, and reintroduction causes recurrence of symptoms. Overfeeding is a well known cause of regurgitation. Although reduced feeding volume decreases reflux frequency [65], care should be exercised to keep the total daily feeding volume at an amount that allows normal growth and development. Infants with inadequate weight gain due to losses from regurgitation may benefit from increasing the caloric density of formula when volume or frequency of feedings is decreased as part of therapy.

Thickening the formula is the single most effective intervention to reduce regurgitation. Rice cereal-thickened formula decreases the volume of regurgitation [3]. Excessive caloric intake is a potential problem with long-term use of feedings thickened at home with rice cereal or cornstarch. Thickening a 20 kcal/oz infant formula with one tablespoon of rice cereal per ounce increases the caloric density to about 34 kcal/oz (~1.1 kcal/mL). Thickening with one tablespoon/2 oz of formula increases the caloric density to about 27 kcal/oz (~0.95 kcal/mL). Commercial antiregurgitation (AR) formulae containing processed rice, corn or potato starch, guar gum or locust bean gum are now commercially available and have been shown in a recent meta-analysis to reduce the frequency and severity of regurgitation and vomiting [66]. The caloric density, osmolarity, protein, calcium, and fatty acid content of AR formulae is tailored to the infant's nutritional needs, whereas a formula with added thickener may provide more calories than needed [67 –69]. *In vitro* studies have shown a decrease in the absorption of micronutrients from formulae commercially thickened with indigestible carbohydrates. The clinical significance of these findings is unclear since a 3-month follow-up study of children on formula thickened with bean gum showed normal growth and nutritional parameters [70]. There are infants with GERD who are unable to gain weight despite conservative measures and in whom nasogastric or nasojejunal feeding may be beneficial [71]. Nasojejunal feeding may also be useful to infants with recurrent reflux-related aspiration pneumonia.

There is substantial evidence that GER is less frequent in prone head-elevated position [3, 4]. Prone sleep positioning is associated with longer restful sleep periods, and supine sleep leads to more frequent arousals and crying [72]. When the Nordic epidemiologic SIDS study demonstrated that the odds ratio of mortality from SIDS was over 10 times higher in prone-sleeping infants and three times higher in side-sleeping infants than in supine infants [73], it became unethical to recommend prone sleeping for most infants. Currently, prone positioning is acceptable only if the infant is observed and awake, particularly in the post-prandial period. Prone positioning may be beneficial in children over 1 year of age with GERD in whom the risk of SIDS is negligible. Esophageal pH and combined MII–pH monitoring show that reflux is quantitatively similar in the left-side–down and prone positions. Measured reflux in these two positions is less than in the right-side–down and supine positions [74, 75]. Based upon these findings, one study recommended that infants be placed right-side–down for the first hour after feeding to promote gastric emptying and thereafter be switched to left-side–down to decrease reflux [75]. These findings notwithstanding, it is important to note that side lying is an unstable position for an infant who may slip unobserved into the prone position. Bolstering an infant with pillows to maintain a side-lying position is not recommended. The semi-supine positioning associated with lying in an infant car seat exacerbates GER [76]. A recently published pilot study evaluating the Multicare-AR Bed® showed that a 40° supine position in a specially developed bed reduced regurgitation, reflux, and crying [77].

A study evaluated the effectiveness of conservative therapy in infants referred to an academic pediatric gastroenterologist practice [78]. Telephone teaching at the time of the referral included feeding modifications (use of a protein-hydrolysate formula thickened with one tablespoon of dry rice cereal per ounce and use of restricted feeding volumes), positioning changes with avoidance of seated and supine positions, and elimination of tobacco smoke exposure. Approximately 25% of the infants had sufficient improvement that no further intervention was needed.

Lifestyle changes in children and adolescents
Most studies investigating recommendations such as dietary modification, avoidance of alcohol, weight loss, positioning changes, avoidance of late night meals, and cessation of smoking have been performed in adults, thus their applicability to children of all ages is uncertain [79]. Current evidence generally does not support or refute the use of specific dietary changes to treat reflux beyond infancy. Expert opinion suggests that children and adolescents with GERD should avoid caffeine, chocolate, alcohol, and spicy foods if they provoke symptoms. It is not known whether any lifestyle changes have an additive benefit in children or adolescents receiving pharmacologic therapy.

The effectiveness of positioning for treatment of GER and GERD in children over 1 year of age has not been studied. Adults who sleep with the head of the bed elevated have fewer, shorter episodes of reflux, and fewer reflux symptoms. Other studies in adults have shown that reflux increases in the right lateral decubitus position [80]. It is likely therefore that adolescents, like adults, may benefit from the left lateral decubitus sleeping position with elevation of the head of the bed.

Medications

Acid suppressants and prokinetic agents are the cornerstone of pharmacotherapy in the treatment of GERD in both adults and children. Over-the-counter antacids (magnesium hydroxide, aluminum hydroxide) are inexpensive, widely available and, if taken in adequate doses, result in decreased esophageal exposure to acid. Despite evidence that high doses of antacid medications are as effective as cimetidine in the treatment of esophagitis in children [81], such medications are not widely used in children because of their poor taste and the need for frequent administration. Significant absorption of aluminum may lead to microcytic anemia, osteopenia, and neurotoxicity in infants.

Histamine 2-receptor antagonists have been shown in multiple studies to be effective for the treatment of pediatric GERD [81–83]. A randomized, double-blind, placebo-controlled, parallel design trial of a single dose of ranitidine (75 mg) showed that the pharmacokinetic and pharmacodymamic properties of ranitidine in children and adults do not differ [84]. Gastric pH increased within 30 min of ingestion and the effect lasted for up to 5 h. Another study measured gastric acid suppression of varying doses of cimetidine (5, 7.5, 10, and 15 mg/kg) [85]. Although all doses of cimetidine increased gastric pH, the duration of response was maintained for a significantly longer period of time in the groups receiving both 10 and 15 mg/kg.

PPIs are the most effective agents for the healing of GER-induced esophagitis in children and their use in children of all ages has steadily increased in the past decade. So far, regulatory agencies have granted approval for use in children for omeprazole, lansoprazole ,and pantoprazole in the United States and omeprazole in Europe. No PPI is approved for use in infants younger than 1 year of age. A study which examined four large healthcare plans in the United Stated found that PPI use rose four-fold from 2000 to 2003 [2]. Almost half of the patients had initiated PPI use by their fourth month of life. Infants younger than 6 months may require a lower per-kilogram dose than older children and adolescents [86], while children aged 1–10 years appear to require a higher dose per kilogram than adolescents and adults [87]. Studies of omeprazole and lansoprazole have shown that they are more efficacious in improving esophagitis, as documented by both endoscopy and histology when compared with histamine 2-receptor antagonists [88, 89]. A double-blind randomized study of infants with a variety of symptoms "typical" of reflux failed to demonstrate superiority of PPI compared to placebo [28]. There is recent evidence that prolonged acid suppression may increase risk for community-acquired pneumonia and gastroenteritis in children, and candidemia and necrotizing enterocolitis in infants [90 –92].

In view of the fact that GERD is due to a defective motor function of the foregut, prokinetic agents would seem the ideal agents for the treatment of children with reflux. Medications that have been used to ameliorate the motility of the upper gastrointestinal tract in children include metoclopramide, cisapride, domperidone, bethanechol, erythromycin, and baclofen. Domperidone and metoclopramide are antidopaminergic agents that improve esophageal function and facilitate gastric emptying. Metoclopramide was found to reduce the reflux index but did not normalize it in a group of infants younger than 12 months of age [93]. A meta-analysis of seven controlled studies of metoclopramide in children aged 1 month to 2 years with symptoms of GER found that metoclopramide reduced daily symptoms but was associated with significant side effects [94]. Long-term use of metoclopramide is indeed limited by the side effects of drowsiness, restlessness, fatigue, dystonic reactions, extrapyramidal movement disorders, and tardive dyskinesia, consequences of its antidopaminergic activity in the central nervous system. The Food and Drug Administration (FDA) has recently released a "black box" warning against its protracted use. Domperidone is not commercially available in the United States but seems to be safer than metoclopramide. A systematic review concluded that there is no robust evidence for the benefit of domperidone in the treatment of young children with GERD [95]. Cisapride is the prokinetic agent with the most convincing evidence of effectiveness in the treatment of childhood GERD [96]. Cisapride was widely used in the 1990s in children with a variety of symptoms suggestive of GER, but is no longer available in most countries except on a protocol basis secondary to its cardiac adverse effects.

Erythromycin mimics the action of the prokinetic hormone motilin, and induces the phase III of the migrating motor complex in normal individuals. Erythromycin accelerates gastric emptying in individuals with gastroparesis, but does not seem to have a beneficial effect on the esophagus and has a limited role in the treatment of pediatric GERD. Bethanechol, a direct cholinergic agent, was not found to be more effective than antacids in controlling GER in children and was noted to be more difficult to administer and to have a higher rate of side effects [97].

Finally, evidence is increasing about the possible benefit of baclofen, a gamma-amino-butyric acid receptor agonist, in decreasing TLESRs in neurologically normal and impaired children [98, 99]. Baclofen seems to ameliorate vomiting, decrease esophageal exposure to acid, and accelerate gastric emptying. A widespread use of baclofen is limited by its side effects, which include dizziness, constipation, fatigue, and a lowering of the threshold for seizures.

Surgery

Surgery is often considered for the child with GERD who has life-threatening symptoms, persistence of symptoms following medical management, or is unable to be weaned from medical therapy. The Nissen fundoplication is the most popular of the many surgical procedures that have been used for the treatment of GERD. Results and complication rates do not appear to vary by procedure. The literature concerning surgical treatment of GERD in children consists of a large number of descriptive studies composed of retrospective case series [100, 101]. Success rates have been reported to range from 57% to 92%. Complication rates vary widely based on definition used and duration of follow-up. The most commonly reported complications include disruption or migration of the wrap into the chest, gas bloat syndrome (early satiety, post-prandial gagging and retching), persistent esophageal stricture, dumping syndrome, small bowel obstruction, infection, and perforation [102]. Laparoscopic fundoplication is associated with decreased morbidity, shortened hospitalization, lower cost, and fewer preoperative complications. However, there is some evidence that children who have received a laparoscopic antireflux surgery may have a higher rate of reoperation compared to those who receive open surgeries, especially in the presence of comorbidities [103]. There are no published pediatric randomized controlled trials comparing medical to surgical treatments or different types of surgical interventions. It seems that the number of antireflux surgeries in children is decreasing relative to other commonly performed operations, although there is tremendous variability on how frequently these surgeries are performed in different freestanding children's hospitals [104].

When chronic esophagitis is the primary indication for fundoplication, an upper endoscopy with biopsies and a prolonged esophageal pH monitoring study should be performed to confirm that the esophagitis is due to GER, rather than other etiologies, such as eosinophilic esophagitis. If surgery is done primarily to prevent airway symptoms, special attention needs to be given to videofluoroscopy, bronchoalveolar lavage, MII–pH monitoring, and radiographic studies in order to verify if reflux is indeed responsible for the symptoms and that aspiration is not solely due to abnormal swallow function.

Total esophagogastric dissociation is a major operation that is gaining popularity in the treatment of GERD in children with neurologic impairment and life-threatening symptoms. Initially performed in children who had experienced one or several unsuccessful fundoplications, it is now being proposed as a primary antireflux procedure in selected children [105]. The esophagogastric dissociation eliminates

all reflux episodes, while allowing gastrostomy tube feedings and a minimal amount of oral feedings. Nutritional and metabolic complications, including dumping syndrome and chronic malabsorption, have been described after this type of surgery, especially after enteral nutrition weaning [106].

Endoluminal gastroplication has been suggested as an alternative to surgical fundoplication in children aged 6 years or older. A group of 16 children with GERD who received this intervention using a flexible endoscopic sewing device (EndoCinch) showed an immediate post-treatment improvement in symptom severity, symptom frequency, and quality of life scores, which persisted up to 3 years after the intervention [107]. Four had recurrent symptoms requiring a repeat procedure 2–24 months postoperatively. Other endoscopic GERD treatments have not been studied in children.

References

1. Nelson SP, Chen EH, Syniar GM, et al. Prevalence of symptoms of gastroesophageal reflux during infancy. A pediatric practice-based survey. Pediatric Practice Research Grouup. *Arch Pediatr Adolesc Med* 1997;151:569–572.
2. Barron JJ, Tan H, Spalding J, et al. Proton pump inhibitor utilization patterns in infants. *J Pediatr Gastroenterol Nutr* 2007;45:421–427.
3. Vandenplas Y, Rudolph CD, Di Lorenzo C, et al. Pediatric gastroesophageal reflux clinical practice guidelines: joint recommendations of the North American Society for Pediatric Gastroenterology, Hepatology, and Nutrition (NASPGHAN) and the European Society for Pediatric Gastroenterology, Hepatology, and Nutrition (ESPGHAN). *J Pediatr Gastroenterol Nutr* 2009;49:498–547.
4. Sherman PM, Hassall E, Fagundes-Neto U, et al. A global, evidence-based consensus on the definition of gastroesophageal reflux disease in the pediatric population. *Am J Gastroenterol* 2009;104:1278–1295.
5. Vandenplas Y. Gastroesophageal reflux. In: Wyllie R, Hyams J, eds. *Paediatric Gastrointestinal and Liver Disease*. Philadelphia: Elsevier, 2011, pp. 232–247.
6. Hegar B, Dewanti NR, Kadim M, et al. Natural evolution of regurgitation in healthy infants. *Acta Paediatr* 2009;98:1189–1193.
7. Nelson SP, Chen EH, Syniar GM, et al. Prevalence of symptoms of gastroesophageal reflux during childhood: a pediatric practice-based survey. Pediatric Practice Research Group. *Arch Pediatr Adolesc Med* 2000;154:150–154.
8. Nelson SP, Chen EH, Syniar GM, et al. One-year follow-up of symptoms of gastroesophageal reflux during infancy. Pediatric Practice Research Group. *Pediatrics* 1998;102:E67.
9. Lee WS, Beattie RM, Meadows N, et al. Gastro-oesophageal reflux: clinical profiles and outcome. *J Paediatr Child Health* 1999;35:568–571.
10. Johnston BT, Carré IJ, Thomas PS, et al. Twenty to 40 year follow up of infantile hiatal hernia. *Gut* 1995;36:809–812.
11. Waring JP, Feiler MJ, Hunter JG, et al. Childhood gastroesophageal reflux symptoms in adult patients. *J Pediatr Gastroenterol Nutr* 2002;35:334–338.

12. Trudgill NJ, Kapur KC, Riley SA. Familial clustering of reflux symptoms. *Am J Gastroenterol* 1999;94:1172–1178.

13. Cameron AJ, Lagergren J, Henriksson C. Gastroesophageal reflux disease in monozygotic and dizygotic twins. *Gastroenterology* 2002;122:55–59.

14. Hu FZ, Preston RA, Post JC. Mapping of a gene for severe pediatric gastroesophageal reflux to chromosome 13q14. *JAMA* 2000;284:325–334.

15. Orenstein SR, Shalaby TM, Barmada MM, *et al*. Genetics of gastroesophageal reflux disease: a review. *J Pediatr Gastroenterol Nutr* 2002;34:506–510.

16. Carre IJ, Johnston BT, Thomas PS, *et al*. Familial hiatal hernia in a large five generation family confirming true autosomal dominant inheritance. *Gut* 1999;45:649–652.

17. Hassall E. Co-morbidities in childhood Barrett's esophagus. *J Pediatr Gastroenterol Nutr* 1997;25:255–260.

18. Omari TI, Benninga MA, Barnett CP, *et al*. Characterization of esophageal body and lower esophageal sphincter motor function in the very premature neonate. *J Pediatr* 1999;135:517–521.

19. Vandenplas Y, Hassall E. Mechanisms of gastroesophageal reflux and gastroesophageal reflux disease. *J Pediatr Gastroenterol Nutr* 2002;35:119–136.

20. St James-Roberts I, Halil T. Infant crying patterns in the first year: normal community and clinical findings. *J Child Psychol Psychiatry* 1991;32:951–968.

21. Zangen S, Di Lorenzo C, Zangen T, *et al*. Rapid maturation of gastric relaxation in newborn infants. *Pediatr Res* 2001;50: 629–632.

22. Di Lorenzo C, Piepsz A, Ham H, *et al*. Gastric emptying with gastro-oesophageal reflux. *Arch Dis Child* 1987;62:449–453.

23. Cucchiara S, Staiano A, Di Lorenzo C, *et al*. Pathophysiology of gastroesophageal reflux and distal esophageal motility in children with gastroesophageal reflux disease. *J Pediatr Gastroenterol Nutr* 1988;7:830–836.

24. Gorenstein A, Cohen AJ, Cordova Z, *et al*. Hiatal hernia in pediatric gastroesophageal reflux. *J Pediatr Gastroenterol Nutr* 2001;33:554–557.

25. Levine A, Milo T, Broide E, *et al*. Influence of Helicobacter pylori eradication on gastroesophageal reflux symptoms and epigastric pain in children and adolescents. *Pediatrics* 2004;113:54–58.

26. Vandenplas Y, Koletzko S, Isolauri E, *et al*. Guidelines for the diagnosis and management of cow's milk protein allergy in infants. *Arch Dis Child* 2007;92:902–908.

27. Moore DJ, Tao BS, Lines DR, *et al*. Double-blind placebo-controlled trial of omeprazole in irritable infants with gastroesophageal reflux. *J Pediatr* 2003;143:219–223.

28. Orenstein SR, Hassall E, Furmaga-Jablonska W, *et al*. Multicenter, double-blind, randomized, placebo-controlled trial assessing the efficacy and safety of proton pump inhibitor lansoprazole in infants with symptoms of gastroesophageal reflux disease. *J Pediatr* 2009;154:514–520.

29. Gilger MA, El-Serag HB, Gold BD, *et al*. Prevalence of endoscopic findings of erosive esophagitis in children: a population-based study. *J Pediatr Gastroenterol Nutr* 2008;47:141–146.

30. Malcolm WF, Gantz M, Martin RJ, *et al*. Use of medications for gastroesophageal reflux at discharge among extremely low birth weight infants. *Pediatrics* 2008;121:22–27.

31. Furuta GT, Liacouras CA, Collins MH, *et al*. Eosinophilic esophagitis in children and adults: a systematic review and consensus recommendations for diagnosis and treatment. *Gastroenterology* 2007;133:1342–1363.

32. Merwat SN, Spechler SJ. Might the use of acid-suppressive medications predispose to the development of eosinophilic esophagitis? *Am J Gastroenterol* 2009;104:1897–1902.

33. Sheikh S, Stephen T, Howell L, *et al*. Gastroesophageal reflux in infants with wheezing. *Pediatr Pulmonol* 1999;28:181–186.

34. Molle LD, Goldani HA, Fagondes SC, *et al*. Nocturnal reflux in children and adolescents with persistent asthma and gastroesophageal reflux. *J Asthma* 2009;46:347–350.

35. Ramaiah RN Stevenson M, McCallion WA. Hypopharyngeal and distal esophageal pH monitoring in children with gastroesophageal reflux and respiratory symptoms. *J Pediatr Surg* 2005;40:1557–1561.

36. Ayazi S, Lipham JC, Hagen JA, *et al*. A new technique for measurement of pharyngeal pH: normal values and discriminating pH threshold. *J Gastrointest Surg* 2009;13:1422–1429.

37. Starosta V, Kitz R, Hartl D, *et al*. Bronchoalveolar pepsin, bile acids, oxidation, and inflammation in children with gastroesophageal reflux disease. *Chest* 2007;132:1557–1564.

38. Ravelli AM, Panarotto MB, Verdoni L, *et al*. Pulmonary aspiration shown by scintigraphy in gastroesophageal reflux-related respiratory disease. *Chest* 2006;130:1520–1526.

39. Gleeson K, Eggli DF, Maxwell SL. Quantitative aspiration during sleep in normal subjects. *Chest* 1997;111:1266–1272.

40. Morigeri C, Bhattacharya A, Mukhopadhyay K, *et al*. Radionuclide scintigraphy in the evaluation of gastroesophageal reflux in symptomatic and asymptomatic pre-term infants. *Eur J Nucl Med Mol Imaging* 2008;35:1659–1665.

41. Brodzicki J, Trawińska-Bartnicka M, Korzon M. Frequency, consequences and pharmacological treatment of gastroesophageal reflux in children with cystic fibrosis. *Med Sci Monit* 2002;8:CR529–537.

42. Wenzl TG, Schenke S, Peschgens T, *et al*. Association of apnea and nonacid gastroesophageal reflux in infants: Investigations with the intraluminal impedance technique. *Pediatr Pulmonol* 2001;31:144–149.

43. Frankel EA, Shalaby TM, Orenstein SR. Sandifer syndrome posturing: relation to abdominal wall contractions, gastroesophageal reflux, and fundoplication. *Dig Dis Sci* 2006;51: 635–640.

44. Bothwell MR, Parsons DS, Talbot A, *et al*. Outcome of reflux therapy on pediatric chronic sinusitis. *Otolaryngol Head Neck Surg* 1999;121:255–262.

45. Contencin P, Narcy P. Gastropharyngeal reflux in infants and children. A pharyngeal pH monitoring study. *Arch Otolaryngol Head Neck Surg* 1992;118:1028–1030.

46. Gibson WS Jr, Cochran W. Otalgia in infants and children-a manifestation of gastroesophageal reflux. *Int J Pediatr Otorhinolaryngol* 1994;28:213–218.

47. Salvatore S, Hauser B, Vandemaele K, *et al*. Gastroesophageal reflux disease in infants: how much is predictable with questionnaires, pH-metry, endoscopy and histology? *J Pediatr Gastroenterol Nutr* 2005;40:210–215.

48. Stanford EA, Chambers CT, Craig KD. The role of developmental factors in predicting young children's use of a self-report scale for pain. *Pain* 2006;120:16–23.

49. Orenstein SR, Shalaby TM, Cohn JF. Reflux symptoms in 100 normal infants: diagnostic validity of the infant gastroesopha-

geal reflux questionnaire. *Clin Pediatr (Phila)* 1996;35:607–614.

50. Kleinman L, Rothman M, Strauss R, *et al*. The infant gastroesophageal reflux questionnaire revised: development and validation as an evaluative instrument. *Clin Gastroenterol Hepatol* 2006;4:588–596.

51. Jang HS, Lee JS, Lim GY, *et al*. Correlation of color Doppler sonographic findings with pH measurements in gastroesophageal reflux in children. *J Clin Ultrasound* 2001;29:212–217.

52. Vieth M, Haringsma J, Delarive J, *et al*. Red streaks in the oesophagus in patients with reflux disease: is there a histomorphological correlate? *Scand J Gastroenterol* 2001;36:1123–1127.

53. Spechler SJ, Genta RM, Souza RF. Thoughts on the complex relationship between gastroesophageal reflux disease and eosinophilic esophagitis. *Am J Gastroenterol* 2007;102:1301–1306.

54. Hill DJ, Heine RG, Cameron DJ, *et al*. Role of food protein intolerance in infants with persistent distress attributed to reflux esophagitis. *J Pediatr* 2000;136:641–647.

55. Orenstein SR, Shalaby TM, Kelsey SF, *et al*. Natural history of infant reflux esophagitis: symptoms and morphometric histology during one year without pharmacotherapy. *Am J Gastroenterol* 2006;101:628–640.

56. Tuttle SG, Grossman MI. Detection of gastro-esophageal reflux by simultaneous measurement of intraluminal pressure and pH. *Proc Soc Exp Biol Med* 1958;98:225–227.

57. Vandenplas Y, Franckx-Goossens A, Pipeleers-Marichal M, *et al*. Area under pH 4: advantages of a new parameter in the interpretation of esophageal pH monitoring data in infants. *J Pediatr Gastroenterol Nutr* 1989;9:34–39.

58. Rosen R, Lord C, Nurko S. The sensitivity of multichannel intraluminal impedance and the pH probe in the evaluation of gastroesophageal reflux in children. *Clin Gastroenterol Hepatol* 2006;4:167–172.

59. Peter CS, Sprodowski N, Ahlborn V, *et al*. Inter- and intraobserver agreement for gastroesophageal reflux detection in infants using multiple intraluminal impedance. *Biol Neonate* 2004;85:11–14.

60. Dalby K, Nielsen RG, Markoew S, *et al*. Reproducibility of 24-hour combined multiple intraluminal impedance (MII) and pH measurements in infants and children. Evaluation of a diagnostic procedure for gastroesophageal reflux disease. *Dig Dis Sci* 2007;52:2159–2165.

61. Orel R, Brecelj J, Homan M, *et al*. Treatment of oesophageal bile reflux in children: the results of a prospective study with omeprazole. *J Pediatr Gastroenterol Nutr* 2006;42:376–383.

62. He Z, O'Reilly RC, Bolling L, *et al*. Detection of gastric pepsin in middle ear fluid of children with otitis media. *Otolaryngol Head Neck Surg* 2007;137:59–64.

63. Mattioli G, Sacco O, Repetto P, *et al*. Necessity for surgery in children with gastrooesophageal reflux and supraoesophageal symptoms. *Eur J Pediatr Surg* 2004;14:7–13.

64. Numans ME, Lau J, de Wit NJ, *et al*. Short-term treatment with proton-pump inhibitors as a test for gastroesophageal reflux disease: a meta-analysis of diagnostic test characteristics. *Ann Intern Med* 2004;140:518–527.

65. Khoshoo V, Ross G, Brown S, *et al*. Smaller volume, thickened formulas in the management of gastroesophageal reflux in thriving infants. *J Pediatr Gastroenterol Nutr* 2000;31:554–556.

66. Horvath A, Dziechciarz P, Szajewska H. The effect of thickened-feed interventions on gastroesophageal reflux in infants: systematic review and meta-analysis of randomized, controlled trials. *Pediatrics* 2008;122:e1268–1277.

67. Chao HC, Vandenplas Y. Effect of cereal-thickened formula and upright positioning on regurgitation, gastric emptying and weight gain in infants with regurgitation. *Nutrition* 2007;23:23–28.

68. Xinias I, Mouane N, Le Luyer B, *et al*. Cornstarch thickened formula reduces oesophageal acid exposure time in infants. *Dig Liver Dis* 2005;37:23–27.

69. Hegar B, Rantos R, Firmansyah A, *et al*. Natural evolution of infantile regurgitation versus the efficacy of thickened formula. *J Pediatr Gastroenterol Nutr* 2008;47:26–30.

70. Levtchenko E, Hauser B, Vandenplas Y. Nutritional value of an "anti-regurgitation" formula. *Acta Gastroenterol Belg* 1998;61:285–287.

71. Ferry GD, Selby M, Pietro TJ. Clinical response to short-term nasogastric feeding in infants with gastroesophageal reflux and growth failure. *J Pediatr Gastroenterol Nutr* 1983;2:57–61.

72. Vandenplas Y, Hauser B. Gastro-oesophageal reflux, sleep pattern, apparent life threatening event and sudden infant death. The point of view of a gastroenterologist. *Eur J Pediatr* 2000;159:726–729.

73. Oyen N, Markestad T, Skaerven R, *et al*. Combined effects of sleeping position and prenatal risk factors in sudden infant death syndrome: the Nordic Epidemiological SIDS Study. *Pediatrics* 1997;100:613–621.

74. Omari TI, Rommel N, Staunton E, *et al*. Paradoxical impact of body positioning on gastroesophageal reflux and gastric emptying in the premature neonate. *J Pediatr* 2004;145:194–200.

75. van Wijk MP, Benninga MA, Dent J, *et al*. Effect of body position changes on postprandial gastroesophageal reflux and gastric emptying in the healthy premature neonate. *J Pediatr* 2007;151:585–590, 590 e1–2.

76. Orenstein SR, Whitington PF, Orenstein DM. The infant seat as treatment for gastroesophageal reflux. *N Engl J Med* 1983;309:760–763.

77. Vandenplas Y, De Schepper J, Verheyden S, *et al*. A preliminary report on the efficacy of the Multicare AR-Bed in 3-week-3-month-old infants on regurgitation, associated symptoms and acid reflux. *Arch Dis Child* 2010;95:26–30.

78. Shalaby TM, Orenstein SR. Efficacy of telephone teaching of conservative therapy for infants with symptomatic gastroesophageal reflux referred by pediatricians to pediatric gastroenterologists. *J Pediatr* 2003;142:57–61.

79. Kaltenbach T, Crockett S, Gerson LB. Are lifestyle measures effective in patients with gastroesophageal reflux disease? An evidence-based approach. *Arch Intern Med* 2006;166:965–971.

80. Meining A, Classen M. The role of diet and lifestyle measures in the pathogenesis and treatment of gastroesophageal reflux disease. *Am J Gastroenterol* 2000;95:2692–2697.

81. Cucchiara S, Staiano A, Romaniello G, *et al*. Antacids and cimetidine treatment for gastro-oesophageal reflux and peptic oesophagitis. *Arch Dis Child* 1984;59:842–847.

82. Orenstein SR, Shalaby TM, DeVandry SN, *et al*. Famotidine for infant gastrooesopheal reflux : a multi-centre, randomized, placebo-controlled, withdrawal trial. *Aliment Pharmacol Ther* 2003;17:1–11.

83. Orenstein SR, Gremse DA, Pantaleon CD, *et al.* Nizatidine for the treatment of pediatric gastroesophageal reflux symptoms: an open-label, multiple-dose, randomized, multicenter clinical trial in 210 children. *Clin Ther* 2005;27:472–483.

84. Orenstein SR, Blumer JL, Fassel HM, *et al.* Rantidine, 75mg, over-the-counter does: pharmacokinetic and pharmacodynamic effects in children with symptoms of gastrooesophageal reflux. *Aliment Pharmacol Ther* 2002;16:899–907.

85. Lambert J, Mobassaleh M, Grand RJ. Efficacy of cimetidine for gastric acid suppression in pediatric patients. *J Pediatr* 1992;120:474–478.

86. Omari TI, Haslam RR, Lundborg P, *et al.* Effect of omeprazole on acid gastroesophageal reflux and gastric acidity in preterm infants with pathological acid reflux. *J Pediatr Gastroenterol Nutr* 2007;44:41–44.

87. Andersson T, Hassall E, Lundborg P, *et al.* Pharmacokinetics of orally administered omeprazole in children. International Pediatric Omeprazole Pharmacokinetic Group. *Am J Gastroenterol* 2000;95:3101–3106.

88. Fiedorek S, Tolia V, Gold BD, *et al.* Efficacy and safety of lansoprazole in adolescents with symptomatic erosive and non-erosive gastroesophageal reflux disease. *J Pediatr Gastroenterol Nutr* 2005;40:319–327.

89. Tolia V, Fitzgerald J, Hassall E, *et al.* Safety of lansoprazole in the treatment of gastroesophageal reflux disease in children. *J Pediatr Gastroenterol Nutr* 2002;35 (Suppl 4):S300–307.

90. Canani RB, Cirillo P, Roggero P, *et al.* Therapy with gastric acidity inhibitors increases the risk of acute gastroenteritis and community-acquired pneumonia in children. *Pediatrics* 2006;117:e817–820.

91. Saiman L, Ludington E, Dawson JD, *et al.* Risk factors for Candida species colonization of neonatal intensive care unit patients. *Pediatr Infect Dis J* 2001;20:1119–1124.

92. Guillet R, Stoll BJ, Cotten CM, *et al.* Association of H2-blocker therapy and higher incidence of necrotizing enterocolitis in very low birth weight infants. *Pediatrics* 2006;117:e137–142.

93. Tolia V, Calhoun J, Kuhns L, *et al.* Randomized, prospective double-blind trial of metoclopramide and placebo for gastroesophageal reflux in infants. *J Pediatr* 1989;115:141–5.

94. Craig WR, Hanlon-Dearman A, Sinclair C, *et al.* Metoclopramide, thickened feedings, and positioning for gastroesophageal reflux in children under two years. *Cochrane Database Syst Rev* 2004:CD003502.

95. Pritchard DS, Baber N, Stephenson T. Should domperidone be used for the treatment of gastro-oesophageal reflux in children? Systematic review of randomized controlled trials in children aged 1 month to 11 years old. *Br J Clin Pharmacol* 2005;59:725–729.

96. Dalby-Payne JR, Morris AM, Craig JC. Meta-analysis of randomized controlled trials on the benefits and risks of using cisapride for the treatment of gastroesophageal reflux in children. *J Gastroenterol Hepatol* 2003;18:196–202.

97. Levi P, Marmo F, Saluzzo C, *et al.* Bethanechol versus antiacids in the treatment of gastroesophageal reflux. *Helv Paediatr Acta* 1985;40:349–359.

98. Omari TI, Benninga MA, Sansom L, *et al.* Effect of baclofen on esophagogastric motility and gastroesophageal reflux in children with gastroesophageal reflux disease: a randomized controlled trial. *J Pediatr* 2006;149:468–474.

99. Kawai M, Kawahara H, Hirayama S, *et al.* Effect of baclofen on emesis and 24-hour esophageal pH in neurologically impaired children with gastroesophageal reflux disease. *J Pediatr Gastroenterol Nutr* 2004;38:317–323.

100. Fonkalsrud EW, Ashcraft KW, Coran AG, *et al.* Surgical treatment of gastroesophageal reflux in children: a combined hospital study of 7467 patients. *Pediatrics* 1998;101:419–422.

101. Mathei J, Coosemans W, Nafteux P, *et al.* Laparoscopic Nissen fundoplication in infants and children: analysis of 106 consecutive patients with special emphasis in neurologically impaired vs. neurologically normal patients. *Surg Endosc* 2008;22:1054–1059.

102. Caniano DA, Ginn-Pease ME, King DR. The failed antireflux procedure: analysis of risk factors and morbidity. *J Pediatr Surg* 1990;25:1022–1025, discussion 1025–1026.

103. Diaz DM, Gibbons TE, Heiss K, *et al.* Antireflux surgery outcomes in pediatric gastroesophageal reflux disease. *Am J Gastroenterol* 2005;100:1844–1852.

104. Goldin AB, Garrison M, Christakis D. Variations between hospitals in antireflux procedures in children. *Arch Pediatr Adolesc Med* 2009;163:658–663.

105. Goyal A, Khalil B, Choo K, *et al.* Esophagogastric dissociation in the neurologically impaired: an alternative to fundoplication? *J Pediatr Surg* 2005;40:915–918; discussion 918–919.

106. Madre C, Serhal L, Michaud L, *et al.* Prolonged enteral feeding is often required to avoid long-term nutritional and metabolic complications after esophagogastric dissociation. *J Pediatr Gastroenterol Nutr* 2010;50:280–286.

107. Thomson M, Antao B, Hall S, *et al.* Medium-term outcome of endoluminal gastroplication with the EndoCinch device in children. *J Pediatr Gastroenterol Nutr* 2008;46:172–177.

32 Surgical Treatment of Gastroesophageal Reflux Disease

Christy M. Dunst and Lee L. Swanstrom

Division of GI and MIS Surgery, The Oregon Clinic, Portland, OR, USA

Background

Gastroesophageal reflux disease (GERD) is defined by the failure of the reflux barrier to prevent escape of toxic gastric contents into the esophagus. This is largely an anatomic and physiologic problem theoretically lending itself to surgical repair. Surgical intervention in the process of gastroesophageal reflux has a long history, but with variable importance and results. Initial attempts to surgically treat reflux were reported in the 1950s and concentrated on correction of the gross anatomic derangements, such as associated hiatal hernias and strictures [1]. Unfortunately, these early attempts were either prone to failure, as in the case of hiatal hernia repair alone, or prone to high rates of severe complications, such as with operative stricturoplasty. As surgical physiologists began to better understand and define the complex relationship between the lower esophageal sphincter (LES), diaphragm, and gastric function, an era of experimental procedures began, which attempted to restore normal anatomy and physiology. Still, as often happens, it was Rudolf Nissen's serendipitous discovery that wrapping the LES with proximal stomach resulted in a normal functioning reflux barrier that gave a practical and reproducible procedure for the cure of GERD [2].

The decades of the 1960s and 1970s saw a remarkable development of surgical treatments for reflux disease that was fostered by the increasing incidence of the problem in the general population, improved understanding of the physiology of the foregut, and the lack of effective medical treatment for GERD. Numerous surgical innovators sought to improve on Nissen's original procedure by creating variations of antireflux procedures and approaches, which they advocated to better address the increasingly sophisticated understanding of the pathophysiology of the disease. These innovations were, as was common with the times, usually eponymously named: Belsey, Toupet, Rosetti, Hill, Lortat-Jacob, Lind, Dor, Guarner, Boix-Ochoa, etc. Many of these procedures are no longer practiced, having faded when their originator disappeared, but others have found specific uses and are still practiced today.

By the end of the 1970s, antireflux operations were one of the most common upper gastrointestinal surgeries performed in the developed world. Over 40 000 procedures were performed annually in the United States, with the majority being either the Nissen or Belsey mark IV procedures. These original operations were performed through large incisions, in either the abdomen or chest respectively, and were associated with a certain, unavoidable morbidity. Consequently, antireflux surgery was often reserved for patients with complications of GERD. Patients with milder forms of the disease were left with few therapeutic options as peptic medications of the time were essentially non-existent, consisting of little besides oral antacids. The ineffectiveness of antacid therapy compared to antireflux surgery was demonstrated in a prospective trial by Behar *et al.* in 1975 [3]. The advent of histamine 2-receptor antagonists (H$_2$RAs) in 1976 was heralded with much enthusiasm by GERD sufferers and clinicians alike. By inhibiting acid production at the gastric parietal cells level, these medications were much more useful for the treatment of occasional heartburn. When compared with the then standard-of-care fundoplication, H$_2$RAs were quickly proven to be less effective than antireflux surgery at treating both the symptoms and early complications of GERD [4] Finally, in 1989, a much more potent medication that blocked acid production was introduced (omeprazole). Proton pump inhibitors (PPIs) have been shown not only to control symptoms of GERD, but to also heal esophagitis and its associated inflammatory cellular changes. Their superiority to H$_2$RAs has been well documented [5–8]. They have few major side effects and are well tolerated by most patients. PPIs represented a major competitor to open fundoplications and, understandably, were quickly embraced, dramatically altering the concept of GERD treatment from one of restoring the normal LES barrier with the goal of palliating symptoms by acid suppres-

The Esophagus, Fifth Edition. Edited by Joel E. Richter, Donald O. Castell.
© 2012 Blackwell Publishing Ltd. Published 2012 by Blackwell Publishing Ltd.

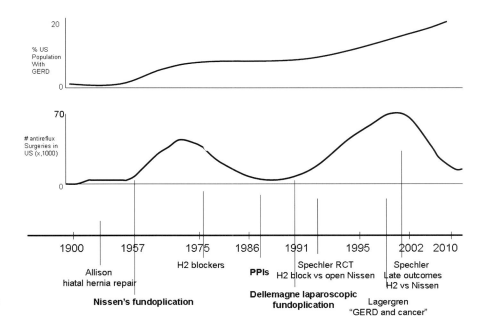

Figure 32.1 Historical events impacting trends in antireflux surgery. PPI, proton pump inhibitor.

sion. The effective symptom control of these medications and the morbidity of open surgery for GERD quickly shifted the paradigm of treatment: within a year of the introduction of the PPI there were fewer than 8000 antireflux surgeries performed in the United States, in spite of the exponentially increasing numbers of patients with the complaint of troublesome reflux (Figure 32.1).

In 1991 a minimally invasive approach to antireflux surgery was described by Dellemagne *et al.* using the newly described modality of videolaparoscopy [9]. There followed a rapid adoption of this less invasive approach by the new generation of "minimally invasive" surgeons and numbers of antireflux surgeries once again steadily increased over the next decade. By 2002 it was estimated that there were approximately 62 000 antireflux surgeries per year in the United States. This dramatic increase was due to several factors: the tremendous success of laparoscopic cholecystectomy created excitement in the medical and patient community for "keyhole surgery" in general; publication of Spechler's VA-based, randomized comparison of medical (H_2RAs) and surgical treatment (open fundoplication) showing superior results with surgery [4]; the expense of proprietary PPIs; increasing public awareness of the connection between GERD and esophageal cancer [10]; excellent early results in the literature with laparoscopic fundoplication; and the fact that surgical leaders were advocating "best practices" to the surgeons interested in antireflux surgery. Unfortunately, this trend did not continue and, since 2002, there has been a steady decline in the numbers of antireflux surgeries being performed. The reason for this is also multifactorial: PPIs became generic and the cost of medical treatment became more affordable; long-term results of antireflux surgery were called into question, primarily based on

Spechler's follow-up to his original study showing that up to 60% of surgical patients were back on peptic medication at 10 years [11]; and the variable quality in outcomes between centers of excellence—which typically report 85–95% long-term success rates—and lower volume surgeons with perhaps less successful outcomes [12]. Currently, it is estimated that there are around 20 000 antireflux surgeries performed each year in the United States, an almost insignificant number in a nation with 60 million GERD sufferers.

In spite of this, surgery remains, at least theoretically, the best treatment for GERD; offering the ability to restore the normal antireflux barrier of the gastroesophageal junction (GEJ) without manipulating the complex secretory functions of the stomach. Essentially, all antireflux surgery today is performed laparoscopically with very minimal operative morbidity (<0.001%) and very short hospital stays (0–2 days). Much current research is focused on even less invasive approaches to reconstructing the LES using technologies like implants and endoluminal suturing.

Today, deciding which GERD patients should receive surgery and which surgery (and by whom) to ensure the most optimal results, is a fairly complex task. It is, however, also one that lends itself to being approached by evidence-based treatment algorithms, which we aim to present here.

Patient selection

Indications for surgery most commonly include refractory symptoms despite adequate proton pump inhibition, dissatisfaction with medical management or patient choice. There are many non-objective reasons for patient dissatisfaction, including factors such as patient finances, insurance coverage policies, availability of surgical expertise, and past experience with antireflux surgery either on the part of the patient or the referring physician [13]. Many of these are outside the control of treating physicians, but still there are basic guidelines that at least can be used when considering offering surgical referral to patients considered to be medical treatment failures.

However, deciding who should be referred for reflux surgery is not always simple. Some have opined that there is no reason to ever choose antireflux surgery over chronic medical therapy [14]. At the same time, the same experts described inadequate results with PPIs in up to 40–60% of patients [15, 16]. PPIs are highly effective for palliation of many reflux symptoms and for prevention of some of the complications of uncontrolled esophageal acid exposure. None the less, they are not universally successful. A patient survey performed by the American Gastroenterological Association (AGA) and released on their website in 2008 showed that 30% of GERD patients were marginally satisfied or totally dissatisfied by their PPI therapy [17].

As with any chronic medical therapy, patient compliance is always an issue and many patients simply cannot or will not take PPIs on an ongoing basis. This may be due to the appreciable cost of these medications ($US24–120/month), forgetfulness, or a philosophical problem with the need to take a daily medication for the rest of one's life. It is also widely reported that the need to take PPIs with food is not widely known by patients and even prescribing physicians, so their efficacy may not always be maximized. Finally, many patients are disturbed by recent reports of deleterious side effects of PPIs. These include osteoporosis and associated fractures, weight gain, arthritis, vitamin deficiencies, reduced iron absorption, chronic diarrhea, medication interactions, etc., which, while rare, are concerning to many patients [18].

It is strongly recommended that all GERD patients have a trial of maximized medical treatment before considering surgery, with dose escalation if needed and a twice-daily regimen for complications of the reflux. Response to medication can be an important prognostic measure for surgical success or indicate possible alternative diagnoses for symptoms. It also gives the patient a fair comparison of their quality of life if they should go on to choose surgery. Factors known to be associated with improved outcomes after surgery include the presence of typical symptoms (heartburn, regurgitation, and/or dysphagia), documented abnormal acid exposure on pH testing, and symptom response to PPIs [19, 20]. An ideal population then, for surgical referral, is patients who have a good symptomatic response to their pH documented reflux but who are unwilling to take medication for whatever reasons. That said, failure of medical therapy, defined most simply as patient dissatisfaction, is reason enough to seek surgical consultation to discuss options. A more cautious approach should be taken with

patients who claim to experience no benefit with high-dose PPIs. These patients should be referred to surgery only after they have abnormal pH or impedance confirmation of reflux or present with complications of reflux (strictures, esophagitis, etc.) while on maximal medical therapy. These patients only do well with surgery if they have objective confirmation of reflux and extensive counseling.

Side effects of antireflux surgery

Potential side effects of antireflux surgery must be thoroughly discussed with the patient in order for them to make an informed decision. The most common and expected side effects of laparoscopic fundoplication include transient dysphagia, early satiety, and gas-related symptoms. Some degree of dysphagia due to post-surgical edema is expected in all patients for the first 2–6 weeks after surgery and this will resolve in nearly all by 3 months [21–23]. A small percentage of patients will require endoscopic dilation for persistent dysphagia and about 1% will require reoperation [24]. A modified diet, or post-fundoplication diet, consisting of puréed or soft foods is generally recommended until the dysphagia resolves. Maintaining adequate nutrition during this time should be emphasized and it is not uncommon for patients to lose 5–10 lb after surgery.

Early satiety is common and is probably secondary to surgical manipulation of the gastric fundus, which acts as a satiety regulator in the normal individual. It is seldom a major complaint of patients and usually resolves after 3–6 months.

Postoperative complaints of bloating and flatulence are common for the first few months after surgery due to conditioned aerophagia associated with gastroesophageal reflux. Gastroesophageal reflux results in an increased frequency of swallowing, which neutralizes the distal esophagus with alkaline saliva. Since air is propelled into the stomach with each swallow, bloating and repetitive belching typically accompany GERD. After fundoplication there is a transient inability to belch and the swallowed air leads to the sensation of bloating. This improves with time but can be unpredictable. Reassurance, avoidance of carbonated beverages, and simethicone are the mainstays of treatment. Biofeedback mechanisms have been used to retrain patients to decrease the frequency of swallowing after antireflux surgery, with some success [25]. Curiously, a prospective randomized trial of patients with GERD showed a similar incidence of these symptoms in those on medical therapy and those after fundoplication [11]. On rare occasions this condition is severe enough to require intervention for acute gastric distention (gas-bloat syndrome). If acute gas bloat does occur, it usually responds to decompression and conservative measures. The natural, long-term evolution of "gas-bloat syndrome" is unknown, but it mostly resolves within the first year after surgery.

Importantly, satisfaction with the surgery remains high regardless of the presence or severity of these expected postoperative side effects [26–28]. It is imperative that the surgeon thoroughly reviews dysphagia and gas-bloat expectations with patients before surgery. A properly informed patient will decide whether or not the impact that their reflux symptoms have on their lifestyle warrants surgical intervention. Overall, properly selected patients in this group enjoy excellent surgical outcomes with relief of their reflux symptoms and patient satisfaction rates of over 90% in multiple studies.

Special circumstances: atypical reflux and abnormal impedance

While most patients' complaints are related to the pain from acid-related tissue damage, some have symptoms mostly from positional reflux and are unaffected by acid neutralization. Acid suppression alters the pH of the gastric refluxate and may even decrease its volume to some degree, but does nothing to restore the integrity of the LES or affect the other elements involved in GERD, such as esophageal clearance or delayed gastric emptying (DGE). Some patients have persistent troublesome reflux symptoms despite adequate acid suppression. The most straightforward example of this scenario is patients who suffer from refractory positional regurgitation, often in the setting of a hiatal hernia. Sleep disruption due to severe positional regurgitation can be a significant quality-of-life issue and many will present with frank aspiration. These patients have a clear anatomic problem that only surgery can treat. Aspiration of gastric juice is toxic and can lead to severe end-stage lung disease from chronic pneumonia and pulmonary fibrosis. It has recently been advocated that GERD be identified and surgically treated in patients who are candidates for lung transplant as such reflux, symptomatic or not, has been implicated in transplant failure [29]. Therefore, patients who relate a history of unremitting volume regurgitation should be evaluated for underlying esophageal or gastric dysmotility, but, in general, make good candidates for surgical referral. Not surprisingly, these patients are some of the most satisfied with antireflux surgery.

However, sometimes the decision to refer for surgery is not so clear. Some reflux patients will present with symptoms ranging from sore throat, throat clearing, and laryngitis to exacerbation of reactive airway disease and chronic cough. More obscure symptoms, such as dental erosions, globus sensation, sinus issues, and halitosis may also have a reflux etiology. These patients may or may not have abnormal acid exposure in the distal esophagus, especially on therapy, but their symptoms may still be manifestations of GERD. It is not unusual for these complaints to not respond to medical therapy. One hypothesis is that the chronic onslaught of toxic reflux and the secondary inflammation causes atypical symptoms and that a lack of temporal symptom correlation does not rule out GERD. This is likely true and may partly explain the historic difficulty of correctly selecting atypical symptom patients for antireflux surgery. Such atypical symptoms can be difficult to treat

with antireflux surgery as they can also be due to primary pulmonary and pharyngeallaryngeal causes. Conventional pH testing is not reliable in differentiating between patients whose atypical symptoms are reflux related and those whose are not [30]. Even when the only objective finding is abnormal acid exposure in the esophagus, successful treatment of these symptoms is difficult to predict. Surgery is particularly controversial for these cases and in the past was advocated only as a "last ditch" attempt—and then with only a 55% success rate [31]. On the other hand, there is often little else to offer these patients since medications are ineffective and they often do come to surgery. It is important to caution patients in these cases that surgery may result in no or only a partial improvement of such atypical symptoms.

The hypothesis for failure of antireflux surgery in these patients is that their symptoms were not actually caused by reflux. Therefore, it is actually a failure of the diagnostic tests used. Early enthusiasm for the role of proximal esophageal pH monitoring to aid in the diagnosis of atypical reflux symptoms rather fell out of favor due to inconsistent results and poor predictive value [32, 33]. Only recently have normal values for proximal acid exposure been published, making it possible that this modality will prove more useful in the future [34]. A combination of still newer test modalities and more targeted patient selection has recently shown an improvement for surgical outcomes for these problems. Twenty-four hour impedance data have identified a group of these hard to pinpoint patients who do well with surgery; namely those with a high correlation between symptoms and acid/non-acid reflux events [35, 36]. Allen and Anvari reported a 71% symptom resolution at 5 years for patients with chronic cough and pulmonary issues after antireflux surgery based on impedance testing [37]. A specialized laryngeal–pharyngeal reflux pH detection system has been developed as another diagnostic tool with documented normal values (Dx-pH; Restech Corporation, San Diego, CA, USA) [38]. The Dx-pH system seems to be fairly specific at identifying abnormal acid exposure in the pharynx [39]. While we do not yet have enough data to clearly advocate its use routinely, Dx-pH testing may prove very useful in differentiating atypical reflux symptoms. Unfortunately, it is likely that, no matter what test is done, extraesophageal symptoms will be difficult to sort out due to the multifactorial nature of the etiology of these atypical types of symptoms.

Ultimately, it is the responsibility of the surgeon to decide if antireflux surgery will improve the patient's quality of life. Such a decision should be based on a comprehensive evaluation of all the objective data. Whether it is break-through heartburn, troublesome regurgitation, oropharyngeal and pulmonary manifestations, or a symptomatic hiatal hernia, further evaluation is warranted in these circumstances.

A summary of the indications for referral for antireflux surgery is listed in Table 32.1.

Table 32.1 Relative indications for referral for antireflux surgery.

Indication	Medical therapy	Antireflux surgery
Good response with PPI	++	+
Non-response to PPI therapy (proven GERD)	–	++
Complications in spite of a symptomatic response to PPIs (strictures, esophagitis, bleeding, aspiration)	–	++
Positional volume reflux symptoms	–	++
Inability to afford PPIs	–	+
Refusal to take long-term PPIs	–	+
Intolerable side effects of PPIs	+	++
Lung transplant candidate	+	++

PPI, proton pump inhibitor; GERD, gastroesophageal reflux disease.

Table 32.2 Comprehensive preoperative foregut evaluation for antireflux surgery.

Esophagogastroduodenoscopy with biopsies
Esophageal manometry
24–48-h pH testing
24-h multichannel intralumenal impedance (MII) with symptom correlation
Barium esophagram
Gastric emptying study (scintigraphy or capsule)

Preoperative testing for antireflux surgery

A trial of acid suppression is often considered an important diagnostic test. A good response to PPIs has been shown to correlate with a good response to antireflux surgery. On the other hand, if medication fails to provide relief, it may indicate a more complicated foregut problem, such as hiatal hernias, motility disorders of the stomach or esophagus, diverticulum, or simply that the medication does not work for that particular patient. These patients may well be good candidates for antireflux surgery, but only after more extensive testing. When considering surgery for reflux, it is imperative that a comprehensive foregut evaluation, in addition to standard history and physical and selective cardiopulmonary evaluation, is obtained to ensure that the patient is a good candidate and to help to choose the best surgical therapy.

Preoperative evaluation should focus on specific anatomic and functional details that might impact surgical selection and therefore operative planning and patient counseling. The components of a comprehensive preoperative foregut evaluation are discussed below (Table 32.2).

Esophagogastroduodenoscopy with biopsies

The role of endoscopy in preoperative planning differs from standard esophagogastroduodenoscopy in that it should focus on careful anatomic detail to provide information that will be helpful in surgical selection. In the era of powerful antisecretory medications, the absence of endoscopic esophagitis is less important, but certainly this finding in the face of ongoing medication suggests medical failure. Careful attention to the GEJ is important for selection of the appropriate operation. First, measurements of the squamocolumnar junction (SCJ), or Z-line, in relation to the GEJ identifies the length of columnar metaplasia. Biopsies at the SCJ are required to confirm or refute the presence of intestinal metaplasia (IM). If there is no measurable segment of columnar-lined esophagus, gastric biopsies should also be obtained to help differentiate reflux-related IM from gastric IM, since reflux IM will need scheduled interval surveillance. If there is more that 1 cm difference between the SCJ and the GEJ, standard Barrett's surveillance biopsies should be done. It is important to obtain these biopsies prior to antireflux surgery because the surgery will alter the anatomy at the GEJ and may make it more difficult to evaluate in the future. Next, measurements of the GEJ and diaphragm are obtained to document the presence, size and type of hiatal hernia, and these can alert the surgeon to the possibility of a shortened esophagus. A redundant, dilated or tortuous esophagus should also be noted in this regard. A retroflex view of the proximal stomach and GEJ is used to further characterize both the integrity of the reflux barrier and to confirm the type of hiatal hernia. Axial hiatal hernias should be differentiated from paraesophageal hernias by the degree of herniated fundus. It is very helpful to categorize the gastroesophageal flap valve, or musculomucosal fold that comprises the angle of HIS, according to the Hill classification [40].

Esophageal manometry

All patients undergoing antireflux surgery need to have their esophageal motility evaluated. This can be accomplished using water-perfused motility catheters or high-resolution solid-state manometry systems. Although some studies show excellent correlation between motility studies and videoesophagram in determining peristaltic function, X-rays should not replace manometric testing in most centers. Manometry is critical in order to rule out achalasia or other motility disturbances (such as intraoperative esophageal manometry, non-relaxing LES or esophageal spasm), which may lead to dysphagia after surgery. The presence or absence of a manometrically defective LES is less important. The necessity for tailoring the fundoplication based on the motility is controversial, but no one would argue that failure to identify a patient with achalasia, and performing a full fundoplication on them, would have potentially devastating consequences. It has been shown that a distal esophageal contraction amplitude of at least

25 mmHg is required to overcome the resistance created by a full fundoplication, and that patients with weaker esophageal function may have more postoperative dysphagia. Similarly, poor peristaltic function is thought to negatively impact outcomes. Ineffective esophageal motility (>30% of swallows with contraction amplitude <30 mmHg) in the distal esophagus has been used as an indication for partial fundoplication. Recent data suggest that this value should be raised to 50%, which may be more clinically relevant to fundoplication selection [41]. If dysmotility is secondary to chronic reflux, it has been documented that peristaltic function may improve after an effective antireflux surgery. Patients with abnormal esophageal motility still need to be appropriately counseled about their potentially increased risk of postoperative dysphagia.

24–48-h pH testing

The definitive diagnostic test to confirm abnormal gastroesophageal reflux remains the distal esophageal pH test. Both traditional catheters and newer wireless devices have been validated as methods to objectively document acid exposure in the distal esophagus [42, 43]. Society guidelines recommend all patients undergo pH testing off antisecretory medications prior to antireflux surgery to confirm abnormal acid exposure. Proximal esophageal or pharyngeal pH testing may be helpful in select patients with atypical symptoms. Twenty-four hour pH testing on PPI can occasionally be helpful in patients with refractory heartburn, as it will sometimes reveal abnormal acid exposure despite medication. Unfortunately, even this is not straightforward as studies have confirmed that as many as 33% of asymptomatic patients will continue to have abnormal pH on standard-dose therapy [44]. The role of symptom correlation will likely become more important in patients with continued heartburn and incomplete acid suppression.

24-h Multichannel intralumenal impedance with symptom correlation

For most patients seeking surgery, inadequate acid suppression is not the issue as the current powerful antisecretory medications are highly effective. Instead, non-acid reflux is becoming more widely recognized as a clinical entity [45, 46]. Severe regurgitation despite PPI represents an extreme example of "symptomatic non-acid reflux." Still others will describe "heartburn" despite documented acid suppression. These patients are often labeled "sensitive esophagus" or functional heartburn. Esophageal impedance monitoring is effective at detecting non-acid reflux events and it has been shown that if symptoms correlate with non-acid reflux events, this is a group of patients who will respond well to surgery even in the absence of severe regurgitation symptoms [35]. Not every patient referred for antireflux surgery needs to have this specialized test, but it can be helpful in patients with classic symptoms and normal pH testing or

with atypical symptoms. It has been proposed that the sensation of the refluxed non-acid fluid bolus is responsible for refractory epigastric symptoms in some patients. This test can be done on antacid medications to evaluate persistent symptoms using the symptom index (number of symptoms associated with reflux divided by the number of symptoms). Caution is advised if this test is the only abnormality identified for a patient undergoing a comprehensive preoperative evaluation for reflux surgery. Overall, impedance testing is evolving as an important tool for the diagnosis and treatment of refractory or complicated GERD.

Barium esophagram

A barium esophagram should be obtained in all patients with atypical symptoms, including chronic cough, halitosis, sore throat, and aspiration. This test will rule out anatomic abnormalities that can be missed with other tests, such as diverticulum, proximal reflux, and rarely, esophagopulmonary fistula. Furthermore, esophageal length and hiatal hernia reduction can be estimated, which aids in proper preoperative planning. This test, however, is extremely dependent on the quality and dedication of the radiology department.

Gastric emptying study

An often overlooked cause of GER is DGE. While gastric outlet obstruction leading to reflux is easily diagnosed with other tests, DGE secondary to gastroparesis can be easily missed. Gastric emptying tests should be obtained in all reflux patients with significant symptoms of gas bloat, nausea or vomiting (as opposed to positional reflux) prior to surgery. Standard testing includes a 4-h nuclear gastric emptying scintigraphy [47].

Gastric emptying scintigraphy methods vary widely between centers. It has been documented that as many as 17–29% of gastroparetic patients can be underdiagnosed based on insufficient testing measures [48, 49]. The most common error in testing is failure to continue the measurements out to the 4-h time point, with most reporting only a 2-h percentage emptying or an extrapolated half-life. Other common variations include using non-standardized test meals and inconsistent patient physical activity between time points. A consensus report outlines the recommended standard gastric emptying scintigraphy protocol that should be followed to decrease these errors [47, 50, 51]. The protocol, often referred to as the Tougas protocol, defines a standardized radiolabeled low-fat egg-white meal with imaging at 0, 1, 2, and 4 h after meal ingestion. Abnormal values for quantitative emptying are greater than 90%, greater than 60%, greater than 30%, and greater than 10% of retained meal at each time point, respectively. If gastric emptying is implicated in gastroesophageal reflux, this must be taken into consideration in surgical planning. Severe emptying problems should be addressed surgically with the addition of a gastric emptying procedure or even with a subtotal gastrectomy in the case of the morbidly obese or reoperative patient.

Standard gastroesophageal reflux disease surgery

Laparoscopic Nissen fundoplication is the current gold standard surgical therapy for gastroesophageal reflux. The procedure involves creating a 360-degree "wrap" of the

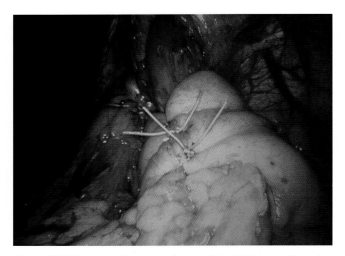

Figure 32.2 Intraoperative image of a completed 360-degree (Nissen) fundoplication.

gastric fundus around the GEJ, performed over a large esophageal bougie under general anesthesia [52, 53] (Figure 32.2). The wrap prevents unfolding of the LES and is an effective barrier against all gastric contents. Most patients will require less than a 24-h hospital stay and will have minimal pain. Objective control of gastroesophageal reflux with normalization of 24-h acid exposure has been demonstrated for between 83% and 100% of patients following laparoscopic fundoplication [21, 28, 52, 54–58] (Table 32.3).

It is not unusual for patients with long-standing reflux—or a history of reflux—to present with hiatal hernias. Though they are often asymptomatic, hiatal hernias can sometimes create problems due to anatomic distortion ranging from mild dysphagia to non-cardiac chest pain and even to strangulation if they become large enough. Hiatal hernia repair is therefore a routine part of any antireflux surgery and involves closure of the diaphragmatic crura around the esophagus.

Gastroesophageal reflux disease associated with esophageal motility disorders

Esophageal motility disorders are not a contraindication to surgical treatment of reflux, but call for extra care and sometimes alteration of the surgical approach. Motility is primarily a concern if the patient presents with complaints of dysphagia or has other evidence of delayed esophageal clearance such as esophageal regurgitation. Standard esophageal manometry is an essential test to define motility disorders

Table 32.3 Objective outcomes of laparoscopic antireflux surgery.

Study	Number of patients in study	Number of patients with objective data	Median follow-up (months)	Outcome assessment method	Clinical success (%)	Normal postoperative pH (%)
Hinder et al. 1994 [52]	198	51	12	Questionnaire, selected pH, manometry	97	88
Gotley et al. (19960 [56]	170	10	12	Questionnaire, selected pH		100
Peters et al. (1988) [55]	100	28	21	Questionnaire, pH, manometry, EGD	95	93
Eubanks et al. (2002) [57]	212	189	3	Questionnaire, pH, manometry	93	83
Anvari et al. (2003) [21]	181	181	60	Questionnaire, pH, manometry, some EGD	86	95
Ackroyd et al. (2004) [58]	52	42	12	Questionnaire, pH, manometry, EGD		98
Fein et al. (20080 [54]	88	74	24-60	Questionnaire, pH, manometry, EGD	87	70
Shaw et al. (2010) [28]	50	41	3	Questionnaire, pH, manometry		93

EGD, esophagogastroduodenoscopy.

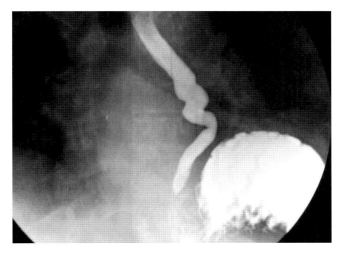

Figure 32.3 Barium esophagram demonstrating a large paraesophageal hiatal hernia. The accordian shape of the esophagus suggests adequate length after surgical reduction.

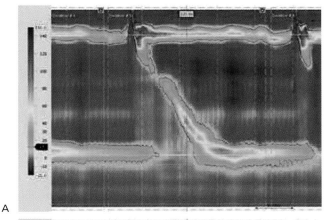

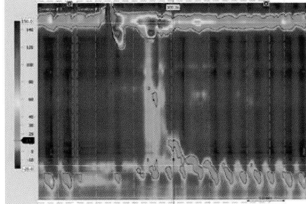

Figure 32.4 High-resolution manometry demonstrating (A) normal esophageal pressures and (B) functional esophageal damage due to chronic injury compared to normal. Note the low amplitude contractions and defective lower esophageal sphincter.

and should be performed on all patients prior to surgery. For the surgeon, manometric motility disorders can be classed into two main categories: acquired or primary. Acquired motility disorders are typically a result of the anatomic distortion from large hiatal hernias ("accordion" esophagus) or damage from chronic acid reflux. It is somewhat unusual for acquired dysmotility patients to have major dysphagia. The accordion esophagus of large hiatal hernias can have a non-specific motility pattern, often characterized by short inter-sphincteric length and an intrathoracic LES (Figure 32.3) Surgical reduction of the GEJ into the abdomen will often correct this type of motility disorder.

Damage due to chronic injury often shows a typical pattern characterized by antegrade peristalsis, but with progressively decreasing amplitudes of contraction and a weak LES (Figure 32.4). These patients respond well to anti-reflux surgery and multiple studies have shown no increase in dysphagia [59] and a gradual improvement in their postoperative peristaltic strength as the esophagitis heals [60].

Primary motility disorders are due to intrinsic neuromotor dysfunction and tend to be more significant and often progressive. These include the named dysmotility disorders (achalasia, diffuse esophageal spasm, nutcracker, hypertensive LES, ineffective esophageal motility, and profound motility absence, as seen with connective tissue disorders like scleroderma). It is not unusual for these patients to present with a primary symptom of heartburn or regurgitation as well as dysphagia, although they do not in fact often have gastroesophageal reflux. Surgery for these disorders is indicated instead to relieve esophageal outlet obstruction or spasm and usually involves a myotomy (surgical muscle division). If the myotomy extends across the LES (for achalasia, hypertensive LES or occasionally for very symptomatic nutcracker or diffuse esophageal spasm), there will be a high

incidence of subsequent gastroesophageal reflux and a non-obstruction or partial fundoplication is usually added.

Partial fundoplications are modifications of the standard 360-degree wrap specifically designed to provide less esophageal outflow restriction. This is accomplished by leaving varying degrees of the esophageal wall unreinforced, which acts as a sort of "hinge" when a food bolus passes through. It also serves to soften the pressure profile of the reconstructed LES (Figure 32.5). The most common partial fundoplications performed are the Toupet, which is a 270-degree posterior wrap, and the Dor fundoplication, which is a 180-degree wrap placed anteriorly that is mostly used only as an adjunct to a esophageal myotomy (Figure 32.6).

For patients with reflux in association with a severely hypomotile or amotile esophagus and a hypotensive LES (scleroderma esophagus or other profound primary disorders); a partial fundoplication is also indicated as a 360degree wrap can cause early dysphagia or, if tolerated early on, late esophageal failure with progressive esophageal body dilatation and recurrent dysphagia [61].

Gastroesophageal reflux disease with large hiatal hernias

Hiatal hernias are classified based on the location of the GEJ with respect to the diaphragmatic hiatus, as well as the proportion of involved fundus. Type I, or axial, hernias refer to relatively small hernias with cephalad migration of the GEJ into the mediastinum over a length of at least 2 cm. The surrounding connective tissue that anchors the GEJ to the hiatus, the phrenoesophageal ligament, becomes attenuated and the hiatal diameter begins to enlarge as the size of the hernia grows. Small hernias are treated in a similar way as in routine antireflux repairs. Type II, or true paraesophageal, hernias, are defined by the herniation of a portion of the fundus into the mediastinum with a normal intra-abdominal location of the GEJ. Type III hiatal hernias are combination hernias in which both the GEJ and portion of the fundus reside in the mediastinum. Giant paraesophageal hiatal hernia is a subjective term to describe the situation when at least 30–50% of the stomach is involved in the hernia with or without organoaxial rotation (Figure 32.7). When a majority of the stomach herniates above the diaphragm, and is associated with other abdominal organs, it is known as a type IV hernia. Types II–IV are associated with a defined hernia sac that must be fully excised from the mediastinum for a complete repair. Type III and IV hernias usually have a markedly enlarged hiatus, adding to the complexity of the operation. Symptomatic giant hiatal hernias should be surgically repaired when at all possible as they have a significant (5–30%) risk of catastrophic strangulation.

Large hiatal hernias may present with a variety of symptoms, such as atypical chest pain, epigastric or upper abdominal pain possibly radiating to the left subcostal region, dysphagia, decreased exercise tolerance, regurgitation, aspi-

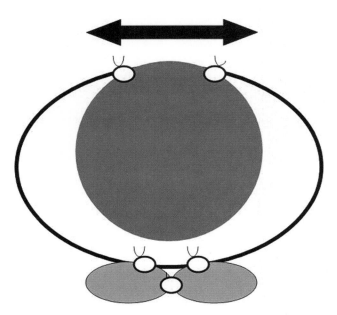

Figure 32.5 Partial fundoplication.

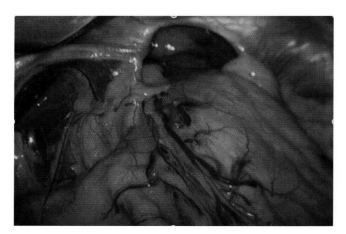

Figure 32.7 Intraoperative image of a giant paraesophageal hiatal hernia.

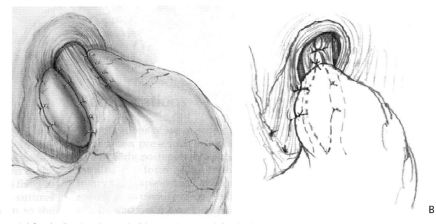

A

B

Figure 32.6 (A) Posterior partial fundoplication (Toupet). (B) Anterior partial fundoplication (Dor).

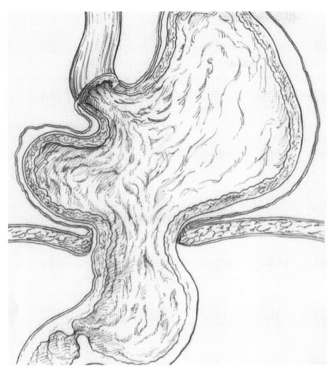

Figure 32.8 "Hour glass" deformity of giant paraesophageal hiatal hernia.

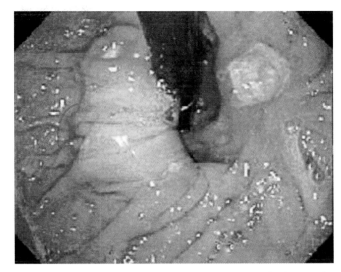

Figure 32.9 Endoscopic image depicting Cameron's gastric ulcers at the hiatus of a large hiatal hernia.

Table 32.4 Surgical principles of large hiatal hernia repair.

Extensive esophageal mobilization via high mediastinal dissection to maximize intra-abdominal esophageal length
Reduction and excision of hernia sac
Careful crural dissection with preservation of overlying fascia
Recognition of the foreshortened esophagus and performance of esophageal lengthening when necessary
Tension-free crural closure

ration, and gastric outlet obstruction. These symptoms are due to either angulation of the distal esophagus, mediastinal trapping creating an "hour glass" deformity, or simply as a result of occupying thoracic space (Figure 32.8). Large hiatal hernias also put the patient at risk for the development of mechanical ulcerations (Cameron's ulcers) caused by localized trauma to the gastric mucosa by the motion of the crura (Figure 32.9). Cameron's ulcers are a common cause of chronic anemia in the older population and should always be suspected when the bleeding source is non-colonic and there is a large hiatal hernia. Such ulcers seldom respond to medical therapy and are another good indication for surgical intervention [62]. GERD may or may not be part of the symptom profile in the presentation of large hiatal hernias. Rarely, large hiatal hernias will present with life-threatening complications such as frank hemorrhage, torsion, gastric ischemia, necrosis, and perforation. Patients with a history of early symptoms should be considered for surgery to avoid such catastrophic consequences [63–67].

Repair of large hiatal hernias can be successfully performed with excellent results and improved quality of life for most patients [68–70]. Truly asymptomatic hiatal hernias may not need to be repaired, but giant ones are rarely asymptomatic to the careful historian and should be referred to an experienced surgeon. It is generally accepted that repair of large hiatal hernias is much more technically challenging than other antireflux procedures, and a large opera-

tive experience and knowledge of anatomic variables is needed to optimize outcomes.

Surgical repair of large hiatal hernias has traditionally been through a large thoracic or upper abdominal incision. Early publications comparing open to laparoscopic approaches suggested superiority of the open technique despite the accompanying incisional morbidity [71]. However, with experience and precise adaptation of sound surgical principles learned from the open approach (Table 32.4) [72], repair of large hiatal hernias is now preferentially performed laparoscopically with excellent results, including shorter hospital stays and minimal postoperative pain.

An important technical aspect of the repair of a hiatal hernia of any size is the diaphragmatic closure as recurrences are largely related to its failure. This continues to be the Achilles heel of repair of large hiatal/paraesophageal hernias and in large part accounts for the 2–50% recurrence rates reported in the literature [70, 71, 73–75]. Fortunately, most recurrences are small and do not require intervention [68].

The crural muscle in patients with hiatal hernias has been found to have varying degrees of underlying structural abnormalities [76], which may account for intrinsic weakness and diaphragmatic closure failures. Because of this, various mesh reinforcements have been incorporated into crural repairs over the years to try to minimize recurrences [77, 78]. Initially these repairs used prosthetic meshes and severe complications were observed, such as refractory dysphagia, erosion, and even pericardial tamponade [79]. More recently, biologic mesh has been shown to be a safer alternative and to decrease short-term recurrence rates to less than 10%, with a good safety profile [74, but superior long-term durability has not been definitively demonstrated. One reason for this may be the variability in technique. Biologic mesh is known to incorporate into tissues it is in close contact with. We have previously published our technique of biologic mesh placement, which involves incorporation of mesh into the sutured crural closure to maximize mesh–crural contact and optimize its effectiveness (Figure 32.10) [80]. Absorbable synthetic mesh has also been successfully used [69].

In certain circumstances where the diaphragmatic anatomy is particularly unfavorable, more complex repairs are warranted, e.g. diaphragmatic relaxing incisions to decrease tension and mobilization of the left lobe of the liver to strengthen the crural closure with or without mesh. The latter technique, known as the hepatic shoulder maneuver, mobilizes the left lobe of the liver and places it over the repair behind the GEJ [81].

The existence of the truly foreshortened esophagus is widely debated, but there is no doubt that it can be physically difficult to reduce some large hiatal hernias. A goal of hiatal hernia surgery is to achieve at least 2–3 cm of tension-free intra-abdominal esophageal length after mobilization and reduction of the hernia sac. In 2–20% of cases this cannot be accomplished in spite of extensive mediastinal mobilization, and surgeons should always be prepared to perform an esophageal lengthening procedure (Collis gastroplasty) when necessary. Esophageal lengthening can be achieved using a laparoscopic stapler with or without accompanying wedge gastrectomy [70, 82, 83] (Figure 32.11).

A tailored antireflux procedure is a standard part of paraesophageal hiatal hernia repair for most esophageal surgeons. However, there is still some controversy surrounding the addition of a fundoplication in all patients. Clearly a fundoplication is indicated for patients with a history of GERD. However, many patients with giant paraesophageal hernias have otherwise normal GEJ anatomy and no reflux. For them, the problem is purely a diaphragmatic disease and the addition of a full 360-degree fundoplication may be unnecessary. Proponents argue that the fundoplication serves to buttress the repair against the diaphragm to help prevent recurrences and therefore is indicated regardless of reflux disease. Indeed, up to an 80% recurrence rate has been reported in a small number of patients who had paraesophageal hernia repairs without fundoplication [84]. Still, some investigators argue that fundoplication is unnecessary and itself may be a risk factor for recurrence [85, 86]. A second proposed reason to add a fundoplication is that the extensive dissection required to reduce the hiatal hernia will significantly disrupt the components of the gastroesophageal anatomy, resulting in a defective barrier mechanism regardless of whether or not it was intact before surgery. Despite these controversies, fundoplication has been demonstrated to be a safe adjunct to the operation and is widely advocated to rebuild the GEJ and help decrease recurrence of paraesophageal hiatal hernias [70, 84, 87, 88].

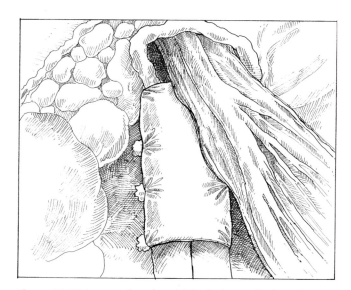

Figure 32.10 Incorporation of mesh into diaphragmatic closure to maximize tissue–mesh apposition and ingrowth.

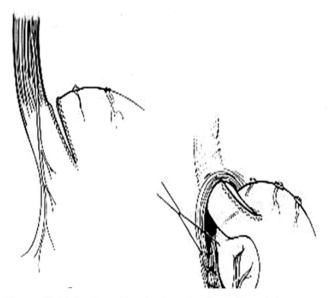

Figure 32.11 Esophageal lengthening using the Collis stapled technique.

Gastroesophageal reflux disease with gastroparesis

An estimated 20–40% of patients presenting for surgical evaluation of GERD will have underlying symptoms suggestive of gastroparesis [89]. Gastroparesis is a chronic digestive disorder defined as severe and life-altering nausea, vomiting, bloating, and abdominal pain in the setting of objective DGE. The etiology is most often idiopathic but it has also been associated with severe diabetes. Patients with gastroparesis often have chronic gastric distention, which can lead to secondary or overflow reflux and regurgitation. Gastric distention leads to unfolding of the LES, resulting in incompetence and gastroesophageal reflux. This phenomenon has been documented manometrically as transient lower esophageal sphincter relaxations (TLESRs) or shortenings. With time, chronic distention and reflux may lead to permanent anatomic and functional deterioration of the gastroesophageal reflux barrier.

Symptoms of bloating, nausea, and "emesis" are common in GERD patients due to reactive hyper-swallowing and aerophagia, and can be difficult to distinguish from underlying gastroparesis. For patients with these symptoms a radionuclide gastric emptying test is important and will provide objective evidence of gastroparesis in approximately 50% of patients with symptoms. The majority of GERD patients with DGE will have a significant improvement in their gastric symptoms if a gastric drainage procedure is performed in combination with an antireflux procedure [89–91]. A pyloroplasty helps decrease symptoms and improves gastric emptying in patients with dysfunctional gastric motility by ablating the impaired or uncoordinated pyloric outlet. On the other hand, a fundoplication alone in a patient with gastroparesis may actually worsen the severity of gas bloat and lead to early failure of the wrap [92–96]. There is evidence that the reduction of fundic volume involved with a fundoplication may improve gastric emptying to some degree even without a pyloroplasty [97, 98]. It has therefore been hypothesized that patients with delayed proximal emptying only, as opposed to antral, would make up the category of patients who benefit from fundoplication alone. However, these patients are hard to diagnose preoperatively. In general, patients who have objective findings of DGE on scintigraphy who undergo a Nissen alone have more dyspeptic symptoms than patients who undergo combined Nissen and pyloroplasty or Nissen with a decompressing gastrostomy. The symptomatic failure rate in gastroparetic patients treated with fundoplication alone can also be as high as 25% [89]. The addition of a pyloroplasty or gastric tube to a fundoplication in patients with both GERD and gastroparesis leads to improved outcomes [89–91]. Therefore, reflux patients with suspected gastroparetic symptoms should undergo formal gastric emptying scintigraphy and additional gastric drainage procedures considered for patients with objective findings of gastroparesis.

Laparoscopic pyloroplasty can be performed safely in conjunction with an antireflux procedure in patients with gastroparesis. It is inherently more appealing than a gastric decompression tube due to the lack of an external appliance. However, it is associated with more postoperative diarrhea than a gastric tube or Nissen alone. The procedure is performed without additional laparoscopic trocars. The pylorus is mobilized to decrease tension on the suture line, and then divided full-thickness longitudinally for a distance of 5 cm. The opening is then closed transversely (Heineke–Mikulicz) using running absorbable monofilament sutures. This serves to both divide the sphincter and physically widen the gastric outlet. An intraoperative endoscopic methylene blue or air leak test can be performed to ensure integrity of the suture closure (Figure 32.12). These patients also typically go home the following day.

Gastroesophageal reflux disease and the obese

Obesity has a long association with reflux disease, although it is controversial whether the relationship is truly causal. There is certainly a high prevalence of GERD symptoms in the morbidly obese and it is well documented that obesity increases the risk of having GERD three to six fold, varying somewhat with sex and degree of obesity [99]. With the growing epidemic of morbid obesity in the developed world, dealing with gastroesophageal reflux in the obese is inevitable. The refluxing obese patient requires careful counseling regarding their options: chronic medical therapy, antireflux surgery or a radical bariatric surgical procedure such as a gastric bypass. What is clear is that the age-old primary

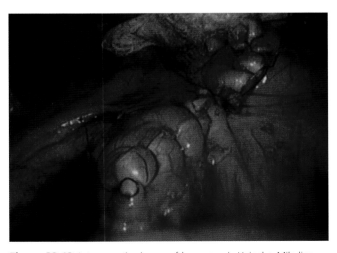

Figure 32.12 Intraoperative image of laparoscopic Heineke–Mikulicz pyloroplasty.

treatment recommendation to GERD patients to "lose weight" is hopeless advice as 96% of obese patients are unable to lose appreciable weight with dieting [100, 101].

There are several conflicting issues when dealing with the obese GERD patient. While most evidence supports acceptable outcomes when fundoplications are performed in these patients, there is some evidence that standard antireflux surgery may have a slightly higher failure rate in the morbidly obese. Anvari *et al.* showed equal outcomes in a case-match series of Nissen fundoplications in patients with body mass indices (BMIs) greater than 35 and under 35. They showed 98% normal postoperative pH for both groups at 4-year follow-up [99]. Delasi *et al.* and Fraser *et al.* also showed that the failure rate was not higher when antireflux was performed in the morbidly obese [100, 101]. On the other hand, Perez *et al.* showed a 4.5% versus 31% recurrence rate between normal weight and morbidly obese patients, although "recurrence" was not well defined and was mostly subjective [102].

The alternative surgical procedure is the Roux-en-Y gastric bypass, which remains the most common and "gold standard" treatment for morbid obesity (BMI > 35) (Figure 32.13). While there are several other alternative bariatric procedures—the lap band, gastric sleeves, vertical banded gastroplasties—these are less successful treatments for obesity and are discouraged in GERD patients as they tend to be GERD inducing or exacerbating procedures. The standard gastric bypass, in contrast, is a fairly effective antireflux procedure [103].

The obese GERD patient is therefore faced with deciding between a low morbidity, effective antireflux treatment that does nothing for their obesity and related comorbidities, and a higher risk (0.5% mortality vs 0.01% for Nissen) equally effective reflux surgery that results in weight loss but requires a dramatic change in lifestyle. For the morbidly obese, deciding which GERD surgery to choose requires care, aided by extensive counseling by their caregivers and surgeons. If patients do decide on a bariatric treatment, they should be referred to a high-volume bariatric center as optimal outcomes depend on experience and a team approach to the patient. Reassuringly, whichever the choice, there is a high likelihood of relieving their reflux complaint.

Recurrent gastroesophageal reflux disease following surgery

Occasionally, postoperative patients will complain of recurrent symptoms raising the suspicion that their antireflux surgery has failed. Long-term follow-up of laparoscopic fundoplications shows between an 85 and 95% symptomatic and objective cure rate over 10 years in expert hands [23, 104, 105]. It is recommended that any patient who complains of symptoms after surgery be aggressively evaluated before assuming that they truly have a failed surgery.

Several studies have shown that in the postoperative period, symptoms have a poor correlation to wrap failure. Khajanchee *et al.* showed that 71% of postoperative patients who complained of reflux in fact had normal endoscopies and pH studies [106]. Lord *et al.* reported that only 23% of postoperative patients who complained of recurrent gastroesophageal reflux had positive pH studies and only 24% of postoperative patients taking medications had objective evidence of reflux. They also described that retroflexed endoscopic views of the wrap were valuable and a disrupted appearing wrap had a 56-fold increased risk of having abnormal pH studies [107]. Similar results were described by Thompson *et al.*, with normal pH studies in 74% of a group of postoperative patients complaining of gastroesophageal reflux. They found predictive risk factors in this group for actual reflux: having had a partial fundoplication ($P = 0.039$), onset of symptoms 6 months or more after surgery ($P < .001$), and a good symptom response when antireflux medication was recommended ($P = .015$) [108]. Therefore, at a bare minimum, such patients should have an esophagogastroduodenoscopy and a 24-h pH study before making any conclusions about the status of their repair.

For those patients who do have positive postoperative studies, treatment options include resumption of medical therapy or consideration of reoperative surgery. In our expe-

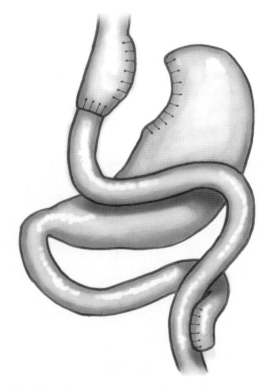

Figure 32.13 Standard Roux-en-Y gastric bypass. The bypassed stomach and long Roux limb distancing the biliary drainage serves well as an antireflux surgery.

rience, patients who have had good results from antireflux surgery but have later failed strongly prefer a second surgery over resumption of medical treatment. If surgery is considered, comprehensive testing is indicated to try to determine the cause of failure so it can be specifically addressed. Commonly ordered assessments are esophageal motility to rule out a tight or non-relaxing wrap or a missed dysmotility; endoscopy or upper gastrointestinal X-rays to rule out wrap herniation; and gastric emptying studies to assess the role of DGE in the recurrence.

Reoperative surgeries are an order of magnitude more difficult, particularly if the first surgery was an open one. Many studies have shown that redo surgeries can be safely done laparoscopically and that good results can be obtained, although not with the rate of success seen for first-time repairs. Furnee *et al.*, in a review of 4584 reoperative fundoplications from 81 peer-reviewed studies, showed a 15% complication rate, 0.9% mortality, and 81% symptomatic success, the latter somewhat lower than typically reported for first-time repairs. Objective testing in these patients confirmed success in 86% of laparoscopically-revised patients versus 78% for those done with an open procedure [109].

Several studies have compared the outcomes between first time and reoperative fundoplications. In our experience, multiple reinterventions show progressively worse outcomes, with more than three revisionary operations frequently ending with gastrectomy or even esophagectomy [110] (Figure 32.14). Without a doubt, a patient who desires a reoperation for their GERD should only be operated on at a high-volume center with an extensive experience with both the evaluation and surgery of these patients.

Future of gastroesophageal surgery

Gastroesophageal reflux is an exceedingly common disease with millions of people taking potent antacid medications. It is well documented that as many as 40% of these patients are unsatisfied with the results [111, 112] of medical management, but yet many are not appropriate candidates for laparoscopic antireflux surgery for a variety of reasons. Consequently, the quest for less invasive alternatives has been undertaken by many. Unfortunately, despite various endoscopic suturing devices, injectables or ablative procedures, none has been shown to be effective enough to be uniformly recommended to patients or for insurance companies to support. The best objective results for these less invasive reflux therapies have been short-term normalization of esophageal pH in 50% [113], a far cry from the 85% or greater long-term success of traditional antireflux surgery. Interestingly, results of sham procedures have demonstrated a 50% placebo effect on reflux symptoms, making it imperative to judge these therapies on objective data [114, 115]. Newer implantable devices, such as the Linx magnetic collar (Torax Medical, Shoreville, MN, USA) show early promise and may be a less invasive laparoscopic procedure with greater surgical reproducibility (see Chapter 26 for a full review on these procedures).

Conclusions

Antireflux surgery is an effective treatment for GERD with careful patient selection. While medication remains the treatment mainstay for the vast numbers of reflux patients worldwide, laparoscopic antireflux surgery can provide a better quality of life with good cost-effectiveness over the long term for many GERD patients. The key to success is selection of good surgical candidates, choosing the right surgeon, and a surgical approach that is meticulous, evidence based, and able to be adapted to each individual's peculiar physiology, psychology and needs. There should be no "cutting of corners" in the evaluation of patients considering surgery—while the laparoscopic Nissen fundoplication

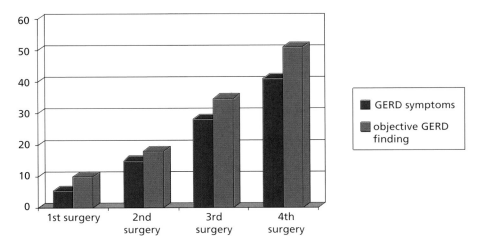

Figure 32.14 Outcomes after revision antireflux surgery. GERD, gastroesophageal reflux surgery.

is a good surgery in most reflux patients, there are 15% of patients who will have findings on preoperative endoscopy, 24-h pH, or motility testing that call for a modification of this "gold standard" procedure. As long as the gastroenterologist or primary care physician has access to surgeons who follow these precepts, they should have no concerns about referring patients for a discussion regarding the "surgical options." The majority of procedures are performed laparoscopically with minimal hospital stays and comorbidity, and there are new developments that may make the surgical approach even less traumatic. Patient satisfaction, always the most important endpoint of treatment, is over 90% with laparoscopic surgery.

References

1. Allison PR. Reflux esophagitis, sliding hiatal hernia, and the anatomy of repair. *Surg Gynecol Obstet* 1951;92:419–431.

2. Nissen R. A simple operation for control of reflux esophagitis. *Schweiz Med Wochenschr* 1956;86:590–592.

3. Behar J, Sheahan D, Biancani P, Spiro H, Storer E. Medical ands-Surgical management of reflux esophagitis, a 38-month report on a prospective clinical trial. *N Engl J Med* 1975;293:263–268.

4. Spechler S. Comparison of medical and surgical therapy for complicated gastroesophageal reflux disease in veterans. The Department of Veterans Affairs Gastroesophageal Reflux Disease Study Group [see comments]. *N Engl J Med* 1992;326: 786–792.

5. Smith P, Graeme D, Cockel R, *et al.* A comparison of omeprazole and ranitidine in the prevention and recurrence of benign esophageal stricture. *Gastroenterology* 1994;107:1312–1318.

6. Sontag SJ, Kogut DG, Fleischmann R, *et al.* Lansoprazole heals erosive reflux esophagitis resistant to histamine H2-receptor antagonist therapy. *Am J Gastroenterol* 1997;92:429–437.

7. Richter J, Campbell D, Kahrilas P, Huang B, Fludas C. Lansoprazole compared with ranitidine for the treatment of non-erosive gastroesophageal reflux disease. *Arch Intern Med* 2000;160:1803–1809.

8. Klinkenberg-Knol E, Festen H, Jansen J, *et al.* Long-term treatment with omeprazole for refractory reflux esophagitis: efficacy and safety [see comments]. *Ann Intern Med* 1994;121: 161–167.

9. Dallemagne B, Weerts JM, Jehaes C, Markiewicz S, Lombard R. Laparoscopic Nissen fundoplication: preliminary report. *Surg Laparosc Endosc* 1991;3:138–143.

10. Lagergren J, Bergström R, Lindgren A, Nyrén O. Symptomatic gastroesophageal reflux as a risk factor for esophageal adenocarcinoma. *N Engl J Med* 1999;340:825–831.

11. Spechler SJ, Lee E, Ahnen D, *et al.* Long-term outcome of medical and surgical therapies for gastroesophageal reflux disease: follow-up of a randomized controlled trial. *JAMA* 2001;285:2331–2338.

12. Carlson M, Frantzides CT. Complications and results of primary minimally invasive antireflux procedures: a review of 10,735 reported cases. *J Am Coll Surg* 2001;193:428–439.

13. Chey WD, Mody RR, Izat E. Patient and physician satisfaction with proton pump inhibitors (PPIs): Are there opportunities for improvement? *Dig Dis Sci* 2010;55:3415–3422.

14. Spechler SJ. Medical or invasive therapy for GERD: an acidulous analysis. *Clin Gastroenterol Hepatol* 2003;2:81–88.

15. Spechler SJ. Surgery for gastroesophageal reflux disease: esophageal impedance to progress? *Clin Gastroenterol Hepatol* 2009;7:1264–1265.

16. Dean BB, Gano AD, Knight K, *et al.* Effectiveness of proton pump inhibitiors in nonerosive reflux disease. *Clin Gastroenterol Hepatol* 2004;2:654–655.

17. http://www.gastro.org/wmspage.cfm?parm1=6321

18. Ali T, Roberts DN, Tierney WM. Long-term safety concerns with proton pump inhibitors. *Am J Med* 2009;122:896–903.

19. Campos GM, Peters JH, DeMeester TR, *et al.* Multivariate analysis of factors predicting outcome after laparoscopic Nissen fundoplication. *J Gastrointest Surg* 1999;3:292–300.

20. Khajanchee YS, Hong D, Hansen PD, Swanstrom LL. Outcomes of antireflux surgery in patients with normal preoperative 24-hour pH test results. *Am J Surg* 2004;187:599–603.

21. Anvari M, Allen C. Five-year comprehensive outcomes evaluation in 181 patients after laparoscopic Nissen fundoplication. *J Am Coll Surg* 2003;196:51–57; discussion 57–58; author reply 58–59.

22. Blom D, Peters JH, DeMeester TR, *et al.* Physiologic mechanism and preoperative prediction of new-onset dysphagia after laparoscopic Nissen fundoplication. *J Gastrointest Surg* 2002;6: 22–27; discussion 27–28.

23. Zaninotto G, Portale G, Costantini M, *et al.* Long-term results (6-10 years) of laparoscopic fundoplication. *J Gastrointest Surg* 2007;11:1138–1145.

24. Malhi-Chowla N, Gorecki P, Bammer T, Achem SR, Hinder RA, Devault KR. Dilation after fundoplication: timing, frequency, indications, and outcome. *Gastrointest Endosc* 2002;55:219–223.

25. Swanstrom L, Wayne R. Spectrum of gastrointestinal symptoms after laparoscopic fundoplication. *Am J Surg* 1994;167:538–541.

26. Triponez F, Dumonceau JM, Azagury D, *et al.* Reflux, dysphagia, and gas bloat after laparoscopic fundoplication in patients with incidentally discovered hiatal hernia and in a control group. *Surgery* 2005;137:235–242.

27. Hazan TB, Gamarra FN, Stawick L, Maas LC. Nissen fundoplication and gastrointestinal-related complications: a guide for the primary care physician. *South Med J.* 2009; 102(10): 1041–5.

28. Shaw JM, Bornman PC, Callanan MD, Beckingham IJ, Metz DC. Long-term outcome of laparoscopic Nissen and laparoscopic Toupet fundoplication for gastroesophageal reflux disease: a prospective, randomized trial. *Surg Endosc* 2010;24:924–932.

29. King BJ, Iyer H, Leidi AA, Carby MR. Gastroesophageal reflux in bronchiolitiis obliterans syndrom: a new perspective. *J Art Lung Transplant* 2009;28:870–875.

30. Oelschlager BK, Chang L, Pope CE 2nd, Pellegrini CA. Typical GERD symptoms and esophageal pH monitoring are not enough to diagnose pharyngeal reflux. *J Surg Res* 2005;128: 55–60.

31. Hamdy E, El-Shahawy M, Abd El Shoubary M, *et al.* Response of atypical symptoms of GERD to antireflux surgery. *Hepatogastroenterology* 2009;56:403–406.

32. Cool M, Peolmans J, Feenstra L, *et al.* Charachteristics and clinical relevance of proximal esophageal pH monitoring. *Am J Gastroenterol* 2004;99:2317–2323.

33. Wo JM, Koopman J, Harrell SP, *et al.* Double Blind placebo controlled trial with single-dose pantoprazole for laryngopharyngeal reflux. *Am J Gastroenterol* 2006;101:1972–1978.

34. Ayazi S, Hagen JA, Zehetner J, *et al.* Proximal esophageal pH monitoring: improved definition of normal values and determination of a composite pH score. *J Am Coll Surg* 2010;210: 345–350.

35. Mainie I, Tutuian R, Agrawal A, Adams D, Castell DO. Combined multichannel intraluminal impedance-pH monitoring to select patients with persistent gastro-oesophageal reflux for laparoscopic Nissen fundoplication. *Br J Surg* 2006;93: 1483–1487.

36. Sifrim D, Dupont L, Blondeau K, Zhang X, Tack J, Janssens J. Weakly acidic reflux in patients with chronic unexplained cough during 24 hour pressure, pH and impedance monitoring. *Gut* 2004;54:449–454.

37. Allen CJ, Anvari M. Does laparoscopic fundoplication provide long-term control of gastroesophageal reflux related cough? *Surg Endosc* 2004;18:633–637.

38. Ayazi S, Lipham JC, Hagen JA, *et al.* A new technique for measurement of pharyngeal pH: normal values and discriminating pH threshold. *J Gastrointest Surg* 2009;13:1422–1429.

39. Wiener GJ, Tsukashima R, Kelly C, *et al.* Oropharyngeal pH Monitoring for the detection of liquid and aerosolized supraesophageal gastric reflux. *J Voice* 2009;23:498–504.

40. Hill LD, Kozarek RA, Kraemer SJ, *et al.* The gastroesophageal flap valve:in vitro and in vivo observations. *Gastrointest Endosc* 1996;44:541–547.

41. Blonski W, Vela M, Safder A, Hila A, Castell DO. Revised criterion for diagnosis of ineffective esophageal motility is associated with more frequent dysphagia and greater bolus transit abnormalities. *Am J Gastroenterol* 2008;103:699–704.

42. Ayazi S, Lipham JC, Portale G, *et al.* Bravo catheter-free pH monitoring: normal values, concordance, optimal diagnostic thresholds, and accuracy. *Clin Gastroenterol Hepatol* 2009;7: 60–67.

43. Johnson LF, Demeester TR. Twenty-four-hour pH monitoring of the distal esophagus. A quantitative measure of gastroesophageal reflux. *Am J Gastroenterol* 1974;62:325–332.

44. Grigolon A, Cantù P, Savojardo D, Conte D, Penagini R. Esophageal acid exposure on proton pump inhibitors in unselected asymptomatic gastroesophageal reflux disease patients. *J Clin Gastroenterol* 2008;42:969–973.

45. Zerbib F, Roman S, Ropert A, *et al.* Esophageal pH-Impedance monitoring and symptom analysis in GERD: a study in patients off and on therapy. *Am J Gastroenterol* 2006;101:1956–1963.

46. Hila A, Agrawal A, Castell DO. Combined multichannel intraluminal impedance and pH esophageal testing compared to pH alone for diagnosing both acid and weakly acidic gastroesophageal reflux. *Clin Gastroenterol Hepatol* 2007;5:172–177.

47. Abell TL, Camilleri M, Donohoe K, *et al.* Consensus recommendations for gastric emptying scintigraphy: a joint report of the American Neurogastroenterology and Motility Society and the Society of Nuclear Medicine. *Am J Gastroenterol* 2008;103: 753–763.

48. Guo JP, Maurer AH, Fisher RS, Parkman HP. Extending gastric emptying scintigraphy from two to four hours detects more patients with gastroparesis. *Dig Dis Sci* 2001;46:24–29.

49. Ziessman HA, Bonta DV, Goetze S, Ravich WJ. Experience with a simplified, standardized 4-hour gastric-emptying protocol. *J Nucl Med* 2007;48:568–572.

50. Tougas G, Chen Y, Coates G, *et al.* Standardization of a simplified scintigraphic methodology for the assessment of gastric emptying in a multicenter setting. *Am J Gastroenterol* 2000;95:78–86.

51. Tougas G, Eaker EY, Abell TL, *et al.* Assessment of gastric emptying using a low fat meal: establishment of international control values. *Am J Gastroenterol* 2000;95:1456–1462.

52. Hinder RA, Filipi CJ, Wetscher G, Neary P, DeMeester TR, Perdikis G. Laparoscopic Nissen fundoplication is an effective treatment for gastroesophageal reflux disease. *Ann Surg* 1994;220:472–481; discussion 481–483.

53. Patterson EJ, Herron DM, Hansen PD, Ramzi N, Standage BA, Swanstrom LL. Effect of an esophageal bougie on the incidence of dysphagia following nissen fundoplication: a prospective, blinded, randomized clinical trial. *Arch Surg* 2000;135: 1055–1061; discussion 1061–1062.

54. Fein M, Bueter M, Thalheimer A, *et al.* Ten-year outcome of laparoscopic antireflux surgery. *J Gastrointest Surg* 2008;12: 1893–1899.

55. Peters JH, DeMeester TR, Crookes P, *et al.* The treatment of gastroesophageal reflux disease with laparoscopic Nissen fundoplication: prospective evaluation of 100 patients with "typical" symptoms. *Ann Surg* 1998;228:40–50.

56. Gotley DC, Smithers BM, Rhodes M, Menzies B, Branicki FJ, Nathanson L. Laparoscopic Nissen fundoplication—200 consecutive cases. *Gut* 1996;38:487–491.

57. Eubanks TR, Omelanczuk P, Richards C, Pohl D, Pellegrini CA. Outcomes of laparoscopic antireflux procedures. *Am J Surg* 2000;179:391–395.

58. Ackroyd R, Watson DI, Majeed AW, Troy G, Treacy PJ, Stoddard CJ. Randomized clinical trial of laparoscopic versus open fundoplication for gastro-oesophageal reflux disease. *Br J Surg* 2004;91:975–982.

59. Novitsky YW, Wong J, Kercher KW, Litwin DE, Swanstrom LL, Heniford BT. Severely disordered esophageal peristalsis is not a contraindication to laparoscopic Nissen fundoplication. *Surg Endosc* 2007;21:950–954.

60. Biertho L, Sebajang H, Allen C, Anvari M. Does laparoscopic Nissen fundoplication lead to chronic gastrointestinal dysfunction? *Surg Endosc* 2006;20:1360–1363.

61. Topart P, Deschamps C, Taillefer R, Duranceau CA. Long-term effect of total fundoplication on the myotomized esophagus. *Ann Thorac Surg* 1992;54:1046–1051.

62. Hayden JD, Jamieson GG. Effect on iron deficiency anemia of laparoscopic repair of large paraesophageal hernias. *Dis Esophagus* 2005;18:329–331.

63. Hwang J, Weigel TL. Acute esophageal necrosis: "black esophagus". *JSLS* 2007;11:165–167.

64. Maruyama T, Fukue M, Imamura F, Nozue M. Incarcerated paraesophageal hernia associated with perforation of the fundus of the stomach: report of a case. *Surg Today* 2001;31: 454–457.

65. Polomsky M, Hu R, Sepesi B, *et al.* A population-based analysis of emergent vs. elective hospital admissions for an intrathoracic stomach. *Surg Endosc* 2010;24:1250–1255.

66. Polomsky M, Jones CE, Sepesi B, *et al.* Should elective repair of intrathoracic stomach be encouraged? *J Gastrointest Surg* 2010;14:203–210.

67. Salameh B, Pallati PK, Mittal SK. Incarcerated intrathoracic stomach with antral ischemia resulting in gastric outlet obstruction: a case report. *Dis Esophagus* 2008;21:189–191.

68. Low DE, Unger T. Open repair of paraesophageal hernia: reassessment of subjective and objective outcomes. *Ann Thorac Surg* 2005;80:287–294.

69. Zehetner J, Lipham JC, Ayazi S, *et al.* A simplified technique for intrathoracic stomach repair: laparoscopic fundoplication with Vicryl mesh and BioGlue crural reinforcement. *Surg Endosc* 2010;24:675–679.

70. Luketich JD, Nason KS, Christie NA, *et al.* Outcomes after a decade of laparoscopic giant paraesophageal hernia repair. *J Thorac Cardiovasc Surg* 2010;139:395–404, e1.

71. Hashemi M, Peters JH, DeMeester TR, *et al.* Laparoscopic repair of large type III hiatal hernia: objective followup reveals high recurrence rate. *J Am Coll Surg* 2000;190:553–560; discussion 560–561.

72. Maziak DE, Todd TR, Pearson FG. Massive hiatus hernia: evaluation and surgical management. *J Thorac Cardiovasc Surg* 1998;115:53–60; discussion 61–62.

73. Nason KS, Luketich JD, Qureshi I, *et al.* Laparoscopic repair of giant paraesophageal hernia results in long-term patient satisfaction and a durable repair. *J Gastrointest Surg* 2008;12:2066–2075; discussion 2075–2077.

74. Oelschlager BK, Pellegrini CA, Hunter J, *et al.* Biologic prosthesis reduces recurrence after laparoscopic paraesophageal hernia repair: a multicenter, prospective, randomized trial. *Ann Surg* 2006;244:481–490.

75. Yano F, Stadlhuber RJ, Tsuboi K, Gerhardt J, Filipi CJ, Mittal SK. Outcomes of surgical treatment of intrathoracic stomach. *Dis Esophagus* 2009;22:284–288.

76. Fei L, del Genio G, Rossetti G, *et al.* Hiatal hernia recurrence: surgical complication or disease? Electron microscope findings of the diaphragmatic pillars. *J Gastrointest Surg* 2009;13:459–464.

77. Granderath FA, Carlson MA, Champion JK, *et al.* Prosthetic closure of the esophageal hiatus in large hiatal hernia repair and laparoscopic antireflux surgery. *Surg Endosc* 2006;20:367–379.

78. Granderath FA, Schweiger UM, Kamolz T, Asche KU, Pointner R. Laparoscopic Nissen fundoplication with prosthetic hiatal closure reduces postoperative intrathoracic wrap herniation: preliminary results of a prospective randomized functional and clinical study. *Arch Surg* 2005;140:40–48.

79. Stadlhuber RJ, Sherif AE, Mittal SK, *et al.* Mesh complications after prosthetic reinforcement of hiatal closure: a 28-case series. *Surg Endosc* 2009;23:1219–1226.

80. Diwan TS, Martinec DV, Ujiki MB, Dunst CM, Swanstrom LL. A simplified technique for placement of biologic mesh in paraesophageal hernia repair (PEH). *Surg Endosc* 2010;24:221–222.

81. Quilici PJ, McVay C, Tovar A. Laparoscopic antireflux procedures with hepatic shoulder technique for the surgical management of large paraesophageal hernias and gastroesophageal reflux disease. *Surg Endosc* 2009;23:2620–2623.

82. Houghton SG, Deschamps C, Cassivi SD, Nichols FC, Allen MS, Pairolero PC. The influence of transabdominal gastroplasty: early outcomes of hiatal hernia repair. *J Gastrointest Surg* 2007;11:101–106.

83. Whitson BA, Hoang CD, Boettcher AK, Dahlberg PS, Andrade RS, Maddaus MA. Wedge gastroplasty and reinforced crural repair: important components of laparoscopic giant or recurrent hiatal hernia repair. *J Thorac Cardiovasc Surg* 2006;132:1196–1202 e3.

84. Swanstrom LL, Jobe BA, Kinzie LR, Horvath KD. Esophageal motility and outcomes following laparoscopic paraesophageal hernia repair and fundoplication. *Am J Surg* 1999;177:359–363.

85. Furnee EJ, Draaisma WA, Simmermacher RK, Stapper G, Broeders IA. Long-term symptomatic outcome and radiologic assessment of laparoscopic hiatal hernia repair. *Am J Surg* 2010;199:695–701.

86. Morris-Stiff G, Hassn A. Laparoscopic paraoesophageal hernia repair: fundoplication is not usually indicated. *Hernia* 2008;12:299–302.

87. Casabella F, Sinanan M, Horgan S, Pellegrini CA. Systematic use of gastric fundoplication in laparoscopic repair of paraesophageal hernias. *Am J Surg* 1996;171:485–489.

88. Wiechmann RJ, Ferguson MK, Naunheim KS, *et al.* Laparoscopic management of giant paraesophageal herniation. *Ann Thorac Surg* 2001;71:1080–1086; discussion 1086–1087.

89. Khajanchee YS, Dunst CM, Swanstrom LL. Outcomes of Nissen fundoplication in patients with gastroesophageal reflux disease and delayed gastric emptying. *Arch Surg* 2009;144:823–828.

90. Masqusi S, Velanovich V. Pyloroplasty with fundoplication in the treatment of combined gastroesophageal reflux disease and bloating. *World J Surg* 2007;31:332–336.

91. Van Sickle KR, McClusky DA, Swafford VA, Smith CD. Delayed gastric emptying in patients undergoing antireflux surgery: analysis of a treatment algorithm. *J Laparoendosc Adv Surg Tech A* 2007;17:7–11.

92. Maddern GJ, Jamieson GG, Chatterton BE, Collins PJ. Is there an association between failed antireflux procedures and delayed gastric emptying? *Ann Surg* 1985;202:162–165.

93. Alexander F, Wyllie R, Jirousek K, Secic M, Porvasnik S. Delayed gastric emptying affects outcome of Nissen fundoplication in neurologically impaired children. *Surgery* 1997;122:690–697; discussion 697–698.

94. Brown RA, Wynchank S, Rode H, Millar AJ, Mann MD. Is a gastric drainage procedure necessary at the time of antireflux surgery? *J Pediatr Gastroenterol Nutr* 1997;25:377–380.

95. Dunn JC, Lai EC, Webber MM, Ament ME, Fonkalsrud EW. Long-term quantitative results following fundoplication and antroplasty for gastroesophageal reflux and delayed gastric emptying in children. *Am J Surg* 1998;175:27–29.

96. Cogliandolo A, Gulino FM, Mezzasalma F, Pidoto R, Micali B. [Reflux esophagitis. What factors influence the choice of antireflux surgery?] *Ann Ital Chir* 1993;64:29–33.

97. Farrell TM, Richardson WS, Halkar R, *et al.* Nissen fundoplication improves gastric motility in patients with delayed gastric emptying. *Surg Endosc* 2001;15:271–274.

98. Bais JE, Samsom M, Boudesteijn EA, van Rijk PP, Akkermans LM, Gooszen HG. Impact of delayed gastric emptying on the outcome of antireflux surgery. *Ann Surg* 2001;234:139–146.

99. Nilsson M, Johnsen R, Ye W, *et al*. Obesity and estrogen as risk factors for GERD symptoms. *JAMA* 2003;290:66–72.

100. Stern L, Iqba lN, Seshadri P, *et al*. The effects of low carbohydrate versus conventional eight loss diets in severely obese adults: One year follow-up of a randomized trial. *Ann Intern Med* 2004;140:778–785.

101. Anderson T, Stokholm KH, Backer OG, Quaade F. Long term (5 year) results after horizontal gastroplasty or very low calorie diet for morbid obesity. *Int J Obes* 1988;12:277–284.

102. Perez AR, Moncure AC, Rattner DW. Obesity adversely affects the outcomes of antirefluxoperations. *Surg Endosc* 2001;15:986–989.

103. Patterson EJ, Davis DG, Khajanchee Y, Swanstrom LL. Comparison of objective outcomes following laparoscopic Nissen fundoplication versus laparoscopic gastric bypass in the morbidly obese with heartburn. *Surg Endosc* 2003;17:1561–1565.

104. Salminen PT, Hiekkanen HI, Rantala AP, Ovaska JT. Comparison of long term outcome of laparoscopic and conventional Nissen fundoplication: a prospective randomized study with an 11 year follow-up. *Ann Surg* 2007;246:201–206.

105. Dallemagne B, Weerts J, Markiewicz S, *et al*. Clinical results of laparoscopic fundoplication at 10 years after surgery. *Surg Endosc* 2006;20:159–165.

106. Khajanchee YS, O'Rourke RW, Lockhart B, Patterson EJ, Hansen PD, Swanstrom LL. Postoperative symptoms and failure after antireflux surgery. *Arch Surg* 2002;137:1008–1013; discussion 1013–1014.

107. Lord RV, Kaminski A, Oberg S, *et al*. Absence of gastroesophageal reflux disease in a majority of patients taking acid suppression medications after Nissen fundoplication. *J Gastrointest Surg* 2002;6:3–9; discussion 10.

108. Thompson SK, Jamieson GG, Myers JC, Chin KF, Watson DI, Devitt PG. Recurrent heartburn after laparoscopic fundoplication is not always recurrent reflux. *J Gastrointest Surg* 2007;11:642–647.

109. Furnee EJ, Draaisma WA, Broeders IA, Gooszen HG. Surgical reintervention after failed antireflux surgery: a systematic review of the literature. *J Gastrointest Surg* 2009;13:1539–1549.

110. Khajanchee YS, O'Rourke R, Cassera MA, Gatta P, Hansen PD, Swanstrom LL. Laparoscopic reintervention for failed antireflux surgery: subjective and objective outcomes in 176 consecutive patients. *Arch Surg* 2007;142:785–901; discussion 791-2.

111. Fass R. Proton-pump inhibitor therapy in patients with gastro-oesophageal reflux disease: putative mechanisms of failure. *Drugs* 2007;67:1521–1530.

112. Inadomi JM, McIntyre L, Bernard L, Fendrick AM. Step-down from multiple- to single-dose proton pump inhibitors (PPIs): a prospective study of patients with heartburn or acid regurgitation completely relieved with PPIs. *Am J Gastroenterol* 2003;98:1940–1944.

113. Chen D, Barber C, McLoughlin P, Thavaneswaran P, Jamieson GG, Maddern GJ. Systematic review of endoscopic treatments for gastro-oesophageal reflux disease. *Br J Surg* 2009;96:128–136.

114. DeVault KR, Hinder RA, Floch N. Endoscopic treatment of reflux: a quest for the holy grail of reflux? *J Clin Gastroenterol* 2005;39:179–180.

115. Hogan WJ. Clinical trials evaluating endoscopic GERD treatments: is it time for a moratorium on the clinical use of these procedures? *Am J Gastroenterol* 2006;101:437–439.

33 Obesity and Gastroesophageal Reflux Disease

Frank Friedenberg
Temple University Hospital, Philadelphia, PA, USA

Introduction

Obesity, defined as a body mass index (BMI) of $30\,kg/m^2$ or greater, has become a significant health problem in the United States. The prevalence of obesity from 1980 to 2004 increased from 15% to 33% in adults, and from 6% to 19% in children [1]. Accumulating epidemiologic and physiologic data have demonstrated that obesity is an important risk factor for the development of gastroesophageal reflux disease (GERD). Endoscopic data, primarily from Asia, have supported the link between these two disorders. Strengthening the association has been the identification that weight loss, either in the form of a structured diet or bariatric surgery, can have remarkable benefits for GERD sufferers.

Is the link between obesity and reflux as simple as increased external pressure on the stomach creating a refluxogenic milieu? This likely is important; however, visceral fat is metabolically active tissue, capable of modulating several cytokines, including tumor necrosis factor-alpha (TNF-α). Additionally, serum levels of estrogen, ghrelin, and adiponectin may influence the propensity to reflux through an endocrine pathway. Alterations in peptide levels may explain esophageal motor disturbances identified in obesity that appear to improve after bariatric surgery.

Of concern has been the emerging link between obesity and Barrett's esophagus and esophageal adenocarcinoma. The incidence of esophageal adenocarcinoma has risen substantially over the past 20 years and perhaps represents an additional adverse health consequence of obesity. The link may be through the promotion of reflux by obesity; however, other factors such as diet, tobacco, and alcohol, and genetic susceptibility are likely to be important.

The treatment of obesity has evolved substantially. A low-calorie diet independent of carbohydrate content in conjunction with regular exercise will reliably lead to weight loss. For those with severe obesity and associated comorbidities, bariatric surgery has become routine. Surgical management of obese patients with severe reflux has evolved from fundoplication to gastric bypass, which provides benefit for both disorders. Use of laparoscopic banding for obesity continues to increase. In the past, there was a concern that this procedure was refluxogenic, although newer devices and modification of previous surgical techniques may be overcoming this important limitation.

Epidemiologic link

Gastroesophageal reflux disease and obesity

With rare exception, epidemiologic studies (primarily cross-sectional) have demonstrated that the prevalence of GERD is considerably higher in obese individuals relative to the non-obese. Moreover, there appears to be a dose–response relationship with higher degrees of obesity being a greater risk for the presence of GERD. In 2000, a supplemental GERD questionnaire was added to the ongoing Nurses' Health Study. Jacobson *et al.* analyzed subjects who reported GERD symptoms at least weekly and found a near linear increase in the adjusted odds ratio (OR) for reflux symptoms for each BMI strata [2]. Interestingly, even for those participants with a BMI in the upper range of normal (22.5–$24.9\,kg/m^2$), the risk was elevated relative to a control group having a BMI in the range of 20.0–$22.4\,kg/m^2$ [2] (Figure 33.1). Recently, results from the Kaiser Permanente MultiPhasic Health Check-Up cohort were reported [3]. Of 80 110 insurance members, the prevalence of GERD was 11%. Increasing abdominal diameter and increasing BMI were found to be associated with GERD. Interestingly, the association between BMI and GERD was much stronger among white as compared to black members [3].

Smaller studies in the United States have confirmed the findings of larger studies. El-Serag *et al.* interviewed 453 employees at their hospital [4]. A surprisingly large number

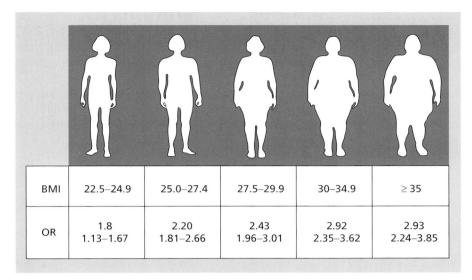

BMI	22.5–24.9	25.0–27.4	27.5–29.9	30–34.9	≥ 35
OR	1.8 1.13–1.67	2.20 1.81–2.66	2.43 1.96–3.01	2.92 2.35–3.62	2.93 2.24–3.85

Figure 33.1 Relationship between risk of GERD and body mass index. BMI, body mass index in kg/m^2; OR, odds ratio. 95% confidence interval shown below OR.

(118 or 26%) had GERD on at least a weekly basis, manifested as either heartburn or regurgitation. The authors invited all 453 employees to undergo an upper endoscopy and 196 (43.3%) agreed to the examination. They found that increasing levels of obesity were associated with a greater likelihood of GERD ($P = .004$ for trend), and a greater likelihood of having esophagitis on endoscopy ($P = .04$) [4]. Two small cohort studies from Olmstead County, MN, USA have evaluated the relationship between obesity and GERD. The first identified obesity as a risk factor for the initial development of GERD as well as the persistence of symptoms [5]. The second study evaluated the role of body weight, diet, and exercise on the presence of GERD, and found that BMI was associated with GERD (OR 1.9) independent of diet and energy expenditure [6].

The epidemiologic relationship between obesity and GERD has also been identified in non-US populations. For example, in the German National Health Interview and Examination Survey, the OR for GERD was 1.8 for overweight individuals and 2.6 for obese participants [7]. In England, the Bristol Helicobacter Project found that obesity was associated with the frequency of heartburn (OR 2.91) and acid regurgitation (OR 2.23), but found no relationship between body weight and the severity of symptoms [8]. In Spain, a telephone survey of 2500 subjects revealed that the annual prevalence of GERD was 31.6% with 9.8% of subjects having symptoms at least weekly [9]. GERD symptoms were associated with being overweight (OR 1.53) or obese (OR 1.74). Additionally, patients with GERD symptoms for 10 years or longer were much more likely to be obese (OR 1.92) [9]. In a separate publication by this group using the same population, they reported that a weight gain of more than 5 kg in the past year predisposed to the development

of "new" GERD (OR 3.0 vs those with no weight gain) [10]. In Norway, Nilson *et al.* conducted nationwide surveys during 1984–1986 (n = 74 599) and 1995–1997 (n = 65 363) [11]. They found that for severely obese men (BMI > 35 kg/m^2) the OR for reflux was 3.3, while the OR for severely obese women was 6.3 [11]. Women who were premenopausal and those who were post-menopausal but taking hormone replacement therapy were at an increased risk for GERD relative to untreated post-menopausal women ($P < .001$) [11].

There is emerging data from Asia confirming the findings seen in Western populations. Kang *et al.* prospectively examined 2457 subjects who underwent upper endoscopy at a single center in Korea [12]. They found a linear relationship between higher strata of BMI and the presence of erosive esophagitis ($P = .002$ for trend). In a nested case–control study from Shanghai, Ma *et al.* found an association between obesity and dwelling in an urban environment with the prevalence of GERD [13]. These studies, along with a study by Rosaida *et al.*, have thus far demonstrated that obesity is a risk factor for GERD in Asian populations [14].

A single study of relatively modest size (n = 820) from Sweden failed to identify a relationship between increasing levels of body weight and GERD symptoms [15]. The individuals included were primarily males (~85%) of advanced age (mean age 66 years). Individuals reported their height and weight at age 20 years and 20 years before the interview. Subjects were asked their lifetime history of reflux symptoms excluding the 5 years prior to the interview. The authors found that among those who had ever been overweight or obese, the adjusted OR for GERD was 0.99 (95% CI 0.66–1.47). They also found no association between obesity and the severity of reflux symptoms [15].

Whether a change in weight effects GERD symptoms has not been studied extensively. Cremoni *et al.* surveyed 673 individuals and found that neither a weight increase or decrease by 10 lb was associated with persistent, new onset, or disappearing GERD [5]. However, Rey *et al.* interviewed 2500 individuals and found that those with a weight gain over 5 kg demonstrated a nearly three-fold higher (OR 2.7; 95% CI 1.4–5.4) risk of new GERD symptoms [10]. Similarly, Jacobson *et al.*, in selected individuals from the Nurses' Health Study, reported an increase in BMI of more than 3.5 kg/m² as compared with no weight changes, and this was associated with an increased risk of frequent symptoms of reflux (OR 2.8; 95% CI 1.6–4.8) [2]. As will be discussed, bariatric surgery can result in a benefit in individuals with GERD symptoms, although the efficacy may vary considerably depending on the procedure utilized.

In summary, the majority of data as reported in population-based samples, demonstrates an association between increasing levels of obesity and reflux disease. This association appears to be consistent in both Western and Eastern populations. Although the data are limited, the relationship may not be as strong in certain populations, such as African Americans and post-menopausal females. Weight gain during adulthood appears to be an important precipitant of GERD.

Complications of gastroesophageal reflux disease and obesity

There is accumulating data that obesity is associated with complications related to long-standing GERD, such as erosive esophagitis, Barrett's esophagus, and esophageal adenocarcinoma [4, 16–20]. In a large endoscopic study, El-Serag *et al.* reported that relative to those with no erosions, those with erosive esophagitis were more likely to be overweight (39% vs 26%) or obese (41% vs 32%; *P* = .04) [4]. Likewise, in an endoscopic study of over 3000 participants in Korea, Lee *et al.* found an OR of 3.3 (95% CI 1.79–6.11) for EE in individuals with a BMI greater than 30 compared to normal-weight participants [21]. A meta-analysis concluded that mucosal injury appears to be more likely with increasing levels of obesity [22]

With reference to Barrett's esophagus, Stein *et al.* from the Southern Arizona VA System found that for each 5-unit increase in BMI, the risk of Barrett's esophagus increased by 35% relative to control patients without Barrett's esophagus undergoing diagnostic endoscopy [16]. El-Serag *et al.* utilized abdominal computed tomography (CT) imaging to demonstrate that increased amounts of visceral adipose tissue rather than subcutaneous adipose tissue were associated with Barrett's esophagus [17].

However, not all studies have found an association between BMI and Barrett's esophagus. An Australian study found that weekly GERD symptoms and smoking, but not BMI (OR 2.1; 95% CI 0.7–6.4) were independent risks for

the presence of Barrett's esophagus [23]. Similarly, a study from a tertiary center in Canada failed to demonstrate an association between obesity and Barrett's esophagus, but did find an association with esophageal adenocarcinoma [19]. This group used a food questionnaire and found that vitamin C was protective against the development of both Barrett's esophagus and esophageal adenocarcinoma [19]. Gerson *et al.* also failed to find an association between Barrett's esophagus and BMI in a large, multicenter study from the United States [24].

It has been proposed that excessive fat in the waist region (central obesity) rather than overall BMI is the most important risk for Barrett's esophagus and this may explain the negative findings in the above studies. For example, Corley *et al.* utilized Kaiser Permanente data from Northern California and found that a larger abdominal circumference (measured at the iliac crest with the abdomen relaxed), independent of BMI, was associated with Barrett's esophagus. Those individuals with an abdominal circumference greater than 80 cm had an OR of 2.24 for the presence of Barrett's esophagus [25]. Another study from four US gastroenterology clinics also demonstrated that central adiposity rather than BMI was associated with the presence of Barrett's esophagus, particularly long-segment disease [26]. Edelstein *et al.* found that for individuals in the highest category of waist-to-hip ratio, the adjusted OR for Barrett's esophagus was 2.4, and 4.3 for long-segment Barrett's esophagus [26].

Adipocytes secrete a variety of compounds, including numerous cytokines, adiponectin, leptin, and estrogen (Figure 33.2) [27]. A proposed link between obesity and metaplasia/neoplasia is via altered secretion of adiponectin and leptin [28]. Adiponectin is a protein that has anti-inflammatory and immunomodulatory functions and stimulates apoptosis [29]. Secretion of this adipokine decreases in obesity. Leptin is secreted by adipocytes and gastric chief cells, and has been shown to have mitogenic properties and to induce proliferation in a number of human cell lines,

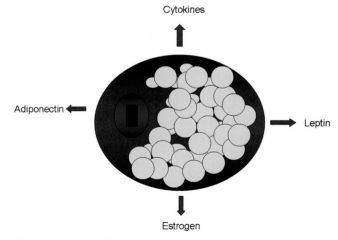

Figure 33.2 Metabolic products of a human fat cell.

including esophageal cancer cells. Plasma leptin levels are exponentially related to total adipose mass [27]. Kendall *et al.* found that in male Barrett's esophagus patients plasma leptin levels were significantly higher relative to healthy controls. Those subjects with a leptin level in the highest quartile had an OR of 3.3 for the presence of Barrett's esophagus [28]. It is noteworthy that in men leptin is secreted equally by omental and peripheral adipocytes, and levels can reach very high values in those with central obesity. In obese females it is primarily secreted by peripheral adipocytes. This may explain why central obesity (seen more often in men) is associated with Barrett's esophagus. The same study failed to demonstrate an association between adiponectin levels and the presence of Barrett's esophagus. A more recent study found an inverse association between plasma adiponectin levels and Barrett's esophagus [30]. Adjustment for central obesity but not BMI significantly influenced the relationship. Thus, the available data suggest that central obesity has the greatest influence on circulating adipokine levels which, in turn, appears to be associated with Barrett's esophagus either directly (leptin) or inversely (adiponectin).

The incidence of adenocarcinoma of the esophagus has been rising. There are limited data to support a genetic susceptibility to these cancers [31]. A number of studies have examined the relationship between obesity and esophageal adenocarcinoma. There is some limitation in review of this data as "junctional" adenocarcinomas are usually included along with esophageal adenocarcinoma as a combined endpoint. In 1998, a National Cancer Institute study by Chow *et al.* found that there was an association between increasing strata of BMI and esophageal cancer, particularly among younger individuals and those who were non-smokers [32]. A Swedish study identified an association between esophageal adenocarcinoma and an individual's BMI 20 years prior to the development of malignancy [33]. Obese persons (BMI > 30 kg/m^2) had an OR of 16.2 (95% CI 6.3–41.4) for the development of adenocarcinoma compared with the leanest individuals (BMI < 22 kg/m^2). Data from Olmstead County, MN, USA did not find a relationship (OR 1.7; 95% CI 0.4–7.0) for obesity (using a cut-off BMI of >30 kg/m^2) as a risk for esophageal adenocarcinoma. However, the population attributable risk (PAR; proportion of occurrences in the population that may be preventable if a factor were totally eliminated) for obesity when combined with age as a cofactor was 14.5%. A more dramatic finding was that reported by Engel *et al.* who used a population-based database to determine that the PAR from increased weight (using a BMI of <23.1 kg/m^2 as the reference) rose steadily from 5.4% (BMI 23.2–25.1 kg/m^2) all the way to 21.3% (BMI 27.3–40.2 kg/m^2) [34].

Perhaps the most persuasive study to date is that by Whiteman *et al.* Using an Australian cancer registry, they found that severe obesity (BMI ≥ 40 kg/m^2) conferred a greater than six-fold increased risk of cancer [20]. This rela-

tionship was only modestly attenuated by gender, age, the presence of GERD, and smoking. They found a synergistic relationship between obesity and GERD, in that the risk of cancer was increased substantially (OR 16.5; 95% CI 8.9–30.6) in patients with both risk factors compared to those with obesity alone (OR 2.2; 95% CI 1.1–4.3) or GERD alone (OR 5.6; 95% CI 2.8–11.3) [20].

In summary, there appear to be substantial and consistent epidemiologic data supporting the role of increasing levels of obesity and esophageal adenocarcinoma. The presence of reflux likely functions as a synergistic cofactor for this malignancy.

Pathophysiologic mechanisms

Several pathophysiologic abnormalities that could lead to prolonged esophageal acid exposure have been found to occur more frequently in obese individuals than in their normal-weight counterparts (Table 33.1). Many of these disturbances have been identified in the severely obese (BMI > 35 kg/m^2) and may not apply to those with lesser degrees of obesity. Many of these abnormalities have been identified in patients scheduled for bariatric surgery and comparison data are available postoperatively, although this information is less than ideal. Most surgeons will repair a hiatal hernia at the time of surgery and the anatomy of the proximal stomach is severely altered with gastric bypass or laparoscopic banding procedures. The following section will review data accumulated on the esophagogastric physiologic disturbances identified in the obese.

Esophageal motor abnormalities
In a very large study that included 345 patients selected for bariatric surgery, esophageal manometry revealed that 85 (25.6%) had abnormal motility findings [35]. Common

Table 33.1 Potential pathophysiologic disturbances in obesity which could lead to gastroesophageal reflux.

Abnormality	Consequence
Esophagus	Ineffective acid clearance
Ineffective contractions, Nutcracker esophagus	
Increased frequency of TRLES	Promotes acid reflux
Hypotensive LES	Promotes acid reflux
Hiatal hernia	Promotes acid reflux, ineffective acid clearance
Stomach	
Delayed gastric emptying	Promotes acid reflux
Increased intragastric pressure	Promotes acid reflux

findings included nutcracker esophagus in 16 patients (19%) and non-specific motility disorder in 14 patients (16%) [35]. Koppman *et al.* studied 116 obese patients selected for bariatric surgery and found that 46 (40%) had abnormal manometric findings. Their study also found the most common abnormalities to be non-specific motility disorder and nutcracker esophagus [36]. Jaffin *et al.* studied 152 presurgery patients and found that 61% had a motility disorder, including hypotensive lower esophageal sphincter (LES) pressure (41%), nutcracker esophagus (24%), and non-specific motility disorders (22%) [37]. Interestingly, most patients evaluated in these three studies were asymptomatic and did not complain of dysphagia or chest pain.

Two studies have focused specifically on morbidly obese presurgical patients with symptoms of GERD and excluded those who were asymptomatic. One of these studies investigated 61 patients and found that 20 (32.8%) had abnormal manometric results involving the esophageal body, with the most frequent finding being non-specific motor disorder [38]. The second study used manometry, 24-h pH measurement, and esophageal impedance to compare 10 normal-weight, asymptomatic subjects (control group I), 22 non-obese (BMI < 35 kg/m²) GERD patients (control group II), and 22 obese, GERD patients [39]. All of the normal-weight, asymptomatic individuals had normal acid exposure, esophageal motility, and bolus transit. There were a total of 10 patients among both GERD groups with abnormal manometric findings, which included ineffective esophageal motility (n = 4), nutcracker esophagus (n = 4), hypertensive LES pressure (>50 mmHg) (n = 1), and diffuse esophageal spasm (n = 1). The only difference between the obese and non-obese GERD groups was that the obese subjects had a lower rate of esophageal clearance (66% complete bolus transit vs 88% complete bolus transit, respectively; P = 0.04) [39]. This study confirmed the high prevalence of motility disorders among patients with GERD and also suggests that when GERD is associated with obesity, these abnormalities are more likely to lead to functional impairment.

Lower esophageal sphincter abnormalities

A hypotensive LES (<10 mmHg) is a clear risk factor for the development of GERD, and the correlation between BMI and LES pressure has been extensively investigated. One study focused on 64 consecutive patients with symptoms of weekly heartburn and/or regurgitation. BMI was calculated and the patients were divided into three groups: group A (n = 23) had a BMI of less than 25 kg/m²; group B (n = 25) had a BMI of greater than 25 and less than 30 kg/m²; and group C (n = 16) had a BMI greater than 30 kg/m². The authors found a strong inverse relationship (P < .001) between BMI and LES pressure; i.e. as BMI increased, LES pressure decreased significantly [40]. Also, the proportion of patients with severe reflux symptoms was significantly higher among both the over-

weight (32%) and obese patients (43.8%) versus normal-weight GERD patients (8.7%) [40]. Contrary to this, Fisher *et al.* investigated 30 morbidly obese patients with manometry and esophageal pH monitoring and observed no relationship between LES pressure and BMI. However, they did find a correlation between rising BMI and both increased acid exposure and number of reflux episodes [41].

Transient lower esophageal sphincter relaxations in obesity

Transient LES relaxations (TLESRs) allow acid reflux regardless of the resting LES pressure and can become pathologic if accompanied by recurrent reflux of gastric contents into the esophagus [42]. The main stimulus for generating TLESRs is gastric distention, particularly from the response of stretch receptors in the proximal stomach [43, 44]. A study investigating the association between TLESRs and obesity compared three groups of subjects [45]. Overall, 28 obese, 28 overweight, and 28 normal subjects completed upper endoscopy, manometry, and pH recordings for both the fasting and postprandial periods. Overweight and obese individuals were found to have a significantly higher rate of TLESRs during the 2-h period after meal ingestion. Also, the proportion of TLESRs accompanied by acid reflux and the total acid exposure were significantly higher in obese and overweight subjects. A direct correlation between BMI, number of TLESRs, and number of TLESRs associated with acid reflux was identified [45].

Hiatal hernia

In a study by Sutter *et al,*. 181 of 345 (52.6%) morbidly obese patients selected for bariatric surgery were diagnosed with a hiatal hernia. In the patients with a hiatal hernia, findings of either esophagitis (47.5% vs 15.8%) or abnormally low distal esophageal pH (7.4% vs 5.1%) were significantly more common than in those without hernias [35]. Similar results were reported in a study of 31 obese patients referred for bariatric surgery in which eight patients (26%) had evidence of a hiatal hernia. Among those patients with abnormal acid exposure, there was a significantly higher prevalence of hiatal hernia (42% vs 8.3%) [46]. A recent report by Pandolfino *et al.* provides evidence that the pressure morphology along the gastroesophageal junction (GEJ) is altered with obesity in a manner supporting the formation of a hiatal hernia [47]. Manometric studies were performed on 285 patients. They found that both intragastric pressure (r = 0.55) and the gastroesophageal pressure gradient (r = 0.37) strongly correlated with increasing levels of BMI [47]. In addition, there was a modest, but statistically significant correlation between the magnitude of separation of the components of the GEJ (diaphragmatic crus, LES) and BMI (r = 0.17; P < .005) [47].

Elevated intra-abdominal and intragastric pressure

An obvious consequence of obesity, particularly central obesity, is the transmission of the gravitational force of this mass on the abdominal cavity. A pressure rise within the abdominal cavity could lead to a rise in intragastric pressure, which would predispose to GERD. Lambert *et al.* studied 45 morbidly obese subjects with an indwelling urinary manometry catheter. Readings were considered to represent the pressure within the intra-abdominal cavity [48]. The authors demonstrated that intra-abdominal pressure was significantly higher in this group compared to a normal-weight control group (12 ± 0.8 vs $0 \pm 2\,cmH_2O$). Using similar methodology, this finding was subsequently confirmed by Varela *et al.* [49]. El-Serag *et al.*, using an intragastric manometry catheter, demonstrated a correlation between increasing intragastric pressure and increasing BMI ($r = 0.11$; $P = .05$) [50]. Pandolfino *et al.* demonstrated that waist circumference correlated significantly with intragastric pressure and the pressure gradient between the stomach and esophagus [47]. In a study of 31 morbidly obese patients referred for bariatric surgery and eight healthy volunteers, a barostat (highly compliant balloon) was used to measure proximal gastric compliance and tone [46]. Minimal distending pressure (MDP, defined as the first pressure inducing an intragastric volume >30 mL) was significantly higher in obese patients compared with lean healthy controls (11.8 ± 2.2 vs $6.4 \pm 3.0\,mmHg$; $P < .001$). Higher MDP was thought to be due to the external pressure induced by central obesity. Additional studies in this area are needed to confirm these preliminary findings.

Gastric abnormalities

It has been proposed that an increase in gastric contents due either to a more capacious stomach or refluxogenic delayed gastric emptying. Three studies looking at gastric capacity have been performed in obese subjects. One group evaluated gastric capacity by filling a gastric balloon at a rate of 100 mL/min until the maximal tolerated volume (MTV) was reached. They found that obese subjects had a significantly larger gastric capacity than lean individuals (1925 ± 175 vs $1100 \pm 185\,mL$; $P = .02$) [51]. These results were seen in another study of similar design, which found that the mean MTV was significantly greater in an obese group relative to lean controls (1763 ± 70 vs $1000 \pm 67\,mL$) [52]. Chiloiro *et al.* performed ultrasound examinations of 109 school-aged children and found a correlation between the cross-sectional area of the antrum and BMI ($r = 0.44$; $P < .0001$) [53]. In total, these studies suggest that gastric capacity is significantly larger in obese individuals.

The data with respect to gastric emptying in obese subjects have been conflicting. At least three studies have documented an acceleration of gastric emptying in obese individuals [54–56]. However, the group led by Horowitz *et al.* has failed to confirm this finding [57, 58]. It should be noted that most of these studies are over 20 years old and did not use standardized nuclear imaging techniques. Further studies are needed to clarify the relationship between gastric emptying and obesity.

Medical management of gastroesophageal reflux disease in obese patients

The relationship between weight gain and increases in GERD symptoms is well documented [5, 10]. Only three studies to date have examined the effect of weight loss through dieting on GERD symptoms [59–61]. Kjellin *et al.* examined 20 obese patients with reflux defined by abnormal 24-h pH study and GERD symptoms requiring daily acid-suppression medication [61]. Patients were randomized to treatment with either a very low-caloric diet (VLCD) or no change in diet. After 6 months, the treatment group had lost an average of 10.8 kg, whereas the control group had gained 0.6 kg. The authors found no reduction in reflux according to pH measurement and no significant changes in reflux symptoms. Further, the control group was then prescribed the VLCD and lost an average of 9.7 kg, but similarly, reflux parameters remained unchanged, and all patients from both groups, except for one, remained dependent on daily medication.

Frederiksen *et al.*, using serial 24-h pH measurements, studied morbidly obese patients consuming a prescribed liquid VLCD pre- and post-vertical banded gastroplasty [60]. While on the VLCD prior to surgery, 12 patients lost weight and three gained weight. All patients lost weight after surgery. There were no significant changes in acid exposure time from baseline compared with 10–14 days following the start of the diet or three weeks after surgery while still on the modified diet.

In contrast, Fraser-Moodie *et al.* examined 34 patients with a BMI greater than $23\,kg/m^2$ who experienced frequent symptoms of gastroesophageal reflux for at least the previous 6 months [59]. Patients were provided with dietary advice to lose weight, but were asked to make no other changes in lifestyle. Their weight and symptom scores were assessed 2, 18, and 26 weeks after enrollment. Twenty-seven patients lost weight, with a mean loss of 4 kg. Weight loss was associated with reduced reflux symptoms by a mean of 75% from baseline using the modified DeMeester questionnaire. Nine patients became asymptomatic, three gained weight and had a worsening of their symptoms, and four gained weight but still improved their symptom score. No patient who experienced weight loss had a worsening of symptoms. The major limitation of this study is the lack of a structured weight loss protocol or prescribed caloric recommendations. It is possible that a change in diet, away from meals consisting of high fat and high caloric density, independent of weight loss, was the mechanism by which patients experienced amelioration of their symptoms [62, 63].

Surgical management of gastroesophageal reflux disease in obese patients

There has been a growing body of literature on the impact of surgical techniques for weight loss on acid reflux disease and symptoms. Bariatric procedures are classified as either restrictive [intragastric balloons, sleeve gastrectomy, and laparoscopic adjustable gastric banding (LAGB)], malabsorptive (biliopancreatic diversion with duodenal switch), or combined [proximal Roux-en-Y gastric bypass (RYGBP)]. Many studies looking at the effect of bariatric surgery on GERD symptoms have been retrospective and uncontrolled, and included relatively few participants. Analysis of results from many trials is also confounded by the common practice of repairing obvious hiatal hernias during surgery. In this section, only trials of LAGB and RYGBP will be discussed as they are the most common procedures performed currently in the United States.

In LAGB a band device is placed around the fundus of the stomach immediately below the GEJ and a subcutaneous reservoir is used to adjust the band size (Figure 33.3A). The resulting pouch dramatically reduces the functional capacity of the stomach. Dixon et al. studied 48 symptomatic patients preoperatively who had either erosive esophagitis (n = 18) or the requirement for frequent reflux treatment with antisecretory therapy (n = 30) [64]. After LAGB, 14 patients (77.8%) with erosive esophagitis and 22 (73.3%) on frequent medication had complete resolution of symptoms within 21 days of surgery. Iovino et al. identified 16 obese patients with abnormal esophageal acid exposure prior to

LAGB [65]. Heartburn and regurgitation scores improved dramatically with LAGB at the expense of increased dysphagia symptoms. Compared to before surgery, there was a dramatic decrease in the duration of time that the esophageal pH was below 4.0 for the study group after LAGB (8.2 vs 2.2 %; P < .01).

Tolonen et al. examined 31 symptomatic obese patients pre- and post-LAGB with upper endoscopy and 24 pH studies [66]. Nearly all patients on both pre- and postoperative upper endoscopy had a normal examination or only minor mucosal breaks. Hiatal hernias were frequently found prior to surgery and corrected during surgery. Nevertheless, the number of reflux episodes (44.6 down to 22.09; P < .001) and total reflux time (9.5% down to 3.5%; P < .001) improved dramatically from the preoperative to postoperative period. This corresponded with a significant decrease in the DeMeester score (38.5 down to 18.6; P = .03).

A study from Germany failed to demonstrate an improvement in GERD parameters following LAGB [67]. Despite impressive weight loss and a relatively low rate of complications (9.7%), the authors noted a significant increase in the presence of erosive esophageal changes postoperatively (30%; preoperative prevalence 16.7%) and pH parameters worsened as well (% time pH < 4 increased from 4.3% to 7.9%). De Jong et al. reported similar findings in 29 patients undergoing LAGB [68]. They found that symptoms of reflux frequently developed at 6 months postoperatively. They concluded that in many patients, LAGB initially reduces symptoms of GERD but, over time, symptoms increase toward baseline or beyond. This increase is likely due to slippage of the band distally, creating an acid reservoir above the band.

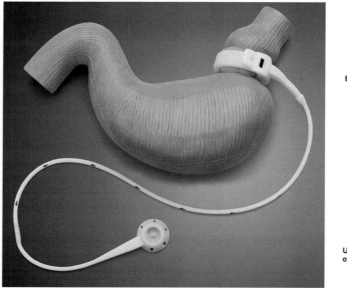
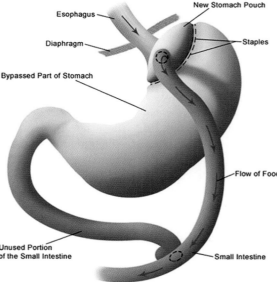

Figure 33.3 (A) Adjustable gastric band. A subcutaneous port is shown which can be accessed to adjust restriction of band. (B) Anatomic changes after Roux-en-Y gastric bypass procedure.

RYGBP involves stapling of the stomach to create a small (≤30 mL) upper gastric pouch (Figure 33.3B) [69]. A Roux limb of jejunum is then anastomosed to the gastric pouch, bypassing considerable absorptive surface area. Again, usually a repair of a concomitant hiatal hernia is performed. RYGBP may be successful at reducing GERD symptoms by diverting bile away from the esophagus [70, 71], eliminating acid production in the gastric pouch [71], or reducing the volume of acid refluxate [72]. Ortega et al. evaluated 40 patients before and after RYGBP [73]. Overall, 57.5% of obese patients had a study positive for reflux (pH < 4 for ≥4% of the total study time) preoperatively, which dropped to 10% after 3 months, and was present in 15% after 1 year (P < .05).

Another study which analyzed GERD in a prospective method with objective data was performed by Mejia-Rivas et al. [74]. This group looked at 20 patients who had a BMI of 48.5 ± 6.2 and 33.2 ± 4.5 kg/m^2 before and after RYGBP, respectively. Esophageal acid exposure improved significantly after RYGBP. For the group, the percentage of time at pH below 4 was 10.7 ± 6.7% before and 1.6 ± 1.2% after the surgical procedure (P < .001) [74].

In summary, surgical management of morbid obesity is usually approached by either LAGB or RYGBP. Although less invasive, LAGB has the potential to increase the possibility of GERD by the creation of an acid reservoir above the band should it begin to slip distally. In patients with severe GERD preoperatively, consideration should be given to performing RYGBP, which is likely to substantially improve symptoms.

Future areas of research and gaps in our knowledge

Future studies that examine the effects of dietary modification for weight loss on GERD are needed. Studies should include larger patient numbers, control for confounding variables (such as baseline weight, hiatal hernia, medication use), a clearly defined dietary plan, and detailed assessment of lifestyle factors. Until this is accomplished, no conclusions on the effects of weight loss on GERD, independent of surgery, can be made. Much more information is needed on the effect of leptin and adiponectin released from adipocytes. Preliminary data indicate that alterations in the circulating levels of these proteins in obesity (increase in leptin, decrease in adiponectin) may increase the risk of Barrett's esophagus and esophageal adenocarcinoma. Improvements in the materials and surgical methods used in LAGB are needed such that band slippage becomes a less frequent complication.

Conclusions

Epidemiologic studies strongly suggest that the prevalence of GERD is increasing and the major contributing factor to this trend is the rising prevalence of obesity. Central obesity has now been linked to the development of long-segment Barrett's esophagus and esophageal adenocarcinoma. Common bariatric procedures including laparoscopic banding and gastric bypass have demonstrated good results in ameliorating the symptoms of reflux. However, only a few studies have recorded objective data in the form of endoscopy or pH studies to document improvement after surgery. The findings for weight loss through diet alone have been conflicting. Prospective trials with adequate controls are needed.

References

1. Ogden CL, Yanovski SZ, Carroll MD, et al. The epidemiology of obesity. Gastroenterology 2007;132:2087–2102.
2. Jacobson BC, Somers SC, Fuchs CS, et al. Body-mass index and symptoms of gastroesophageal reflux in women. N Engl J Med 2006;354:2340–2348.
3. Corley DA, Kubo A, Zhao W. Abdominal obesity, ethnicity and gastro-oesophageal reflux symptoms. Gut 2007;56:756–762.
4. El-Serag HB, Graham DY, Satia JA, et al. Obesity is an independent risk factor for GERD symptoms and erosive esophagitis. Am J Gastroenterol 2005;100:1243–1250.
5. Cremonini F, Locke GR,3rd, Schleck CD, et al. Relationship between upper gastrointestinal symptoms and changes in body weight in a population-based cohort. Neurogastroenterol Motil 2006;18:987–994.
6. Nandurkar S, Locke GR 3rd, Fett S, et al. Relationship between body mass index, diet, exercise and gastro-oesophageal reflux symptoms in a community. Aliment Pharmacol Ther 2004;20:497–505.
7. Nocon M, Labenz J, Willich SN. Lifestyle factors and symptoms of gastro-oesophageal reflux—a population-based study. Aliment Pharmacol Ther 2006;23:169–174.
8. Murray L, Johnston B, Lane A, et al. Relationship between body mass and gastro-oesophageal reflux symptoms: The Bristol helicobacter project. Int J Epidemiol 2003;32:645–650.
9. Diaz-Rubio M, Moreno-Elola-Olaso C, Rey E, et al. Symptoms of gastro-oesophageal reflux: Prevalence, severity, duration and associated factors in a Spanish population. Aliment Pharmacol Ther 2004;19:95–105.
10. Rey E, Moreno-Elola-Olaso C, Artalejo FR, et al. Association between weight gain and symptoms of gastroesophageal reflux in the general population. Am J Gastroenterol 2006;101:229–233.
11. Nilsson M, Johnsen R, Ye W, et al. Obesity and estrogen as risk factors for gastroesophageal reflux symptoms. JAMA 2003;290:66–72.
12. Kang MS, Park DI, Oh SY, et al. Abdominal obesity is an independent risk factor for erosive esophagitis in a Korean population. J Gastroenterol Hepatol 2007;22:1656–1661.
13. Ma XQ, Cao Y, Wang R, et al. Prevalence of, and factors associated with, gastroesophageal reflux disease: A population-based study in Shanghai, china. Dis Esophagus 2009;22:317–322.

14. Rosaida MS, Goh KL. Gastro-oesophageal reflux disease, reflux oesophagitis and non-erosive reflux disease in a multiracial asian population: A prospective, endoscopy based study. *Eur J Gastroenterol Hepatol* 2004;16:495–501.

15. Lagergren J, Bergstrom R, Nyren O. No relation between body mass and gastro-oesophageal reflux symptoms in a swedish population based study. *Gut* 2000;47:26–29.

16. Stein DJ, El-Serag HB, Kuczynski J, et al. The association of body mass index with Barrett's oesophagus. *Aliment Pharmacol Ther* 2005;22:1005–1010.

17. El-Serag HB, Kvapil P, Hacken-Bitar J, et al. Abdominal obesity and the risk of Barrett's esophagus. *Am J Gastroenterol* 2005;100: 2151–2156.

18. Freeman HJ. Risk of gastrointestinal malignancies and mechanisms of cancer development with obesity and its treatment. *Best Pract Res Clin Gastroenterol* 2004;18:1167–1175.

19. Veugelers PJ, Porter GA, Guernsey DL, et al. Obesity and lifestyle risk factors for gastroesophageal reflux disease, Barrett esophagus and esophageal adenocarcinoma. *Dis Esophagus* 2006;19:321–328.

20. Whiteman DC, Sadeghi S, Pandeya N, et al. Combined effects of obesity, acid reflux and smoking on the risk of adenocarcinomas of the oesophagus. *Gut* 2008;57:173–180.

21. Lee HL, Eun CS, Lee OY, et al. Association between GERD-related erosive esophagitis and obesity. *J Clin Gastroenterol* 2008;42:672–675.

22. Hampel H, Abraham NS, El-Serag HB. Meta-analysis: Obesity and the risk for gastroesophageal reflux disease and its complications. *Ann Intern Med* 2005;143:199–211.

23. Smith KJ, O'Brien SM, Smithers BM, et al. Interactions among smoking, obesity, and symptoms of acid reflux in Barrett's esophagus. *Cancer Epidemiol Biomarkers Prev* 2005;14: J2481–2486.

24. Gerson LB, Ullah N, Fass R, et al. Does body mass index differ between patients with Barrett's oesophagus and patients with chronic gastro-oesophageal reflux disease? *Aliment Pharmacol Ther* 2007;25:1079–1086.

25. Corley DA, Kubo A, Levin TR, et al. Abdominal obesity and body mass index as risk factors for Barrett's esophagus. *Gastroenterology* 2007;133:34–41; quiz 41.

26. Edelstein ZR, Farrow DC, Bronner MP, et al. Central adiposity and risk of Barrett's esophagus. *Gastroenterology* 2007;133: 403–411.

27. Weigle DS. Leptin and other secretory products of adipocytes modulate multiple physiological functions. *Ann Endocrinol (Paris)* 1997;58:132–136.

28. Kendall BJ, Macdonald GA, Hayward NK, et al. Leptin and the risk of Barrett's oesophagus. *Gut* 2008;57:448–454.

29. Kelesidis I, Kelesidis T, Mantzoros CS. Adiponectin and cancer: A systematic review. *Br J Cancer* 2006;94:1221–1225.

30. Rubenstein JH, Dahlkemper A, Kao JY, et al. A pilot study of the association of low plasma adiponectin and Barrett's esophagus. *Am J Gastroenterol* 2008;103:1358–1364.

31. Chak A, Falk G, Grady WM, et al. Assessment of familiality, obesity, and other risk factors for early age of cancer diagnosis in adenocarcinomas of the esophagus and gastroesophageal junction. *Am J Gastroenterol* 2009;104:1913–1921.

32. Chow WH, Blot WJ, Vaughan TL, et al. Body mass index and risk of adenocarcinomas of the esophagus and gastric cardia. *J Natl Cancer Inst* 1998;90:150–155.

33. Lagergren J, Bergstrom R, Nyren O. Association between body mass and adenocarcinoma of the esophagus and gastric cardia. *Ann Intern Med* 1999;130:883–890.

34. Engel LS, Chow WH, Vaughan TL, et al. Population attributable risks of esophageal and gastric cancers. *J Natl Cancer Inst* 2003;95:1404–1413.

35. Suter M, Dorta G, Giusti V, et al. Gastro-esophageal reflux and esophageal motility disorders in morbidly obese patients. *Obes Surg* 2004;14:959–966.

36. Koppman JS, Poggi L, Szomstein S, et al. Esophageal motility disorders in the morbidly obese population. *Surg Endosc* 2007;21:761–764.

37. Jaffin BW, Knoepflmacher P, Greenstein R. High prevalence of asymptomatic esophageal motility disorders among morbidly obese patients. *Obes Surg* 1999;9:390–395.

38. Hong D, Khajanchee YS, Pereira N, et al. Manometric abnormalities and gastroesophageal reflux disease in the morbidly obese. *Obes Surg* 2004;14:744–749.

39. Quiroga E, Cuenca-Abente F, Flum D, et al. Impaired esophageal function in morbidly obese patients with gastroesophageal reflux disease: Evaluation with multichannel intraluminal impedance. *Surg Endosc* 2006;20(5):739–743.

40. Kouklakis G, Moschos J, Kountouras J, et al. Relationship between obesity and gastroesophageal reflux disease as recorded by 3-hour esophageal pH monitoring. *Rom J Gastroenterol* 2005;14:117–121.

41. Fisher BL, Pennathur A, Mutnick JL, et al. Obesity correlates with gastroesophageal reflux. *Dig Dis Sci* 1999;44:2290–2294.

42. Xing J, Chen JD. Alterations of gastrointestinal motility in obesity. *Obes Res* 2004;12:1723–1732.

43. Kahrilas PJ, Shi G, Manka M, et al. Increased frequency of transient lower esophageal sphincter relaxation induced by gastric distention in reflux patients with hiatal hernia. *Gastroenterology* 2000;118:688–695.

44. Penagini R, Carmagnola S, Cantu P, et al. Mechanoreceptors of the proximal stomach: Role in triggering transient lower esophageal sphincter relaxation. *Gastroenterology* 2004;126:49–56.

45. Wu JC, Mui LM, Cheung CM, et al. Obesity is associated with increased transient lower esophageal sphincter relaxation. *Gastroenterology* 2007;132:883–889.

46. Iovino P, Angrisani L, Galloro G, et al. Proximal stomach function in obesity with normal or abnormal oesophageal acid exposure. *Neurogastroenterol Motil* 2006;18:425–432.

47. Pandolfino JE, El-Serag HB, Zhang Q, et al. Obesity: A challenge to esophagogastric junction integrity. *Gastroenterology* 2006;130: 639–649.

48. Lambert DM, Marceau S, Forse RA. Intra-abdominal pressure in the morbidly obese. *Obes Surg* 2005;15:1225–1232.

49. Varela JE, Hinojosa M, Nguyen N. Correlations between intra-abdominal pressure and obesity-related co-morbidities. *Surg Obes Relat Dis* 2009;5:524–528.

50. El-Serag HB, Tran T, Richardson P, et al. Anthropometric correlates of intragastric pressure. *Scand J Gastroenterol* 2006;41: 887–891.

51. Geliebter A. Gastric distension and gastric capacity in relation to food intake in humans. *Physiol Behav* 1988;44:665–668.

52. Granstrom L, Backman L. Stomach distension in extremely obese and in normal subjects. *Acta Chir Scand* 1985;151:367–370.

53. Chiloiro M, Caroli M, Guerra V, *et al.* Gastric emptying in normal weight and obese children–an ultrasound study. *Int J Obes Relat Metab Disord* 1999;23:1303–1306.

54. Zahorska-Markiewicz B, Jonderko K, Lelek A, *et al.* Gastric emptying in obesity. *Hum Nutr Clin Nutr* 1986;40:309–313.

55. Wright RA, Krinsky S, Fleeman C, *et al.* Gastric emptying and obesity. *Gastroenterology* 1983;84:747–751.

56. Tosetti C, Corinaldesi R, Stanghellini V, *et al.* Gastric emptying of solids in morbid obesity. *Int J Obes Relat Metab Disord* 1996;20:200–205.

57. Horowitz M, Collins PJ, Cook DJ, *et al.* Abnormalities of gastric emptying in obese patients. *Int J Obes* 1983;7:415–421.

58. Maddox A, Horowitz M, Wishart J, *et al.* Gastric and oesophageal emptying in obesity. *Scand J Gastroenterol* 1989;24: 593–598.

59. Fraser-Moodie CA, Norton B, Gornall C, *et al.* Weight loss has an independent beneficial effect on symptoms of gastro-oesophageal reflux in patients who are overweight. *Scand J Gastroenterol* 1999;34:337–340.

60. Frederiksen SG, Johansson J, Johnsson F, *et al.* Neither low-calorie diet nor vertical banded gastroplasty influence gastro-oesophageal reflux in morbidly obese patients. *Eur J Surg* 2000;166:296–300.

61. Kjellin A, Ramel S, Rossner S, *et al.* Gastroesophageal reflux in obese patients is not reduced by weight reduction. *Scand J Gastroenterol* 1996;31:1047–1051.

62. El-Serag HB, Satia JA, Rabeneck L. Dietary intake and the risk of gastro-oesophageal reflux disease: A cross sectional study in volunteers. *Gut* 2005;54:11–17.

63. Fox M, Barr C, Nolan S, *et al.* The effects of dietary fat and calorie density on esophageal acid exposure and reflux symptoms. *Clin Gastroenterol Hepatol* 2007;5:439–444.

64. Dixon JB, O'Brien PE. Gastroesophageal reflux in obesity: The effect of lap-band placement. *Obes Surg* 1999;9:527–531.

65. Iovino P, Angrisani L, Tremolaterra F, *et al.* Abnormal esophageal acid exposure is common in morbidly obese patients and improves after a successful lap-band system implantation. *Surg Endosc* 2002;16:1631–1635.

66. Tolonen P, Victorzon M, Niemi R, *et al.* Does gastric banding for morbid obesity reduce or increase gastroesophageal reflux? *Obes Surg* 2006;16:1469–1474.

67. Gutschow CA, Collet P, Prenzel K, *et al.* Long-term results and gastroesophageal reflux in a series of laparoscopic adjustable gastric banding. *J Gastrointest Surg* 2005;9:941–948.

68. de Jong JR, van Ramshorst B, Timmer R, *et al.* Effect of laparoscopic gastric banding on esophageal motility. *Obes Surg* 2006;16:52–58.

69. DeMaria EJ. Bariatric surgery for morbid obesity. *N Engl J Med* 2007;356:2176–2183.

70. Frezza EE, Ikramuddin S, Gourash W, *et al.* Symptomatic improvement in gastroesophageal reflux disease (GERD) following laparoscopic Roux-en-Y gastric bypass. *Surg Endosc* 2002;16:1027–1031.

71. Cobey F, Oelschlager B. Complete regression of Barrett's esophagus after Roux-en-Y gastric bypass. *Obes Surg* 2005;15: 710–712.

72. Smith SC, Edwards CB, Goodman GN. Symptomatic and clinical improvement in morbidly obese patients with gastroesophageal reflux disease following Roux-en-Y gastric bypass. *Obes Surg* 1997;7:479–484.

73. Ortega J, Escudero MD, Mora F, *et al.* Outcome of esophageal function and 24-hour esophageal pH monitoring after vertical banded gastroplasty and Roux-en-Y gastric bypass. *Obes Surg* 2004;14:1086–1094.

74. Mejia-Rivas MA, Herrera-Lopez A, Hernandez-Calleros J, *et al.* Gastroesophageal reflux disease in morbid obesity: The effect of Roux-en-Y gastric bypass. *Obes Surg* 2008;18:1217–1224.

V Malignant Disease

34 Tumors of the Esophagus

Susana Gonzalez[1] and Charles J. Lightdale[2]

[1]Mount Sinai School of Medicine, New York, NY, USA
[2]Columbia University Medical Center, New York, NY, USA

Introduction

Worldwide, esophageal cancer is the eighth most common incident cancer, with about 400 000 new cases diagnosed in 2002, and the sixth most common cause of death [1]. In 2009 in the United States, 16 470 new cases of esophageal cancer were reported, with 12 940 males affected, and a total of 14 530 deaths, 11 490 of whom were male [2]. Despite advances in technology used for screening, diagnosis, and treatment, mortality remains elevated. In fact, among men in the United States, it is one of a few cancers that has an increasing death rate [2]. For all patients with esophageal cancer, the 5-year survival rate is about 20%. The two most common histopathologic subtypes of esophageal cancer are squamous cell carcinoma and adenocarcinoma.

Malignant esophageal cancers

This section will focus on the epidemiology, pathogenesis, clinical presentation and diagnosis, staging, and endoscopic therapies for malignant esophageal cancers.

Epidemiology

There is remarkable geographic variation in the incidence of esophageal cancer. The Asian esophageal cancer belt, which spans North–Central China to Iran, has the highest incidences of esophageal squamous cell carcinoma, with some locations having an incidence as high as 100 per 100 000 persons, with men and women having similar incidence rates [3, 4]. Esophageal squamous cell carcinoma was once also the dominant subtype of esophageal cancer in the Western world. However, over the last 30 years, there has been a major shift, with a large increase in adenocarcinoma and a modest decline in squamous cell carcinoma [5–7]. Despite these changes, squamous cell carcinoma remains the predominant subtype among African Americans and Hispanics, while adenocarcinoma is more predominant in Caucasian males [8–10]. Gender disparities also exist with squamous cell carcinoma, which occurs 3–4 times more often in men than women, and adenocarcinoma which is 6–8 times more likely in men than women [5].

Pathogenesis

Certain risk factors are associated with the development of esophageal cancer (Table 34.1). Alcohol and tobacco consumption have long been known to be a major cause of esophageal cancer. Tobacco use is more strongly associated with squamous cell cancer of the esophagus than with adenocarcinoma. Studies have shown that smokers have a 3–7-fold increased risk of squamous cell cancer [11–15]. An exception to this finding is the Asian esophageal cancer belt where tobacco use is only mildly associated with an increased risk of squamous cell cancer [16–18]. Tobacco use has also been associated with esophageal adenocarcinoma, increasing the risk nearly two-fold [19–27]. Heavy alcohol use, more than three drinks/day, has been associated with a 3–5-fold increased risk of squamous cell carcinoma [15, 28–30]. It has also been suggested that mutations in aldehyde dehydrogenase, which are responsible for the flushing response in the Asian population, may be associated with an increased risk of squamous cell carcinoma [31, 32]. On the other hand, there is little evidence for an increased risk of esophageal adenocarcinoma with alcohol consumption [15, 19–21, 23, 24, 26, 33].

Dietary and nutritional factors play a role in the pathogenesis of esophageal cancer. Diets that have low intake of fresh fruits and vegetables increase the risk of squamous cell carcinoma more than adenocarcinoma [34–36]. In addition, the direct effect of carcinogen compounds, such as nitrosamines and acetylaldehyde, have been associated with increased rates of esophageal cancer [37, 38].

While human papilloma virus (HPV) subtypes 16 and 18 play an important role in the etiology of oropharyngeal and other cancers, the role of HPV in esophageal cancer remains

The Esophagus, Fifth Edition. Edited by Joel E. Richter, Donald O. Castell.
© 2012 Blackwell Publishing Ltd. Published 2012 by Blackwell Publishing Ltd.

Table 34.1 Risk factors for esophageal cancer by histologic subtype.

Adenocarcinoma	Squamous cell carcinoma (SCC)
Tobacco (less risk than for SCC)	Tobacco and alcohol use
GERD	Dietary factors
	Low intake of fresh fruits and vegetables
Obesity	Native of the Asian esophageal cancer belt
Barrett's esophagus	Achalasia
	Caustic injury
	Tylosis
	Plummer–Vinson syndrome
	Head and neck cancer

GERD, gastroesophageal reflux disease.

controversial. It is possible that differences in study design and geographic variation have led to some studies finding positive associations between HPV and esophageal cancer [39–41], while other studies have found no association [42–45]. Given these inconsistent results, further evidence is needed to determine what role, if any, HPV has in esophageal cancer.

There is, however, consistent evidence that infection with *Helicobacter pylori* is protective against esophageal adenocarcinoma. Colonization with *H. pylori* was associated with about a 50% reduction in risk of development of esophageal adenocarcinoma, but no association with esophageal squamous cell carcinoma [46–48].

Several predisposing conditions have been associated with esophageal cancer. A 2–3-fold increased risk in esophageal adenocarcinoma has been observed in a dose–response pattern in overweight and obese individuals. [27, 49–54]. Gastroesophageal acid reflux is associated with an increased risk of esophageal adenocarcinoma. Lagergren *et al.* performed a case–control study in Sweden and found a dose–response association of frequency and duration of reflux leading to a greater risk of esophageal adenocarcinoma [55]. This study found that in individuals with recurrent symptoms of reflux, the odds ratio was 7.7 (95% CI 5.3–11.4) for esophageal adenocarcinoma. In individuals with more frequent, more severe, and longer lasting symptoms of reflux, the odds ratio was 43.5 (95% CI 18.3–103.5) for esophageal adenocarcinoma and the risk of esophageal squamous cell carcinoma was not associated with reflux (odds ratio 1.1; 95% CI 0.7–1.9) [55]. Since this study, several other studies have confirmed a dose–response association between reflux and esophageal adenocarcinoma, but with slightly decreased relative risk [27, 49, 56, 57]. In addition, reflux is strongly associated with the development of Barrett's esophagus, a condition in which the normal esophageal squamous

epithelium is replaced by metaplastic columnar mucosa [58–60]. The mucosal damage inflicted by gastroesophageal acid reflux is postulated to be the inciting factor in this histologic transition [61]. In patients with Barrett's esophagus, the annual rate of progression from non-dysplastic to esophageal adenocarcinoma is 0.5–1% per patient-year [62]. Screening patients for Barrett's esophagus remains controversial, while surveillance of these patients is indicated at intervals determined by the degree of dysplasia [63, 64].

Achalasia is an esophageal motility disorder in which there is loss of the lower esophageal sphincter relaxation and aperistalsis in the distal esophagus. Several studies have shown up to a 10-fold increased risk of both esophageal squamous cell cancer and adenocarcinoma in patients with achalasia [65–68]. Tylosis is an autosomal dominantly inherited disorder with a genetic defect in the 17q25 region that leads to hyperkeratosis of the palms and soles. Patients with tylosis have an increased risk of esophageal squamous cell carcinoma by the age of 65 years [69]. Plummer–Vinson syndrome which is characterized by dysphagia, iron-deficiency anemia, and esophageal webs, and chronic strictures from acid or lye ingestion have also been associated with an increased risk of esophageal cancer [70, 71]. In addition, patients with oral and oropharyngeal squamous cell cancer have been shown to have synchronous and metachronous squamous cell cancer of the esophagus [72, 73]. Screening endoscopy is recommended in these patients.

Clinical presentation and diagnosis

Unfortunately, despite screening in endemic areas of high-risk individuals and surveillance programs for patients with Barrett's esophagus, the majority of patients newly diagnosed with esophageal cancer present late in the course of their disease. Usually, it is not until the tumor is large enough to cause a mechanical obstruction that symptoms such as dysphagia, anorexia, and weight loss develop. Additional signs and symptoms include anemia, gastrointestinal bleeding, gastroesophageal reflux, nausea, vomiting, odynophagia, and chest pain. Cough and recurrent pneumonia may indicate an esophagopulmonary fistula or recurrent aspiration. Hoarseness may indicate involvement of the recurrent laryngeal nerve. Bony pain may signal the development of bone metastases.

At presentation, a thorough history, including assessment of risk factors such as reflux duration and severity, and tobacco and alcohol use should be performed. Physical examination may provide additional clues if lymphadenopathy, hepatomegaly, or cachexia is noted. Laboratory analysis may reveal an iron-deficiency anemia and hypoalbuminemia. Endoscopy is the mainstay in the diagnosis of esophageal cancer. It allows direct visualization of the tumor, as well as an opportunity to perform tissue biopsy for diagnosis. Early lesions may appear as a superficial ulcer, while

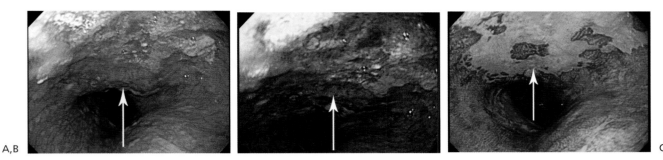

Figure 34.1 Endoscopic examination of a squamous cell carcinoma. (A) View of a squamous cell carcinoma with white light endoscopy (arrow indicates lesion). (B) Narrow-band imaging view of the same squamous cell carcinoma (arrow indicates lesion). (C) View of the same squamous cell carcinoma with Lugol's solution (arrow indicates lesion).

advanced lesions may appear friable, polypoid, exophytic, ulcerated, and stenotic. Biopsies are essential and at least six should be obtained from both the center and the edges of the tumor [74]. In the case of a tight stricture, the endoscopist should consider using a smaller diameter endoscope [75].

Chromoendoscopy with Lugol's solution and toluidine blue have been found to be useful in the detection of early squamous cell carcinomas of the esophagus [76]. Lugol's solution has an affinity for glycogen and the malignant cells in squamous cell cancer are depleted of glycogen, which results in an absence of staining seen on endoscopy [77] (Figure 34.1). On the other hand, toluidine blue stains cell nuclei and therefore malignant cells with increased mitotic activity will avidly absorb the dye, resulting in a blue discoloration [78]. Methylene blue has been studied in the detection of Barrett's esophagus; however, there is not enough evidence to support its use [79]. Narrow-band imaging (NBI) enhances the imaging of mucosal and glandular changes and the visualization of abnormal vascular patterns without using dyes. Optical filters can be enabled or disabled during endoscopy and allow limited wavelengths of light, specifically blue light at 390–445-nm bandwith and green light at 530–550-nm bandwith. These wavelengths can only penetrate superficially and therefore enhance the visualization of the superficial mucosal layer [80]. It has shown promising results in the detection of dysplasia in Barrett's esophagus, but classifications of patterns seen with NBI have not yet been standardized, therefore limiting its use in clinical practice. Further promising new imaging techniques, such as confocal laser endomicroscopy, optical coherence tomography, and light scattering spectroscopy, are still under investigation.

Staging of esophageal cancer

Accurate staging of esophageal cancer remains crucial in determining prognosis and guiding individual therapy. Prognosis of individuals with advanced stage and distant lymph node metastases have far lower rates of survival compared to patients without distant metastases or regional lymph node metastases [81–87]. Therefore, accurate staging will assist in identifying those patients in whom surgery would not be indicated and who should receive palliative treatment. Esophageal cancer is staged according to the American Joint Commission for Cancer (AJCC)/Union for International Cancer Control (UICC) TNM classification system, where T refers to depth of tumor invasion, N to the presence or absence of regional lymph node metastases, and M to the presence or absence of distant metastases (Tables 34.2 and 34.3). The most recent edition of this has undergone changes, including the addition of histologic grade to the staging system to more accurately prognosticate survival [88]. Endoscopy alone has previously been shown to provide some indirect information regarding the stage of esophageal cancer. Several studies found that tumors greater than 5 cm in length and with malignant stenoses were very likely to be a T3 or T4 lesion [89–91]. In addition, patients with T3 tumors were more likely to have regional lymph node metastases [92].

Presently, the most commonly used imaging modalities for staging esophageal cancer include computed tomography (CT), endoscopic ultrasound, and [^{18}F]fluoro-2-deoxy-D-glucose positron emission tomography (FDG-PET). The aim of the initial staging work-up is to determine any distal metastatic disease. Therefore, a CT scan of the chest and abdomen is usually the initial test in assessing metastasis or invasion of other organs [93]. Endoscopic ultrasound (EUS) is employed to determine the depth of tumor invasion and the presence of malignant regional and celiac lymph nodes. EUS accuracy for T staging is about 90% [94]. Early T1 esophageal cancers are usually seen on endoscopy as small mucosal defects or nodules. Using EUS, T1 tumors are localized either to the lamina propria (T1a) or submucosa (T1b) (Figure 34.2). T2 tumors involve the muscularis propria, but do not invade through the wall of the esophagus, while T3 and T4 tumors are extraesophageal (Figure 34.3). Lymph node involvement is designated as N0, no involvement, or N1, for an involved lymph node. EUS features that are

Table 34.2 Staging of esophageal cancer (reproduced courtesy of the American Joint Committee on Cancer (AJCC) [88], with permission).

Stage	Anatomic stage/prognostic groups				
	T	N	M	Grade	Tumor location**
*Squamous cell carcinoma**					
0	Tis (HGD)	N0	M0	1, X	Any
IA	T1	N0	M0	1, X	Any
IB	T1	N0	M0	2–3	Any
	T2–3	N0	M0	1, X	Lower, X
IIA	T2–3	N0	M0	1, X	Upper, middle
	T2–3	N0	M0	2–3	Lower, X
IIB	T2–3	N0	M0	2–3	Upper, middle
	T1–2	N1	M0	Any	Any
IIIA	T1–2	N2	M0	Any	Any
	T3	N1	M0	Any	Any
	T4a	N0	M0	Any	Any
IIIB	T3	N2	M0	Any	Any
IIIC	T4a	N1-2	M0	Any	Any
	T4b	Any	M0	Any	Any
	Any	N3	M0	Any	Any
IV	Any	Any	M1	Any	Any
Adenocarcinoma	T	N	M	Grade	
0	Tis (HGD)	N0	M0	1,X	
IA	T1	N0	M0	1–2, X	
IB	T1	N0	M0	3	
	T2	N0	M0	1–2, X	
IIA	T2	N0	M0	3	
IIB	T3	N0	M0	Any	
	T1–2	N1	M0	Any	
IIIA	T1–2	N2	M0	Any	
	T3	N1	M0	Any	
	T4a	N0	M0	Any	
IIIB	T3	N2	M0	Any	
IIIC	T4a	N1–2	M0	Any	
	T4b	Any	M0	Any	
	Any	N3	M0	Any	
IV	Any	Any	M1	Any	

*Or mixed histology including a squamous component or not otherwise specified (NOS).
**Location of the primary cancer site is defined by the position of the upper (proximal) edge of the tumor in the esophagus.

Table 34.3 Histologic grading of esophageal cancer (reproduced courtesy of the American Joint Committee on Cancer (AJCC) [88], with permission).

Gx	Grade cannot be assessed—stage grouping as G1
G1	Well differentiated
G2	Moderately differentiated
G3	Poorly differentiated
G4	Undifferentiated—stage grouping as G3 squamous

suggestive of lymph node involvement with malignancy include a hypoechoic structure, sharply demarcated borders, rounded contour, and size greater than 1 cm [95]. The presence of these four features allows 100% accuracy in the detection of malignancy. However, the presence of all four features is usually only seen in about 25% of cases, making it difficult to accurately assess the remaining cases. The addition of fine needle aspiration (FNA) to EUS has increased the accuracy of nodal staging. EUS–FNA staging of lymph

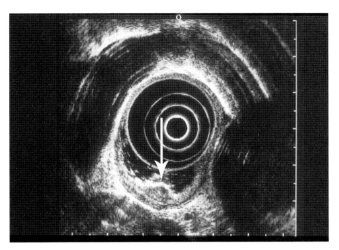

Figure 34.2 Endoscopic ultrasound examination demonstrates a T1N0 lesion (arrow indicates lesion).

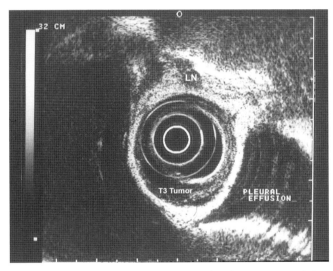

Figure 34.3 Endoscopic ultrasound examination demonstrates a T3N1 lesion and a pleural effusion is identified suggesting M1 disease.

nodes has a reported sensitivity and specificity of 80–90% [96–98]. A limitation to this test is a scenario in which the needle would have to traverse the primary tumor to reach the lymph node and could therefore yield a false-positive result. However, whenever feasible, the endosonographer should incorporate FNA into the EUS [99].

Malignant stenoses, which occur in about 30% of cases, pose a challenge when attempting to perform EUS staging. As previously mentioned, most patients who present with a malignant stenosis have stage III–IV disease. In 1997, Hiele *et al.* found that patients with a non-traversable stricture had a median survival of about 10 months, while those patients with traversable strictures had a median survival of about 20 months [100]. Failure to traverse a stricture is associated

with decreased accuracy of EUS staging. Early studies that assessed dilation of malignant esophageal strictures prior to EUS had rates of perforation as high as 24% [90]. Wallace *et al.* performed dilations in 42 patients prior to EUS staging and found that dilation to 14–16 mm allowed for successful completion of 87% of procedures compared to 36% completion with dilation less than 14 mm. In addition, 19% of patients with malignant strictures had advanced disease that was detected as a result of dilation [101]. There were no perforations in their study. Furthermore, in a recent multicenter retrospective review of 272 EUS cases, dilations were performed with through the scope balloons in 73 cases with two perforations, one of which occurred without dilation [102]. An alternative method of traversing a malignant stricture is to use small radial mini-probes that can be passed through the biopsy channel of an endoscope. However, these instruments are limited in that they are incapable of performing FNA and have a limited depth of penetration [103].

FDG-PET and CT are more commonly used to assess for the presence of malignant lymph nodes and distant metastases. A study evaluating 75 patients with newly diagnosed esophageal cancer with PET, CT, and EUS found that, while EUS was superior over PET and CT at local tumor staging, CT and PET had better sensitivity and specificity than EUS in detecting distant metastases [104]. Furthermore, the results of a meta-analysis aimed at comparing the diagnostic performance of EUS, CT, and FDG-PET suggest that each modality may have a distinctive role in the detection of metastases [105]. For regional lymph node metastases, random effects pooled sensitivities of EUS, CT, and FDG-PET were 0.80 (95% CI 0.75–0.84), 0.50 (0.41–0.60), and 0.57 (0.43–0.70), respectively, and specificities were 0.70 (0.65–0.75), 0.83 (0.77–0.89), and 0.85 (0.76–0.95), respectively. For detection of celiac lymph node metastases by EUS, sensitivity and specificity were 0.85 (0.72–0.99) and 0.96 (0.92–1.00), respectively. For abdominal lymph node metastases by CT, sensitivity and specificity were 0.42 (0.29–0.54) and 0.93 (0.86–1.00), respectively. For distant metastases, sensitivity and specificity were 0.71 (0.62–0.79) and 0.93 (0.89–0.97) for FDG-PET and 0.52 (0.33–0.71) and 0.91 (0.86–0.96) for CT, respectively. Diagnostic performance of FDG-PET for distant metastases was significantly higher than that of CT, which was not significantly affected by study and patient characteristics. Integrated PET–CT has an advantage over PET alone due to improvement in spatial resolution. This imaging modality allows the metabolic information obtained by PET to be localized to the anatomic CT images. Data are still emerging regarding the role of PET–CT in the staging evaluation of esophageal cancer; however, because of its improved spatial resolution, many centers now prefer PET–CT to PET alone.

Endoscopic ultrasound restaging after chemoradiotherapy

The value of EUS in assessing response to chemoradiation therapy is less well-defined than its role in the initial staging of disease. Isenberg *et al.* found that EUS T staging accuracy after chemoradiation was only 43% and that reduction in maximal cross-sectional area of tumor appeared to be a more useful measure for assessing response to neoadjuvant therapy [106]. This decrease in sensitivity is thought to be due to inflammation and fibrosis that distort the intrawall layers of the esophagus and cause artifact on EUS. In a study of 83 patients with locoregional esophageal adenocarcinoma who were treated with chemoradiation and surgical resection, EUS did not retain its usefulness as a restaging modality [107]. The sensitivities of EUS for the individual T classifications were 0% for T0 tumors, 19% for T1 tumors, 27% for T2 tumors, 52% for T3 tumors, and 0% for T4 tumors. In 42 of 83 patients, the tumor classification was over-classified and 15 of 83 were under-classified. The sensitivity of EUS for N classification was 48% for N0 disease and 52% for N1 disease. Furthermore, patients with residual cancer in lymph nodes after preoperative chemoradiation have been shown to have a significantly lower survival rate than patients with no residual tumor in lymph nodes [108]. The authors concluded that EUS-guided FNA may be helpful in identifying residual tumor in lymph nodes and to select patients who benefit maximally from surgery. Further studies are needed to demonstrate a benefit of EUS for this indication.

Endoscopic treatment of esophageal cancer

Historically, esophagectomy was the mainstay in the treatment of superficial esophageal cancer (T0, Tis, or T1a) with high cure rates, but at the cost of significant morbidity and mortality. Endoscopic therapy has aimed at providing a cure, while preserving the patient's esophagus. The most important prognostic factor in determining candidacy for

endoscopic treatment is the determination of submucosal invasion, or T1b disease. A more comprehensive subclassification scheme to determine prognosis has been published that divides mucosa tumors into three types (M1, M2, M3) depending on depth of invasion, as well as a classification based on invasion into the submucosa (SM1, SM2, SM3) (Table 34.4) [109, 110]. Tumors confined to the epithelial layer or lamina propria are not associated with lymph node metastases, while tumors invading into but not through the muscularis mucosa have a risk of nodal metastasis of 8% [109]. All submucosal tumors have an increased risk of lymph node metastasis [111–115]. Therefore, patients with disease limited to the epithelium and lamina propria should be the only ones considered for endoscopic therapy. Tumor histology may also play an important role given that well-differentiated tumors are usually limited to the mucosa (92.7 %), in contrast to moderately and poorly differentiated carcinomas (73.7 % and 22.7 %, respectively) [116].

Endoscopic mucosal resection (EMR) excises the neoplastic epithelium and allows for a definitive histologic diagnosis (Figure 34.4). A large prospective study investigating the

Table 34.4 Subclassification of T1 esophageal cancers.

Tis	M1: Limited to epithelial layer
T1a	M2: Invades the lamina propria
	M3: Invades into but not through the muscularis mucosa
T1b	SM1: Penetrates the shallowest one-third of the submucosa
	SM2: Penetrates the intermediate one-third of the submucosa
	SM3: Penetrates the deepest one-third of the submucosa

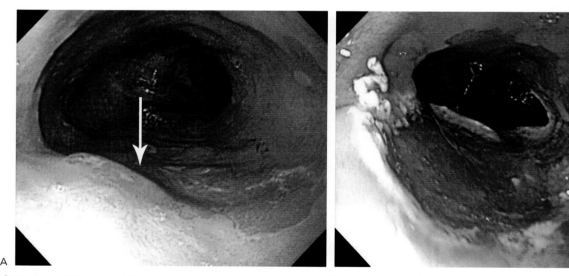

Figure 34.4 Endoscopic examination in a patient with long-segment Barrett's esophagus. (A) On white light examination, a slightly raised nodular lesion (arrow) is seen in a long segment of Barrett's esophagus. (B) Endoscopic mucosal resection of nodular lesion was performed. Pathologic examination demonstrated an intramucosal adenocarcinoma.

efficacy and safety of endoscopic mucosal resection in 486 patients with Barrett's esophagus, 61 with high-grade intraepithelial neoplasia and 288 with mucosal adenocarcinoma, has shown that endoscopic therapy was highly effective and safe, with an excellent long-term survival rate [117]. Endoscopic resection was performed in 279 patients, photodynamic therapy (PDT) in 55, EMR/PDT in 13, and two patients received argon plasma coagulation. Complete response (CR) was achieved in 96.6% and surgery was necessary in 3.7% after endoscopic therapy failed. Metachronous lesions developed during the follow-up in 21.5% of the patients, but none died of esophageal cancer. The calculated 5-year survival rate was 84%. Randomized trials comparing EMR versus esophagectomy are lacking, but the available evidence from retrospective reviews has shown that the success rate of EMR is comparable to surgical resection [118, 119]. Potential EMR complications include bleeding and perforation. EMR specimen resection size is limited to about 2 cm. Endoscopic submucosal dissection (ESD) is a novel technique that allows *en-bloc* tissue resection regardless of size. Data are emerging regarding the role of ESD in the treatment of superficial esophageal cancer.

In patients with Barrett's esophagus, ablative therapies are recommended to eliminate all malignant potential after EMR. PDT and argon plasma coagulation have been used for this purpose, but both have had high rates of recurrent neoplasia, residual intestinal metaplasia, and stenosis [120, 121]. In addition, PDT is associated with a significant photosensitivity. Two newer modalities that appear very promising include radiofrequency ablation and cryotherapy.

The treatment of lesions that are T1b or greater is beyond the scope of this chapter. However, these patients benefit from a multidisciplinary team approach that includes a medical oncologist, radiation-oncologist, thoracic surgeon, in addition to a gastroenterologist. Treatment will depend on a patient's medical comorbidities to determine if they are able to tolerate chemoradiation therapy and/or surgery.

Palliation of unresectable esophageal cancer

In patients who need palliation of dysphagia, there are several treatment options, including dilation, laser therapy, injection therapy, PDT, and stenting. The modality of choice depends on the individual clinical scenario. Esophageal dilation with through the scope balloons or wire-guided bougies can provide temporary relief of dysphagia and have a low rate of perforation; however, repeat dilations are usually required [122, 123]. Laser therapy with neodymium–yttrium–aluminum–garnet (Nd:YAG) has been used for palliative treatment for esophageal cancer. In a study assessing Nd:YAG laser therapy in patients with advanced esophageal cancer, about 70% of patients treated with laser therapy had a functional success with the ability to ingest all necessary calories and leave the hospital for home. Limitations to laser therapy include the need for repeat sessions, high cost, and

high risk of perforation [124, 125]. PDT uses a photosensitizing agent that has an affinity for malignant tissue in combination with a low-power laser. When the laser treatment is applied, ischemic damage occurs to the malignant tissue. Studies have found PDT to be comparable or superior to Nd:YAG laser therapy; however, its significant photosensitivity is a limitation [126].

Placing self-expandable metal stents (SEMS) for palliation of malignant esophageal strictures has become standard of care (Figure 34.5). Covered SEMS are replacing uncovered SEMS in the treatment of malignant strictures. Covered SEMS have become particularly useful in the management of esophagopulmonary fistulae [127]. Uncovered SEMS led to problems of tumor ingrowth and recurrent dysphagia. In addition to tumor ingrowth, potential complications of using SEMS include stent migration, chest pain, reflux (in stents placed at the gastroesophageal junction), perforation, fistula development, intestinal obstruction after migration, hemorrhage, and stent fracture [128]. Removable stents are also becoming available and may play a role in relieving dysphagia in operative candidates. SEMS are typically placed with endoscopic or fluoroscopic guidance or both. Dilation prior to stent placement may be necessary in some cases.

Other malignancies of the esophagus

Other esophageal malignancies are rare. Metastatic disease from breast cancer and melanoma may be found in the esophagus. Hodgkin's and non-Hodgkin's lymphoma can also involve the esophagus. Reports of other rare tumors include adenoid cystic carcinoma, solitary plasmacytoma, sarcoma, and small cell carcinoma.

Conclusions

The epidemiology of esophageal cancer has changed significantly over the last 30 years with adenocarcinoma becoming much more common than squamous cell carcinoma in the Western world. At presentation, most cases are already advanced. Risk factors can be gleaned from a patient's history. Endoscopy remains a cornerstone in the diagnosis, while endoscopic ultrasound aids in staging and guiding individual therapy. Endoscopic treatment of early esophageal cancers has progressed with EMR and the development of ESD. For patients with unresectable cancer, palliation with various endoscopic treatments and SEMS is available.

Benign tumors of the esophagus:

Benign esophageal tumors are rare (Table 34.5). They are usually asymptomatic and discovered incidentally on endoscopy for evaluation for an unrelated problem. Their premalignant potential is usually very low. This section focuses on the clinical presentation, diagnosis, histopathology and

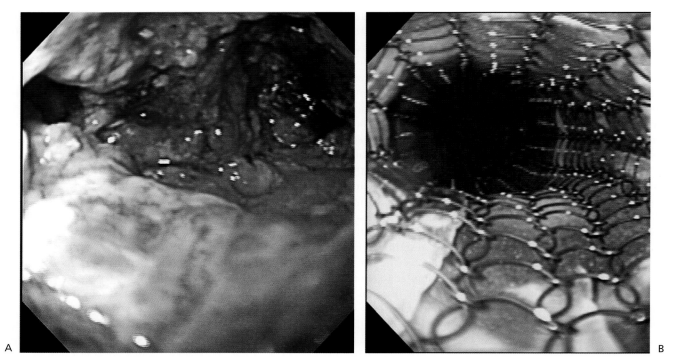

Figure 34.5 Endoscopic examination in a patient with dysphagia and weight loss. (A) Endoscopy demonstrates an obstructing lesion; biopsies confirmed this to be a squamous cell carcinoma. (B) Self-expanding metal stent placement in obstructing squamous cell carcinoma.

Table 34.5 Common benign esophageal tumors.

Tumor type	Treatment
Fibrovascular polyps	Observation; endoscopic resection or surgery for symptomatic polyps
Granular cell tumors	Endoscopic resection due to malignant potential
Papillomas	Observation; endoscopic resection if symptomatic
Leiomyomas	Expectant management with endoscopic ultrasound q 1–2 years; surgery with unremitting symptoms, tumor growth or ulceration

management of some of the more common benign esophageal neoplasms.

Fibrovascular polyps

These lesions are rare, accounting for about 0.5–1% of all benign esophageal lesions. They are commonly found in the proximal esophagus and usually attach at the inferior aspect of the cricopharyngeus. They are generally asymptomatic, but can undergo traction and elongation as a result of peristalsis. Patients with large lesions can experience dysphagia, chronic cough, nausea and vomiting. The fibrovascular polyp contains a mixture of fibrous, vascular, and adipose tissue covered by squamous epithelium. About 75% of cases have been reported in men in their 50s and 60s [129].

Symptomatic polyps should be resected. Endoscopic resection using a snare and EUS has been reported [129]. EUS is utilized to exclude the presence of a large vessel in the stalk of the polyp. Surgical resection may be required if there is a feeding vessel.

Granular cell tumors

Granular cell tumors represent about 1% of benign esophageal tumors. About 60% of cases have been reported in men with a mean age of diagnosis of 45 years [130]. About one-third of patients will report dysphagia with the remainder being asymptomatic. These lesions appear pale and have normal overlying mucosa, but are firm to the touch with a forceps (Figure 34.6). Biopsy forceps can be used to make a diagnosis. On histologic examination, these lesions are comprised of nests of cells with eosinophilic granules and stain positive for S-100 protein [131, 132]. Although low, granular cell tumors do have malignant potential. This is most commonly seen in large tumors (>4 cm) or those that exhibit growth [130]. Therefore these tumors should undergo endoscopic resection.

Papillomas

These are usually small, less than 1 cm, whitish-pink, wart-like exophytic projections and are found in the distal

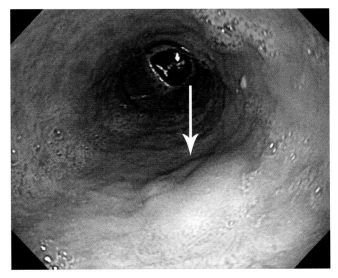

Figure 34.6 Granular cell tumor (arrow indicates lesion).

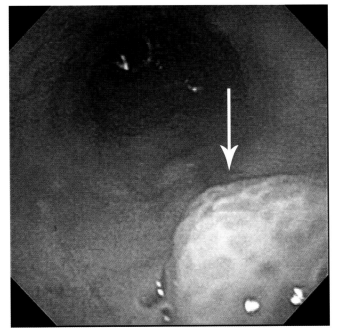

Figure 34.7 Squamous papilloma (arrow indicates lesion).

esophagus (Figure 34.7). The majority are solitary, but patients have been described with more than 10 lesions [133]. Patients are usually asymptomatic, although large lesions can cause dysphagia. The pathogenesis of papillomas remains controversial. Some investigators have found them to be a result of inflammation in the distal esophagus, such as reflux or other mucosal irritants, and others have documented HPV in papillomas [134, 135]. Histologically, they

are finger-like projections of connective tissue covered with hyperplastic squamous epithelium. Asymptomatic lesions can be observed. However, large lesions may need to be removed endoscopically, with endoscopic mucosal resection [133].

Esophageal leiomyomas

Leiomyomas are the most common benign tumor of the esophagus and account for about two-thirds of all benign esophageal tumors. The incidence of leiomyoma reported in autopsy series ranged from 0.005% to 5.1% [136, 137]. They can occur at any age, but the peak incidence is in the third to fifth decades and they occur most commonly in men.

Leiomyomas can occur in all parts of the esophagus, but are most common in the distal third of the esophagus. About 80% are located intramurally, originating in the muscularis propria. Up to 13% of these intramural lesions can have annular morphology [138]. Leiomyomas are very slow growing tumors and the majority, 93%, are less than 15 cm in size. There has been no correlation found between symptoms and size of the tumor. Dysphagia is the most common symptoms, but patients may also report retrosternal pain. On endoscopy, the tumor may project into the lumen, is freely movable, and has normal and intact overlying mucosa. Endoscopic biopsy is contraindicated as this can risk secondary infection, bleeding, and perforation [139]. EUS is helpful in determining the layer of origin, and the addition of FNA can obtain cytology to confirm the diagnosis. On histology, these tumors have low cellularity, and are comprised of interlacing bundles of smooth muscle cells with absent mitoses. Immunohistochemical staining will demonstrate positivity for desmin and smooth muscle actin. They will stain negative for CD34 and CD117, thereby distinguishing a leiomyoma from a gastrointestinal stromal tumor [139]. The risk of malignant transformation of these tumors is incredibly low, with very few case reports in the literature of transformation to leiomyosarcomas. In addition, as they are very slow growing tumors, in asymptomatic individuals expectant management with EUS every 1–2 years is recommended. Surgery is reserved for symptomatic patients with unremitting symptoms or a progressive increase in tumor size and ulceration of the tumor.

Other benign esophageal lesions

On endoscopy, other commonly encountered esophageal lesions include glycogen acanthoses, which appear as uniformly round elevations in the mucosa and have hyperplastic squamous epithelium with abundant intracellular glycogen on histology. Inlet patches are usually found in the upper esophagus and appear as a discrete patch of mucosa that has a similar appearance to gastric mucosa. Esophageal lipomas will appear pale or yellow with normal overlying mucosa. When probed with biopsy forceps, they will create an indentation often known as the "pillow sign." On EUS, these lesions are seen arising from the submucosa. Hemangiomas will have a blue–purple hue and, if large, can appear cystic.

Conclusions

Benign esophageal tumors are rare. The majority of these lesions have no malignant potential and can be observed in asymptomatic patients. EUS can assist in establishing the nature of these lesions by determining the originating gastrointestinal tract layer. Furthermore, the sonographic characteristics of the lesion can aid in an accurate diagnosis.

References

1. Parkin DM, Bray F, Ferlay J, Pisani P. Global cancer statistics, 2002. *CA Cancer J Clin* 2005;55:74–108.

2. Jemal A, Siegel R, Ward E, Hao Y, Xu J, Thun MJ. Cancer statistics, 2009. *CA Cancer J Clin* 2009;59:225–249.

3. Umar SB, Fleischer DE. Esophageal cancer: epidemiology, pathogenesis and prevention. *Nat Clin Pract Gastroenterol Hepatol* 2008;5:517–526.

4. Hongo M, Nagasaki Y, Shoji T. Epidemiology of esophageal cancer: Orient to Occident. Effects of chronology, geography and ethnicity. *J Gastroenterol Hepatol* 2009;24:729–735.

5. Blot WJ, Devesa SS, Kneller RW, Fraumeni JF Jr. Rising incidence of adenocarcinoma of the esophagus and gastric cardia. *JAMA* 1991;265:1287–1289.

6. Pera M, Cameron AJ, Trastek VF, Carpenter HA, Zinsmeister AR. Increasing incidence of adenocarcinoma of the esophagus and esophagogastric junction. *Gastroenterology* 1993;104:510–513.

7. Devesa SS, Blot WJ, Fraumeni JF Jr. Changing patterns in the incidence of esophageal and gastric carcinoma in the United States. *Cancer* 1998;83:2049–2053.

8. Baquet CR, Commiskey P, Mack K, Meltzer S, Mishra SI. Esophageal cancer epidemiology in blacks and whites: racial and gender disparities in incidence, mortality, survival rates and histology. *J Natl Med Assoc* 2005;97:1471–1478.

9. Greenstein AJ, Litle VR, Swanson SJ, *et al.* Racial disparities in esophageal cancer treatment and outcomes. *Ann Surg Oncol* 2008;15:881–888.

10. Trivers KF, Sabatino SA, Stewart SL. Trends in esophageal cancer incidence by histology, United States, 1998-2003. *Int J Cancer* 2008;123:1422–1428.

11. Doll R, Peto R, Wheatley K, Gray R, Sutherland I. Mortality in relation to smoking: 40 years' observations on male British doctors. *Br Med J* 1994;309:901–911.

12. Carstensen JM, Pershagen G, Eklund G. Mortality in relation to cigarette and pipe smoking: 16 years' observation of 25 000 Swedish men. *J Epidemiol Community Health* 1987;41:166–172.

13. McLaughlin JK, Hrubec Z, Blot WJ, Fraumeni JF Jr. Smoking and cancer mortality among U.S. veterans: a 26-year follow-up. *Int J Cancer* 1995;60:190–193.

14. Ishikawa A, Kuriyama S, Tsubono Y, *et al.* Smoking, alcohol drinking, green tea consumption and the risk of esophageal cancer in Japanese men. *J Epidemiol* 2006;16:185–192.

15. Freedman ND, Abnet CC, Leitzmann MF, *et al.* A prospective study of tobacco, alcohol, and the risk of esophageal and gastric cancer subtypes. *Am J Epidemiol* 2007;165:1424–1433.

16. Tran GD, Sun XD, Abnet CC, *et al.* Prospective study of risk factors for esophageal and gastric cancers in the Linxian general population trial cohort in China. *Int J Cancer* 2005;113:456–463.

17. Nasrollahzadeh D, Kamangar F, Aghcheli K, *et al.* Opium, tobacco, and alcohol use in relation to oesophageal squamous cell carcinoma in a high-risk area of Iran. *Br J Cancer* 2008;98:1857–1863.

18. Cook-Mozaffari PJ, Azordegan F, Day NE, Ressicaud A, Sabai C, Aramesh B. Oesophageal cancer studies in the Caspian Littoral of Iran: results of a case-control study. *Br J Cancer* 1979;39:293–309.

19. Brown LM, Silverman DT, Pottern LM, *et al.* Adenocarcinoma of the esophagus and esophagogastric junction in white men in the United States: alcohol, tobacco, and socioeconomic factors. *Cancer Causes Control* 1994;5:333–340.

20. Vaughan TL, Davis S, Kristal A, Thomas DB. Obesity, alcohol, and tobacco as risk factors for cancers of the esophagus and gastric cardia: adenocarcinoma versus squamous cell carcinoma. *Cancer Epidemiol Biomarkers Prev* 1995;4:85–92.

21. Gammon MD, Schoenberg JB, Ahsan H, *et al.* Tobacco, alcohol, and socioeconomic status and adenocarcinomas of the esophagus and gastric cardia. *J Natl Cancer Inst* 1997;89:1277–1284.

22. Lagergren J, Bergstrom R, Lindgren A, Nyren O. The role of tobacco, snuff and alcohol use in the aetiology of cancer of the oesophagus and gastric cardia. *Int J Cancer* 2000;85:340–346.

23. Cheng KK, Sharp L, McKinney PA, *et al.* A case-control study of oesophageal adenocarcinoma in women: a preventable disease. *Br J Cancer* 2000;83:127–132.

24. Wu AH, Wan P, Bernstein L. A multiethnic population-based study of smoking, alcohol and body size and risk of adenocarcinomas of the stomach and esophagus (United States). *Cancer Causes Control* 2001;12:721–732.

25. Chen H, Ward MH, Graubard BI, *et al.* Dietary patterns and adenocarcinoma of the esophagus and distal stomach. *Am J Clin Nutr* 2002;75:137–144.

26. Veugelers PJ, Porter GA, Guernsey DL, Casson AG. Obesity and lifestyle risk factors for gastroesophageal reflux disease, Barrett esophagus and esophageal adenocarcinoma. *Dis Esophagus* 2006;19:321–328.

27. Whiteman DC, Sadeghi S, Pandeya N, *et al.* Combined effects of obesity, acid reflux and smoking on the risk of adenocarcinomas of the oesophagus. *Gut* 2008;57:173–180.

28. Boffetta P, Garfinkel L. Alcohol drinking and mortality among men enrolled in an American Cancer Society prospective study. *Epidemiology* 1990;1:342–348.

29. Brown LM, Hoover RN, Greenberg RS, *et al.* Are racial differences in squamous cell esophageal cancer explained by alcohol and tobacco use? *J Natl Cancer Inst* 1994;86:1340–1345.

30. Brown LM, Hoover R, Silverman D, *et al.* Excess incidence of squamous cell esophageal cancer among US Black men: role of social class and other risk factors. *Am J Epidemiol* 2001;153:114–122.

31. Yokoyama T, Yokoyama A, Kato H, *et al*. Alcohol flushing, alcohol and aldehyde dehydrogenase genotypes, and risk for esophageal squamous cell carcinoma in Japanese men. *Cancer Epidemiol Biomarkers Prev* 2003;12:1227–1233.

32. Brooks PJ, Enoch MA, Goldman D, Li TK, Yokoyama A. The alcohol flushing response: an unrecognized risk factor for esophageal cancer from alcohol consumption. *PLoS Med* 2009;6:e50.

33. Kabat GC, Ng SK, Wynder EL. Tobacco, alcohol intake, and diet in relation to adenocarcinoma of the esophagus and gastric cardia. *Cancer Causes Control* 1993;4:123–132.

34. Wiseman M. The second World Cancer Research Fund/American Institute for Cancer Research expert report. Food, nutrition, physical activity, and the prevention of cancer: a global perspective. *Proc Nutr Soc* 2008;67:253–256.

35. Freedman ND, Park Y, Subar AF, *et al*. Fruit and vegetable intake and esophageal cancer in a large prospective cohort study. *Int J Cancer* 2007;121:2753–2760.

36. Gonzalez CA, Pera G, Agudo A, *et al*. Fruit and vegetable intake and the risk of stomach and oesophagus adenocarcinoma in the European Prospective Investigation into Cancer and Nutrition (EPIC-EURGAST). *Int J Cancer* 2006;118:2559–2566.

37. Jakszyn P, Gonzalez CA. Nitrosamine and related food intake and gastric and oesophageal cancer risk: a systematic review of the epidemiological evidence. *World J Gastroenterol* 2006;12: 4296–4303.

38. Yokoyama A, Omori T. Genetic polymorphisms of alcohol and aldehyde dehydrogenases and risk for esophageal and head and neck cancers. *Alcohol* 2005;35:175–185.

39. Dillner J, Knekt P, Schiller JT, Hakulinen T. Prospective seroepidemiological evidence that human papillomavirus type 16 infection is a risk factor for oesophageal squamous cell carcinoma. *Br Med J* 1995;311:1346.

40. Bjorge T, Dillner J, Anttila T, *et al*. Prospective seroepidemiological study of role of human papillomavirus in non-cervical anogenital cancers. *Br Med J* 1997;315:646–649.

41. Han C, Qiao G, Hubbert NL, *et al*. Serologic association between human papillomavirus type 16 infection and esophageal cancer in Shaanxi Province, China. *J Natl Cancer Inst* 1996;88:1467–1471.

42. Lagergren J, Wang Z, Bergstrom R, Dillner J, Nyren O. Human papillomavirus infection and esophageal cancer: a nationwide seroepidemiologic case-control study in Sweden. *J Natl Cancer Inst* 1999;91:156–162.

43. Van Doornum GJ, Korse CM, Buning-Kager JC, *et al*. Reactivity to human papillomavirus type 16 L1 virus-like particles in sera from patients with genital cancer and patients with carcinomas at five different extragenital sites. *Br J Cancer* 2003;88: 1095–1100.

44. Kamangar F, Qiao YL, Schiller JT, *et al*. Human papillomavirus serology and the risk of esophageal and gastric cancers: results from a cohort in a high-risk region in China. *Int J Cancer* 2006;119:579–584.

45. Gao GF, Roth MJ, Wei WQ, *et al*. No association between HPV infection and the neoplastic progression of esophageal squamous cell carcinoma: result from a cross-sectional study in a high-risk region of China. *Int J Cancer* 2006;119:1354–1359.

46. Islami F, Kamangar F. Helicobacter pylori and esophageal cancer risk: a meta-analysis. *Cancer Prev Res (Phila Pa)* 2008;1:329–338.

47. Rokkas T, Pistiolas D, Sechopoulos P, Robotis I, Margantinis G. Relationship between Helicobacter pylori infection and esophageal neoplasia: a meta-analysis. *Clin Gastroenterol Hepatol* 2007;5:1413–1417, e1–2.

48. Zhuo X, Zhang Y, Wang Y, Zhuo W, Zhu Y, Zhang X. Helicobacter pylori infection and oesophageal cancer risk: association studies via evidence-based meta-analyses. *Clin Oncol (R Coll Radiol)* 2008;20:757–762.

49. Anderson LA, Watson RG, Murphy SJ, *et al*. Risk factors for Barrett's oesophagus and oesophageal adenocarcinoma: results from the FINBAR study. *World J Gastroenterol* 2007;13:1585–1594.

50. Hampel H, Abraham NS, El-Serag HB. Meta-analysis: obesity and the risk for gastroesophageal reflux disease and its complications. *Ann Intern Med* 2005;143:199–211.

51. Kubo A, Corley DA. Body mass index and adenocarcinomas of the esophagus or gastric cardia: a systematic review and meta-analysis. *Cancer Epidemiol Biomarkers Prev* 2006;15: 872–878.

52. Abnet CC, Freedman ND, Hollenbeck AR, Fraumeni JF Jr, Leitzmann M, Schatzkin A. A prospective study of BMI and risk of oesophageal and gastric adenocarcinoma. *Eur J Cancer* 2008;44:465–471.

53. Corley DA, Kubo A, Zhao W. Abdominal obesity and the risk of esophageal and gastric cardia carcinomas. *Cancer Epidemiol Biomarkers Prev* 2008;17:352–358.

54. Corley DA. Obesity and the rising incidence of oesophageal and gastric adenocarcinoma: what is the link? *Gut* 2007;56: 1493–1494.

55. Lagergren J, Bergstrom R, Lindgren A, Nyren O. Symptomatic gastroesophageal reflux as a risk factor for esophageal adenocarcinoma. *N Engl J Med* 1999;340:825–831.

56. Farrow DC, Vaughan TL, Sweeney C, *et al*. Gastroesophageal reflux disease, use of H2 receptor antagonists, and risk of esophageal and gastric cancer. *Cancer Causes Control* 2000;11: 231–238.

57. Wu AH, Tseng CC, Bernstein L. Hiatal hernia, reflux symptoms, body size, and risk of esophageal and gastric adenocarcinoma. *Cancer* 2003;98:940–948.

58. Lieberman DA, Oehlke M, Helfand M. Risk factors for Barrett's esophagus in community-based practice. GORGE consortium. Gastroenterology Outcomes Research Group in Endoscopy. *Am J Gastroenterol* 1997;92:1293–1297.

59. Enzinger PC, Mayer RJ. Esophageal cancer. *N Engl J Med* 2003;349:2241–2252.

60. Sharma P. Clinical practice. Barrett's esophagus. *N Engl J Med* 2009;361:2548–2556.

61. Spechler SJ. Clinical practice. Barrett's esophagus. *N Engl J Med* 2002;346:836–842.

62. Shaheen N, Ransohoff DF. Gastroesophageal reflux, barrett esophagus, and esophageal cancer: scientific review. *JAMA* 2002;287:1972–1981.

63. Wang KK, Wongkeesong M, Buttar NS. American Gastroenterological Association technical review on the role of the gastroenterologist in the management of esophageal carcinoma. *Gastroenterology* 2005;128:1471–1505.

64. Hirota WK, Zuckerman MJ, Adler DG, *et al*. ASGE guideline: the role of endoscopy in the surveillance of premalignant conditions of the upper GI tract. *Gastrointest Endosc* 2006;63: 570–580.

65. Wychulis AR, Woolam GL, Andersen HA, Ellis FH Jr. Achalasia and carcinoma of the esophagus. *JAMA* 1971;215:1638–1641.

66. Meijssen MA, Tilanus HW, van Blankenstein M, Hop WC, Ong GL. Achalasia complicated by oesophageal squamous cell carcinoma: a prospective study in 195 patients. *Gut* 1992;33:155–158.

67. Streitz JM, Jr., Ellis FH Jr, Gibb SP, Heatley GM. Achalasia and squamous cell carcinoma of the esophagus: analysis of 241 patients. *Ann Thorac Surg* 1995;59:1604–1609.

68. Zendehdel K, Nyren O, Edberg A, Ye W. Risk of esophageal adenocarcinoma in achalasia patients, a retrospective cohort study in Sweden. *Am J Gastroenterol* 2011;106:57–61.

69. Iwaya T, Maesawa C, Ogasawara S, Tamura G. Tylosis esophageal cancer locus on chromosome 17q25.1 is commonly deleted in sporadic human esophageal cancer. *Gastroenterology* 1998;114:1206–1210.

70. Hoffman RM, Jaffe PE. Plummer-Vinson syndrome. A case report and literature review. *Arch Intern Med* 1995;155:2008–2011.

71. Shimizu M, Ban S, Odze RD. Squamous dysplasia and other precursor lesions related to esophageal squamous cell carcinoma. *Gastroenterol Clin North Am* 2007;36:797–811, v–vi.

72. Ina H, Shibuya H, Ohashi I, Kitagawa M. The frequency of a concomitant early esophageal cancer in male patients with oral and oropharyngeal cancer. Screening results using Lugol dye endoscopy. *Cancer* 1994;73:2038–2041.

73. Muto M, Hironaka S, Nakane M, Boku N, Ohtsu A, Yoshida S. Association of multiple Lugol-voiding lesions with synchronous and metachronous esophageal squamous cell carcinoma in patients with head and neck cancer. *Gastrointest Endosc* 2002;56:517–521.

74. Lal N, Bhasin DK, Malik AK, Gupta NM, Singh K, Mehta SK. Optimal number of biopsy specimens in the diagnosis of carcinoma of the oesophagus. *Gut* 1992;33:724–726.

75. Mulcahy HE, Fairclough PD. Ultrathin endoscopy in the assessment and treatment of upper and lower gastrointestinal tract strictures. *Gastrointest Endosc* 1998;48:618–620.

76. Davila RE. Chromoendoscopy. *Gastrointest Endosc Clin N Am* 2009;19:193–208.

77. Freitag CP, Barros SG, Kruel CD, *et al*. Esophageal dysplasias are detected by endoscopy with Lugol in patients at risk for squamous cell carcinoma in southern Brazil. *Dis Esophagus* 1999;12:191–195.

78. Herlin P, Marnay J, Jacob JH, Ollivier JM, Mandard AM. A study of the mechanism of the toluidine blue dye test. *Endoscopy* 1983;15:4–7.

79. Kaltenbach T, Sano Y, Friedland S, Soetikno R. American Gastroenterological Association (AGA) Institute technology assessment on image-enhanced endoscopy. *Gastroenterology* 2008;134:327–340.

80. Shahid MW, Wallace MB. Endoscopic imaging for the detection of esophageal dysplasia and carcinoma. *Gastrointest Endosc Clin North Am* 2010;20:11–24, v.

81. DeMeester TR. Esophageal carcinoma: current controversies. *Semin Surg Oncol* 1997;13:217–233.

82. Fockens P, Kisman K, Merkus MP, van Lanschot JJ, Obertop H, Tytgat GN. The prognosis of esophageal carcinoma staged irresectable (T4) by endosonography. *J Am Coll Surg* 1998;186: 17–23.

83. Korst RJ, Rusch VW, Venkatraman E, *et al*. Proposed revision of the staging classification for esophageal cancer. *J Thorac Cardiovasc Surg* 1998;115:660–669; discussion 669–670.

84. Berdejo L. Transhiatal versus transthoracic esophagectomy for clinical stage I esophageal carcinoma. *Hepatogastroenterology* 1995;42:789–791.

85. Law SY, Fok M, Wong J. Pattern of recurrence after oesophageal resection for cancer: clinical implications. *Br J Surg* 1996; 83:107–111.

86. Stark SP, Romberg MS, Pierce GE, *et al*. Transhiatal versus transthoracic esophagectomy for adenocarcinoma of the distal esophagus and cardia. *Am J Surg* 1996;172:478–481; discussion 481–482.

87. Pommier RF, Vetto JT, Ferris BL, Wilmarth TJ. Relationships between operative approaches and outcomes in esophageal cancer. *Am J Surg* 1998;175:422–425.

88. Edge SE, Byrd DR, Carducci MA, eds. *AJCC Cancer Staging Manual*, 7th edn. New York: Springer, 2010.

89. Bhutani MS, Barde CJ, Markert RJ, Gopalswamy N. Length of esophageal cancer and degree of luminal stenosis during upper endoscopy predict T stage by endoscopic ultrasound. *Endoscopy* 2002;34:461–463.

90. Van Dam J, Rice TW, Catalano MF, Kirby T, Sivak MV Jr. High-grade malignant stricture is predictive of esophageal tumor stage. Risks of endosonographic evaluation. *Cancer* 1993;71: 2910–2917.

91. Vickers J, Alderson D. Influence of luminal obstruction on oesophageal cancer staging using endoscopic ultrasonography. *Br J Surg* 1998;85:999–1001.

92. Rice TW, Zuccaro G Jr, Adelstein DJ, Rybicki LA, Blackstone EH, Goldblum JR. Esophageal carcinoma: depth of tumor invasion is predictive of regional lymph node status. *Ann Thorac Surg* 1998;65:787–792.

93. Saunders HS, Wolfman NT, Ott DJ. Esophageal cancer. Radiologic staging. *Radiol Clin North Am* 1997;35:281–294.

94. Rosch T. Endosonographic staging of esophageal cancer: a review of literature results. *Gastrointest Endosc Clin N Am* 1995;5:537–547.

95. Catalano MF, Sivak MV Jr, Rice T, Gragg LA, Van Dam J. Endosonographic features predictive of lymph node metastasis. *Gastrointest Endosc* 1994;40:442–446.

96. Giovannini M, Seitz JF, Monges G, Perrier H, Rabbia I. Fine-needle aspiration cytology guided by endoscopic ultrasonography: results in 141 patients. *Endoscopy* 1995;27:171–177.

97. Wiersema MJ, Vilmann P, Giovannini M, Chang KJ, Wiersema LM. Endosonography-guided fine-needle aspiration biopsy: diagnostic accuracy and complication assessment. *Gastroenterology* 1997;112:1087–1095.

98. Vazquez-Sequeiros E, Wiersema MJ, Clain JE, *et al*. Impact of lymph node staging on therapy of esophageal carcinoma. *Gastroenterology* 2003;125:1626–1635.

99. Jacobson BC, Chak A, Hoffman B, *et al*. Quality indicators for endoscopic ultrasonography. *Am J Gastroenterol* 2006;101: 898–901.

100. Hiele M, De Leyn P, Schurmans P, *et al.* Relation between endoscopic ultrasound findings and outcome of patients with tumors of the esophagus or esophagogastric junction. *Gastrointest Endosc* 1997;45:381–386.

101. Wallace MB, Hawes RH, Sahai AV, Van Velse A, Hoffman BJ. Dilation of malignant esophageal stenosis to allow EUS guided fine-needle aspiration: safety and effect on patient management. *Gastrointest Endosc* 2000;51:309–313.

102. Jacobson BC, Shami VM, Faigel DO, *et al.* Through-the-scope balloon dilation for endoscopic ultrasound staging of stenosing esophageal cancer. *Dig Dis Sci* 2007;52:817–822.

103. Hunerbein M, Ghadimi BM, Haensch W, Schlag PM. Transendoscopic ultrasound of esophageal and gastric cancer using miniaturized ultrasound catheter probes. *Gastrointest Endosc* 1998;48:371–375.

104. Lowe VJ, Booya F, Fletcher JG, *et al.* Comparison of positron emission tomography, computed tomography, and endoscopic ultrasound in the initial staging of patients with esophageal cancer. *Mol Imaging Biol* 2005;7:422–430.

105. van Vliet EP, Heijenbrok-Kal MH, Hunink MG, Kuipers EJ, Siersema PD. Staging investigations for oesophageal cancer: a meta-analysis. *Br J Cancer* 2008;98:547–557.

106. Isenberg G, Chak A, Canto MI, *et al.* Endoscopic ultrasound in restaging of esophageal cancer after neoadjuvant chemoradiation. *Gastrointest Endosc* 1998;48:158–163.

107. Kalha I, Kaw M, Fukami N, *et al.* The accuracy of endoscopic ultrasound for restaging esophageal carcinoma after chemoradiation therapy. *Cancer* 2004;101:940–947.

108. Agarwal B, Swisher S, Ajani J, *et al.* Endoscopic ultrasound after preoperative chemoradiation can help identify patients who benefit maximally after surgical esophageal resection. *Am J Gastroenterol* 2004;99:1258–1266.

109. Endo M, Yoshino K, Kawano T, Nagai K, Inoue H. Clinicopathologic analysis of lymph node metastasis in surgically resected superficial cancer of the thoracic esophagus. *Dis Esophagus* 2000;13:125–129.

110. Shimada H, Nabeya Y, Matsubara H, *et al.* Prediction of lymph node status in patients with superficial esophageal carcinoma: analysis of 160 surgically resected cancers. *Am J Surg* 2006;191:250–254.

111. Fujita H, Sueyoshi S, Yamana H, *et al.* Optimum treatment strategy for superficial esophageal cancer: endoscopic mucosal resection versus radical esophagectomy. *World J Surg* 2001;25:424–431.

112. Liu L, Hofstetter WL, Rashid A, *et al.* Significance of the depth of tumor invasion and lymph node metastasis in superficially invasive (T1) esophageal adenocarcinoma. *Am J Surg Pathol* 2005;29:1079–1085.

113. Westerterp M, Koppert LB, Buskens CJ, Tilanus HW, ten Kate FJ, Bergman JJ, et al. Outcome of surgical treatment for early adenocarcinoma of the esophagus or gastro-esophageal junction. *Virchows Arch* 2005;446:497–504.

114. Araki K, Ohno S, Egashira A, Saeki H, Kawaguchi H, Sugimachi K. Pathologic features of superficial esophageal squamous cell carcinoma with lymph node and distal metastasis. *Cancer* 2002;94:570–575.

115. Ancona E, Rampado S, Cassaro M, *et al.* Prediction of lymph node status in superficial esophageal carcinoma. *Ann Surg Oncol* 2008;15:3278–3288.

116. Vieth M, Ell C, Gossner L, May A, Stolte M. Histological analysis of endoscopic resection specimens from 326 patients with Barrett's esophagus and early neoplasia. *Endoscopy* 2004;36:776–781.

117. Pech O, Behrens A, May A, *et al.* Long-term results and risk factor analysis for recurrence after curative endoscopic therapy in 349 patients with high-grade intraepithelial neoplasia and mucosal adenocarcinoma in Barrett's oesophagus. *Gut* 2008;57:1200–1206.

118. Prasad GA, Wu TT, Wigle DA, *et al.* Endoscopic and surgical treatment of mucosal (T1a) esophageal adenocarcinoma in Barrett's esophagus. *Gastroenterology* 2009;137:815–823.

119. Das A, Singh V, Fleischer DE, Sharma VK. A comparison of endoscopic treatment and surgery in early esophageal cancer: an analysis of surveillance epidemiology and end results data. *Am J Gastroenterol* 2008;103:1340–1345.

120. Overholt BF, Panjehpour M, Halberg DL. Photodynamic therapy for Barrett's esophagus with dysplasia and/or early stage carcinoma: long-term results. *Gastrointest Endosc* 2003;58:183–188.

121. Peters F, Kara M, Rosmolen W, *et al.* Poor results of 5-aminolevulinic acid-photodynamic therapy for residual high-grade dysplasia and early cancer in barrett esophagus after endoscopic resection. *Endoscopy* 2005;37:418–424.

122. Boyce HW, Jr. Palliation of Dysphagia of Esophageal Cancer by Endoscopic Lumen Restoration Techniques. *Cancer Control* 1999;6:73–83.

123. Hernandez LV, Jacobson JW, Harris MS. Comparison among the perforation rates of Maloney, balloon, and savary dilation of esophageal strictures. *Gastrointest Endosc* 2000;51:460–462.

124. Mellow MH, Pinkas H. Endoscopic laser therapy for malignancies affecting the esophagus and gastroesophageal junction. Analysis of technical and functional efficacy. *Arch Intern Med* 1985;145:1443–1446.

125. Haddad NG, Fleischer DE. Endoscopic laser therapy for esophageal cancer. *Gastrointest Endosc Clin North Am* 1994;4:863–874.

126. Lightdale CJ, Heier SK, Marcon NE, *et al.* Photodynamic therapy with porfimer sodium versus thermal ablation therapy with Nd:YAG laser for palliation of esophageal cancer: a multicenter randomized trial. *Gastrointest Endosc* 1995;42:507–512.

127. Ross WA, Alkassab F, Lynch PM, *et al.* Evolving role of self-expanding metal stents in the treatment of malignant dysphagia and fistulas. *Gastrointest Endosc* 2007;65:70–76.

128. Simmons DT, Baron TH. Endoluminal palliation. *Gastrointest Endosc Clin North Am* 2005;15:467–484, viii.

129. Avezzano EA, Fleischer DE, Merida MA, Anderson DL. Giant fibrovascular polyps of the esophagus. *Am J Gastroenterol* 1990;85:299–302.

130. Orlowska J, Pachlewski J, Gugulski A, Butruk E. A conservative approach to granular cell tumors of the esophagus: four case reports and literature review. *Am J Gastroenterol* 1993;88:311–315.

131. Brady PG, Nord HJ, Connar RG. Granular cell tumor of the esophagus: natural history, diagnosis, and therapy. *Dig Dis Sci* 1988;33:1329–1333.

132. Stefansson K, Wollmann RL. S-100 protein in granular cell tumors (granular cell myoblastomas). *Cancer* 1982;49:1834–1838.

133. Carr NJ, Monihan JM, Sobin LH. Squamous cell papilloma of the esophagus: a clinicopathologic and follow-up study of 25 cases. *Am J Gastroenterol* 1994;89:245–248.

134. Szanto I, Szentirmay Z, Banai J, *et al*. [Squamous papilloma of the esophagus. Clinical and pathological observations based on 172 papillomas in 155 patients]. *Orv Hetil* 2005;146:547–552.

135. Syrjanen KJ. HPV infections and oesophageal cancer. *J Clin Pathol* 2002;55:721–728.

136. Seremetis MG, Lyons WS, deGuzman VC, Peabody JW, Jr. Leiomyomata of the esophagus. An analysis of 838 cases. *Cancer* 1976;38:2166–2177.

137. Postlethwait RW, Musser AW. Changes in the esophagus in 1,000 autopsy specimens. *J Thorac Cardiovasc Surg* 1974;68: 953–956.

138. Hatch GF 3rd, Wertheimer-Hatch L, Hatch KF, *et al*. Tumors of the esophagus. *World J Surg* 2000;24:401–411.

139. Lee LS, Singhal S, Brinster CJ, *et al*. Current management of esophageal leiomyoma. *J Am Coll Surg* 2004;198:136–146.

35 Surgery for Cancer of the Esophagus and Gastroesophageal Junction

Thomas W. Rice

Department of Thoracic and Cardiovascular Surgery, Cleveland Clinic, Cleveland, OH, USA

Introduction

Surgery for carcinoma of the esophagus and gastroesophageal junction (GEJ) evolved from cervical esophageal bypass for palliation of dysphagia to curative resection and reconstruction in a little over 130 years. Early surgery carried significant morbidity and mortality with minimal hope for cure. This led to the use of radiation as definitive, yet palliative, therapy. With advances in diagnosis and staging, better preoperative evaluation and preparation, alternative surgical techniques, and improved postoperative care, surgery is now the principal curative therapy for esophageal cancer.

Although these evolutionary changes seem only natural, they were not direct or easy. Innovative therapy or technique always gives rise to controversy. Manuscripts and dissertations address topics such as best therapy for a specific cancer, criteria for a good surgical candidate, optimal surgical technique, qualifications needed to perform surgery, and role of adjuvant therapy. Despite uncertainties, surgical management of cancer of the esophagus and GEJ must begin with accurate assessment of both the cancer and the patient.

The cancer

Diagnosis

Clinical diagnosis of esophageal carcinoma includes history, physical examination, barium esophagram, and esophagoscopy. Solid dysphagia in a middle-aged to older white man with a long-standing history of reflux and a known hiatal hernia is the classic presentation in the Western hemisphere. A second presentation is increasingly seen, that of a middle-aged white male with sudden onset of solid dysphagia without gastroesophageal reflux disease (GERD) or hiatal hernia. These clinical diagnoses of these patients are adeno-carcinoma of the distal esophagus (classic presentation) or GEJ/gastric cardia (second presentation). Typically, physical examination reveals a robust middle-aged to older white man with potential comorbidities, without weight loss, and without clinically detectable metastases to non-regional lymph nodes (supraclavicular) or distant sites (e.g. liver, pleura). In contradistinction, squamous cell carcinoma is found in the mid-thoracic esophagus in middle-aged non-white men, usually from an endemic area and a lower socio-economic class. History is typically of dysphagia, weight loss, and heavy smoking and drinking, and examination usually reveals an advanced-stage carcinoma.

In most centers, flexible fiberoptic videoesophagoscopy (Figure 35.1) has replaced the barium esophagram (Figure 35.2) as the first investigation in the evaluation of dysphagia and the clinical diagnosis of esophageal carcinoma. However, in patients with esophageal carcinoma, reports show that the modern barium esophagram detects a lesion in 98% of barium studies, is suggestive or diagnostic of esophageal carcinoma in 96%, and has an estimated positive predictive value of 42% [1]. For many physicians outside the Western world, the barium esophagram remains the principal test for clinical diagnosis of esophageal carcinoma. However, today the clinical diagnosis of cancer of the esophagus and GEJ requires tissue confirmation, which is not obtained by barium esophagram.

For the pathologic diagnosis of esophageal carcinoma, flexible esophagoscopy is the procedure of choice. Cytology brushings followed by multiple biopsies are diagnostic in most patients (Figures 35.3 and 35.4). Useful in the diagnosis of malignant strictures that are not endoscopically accessible are endoscopic esophageal ultrasound (EUS) and fine-needle aspiration (EUS FNA) of the abnormal esophageal wall [2]. FNA or open biopsy of distant metastases can provide both a pathologic diagnosis and crucial staging.

In North America, patients with a columnar-lined esophagus should have esophagoscopy and biopsy (four-quadrant

The Esophagus, Fifth Edition. Edited by Joel E. Richter, Donald O. Castell.
© 2012 Blackwell Publishing Ltd. Published 2012 by Blackwell Publishing Ltd.

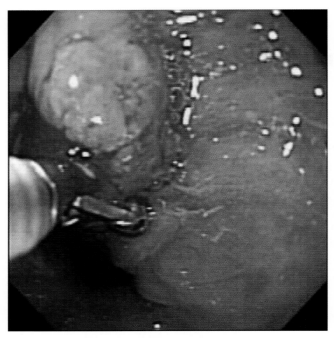

Figure 35.1 Esophagoscopy and biopsy following brush cytology of a malignant esophageal stricture.

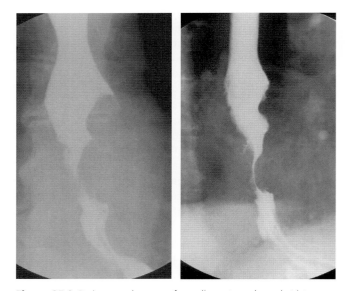

Figure 35.2 Barium esophagram of a malignant esophageal stricture. This long, irregular stricture has mucosal destruction and irregular filling defects obstructing the esophageal lumen. It occurs above a hiatal hernia.

biopsies every 2 cm) every 3 years. Surveillance of these high-risk groups allows diagnosis of early-stage disease in asymptomatic patients and is cost-effective compared with other cancer surveillance programs [3, 4].

Staging

Staging of cancer of the esophagus and GEJ has been extensively changed and improved in the seventh edition of the

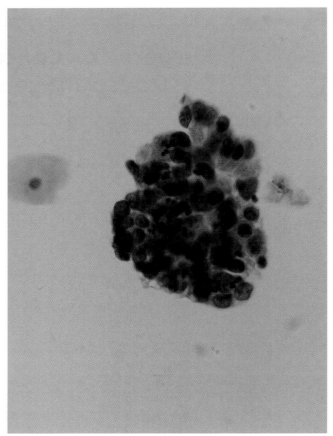

Figure 35.3 Cytology of adenocarcinoma. Cells were obtained from brushings of Barrett's esophagus. Clusters of neoplastic cells with hyperchromatic, pleomorphic nuclei and loss of polarity, but retained columnar configuration and cytoplasmic mucin.

American Joint Committee on Cancer (AJCC)/Union for International Cancer Control (UICC) Cancer Staging Manuals [5, 6]. Changes address problems of empiric stage grouping and lack of harmonization with stomach cancer. This was accomplished by assembling worldwide data and using modern machine learning techniques for data-driven staging [7–10]. Improvements include new definitions of Tis, T4, regional lymph node, N classification, and M classification, and addition of the non-anatomic cancer characteristics: histopathologic cell type, histologic grade, and tumor location. Stage groupings were constructed by adherence to principles of staging, including monotonic decreasing survival with increasing stage group, distinct survival between groups, and homogeneous survival within groups.

Depth of tumor invasion classifies the primary tumor (T) (Table 35.1 and Figure 35.5). Tis tumors are intraepithelial malignancies confined to the epithelium without invasion of the basement membrane and are now termed *high-grade dysplasia*. Tis includes all non-invasive neoplastic epithelium that was previously called carcinoma *in situ*. T1 tumors

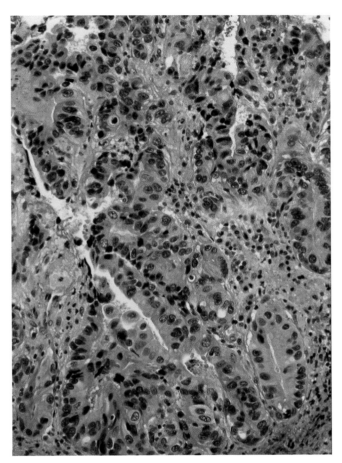

Figure 35.4 Intramucosal adenocarcinoma: Neoplastic glands infiltrate the lamina propria, but do not invade beyond the muscularis mucosa.

breach the basement membrane to invade the lamina propria, muscularis mucosa, or the submucosa, but do not invade beyond the submucosa. T1 tumors may be subclassified into T1a, tumors that invade only the mucosa, and T1b, tumors that invade the submucosa [11]. T2 tumors invade into but not beyond the muscularis propria. T3 tumors invade beyond the esophageal wall into the periesophageal tissue, but do not invade adjacent structures. T4 tumors directly invade structures in the vicinity of the esophagus. T4 has been subclassified as T4a and T4b; T4a tumors are resectable cancers invading adjacent structures, such as pleura, pericardium, or diaphragm. T4b tumors are unresectable cancers invading other adjacent structures, such as aorta, vertebral body, or trachea.

A regional lymph node has been redefined to include any paraesophageal lymph node extending from cervical nodes to celiac nodes (Table 35.1 and Figure 35.5). Data analyses support convenient coarse groupings of number of cancer-positive nodes [7–9]. Regional lymph node (N) classification comprises N0 (no cancer-positive nodes), N1 (one or two), N2 (three to six), and N3 (seven or more). N classifications

Table 35.1 Seventh edition AJCC/UICC staging of cancer of the esophagus and gastroesophageal junction.

T: Primary tumor

TX	Tumor cannot be assessed	
T0	No evidence of tumor	
Tis	High-grade dysplasia	
T1	Tumor invades the lamina propria, muscularis mucosa, or submucosa. It does not breach the submucosa	
T2	Tumor invades into but not beyond the muscularis propria	
T3	Tumor invades the paraesophageal tissue, but does not invade adjacent structures	
T4	T4a	Resectable tumor invades adjacent structures, such as pleura, pericardium, diaphragm
	T4b	Unresectable tumor invades adjacent structures, such as aorta, vertebral body, trachea

N: Regional lymph nodes

Any periesophageal lymph node from cervical lymph nodes to celiac node

NX	Regional lymph nodes cannot be assessed
N0	No regional lymph node metastases
N1	One to two positive regional lymph nodes
N2	Three to six positive regional lymph nodes
N3	Seven or more positive regional lymph nodes

M: Distant metastasis

M0	No distant metastases
M1	Distant metastases

Non-anatomic cancer characteristics

Histopathologic cell type:
  Adenocarcinoma
  Squamous cell carcinoma

Histologic grade:

G1	Well differentiated
G2	Moderately differentiated
G3	Poorly differentiated
G4	Undifferentiated

Tumor location:

Upper thoracic	20–25 cm from incisors
Middle thoracic	>25–30 cm from incisors
Lower thoracic	>30–40 cm from incisors
Gastroesophageal junction (GEJ):	Includes cancers whose epicenter is in the distal thoracic esophagus, GEJ, or within the proximal 5 cm of the stomach (cardia) that extend into the GEJ or esophagus and are stage grouped similar to adenocarcinoma of the esophagus

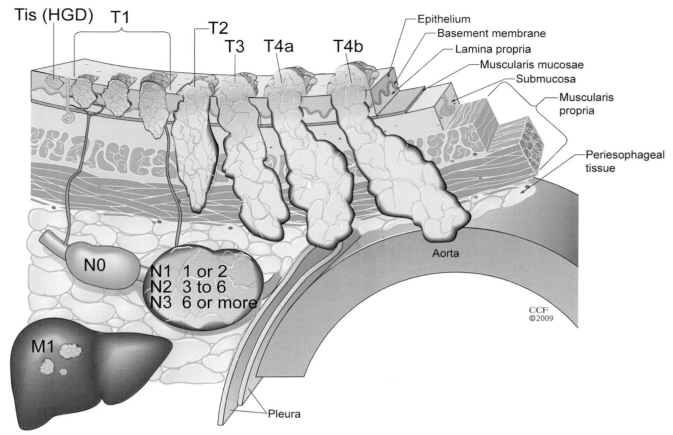

Figure 35.5 Seventh edition TNM classification. T is classified as Tis: high-grade dysplasia; T1: cancer invades lamina propria, muscularis mucosae, or submucosa; T2: cancer invades muscularis propria; T3: cancer invades adventitia; T4a: resectable cancer invades adjacent structures such as pleura, pericardium, or diaphragm; and T4b: unresectable cancer invades other adjacent structures, such as aorta, vertebral body, or trachea. N is classified as N0: no regional lymph node metastasis; N1: regional lymph node metastases involving one to two nodes; N2: regional lymph node metastases involving three to six nodes; and N3: regional lymph node metastases involving seven or more nodes. M is classified as M0: no distant metastasis; and M1: distant metastasis.

for cancers of the esophagus and GEJ are identical to stomach cancer N classifications.

The subclassifications M1a and M1b have been eliminated, as has MX (Table 35.1). Distant metastases are simply designated M0, no distant metastasis, and M1, distant metastasis.

Three non-anatomic cancer characteristics—histopathologic cell type, histologic grade, and tumor location—are necessary for staging (Table 35.1). Since the AJCC/UICC seventh edition staging of cancer of the esophagus and GEJ is based on cancers arising from the epithelium, histopathologic cell type is either adenocarcinoma or squamous cell carcinoma. Because the data indicate that squamous cell carcinoma has a poorer prognosis than adenocarcinoma, a tumor of mixed histopathologic type is staged as squamous cell carcinoma. Non-mucosal cancers arising in the wall are classified according to their cell of origin.

The non-anatomic cancer characteristic histologic grade is categorized as G1, well differentiated; G2, moderately differentiated; G3, poorly differentiated; or G4, undifferentiated (Table 35.1). Because the data indicate that squamous cell carcinoma has a poorer prognosis than adenocarcinoma, G4, undifferentiated cancers, are staged similarly to G3 squamous cell carcinoma.

Tumor location is defined by position of the upper end of the cancer in the esophagus. It is best expressed as the distance from the incisors to the proximal edge of the tumor, and conventionally by its location within broad regions of the esophagus. Typical esophagoscopy measurements of cervical esophageal cancer measured from the incisors is from 15 to less than 20 cm (Figure 35.6). If esophagoscopy is not available, location can be assessed by computed tomography (CT). If thickening of the esophageal wall begins above the sternal notch, location is cervical. Typical esophagoscopy measurements of upper thoracic esophageal cancer from the incisors is from 20 to less than 25 cm (Figure 35.6). CT location of an upper thoracic cancer is esophageal wall

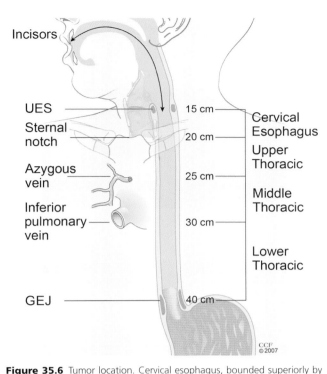

Figure 35.6 Tumor location. Cervical esophagus, bounded superiorly by the cricopharyngeus and inferiorly by the sternal notch, is typically 15–20 cm from the incisors at esophagoscopy. Upper thoracic esophagus, bounded superiorly by the sternal notch and inferiorly by the azygos arch, is typically greater than 20–25 cm from the incisors at esophagoscopy. Middle thoracic esophagus, bounded superiorly by the azygos arch and inferiorly by the inferior pulmonary vein, is typically greater than 25–30 cm from the incisors at esophagoscopy. Lower thoracic esophagus, bounded superiorly by the inferior pulmonary vein and inferiorly by the lower esophageal sphincter, is typically greater than 30–40 cm from the incisors at esophagoscopy; it includes cancers whose epicenter is within the proximal 5 cm of the stomach and that extend into the gastroesophageal junction (GEJ) or lower thoracic esophagus. UES, upper esophageal sphincter.

Adenocarcinoma

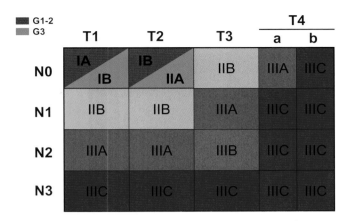

Figure 35.7 Stage groupings for M0 adenocarcinoma by T and N classification and histologic grade (G).

thickening that begins between the sternal notch and azygos vein. Typical esophagoscopy measurements of middle thoracic esophageal cancer from the incisors is from 25 to less than 30 cm (Figure 35.6). CT location is wall thickening that begins between the azygos vein and inferior pulmonary vein. Typical esophagoscopy measurements of lower thoracic esophageal cancer from the incisors is from 30 to 40 cm (Figure 35.6). CT location is wall thickening that begins below the inferior pulmonary vein. The abdominal esophagus is included in the lower thoracic esophagus. Cancers whose epicenter is in the lower thoracic esophagus, GEJ, or within the proximal 5 cm of the stomach (cardia) that extend into the GEJ or esophagus (Siewert III) are staged as adenocarcinoma of the esophagus. All other cancers with an epicenter in the stomach greater than 5 cm distal to the GEJ, or those within 5 cm of the GEJ, but not extending into it

or the esophagus, are staged grouped using the gastric (non-GEJ) cancer staging system [5].

TNM descriptors are grouped into stages to assemble subgroups with similar behavior and prognosis. Stages 0 and IV are by definition (not data driven) TisN0M0 and Tany Nany M1, respectively. Stage groupings for M0 adenocarcinoma are shown in Figure 35.7. For T1N0M0 and T2N0M0 adenocarcinoma, subgrouping is by histologic grade, G1and G2 (not G3) versus G3. The difference in survival between adenocarcinoma and squamous cell carcinoma was best managed by separate stage groupings for stages I and II.

Stage groupings for M0 squamous cell carcinoma are shown in Figure 35.8. For T1N0M0 squamous cell carcinoma, subgrouping is by histologic grade: G1 versus all other G (Figure 35.8A). For T2N0M0 and T3N0M0 squamous cell carcinoma, stage grouping is by histologic grade and location (Figure 35.8A). The four combinations range from G1 lower thoracic squamous cell carcinoma (stage IB), which has the best survival, to G2–G4 upper and middle thoracic squamous cell carcinomas (stage IIB), which have the worst. G2–G4 lower thoracic squamous cell carcinomas and G1 upper and middle thoracic squamous cell carcinomas are grouped together (stage IIA) with intermediate survival.

Stage 0, III, and IV adenocarcinoma (Figure 35.7) and squamous cell carcinoma (Figure 35.8B) are stage grouped identically. Adenosquamous carcinomas are staged as squamous cell carcinoma.

Clinical staging

Clinical staging is based on evidence before primary therapy. It involves esophagoscopy with biopsy, EUS, EUS-FNA, CT, [18F]fluoro-2-deoxy-D-glucose positron emission tomography (FDG-PET) for assessment of T, N, M, and G classifications, histopathologic type, and cancer location. These

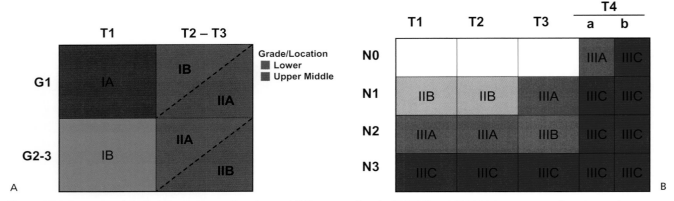

Figure 35.8 Stage groupings for M0 squamous cell carcinoma. (A) Stage groupings for T1N0M0 and T2-3N0M0 squamous cell carcinomas by histologic grade (G) and cancer location. (B) Stage groupings for all other M0 squamous cell carcinomas.

investigations may be supplemented by cervical lymph node biopsy, bronchoscopy, endoscopic bronchial ultrasound (EBUS) and EBUS-FNA, mediastinoscopy, thoracoscopy, laparoscopy, and ultrasound- or CT-directed percutaneous biopsy. Clinical stage provides the baseline for treatment evaluation and rational treatment decisions. The seventh edition of the AJCC staging form for cancer of the esophagus and GEJ requires description of clinical staging used in treatment planning.

Determination of non-anatomic cancer characteristics

Esophagoscopy and biopsy are necessary to determine non-anatomic cancer characteristics. As well as location, which is defined as the distance to the proximal edge of the cancer from incisors, the seventh edition staging form requires the site-specific factor distance to the distal edge of the cancer from incisors be recorded [5]. This will allow esophageal cancer length to be calculated. Histopathologic cell type and histologic grade are determined from pathologic assessment of biopsies.

Determination of cT

EUS is the only clinical tool that provides detailed examination of the esophageal wall. It is the procedure of choice for determining cT (depth of tumor penetration). The muscularis propria (fourth ultrasound layer) is vital in differentiating T1, T2, and T3 tumors (Figure 35.9). Tumors are defined as cT1 if there is no invasion of the muscularis propria (fourth ultrasound layer); cT2, if invasion is into the muscularis propria; or cT3, if invasion is beyond the muscularis propria. EUS evaluates the interface between the primary tumor and adjacent structures. If invasion is detected, the tumor is cT4. In a review of 21 series, the accuracy of EUS for T determination was 84% [12]. Accuracy is not constant and varies with T. In this meta-analysis, accuracy for T1 carcinomas was 83.5% with 16.5% of tumors overstaged; accuracy for T2

was 73% with 10% understaged and 17% overstaged; accuracy for T3 was 89% with 5% understaged and 6% overstaged; and accuracy for T4 was 89% with 11% understaged. A review of the literature shows variation in accuracy with T: 75–82% for T1, 64–85% for T2, 89–94% for T3, and 88–100% for T4 [12]. The most unreliable of cT EUS determinations is for cT2 [13–17]. A meta-analysis of 27 articles demonstrates EUS as being highly effective in the differentiation of T1 and T2 from T3 and T4 cancers [18].

EUS and esophagoscopy are complementary and should be performed together. A malignant stricture that prohibits passage of the examining instrument is highly predictive of an advanced stage cancer [19–21]. A tumor length greater than 5 cm is predictive of T3 cancers with 89% sensitivity, 92% specificity, 89% positive predictive value, and 92% negative predictive value [21].

Exclusion of cT4 cancers, demonstrated by the preservation of fat planes between an esophageal cancer and adjacent structures, is the only role of CT in the determination of cT (Figure 35.10). Contiguous soft tissues provide radiographic contrast necessary to define the esophagus; however, these planes may be absent in cachectic patients. In normal patients, fat between an esophageal cancer and aorta, trachea, left main bronchus, or pericardium may be absent. Physiologic absence of fat planes complicates the assessment of invasion of adjacent structures. Alternative CT criteria have been proposed to predict T4 status. Aortic invasion is suggested by an arc of contact between the tumor and the aorta greater than 90 degrees, although this is not an absolute confirmation of a T4 tumor. Thickening or indentation of the normally flat or slightly convex posterior membranous wall of the intrathoracic trachea or left main bronchus is suggestive of airway invasion. On occasion, tumor in the airway lumen or a fistula between the esophagus and airway may be visualized; however, bronchoscopic confirmation with biopsy is necessary. Pericardial invasion is suspected if pericardial thickening, pericardial effusion, or indentation of

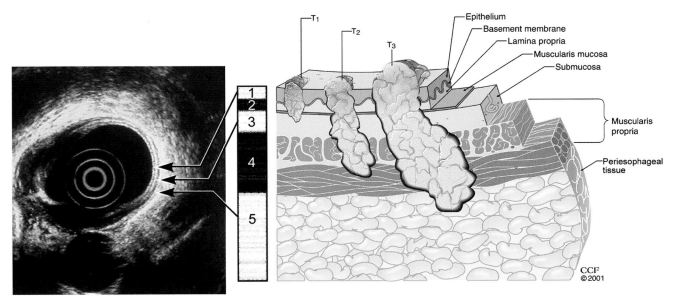

Figure 35.9 Esophageal wall is visualized as five alternating layers of differing echogenicity by esophageal ultrasound (EUS). The first layer is hyperechoic (white) and represents the superficial mucosa (epithelium and lamina propria). The second layer is hypoechoic (black) and represents the deep mucosa (muscularis mucosa). The third layer is hyperechoic and represents the submucosa. The forth ultrasound layer is hypoechoic and represents the muscularis mucosa. This layer (muscularis propria) is critical in differentiating T1, T2, and T3 tumors. The fifth ultrasound layer is hyperechoic and represents the periesophageal tissue. The thickness of the EUS layers is not equal to the actual thickness of the anatomic layers.

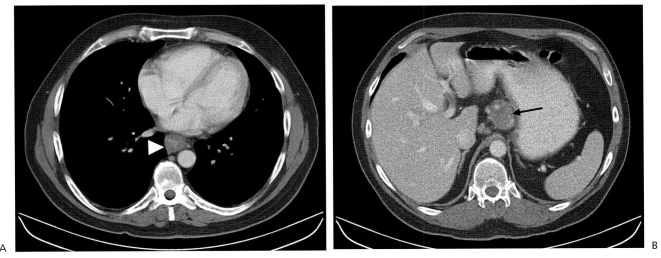

Figure 35.10 (A) Non-specific CT finding of esophageal cancer (arrowhead) is thickening of the esophageal wall. CT does not discriminate between cTis, cT1, cT2, and cT3 tumors. Preservation of periesophageal fat excludes cT4 cancer. In this study, preservation of fat planes excludes invasion of the prevertebral fascia, aorta, and pericardium. (B) In this same patient, an enlarged celiac axis lymph node (arrow) is seen.

the heart with loss of the pericardial fat plane at the level of the tumor is seen. Magnetic resonance imaging (MRI) offers no significant advantage over CT.

With FDG-PET, FDGFDG is reported to accumulate in 92–100% of esophageal cancers [22, 23]. FDG-PET and other imaging modalities do not provide definition of the esophageal wall or paraesophageal tissue and, therefore, have no value in the determination of cT.

Theoretically, thoracoscopy could exclude a cT4 tumor, but requires dissection of the primary tumor and the adjacent structure thought to be invaded. Although mentioned as a possible staging tool for cT4 detection [24, 25], the only documentation of T4 is the detection of cT4 disease in 14% of patients undergoing thoracoscopy and laparoscopy for regional lymph node staging [26].

Bronchoscopy did not improve clinical staging of esophageal cancers at or above the tracheal carina after EUS determination of T [27].

Determination of cN

EUS evaluates nodal size, shape, border, and internal echo characteristics in regional lymph node assessment. In a retrospective review of 100 EUS examinations, determination of N was 89% sensitive, 75% specific, and 84% accurate [28]. Positive predictive value of EUS for N+ disease was 86%; negative predictive value was 79%. A meta-analysis of 21 series reported EUS as being 77% accurate for N, 69% for N0, and 89% for N+ [12]. EUS FNA further refines clinical staging by adding tissue sampling to endosonography findings. In a multicenter study, 171 patients had EUS FNA of 192 lymph nodes [29]. EUS FNA for determination of lymph node status was 92% sensitive , 93% specific, 100% positively predictive, and 86% negatively predictive. Combined EUS and EUS FNA assessment of celiac lymph nodes was 72% sensitive, 97% specific, 95% positively predictive, and 82% negatively predictive [30]. FNA confirmed positive EUS celiac lymph nodes in 88% of patients. More recent experience of this group reported 98% accuracy of EUS FNA detection of malignant celiac lymph nodes [31].

Subclassification of N+ requires determination of the number of regional lymph nodes containing metastases (positive nodes). EUS can accurately determine number of positive regional lymph nodes and this clinical assessment is predictive of survival [32–34].

An enlarged lymph node on CT suggests nodal metastasis (Figure 35.10B). The short axis of these nodes is easily measured; intrathoracic and abdominal lymph nodes greater than 1 cm are enlarged. Supraclavicular lymph nodes with a short axis greater than 0.5 cm and retrocrural lymph nodes greater than 0.6 cm are pathologic [35]. However, the probability is small that cN status can be determined by lymph node size alone [36]. Normal-sized nodes that contain metastatic deposits and metastatic nodes in direct contact with the tumor may be indistinguishable from the primary tumor. These result in false-negative examinations and influence the sensitivity and negative predictive value. All enlarged lymph nodes may not be malignant. Inflammatory nodes are the most common cause of a false-positive examination and of lower specificity and positive predictive value. CT assessment of lymph nodes varies with anatomic site; accuracies of 61–96%, sensitivities of 8–75%, and specificities of 60–98% were reported for cervical, mediastinal, and abdominal nodes [37]. MRI offers no important advantage over CT.

Physiologic evaluation of esophageal carcinoma provided by FDG-PET relies not only on size of the metastatic deposit but also on the intensity of FDG uptake and decay.

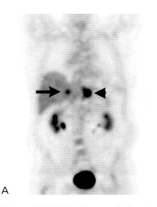
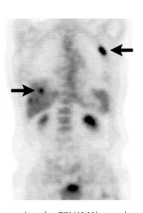

Figure 35.11 Positron emission tomography of a T3N1M1b esophageal cancer. (**A**) Primary tumor and regional lymph nodes cannot be differentiated and appear as one large mass (arrowhead). (A, B) There are two sites of metastases (arrows), two metastases in the liver and one in the left rib. The kidneys excrete and the bladder stores 2-[^{18}F]-fluoro-2-deoxy-D-glucose (FDG).

Theoretically, it is possible to identify microscopic metastases if glucose metabolism is sufficient to concentrate large quantities of FDG. FDG-PET cannot differentiate adjacent N+ from the primary tumor [22] (Figure 35.11). FDG-PET is least sensitive in the assessment of lymph nodes in the mid and lower thoracic esophagus [38]. The accuracy of FDG-PET in the detection of lymph node metastases from esophageal carcinomas is variable, ranging from 37% to 90% [23, 39–42]. Compared with detection of lymph node metastases in lung cancer, FDG-PET is much less accurate in esophageal carcinoma [43]. Because of its high sensitivity, the main role of FDG-PET is confirmation of cN0 status [44]. PET can determine number of positive regional lymph nodes and this clinical subclassification of N+ is predictive of survival [45].

Thoracoscopic and laparoscopic staging have been used to evaluate regional lymph node status. A combination of thoracoscopic and laparoscopic staging is 94% accurate in detecting lymph node metastases [26]. For thoracic lymph nodes, sensitivity, specificity, and positive predictive value are 63%, 100%, and 100%, respectively. For abdominal lymph nodes, sensitivity, specificity, and positive predictive value are 85%, 100%, and 100%, respectively. Of 88 patients entered into the study, thoracoscopy was performed in 82 (93%), laparoscopy in 55 (63%), and both in 49 (57%). Induction chemoradiotherapy was administered to 34 (39%) patients. These procedures are not without serious morbidity [46] and the possibility of port-site metastasis [47]. Only 47 (53%) of patients underwent resection, making comparative pathologic stage available in only 13 (15%) patients. The best operative time and hospital stay reported are 3.6 h and 1.8 days, respectively [48].

Determination of cM

In patients with recently diagnosed esophageal carcinoma, metastases were found in the liver in 35%, in the lung in

20%, in the bone in 9%, in the adrenal gland in 2%, in the brain in 2%, and 1% in each of the pericardium, pleura, soft tissues, stomach, pancreas, and spleen [49]. Except for the brain, CT scanning of the esophagus includes all or a portion of all other sites. Contrast-enhanced CT scanning with imaging during the portal venous phases of contrast distribution provides both screening for and diagnosis of masses in these areas.

Hepatic metastases appear as ill-defined, low-density lesions of variable size (Figure 35.12). Conventional CT imaging (dynamic incremental scanning with intravenous bolus contrast enhancement) is excellent in the detection of hepatic metastases greater than 2 cm [50]. Sensitivity is 70–80% [35]. Although no study is available for esophageal cancer, spiral CT produced similar results to conventional CT in the detection of colorectal liver metastases; sensitivity of 76% and a positive predictive value of 90% have been reported [51]. CT frequently does not recognize subcentimeter metastases; they are the main cause of false-negative examinations and the low sensitivity of CT in the detection

of liver metastases. To distinguish benign from malignant nodules, ultrasound is used for diagnosis of benign cysts and MRI for hemangiomas. Adrenal metastases cause heterogeneous focal enlargement of the adrenal gland. Contrast-enhanced CT is a sensitive but non-specific screening tool for adrenal masses. Non-contrast CT, MRI, percutaneous FNA, or laparoscopy may be required to confirm the nature of these nodules.

In a cohort of patients with predominate squamous cell carcinoma of the esophagus, solitary lung metastases were rare at diagnosis of the primary cancer and were likely to be benign nodules or synchronous primary lung cancer [52]. Although multiple lung metastases were uncommon at diagnosis, they became more common during the late stages of the disease (Figure 35.12). Many were not visualized by chest radiograph. CT is very sensitive in the detection of pulmonary nodules; however, histologic confirmation of these abnormalities is required if their presence alone determines therapy.

The presence of ascites, pleural effusion, or nodules in the omentum or pleura suggests metastases to these mesothelial-lined surfaces. Laparoscopy or thoracoscopy confirms these findings.

Brain metastases are reported in 2–4% of patients presenting with esophageal carcinoma [49, 53]. They tend to occur in patients with large adenocarcinoma of the GEJ with local invasion or metastases to lymph nodes. Pretreatment CT of the brain may be reasonable in these patients.

Despite improved technology, CT is only 37–66% sensitive in screening for distant metastases in patients with esophageal cancer [39, 40, 43, 54]. FDG-PET is superior to CT in detecting M1 disease. In 91 patients undergoing 100 FDG-PET studies, distant metastatic disease was detected in 39 scans at 51 sites [43]. Seventy distant metastases were confirmed by biopsy or at resection. The sensitivity of FDG-PET was 69%, specificity 93%, and overall accuracy 84%. In this series, the sensitivity of CT was 46%, specificity 74%, and accuracy 63%. FDG-PET failed to diagnose distant metastases in the liver in 10 patients, pleura in four patients, lung in two patients, and peritoneum in one patient. All metastases were less than 1 cm in diameter. Of 21 false-negative CT scans, FDG-PET identified distant metastases in 11 (62%); of 12 false-negative FDG PET scans, CT was accurate in four (33%). These mature results are less favorable than in an earlier report by the same group in which sensitivity of FDG-PET in detection of distant metastases was 88%, specificity 93%, and accuracy 91% [41].

Five (71%) of seven patients with distant metastatic disease were diagnosed by FDG-PET [22]. A liver metastasis less than 1 cm in diameter was not visualized and a pancreatic metastasis was misinterpreted as a left gastric lymph node metastasis. There were no false-positive examinations in 36 patients. Over a similar time period, the same group reported 17 distant metastases in 59 patients with FDG-PET.

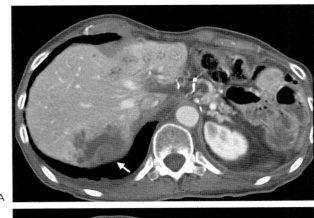

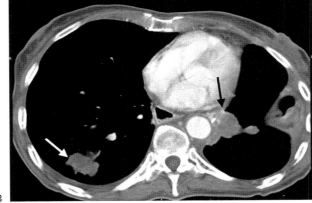

Figure 35.12 (A) CT of a hepatic metastasis appears as ill-defined, low-density lesion in the posterior portion of the right lobe (arrow). (B) CT of a pulmonary metastasis in the right lower lobe (white arrow) and mediastinal lymph nodes (black arrow) in the same patient with diffusely metastatic esophageal carcinoma.

There were no false-negative examinations; however, transhiatal esophagectomy was commonly used to obtain pathologic stage [39].

FDG-PET detects radiographically occult distant metastatic disease in 10–20% of patients with esophageal cancer [39–41, 43]. The combination of FDG-PET and CT has a diagnostic accuracy of 80–92% [39, 40] and avoids unnecessary surgery in 90% [40]. FDG-PET provides additional staging information in 22% of patients, upstaging 15% and downstaging 7% [44].

Laparoscopy is reported to change therapy in 10% of patients, allowing resection in 2% who are overstaged and avoiding resection in 8% with undetected M1 disease [55]. The sensitivities of laparoscopy in detecting peritoneal and liver metastases are 71% and 86%, respectively. Heath *et al.* reported that laparoscopy changed the treatment in 17% [56]. Laparoscopic ultrasonography does not improve staging by laparoscopy alone [57, 58].

EUS has limited value in screening for distant metastases (M1). The distant organ must be in direct contact with the upper gastrointestinal tract for EUS to be useful (e.g. the left lateral segment of the liver and retroperitoneum).

Role of clinical staging
Esophagoscopy with biopsy, EUS, EUS FNA, and CT PET are mainstays in clinical staging of esophageal carcinoma. No single test is sufficient and these investigations are complimentary [59–62]. Results of these studies determine the necessity for invasive staging techniques such as thoracoscopy and laparoscopy and direct their use. Clinical stage is highly predictive of pathologic stage and outcome (Figures 35.13 and 35.14) and is key in determining therapy. However, equally important to decision-making is the assessment of the patient.

The patient

Patient assessment, selection, and preoperative preparation are crucial in reducing postoperative morbidity and mortality, and ensuring improved survival following surgery for esophageal cancer.

General condition
The patient's overall state of health, although hard to define or quantify, significantly influences outcome. The amalgam of history and physical examination, a surgeon's accumulated experience, clinical acumen, and "feeling" about the patient often form the entire assessment of general health. However, quantification of a patient's general condition by the preoperative Karnofsky index can accurately predict

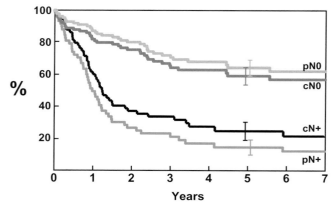

Figure 35.14 Kaplan–Meier survival estimates of 230 clinically-staged patients undergoing surgery alone for esophageal cancer. cN is the clinically determined regional lymph node status; pN is the pathologic regional lymph node status determined by examination of the resection specimen.

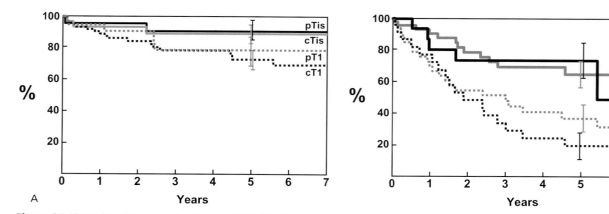

Figure 35.13 Kaplan–Meier survival estimates of 153 clinically-staged patients undergoing surgery alone for esophageal cancer. (A) N0M0 cancers confined to the esophageal wall. (B) N0M0 cancers invading beyond the esophageal wall. cT is the clinically determined depth of tumor invasion; pT is the pathologic depth of tumor invasion determined by examination of the resected tumor.

outcome [63]. Patients with a score of less than 80 are more likely to have a complicated or lethal postoperative course.

Key to successful postoperative recovery is the cooperation of the patient in their care. Subtle impairment that affects intellect or cooperation, and which may be overlooked in the preoperative assessment of the elderly or alcoholic patient, may be of prime significance during the postoperative course. A simple grading of the patient's ability to cooperate as either good or poor is predictive of outcome [63]. Bartel *et al.* proposed the classification of a patient's general condition as normal (Kanofsky index >80 and "good" cooperation), compromised (Karnofsky index <80 or "poor" cooperation), and severely impaired (Karnofsky index <80 and "poor" cooperation).

Age

Survival following surgery for esophageal cancer is inversely related to age. The effect of age is best appreciated in patients with superficial adenocarcinoma because the overwhelming effect of esophageal cancer on survival is minimized in early-stage cancers [64]. In these patients, increasing age is an independent predictor of decreasing survival. However, compared with age-matched cohorts, survival improves with age (Figure 35.15). Although uncommon, a cancer death in a younger patient with superficial esophageal adenocarcinoma is significant compared to age-matched patients who are unlikely to die of any cause. As patients age, the incidence of death from other causes increases; thus, in the highly selected "good risk" elderly patients chosen for resection of "good prognosis" superficial esophageal adenocarcinoma, survival is similar to their contemporaries without cancer.

Preoperative risk factors, advanced stage cancers, postoperative morbidity and mortality, and late deaths are variably reported to occur more frequently in elderly patients undergoing esophagectomy [65–76]. In these reports, age is not analyzed as a continuum, but rather as artificially picked cut-offs (e.g. 65, 70, 75, and 80 years), making incorporation of these data into practice difficult. However, despite the variable definitions of "elderly," comparisons of unmatched but highly selected groups of young and old patients undergoing surgery indicate that similar palliation and survival can be achieved regardless of age. However, population-based outcomes after high-risk cancer operations (esophagus, lung, and pancreas) are considerably worse than in case series and published survival statistics [77]. Increasing age is a relative contraindication to surgery; it is an indicator of comorbidity and poor general condition. In carefully chosen elderly patients with early-stage cancers, surgery with curative intent may be indicated. In high-risk elderly patients or elderly patients with advanced-stage cancers, non-surgical palliation may be optimum.

Race

African Americans (blacks) have higher mortality than whites from esophageal cancer. In an analysis of the SEER database of T0–T2 N0 esophageal cancer, 5-year survival was 37% for black patients and 60% for white patients (*P* < 0001) [78]. Blacks were more likely to have advanced stage and squamous cell cancers and they were less likely to undergo surgery. Black race in a multivariable analysis of these data controlled for age, sex, marital status, histopathologic cell type, and tumor location was associated with worse survival. This association was lost when cancer stage and treatment modalities of surgery and radiotherapy were added to the analysis.

Histologic cell type

In contrast to patients with adenocarcinoma, those with squamous cell carcinoma have higher alcohol and tobacco consumptions, and greater impairment of pulmonary and hepatic functions [79]. Patients with adenocarcinoma are generally better educated, are from a higher socioeconomic stratum, and are more likely to be overweight (up to 50% of patients), and suffer cardiovascular impairment. In either cell type, incidence in men predominates. Although these are profiles and do not apply to individual patients, they highlight potential comorbidities and postoperative complications that should be considered when tissue diagnosis of esophageal carcinoma is made.

Pulmonary function

Pulmonary complications are common following esophagectomy. In a large retrospective series, they occurred in 20–35% of patients [80]. In a small prospective study of 20 patients, 50% developed pulmonary complications, defined as temperature greater than 38° C and pulmonary infiltrate documented radiographically [81]. In a recent review,

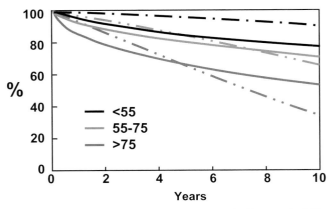

Figure 35.15 Survival within age groups compared with a matched US population. The dot–dash curve is the matched survival among patients younger than 55 years of age. The dash–dot–dot–dash curve is the population life table for patients between the ages of 55 and 75 years. The lowest dash–dot–dot–dash curve is for the matched population older than 75 years of age (reproduced from Rice *et al.*, [64], with permission).

pulmonary complications occurred in 15–40% of patients, and are associated with a 4.5-fold increase in morbidity and mortality, leading to 45% of all deaths post esophagectomy [82]. Pulmonary complications, defined by atelectasis, pleural effusion, or pneumothorax on chest radiograph, are a universal occurrence in patients undergoing esophagectomy for cancer [83, 84]. Increasing age (OR 1.31; 95% CI 0.99–1.74; $P = .06$) and impaired pulmonary function, measured by decreased percentage forced expiratory volume in 1 s (FEV_1) (OR 1.21; 95% CI 1.07–1.38; $P = .003$), are identified as independent predictors of major pulmonary complications [80]. In addition, Avendano *et al.* found patients receiving preoperative chemoradiotherapy more likely to experience postoperative complications [84].

Improvement in operative mortality in current esophageal surgery is primarily the result of reducing pulmonary complications [85]. Long-term (10-year) survival in patients with superficial esophageal adenocarcinoma decreases exponentially with a decrease in preoperative FEV_1 of less than 2 L [64] (Figure 35.16). Reducing pulmonary complications following thoracic surgery is tantamount to improving outcome.

Preoperative assessment of all patients considered for esophagectomy should include pulmonary function testing and arterial blood gases. Smoking cessation for a period of 4–8 weeks before surgery has been shown to reduce postoperative morbidity in major pulmonary resections [86, 87]. Reversible airway disease and bronchitis should be aggressively treated. Pulmonary rehabilitation may be beneficial, especially in patients with early-stage cancer who have time before surgery for this valuable therapy.

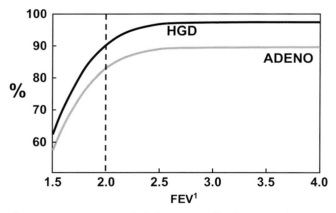

Figure 35.16 Ten-year survival of two types of patients, according to forced expiratory volume (FEV). One patient group has high-grade dysplasia (HGD) on preoperative biopsy, the other invasive adenocarcinoma (ADENO). Both are in a Barrett's esophagus surveillance program, and both would have a planned transhiatal esophagectomy. Note the evident differences (non-overlapping lower and upper confidence limits) below FEV_1 of approximately 2 L (reproduced from Rice *et al.*, [64], with permission).

Cardiovascular function

Dysrhythmias are common following esophagectomy, reported to occur in as many as 60% of patients [88]. The prevalence in most series ranges from 10% to 25%. Supraventricular arrhythmias are associated with a significant increase in postoperative morbidity and mortality [65]. However, arrhythmias are not the cause of death, but a marker for lethal complications. Predictors of supraventricular arrhythmias are increasing age and poor pulmonary function measured by preoperative theophylline use and a low diffusing capacity for carbon monoxide [65]. Maximal oxygen uptake during exercise testing correlates with postoperative pulmonary complications and cardiac dysrhythmias [89]. The preoperative maneuvers used to reduce pulmonary complications may have a similar effect on cardiac dysrhythmias.

Coronary artery disease is a common finding in patients with carcinoma of the esophagus [90], although myocardial infarction is uncommon. In octogenarians undergoing esophagectomy, myocardial infarction occurs in only 3% of patients [91]. Preoperative predictors of infarction have not been identified. This is most likely due to careful patient selection based on preoperative cardiac evaluation along with pre-esophagectomy intervention in resectable patients with significant coronary artery disease.

As many as 11% of postoperative deaths are attributed to cardiac causes [85]. Simple assessment of cardiac risk by a cardiologist as normal, increased, or high is a strong predictor of postoperative mortality [92].

Other organ systems

Cirrhosis is a contraindication to esophagectomy. In a small series of 18 patients with cirrhosis (11 patients were Child A and seven were Child B), operative morbidity was 83% and mortality was 17% [93]. Patients with Child B and Child C cirrhosis were reported to have a operative mortality of 50% and 100%, respectively, following esophagectomy [94]. Impaired hepatic function assessed by serum albumin, serum bilirubin, partial thromboplastin time, aminopyrine breath test, and the presence or absence of cirrhosis is a predictor of hospital mortality [63, 90].

In other surgical series, comorbidities such as diabetes, renal dysfunction, and peripheral vascular disease were not associated with an increase in either morbidity or mortality. However, in individual patients, recognition, assessment, and treatment of comorbidities are essential in improving outcome.

Preoperative risk score

Stein *et al.* developed a composite score for assessing risk of postoperative mortality after esophagectomy [90]. Four factors (patient's general status and cardiac, pulmonary, and hepatic functions) are rated as 1 for normal, 2 for compromised, or 3 for severely impaired. These are weighted and summed to produce scores ranging from 11 to 33 (Table 35.2). Scores of less than 18 are associated with low mortality and allow patients to be considered for aggressive therapy, including extensive resection or multimodality therapy. Scores greater than 21 are predictive of excessive mortality. Using this tool, the authors excluded 30% of patients with otherwise resectable tumors from surgery. This resulted in a decreased operative mortality from 10% before initiation of this system to 2% after its inception.

The operation

Operation for cancer of the esophagus and GEJ requires resection and reconstruction. Because each component

influences the other, one cannot be performed separately without consideration of the other.

Resection

Primary tumor

The extent of resection is determined by characteristics of the primary tumor and details of reconstruction (Figure 35.17). In 3% of patients, the existence of cancer 10.5 cm proximal to visible tumor led to adoption of a 12-cm proximal margin for esophagectomy [95]. A proximal margin of less than 5 cm from the primary tumor is associated with a 20% chance of local recurrence. If the margin is 5–10 cm, recurrence is reduced to 8% [96]. Mean length from the tumor to the resection margin is 2.7 cm in patients with anastomotic recurrence and 4.4 cm in patients without recurrence ($P = .007$) [97]. Casson *et al.* recommended a macroscopic margin of 5 cm beyond the primary tumor to achieve a consistently negative distal resection margin [98]. Compared with esophagogastrectomy, total thoracic esophagectomy with cervical esophagogastric anastomosis increases the length from the tumor to the proximal resection margin and decreases the incidence of anastomotic recurrence [99].

Accumulated experience with superficial carcinoma provides useful data to guide extent of resection. Subepithelial extension of primary tumor (defined as lymphatic, vascular or ductal permeation, intramural metastases, or direct

Table 35.2 Composite preoperative score (reproduced from Stein *et al.* [90], with permission).

Factor	Score	Weight	Minimum	Maximum
General status	1–3	4	4	12
Cardiac function	1–3	3	3	9
Pulmonary function	1–3	2	2	6
Hepatic function	1–3	2	2	6
Composite score			11	33

Score: 1, normal; 2, compromised; 3, severely impaired.

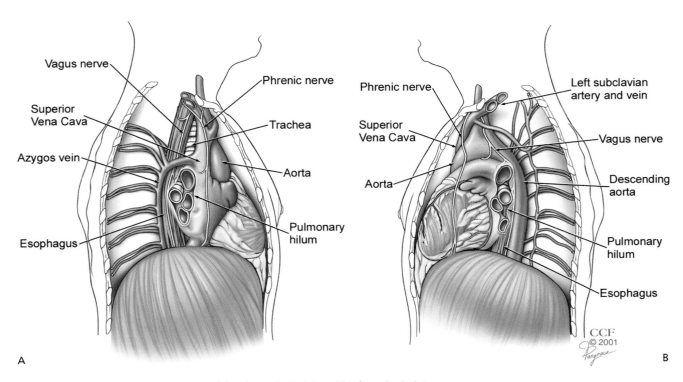

Figure 35.17 Thoracic esophageal resection. (A) Right mediastinal view. (B) Left mediastinal view.

invasion) is related to depth of tumor invasion [100]. Only 4% of patients with tumors limited to the mucosa, 37% with submucosal invasion, and 46% with muscularis propria invasion have subepithelial extension. Risk of a positive resection margin is similarly related to depth of invasion [101]. To ensure a less than 5% chance of a positive resection margin, a length from tumor to resection margins greater than 10 mm is required for tumors confined to the esophageal wall, and greater than 30 mm for those invading beyond the esophageal wall.

Anastomotic recurrence is reported in 10% of patients with positive margins (R1 resection has microscopic positive margin, R2 resection has macroscopic positive margin) and 5% of patients with negative margins (RO resection) (P = .15). Of 463 patients undergoing esophagectomy, 12 (3%) experienced an anastomotic recurrence [102]. Ten anastomotic recurrences were in patients with negative margins. In 16 patients with positive margins, distant metastases developed in 11 and anastomotic recurrence developed in two. Only in patients without regional lymph node metastases or with low burden of regional lymph node metastases (<25% of nodes positive) is survival decreased by a positive resection margin [103].

Lateral extent of the resection should include the periesophageal tissue and may include the pleura and pericardium. Preservation of the spleen is recommended, because splenectomy at esophagectomy for cancer is associated with increased septic complications (pneumonia, intra-abdominal abscess, postoperative sepsis, and anastomotic leak) and postoperative mortality (36% vs 8%; P < .01) [104]. Invasion of the trachea, aorta, vertebral bodies, lung, or heart precludes resection (Figure 35.17).

If it is planned that the stomach is to be reconstructed, a cervical anastomosis may provide the best long-term func-

tional results. A low intrathoracic esophagogastric anastomosis has long been known to be unsatisfactory, because of excessive gastroesophageal reflux [105]. One year after esophagectomy, patients with cervical anastomosis reported less reflux than those with intrathoracic anastomosis [106]. Both reflex symptoms (4% vs 50%; P = .0001) and esophagitis (8% vs 53%; P = .0001) are less severe in patients with cervical anastomosis. Although 86% of patients experienced excellent or very good late functional results, only 6% of patients who underwent cervical anastomosis had a Visick score of 3 or 4 versus 23% in patients with an intrathoracic anastomosis. Long-term function and quality-of-life assessment following esophagectomy identifies cervical anastomosis as a predictor of reduced reflux symptoms [107].

Considerations of resection of the primary tumor and particulars of reconstruction lead most surgeons to perform a thoracic esophagectomy with cervical or high intrathoracic anastomosis for thoracic esophageal cancers and cancers of the GEJ. For true gastric tumors invading the esophagus, distal esophagectomy and total gastrectomy may produce the best results [108, 109]. Squamous cell cancers of the cervical esophagus are generally unresectable because of location, but pharyngolaryngoesophagectomy may be considered in select patients. Alternatively, a limited resection with jejunal replacement may be used.

Regional lymph nodes

Unlike other tubular gastrointestinal organs or the lung, where lymphatic drainage is centripetal to the root of the mesentery or hilum, respectively, esophageal lymphatic drainage is longitudinal (Figure 35.18); i.e. lymphatic metastases develop orthogonal to tumor invasion [110]. Implications of the longitudinal nature of lymphatic drainage are that anatomic location of the primary cancer and

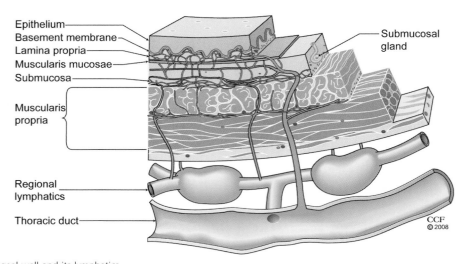

Figure 35.18 Esophageal wall and its lymphatics.

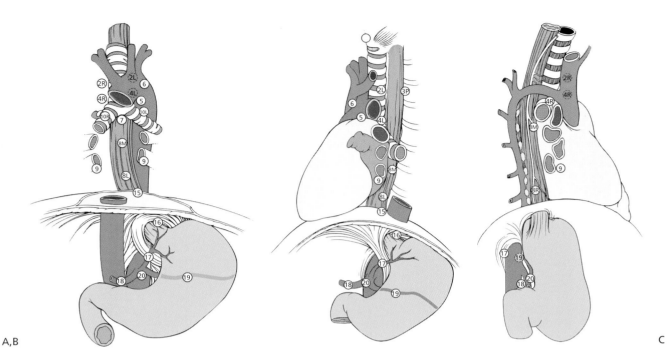

Figure 35.19 Lymph node map for esophageal cancer. (A) Anterior view. (B) Left lateral view. (C) Right lateral view. Lymph node stations: 1, pretracheal; 2R, right paratracheal; 2L, left paratracheal; 3P, posterior mediastinal; 4R, right tracheobronchial angle; 4L, left tracheobronchial; 5, aortopulmonary; 6, anterior mediastinal; 7, subcarinal; 8M, middle paraesophageal; 8L, lower paraesophageal; 9, inferior pulmonary ligament; 10, hilar; 15, diaphragmatic; 16, paracardial; 17, left gastric; 18, common hepatic; 19, splenic; 20, celiac.

location of the nodes to which lymphatics drain from that cancer may not coincide. For this reason, the definition of a regional lymph node now includes any periesophageal lymph node extending from cervical to celiac nodes (Figure 35.19) [5].

Although regional lymph nodes may be found scattered in the region of the extramural lymphatic network, they are generally concentrated. The majority of cervical lymph nodes are located about the recurrent laryngeal nerves and the carotid sheath. The major thoracic hub is located in the region of the tracheobronchial bifurcation and pulmonary hilum. These nodes drain both the esophagus and the lung, and the direction of lymph flow may be either cephalad or caudad. Below this, most lymph flow proceeds caudad. The major abdominal hub of regional lymph nodes is located at the GEJ, cardia, and lesser omentum. In contrast to the thoracic hub, it is more diffuse.

There are marked differences in the adventitial lymphatic system according to the side of the esophagus on which the lymphatic is found [111]. Lymphatic drainage from the right side of the esophagus is longitudinal and multistationed; longitudinal lymphatics are less well developed on the left side of the esophagus and frequently drain into the thoracic duct [111]. Existence of direct routes from mural and extramural lymphatics to the thoracic duct, without relay through regional lymph nodes, has been documented [112–114]; however, the exact patterns and occurrence of these pathways are highly variable.

It is a revolutionary concept that the esophagus comprises a single region drained by a lymphatic system that is not uniformly distributed, but it is a reality. The clinical implications of this redefinition are important for extent of lymphadenectomy.

Lymphadenectomy is a standard component of esophagectomy, but how extensive it should be for accurate cancer staging and to maximize survival is controversial. Only one study has examined the number of resected lymph nodes necessary to adequately predict positive lymph node classification (pN+) [115]. Although the sensitivity of classifying pN+ continued to improve up to 100 nodes examined, maximum increase of sensitivity occurred from zero to six nodes, and over 90% sensitivity was reached at 12.

Many recent studies have attempted to identify a specific number of lymph nodes that should be resected and examined to maximize survival (Table 35.3). These analyses examine goodness of fit or *P* values to test for a statistically significant effect of number of resected lymph nodes on survival. It is evident that no single number exists, but a range from greater than 10 to greater than 40 nodes was identified, depending on data source and method of analysis

Table 35.3 Number of lymph nodes resected to maximize survival (reproduced from Rice TW, Blackstone EH. Extent of lymph node dissection in esophageal cancer. In: Ferguson MK, ed. *Difficult Decisions in Thoracic Surgery*, 2nd edn. London: Springer, 2011, in press.)

Study	Source	Number of patients	Analysis	Number of lymph nodes	Grade
Twine *et al.* [116]	SI	237	MVA	>10	2A
Altorki1 *et al.* [117]	SI	264	MVA	>40 (stages I-II) >16 (stages III-IV)	2A
Rizk *et al.* [118]	SI	336	RPA	≥18	2A
Greenstein *et al.* [119]	SEER	977	MVA	≥18	1C
Groth *et al.* [120]	SEER	4882	RPA	>30	1B
Schwarz *et al.* [121]	SEER	5620	MVA	>30	1B
Chen *et al.* [122]	NODB	3144	MVA	12	1C
Peyre *et al.* [123]	International database	2303	MVA	23	1B

MVA, multivariable analysis; NODB, National Oncology Database; RPA, recursive partitioning analysis; SEER, Surveillance, Epidemiology and End Results program; SI, single institution.

[116–123]. Evidence from these studies, however, indicates that the number is greater than the typical US experience of 13 ± 9 nodes resected, as recently reported by the American College of Surgeons study group [124].

Rizk *et al.* used the modern machine learning technique random forests analysis in analyzing data from the Worldwide Esophageal Cancer Collaboration (WECC) [10] to identify the optimal lymphadenectomy to maximize 5-year survival [125]. This technique allows complex interactions among variables to be identified and can account for non-linear relationships, such as between T and N classifications. The recommendations based on this unique analysis are to resect a minimum of 10 lymph nodes for T1 cancers, 20 for T2, and 30 for T3.

Beyond a finite number of regional nodes, complications may limit the benefit of more extensive lymphadenectomy. Lymphadenectomy of more than 60 nodes was identified in a multivariable analysis of a single-center experience as an independent predictor of airway injury, as measured by postoperative tracheobronchial erosions, ulcers, and fistulae [126].

The anatomic extent of lymph node dissection is contentious. The possibility of cervical lymph node metastases from esophageal cancers has prompted use of three-field lymphadenectomy, which has variable definitions but includes a "two-field" lymphadenectomy (which also has a variable definition) and cervical dissection of lymph nodes in the region of recurrent laryngeal nerves, carotid artery and internal jugular vein, and supraclavicular nodes. The seminal paper of Akiyama *et al.* cited an occurrence of cervical nodal metastases of 46%, 29%, and 27% for primary squamous cell carcinomas of the upper, middle, and lower thoracic esophagus, respectively [127]. This analysis of a single-institution experience of 717 patients with R0 resections from a series of 913 esophagectomies for esophageal cancer has been the main evidence supporting three-field lymphadenectomy. The reported 5-year survival difference of 55% for three-field lymphadenectomy versus 38% for two-field lymphadenectomy ($P = .0013$) is attributed to lymphadenectomy extent. However, there is a temporal bias, because 393 patients underwent two-field lymphadenectomy from 1973 to 1984 and 324 underwent three-field lymphadenectomy from 1984 to 1993. This is also an unmatched comparison of highly selected patients whose characteristics are unstated and may differ between groups. The authors admit that the apparent effect on survival might be explained by stage migration in patients undergoing more extensive lymphadenectomy. This experience has prompted many single-institution studies that report "better than expected" results using three-field lymphadenectomy.

Kato *et al.* randomized surgeons who performed either three- or two-field lymphadenectomy to treat 150 esophageal cancer patients [128]. Compared with the two-field group, three-field patients were younger ($P < .05$) and had better 3-year survival (48% vs 34%; $P < .01$), respectively. The magnitude of improved lymph node staging was readily apparent. In the three-field group, 43 patients were cN+, 49 were pN+, 69 ± 6.9 nodes were resected, and 3.7 ± 6.8 nodes were positive; in two-field patients, these data were 46, 48, 36.4 ± 17.6, and 3.2 ± 4.3, respectively. Characteristics of the surgeons were not stated, but in-hospital mortality was five times greater for surgeons performing two-field lymphadenectomy ($P < .05$). In a nationwide survey conducted by the Japanese Society for Esophageal Diseases, 1791 patients underwent three-field lymphadenectomy and 2799 two-field lymphadenectomy. Survival analysis demonstrated a difference at 5 years of 34% versus 27%, respectively, but this difference was not seen in early- or advanced-stage patients [129]. These studies are two excellent examples of the three-field lymphadenectomy literature. The purported therapeutic benefit of three-field lymphadenectomy is just as possibly the result of patient selection, surgeon experience, and improved staging. No randomized studies have been performed to provide high-grade evidence for or against the necessity of three-field lymphadenectomy.

For upper thoracic and cervical esophageal cancers, a cervical dissection is required to sample lymph nodes directly in the region of the cancer. For accurate staging, there is no argument that three-field lymphadenectomy is superior to lesser lymphadenectomy. However, if the patient has been accurately staged with a lesser lymphadenectomy, there may be no need to perform three-field lymphadenectomy for staging. Patients with more than five lymph node metastases; simultaneous cervical, mediastinal, and abdominal metastases; or cervical lymph node metastases from lower thoracic esophageal cancers did not experience a survival benefit from three-field lymphadenectomy [130].

The importance of number of lymph nodes resected versus location of lymph node metastases has been examined in patients undergoing three-field lymphadenectomy [131]. Depth of tumor invasion was the sole predictor of survival; however, in a reanalysis restricted to lymph node factors only, number of lymph node metastases and abdominal lymph node metastases, but not cervical lymph node metastases, were predictors of survival.

Three-field lymphadenectomy may come with a price. In a review of 36 studies of three-field lymphadenectomy, 30-day mortality ranged from 0% to 3.7% and in-hospital mortality from 0% to 10.3% (average 4%) [132]. Complications occurred on average in 45% of patients (range 38–47%). The most frequent complication was sepsis (27%), half of which were secondary to anastomotic leak. In the nationwide Japanese survey, three-field lymphadenectomy was more likely than two-field lymphadenectomy to be compli-cated by recurrent laryngeal nerve palsy; 20% versus 14% ($P < .01$), respectively [129]. Three-field lymphadenectomy was identified in a multivariable analysis of a single-center experience as an independent predictor of airway injury as measured by postoperative tracheobronchial erosions, ulcers, and fistulae [126].

Transhiatal esophagectomy is at the other extreme of lymphadenectomy. A formal lymphadenectomy is not performed, and lymph node sampling is limited to a restricted area accessible only by abdominal and cervical incisions. However, three randomized trials could not demonstrate a survival difference when compared with transthoracic resections (Table 35.4) [133–136]. In subset analysis, patients undergoing transthoracic esophagectomy with 1one to eight nodes positive had better survival than those receiving a transhiatal esophagectomy [135, 136]. Again, this effect ascribed to therapy may also be explained by improved staging of pN1 and pN2 patients.

Reconstruction

The ideal esophageal substitute connects the esophagus to the stomach and replicates esophageal function. The stomach, however, is not an esophageal substitute. The esophagus shortened by resection maintains the upper sphincter and an abbreviated but peristaltic esophageal body. Advancing the stomach bridges the gap between the proximal esophagus and stomach. The stomach is freed from its abdominal attachments by dividing the short gastric and left gastric vasculature. The stomach, based on the right gastro-epiploic and right gastric arteries, is anastomosed to the esophagus. This represents reconstruction of the gastrointestinal tract and not esophageal replacement. Problems with this reconstruction stem from lack of a physiologic lower esophageal sphincter and a denervated intrathoracic stomach. The stomach may, indeed, lose its reservoir function. These difficulties may be overcome by surgical anasto-motic technique, constructing the anastomosis high in the chest or neck and draining the stomach with either a pyloroplasty or pyloromyotomy [137]. A change in eating habits,

Table 35.4 Randomized studies of transhiatal (THE) versus transthoracic (TTE) esophagectomy (reproduced from Rice TW, Blackstone EH. Extent of lymph node dissection in esophageal cancer. In: Ferguson MK, ed. *Difficult Decisions in Thoracic Surgery*, 2nd edn. London: Springer, 2011, in press.)

Study	Source	Number of patients	Differences for THE	Predictors of survival	Grade
Goldminc *et al.* [133]	SI	67	Shorter OR time	Lymph node metastases	2A
Chu *et al.* [134]	SI	39	Shorter OR time Increased OR hypotension	None	2A

Hulsher *et al.* [135]
  Omloo *et al.* [136]
	Two institutions	220	Fewer complications, shorter
			  ICU and hospital stays
			Fewer lymph nodes resected
				TTE provides survival
				  benefit for patients with
				  1 to 8 positive nodes
					1B

ICU, intensive care unit; OR, operating room; SI, single institution.

diet modification, and the use of acid suppression and prokinetic medication [138, 139] may be useful in dealing with postoperative problems of gastric reconstruction. Use of the stomach may result in difficulty with the distal resection margin and completeness of regional and non-regional lymphadenectomy [140]. Excessive gastric resection and denervation may limit the reservoir function of the stomach. A side-to-side anastomosis that uses endostapling technology has reduced anastomotic complications [141–143] (Figure 35.20). Prior fundoplication does not preclude the use of the stomach for esophageal reconstruction [144].

The colon was the first organ used for esophageal replacement. Only recently have long-term results become known. Advantages of colon replacement are few. Adequate length of colon is usually available. Blood supply, although less reliable than for the stomach, is easily assessed and generally adequate. Disadvantages of colon replacement are multiple. Preoperative evaluation and preparation of the colon are more demanding than evaluation or preparation of either the stomach or jejunum because of frequent intrinsic colonic disease and abundant bacterial colonization of the colon. Colon replacement is a more complex operation than either gastric or simple jejunal replacement. Three anastomoses are mandatory to re-establish gastrointestinal continuity in the colon and jejunal replacements; only one anastomosis is required in gastric substitution. Early complication of colonic graft necrosis is uniformly lethal if not recognized early and treated by excision of the colon replacement. There is a propensity to late complications, a result of limited acid resistance of the colonic mucosa, and a tendency of the colon replacement to dilate and form redundant loops. In the largest series with long-term follow-up of 69 patients with long-segment colon interpositions, 10% required anastomotic revision and 25% developed significant colonic redundancy [145].

The colon should be considered for esophageal replacement only in patients in whom the stomach is not available and who have potential for long-term survival with an otherwise functional gastrointestinal tract. The segment of colon used (i.e. right, transverse, or left) and the direction of replacement (i.e. isoperistaltic or antiperistaltic) are determined by the state of the colon and the surgeon's preference and experience.

Jejunum is the replacement of choice following distal esophagectomy and total gastrectomy. The reconstruction may be done as a simple loop with an end-to-side esophagojejunal anastomosis. To protect the esophagus from duodenal reflux, it is best to perform this reconstruction using a Roux-en-Y technique. If the stomach and colon are not available for esophageal reconstruction, then jejunum by default becomes the organ of choice. Mesenteric and not jejunal length is limiting in esophageal reconstruction. The arc of jejunum is based on a radiating arcade of mesenteric vessels, much like a parachute canopy (jejunum) and

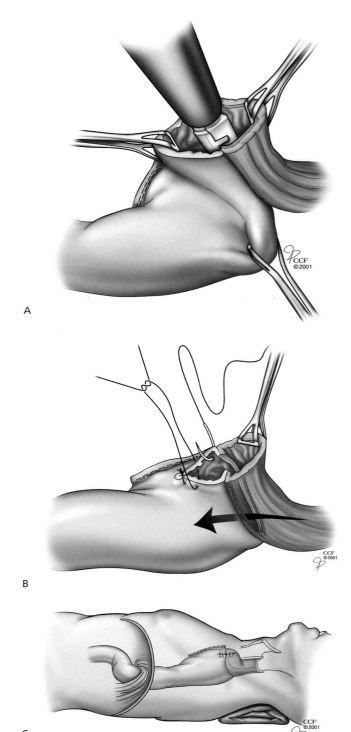

Figure 35.20 Current side-to-side cervical anastomotic technique. (A) Posterior portion of the anastomosis is constructed using a linear endoscopic stapler. (B) The anterior wall of the anastomosis is hand sewn; alternatively, it can be stapled with a standard linear stapler. (C) The anastomosis typically lies in the posterior mediastinum at the thoracic inlet.

shrouds (vessels) [146]. Dividing limbs of the vascular arcade may open the semicircular architecture of the vascular arcade. However, this makes the vasculature dependent on the distal limb of the artery and vein, eliminating the multiple channels of the arcade. In excess, this renders the blood supply inadequate, necessitating "supercharging" of the arterial supply and venous drainage with a microvascular anastomosis of the distal jejunal vessels to native vessels at the proximal anastomotic site [147, 148]. Alternatively, if an adequate length of vascular arcade is chosen, a redundant jejunal reconstruction results, necessitating jejunal resection, with preservation of the arcade in the mid-portion of the jejunal loop [149].

Route

The route of reconstruction can be posterior mediastinal in the bed of the esophagus, transpleural either anterior or posterior to the pulmonary hilum, substernal, or subcutaneous (Figure 35.21). The bed of the esophagus is the preferred route. It is the shortest and most direct route [150] and minimizes angulation of the anastomosis between the esophagus and organ of reconstruction. The thoracic inlet is sufficiently large to accommodate the stomach and colon. It is reported to have a lower incidence of cardiopulmonary and anastomotic complications [151]. However, it may not be available because of incomplete (R1 or R2) resection, previous inflammation, or scarring [152].

The substernal route is used when the posterior mediastinum is not available or when postoperative palliative radiation of the esophageal bed is required. This route usually requires excision of a portion of the manubrium, clavicular head, and first rib to prevent vascular compromise of the organ of reconstruction. Previous or planned anterior mediastinal or cardiac surgery may preclude its use. Transpleural

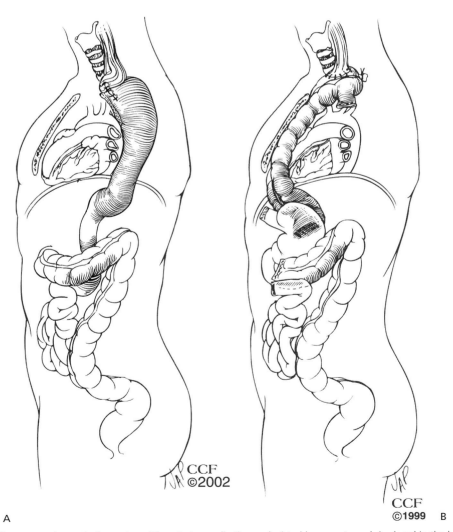

A

B

Figure 35.21 Routes of reconstruction typically used are (A) posterior mediastinum, depicted here as stomach is placed in the bed of the resected esophagus, and (B) substernal, depicted here as the colon is placed in the retrosternal tunnel.

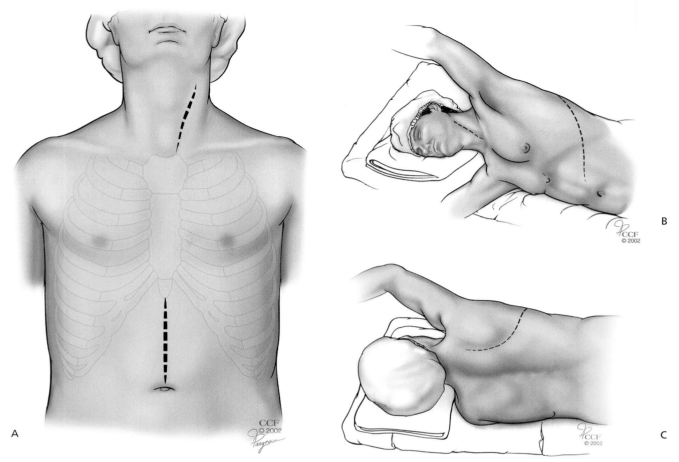

Figure 35.22 Surgical approaches are (A) esophagectomy without thoracotomy (transhiatal)—a midline laparotomy, and left cervical incisions are used; (B) esophagectomy with thoracotomy—thoracoabdominal alone requires a low intrathoracic anastomosis or with simultaneous cervical incision; and (C) right thoracotomy—with laparotomy Ivor–Lewis esophagectomy, with laparotomy and cervical incision McKeown esophagectomy.

and subcutaneous routes of reconstruction are rarely used and only as alternatives if the two principal routes are not available or acceptable.

Approach

Two options exist for open surgery: with thoracotomy (transthoracic) or without (transhiatal) (Figure 35.22). This presents considerable surgical philosophic controversy: should extensive (transthoracic) resection be used to improve long-term survival or should resection be curtailed (transhiatal) to reduce early mortality and morbidity? Thoracotomy allows controlled *en bloc* excision of thoracic esophageal cancers and an intrathoracic lymphadenectomy. Ivor–Lewis (laparotomy and right thoracotomy) or McKeown (laparotomy, right thoracotomy, and cervical incision) approaches are necessary to perform a complete thoracic lymphadenectomy. A left thoracotomy with division of the diaphragm, separate abdominal incision, or as part of a left thoracoabdominal incision, allows excellent exposure of the distal

thoracic esophagus and GEJ. It does, however, limit lymphadenectomy distal to the aortic arch and makes an intrathoracic anastomosis necessary unless a cervical incision is added. A transhiatal esophagectomy requires only an abdominal and thoracic incision. The thoracic esophagus is bluntly dissected through the esophageal hiatus and the cervical incision. This does not permit *en bloc* excision of the cancer or thoracic lymphadenectomy, but a thoracotomy is avoided. Meta-analysis of 24 reports comparing transthoracic and transhiatal esophagectomies shows an increase in pulmonary complications and postoperative mortality with transthoracic esophagectomy. Long-term survival is similar regardless of approach [153]. Randomized studies of transhiatal esophagectomy and esophagectomy with thoracotomy demonstrated similar hospital mortality and survival (overall, disease-free, and quality adjusted) [133–136] (Table 35.4). Operative morbidity was less with a transhiatal approach [135]. However, in patients with superficial esophageal cancer and in whom long-term prognosis is excellent and less dependent on cancer stage, a transhiatal approach is associated with improved survival [64].

Minimally invasive esophagectomy is in evolution and its place in treatment of esophageal cancer is being defined. Three approaches have emerged. The most radical borrows from obesity surgery and is a variant of an Ivor–Lewis esophagectomy [154]. A severely tailored stomach (gastric sleeve), which is constructed at laparoscopy, is anastomosed to the intrathoracic esophagus in the right chest in an end-to-side fashion via thoracoscopy. The anastomotic technique requires further sacrifice of the gastric tube to accomplish reconstruction and may result in a low intrathoracic anastomosis. The second approach reproduces an open McKeown esophagectomy, utilizing right thoracoscopy and laparoscopy for resection [155]. Either laparoscopy or a utility abdominal incision is used to prepare a classic gastric tube, which is then brought to the neck for anastomosis. The third approach is a minimally invasive variant of the transhiatal esophagectomy. Mediastinal dissection is performed transhiatally at laparoscopy [156] and may be assisted by mediastinoscopy performed through the neck incision [157].

Many single-institution studies have demonstrated that minimally invasive esophagectomy is technically feasible and safe, with outcomes similar to open esophagectomy. In highly selected experiences, minimally invasive esophagectomy has decreased blood loss and reduced hospital and ICU stays, but these comparative studies are retrospective and not matched, and no prospective studies have been performed comparing open and minimally invasive esophagectomy [158–160]. Port-site recurrence [161–163] and intracavitary tumor dissemination with pneumoperitoneum [164] are new problems introduced by this approach. It is our responsibility to carefully determine the role of minimally invasive esophagectomy so as not to repeat the laparoscopic experience with the treatment of hiatal hernia/GERD.

Results

Morbidity

Complications are common following esophagectomy. In a multi-institutional study of induction chemoradiotherapy versus surgery, Kelsen *et al.* reported major complications in 26% and minor complications in 31% of 217 patients undergoing surgery alone [165]. Walsh *et al.* reported 50 different complications in 55 patients undergoing resection of esophageal adenocarcinoma [166]. Complications occur during three distinct intervals: intraoperative, postoperative, and late.

Important intraoperative complications include hemorrhage, tracheobronchial injury, hypotension, and arrhythmias. Patients experiencing technical complications have an increased length of stay, associated medical complications, in-hospital mortality, and overall mortality compared to patients who do not [167]. Postoperative complications are dominated by pulmonary morbidity. However, anastomotic leakage, gastric or colonic necrosis, chylothorax, and recurrent laryngeal nerve injury are significant problems that impact outcome. Anastomotic leakage rates as high as 41% have been reported [168]. Although an anastomotic leak may be twice as common following cervical anastomosis as following intrathoracic anastomosis, mortality is three times greater following an intrathoracic leak [169]. Necrosis of the organ of esophageal reconstruction occurs in about 2% of gastric replacements and 10% of colon replacements, and is fatal in 90% [170]. Chylothorax is infrequent, occurring in fewer than 1% of patients, but carries a 50% mortality [168]. Prompt recognition and early surgical intervention with intrathoracic ligation of the thoracic duct are critical to good outcome [171]. Limiting the extent of cervical dissection and attention and care during cervical dissection can reduce the incidence of recurrent laryngeal nerve injury. The impact of this single complication on early and long-term outcome is enormous.

Late complications are dominated by gastrointestinal tract dysfunction. Anastomotic stricture occurs in 10–15% of patients and is successfully treated with dilation [172, 173]. An anastomotic leak is the most reliable predictor of an anastomotic stricture. Dumping, delayed gastric emptying, and reflux can be minimized by careful surgical technique. Gastrointestinal dysfunction can be managed successfully with dietary and lifestyle modifications, and judicious use of acid suppression and prokinetic medications.

Mortality

Postoperative mortality has decreased to a single digit level; most specialty centers have mortality rates less than 5%. Short-term outcome is greatly improved as volume [174–178] (measured by number of esophagectomies, number of operations, and hospital size) and surgeon's experience increase [179, 180]. Increasing volume and experience also decrease length of stay in both the intensive care unit and hospital. However, volume is a crude measure of outcome after esophagectomy and is not the best surrogate for mortality [181].

Long-term outcome is a function of stage and completeness of resection. A survey of 828 hospitals performing 5044 esophagectomies for cancer from 1994 to 1995 report 1-year survival of 71% for stage I, 57% for stage II, 41% for stage III, and 18% for stage IV [182]. More than half these patients received adjuvant therapy. For patients receiving surgery alone, survival is dependent on stage (Figure 35.23).

Recurrence

Following transhiatal esophagectomy used indiscriminately and without staging selection, approximately half the patients developed recurrent cancer during follow-up (median 24–27 months) [183, 184]. Median time to recurrence was 11 months [183, 184]; most were detected by 2

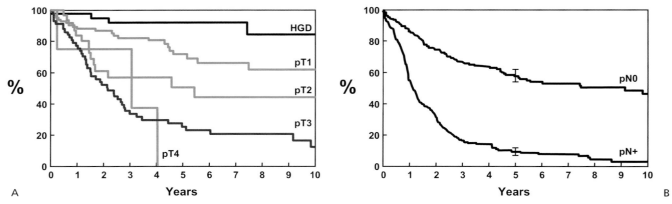

Figure 35.23 Kaplan–Meier survival estimates for (A) 252 N0M0 patients undergoing surgery alone stratified by pT and (B) for 395 patients undergoing surgery alone stratified by pN. HGD, high-grade dysplasia.

years [183]. The prevalence of recurrent carcinoma was similar for adenocarcinoma and squamous cell carcinoma. Recurrences were nearly equal in distribution among locoregional, distant, or both. Cervical lymph node recurrence was seen in only 8% of all patients [184]. Distant recurrences were found in the liver in 38%, in the bone in 25%, and in the lung in 18%. Recurrent carcinomas were associated with lymph node metastases, R1 resection, and poorly differentiated histology.

Data for recurrent cancer following two-field lymphadenectomy are remarkably similar. Forty-eight percent of patients, followed up for a mean of 26 months, experienced recurrent cancer [185]. Median time to recurrence was 12 months. There were no differences between adenocarcinoma and squamous cell carcinoma. Recurrent carcinoma was locoregional in 27% and distant in 18%.

Quality of life

Quality of life (QOL) deteriorates immediately following esophagectomy, but improves over time. Six weeks after surgery, patients reported a lessened QOL compared to that before surgery [186]. In patients who survived for more than 2 years, QOL returned to preoperative level by 9 months. For patients surviving less than 2 years, QOL never returned to preoperative levels. Patients undergoing minimally invasive esophagectomy reported an immediate deterioration of functional aspects of QOL and more symptoms compared to baseline [187]. Most patient experienced improvement by 3 months and returned to baseline by 6 months. At 1 year, 85% had recovered in more than 50% of the health-related QOL (HRQOL) domains. There is a direct relationship between improved QOL and increased survival [188]. As expected, sense of well-being is greater in patients with curative surgery.

Surgical technique may influence QOL. Patients undergoing palliative esophagectomy reported an improvement in diet (measured by type and quantity of food eaten) and

reduction of diet-related symptoms. This benefit was sometimes offset by a significant problem with pain [189]. QOL scores were significantly lower in these patients 6–9 months after esophagectomy than in patients with curative resections. Younger age, female gender, and intrathoracic anastomosis were all associated with decreased QOL [107]. The negative impact of recurrent nerve paralysis was profound and long lasting [190, 191]. The effects of patient education along with the support of other patients on the improvement of QOL are incalculable [192].

Compared to radiation, esophagectomy was twice as likely to improve swallowing and offers a survival advantage [193]. Although surgery was more costly than palliation, cost per month of survival were similar for both modalities [194].

Adjuvant therapy

Four randomized phase III trials comparing induction chemotherapy with cisplatin and fluorouracil and surgery versus surgery alone for esophageal cancer (Table 35.5) produced conflicting results. Law *et al.* reported chemotherapy was safe, resulting in significant downstaging (5% complete response, 36% partial response), and increased curative resections (67% vs 35%) in patients with squamous cell carcinoma [195]. Although survival of responders (median 42.2 months) was superior to the surgical group (median 13.8 months), there were no survival differences between the randomized treatment groups. Kelsen *et al.* reported that chemotherapy and surgery did not improve survival, resectability, or local control [165]. There were no differences between patients with squamous cell carcinoma or with adenocarcinoma [124]. Weight loss was a predictor of poor outcome. The Medical Research Council of England conducted a trial randomizing 802 patients with resectable esophageal cancer [196]. Patients receiving induction chemotherapy had an estimated 21% reduction in the risk of death. Median and 2-year survival was better in patients

Table 35.5 Phase III treatment trials for esophageal carcinoma.

Study	Cell type	Rx1	Rx2	Survival	Positive findings
Law et al. [195]	Squamous	Surg	Che/Surg	Same	↑ Downstaging Rx2 ↑ Curative Resection, Rx2
Kelsen et al. [165]	Both	Surg	Che/Surg	Same	—
Medical Research Council [196]	Both	Surg	Che/Surg	34% vs 43% (2 years, P = .004)	↓ T and N Rx2
Cunningham et al. [197]	Adeno	Surg	Che/Surg	23% vs 36% (5 year, P = .009)	↓ size and stage of resected cancer Rx2
Ando et al. [198]	Squ	Surg	Surg/Che	Same	
Walsh et al. [166]	Adeno	Surg	Che/Rad/Surg	6% vs 32% (3 years, P = .01)	↓ N+ and M1, Rx2
Bosset et al. [199]	Squ	Surg	Che/Rad/Surg	Same	↑ DF survival, Rx2
Urba et al. [200]	Both	Surg	Che/Rad/Surg	Same	↑ survival in responders
Tepper et al. [201]	Both	Surg	Che/Rad/Surg	16% vs 39% (5 year, P = .002)	
Stahl et al. [202]	Squ	Che/Rad	Che/Rad/Surg	24% vs 31% (3 year, P = .02)	↑ local control with addition of surgery
Macdonald et al. [207]	Adeno	Surg	Surg/Che/Rad	27 months vs 36 months (median, P = .005)	
Xiao et al. [208]	Squ	Surg	Surg/Rad	Same	Improved survival in N+

Adeno, adenocarcinoma; Che, chemotherapy; Rad, radiation therapy; Squ, squamous cell carcinoma; Surg, surgery; Rx1, control treatment; Rx2, adjuvant treatment; DF, disease-free.

receiving chemotherapy and surgery versus surgery alone, 512 days versus 405 days, and 43% versus 34%, respectively. This was accomplished without additional adverse events. It is not known whether this survival advantage persists long term. Cunningham et al. reported that chemotherapy and surgery improved survival in patients with adenocarcinoma (hazard ratio for death 0.75; 95% CI 0.60–0.93; P < .001) compared to surgery alone [197]. Five-year survival was 36% versus 23%, respectively (P = .009). Resected cancers were smaller and less advanced in the chemotherapy and surgery group.

Postoperative adjuvant chemotherapy with cisplatin and vindesine offers no survival advantage over surgery alone in patients with squamous cell carcinoma [198] (Table 35.5). Survival was similar even with stratification of N1 disease. The site of cancer recurrence was similar for both groups.

Four randomized phase III trials compared induction chemoradiotherapy and surgery versus surgery alone for esophageal cancer (Table 35.5). Walsh et al. reported patients with adenocarcinoma of the esophagus who received induction chemoradiotherapy (two courses of cisplatin and fluorouracil and 40 Gy of radiation) followed by surgery had an improved survival compared with those who had surgery alone [166]. Survival advantage was evident at 3 years (32% vs 6%; P = .01). Of patients receiving multimodality therapy, 42% had lymph node or distant metastases at surgery, in contrast to 82% of patients treated with surgery alone who had lymph node or distant metastases. The survival of patients treated with surgery only is much worse than expected from previous experience. Bosset et al. treated patients with squamous cell carcinoma of the esophagus with induction chemoradiotherapy (cisplatin and 18.5 Gy) plus surgery and with surgery alone [199]. Although there were no survival differences between the groups, patients receiving induction chemoradiotherapy had longer disease-free survival, longer local disease-free interval, lower rate of cancer-related deaths, and higher rate of curative resections. Multimodality therapy was associated with an increased postoperative mortality. Predictors of reduced survival were weight loss of greater than 5% of body weight, tumors located within 25 cm of the mandibular arch, N1 disease, and an incomplete resection. Urba et al. did a randomized study of induction chemoradiotherapy using cisplatin, 5-fluorouracil and vinblastine, and 45 Gy of radiotherapy [200]. No survival differences were apparent after a median of 8.2 years of follow-up. Tepper et al. reported improved median (4.5 vs 1.8 years, respectively; P = .002) and 5-year (39% vs 16%, respectively) survival in patients receiving chemoradiotherapy and surgery compared to those treated with surgery alone [201]. The addition of surgery to chemoradiotherapy improved local control but not survival in patients with squamous cell carcinoma of the esophagus (Table 35.5) [202]. Meta-analysis of the chemoradiotherapy and surgery literature demonstrates a survival advantage for chemoradiotherapy and surgery compared to surgery alone [203–206].

Macdonald *et al.* demonstrated improved survival in patients receiving postoperative adjuvant chemoradiotherapy (median survival 36 months vs 27 months, respectively; *P* = .005, Table 35.5) [207]. The hazard ratio for death in surgery only patients was 1.35 (95% CI 1.09–1.66; *P* = .005).

A randomized study of postoperative adjuvant radiotherapy performed in China without patient consent demonstrated no survival advantage for the entire study group as a whole [208]. However, in patients with locally advanced cancer (stage IIB and III cancer, sixth edition staging) a survival improvement was gained with adjuvant radiotherapy.

In earlier phase III studies, adjuvant therapy was offered regardless of stage. The conflicting results of many of these early studies are in part the result of non-selective adjuvant therapy.

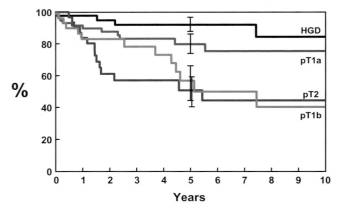

Figure 35.24 Kaplan–Meier survival estimates for N0M0 patients with tumor invasion confined to the esophageal wall. HGD, high-grade dysplasia, T1a, intramucosal cancer, T1b, submucosal cancer (reproduced from Rice *et al.* [11], with permission).

A treatment strategy

A single-treatment strategy for all patients with the spectrum of locoregionally contained esophageal carcinoma is outdated [209, 210]. A tailored, stage-dependent treatment of esophageal cancer is now possible with detection of cancer at an earlier stage by Barrett's surveillance, accurate clinical staging, advanced surgical techniques, and developments of new treatments. Since esophagectomy should be offered in the appropriate patient and done only with curative intent, treatment modifications according to stage are mandatory. One operation for all patients is an obsolete philosophy. It denies individual patients the benefits of personalized procedures and exposes them to unnecessary risk. The optimum operation should be chosen only after investigating both the patient and the cancer.

At one end of the cancer spectrum is high-grade dysplasia and intramucosal cancers. Surgery alone offers excellent survival [64, 211] (Figure 35.24). Regional lymph node metastases do not occur in patients with high-grade dysplasia and are uncommon (<5%) in patients with intramucosal cancer [212]. Radical lymphadenectomy, therefore, is not required and sampling of 10 regional lymph nodes is preferred [125]. In these patients, transhiatal esophagectomy minimizes morbidity and mortality, and should be considered if the tumor can be completely resected through the esophageal hiatus and lymph nodes sampled [64]. For these patients, the toxicity of adjuvant therapy outweighs any small survival advantage [14] (Figure 35.25).

At the opposite end of the cancer spectrum are marginally operable tumors because of either bulky T3 or T4 cancers or significant regional lymph node metastases (Figure 35.26). An incomplete resection (R1 and R2) is likely if surgery is the only treatment option. Surgery alone offers little hope of cure. Induction therapy downstages one-third of these patients and subsequent resection offers responders an

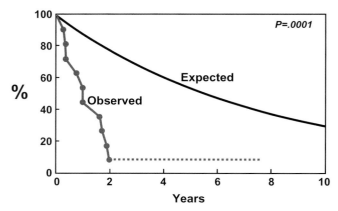

Figure 35.25 Observed and expected survival in patients with cT1N0 and cT2N0 carcinoma receiving induction therapy (reproduced from Rice *et al.* [14], with permission.)

intermediate survival [213, 214] (Figure 35.26). Downstaging may also improve resectability. Survival advantage in responders far outweighs the toxicity of treatment. Non-responders derive no benefit from therapy; however, presently these patients are difficult to identify preoperatively. In non-responders identified after induction therapy, surgery might be avoided and the best choice of palliation offered. In the future, preoperative identification of likely responders will further refine this approach.

Esophageal cancers that lie between these two ends of the spectrum affect many patients who have intermediate survival after surgery alone (see Figures 35.23 and 35.24). Once esophageal cancers have invaded the submucosa (T1b) or muscularis propria (T2), esophagectomy with lymphadenectomy is the procedure of choice for patients clinically staged as T1bN0M0 and T2N0M0. Thoracotomy facilitates the

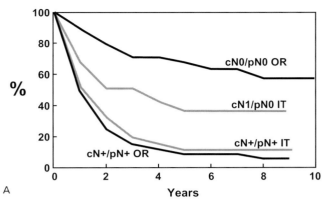

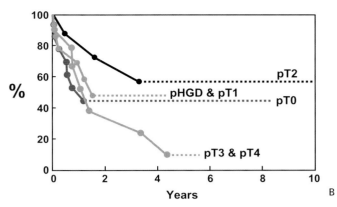

Figure 35.26 Effect of induction therapy. (A) Downstaging (cN1/pN0 IT) produces an intermediate survival compared to pN0 and pN1 patients undergoing surgery alone. Failure to downstage (cN1/pN1 IT) produces similar survival to pN1 patients undergoing surgery alone. (B) For cN1/pN0 patients, inability to achieve synchronous downstaging (pT3 and pT4) fails to impact survival. Synchronous downstaging of T and N homogenizes survival (reproduced from Rice *et al*. [213], with permission).

resection of these larger tumors and allows adequate lymphadenectomy. The incidence of regional lymph node metastases increases exponentially with increasing depth of tumor invasion, with at least 25% of T1b tumors and 50% of T2 tumors metastasizing to regional lymph nodes (N1) [212]. Because EUS accuracy in the determination of N is 80%, lymphadenectomy is mandatory to detect clinically occult N+ disease. The goal of lymphadenectomy is accurate pathologic staging; its impact on survival is controversial. In these patients a minimum of 10 (T1), 20 (T2), and 30 (T3) regional lymph nodes should be resected [125].

Resection followed by postoperative adjuvant therapy may be considered in the following clinical situations: (1) patients with incorrect clinical staging who have resection and are found to have more advanced disease (T3 or N+); and (2) patients with T3 or N+ cancers (few regional nodal metastases) who appear technically resectable (R0 resection possible) and are not candidates for induction therapy. In a propensity-matched study, postoperative adjuvant chemoradiotherapy improved survival in patients with locally advanced esophageal cancer [215] (Figure 35.27).

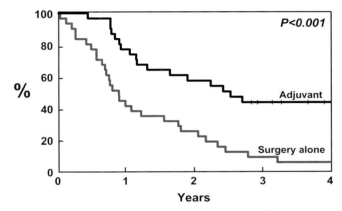

Figure 35.27 Survival in matched patients undergoing either surgery followed by adjuvant therapy or surgery alone. For surgery followed by adjuvant therapy, survival estimates, their standard error, and, in parentheses, number of patients remaining at risk at 1, 2, 3, and 4 years were 77 ± 7.5% (24), 58 ± 8.9% (17), 44 ± 9.0% (10), and 44 ± 9.0% (6), respectively. For surgery alone, these same statistics were 42 ± 8.9% (13), 26 ± 7.9% (8), 9.7 ± 5.3% (3), and 6.4 ± 4.4% (2), respectively (reproduced from Rice *et al*. [215], with permission).

Conclusions

Diagnosis and clinical staging of esophageal carcinoma is afforded by the combination of esophagoscopy and biopsy, EUS FNA, and CT PET scanning. Clinical staging is necessary to plan treatment. Patient selection and preparation are critical to minimizing operative morbidity and mortality. Surgery is the mainstay of curative therapy for esophageal carcinoma. Outcome in early-stage cancer is impacted by the surgical approach. In locally advanced cancer, the effect of stage overshadows operative approach. Surgery alone is unlikely to cure patients with locally advanced esophageal cancer. Recent randomized studies and meta-analysis of

adjuvant therapy report improved survival with this treatment. Multimodality therapy should be considered for select patients with locally advanced esophageal cancer.

References

1. Levine MS, Chu P, Furth EE, *et al*. Carcinoma of the esophagus and esophagogastric junction: sensitivity of radiographic diagnosis. *AJR Am J Roentgenol* 1997;168:1423–1426.
2. Faigel DO, Deveney C, Phillips D, *et al*. Biopsy-negative malignant esophageal stricture: diagnosis by endoscopic ultrasound. *Am J Gastroenterol* 1998;93:2257–2260.

3. Provenzale D, Schmitt C, Wong JB. Barrett's esophagus: a new look at surveillance based on emerging estimates of cancer risk. *Am J Gastroenterol* 1999;94:2043–2053.

4. Streitz JM Jr, Ellis FH Jr, Tilden RL, *et al*. Endoscopic surveillance of Barrett's esophagus: a cost-effectiveness comparison with mammographic surveillance for breast cancer. *Am J Gastroenterol* 1998;93:911–915.

5. American Joint Committee on Cancer. *AJCC Cancer Staging Manual*, 7th edn. New York: Springer, 2010.

6. International Union Against Cancer. *TNM Classification of Malignant Tumors*, 7th edn. Oxford: Wiley-Blackwell, 2009.

7. Rice TW, Rusch VW, Apperson-Hansen C, *et al*. Worldwide Esophageal Cancer Collaboration. *Dis Esoph* 2009;22:1.

8. Ishwaran H, Blackstone EH, Apperson-Hansen C, Rice TW. A novel approach to cancer staging: application to esophageal cancer. *Biostatistics* 2009;10:603–620.

9. Rice TW, Rusch VW, Ishwaran H, Blackstone EH. Cancer of the esophagus and esophagogastric junction: Data-driven staging for the 7th edition of the AJCC cancer staging manual. *Cancer* 2010;116:3763–3773.

10. Rice TW, Blackstone EH, Rusch VW. A cancer staging primer: esophagus and esophagogastric junction. *J Thorac Cardiovasc Surg* 2010;139:527–529.

11. Rice TW, Blackstone EH, Rybicki LA, *et al*. Refining esophageal cancer staging. *J Thorac Cardiovasc Surg* 2003;125:1103–1113.

12. Rosch T. Endosonographic staging of esophageal cancer: a review of literature results. *Gastrointest Endosc Clin North Am* 1995;5:537–547.

13. Saunders HS, Wolfman NT, Ott DJ. Esophageal cancer. Radiologic staging. *Radiol Clin North Am* 1997;35:281–294.

14. Rice TW, Blackstone EH, Adelstein DJ, *et al*. Role of clinically determined depth of tumor invasion in the treatment of esophageal carcinoma. *J Thorac Cardiovasc Surg* 2003;125:1091–1102.

15. Heidemann J, Schilling MK, Schmassmann A, *et al*. Accuracy of endoscopic ultrasonography in preoperative staging of esophageal carcinoma. *Dig Surg* 2000;17:219–224.

16. Rice TW, Mason DP, Murthy SC, *et al*. T2N0M0 esophageal cancer. *J Thorac Cardiovasc Surg*, 2007;133:317–324.

17. Pech O, Günter E, Dusemund F, *et al*. Accuracy of endoscopic ultrasound in preoperative staging of esophageal cancer: results from a referral center for early esophageal cancer. *Endoscopy*. 2010;42:456–461.

18. Kelly S, Harris KM, Berry E, *et al*. A systematic review of the staging performance of endoscopic ultrasound in gastrooesophageal carcinoma. *Gut* 2001;49:534–539.

19. Van Dam J, Rice TW, Catalano MF, *et al*. High-grade malignant stricture is predictive of esophageal tumor stage. Risks of endosonographic evaluation. *Cancer* 1993;71:2910–2917.

20. Pfau PR, Ginsberg GG, Lew RJ, *et al*. Esophageal dilation for endosonographic evaluation of malignant esophageal strictures is safe and effective. *Am J Gastroenterol* 2000;95:2813–2815.

21. Bhutani MS, Barde CJ, Markert RJ, *et al*. Length of esophageal cancer and degree of luminal stenosis during upper endoscopy predict T stage by endoscopic ultrasound. *Endoscopy* 2002;34:461–463.

22. Flanagan FL, Dehdashti F, Siegel BA, *et al*. Staging of esophageal cancer with 18F-fluorodeoxyglucose positron emission tomography. *AJR Am J Roentgenol* 1997;168:417–424.

23. Rankin SC, Taylor H, Cook GJ, *et al*. Computed tomography and positron emission tomography in the pre-operative staging of oesophageal carcinoma. *Clin Radiol* 1998;53:659–665.

24. Krasna MJ. Minimally invasive staging for esophageal cancer. *Chest* 1997;112:191S–194S.

25. Buenaventura P, Luketich JD. Surgical staging of esophageal cancer. *Chest Surg Clin North Am* 2000;10:487–497.

26. Krasna MJ, Mao YS, Sonett J, *et al*. The role of thoracoscopic staging of esophageal cancer patients. *Eur J Cardiothorac Surg* 1999;16 (Suppl 1):S31–S33.

27. Omloo JM, van Heijl M, Bergman JJ, *et al*. Value of bronchoscopy after EUS in the preoperative assessment of patients with esophageal cancer at or above the carina. *J Gastrointest Surg* 2008;12:1874–1879.

28. Catalano MF, Sivak MV Jr, Rice T, *et al*. Endosonographic features predictive of lymph node metastasis. *Gastrointest Endosc* 1994;40:442–446.

29. Wiersema MJ, Vilmann P, Giovannini M, *et al*. Endosonography-guided fine-needle aspiration biopsy: diagnostic accuracy and complication assessment. *Gastroenterology* 1997;112:1087–1095.

30. Reed CE, Mishra G, Sahai AV, *et al*. Esophageal cancer staging: improved accuracy by endoscopic ultrasound of celiac lymph nodes. *Ann Thorac Surg* 1999;67:319–321; discussion 322.

31. Eloubeidi MA, Wallace MB, Reed CE, *et al*. The utility of EUS and EUS-guided fine needle aspiration in detecting celiac lymph node metastasis in patients with esophageal cancer: a single-center experience. *Gastrointest Endosc* 2001;54:714–719.

32. Natsugoe S, Yoshinaka H, Shimada M, *et al*. Number of lymph node metastases determined by presurgical ultrasound and endoscopic ultrasound is related to prognosis in patients with esophageal carcinoma. *Ann Surg* 2001;234:613–618.

33. Chen J, Xu R, Hunt GC, *et al*. Influence of the number of malignant regional lymph nodes detected by endoscopic ultrasonography on survival stratification in esophageal adenocarcinoma. *Clin Gastroenterol Hepatol* 2006;4:573–579.

34. Twine CP, Roberts SA, Rawlinson CE, *et al*. Prognostic significance of the endoscopic ultrasound defined lymph node metastasis count in esophageal cancer. *Dis Esophagus* 2010;23:652–659.

35. van Overhagen H, Becker CD. Diagnosis and staging of carcinoma of the esophagus and gastroesophageal junction, and detection of postoperative recurrence, by computed tomography. In: Meyers M, ed. *Neoplasms of the Digestive Tract. Imaging, Staging and Management*. Philadelphia: Lippincott-Raven, 1998, pp. 31–48.

36. Doi N, Aoyama N, Tokunaga M, *et al*. Possibility of preoperative diagnosis of lymph node metastasis based on morphology. *Hepatogastroenterology* 1999;46:977–980.

37. Chandawarkar RY, Kakegawa T, Fujita H, *et al*. Comparative analysis of imaging modalities in the preoperative assessment of nodal metastasis in esophageal cancer. *J Surg Oncol* 1996;61:214–217.

38. Kato H, Kuwano H, Nakajima M, *et al*. Comparison between positron emission tomography and computed tomography in the use of the assessment of esophageal carcinoma. *Cancer* 2002;94:921–928.

39. Block MI, Patterson GA, Sundaresan RS, *et al*. Improvement in staging of esophageal cancer with the addition of positron emission tomography. *Ann Thorac Surg* 1997;64:770–776; discussion 776–777.

40. Kole AC, Plukker JT, Nieweg OE, *et al*. Positron emission tomography for staging of oesophageal and gastroesophageal malignancy. *Br J Cancer* 1998;78:521–527.

41. Luketich JD, Schauer PR, Meltzer CC, *et al*. Role of positron emission tomography in staging esophageal cancer. *Ann Thorac Surg* 1997;64:765–769.

42. Lerut T, Flamen P, Ectors N, *et al*. Histopathologic validation of lymph node staging with FDG-PET scan in cancer of the esophagus and gastroesophageal junction: a prospective study based on primary surgery with extensive lymphadenectomy. *Ann Surg* 2000;232:743–752.

43. Luketich JD, Friedman DM, Weigel TL, *et al*. Evaluation of distant metastases in esophageal cancer: 100 consecutive positron emission tomography scans. *Ann Thorac Surg* 1999;68:1133–1136.

44. Flamen P, Lerut A, Van Cutsem E, *et al*. The utility of positron emission tomography for the diagnosis and staging of recurrent esophageal cancer. *J Thorac Cardiovasc Surg* 2000;120:1085–1092.

45. Choi JY, Lee KH, Shim YM, *et al*. Improved detection of individual nodal involvement in squamous cell carcinoma of the esophagus by FDG PET. *J Nucl Med* 2000;41:808–815.

46. Gilbert TB, Goodsell CW, Krasna MJ. Bronchial rupture by a double-lumen endobronchial tube during staging thoracoscopy. *Anesth Analg* 1999;88:1252–1253.

47. Freeman RK, Wait MA. Port site metastasis after laparoscopic staging of esophageal carcinoma. *Ann Thorac Surg* 2001;71:1032–1034.

48. Luketich JD, Schauer P, Landreneau R, *et al*. Minimally invasive surgical staging is superior to endoscopic ultrasound in detecting lymph node metastases in esophageal cancer. *J Thorac Cardiovasc Surg* 1997;114:817–821.

49. Quint LE, Hepburn LM, Francis IR, *et al*. Incidence and distribution of distant metastases from newly diagnosed esophageal carcinoma. *Cancer* 1995;76:1120–1125.

50. Wernecke K, Rummeny E, Bongartz G, *et al*. Detection of hepatic masses in patients with carcinoma: comparative sensitivities of sonography CT, and MR imaging. *Am J Roentgenol* 1991;157:731–739.

51. Valls C, Lopez E, Guma A, *et al*. Helical CT versus CT arterial portography in the detection of hepatic metastasis of colorectal carcinoma. *AJR Am J Roentgenol* 1998;170:1341–1347.

52. Margolis ML, Howlett P, Bubanj R. Pulmonary nodules in patients with esophageal carcinoma. *J Clin Gastroenterol* 1998;26:245–248.

53. Gabrielsen TO, Eldevik OP, Orringer MB, *et al*. Esophageal carcinoma metastatic to the brain: clinical value and cost-effectiveness of routine enhanced head CT before esophagectomy. *AJNR Am J Neuroradiol* 1995;16:1915–1921.

54. O'Brien MG, Fitzgerald EF, Lee G, *et al*. A prospective comparison of laparoscopy and imaging in the staging of esophagogastric cancer before surgery. *Am J Gastroenterol* 1995;90:2191–2194.

55. Bonavina L, Incarbone R, Lattuada E, *et al*. Preoperative laparoscopy in management of patients with carcinoma of the esophagus and of the esophagogastric junction. *J Surg Oncol* 1997;65:171–174.

56. Heath EI, Kaufman HS, Talamini MA, *et al*. The role of laparoscopy in preoperative staging of esophageal cancer. *Surg Endosc* 2000;14:495–499.

57. Bemelman WA, van Delden OM, van Lanschot JJ, *et al*. Laparoscopy and laparoscopic ultrasonography in staging of carcinoma of the esophagus and gastric cardia. *J Am Coll Surg* 1995;181:421–425.

58. Romijn MG, van Overhagen H, Spillenaar Bilgen EJ, *et al*. Laparoscopy and laparoscopic ultrasonography in staging of oesophageal and cardial carcinoma. *Br J Surg* 1998;85:1010–1012.

59. Wakelin SJ, Deans C, Crofts TJ, *et al*. A comparison of computerised tomography, laparoscopic ultrasound and endoscopic ultrasound in the preoperative staging of oesophago-gastric carcinoma. *Eur J Radiol.* 2002;41:161–167.

60. Weaver SR, Blackshaw GR, Lewis WG, *et al*. Comparison of special interest computed tomography, endosonography and histopathological stage of oesophageal cancer. *Clin Radiol.* 2004;59:499–504.

61. Blackshaw G, Lewis WG, Hopper AN, *et al*. Prospective comparison of endosonography, computed tomography, and histopathological stage of junctional oesophagogastric cancer. *Clin Radiol.* 2008;63:1092–1098.

62. Walker AJ, Spier BJ, Perlman SB, *et al*. Integrated PET/CT fusion imaging and endoscopic ultrasound in the pre-operative staging and evaluation of esophageal cancer. *Mol Imaging Biol* 2010;13:166–171.

63. Bartels H, Stein HJ, Siewert JR. Risk analysis in esophageal surgery. *Recent Results Cancer Res* 2000;155:89–96.

64. Rice TW, Blackstone EH, Goldblum JR, *et al*. Superficial adenocarcinoma of the esophagus. *J Thorac Cardiovasc Surg* 2001;122:1077–1090.

65. Amar D, Burt ME, Bains MS, *et al*. Symptomatic tachydysrhythmias after esophagectomy: incidence and outcome measures. *Ann Thorac Surg* 1996;61:1506–1509.

66. Thomas P, Doddoli C, Neville P, et al. Esophageal cancer resection in the elderly. *Eur J Cardiothorac Surg* 1996;10:941–946.

67. Chino O, Makuuchi H, Machimura T, *et al*. Treatment of esophageal cancer in patients over 80 years old. *Surg Today* 1997;27:9–16.

68. Alexiou C, Beggs D, Salama FD, *et al*. Surgery for esophageal cancer in elderly patients: the view from Nottingham. *J Thorac Cardiovasc Surg* 1998;116:545–553.

69. Ellis FH Jr, Williamson WA, Heatley GJ. Cancer of the esophagus and cardia: does age influence treatment selection and surgical outcomes? *J Am Coll Surg* 1998;187:345–351.

70. Poon RT, Law SY, Chu KM, *et al*. Esophagectomy for carcinoma of the esophagus in the elderly: results of current surgical management. *Ann Surg* 1998;227:357–364.

71. Kinugasa S, Tachibana M, Yoshimura H, *et al*. Esophageal resection in elderly esophageal carcinoma patients: improvement in postoperative complications. *Ann Thorac Surg* 2001;71:414–418.

72. Fontes PR, Nectoux M, Escobar AG, *et al*. Is age a risk factor for esophagectomy? *Int Surg* 2001;86:94–96.

73. Sabel MS, Smith JL, Nava HR, *et al.* Esophageal resection for carcinoma in patients older than 70 years. *Ann Surg Oncol* 2002;9:210–214.

74. Moskovitz AH, Rizk NP, Venkatraman E, *et al.* Mortality increases for octogenarians undergoing esophagogastrectomy for esophageal cancer. *Ann Thorac Surg* 2006;82:2031–2036.

75. Ruol A, Portale G, Castoro C, *et al.* Management of esophageal cancer in patients aged over 80 years. *Eur J Cardiothorac Surg* 2007;32:445–448.

76. Braiteh F, Correa AM, Hofstetter WL, *et al.* Association of age and survival in patients with gastroesophageal cancer undergoing surgery with or without preoperative therapy. *Cancer* 2009;115:4450–4458.

77. Finlayson E, Fan Z, Birkmeyer JD. Outcomes in octogenarians undergoing high-risk cancer operation: a national study. *J Am Coll Surg* 2007;205:729–734.

78. Greenstein AJ, Litle VR, Swanson SJ, *et al.* Racial disparities in esophageal cancer treatment and outcomes. *Ann Surg Oncol* 2008;15:881–888.

79. Bollschweiler E, Schroder W, Holscher AH, *et al.* Preoperative risk analysis in patients with adenocarcinoma or squamous cell carcinoma of the oesophagus. *Br J Surg* 2000; 87:1106–1110.

80. Ferguson MK, Durkin AE. Preoperative prediction of the risk of pulmonary complications after esophagectomy for cancer. *J Thorac Cardiovasc Surg* 2002;123:661–669.

81. Crozier TA, Sydow M, Siewert JR, *et al.* Postoperative pulmonary complication rate and long-term changes in respiratory function following esophagectomy with esophagogastrostomy. *Acta Anaesthesiol Scand* 1992;36:10–15.

82. Feeney C, Hussey J, Carey M, Reynolds J. Assessment of physical fitness for esophageal surgery, and targeting interventions to optimize. *Dis Esophagus* 2010;23:529–539.

83. Gillinov AM, Heitmiller RF. Strategies to reduce pulmonary complications after transhiatal esophagectomy. *Dis Esophagus* 1998;11:43–47.

84. Avendano CE, Flume PA, Silvestri GA, *et al.* Pulmonary complications after esophagectomy. *Ann Thorac Surg* 2002;73: 922–926.

85. Whooley BP, Law S, Murthy SC, *et al.* Analysis of reduced death and complication rates after esophageal resection. *Ann Surg* 2001;233:338–344.

86. Vaporciyan AA, Merriman KW, Ece F, *et al.* Incidence of major pulmonary morbidity after pneumonectomy: association with timing of smoking cessation. *Ann Thorac Surg* 2002;73:420–425; discussion 425–426.

87. Nakagawa M, Tanaka H, Tsukuma H, *et al.* Relationship between the duration of the preoperative smoke-free period and the incidence of postoperative pulmonary complications after pulmonary surgery. *Chest* 2001;120:705–710.

88. Ritchie AJ, Whiteside M, Tolan M, *et al.* Cardiac dysrhythmia in total thoracic oesophagectomy. A prospective study. *Eur J Cardiothorac Surg* 1993;7:420–422.

89. Nagamatsu Y, Shima I, Yamana H, *et al.* Preoperative evaluation of cardiopulmonary reserve with the use of expired gas analysis during exercise testing in patients with squamous cell carcinoma of the thoracic esophagus. *J Thorac Cardiovasc Surg* 2001;121:1064–1068.

90. Stein HJ, Brucher BL, Sendler A, *et al.* Esophageal cancer: patient evaluation and pre-treatment staging. *Surg Oncol* 2001; 10:103–111.

91. Naunheim KS, Hanosh J, Zwischenberger J, *et al.* Esophagectomy in the septuagenarian. *Ann Thorac Surg* 1993;56:880–883; discussion 883–884.

92. Bartels H, Stein HJ, Siewert JR. Preoperative risk analysis and postoperative mortality of oesophagectomy for resectable oesophageal cancer. *Br J Surg* 1998;85:840–844.

93. Tachibana M, Kotoh T, Kinugasa S, *et al.* Esophageal cancer with cirrhosis of the liver: results of esophagectomy in 18 consecutive patients. *Ann Surg Oncol* 2000;7:758–763.

94. Lu MS, Liu YH, Wu YC, *et al.* Is it safe to perform esophagectomy in esophageal cancer patients combined with liver cirrhosis. *Interactive Cardiovasc Thorac Surg* 2005;4:423–425.

95. Miller C. Carcinoma of thoracic oesophagus and cardia. A review of 405 cases. *Br J Surg* 1962;49:507–522.

96. Tam PC, Siu KF, Cheung HC, *et al.* Local recurrences after subtotal esophagectomy for squamous cell carcinoma. *Ann Surg* 1987;205:189–194.

97. Law S, Àrcilla C, Chu KM, *et al.* The significance of histologically infiltrated resection margin after esophagectomy for esophageal cancer. *Am J Surg* 1998;176:286–290.

98. Casson AG, Darnton SJ, Subramanian S, *et al.* What is the optimal distal resection margin for esophageal carcinoma? *Ann Thorac Surg* 2000;69:205–209.

99. McManus K, Anikin V, McGuigan J. Total thoracic oesophagectomy for oesophageal carcinoma: has it been worth it? *Eur J Cardiothorac Surg* 1999;16:261–265.

100. Kuwano H, Masuda N, Kato H, *et al.* The subepithelial extension of esophageal carcinoma for determining the resection margin during esophagectomy: a serial histopathologic investigation. *Surgery* 2002;131:S14–S21.

101. Tsutsui S, Kuwano H, Watanabe M, *et al.* Resection margin for squamous cell carcinoma of the esophagus. *Ann Surg* 1995;222: 193–202.

102. Kato H, Tachimori Y, Watanabe H, *et al.* Anastomotic recurrence of oesophageal squamous cell carcinoma after transthoracic oesophagectomy. *Eur J Surg* 1998;164:759–764.

103. Dexter SP, Sue-Ling H, McMahon MJ, *et al.* Circumferential resection margin involvement: an independent predictor of survival following surgery for oesophageal cancer. *Gut* 2001;48: 667–670.

104. Kyriazanos ID, Tachibana M, Yoshimura H, *et al.* Impact of splenectomy on the early outcome after oesophagectomy for squamous cell carcinoma of the oesophagus. *Eur J Surg Oncol* 2002;28:113–119.

105. Jeyasingham K. Long-term results of colon replacement. In: Pearson FG, Cooper JD, Deslauriers J, *et al.*, eds. *Esophageal Surgery*, 2nd edn. Philadelphia: Churchill Livingstone, 2002, pp. 931–937.

106. De Leyn P, Vansteenkiste J, Deneffe G, *et al.* Result of induction chemotherapy followed by surgery in patients with stage IIIA N2 NSCLC: importance of pre-treatment mediastinoscopy. *Eur J Cardiothorac Surg* 1999;15:608–614.

107. McLarty AJ, Deschamps C, Trastek VF, *et al.* Esophageal resection for cancer of the esophagus: long-term function and quality of life. *Ann Thorac Surg* 1997;63:1568–1572.

108. Siewert JR, Stein HJ. Adenocarcinoma of the gastroesophageal junction. Classification, pathology and extent of resection. *Dis Esophagus* 1996;9:173–182.

109. Stein HJ, Feith M, Siewert JR. Individualized surgical strategies for cancer of the esophagogastric junction. *Ann Chir Gynaecol* 2000;89:191–198.

110. Akiyama H, Tsurumaru M, Kawamura T, Ono Y. Principles of surgical treatment for carcinoma of the esophagus: analysis of lymph node involvement. *Ann Surg* 1981;194: 438–446.

111. Saito H, Sato T, Miyazaki M. Extramural lymphatic drainage from the thoracic esophagus based on minute cadaveric dissections: fundamentals for the sentinel node navigation surgery for the thoracic esophageal cancers. *Surg Radiol Anat* 2007;29:531–542.

112. Riquet M, Le Pimpec Barthes F, Souilamas R, Hidden G. Thoracic duct tributaries from intrathoracic organs. *Ann Thorac Surg* 2002;73:892–898.

113. Kuge K, Murakami G, Mizobuchi S, *et al.* Submucosal territory of the direct lymphatic drainage system to the thoracic duct in the human esophagus. *J Thorac Cardiovasc Surg* 2003;125: 1343–1349.

114. Murakami G, Sato I, Shimada KC, *et al.* Direct lymphatic drainage from the esophagus into the thoracic duct. *Surg Radiol Anat* 1994;16:399–407.

115. Dutkowski P, Hommel G, Böttger T, *et al.* How many lymph nodes are needed for an accurate pN classification in esophageal cancer? Evidence for a new threshold value. *Hepatogastroenterology* 2002;49:176–180.

116. Twine CP, Lewis WG, Morgan MA, *et al.* The assessment of prognosis of surgically resected oesophageal cancer is dependent upon the number of lymph nodes examined pathologically. *Histopathology* 2008;55:46–52.

117. Altorki NK, Zhou XK, Stiles B, *et al.* Total number of resected lymph nodes predicts survival in esophageal cancer. *Ann Surg* 2008;248:221–226.

118. Rizk N, Venkatraman E, Park B, *et al.* The prognostic importance of the number of involved lymph nodes in esophageal cancer: implications for revisions of the American Joint Committee on Cancer staging system. *J Thorac Cardiovasc Surg* 2006;132:1374–1381.

119. Greenstein AJ, Litle VR, Swanson SJ, *et al.* Effect of the number of lymph nodes sampled on postoperative survival of lymph node-negative esophageal cancer. *Cancer* 2008;112: 1239–1246.

120. Groth SS, Virnig BA, Whitson BA, *et al.* Determination of the minimum number of lymph nodes to examine to maximize survival in patients with esophageal carcinoma: data from the Surveillance Epidemiology and End Results database. *J Thorac Cardiovasc Surg* 2010;139:612–620.

121. Schwarz RE, Smith DD. Clinical impact of lymphadenectomy extent in resectable esophageal cancer. *J Gastrointest Surg* 2007;11:1384–1393.

122. Chen YJ, Schultheiss TE, Wong JY, Kernstine KH. Impact of the number of resected and involved lymph nodes on esophageal cancer survival. *J Surg Oncol* 2009;100:127–132.

123. Peyre CG, Hagen JA, DeMeester SR, *et al.* The number of lymph nodes removed predicts survival in esophageal cancer: an international study on the impact of extent of surgical resection. *Ann Surg* 2008;248:549–556.

124. Veeramachaneni NK, Zoole JB, Decker PA, *et al.* Lymph node analysis in esophageal resection: American College of Surgeons Oncology Group Z0060 trial. *Ann Thorac Surg* 2008;86: 418–421.

125. Rizk NP, Ishwaran H, Rice TW, *et al.* Optimum lymphadenectomy for esophageal cancer. *Ann Surg* 2009;250:1–5.

126. Maruyama K, Motoyama S, Sato Y. Tracheobronchial lesions following esophagectomy: erosions, ulcers, and fistulae, and the predictive value of lymph node-related factors. *World J Surg* 2009;33:778–784.

127. Akiyama H, Tsurumaru M, Udagawa H, Kajiyama Y. Radical lymph node dissection for cancer of the thoracic esophagus. *Ann Surg* 1994;220:364–372.

128. Kato H, Watanabe H, Tachimori Y, Iizuka T. Evaluation of neck node dissection for thoracic esophageal carcinoma. *Ann Thorac Surg* 1991;51:931–935.

129. Isono K, Sato H, Nakayama K. Results of a nationwide study on the three-field lymph node dissection of esophageal cancer. *Oncology* 1991;48:411–420.

130. Nishimaki T, Suzuki T, Suzuki S, *et al.* Outcomes of extended radical esophagectomy for thoracic esophageal cancer. *J Am Coll Surg* 1998;186:306–312.

131. Shimada H, Okazumi S, Matsubara H, *et al.* Impact of the number and extent of positive lymph nodes in 200 patients with thoracic esophageal squamous cell carcinoma after three-field lymph node dissection. *World J Surg* 2006;30: 1441–1449.

132. Tachibana M, Kinugasa S, Yoshimura H, *et al.* Extended esophagectomy with 3-field lymph node dissection for esophageal cancer. *Arch Surg* 2003;138:1383–1389.

133. Goldminc M, Maddern G, Le Prise E, *et al.* Oesophagectomy by a transhiatal approach or thoracotomy: a prospective randomized trial. *Br J Surg* 1993;80:367–370.

134. Chu KM, Law SY, Fok M, Wong J. A prospective randomized comparison of transhiatal and transthoracic resection for lower-third esophageal carcinoma. *Am J Surg* 1997; 174:320–324.

135. Hulscher JB, van Sandick JW, de Boer AG, *et al.* Extended transthoracic resection compared with limited transhiatal resection for adenocarcinoma of the esophagus. *N Engl J Med* 2002;347:1662–1669.

136. Omloo JM, Lagarde SM, Hulscher JB, *et al.* Extended transthoracic resection compared with limited transhiatal resection for adenocarcinoma of the mid/distal esophagus: five-year survival of a randomized clinical trial. *Ann Surg* 2007; 246:992–1000.

137. Law S, Cheung MC, Fok M, *et al.* Pyloroplasty and pyloromyotomy in gastric replacement of the esophagus after esophagectomy: a randomized controlled trial. *J Am Coll Surg* 1997;184: 630–636.

138. Gutschow CA, Collard JM, Romagnoli R, *et al.* Bile exposure of the denervated stomach as an esophageal substitute. *Ann Thorac Surg* 2001;71:1786–1791.

139. Nakabayashi T, Mochiki E, Garcia M, *et al.* Gastropyloric motor activity and the effects of erythromycin given orally after esophagectomy. *Am J Surg* 2002;183:317–323.

140. Schroder W, Baldus SE, Monig SP, *et al.* Lesser curvature lymph node metastases with esophageal squamous cell carcinoma: implications for gastroplasty. *World J Surg* 2001;25: 1125–1128.

141. Singh D, Maley RH, Santucci T, *et al.* Experience and technique of stapled mechanical cervical esophagogastric anastomosis. *Ann Thorac Surg* 2001;71:419–424.

142. Orringer MB, Marshall B, Iannettoni MD. Eliminating the cervical esophagogastric anastomotic leak with a side-to-side stapled anastomosis. *J Thorac Cardiovasc Surg* 2000;119:277–288.

143. Ercan S, Rice TW, Murthy SDC, *et al.* Does esophagogastric anastomotic technique influence the outcome of patients with esophageal xcancer? *J Thorac Cardiovasc Surg* 2005;129:623–631.

144. Casson AG, Madani K, Mann S, *et al.* Does previous fundoplication alter the surgical approach in esophageal adenocarcinoma. *Eur J Cardiothoracic Surg* 2008;34:1097–1101.

145. Jeyasingham K, Lerut T, Belsey RH. Revisional surgery after colon interposition for benign oesophageal disease. *Dis Esophagus* 1999;12:7–9.

146. Hiebert CA, Bredenberg CE. Selection and placement of conduits. In: Pearson FG, Cooper JD, Deslauriers J, *et al.*, eds. *Esophageal Surgery*, 2nd edn. Philadelphia: Churchill Livingstone, 2002, pp. 794–801.

147. Fujita H, Yamana H, Sueyoshi S, *et al.* Impact on outcome of additional microvascular anastomosis-supercharge-on colon interposition for esophageal replacement: comparative and multivariate analysis. *World J Surg* 1997;21:998–1003.

148. Golshani SD, Lee C, Cass D, *et al.* Microvascular "supercharged" cervical colon: minimizing ischemia in esophageal reconstruction. *Ann Plast Surg* 1999;43:533–538.

149. Wong J. The use of small bowel for oesophageal replacement following oesophageal resection. In: Jamieson GG, ed. *Surgery of the Esophagus*. New York: Churchill Livingstone, 1988, pp. 749–760.

150. Maillard JN, Hay JM. Surgical anatomy of available routes for oesophageal bypass. In: Jamieson GG, ed. *Surgery of the Esophagus*. New York: Churchill Livingstone, 1988, pp. 721–726.

151. Urschel JD. Does the interponat affect outcome after esophagectomy for cancer? *Dis Esophagus* 2001;14:124–130.

152. DiPierro FV, Rice TW, DeCamp MM, *et al.* Esophagectomy and staged reconstruction. *Eur J Cardiothorac Surg* 2000;17:702–709.

153. Hulscher JB, Tijssen JG, Obertop H, *et al.* Transthoracic versus transhiatal resection for carcinoma of the esophagus: a metaanalysis. *Ann Thorac Surg* 2001;72:306–313.

154. Nguyen NT, Follette DM, Lemoine PH, *et al.* Minimally invasive Ivor Lewis esophagectomy. *Ann Thorac Surgery* 2001;72: 593–596.

155. Luketich JD, Alvelo-Rivera M, Buenaventura PO, *et al.* Minimally invasive esophagectomy: outcome in 222 patients. *Ann Thorac Surg* 2003;238:486–495.

156. Benzoni E, Bresadola V, Terrosu G, *et al.* Minimally invasive esophagectomy: a comparative study of transhiatal laparoscopic right transthoracic esophagectomy. *Surg Laparosc Endosc Percutan Tech* 2008;2:178–187.

157. Bonavina L, Incarbone R, Bona D, Peracchia A. Esophagectomy via laparoscopy and transmediastinal endodissection *J Laparoendosc Adv Surg Tech* 2004;14:13–16.

158. Biere SS, Cuesta MA, van der Peet DL. Minimally invasive versus open esophagectomy for cancer: a systematic review and meta-analysis. *Minerva Chirurgica* 2009;64:121–133.

159. Verhage RJ, Hazebroek EJ, Boone J, Van Hillegersberg R. Minimally invasive esophagectomy compared to open procedures in esophagectomy for cancer: a systematic review of the literature. *Minerva Chir* 2009;64:135–146.

160. Smithers BM. Minimally invasive esophagectomy: an overview. *Exp Rev Gastroenterol Hepatol* 2010;4:91–99.

161. Dixit AS, Martin CJ, Flynn P Port-site recurrence after thoracoscopic resection of oesophageal cancer. *Aust NZ J Surg* 1997;67:148–149.

162. Ziprin P, Ridgway PF, Peck DH, *et al.* The theories and realities of port-site metastases: a critical appraisal. *J Am Coll Surg* 2002;195:395–408.

163. Yamamoto S, Kawahara K, Maekawa T, *et al.* The port site recurrence after a thoracoscopic and video-assisted esophagectomy for advanced esophageal cancer. *J Thorac Oncol* 2009;4: 131–134.

164. Segalin A. Parietal seeding of esophageal cancer after thoracoscopic resection. *Dis Esophagus* 1994;7:64–65.

165. Kelsen DP, Ginsberg R, Pajak TF, *et al.* Chemotherapy followed by surgery compared with surgery alone for localized esophageal cancer. *N Engl J Med* 1998;339:1979–1984.

166. Walsh TN, Noonan N, Hollywood D, *et al.* A comparison of multimodal therapy and surgery for esophageal adenocarcinoma. *N Engl J Med* 1996;335:462–467.

167. Rizk NP, Bach PB, Schrag D, *et al.* The impact of complications on outcomes after resection for esophageal and gastroesophageal junction carcinoma. *J Am Coll Surg.* 2004;198: 42–50.

168. Bains MS. Complications of abdominal right-thoracic (Ivor Lewis) esophagectomy. *Chest Surg Clin North Am* 1997;7:587–598; discussion 598–599.

169. Muller JM, Erasmi H, Stelzner M, *et al.* Surgical therapy of oesophageal carcinoma. *Br J Surg* 1990;77:845–857.

170. Horvath OP, Lukacs L, Cseke L. Complications following esophageal surgery. *Recent Results Cancer Res* 2000;155:161–173.

171. Cerfolio RJ, Allen MS, Deschamps C, *et al.* Postoperative chylothorax. *J Thorac Cardiovasc Surg* 1996;112:1361–1365; discussion 1365–1366.

172. Gandhi SK, Naunheim KS. Complications of transhiatal esophagectomy. *Chest Surg Clin North Am* 1997;7:601–610; discussion 611–612.

173. Sherry KM. How can we improve the outcome of oesophagectomy? *Br J Anaesth* 2001;86:611–613.

174. Birkmeyer JD, Siewers AE, Finlayson EV, *et al.* Hospital volume and surgical mortality in the United States. *N Engl J Med* 2002;346:1128–1137.

175. Kuo EY, Chang Y, Wright CD. Impact of hospital volume on clinical and economic outcomes for esophagectomy. *Ann Thorac Surg* 2001;72:1118–1124.

176. Swisher SG, Deford L, Merriman KW, *et al.* Effect of operative volume on morbidity, mortality, and hospital use after

esophagectomy for cancer. *J Thorac Cardiovasc Surg* 2000;119: 1126–1132.

177. van Lanschot JJ, Hulscher JB, Buskens CJ, *et al*. Hospital volume and hospital mortality for esophagectomy. *Cancer* 2001;91:1574–1578.

178. Dimick JB, Pronovost PJ, Cowan JA, *et al*. Surgical volume and quality of care for esophageal resection: do high-volume hospitals have fewer complications? *Ann Thorac Surg* 2003;75: 337–341.

179. Matthews HR, Powell DJ, McConkey CC. Effect of surgical experience on the results of resection for oesophageal carcinoma. *Br J Surg* 1986;73:621–623.

180. Miller JD, Jain MK, de Gara CJ, *et al*. Effect of surgical experience on results of esophagectomy for esophageal carcinoma. *J Surg Oncol* 1997;65:20–21.

181. Rice TW, Blackstone EH. Esophagectomy volume threshold as a criterion for centers of excellence: causation or cause, strategy or strategem? *J Thorac Cardiovasc Surg* 2009;137: 10–12.

182. Daly JM, Fry WA, Little AG, *et al*. Esophageal cancer: results of an American College of Surgeons Patient Care Evaluation Study. *J Am Coll Surg* 2000;190:562–572; discussion 572–573.

183. van Sandick JW, van Lanschot JJ, ten Kate FJ, *et al*. Indicators of prognosis after transhiatal esophageal resection without thoracotomy for cancer. *J Am Coll Surg* 2002;194:28–36.

184. Hulscher JB, van Sandick JW, Tijssen JG, *et al*. The recurrence pattern of esophageal carcinoma after transhiatal resection. *J Am Coll Surg* 2000;191:143–148.

185. Dresner SM, Griffin SM. Pattern of recurrence following radical oesophagectomy with two-field lymphadenectomy. *Br J Surg* 2000;87:1426–1433.

186. Blazeby JM, Farndon JR, Donovan J, *et al*. A prospective longitudinal study examining the quality of life of patients with esophageal carcinoma. *Cancer* 2000;88: 1781–1787.

187. Parameswaran R, Blazeby JM, Hughes R, *et al*. Health-quality of life after minimally invasive esophagectomy. *Br J Surg* 2010;97:525–531.

188. Blazeby JM, Brookes ST, Alderson D. The prognostic value of quality of life scores during treatment for oesophageal cancer. *Gut* 2001;49:227–230.

189. Branicki FJ, Law SY, Fok M, *et al*. Quality of life in patients with cancer of the esophagus and gastric cardia: a case for palliative resection. *Arch Surg* 1998;133:316–322.

190. Baba M, Aikou T, Natsugoe S, *et al*. Quality of life following esophagectomy with three-field lymphadenectomy for carcinoma, focusing on its relationship to vocal cord palsy. *Dis Esophagus* 1998;11:28–34

191. Baba M, Natsugoe S, Shimada M, *et al*. Does hoarseness of voice from recurrent nerve paralysis after esophagectomy for carcinoma influence patient quality of life? *J Am Coll Surg* 1999;188:231–236.

192. Kirby JD. Quality of life after oesophagectomy: the patients' perspective. *Dis Esophagus* 1999;12:168–171.

193. Badwe RA, Sharma V, Bhansali MS, *et al*. The quality of swallowing for patients with operable esophageal carcinoma: a randomized trial comparing surgery with radiotherapy. *Cancer* 1999;85:763–768.

194. Farndon MA, Wayman J, Clague MB, *et al*. Cost-effectiveness in the management of patients with oesophageal cancer. *Br J Surg* 1998;85:1394–1398.

195. Law S, Fok M, Chow S, *et al*. Preoperative chemotherapy versus surgical therapy alone for squamous cell carcinoma of the esophagus: a prospective randomized trial. *J Thorac Cardiovasc Surg* 1997;114:210–217.

196. Medical Research Council Oesophageal Cancer Working Group. Surgical resection with or without preoperative chemotherapy in oesophageal cancer: a randomised controlled trial. *Lancet* 2002;359:1727–1733.

197. Cunningham D, Allum WH, Stenning SP, *et al*. Perioperative chemotherapy versus surgery alone for respectable gastroesophageal cancer. *N Engl J Med* 2006;355:11–20.

198. Ando N, Lizuka T, Kakegawa T, *et al*. A randomized trial of surgery with and without chemotherapy for localized squamous carcinoma of the thoracic esophagus: the Japan Clinical Oncology Group Study. *J Thorac Cardiovasc Surg* 1997;114: 205–209.

199. Bosset JF, Gignoux M, Triboulet JP, *et al*. Chemoradiotherapy followed by surgery compared with surgery alone in squamous-cell cancer of the esophagus. *N Engl J Med* 1997; 337:161–167.

200. Urba SG, Orringer MB, Turrisi A, *et al*. Randomized trial of preoperative chemoradiation versus surgery alone in patients with locoregional esophageal carcinoma. *J Clin Oncol* 2001;19: 305–313.

201. Tepper J, Krasna MJ, Niedzwiecki D, *et al*. Phase III trial of trimodality therapy with cisplatin, Fluorouracil, radiotherapy and surgery compard with surgery alone for esophageal cencer: CALGB 9781. *J Clin Oncol* 2008;26:1086–1092.

202. Stahl M, Stuschke M, Lehmann N, *et al*. Chemoradiation with and without surgery in patients with locally advanced squamous cell carcinoma of the esophagus. *J Clin Oncol* 2005;23: 2310–2317.

203. Urschel JD, Vasan H. A meta-analysis of randomized controlled trials that compared neoadjuvant chemoradiation and surgery to surgery alone for respectable esophageal cancer. *Am J Surg* 2003;185:538–543.

204. Fiorica F, Di Bona D, Schepis F, *et al*. Preoperative chemoradiotherapy for esophageal cancer: a systematic review and meta-analysis. *Gut* 2004;53:925–930.

205. Greer SE, Goodney PP, Sutton JE, Birkmeyer. Neoadjuvant chemoradiotherapy for esophageal carcinoma: a meta-analysis. *Surgery* 2005;137:172–177.

206. Jin H, Zhu H, Ling T, *et al*. Neoadjuvant chemoradiotherapy for resectable esophageal carcinoma: a meta-analysis. *World J Gastroenterology* 2009;15:5983–5991.

207. Macdonald JS, Smalley SR, Benedetti J, *et al*. Chemoradio therapy after surgery compared with surgery alone for adenocarcinoma of the stomach and gastroesophageal junction. *N Engl J Med* 2001;345:725–730.

208. Xiao ZF, Yang ZY, Liang J, *et al*. Value of radiotherapy after radical surgery for esophageal carcinoma: a report of 495 patients. *Ann Thorac Surg* 2003;75:331–336.

209. Rice TW, Adelstein DJ. Precise clinical staging allows treatment modification of patients with esophageal carcinoma. *Oncology (Huntingt)* 1997;11:58–62.

210. Kitajima M, Kitagawa Y. Surgical treatment of esophageal cancer-the advent of the era of individualization. *N Engl J Med* 2002;347:1705–1709.

211. Rice TW, Murthy SC, Mason DP, *et al*. Esophagectomy for high-grade dysplasia. *Eur J Cardiothoracic Surg* 2011;40:113–119.

212. Rice TW, Zuccaro G Jr, Adelstein DJ, et al. Esophageal carcinoma: depth of tumor invasion is predictive of regional lymph node status. *Ann Thorac Surg* 1998;65:787–792.

213. Rice TW, Blackstone EH, Adelstein DJ, *et al*. N1 esophageal carcinoma: the importance of staging and downstaging. *J Thorac Cardiovasc Surg* 2001;121:454–464.

214. Adelstein DJ, Rice TW, Rybicki LA, *et al*. Mature results from a phase II trial of postoperative concurrent chemoradiotherapy for poor prognosis cancer of the esophagus and gastroesophageal junction. *J Clin Oncol* 2009;4:1264–1269.

215. Rice T, Adelstein D, Chidel M, *et al*. Benefit of postoperative adjuvant chemotherapy in locoregionally advanced esophageal carcinoma. *J Thorac Cardiovasc Surg* 2003; 126:1590–1596.

VI   Miscellaneous

36 Eosinophilic Esophagitis

David A. Katzka

Mayo Clinic College of Medicine, Rochester, MN, USA

Introduction

It is rare that gastroenterologists, let alone, physicians get to explore a new disease. With the description of eosinophilic esophagitis (EoE) within the past two decades, we have such an opportunity. Fortunately, with the partnership of talented investigators and modern technology, more has been learned about EoE within a decade than we learned about many diseases after centuries of study. Indeed, we have strong clues on the pathogenesis and diagnosis, and even some effective treatments. Challenges still remain in several areas. One area is the differentiation of EoE from potential disease masqueraders or contributors, such as gastroesophageal reflux. Another is the treatment of patients and maintenance of remission, without compromising lifestyle with difficult restricted diets, and the potential risks of topical steroids and the real risks of perforation with endoscopic dilation. In this chapter, the triumphs and current controversies in this new disease will be further explored.

Definition

The definition of EoE varies to a large degree depending upon the context discussed in the literature. Many authors strictly define this disease in pathologic terms determined by the number of eosinophils on an esophageal mucosal biopsy seen in a high power field (HPF) (Figure 36.1). In clinical terms, however, EoE is commonly defined by its pathophysiologic mechanisms; namely a disease state where there is esophageal mucosal eosinophil infiltration induced by an allergic response [1, 2]. The complete definition of EoE uses both of these principles, i.e. the coupling of excess eosinophilic infiltration of the esophageal mucosa with appropriate clinical characteristics of the patient that infer allergy as the cause [3].

The general concept of defining pathologic EoE by an excess of eosinophils in the esophageal mucosa is ostensibly simple as the esophageal squamous mucosa is normally devoid of eosinophils. On the other hand, many entities classically are associated with eosinophilic infiltration (Table 36.1). Even more recently, one study documented eosinophilic esophageal infiltration in two patients with achalasia [4]. As a result, investigators wrestle with the concept of whether a certain number of eosinophils/HPF can better define EoE. This is further complicated by a lack of histologic criteria defining this excess of eosinophils; whether this needs to be seen in one, some or all biopsies; should the average or all counts per field be high; and does the specific distribution of eosinophils in the esophagus suggest a different pathophysiology? An example of this uncertainty is the broad range of 15–25 eosinophils/HPF defining the disease in the literature. Independently, several studies have failed to define that higher eosinophil counts seen in all biopsies confirm more serious disease. Furthermore, whereas some studies suggest that eosinophils in the distal esophagus are more consistent with gastroesophageal reflux disease (GERD) [5], no study has demonstrated that the proximal or distal esophageal location of eosinophilia determines specific pathophysiology [6, 7].

Whether assessment for degradation products of eosinophils in the esophageal mucosa is a more accurate means of detecting EoE is another evolving issue in this disease. In inflamed esophageal mucosa, the activated eosinophils may degranulate, reducing the number of stainable whole eosinophils and thereby potentially leading to false-negative stains. In other words, patients may have fewer than the required 15 eosinophils/HPF but still have EoE (Figure 36.2). As a result, some investigators suggest that staining for products of eosinophil degranulation may be more accurate and a useful adjunct for establishing the diagnosis [8, 9]. Indeed, this method may be most helpful in patients with low numbers of esophageal eosinophils/HPF, but with clinical criteria compatible with a diagnosis of EoE. Specific proteins studied include eosinophil-derived protein [8] and Luna eosinophil granule (LEG) stain [9].

The Esophagus, Fifth Edition. Edited by Joel E. Richter, Donald O. Castell.
© 2012 Blackwell Publishing Ltd. Published 2012 by Blackwell Publishing Ltd.

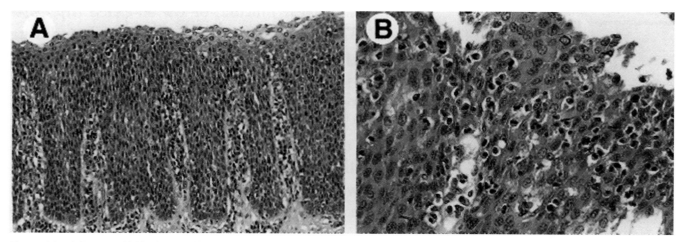

Figure 36.1 (A) Low and (B) high power fields of esophageal biopsy specimen from patient with eosinophilic esophagitis; hematoxylin and eosin staining.

Table 36.1 Disorders associated with esophageal eosinophilia.

Churg–Strauss disease
Esophageal leiomyomatosis
Crohn's disease
Hypereosinophilic syndrome
Periarteritis
Parasitic diseases

Another emerging area of histologic analysis is the ancillary role of other biopsy findings supporting a diagnosis of EoE, particularly when differentiating it from gastroesophageal reflux [10]. These findings include the number of eosinophils, esophageal location of eosinophils, basal cell hyperplasia, spongiosis, and elongation of the rete pegs. Although these findings individually do not reliably discriminate between these two diseases, recent data suggest that compilation of criteria or a scoring system combining histologic variables might be more helpful. For example, one suggested set of histologic criteria consists of major criteria including eosinophilic microabscesses, surface layering of eosinophils associated with surface sloughing of necrotic squamous cells, and peak eosinophil counts greater than 15/HPF. Minor features, which are frequent but less specific, include marked basal cell hyperplasia, lengthening of lamina propria papillae, intercellular edema, and lamina propria fibrosis with chronic inflammation [6]. A more specific proposed scoring system includes criteria such as number of eosinophils/HPF and staining for eosinophil degranulation products [5]. Other recent data suggest that the presence of mast cells may help in differentiating allergy from acid reflux-based disease [9].

Although unlikely to give 100% accuracy, these newer criteria may improve the overall accuracy for defining EoE. At this point, most investigators still define EoE histologically as greater than 15 eosinophils/HPF on any esophageal biopsy. These criteria are in accordance with recent American Gastroenterological Association (AGA) guidelines [7], and serve as a reasonable starting point for making a diagnosis of EoE. Put another way, a clinical diagnosis of EoE based upon histology can only be made in an individual patient when supported by clinical, endoscopic, and perhaps therapeutic criteria.

Pathophysiology

Much has been learned about the pathophysiology of EoE in a relatively short period of time. Since the early clinical descriptions in the 1990s, an elegant pathway both from a clinical and basic science viewpoint has been described, an animal model developed, and a candidate gene identified. Basic science proof of EoE as an allergy-based disease derives from two general models. The first is through the induction and study of this disease in a mouse model developed in the laboratories of Marc Rothenberg [11–15]. These experiments demonstrate the following sequence of events:

1. An initial cutaneous or pulmonary allergic reaction occurs, which "primes" the esophageal mucosa.
2. Upon mucosal exposure to an esophageal allergen derived from air or food, a series of pathways is activated in which (a) allergens initiate a characteristic T-helper cell (Th-2) response with activation of other eosinophil attractants; (b) bone marrow-derived eosinophils migrate to the esophageal mucosa; and (c) a cascade of inflammatory mediators and

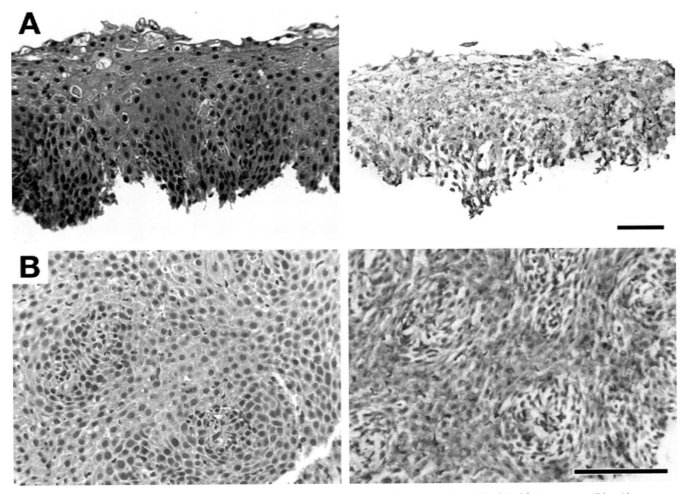

Figure 36.2 (A, B) Left panels, esophageal biopsies with hematoxylin and eosin stain from two patients with clinical features compatible with eosinophilic esophagitis but relatively low eosinophil counts per high power field. Right panels, after staining for an antibody for eosinophil peroxidase, tissue shows obvious evidence of eosinophil degranulation (reproduced from Protheroe *et al.* [8], with permission).

dysregulated T-cell populations are liberated, mounting a general inflammatory response.

3. With chronic exposure, a fibrogenic response occurs which eventually leads to dense collagen deposition and transmural fibrosis [16].

Many other experiments have corroborated this pathway. For example, elevated levels of CD lymphocytes and cytokines, characteristic of the type II allergic reaction are described, in tissue from patients with EoE [17]. Also in human tissue, significant elevations of IL-5, eotaxin, and other eosinophil attractants are well described. Interleukin 5 (IL-5) particularly is an essential component triggering this disease in animal models, as demonstrated by a clear boost in eosinophil recruitment with IL-5 injections and a lack of EoE occurring in an IL-5 knockout mouse (Figure 36.3). In addition to IL-5, other interleukins are likely involved in sustaining the inflammation of EoE. For example, recent

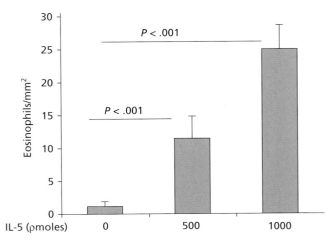

Figure 36.3 Effect of systemic elevations of interleukin 5 (IL-5) on esophageal eosinophil levels after intraperitoneal injection in mouse model (reproduced from Mishra *et al.* [13], with permission).

data report that IL-13 is a potent inducer of IL-5 activity ([18]. Eliciting the interleukins contributing to EoE may help define future therapeutic treatments.

Importantly, animal and human studies show that EoE is a genetic disease mediated by an abnormality in the *eotaxin* gene. In almost 50% of children with EoE, an abnormality of this gene has been identified [19]. The importance of this recognition lies not only in the practical aspects of identifying a potentially genetically-mediated disease, but also the important functional aspects that attend this disease. Specifically, eotaxin is central to the inflammatory response as an eosinophil attractant mediated through interleukin-5.

This is confirmed by increased levels of eotaxin-3, a potent eosinophil attractant in tissue of animal and patients, and by knockout mice models in which loss of the *eotaxin* gene and/or IL-5 mitigates development of the disease [15]. A summary of the proposed pathophysiology of EoE is given in Figure 36.4.

One of the most concerning aspects of EoE is its slow progression to fibrosis. The mechanism, studied in animal models and human tissue, is mediated by a Th2 activation, similar to asthma [20]. In brief, the mucosa becomes infiltrated with eosinophils, mast cells, and T cells, with active proliferation of the epithelium leading to the histologic

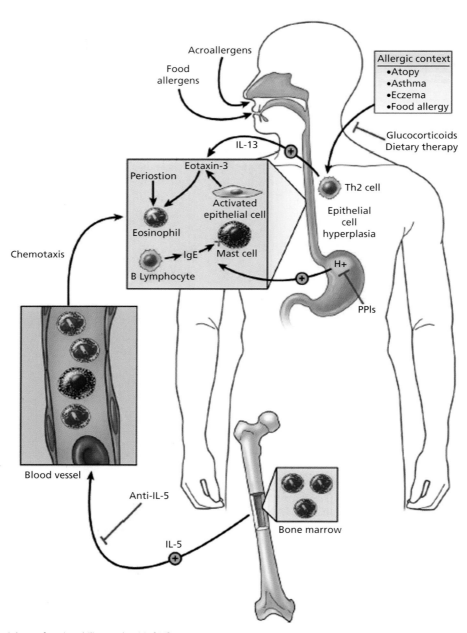

Figure 36.4 Pathophysiology of eosinophilic esophagitis [14].

finding of basal zone hyperplasia. The submucosal lamina propria also becomes infiltrated by inflammatory cells with increased collagen deposition and entrapment of cells and their inflammatory mediators. This leads to a continuous cycle of esophageal remodeling, smooth muscle hyperplasia, and subepithelial fibrosis in chronic EoE [16]. This esophageal fibrosis and stricture formation is not isolated to adults [21]; studies show this fibrotic change may start in childhood [16].

Clinical data

Clinical data support these basic science experiments. For example, in accordance with the priming hypothesis, the occurrence of allergic rhinitis precedes the development of EoE for an average of more than 10 years in patients with EoE [17]. Furthermore, a history of extraesophageal allergy is common in patients with EoE and the disease is more likely to be diagnosed or flare during the allergy season (i.e. spring and summer) [22–24]. EoE in humans is also associated with a characteristic allergic Th2 response [25, 26]. Consistent with the concept that esophageal mucosa exposure to an allergen initiates the inflammatory response, it is well described that identifying and eliminating causative food allergens virtually eliminates the disease [26]. Similarly, the use of an elemental diet, devoid of most food allergens, is nearly 100% effective in reducing symptoms and normalizing esophageal mucosa in children with EoE [27, 28]. Consistent with an inflammatory pathway specific to allergies, medications such as steroids, which are helpful in allergic diseases in general, have been shown in patients to not only ameliorate the disease [29–33], but to inhibit those mediators specifically involved in the EoE pathway [34]. Supporting the genetic etiology of EoE are numerous studies documenting a strong family history of this and other allergic diseases in patients with EoE [35], and a strong predominance in men and in Caucasians when compared to all other races (see below) [7, 21, 28, 36, 37]. Finally, EoE has been reported in association with other genetic diseases such as celiac [38–40] and Crohn's disease [41]. As these diseases are also genetically based, it may suggest a possible overlap in genetic profile or a shared genetic risk for each of these diseases and EoE, although these data are limited.

Epidemiology

As with most new diseases, the description of EoE first started with case reports and small series of patients from specialized medical centers, making the determination of population prevalence speculative at best. The first suggestion that EoE was a common disease came from reports that it was a frequent cause of food impaction[36, 42]; in fact, among patients under the age of 40 years, it is the most common cause of impaction in an emergency room setting [42]. The second data set suggesting a higher prevalence of EoE was a national pathology database demonstrating the presence of the disease in most US states served by this for profit company [37]. These data established EoE as a widespread disease throughout the United States rather than specific to geographic pockets covered by a few medical centers. EoE has been described throughout Europe and in many other countries, including Australia, South Africa, Japan, Puerto Rico, and Iran [43–49]. More recent data found that EoE cases are just as likely to be identified in urban, suburban or rural populations, at least in the Philadelphia area, suggesting a broad population distribution [50]. Finally, there are limited data analyzing prevalence in large populations, but interpretation is subject to the type of population studied. For example, prospective studies of patients undergoing endoscopy for dysphagia found the prevalence for EoE to be 11.9% in Utah [51] and 15% in Olmstead County [52]. In Sweden [47] and West Virginia [53], on the other hand, a prevalence of 0.4% and 0.73%, respectively, was observed in patients undergoing endoscopy for all causes. Finally, a recent study in a military population from Walter Reed demonstrated a 6.5% incidence of EoE in all patients undergoing endoscopy ([54] . The varied incidence ranges among these studies most likely suggests inconsistency in patient population characteristics and relatively small numbers of patients identified. As a result, the true incidence of EoE will require several large population-based studies.

One interesting epidemiologic question is whether the increasing reports of EoE represent increased recognition or a true increase in disease incidence. Most likely, it is a combination of both, but this is difficult to prove. Pathologic databases consistently show an increasing prevalence over the last several decades. The rise in EoE parallels a similar increase in many other allergic diseases [55, 56]. However, the fact that biopsies from decades past misidentified EoE also suggests that increased recognition is an important factor.

At this point, it is safe to say that EoE is a geographically diverse common disease and is likely to become more common as a result of increased recognition and increasing incidence.

The vast majority of EoE studies demonstrate a strong male predominance, with the ratio of males to females varying from 3:1 to 4:1. This seems to hold true even with advancing age beyond childhood. In one study, men still outnumbered women by 3:1 in the seventh decade [37]. Perhaps the only studies with a lower ratio are those where gastroesophageal reflux might be a confounding issue.

The disease predominates in Caucasians with a ratio approaching 9:1 in some studies. Although initially suspected to be an artifact of the early pockets of identified population, a recent study from the ethnically diverse Philadelphia area still consistently demonstrated a high ratio of Caucasians to other races [50].

EoE also tends to be a disease of younger patients; it is most common in children and prevalence falls with age through adulthood [28, 52]. However, patients in their ninth decade and older are described with this disease [37].

Symptoms

Symptoms of EoE vary by age (Figure 36.5; Table 36.2). In toddlers, failure to thrive and vomiting are early disease symptoms. In older children, the most common symptoms are dyspepsia manifested by nausea, vomiting, and heartburn [7, 57]. This is in contrast to adolescents and adults where dysphagia is the most common presenting symptom [58, 59]. In adults, the occurrence of dysphagia is three times more common than all other symptoms combined, followed by heartburn, dyspepsia and chest pain [37]. The occurrence of dysphagia in adults is not surprising given the disease pathophysiology, representing years of inflammation leading to esophageal fibrosis and stricture formation. Esophageal dysmotility secondary to EoE may also be a contributor to dysphagia [60–63]. Patients cope with this

chronic disease by modifying their eating habits to include slow eating, chewing carefully, and avoiding solid food, particularly meats and breads. These subtle symptoms may be present for decades before more overt complaints bring the patient to the physician's attention.

Table 36.2 Symptoms of eosinophilic esophagitis.

Children

Failure to thrive
Nausea
Vomiting
Regurgitation
Dyspepsia
Abdominal pain

Adults

Dysphagia
Heartburn
Chest pain
Regurgitation

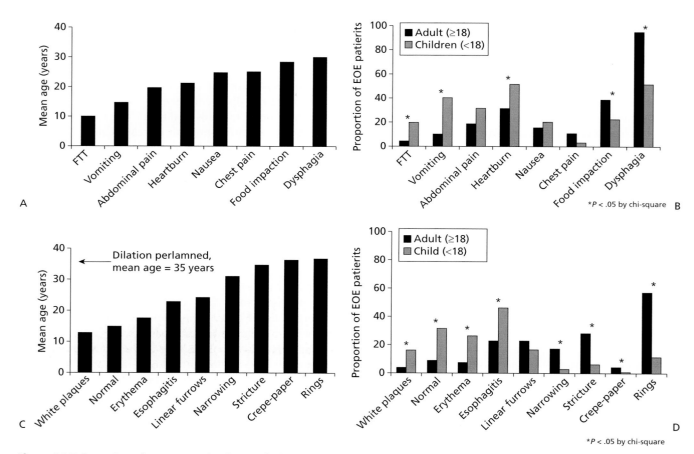

Figure 36.5 Comparison of symptoms and endoscopic findings in children and adults with eosinophilic esophagitis. FTT, (reproduced from Dellon *et al.* [5], with permission).

In contrast to the more subtle presentations of EoE is the catastrophic scenario of food impactions. Although first described in case reports, this is a relatively common presentation. In one case series in 34 patients presenting with food impaction to a community emergency room, 18 (54%) were found to have histologic evidence of EoE [42]. Other large series of patients support the commonality of food impaction in patients with EoE [64]. Food impactions seem to occur in EoE patients with minimal symptoms due to lifestyle changes, when they eat meat too quickly while standing or talking. Another catastrophic presentation is esophageal rupture (Boorhaave's syndrome) resulting from the retching accompanying an impaction. In small series of patients, both children and adults, EoE and Boorhaave's syndrome have been well described [64–68]. One concern in these patients is the appropriate operation to repair these ruptures as the esophagus usually shows extensive fibrosis with strictures. The rents are potentially long, making oversew or patching technically difficult, and potentially leaving esophageal resection as the only viable choice. Fortunately, some patients respond to conservative therapy with antibiotics and nil by mouth for a period of time.

Diagnosis

Although one might think diagnosing EoE is specifically dictated by the finding of eosinophils in the esophageal mucosa, other possible etiologies as well as the potential pitfalls of relying purely on histology have been discussed above. Thus, there is a controversy about the gold standard for this diagnosis. In pursuit of simplicity, the detection of increased levels of either tissue or serum eotaxin-3 would be an attractive and direct means of diagnosing EoE. Unfortunately, this is found in fewer than 50% of children with the disease and data in adults are preliminary (increased expression of eotaxin-3 distinguishes between EoE and GERD [69, 70]. As a result, supporting data coming from endoscopy, radiology, and pathology are often essential to confirming a diagnosis of EoE.

Endoscopy

Endoscopy is helpful in diagnosing EoE, although there is no endoscopic sign completely specific for EoE [71–78] (Figures 36.6–36.9; Table 36.3). In both children and adults, the most common endoscopic finding is linear furrowing. This describes longitudinal thin cracks in the mucosa traversing long distances of the esophagus, usually with several distributed circumferentially around the esophageal lumen. In adults and adolescents, rings and strictures are common and may be of variable length and location in the esophagus, whereas they are uncommon in young children (Figure 36.5). A "white speck" pattern occurs in approximately 15% of children and adults, representing minute conglomerations

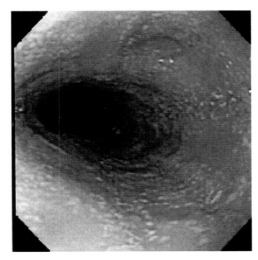
Figure 36.6 Esophageal mucosa with white specks.

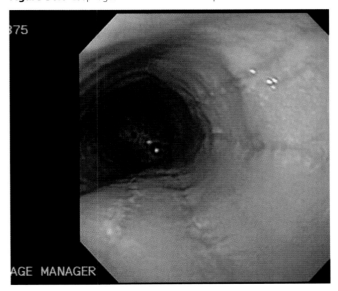
Figure 36.7 Linear furrowing of esophagus.

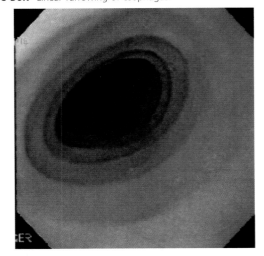
Figure 36.8 Ringed esophagus.

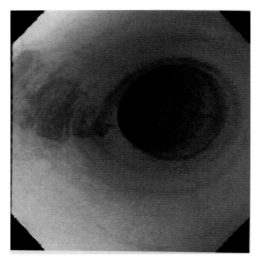

Figure 36.9 Mucosal fragility with crêpe paper appearance and small caliber esophagus.

Table 36.3 Characteristic endoscopic findings of eosinophilic esophagitis.

Linear furrowing
Rings/strictures
White specks
Mucosal fragility

of eosinophils (eosinophilic abscesses). This finding is associated with high numbers of eosinophils in the esophageal mucosa [75, 76].) Another commonly identified endoscopic sign is the "crêpe paper" mucosal appearance. More specifically, the taut mucosa easily tears with a biopsy forceps or with simple passage of the endoscope. Upon scope withdrawal, the endoscopist often sees mucosal tears and blood that was not seen on the initial esophageal intubation. Other endoscopic findings include those typically attributable to peptic esophagitis such as a Schatzki's ring [79] or distal erosive esophagitis [54]. One will also note that even when the mucosa appears completely intact, a "woody" feel to the esophageal lining may still be appreciated. This is not surprising given the early finding on endoscopic ultrasound of submucosal fibrosis in childhood EoE [80]. Although not uniformly observed, some investigators have noted that endoscopic findings of EoE may reverse after therapy. In one EoE study, nearly all rings and all strictures resolved with a 3-month course of fluticasone treatment ([81]. In my practice I rarely see such a robust endoscopic response, but it is encouraging to know that fibrotic lesions may be reversible. Finally, it is important to recognize that 10–23% of patients with EoE, both children and adults, are reported to have a normal appearing esophagus [36, 54],). Thus, if the clinical suspicion is high for EoE, biopsies must be taken to assess the degree of mucosal eosinophilia.

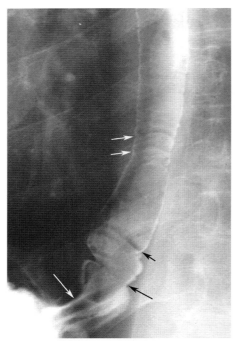

Figure 36.10 Multiple rings (arrows). Radiographic demonstration of multiple esophageal rings in a patient with eosinophilic esophagitis designated by short black and white arrows. Long black arrow demonstrates Schatzki type ring and long white arrow demonstrates gastric folds.

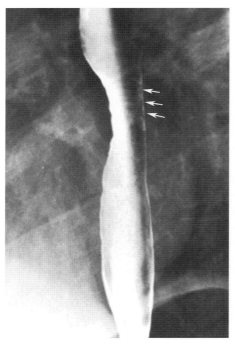

Figure 36.11 Subtle proximal esophageal ring with corrugated pattern (arrows).

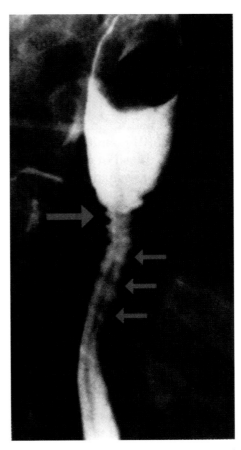

Figure 36.12 Long stricture with corrugated appearance and small caliber esophagus (arrows).

Radiography

Radiography is helpful in supporting a diagnosis of EoE (Figures 36.10–36.12). Although insensitive, particularly for signs of linear furrowing and white specks, barium esophagography may help in imaging rings and strictures. In fact, esophagography may be more sensitive than endoscopy in detecting subtle luminal narrowing. In one study of 14 adult EoE patients, barium swallow detected strictures and/or rings in 10 of them. Esophagography is also particularly helpful in diagnosing the small caliber esophagus seen with EoE [82].) A barium study will not replace endoscopy and biopsies, but among patients with severe dysphagia, the road map obtained with X-rays may help to define the best approach for dilation and potential need for fluoroscopy.

Biopsy sampling and differentiation from gastroesophageal reflux disease

It must be emphasized with endoscopy, that it is necessary to take an adequate number of esophageal biopsies to make a diagnosis of EoE. Gonsalves *et al.* clearly demonstrated that at least five esophageal biopsies, including from both the proximal and distal esophagus, are required to make a histologic diagnosis of EoE, given the patchy distribution of the disease with wide variations in eosinophil counts common

in different biopsies from the same endoscopy [83]. In general, it is recommended that at least two biopsies be taken from the distal, mid, and proximal esophagus. However, histology is not full-proof [84]. Some data suggest that eosinophil counts that approach 50/HPF and higher, and proximal esophageal location may be helpful in making the diagnosis. Similarly, the AGA guidelines [7] that attempt to exclude gastroesophageal reflux by the performance of ambulatory pH monitoring or 2-month treatment with twice-daily proton pump inhibitors (PPIs) prior to biopsy, have not been rigorously studied. Nevertheless, a general consensus among experts is that the diagnosis of EoE is best made by the presence of a group of compatible clinical, demographic, endoscopic, and laboratory criteria [85]. This concept was recently substantiated by investigators from the University of North Carolina [5]. They demonstrated the high predictive accuracy of a scoring system using younger age; symptoms of dysphagia; documented food allergies; observations of esophageal rings, linear furrows, white plaques, or exudates by upper endoscopy; absence of a hiatal hernia on upper endoscopy; a higher maximum eosinophil count; and the presence of eosinophil degranulation on biopsy specimens. In the future, specific clinical and/or histologic scoring systems coupled with esophageal biopsies may be adopted to differentiate eosinophilic esophagitis from GERD. However, currently it is standard treatment to administer a 2-month course of twice-daily PPI therapy and to rebiopsy and/or perform ambulatory pH monitoring off therapy to exclude gastroesophageal reflux. Some proposed algorithms for diagnosing EoE are given in Figure 36.13.

Therapy

Treatment of EoE centers around three general strategies: (1) use of medications to ameliorate the inflammatory response; (2) identification of the food allergens that putatively initiate and sustain the inflammatory response; and (3) mechanical treatment (dilation) of strictures (Table 36.4).

Before discussing the specifics of medical therapy for EoE, a few caveats must be kept in mind. First, one of the most important findings in EoE medical trials is the discovery of a placebo response [33]. Although the precise reason is unclear, case reports suggest that spontaneous remission may coincide with the end of the allergy season [22, 23].

Second, further data suggest highly allergic individuals may respond poorly to dietary or medical therapy. For example, patients with a high number of food allergens are less likely to respond to steroid therapy when compared to patients with EoE and a few or no identifiable allergens [86]. This variable is not accounted for in most studies; thus, one does not know if lack of treatment response represents poor efficacy of an agent or resistance to therapy because a highly immunologic group of patients was studied.

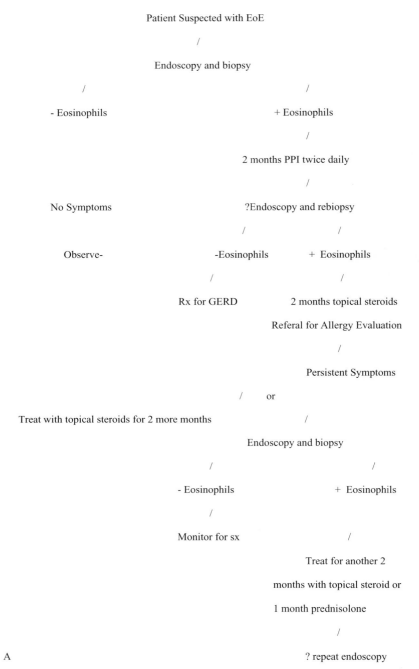

Algorithms for Diagnosis of EoE

Patient Suspected with EoE
/
Endoscopy and biopsy
/   /
- Eosinophils   + Eosinophils
/
2 months PPI twice daily
/
No Symptoms   ?Endoscopy and rebiopsy
/   /
Observe-   -Eosinophils + Eosinophils
/   /
Rx for GERD 2 months topical steroids
Referal for Allergy Evaluation
/
Persistent Symptoms
/ or
Treat with topical steroids for 2 more months /
Endoscopy and biopsy
/   /
- Eosinophils   + Eosinophils
/
Monitor for sx   /
Treat for another 2
months with topical steroid or
1 month prednisolone
/
A   ? repeat endoscopy

Figure 36.13 (A, B) Algorithms for diagnosis of eosinophilic esophagitis (EoE). PPI, proton pump inhibitor; GERD, gastroesophageal reflux disease (B, modified from Dellon *et al.* [5], with permission).

Patient Suspected with EoE*

/

Endoscopy and biopsy

/ /

- eosinophils   + eosinophils

/ /

Rx for GERD or other disorder   Number of Associated

younger age

symptom of dysphagia

documented food allergies

observations of esophageal

rings, linear furrows, white

plaques, or exudates by upper

endoscopy

absence of a hiatal hernia,

a high maximum eosinophil

count

presence of eosinophil

degranulation on bx

/ /

Many   Few

/ /

Steroids   PPI twice daily

For 2 months

/

Endoscopy and biopsy

/ /

- eosinophils   + eosinophils

/ /

Treat for GERD   Treat for EoE

* modified from Dellon et al., ref. 3

B

Figure 36.13 (*continued*)

Table 36.4 Medical therapies for adults with eosinophilic esophagitis.

Steroids

Fluticasone 220–880-μg puffs twice daily for 2 months

Budesonide suspension 3 mg twice daily dissolved in sucralose, twice daily for 2 months

Prednisone tapered over 1 month, starting at 40 mg and tapering by 10 mg weekly

Diet control

Avoidance diet based on RAST, skin prick testing, patch testing

Six-food elimination diet (cow's milk protein, soy, wheat, egg, peanut, and seafood)

Elemental diet for 2 weeks

Other therapies tried but not clearly proven effective

Montelukast

Azathioprine

Mepolizumab

Infliximab

Finally, one of the most important controversies in treating EoE is the desired endpoint. Some investigators suggest that clinical remission should be defined by symptom response. The problem with this endpoint is that many patients have absent or minimal symptoms because of years of behavior accommodation to eating, yet still have significant EoE [87]. As a result, they may remain ostensibly asymptomatic until presenting with a food impaction as their only, yet potentially serious, presentation of EoE. Another possible treatment endpoint is complete elimination of eosinophils from the esophageal mucosa. Although this makes biologic sense, it may be difficult to obtain initially, and more importantly, it may be difficult to sustain on a long-term basis in most patients. At this point, the AGA consensus statement suggests that relief of symptoms should be the main endpoint for treatment. On the other hand, investigators caution against undertreatment in some patients, particularly in those with minimal symptoms but persistent dense eosinophilia of the esophagus as this may portend future complications, such as severe stricture formation and/or recurrent food impaction. Therefore, in our opinion, it is reasonable to try to eliminate EoE completely.

Steroids

The mainstay of medical treatment for EoE is steroids. Steroids are effective in most allergic diseases, and in EoE specifically, steroids inhibit the effects of IL-13, IL-5, and eotaxin,) which, as discussed above, are central to the inflammatory response in EoE. Another potential benefit of steroids is their long-term effect on fibrosis. Some data suggest that steroid therapy can reverse fibrosis and its consequences such as rings and strictures . With more long-term data, this will hopefully be substantiated over time.

The most studied preparation is swallowed fluticasone. Fluticasone has been shown in both uncontrolled and controlled trials to be effective in inducing both symptomatic and histologic remission in EoE. In a classic double-blind controlled trial in children from Indianapolis, fluticasone was 90% effective in inducing complete histologic remission, i.e. total elimination of eosinophils from the esophageal mucosa [33]. Uncontrolled trials in adults have shown similar results [88, 89]. Dosing in adults is two to four 220-μg puffs twice daily for 2 months. Other recent trials demonstrate that budesonide is a reasonable alternative to fluticasone with similar results in small uncontrolled trials [90]. It is particularly well tolerated by children and adults who do not tolerate the inhaled fluticasone preparation.

Specific instructions must be given to patients taking topical steroid preparations. For those taking fluticasone, these include washing the mouth out with and then expectorating the water to prevent fungal infection, avoiding any eating or drinking for at least 30 min after dosing, and reminding the patient to swallow and not inhale the fluticasone. Budesonide must keep it refrigerated and its availability is more limited. Choice of agent can rest on patient tolerance and ease of using a specific preparation.

Oral prednisone is as effective as fluticasone in the treatment of EoE, with some studies suggesting a more rapid response than with topical applications. It should be used in patients with severe symptoms and those not responding to topical esophageal steroid therapy [89]. In adults, a 1-, rather than 2-, month course is used, starting at 40 mg and tapering by 10 mg weekly.

The main side effect of inhaled steroid is esophageal candidiasis, being reported in approximately 5% of EoE patients [33]. A case of candidal esophagitis was reported with swallowed budesonide [90]. One case of herpes esophagitis has been reported [91]. Occasionally patients will report sore throat or hoarseness. The most concerning theoretical side effect with long-term swallowed fluticasone use is bone loss. Using data from patients with asthma, a meta-analysis found that inhaled fluticasone at total daily doses higher than 750 g/day may lead to bone loss [92]) This risk may not be as great with swallowed topical steroids because they are rapidly metabolized by the first-pass effect not present with inhaled steroids.

Another concern with prolonged steroid use is adrenal insufficiency. At least in a trial using budesonide in children, there was no evidence of decreased cortisol levels after a 2-month course [90].

One of the unresolved issues with steroid treatment is how to treat relapses and the frequency with which steroid treatment should be used. This question is clinically relevant given the fact that the 1-year recurrence rate after discontinuing steroids may be as high as 90% [89]. There are occasional patients who remain in histologic remission for years, but often patients relapse both histologically and symptomatically within days to weeks of discontinuing steroids. It is unclear how to manage this latter group, with options including a longer course of topical steroids (2 vs 4 months), use of systemic steroids for rapid relapse, or continuous use of topical steroids, perhaps at a lower dose or on alternating days. No data exist in this area, although anecdotally and through personal communications, all of these strategies are used. More concerning, no data exist on the potential long-term risks of continuous fluticasone therapy relevant to adrenal suppression and osteoporosis

Immunomodulators

As discussed above, IL-5 is central to the pathogenesis of EoE, and also contributes to hypereosinophilic syndrome [93] and eosinophilic gastroenteritis [94], a disease cousin of EoE. As a result, it is not surprising that several investigators have viewed an antagonist to IL-5 as a potential panacea for this disease. Preliminary data in a small series of children [95] were promising with a significant reduction in EoE and symptoms. A larger study in adults [96] also generated data that were encouraging, although not definitive. In 11 adults tested, there was a 67% reduction in eosinophil count and symptoms; however, eosinophil counts still remained high. Although this might seem discouraging, the patients tested were refractory to all other therapies, possibly skewing the results away from a robust response. There were no serious side effects reported with this agent. Clearly, larger studies in more representative patients with EoE are needed.

Finally, small series of patients with EoE have been treated with azathioprine [97] and infliximab [98] without benefit. Additionally, other antiallergy and immunosuppressive medications have also been used in treating EoE. Montelukast, a leukotriene inhibitor, is a commonly used medication for allergies but data are limited in EoE patients [99]. In one study, eight patients with EoE were given montelukast and five had symptomatic response [100]. Unfortunately, improvement in endoscopic features or histology were not assessed. Furthermore, experimental data have also failed to show an alteration in leukotriene levels in EoE, implying that a medication that blocks leukotriene production would be unlikely to have efficacy in EoE [101]. At this point, montelukast cannot be considered as a proven therapy for EoE [7].

Dietary manipulations

Elimination of allergens that trigger the disease is theoretically the most attractive therapy for EoE. This derives from the previously discussed laboratory and clinical data demonstrating that effective elimination of food allergens through an elemental diet eradicates EoE in nearly all pediatric patients. Specifically, Liacouras et al. observed in 361 children over a 10-year period that 98% responded to an elemental diet [28]. Although not well tested in adults, preliminary data also suggest the effectiveness of an elemental diet [102]. Furthermore, aggressive treatment with an elemental diet to the endpoint of normal esophageal mucosa, may allow reintroduction of foods found previously to be intolerant to the patient's esophagus. Unfortunately, use of an elemental diet in adults has practical limitations. Specifically, elemental diets are expensive and unpalatable, often require nasogastric tube administration, and are socially compromising, particularly to teenagers and young adults. If an elemental diet could be developed that obviates some of these problems, it would be an ideal therapy.

Identification and avoidance of food allergens is another theoretically attractive means of treating EoE. Specifically, if allergy testing can identify which food allergens trigger the disease in individual patients, then elimination of these foods could prevent disease occurrence. There are three tests used to achieve this goal. RAST testing (radioallergoabsorbant serum testing) identifies allergens through *in vitro* assays for food-specific IgE antibodies in the serum. Skin prick testing identifies IgE-mediated reactions by causing a wheal and flare response to subdermally injected allergens. Atopy patch testing involves the topical application of a food-containing solution to the skin for 48h. It is helpful in diagnosing non–IgE-mediated food allergy.

Using these tests, many studies have demonstrated a plethora of food allergens in both children and adults with EoE. The range of foods identified may be broad amongst individual patients, both in the type and number of identifiable food allergens [27, 103]. Indeed, some patients have one or two food allergies and others in excess of 30. Furthermore, since each of the food allergen tests uses a different technique, each may reveal a different subset of problematic foods for the patient. As a result, using a combination of these methods seems ideal as the immunologic reactions in EoE are mediated through both IgE and non-IgE related mechanisms. When tested in specific EoE populations, some success has been achieved. For example, Spergel et al. found the use of combined patch and skin testing in 146 children identified food allergens to avoid, leading to elimination of eosinophils and symptoms in 77% of EoE pediatric patients [104]. Unfortunately, other studies are not as encouraging with little data in adults. The lack of consistent usefulness for these methods is not surprising for several reasons. For example, the immunologic mechanisms by which food allergens are identified in the blood or skin do not necessarily reflect what occurs in the esophagus. This can be seen in patients with clear EoE who respond to an elemental diet but have no foods identified by these tests [75]. Conversely other patients may go into histologic remission while consuming foods that yield positive skin or blood testing. Furthermore, the practice of allergy and immunology is such that there is great variability in the type of immunologic tests used to identify food allergens, such that a combination of IgE and non-IgE mediated food allergy is not reliably performed. Finally, it is common to identify many food allergens in EoE patients, such that dietary avoidance would be incompatible with life except for ingesting an elemental diet.

Therefore, therapies restricting some of the more common allergenic foods have been proposed to treat symptoms and partially reduce esophageal eosinophil count. Specifically, one compromise approach tested by Kagalwalla *et al.* [105] was to withdraw the six most commonly identified food allergens in patients with EoE (cow's milk protein, soy, wheat, egg, peanut, and seafood). In this study, the restricted diet produced a significant reduction in both symptoms and EoE. This was also demonstrated in a preliminary study in adults [106]. Unfortunately, resolution of mucosal eosinophilia did not occur, raising the question as to whether partial response is better than no response in preventing histologic fibrogenesis and subsequent stricture formation over time. The answer is not known, but the potential of a graded response in these patients makes intuitive sense.

Esophageal dilation

One of the issues that adult gastroenterologists address more than pediatricians is the treatment of esophageal strictures in EoE patients. The finding of stricture (concordant with the high prevalence of dysphagia) is common in adults, occurring in up to 67% of adults diagnosed with EoE [30, 71]. Several questions must be answered to effectively treat these strictures: (1) Is medical treatment effective and therefore should it be tried first? (2) Is there a specific method of dilation that is more effective for these strictures? (3) What are the risks of complication with dilation? (4) What is the specific endpoint of dilation?

One of the AGA consensus guidelines is first to treat medically, and then to dilate for persistent symptoms. This is based on the following information. First, animal studies find that steroids reverse fibrogenesis in EoE [107]. Second, one study suggests that medical treatment in EoE patients may reduce the need for dilation [108]. Third, a study suggests that patients with active EoE have a greater chance of dilation-induced perforation [109]. Fourth, the clinical experience of some investigators suggests that in time medical treatment may lead to resolution or improvement of strictures in some patients [81]. Finally, one must keep in mind that the symptoms of dysphagia are not all related to mechanical obstruction. Specifically, some have reported that esophageal motility abnormalities may be associated with EoE. Thus, medical treatment of eosinophilic inflammation improves dysphagia irrespective of reduction in stricture diameter. Even though the data are limited, my clinical approach is to avoid the risks by first treating patients with pharmacologic therapies, unless the patient cannot maintain nutrition orally due to the stricture. However, other inves-

tigators feel that initial dilation of a stricture can be justified because of the sustained relief experienced by many patients and the minimal risk if done carefully.

If mechanical dilation is required, there is no comparison data guiding the use of balloon or Savary bougies. As a result, the same general rules for esophageal stricture dilation apply, specifically, using a Savary dilator for long strictures and balloon dilation for shorter strictures, depending on operator comfort. One principle that must be kept in mind is that dilation of EoE strictures needs to be performed more carefully and gradually than for other types of strictures. This was suggested in early studies reporting a higher rate of perforation [110, 111] with one study demonstrating perforation in three of 28 patients undergoing dilation [109] and another study demonstrating perforation in a patient just with passage of the endoscope. This is because the transmural fibrosis in EoE makes "splintering" of the esophageal wall a distinct risk. With this early experience in mind, more recent data suggest that esophageal dilation may be as safe as dilation in other types of esophageal strictures [112], but with two important caveats: the "rule of threes" definitely applies and patients may need more than one session to achieve effective dilation. Patients should also be warned that chest pain is very common, if not expected, after dilation. Finally, even the concept of esophageal perforation is a terrifying one, but it should be noted that most reported perforations have been managed with conservative nonoperative therapy. In other words, the chance of need for surgical repair overall appears to be very small.

Upon embarking on a course of esophageal stricture dilation in patients with EoE, one must decide in advance on the clinical endpoint, which can include symptom relief and/or stricture diameter. Again, no guidelines exist but some general principles might be considered. First, patients typically underestimate their degree of dysphagia. This may encourage the gastroenterologist to dilate more aggressively to achieve greater symptom response, while others may be influenced to dilate more conservatively since less dilation may be needed for adequate symptomatic response. I tend to be a conservative dilator, except in one condition: a history of prior food impaction, particularly in those requiring endoscopic bolus impaction. In these patients, the impaction may represent the one slip made in the face of diligent swallowing accommodation. In these patients, I dilate aggressively to prevent the risk of perforation that may occur with emergent endoscopy and bolus removal or development of spontaneous Boorhaave's syndrome in the presence of acute impaction [113].

Long-term evaluation

One of the major questions asked by patients with EoE is what they can expect in long-term follow-up. This is a particularly relevant issue as this chronic disease is typically diagnosed in young patients who can expect decades of life. One general concern is the premalignant potential of EoE as may be seen with other chronic inflammatory diseases. To date, no cases of cancer have been reported with this disease, though a few case reports of concordant Barrett's esophagus and EoE exist [114, 115]. A more realistic question is whether this disease remits, or conversely, if there is an inexorable course to further inflammation and fibrosis. Furthermore, can long-term treatment alter this course? To date, there is only one long-term study of a small group of adult EoE patients [21]. All patients persisted with EoE, while fibrosis and stricture formation overall progressed. However, most did well; nutrition was not a problem and frequent dilations were uncommon. In children with EoE, the longest follow-up study is 14 years in 620 patients who mostly demonstrated progressive disease, with spontaneous remission in only 11 patients [27]. At the very least, these studies suggest that EoE is a chronic, if not life-long, disease in most patients. Although we do not know the long-term benefits of treatment (or for that matter, not treating), I believe we should lean toward administering effective treatment for both histologic and symptomatic abnormalities.

Conclusions

EoE is a prevalent and new disease. It is clearly established to be an allergy-based disease in genetically predisposed individuals where respiratory or dermatologic conditions prime the esophageal mucosa to react with specific food allergens. This in turn activates a chronic eosinophilic inflammatory process in children, leading to fibrosis and stricture formation in adults. Treatments aimed at this allergic response include the use of topical and systemic steroids, attempts to identify and avoid food allergens, and dilation of symptomatic strictures. Controversy exists in defining appropriate endpoints of therapy (symptomatic vs histologic) and in chronic treatment strategies for what is, in most patients, a relapsing disease. With the great interest in EoE and the application of some remarkably sharp minds and technology, great strides will continue to be made in understanding and treating this fascinating disease.

References

1. Liacouras CA. EoE in children and adults. *J Pediatr Gastroenterol Nutr* 2003;37 (Suppl 1):S23–S28.
2. Lai AL, Girgis S, Liang Y, Carr S, Huynh HQ. Diagnostic criteria for EoE: a 5-year retrospective review in a pediatric population. *J Pediatr Gastroenterol Nutr* 2009;49:63–70.
3. Whitney-Miller CL, Katzka D, Furth EE. Eosinophilic esophagitis: a retrospective review of esophageal biopsy specimens from 1992 to 2004 at an adult academic medical center. *Am J Clin Pathol* 2009;131:788–792.
4. Rodrigo S, Abboud G, Oh D, *et al*. High intraesophageal eosinophil counts in esophageal squamous epithelium are not specific for EoE in adults. *Am J Gastroenterol* 2008;103: 435–442.
5. Dellon E, Gibbs W, Fritchie K, *et al*. Clinical, endoscopic, and histologic findings distinguish eosinophilic esophagitis from gastroesophageal reflux disease. *Clin Gastroenterol Hepatol* 2009;7:1305–1310.
6. Mueller S, Neureiter D, Aigner T, *et al*. Comparison of histological parameters for the diagnosis of eosinophilic oesophagitis versus gastro-oesophageal reflux disease on oesophageal biopsy material. *Histopathology* 2008;53:676–684.
7. Furuta GT, Liacouras CA, Collins MH, *et al*. First International Gastrointestinal Eosinophil Research Symposium (FIGERS) Subcommittees. Eosinophilic esophagitis in children and adults: a systematic review and consensus recommendations for diagnosis and treatment. *Gastroenterology* 2007;133: 1342–1363.
8. Protheroe C, Woodruff S, de Petris G, *et al*. A novel histologic scoring system to evaluate mucosal biopsies from patients with eosinophilic esophagitis. *Clin Gastroenterol Hepatol* 2009;7: 749–755.
9. Lucendo AJ, Bellon T, Lucendo B. The role of mast cells in EoE. *Pediatr Allergy Immunol* 2009;20:512–518.
10. Odze RD. Pathology of EoE: what the clinician needs to know. *Am J Gastroenterol* 2009;104:485–490.
11. Blanchard C, Wang N, Rothenberg ME. Eosinophilic esophagitis: pathogenesis, genetics, and therapy. *J Allergy Clin Immunol* 2006;118:1054–1059.
12. Mishra A, Rothenberg ME. Intratracheal IL-13 induces eosinophilic esophagitis by an IL-5, eotaxin-1, and STAT6-dependent mechanism. *Gastroenterology* 2003;125:1419–1424.
13. Mishra A, Hogan SP, Brandt EB, Rothenberg ME. An etiological role for aeroallergens and eosinophils in experimental esophagitis. *J Clin Invest* 2001;107:83–90.
14. Akei HS, Mishra A, Blanchard C, Rothenberg ME. Epicutaneous antigen exposure primes for experimental eosinophilic esophagitis in mice. *Gastroenterology* 2005;129:985–989.
15. Rothenberg ME. Biology and treatment of eosinophilic esophagitis gastroenterology. *Gastroenterology* 2009;137: 1238–1249.
16. Aceves SS, Ackerman SJ. Relationship between eosinophilic inflammation, tissue remodeling, and fibrosis in EoE. *Immunol Allergy Clin North Am* 2009;29:197–211.
17. Simon D, Marti H, Heer P, *et al*. EoE is frequently associated with IgE-mediated allergic airway diseases. *J Allergy Clin Immunol* 2005;115:1090–1092.
18. Blanchard C, Mingler MK, Vicario M, *et al*. IL-13 involvement in eosionophilic esophagitis: transcriptome analysis and reversibility with glucocorticoids. *J Allergy Clin Immunol* 2007;120:1292–1300.
19. Blanchard C, Wang N, Stringer KF, *et al*. Eotaxin-3 and a uniquely conserved gene-expression profile in eosinophilic esophagitis. *J Clin Invest* 2006;116:536–547.
20. Zhu X, Wang M, Crump CH, Mishra A. An imbalance of esophageal effector and regulatory T cell subsets in experimental EoE mice. *Am J Physiol* 2009;3:G550–558.

21. Straumann A, Spichtin HP, Grize L, *et al.* Natural history of primary EoE: A follow-up of 30 adult patients for up to 11.5 years. *Gastroenterology* 2003;125:1660–1669.

22. Almansa C, Krishna M, Buchner AM, *et al.* Seasonal distribution in newly diagnosed cases of eosinophilic esophagitis in adults. *Am J Gastroenterol* 2009;104:828–833.

23. Wang FY, Gupta SK, Fitzgerald JF. Is there a seasonal variation in the incidence or intensity of allergic eosinophilic esophagitis in newly diagnosed children? *J Clin Gastroenterol* 2007;41:451–453.

24. Sugnanam KK, Collins JT, Smith PK, *et al.* Dichotomy of food and inhalant allergen sensitization in EoE. *Allergy* 2007;62:1257–1260.

25. Straumann A, Bauer M, Fischer B, Blaser K, Simon HU. Idiopathic EoE is associated with a T(H)2-type allergic inflammatory response. *J Allergy Clin Immunol* 2001;108:954–961.

26. Simon D, Marti H, Heer P, Simon HU, Braathen LR, Strauman A. Eosinophilic esophagitis is frequently associated with IgE-mediated allergic airway disease. *J Allergy Clin Immunol* 2005;115:1090–1092.

27. Spergel JM, Brown-Whitehorn TF, Beausoleil JL, *et al.* 14 years of EoE: clinical features and prognosis. *J Pediatr Gastroenterol Nutr* 2009;48:30–36.

28. Liacouras CA, Spergel JM, Ruchelli E, *et al.* Eosinophilic esophagitis: a 10-year experience in 381 children. *Clin Gastroenterol Hepatol* 2005;3:1198–1206.

29. Arora AS, Perrault J, Smyrk TC. Topical corticosteroid treatment of dysphagia due to eosinophilic esophagitis in adults. *Mayo Clin Proc* 2003;78:830–835.

30. Remedios M, Campbell C, Jones DM, Kerlin P. Eosinophilic esophagitis in adults: clinical, endoscopic, histology findings, and response to treatment with fluticasone proprionate. *Gastrointest Endosc* 2006;63:3–12.

31. Aceves SS, Bastian JF, Newbury RO, *et al.* Oral viscous budesonide: A potential new therapy for eosinophilic esophagitis in children. *Am J Gastroenterol* 2007;102:2271–2279.

32. Aceves, SS, Dohil, R, Newbury, RO, *et al.* Topical viscous budesonide suspension for treatment of EoE. *J Allergy Clin Immunol* 2005;116:705–706.

33. Schaefer ET, Fitzgerald JF, Molleston JP, *et al.* Comparison of oral prednisone and topical fluticasone in the treatment of EoE: a randomized trial in children. *Clin Gastroenterol Hepatol* 2008;6:165–173.

34. Lucendo AJ, De Rezende L, Comas C, Caballero T, Bellon T. Treatment with topical steroids downregulates IL-5, eotaxin-1/CCL11, and eotaxin-3/CCL26 gene expression in EoE. *Am J Gastroenterol* 2008;103:2184–2193.

35. Collins MH, Blanchard C, Abonia JP *et al.* Clinical, pathologic, and molecular characterization of familial EoE compared with sporadic cases. *Clin Gastroenterol Hepatol* 2008;6:621–629.

36. Prasad GA, Talley NJ, Romero Y, *et al.* Prevalence and predictive factors of EoE in patients presenting with dysphagia: a prospective study. *Am J Gastroenterol* 2007;102:2627.

37. Kapel RC, Miller JK, Torres C, et al. EoE: a prevalent disease in the United States that affects all age groups. *Gastroenterology* 2008;134:1316–1321.

38. Ooi CY, Day AS, Jackson R, *et al.* Eosinophilic esohagitis in children with celiac disease. *J Gastroenterol Hepatol* 2008;23:1144–1148.

39. Quaglietta L, Coccorullo P, Miele E, *et al.* Eosinophilic oesophagitis and coeliac disease: is there an association? *Aliment Pharmacol Ther* 2007;26:487–493.

40. Verzegnassi F, Bua J, De Angelis P, *et al.* Eosinophilic oesophagitis and coeliac disease: is it just a casual association? *Gut* 2007;56:1029–1030.

41. Suttor VP, Chow C, Turner I. EoE with Crohn's disease: a new association or overlapping immune-mediated enteropathy? *Am J Gastroenterol* 2009;104:794–795.

42. Desai TK, Stecevic V, Chang C-H, *et al.* Association of eosinophilic inflammation with esophageal food impaction in adults. *Gastrointest Endosc* 2005;61:795–801.

43. Velazquez V, Camacho C, Mercado-Quinones AE, Irizarry-Padilla J. Eosinophilic esophagitis and allergies in the pediatric population of Puerto Rico. *Boletin – Asociacion Medica de Puerto Rico* 2009;101:21–22.

44. Furuta, K, Adachi, K, Kowari K, *et al.* A Japanese case of EoE. *J Gastroenterol* 2006;41:706–710

45. Cherian S, Smith NM, Forbes DA. Rapidly increasing prevalence of eosinophilic oesophagitis in Western Australia. *Arch Dis Child* 2006;91:1000–1004.

46. Furuta K, Adachi K, Kowari K, *et al.* A Japanese case of eosinophilic esophagitis. *J Gastroenterol* 2006;41:706–710.

47. Ronkainen J, Talley NJ, Aro P, *et al.* Prevalence of oesophageal eosinophils and eosinophilic oesophagitis in adults: The population-based Kalixanda study. *Gut* 2007;56:615–620.

48. Martin de Carpi J, Gomez Chiari M, Castejon Ponce E, *et al.* Increasing diagnosis of eosinophilic esophagitis in Spain. *Ann Pediatr (Barc)* 2005;62:333–339.

49. Budin C, Villard-Truc F, Rivet C, *et al.* Eosinophilic esophagitis: 3 case reports. *Gastroenterol Clin Biol* 2005;29:73–75.

50 Franciosi JP, Tam V, Liacouras CA, Spergel JM. A case-control study of sociodemographic and geographic characteristics of 335 children with eosinophilic esophagitis. *Clin Gastroenterol Hepatol* 2009;7:415–419.

51. Byrne KR, Panagiotakis PH, Hilden K, Thomas KL, Peterson KA, Fang JC. Retrospective analysis of esophageal food impaction: differences in etiology by age and gender. *Dig Dis Sci* 2007;52:717–721.

52. Prasad GA, Alexander JA, Schleck CD, *et al.* Epidemiology of eosinophilic esophagitis over three decades in Olmsted County, Minnesota. *Clin Gastroenterol Hepatol* 2009;7:1055–1061.

53. Gill R, Durst P, Rewalt M, Elitsur Y. Eosinophilic esophagitis disease in children from West Virginia: a review of the last decade (1995–2004). *Am J Gastroenterol* 2007;102:2281–2285.

54. Veerappan GR, Perry JL, Duncan TJ, *et al.* Prevalence of eosinophilic esophagitis in an adult population undergoing upper endoscopy: a prospective study. *Clin Gastroenterol Hepatol* 2009;7:420–426.

55. Shamssain M. Trends in the prevalence and severity of asthma, rhinitis, and atopic asthma in 6- to 7- and 13- to 14-yr-old children from the north-east of England. *Pediatr Allergy Immunol* 2007;18:149–153

56. Stafford RS, Ma J, Finkelstein SN, *et al.* National trends in asthma visits and asthma pharmacotherapy, 1978–2002. *J Allergy Clin Immunol* 2003;111:729–735.

57. Orenstein SR, Shalaby TM, Di Lorenzo C, *et al.* The spectrum of pediatric Eosinophilic esophagitis beyond infancy: a clinical series of 30 children. *Am J Gastroenterol* 2000;95:1422–1430.

58. Mackenzie SH, Go M, Chadwick B, *et al*. Eosinophilic oesophagitis in patients presenting with dysphagia—a prospective analysis. *Aliment Pharmacol Ther* 2008;28:1140–1146.

59. Croese J, Fairley SK, Masson JW, *et al*. Clinical and endoscopic features of eosinophilic esophagitis in adults. *Gastrointest Endosc* 2003;58:516–522.

60. Bassett J, Maydonovitch C, Perry J, Sobin L, Osgard E, Wong R. Prevalence of esophageal dysmotility in a cohort of patients with esophageal biopsies consistent with eosinophilic esophagitis. *Dis Esophagus* 2009;22:543–548.

61. Korsapati HR, Babaei A, Bhargava V, *et al*. Dysfunction of the longitudinal muscles of the oesophagus in eosinophilic esophagitis. *Gut* 2009;58:1056–1062.

62. Lucendo AJ, Castillo P, Martin-Chavarri S, *et al*. Manometric findings in adult eosinophilic oesophagitis: a study of 12 cases. *Eur J Gastroenterol Hepatol* 2007;19:417–424.

63. Nurko S, Rosen R. Esophageal dysmotility in patients who have eosinophilic esophagitis. *Gastrointest Endosc Clin North Am* 2008;18:73–89.

64. Straumann A, Bussmann C, Zuber M, Vannini S, Simon HU, Schoepfer A. Eosinophilic esophagitis: analysis of food impaction and perforation in 251 adolescent and adult patients. *Clin Gastroenterol Hepatol* 2008;6:598–600.

65. Robles-Medranda C, Villard F, Bouvier R, Dumortier J, Lachaux A. Spontaneous esophageal perforation in eosinophilic esophagitis in children. *Endoscopy* 2008;40 (Suppl 2): E171.

66. Giles H, Smith L, Tolosa D, Miranda MJ, Laman D. Eosinophilic esophagitis: a rare cause of esophageal rupture in children. *Am Surg* 2008;74:750–752.

67. Liguori G, Cortale M, Cimino F, Sozzi M. Circumferential mucosal dissection and esophageal perforation in a patient with eosinophilic esophagitis. *World J Gastroenterol* 2008;14: 803–804.

68. Spiegel A, Wolf DC, Sperber K, Gimenez C. An unusual presentation of eosinophilic esophagitis. *Gastrointest Endosc* 2009;70: 382–383.

69. Konikoff MR, Blanchard C, Kirby C, *et al*. Potential of blood eosinophils, eosinophil-derived neurotoxin, and eotaxin-3 as biomarkers of eosinophilic esophagitis. *Clin Gastroenterol Hepatol* 2006;4:1328.

70. Bhattacharya B, Carlsten J, Sabo E, *et al*. Increased expression of eotaxin-3 distinguishes between eosinophilic esophagitis and gastroesophageal reflux disease. *Hum Pathol* 2007;38: 1744–1753.

71. Croese J, Fairley SK, Masson JW, *et al*. Clinical and endoscopic features of eosinophilic esophagitis in adults. *Gastrointest Endosc* 2003;58:516–522.

72. Aceves SS, Newbury RO, Dohil R, *et al*. Distinguishing eosinophilic esophagitis in pediatric patients: Clinical, endoscopic, and histologic features of an emerging disorder. *J Clin Gastroenterol* 2007;41:252–256.

73. Remedios M, Campbell C, Jones DM, *et al*. Eosinophilic esophagitis in adults: Clinical, endoscopic, histologic findings, and response to treatment with fluticasone propionate. *Gastrointest Endosc* 2006;63:3–12.

74. Muller S, Puhl S, Vieth M, Stolte M. Analysis of symptoms and endoscopic findings in 117 patients with histological diagnoses of eosinophilic esophagitis. *Endoscopy* 2007;39:339–344.

75. Straumann, A, Spichtin, HP, Bucher, KA, *et al*. Eosinophilic esophagitis: Red on microscopy, white on endoscopy. *Digestion* 2004;70:109–116.

76. Lim JR, Gupta SK, Croffie JM, *et al*. White specks in the esophageal mucosa: An endoscopic manifestation of non-reflux eosinophilic esophagitis in children. *Gastrointest Endosc* 2004;59:835–838.

77. Lucendo AJ, Pascual-Turrion JM, Navarro M, *et al*. Endoscopic, bioptic, and manometric findings in eosinophilic esophagitis before and after steroid therapy: a case series. *Endoscopy* 2007;39:765–771.

78. Lai AL, Girgis S, Liang Y, Carr S, Huynh HQ. Diagnostic criteria for eosinophilic esophagitis: a 5-year retrospective review in a pediatric population. *J Pediatr Gastroenterol Nutr* 2009;49: 63–70.

79. Nurko S, Teitelbaum JE, Husain K, *et al*. Association of Schatzki ring with eosinophilic esophagitis in children. *J Pediatr Gastroenterol Nutr* 2004;38;436.

80. Fox VL, Nurko S, Teitelbaum JE, *et al*. High-resolution EUS in children with eosinophilic "allergic" esophagitis. *Gastrointest Endosc* 2003;57:30.

81. Lucendo AJ, Pascual-Turrion JM, Navarro M, *et al*. Endoscopic, bioptic, and manometric findings in eosinophilic esophagitis before and after steroid therapy: a case series. *J Endosc* 2007;39:765–771.

82. White SB, Levine MS, Rubesin SE, Spencer GA, Katzka DA, Lanfer I. The small caliber esophagus: radiographic sign of idiopathic eosinophilic esophagitis. *Radiology* 2010;256: 127–134.

83. Gonsalves N, Policarpio-Nicolas M, Zhang Q, *et al*. Histopathologic variability and endoscopic correlates in adults with eosinophilic esophagitis. *Gastrointest Endosc* 2006;64: 313–319.

84. Ngo P, Furuta GT, Antonioli DA, *et al*. Eosinophils in the esophagus-peptic or allergie eosinophilic esophagitis? Case series of three patients with esophageal eosinophilia. *Am J Gastroenterol* 2006;101;1666.

85. Aceves SS, Newbury RO, Dohil MA, Bastian JF, Dohil R. A symptom scoring tool for identifying pediatric patients with eosinophilic esophagitis and correlating symptoms with inflammation. *Ann Allergy Asthma Immunol* 2009;103: 401–406.

86. Noel RJ, Putnam PE, Collins MH, *et al*. Clinical and immunopathologic effects of swallowed fluticasone for eosinophilic esophagitis. *Clin Gastroenterol Hepatol* 2004;2:568–575.

87. Pentiuk S, Putnam PE, Collins MH, Rothenberg ME. Dissociation between symptoms and histological severity in pediatric eosinophilic esophagitis. *J Pediatr Gastroenterol Nutr* 2009;48:152–160.

88. Helou EF, Simonson J, Arora AS. 3-yr-follow-up of topical corticosteroid treatment for eosinophilic esophagitis in adults. *Am J Gastroenterol* 2008;103:2194–2199.

89. Liacouras CA, Wenner WJ, Brown K, *et al*. Primary eosinophilic esophagitis in children: successful treatment with oral corticosteroids. *J Pediatr Gastroenterol Nutr* 1998;26: 380–385.

90. Aceves SS, Bastian JF, Newbury RO, Dohil R. Oral viscous budesonide: a potential new therapy for eosinophilic esophagitis in children. *Am J Gastroenterol* 2007;102:2271–2279.

91. Lindberg GM, Van Eldik R, Saboorian MH. A case of herpes esophagitis after fluticasone propionate for eosinophilic esophagitis. *Nat Clin Pract Gastroenterol Hepatol* 2008;5: 527–530.

92. Lipworth BJ. Systemic adverse effects of inhaled corticosteroid therapy: a systematic review and meta-analysis. *Arch Intern Med* 1999;159:941–955.

93. Ogbogu PU, Bochner BS, Butterfield JH, *et al.* Hypereosinophilic syndrome: a multicenter, retrospective analysis of clinical characteristics and response to therapy. *J Allergy Clin Immunol* 2009;124:1319–1325.e3.

94. Stone KD, Prussin C. Immunomodulatory therapy of eosinophil-associated gastrointestinal diseases. *Clin Exp Allergy* 2008;38:1858–1865.

95. Stein ML, Collins MH, Villanueva JM, *et al.* Anti-IL-5 (mepolizumab) therapy for eosinophilic esophagitis. *J Allergy Clin Immunol* 2006;118:1312–1319.

96. Straumann A, Conus S, Grzonka P, *et al.* Anti-interleukin-5 antibody treatment (mepolizumab) in active eosinophilic oesophagitis: a randomised, placebo-controlled, double-blind trial. *Gut* 2010;59:21–30.

97. Netzer P, Gschossmann JM, Straumann A, *et al.* Corticosteroid-dependent eosinophilic oesophagitis: azathioprine and 6-mercaptopurine can induce and maintain long-term remission. *Eur J Gastroenterol Hepatol* 2007;19:865.

98. Straumann A, Bussmann C, Conus S, Beglinger C, Simon HU. Anti-TNF-alpha (infliximab) therapy for severe adult eosinophilic esophagitis. *J Allergy Clin Immunol* 2008;122: 425–427.

99. Gawrieh S, Shaker R. Treatment options for eosinophilic esophagitis: montelukast. *Curr Gastroenterol Rep* 2004;6: 189–193.

100. Attwood SE, Lewis CJ, Bronder CS, Morris CD, Armstrong GR, Whittam J. Eosinophilic oesophagitis: a novel treatment using Montelukast. *Gut* 2003;52:181–185.

101. Gupta SK, Peters-Golden M, Fitzgerald JF, *et al.* Cysteinyl leukotriene levels in esophageal mucosal biopsies of children with eosinophilic inflammation: are they all the same? *Am J Gastroenterol* 2006;101:1125–1128.

102. Gonsalves N, Doerfler B, Yang G, Hirano I. A prospective clinical trial of Six food elimination diet or elemental diet in the treatment of adults with eosinophilic gastroenteritis. *Gastroenterology* 2009;S1861.

103. Roy-Ghanta DF, Larosa DF, Katzka DA. Atopic characteristics of adult patients with eosinophilic esophagitis. *Clin Gastroenterol Hepatol* 2008;6:531–535.

104. Spergel JM, Andrews T, Brown-Whitehorn TF, Beausoleil JL, Liacouras CA. Treatment of eosinophilic esophagitis with specific food elimination diet directed by a combination of skin prick and patch tests. *Ann Allergy Asthma Immunol* 2005;95: 336–343.

105. Kagalwalla AF, Sentongo TA, Ritz S, *et al.* Effect of six-food elimination diet on clinical and histologic outcomes in Eosinophilic esophagitis. *Clin Gastroenterol Hepatol* 2006;4: 1097–2002.

106. Gonsalves N, Yang G, Doerfler B, *et al.* A prospective clinical trial of six food elimination diet and reintroduction of causative agents in adults with eosinophilic esophagitis [abstract]. *Gastroenterology* 2008;134:A727.

107. Aceves SS, Newbury RO, Dohil R, Bastian JF, Broide DH. Esophageal remodeling in pediatric eosinophilic esophagitis. *J Allergy Clin Immunol* 2007;119:206–212.

108. Sanjeevi A, Ashwath G, Komorowski R, Massey BT, Shaker R, Hogan WJ. Early recognition and specific medical therapy affects the frequency of esophageal dilatations in patients with eosinophilic esophagitis (EE). *Gastrointest Endosc* 2006;63:AB128.

109. Cohen MS, Kaufman AB, Palazzo JP, Nevin D, Dimarino AJ Jr, Cohen S. An audit of endoscopic complications in adult eosinophilic esophagitis. *Clin Gastroenterol Hepatol* 2007;5: 1149–1153.

110. Francalanci P, De Angelis P, Minnei F, *et al.* Eosinophilic esophagitis and Barrett's esophagus: an occasional association or an overlap disease? Esophageal "double trouble" in two children. *Digestion* 2008;77:16–19.

111. Wolfsen HC. Hemminger LL. Achem SR. Eosinophilic esophagitis and Barrett's esophagus with dysplasia. *Clin Gastroenterol Hepatol* 2007;5:A18.

112. Schoepfer AM, Gschossmann J, Scheurer U, Seibold F, Straumann A. Esophageal strictures in adult eosinophilic esophagitis: dilation is an effective and safe alternative after failure of topical corticosteroids. *Endoscopy* 2008;40:161–164.

113. Cohen MS, Kaufman A, DiMarino AJ Jr, Cohen S. Eosinophilic esophagitis presenting as spontaneous esophageal rupture (Boerhaave's syndrome). *Clin Gastroenterol Hepatol* 2007;5:A24.

114. Nantes O. Jimenez FJ. Zozaya JM, Vila JJ. Increased risk of esophageal perforation in eosinophilic esophagitis. *Endoscopy* 2009;41 (Suppl 2):E177–178.

115. Kaplan M, Mutlu EA, Jakate S, *et al.* Endoscopy in eosinophilic esophagitis: "feline" esophagus and perforation risk. *Clin Gastroenterol Hepatol* 2003;1:433–437.

37 Foreign Bodies

Andrew Y. Wang and David A. Peura

Division of Gastroenterology and Hepatology, University of Virginia Health System, Charlottesville, VA, USA

Introduction

Foreign body ingestion and food impaction are commonly encountered clinical occurrences, which are second only to gastrointestinal bleeding as an endoscopic emergency [1]. The esophagus is the most common site of acute foreign body or food impaction. Esophageal food impactions can be considered a problematic form of ingested foreign material. Therefore, when the term "foreign body" is mentioned in this chapter, it is assumed that esophageal food impactions are also included, unless otherwise specified in the text.

Although the true incidence is difficult to determine, the annual incidence of esophageal food impaction has been estimated at 13.0 per 100 000 [2]. Fortunately, most ingested foreign material will pass through the gastrointestinal tract without serious complication. Eighty to 90% of swallowed objects that reach the stomach will eventually pass uneventfully and require no therapeutic intervention [3]. However, in 10–20% of cases, objects may either become lodged in the esophagus or may pose a significant risk of perforation to the stomach and intestines, and as a result endoscopic intervention will be required. Surgery is necessary in 1% or fewer of cases of ingested foreign bodies [4, 5]. Although mortality from foreign body ingestion is generally low, given its relatively frequent occurrence, approximately 1500–2750 individuals in the United States die each year as a result of ingested foreign bodies [3, 6, 7]. Therefore, it is important to consider every foreign body ingestion as a medical emergency, due to the potential risk of developing a severe, life-threatening complication.

The most common localized complications of foreign body ingestion are associated mucosal changes, including tears, edema, and ulcerations; bleeding; luminal obstruction; respiratory compromise resulting from airway obstruction or aspiration; and perforation [8, 9]. Other proximate complications are usually within the thoracic cavity and are a consequence of migration of the foreign body from the esophagus, compromising different nearby organs [8]. These include arterioesophageal fistulae, aortoesophageal fistulae, mediastinitis, pericarditis, and pericardial effusions [10–14].

The management of patients with esophageal or gastric foreign bodies has shifted over the years from the domain of surgeons and radiologists to that of gastroenterologists. Several factors should be seriously considered when confronted with a patient who has ingested a foreign body, which involve not only the patient's clinical condition but also the type of foreign body that has been ingested [8]. Depending on the scenario, the goal is to either relieve the obstruction and associated symptoms (in the case of an esophageal food impaction) or to remove a potentially dangerous object from the gastrointestinal tract so as to reduce the risk of associated complications.

Several key factors should be considered in assessing an ingested foreign body [3, 5, 8]:

- Type, nature, and number of objects (blunt, sharp, pointed; toxic or non-toxic; single or multiple);
- Location of the foreign body by symptoms or radiography (hypopharynx, esophagus, stomach, small bowel);
- Elapsed time since ingestion (hours, days);
- Presence of symptoms compatible with complete obstruction (inability to manage secretions) or other complications (airway compromise, crepitus, fever);
- Previous esophageal or upper gastrointestinal pathology or surgery;
- If the object needs to be retrieved or can be left alone;
- If the ingested foreign material can be safely managed with available equipment and physician expertise.

Anatomic considerations

Ingested foreign objects can lodge at any level of the gastrointestinal tract, but most commonly they become impacted at regions that are physiologically or pathologically narrowed [3, 15]. This fact may explain why the esophagus is the most common site of foreign body impaction in the gastrointestinal tract, accounting for 75% of all impactions [16].

The adult esophageal lumen can distend to approximately 2 cm in anteroposterior (AP) diameter and up to 3 cm in lateral diameter to accommodate a swallowed bolus. The esophageal wall is composed of four major layers (from innermost to outermost): the mucosa (consisting of the epithelium, lamina propria, and muscularis mucosa), submucosa, muscularis propria, and adventitia [8]. Unlike the remainder of the gastrointestinal tract, the esophagus does not have a serosal layer, but it is surrounded by the adventitia, a thin layer of connective tissue.

The normal esophagus has five physiologic sites of narrowing: (1) upper esophageal sphincter (UES) (including the cricopharyngeus), which is the narrowest point of the gastrointestinal tract (14 mm in diameter, at the level of the C6 vertebra); (2) thoracic inlet (at the level of the T1 vertebra); (3) aortic arch (15–17 mm in diameter, at the level of the T4 vertebra); (4) tracheal bifurcation or left main stem bronchus

(at the level of the T6 vertebra); and (5) lower esophageal sphincter (LES) (16–19 mm in diameter, at the level of the T10–11 vertebrae) [8] (Figure 37.1). Other important areas of physiologic narrowing distal to the esophagus include the pylorus, duodenal sweep, ileocecal valve, and anus. Objects thicker than 2 cm or longer than 5 cm tend to lodge in the stomach [17]. Long foreign bodies (>10 cm in length) tend to hang in the duodenal sweep where perforations may also involve the right kidney [18, 19].

Pathologic narrowing of the esophageal lumen must also be considered in every patient with a retained foreign body. The etiology and frequency of pathologic constriction often varies with age. Congenital conditions, such as vascular rings, resulting in dysphagia or foreign body impaction are rare even in children (Figure 37.2). Whereas children are apt to swallow coins that may lodge in the cervical esophagus, proximal to the cricopharyngeus, they typically will not have a structural lesion. With the evolving understanding of eosinophilic esophagitis, this disease must now be considered in any pediatric or adult patient with dysphagia and food impaction. However, as opposed to adults who typically present with dysphagia or food impaction [20], children with eosinophilic esophagitis can also present with less specific symptoms (e.g. gastroesophageal reflux disease (GERD)-like

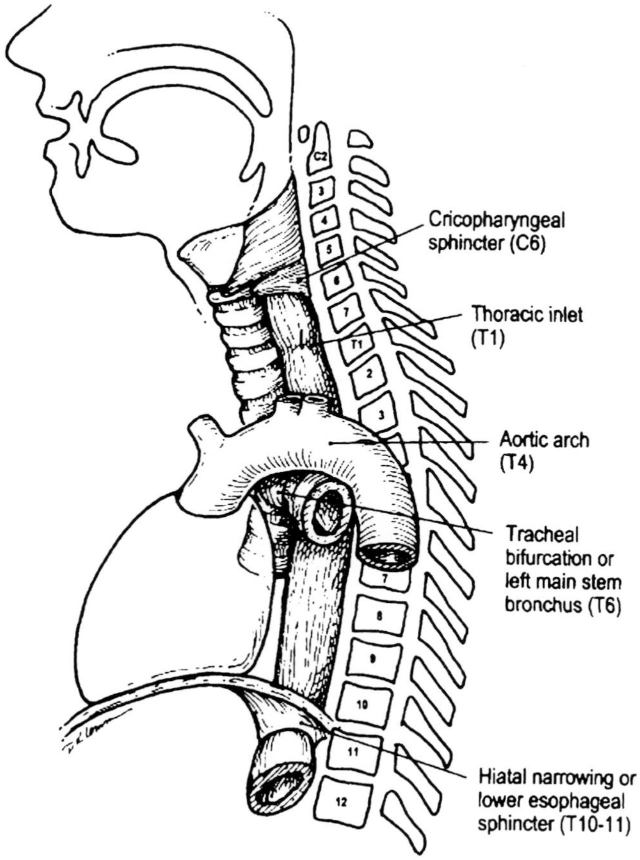

Figure 37.1 Five physiologic sites of narrowing in the esophagus. (reproduced courtesy of Stanley B. Benjamin MD).

Cricopharyngeal sphincter (C6)

Thoracic inlet (T1)

Aortic arch (T4)

Tracheal bifurcation or left main stem bronchus (T6)

Hiatal narrowing or lower esophageal sphincter (T10-11)

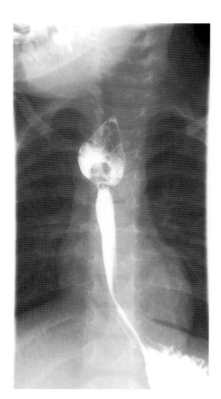

Figure 37.2 A 2-year old girl with a history of a tracheoesophageal fistula repair as an infant presented with an esophageal stricture and an impacted food bolus (reproduced courtesy of Hubert A. Shaffer Jr MD).

symptoms, abdominal pain, or feeding problems), and they typically do not have obstructing rings [21, 22].

In adults, pathologic narrowing of the esophagus is most often due to a peptic stricture or a distal esophageal (Schatzki's) ring [2]. Other causes include strictures from caustic injection, pill esophagitis, eosinophilic esophagitis [23], esophageal webs, cricopharyngeal bars [24], and rarely esophageal intramural pseudodiverticulosis [25, 26]. Pathologic narrowing of the esophagus can also be from an extraluminal cause, such as from a mediastinal mass or bronchogenic carcinoma. Although esophageal malignancies cause stricturing [27], this is a relatively infrequent presentation of esophageal food impaction [3, 4, 28] (Figure 37.3). However, when an esophageal malignancy causes a

circumferential stricture, in most cases this denotes an advanced lesion (T3 or worse).

A right-sided aortic arch without mirror image anatomy of the arteries is a cause of dysphagia lusoria and potential food impaction (Figure 37.4). Typically the point of compression is due to an aberrant origin of the right subclavian artery, which arises from a retroesophageal diverticulum (diverticulum of Kommerell), and contributes to a vascular ring. Patients with a right-sided aortic arch who have mirror-image anatomy of the brachiocephalic vessels (i.e. with the left innominate artery as the first branch off the arch, followed by the right common carotid and subclavian arteries) may also experience dysphagia lusoria, although this is typically due to the descending aorta remaining to the right of

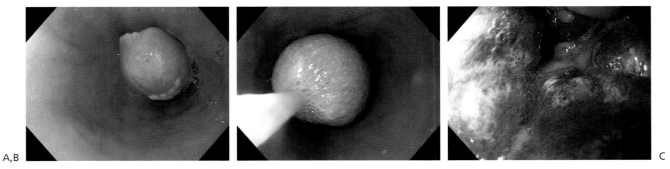

Figure 37.3 An impacted hot dog (A) was removed from the esophagus using a retrieval net (B), which revealed an underlying malignant stricture due to an adenocarcinoma (C).

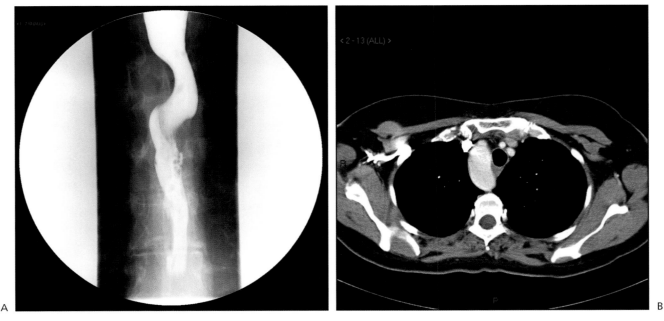

Figure 37.4 Dysphagia lusoria from a right-sided aortic arch as seen on fluoroscopy (A). The esophagus is impinged on one side by the aortic arch and on the other side by the trachea (B) in this patient with mirror-image anatomy (in which left innominate is the first artery to originate from the arch, followed by the right common carotid and subclavian arteries).

midline before reaching the lower thorax. Pediatric patients with a right-sided aortic arch typically present with airway symptomatology in addition to dysphagia or feeding difficulties. Those with primarily esophageal symptomatology tend to be older at presentation [29].

Clinical presentation

Patients who have swallowed a foreign object that results in esophageal impaction can present with a wide array of signs and symptoms. In young children, the history is often unclear as they may be unable to express their symptoms. As the history must often be obtained from a parent or caretaker, the nature of the ingested foreign body is often unknown. In small children, respiratory symptoms frequently predominate over gastrointestinal symptoms because their soft tracheal rings are easily compressed by the esophageal foreign body, leading to compression of the trachea [15]. In infants or children, stridor, persistent cough, drooling, or refusal to take feedings should immediately

raise suspicion for an ingested foreign body and prompt a diagnostic work-up, including radiographic imaging [30]. In contrast, most adults seek medical attention within the first 6 h of impaction, and almost all within the first 24 h [31]. Dysphagia, odynophagaia, sensation of a foreign body, and increased salivation are the most common presenting symptoms associated with esophageal impaction in adults.

The types of objects that children and adults ingest are markedly different. Children are prone to ingest coins, holiday ornaments, small light bulbs, and toys [30, 32]. Esophageal impaction in adults is frequently due to poorly chewed meat that may hang up due to a pathologic or physiologic area of narrowing [2]. In recent years, there have been multiple reports of ingested toothpicks causing perforation and abscesses [33–36]. The types of problematic ingested materials can also differ among different cultures and populations (Table 37.1). One large series from Southern China found that fish bones were the most common cause of esophageal foreign body impactions, representing 38% of ingestions in children and over 50% in adults [37]. Sometimes, attempts by patients to alleviate a foreign body

Table 37.1 Types and locations of ingested foreign bodies in different geographic populations and cultures from recently published studies and abstracts.

		Nijhawan *et al.* (2003) [125] India		Katsinelos *et al.* (2006) [59] Greece		Khorshidi *et al.* (2007) [126] USA		Zhang *et al.* (2009) [37] China	
		Number	%	Number	%	Number	%	Number	%
Type of foreign body	Food boluses (meat)	19	10.3			35	76.1	35	8.0
	Chicken bones							72	16.4
	Fish bones							265	60.4
	Unspecified bones			24	31.2	3	6.5		
	Sharp/pointed	7	3.8	3	3.9				
	Coins	134	72.8	17	22.1				
	Dentures	12	6.5	11	14.3				
	Other	12	6.5	22	28.6	8	17.4	67	15.3
	Total	**184**	**100**	**77**	**100**	**46**	**100**	**439**	**100**
Anatomic location		Not specified				Not specified			
	Pharynx			3	3.9			15	3.4
	Esophagus			20	26.0				
	Upper							305	69.5
	Middle							49	11.2
	Lower							17	3.9
	Stomach			52	67.5			34	7.7
	Duodenum			2	2.6			7	1.6
	Surgical anastomosis							12	2.7
	Total			**77**	**100**			**439**	**100**

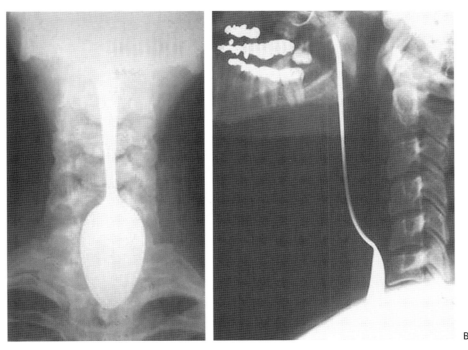

A   B

Figure 37.5 A spoon was inadvertently ingested by a patient who was attempting to dislodge a fish bone from his throat (reproduced from Ramadan and El-Desouky [38], with permission).

impaction can add to the problem, as was the case in a patient who lodged a spoon in his esophagus in an attempt to remove what he thought was an impacted fish bone [38] (Figure 37.5).

Other adult populations in whom the incidence of foreign body ingestion is increased include those with psychiatric disorders, learning disabilities, or impairment due to alcohol ingestion or drug abuse. Incarcerated individuals seeking access to a medical facility as a means of secondary gain represent a group in whom intentional foreign body ingestion can occur. Adults with dentures and dental bridgework are also at increased risk of accidental foreign body ingestion because of compromise of their tactile sensation during swallowing [39].

Although clinically rare, patients with achalasia can certainly present with dysphagia and food impaction. In patients with atypical clinical scenarios for achalasia, in whom occult malignancy may be suspected, psuedoachalasia from an adenocarcinoma in the gastric fundus or from paraneoplastic syndrome must be considered [40].

Diagnostic evaluation

Patient localization of the level of a foreign body impaction is often not reliable [41]. In many instances, the ingestion may go unrecognized or unreported until the onset of symptoms, which may be remote from the time of ingestion [5, 42–44]. Biplanar radiographs are useful as they identify steak bones, most true foreign bodies, and free mediastinal or peritoneal air. Radiographs should be obtained of the chest, abdomen, and pelvis. Biplanar views of the neck should also be obtained if the location of the foreign body is suspected to be in the cervical esophagus or oropharynx [39]. Lateral radiographs may confirm the location in the esophagus and may provide information on the number of objects not readily apparent on PA or AP films, such as ingested coins in children. As the esophagus is wider along its lateral axis as opposed to its AP axis, ingested coins and bottle caps lodged in the esophagus appear round on frontal radiographs and flat on lateral radiographs. Conversely, aspirated coins and bottle caps lodged in the trachea will appear flat on frontal films and round on lateral films (Figure 37.6). Fish bones, chicken bones, and metallic slivers may be difficult to identify despite biplanar views. Plastic and most glass objects may not be radio-opaque at all [5]. Plain films are particularly important when a button battery may have been ingested, which is a true emergency. Radiographs can usually distinguish a coin from a button battery [8].

When plain films are unrevealing, a CT of the neck, thorax, and abdomen may be useful in identifying ingested foreign bodies [45, 46]. In patients with an unrevealing

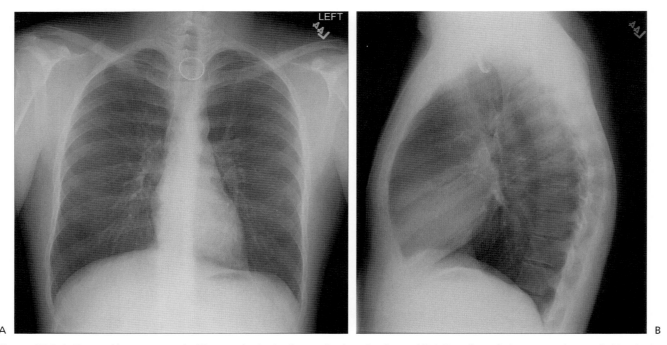

Figure 37.6 A 19-year-old man presented with acute dysphagia after swallowing a bottle cap. (A) A PA radiograph demonstrated a round object in the upper esophagus. (B) A lateral radiograph confirmed that the cap was in the esophagus, as opposed to the trachea. The cap was removed using flexible endoscopy with the assistance of rat-tooth forceps (reproduced courtesy of Hubert A. Shaffer Jr MD).

radiologic work-up, whose signs and symptoms still suggest foreign body retention or esophageal impaction, diagnostic endoscopy is indicated. In patients with a persistent sensation of foreign body ingestion, in whom plain films or even endoscopy has been unrevealing, helical computed tomography (CT) scans [47] and three-dimensional CT reconstruction [48] of the oropharynx and cervical esophagus may play an important role in excluding a small impacted foreign body or localized perforation.

Fluoroscopic contrast studies should not be used routinely to indentify or localize ingested foreign bodies. A water-soluble mixture of sodium amidotrizoate and meglumine amidotrizoate (Gastrografin; Bayer Schering Pharma AG, Germany) is typically the contrast agent of choice if a perforation is suspected, as it is readily absorbed from the mediastinum or pleural space [49]. However, in the case of a food impaction, the use of a sodium amidotrizoate and meglumine amidotrizoate mixture is contraindicated, as it is extremely hypertonic (1900 mOsm/L) and can cause a severe chemical pneumonitis if aspirated into the lung [3, 8]. Low-osmolar non-ionic contrast media, such as iopamidol, metrizamide, or iohexol, are possible alternatives as they may have less tissue reactivity [50]. Barium does not cause chemical pneumonitis; however, pooled barium in the area of an impacted esophageal foreign body will make endoscopic visualization more difficult, and barium can impede endoscopic suction and clog the working channel of the endoscope.

Endoscopic and non-endoscopic interventions

If radiographs identify a foreign body in the hypopharynx, urgent consultation with an otolaryngologist is indicated. Although a gastroenterologist may have success at identifying and removing a hypopharyngeal foreign body, otolaryngologists are better suited to deal with complications in this region if they occur.

The radiology literature is replete with different techniques that have been used to remove esophageal foreign bodies under fluoroscopic guidance. Reported methods include extraction with Foley balloon catheters, suction catheters, and wire baskets [51]. In 1980, Kozarek and Sanowski described a method of treating esophageal food impactions using a modified 34F gastric lavage tube connected to a 120-mL aspiration syringe [52]; however, this method was never widely adopted. The largest radiologic experience has been with Foley catheters, which can be passed either transnasally or orally into the esophagus, past the foreign body, and then withdrawn to deliver the foreign body into the oropharynx where it can be retrieved [1].

Although this technique has a reported success rate of greater than 80% [53, 54], the potential to lose control of the foreign body at the level of the UES and posterior oropharynx puts patients at risk for aspiration and airway obstruction [1, 53]. As a result, we do not advocate this method of foreign body removal in settings where endoscopy is available.

Endoscopic extraction is the method of choice for dealing with esophageal and upper gastrointestinal foreign bodies and food impactions. Rigid endoscopy was formerly the most widely used modality for esophageal foreign body extraction, and it is still effectively used in developing countries to manage foreign bodies in the esophagus [55, 56]. However, since the early 1970s, flexible endoscopy has been used with excellent results worldwide [37], essentially replacing rigid endoscopy, which was associated with a greater risk of complications [16, 57, 58]. Reported success rates using flexible endoscopy to relieve esophageal food impactions and foreign body ingestions exceed 96% [59, 60].

Flexible endoscopy is not only of value diagnostically, but it also offers the opportunity for therapeutic intervention. The endoscopist should always be prepared to extract the foreign object at the time of initial endoscopy. During endoscopy, an examination of the posterior oropharynx should be made, and the esophagus should be intubated using direct visualization. The esophagus should be carefully inspected along its entire extent for mucosal changes, diverticula, areas of intrinsic or extrinsic pathologic narrowing, and masses. If the suspected foreign body is not found in the esophagus, a complete examination of the stomach and duodenum should be performed.

The timing and requirement for diagnostic and therapeutic endoscopy depends on the clinical situation. In the case of a food bolus impaction, if there is any concern that the food bolus remains, then endoscopy is indicated. Patients who cannot handle their own secretions should undergo urgent endoscopy since this suggests a high-grade luminal obstruction. As a general rule, all esophageal food impactions should be relieved within 12–24 h [1, 5].

In the case of an ingested foreign object that has passed the duodenal sweep, endoscopy is not usually required. However, if a potentially dangerous object (e.g. a sharp/pointed object or a button-cell battery) has been ingested and is still within the reach of standard endoscopy or enteroscopy, it should be removed as soon as possible. Since 2001, double-balloon enteroscopy has enabled deep endoscopic evaluation of the small bowel [61]. Single-balloon enteroscopy [62] and rotational enteroscopy [63] are newer options that also permit diagnostic and therapeutic endoscopy of the deep small bowel. Although the capabilities of these deep enteroscopy platforms are still being defined [64], these new technologies now enable the removal of dangerous objects from the deep small bowel, which would otherwise have

been impossible to reach using standard endoscopes and push-enteroscopes. Neumann *et al.* described the removal of a coin that had been lodged in the jejunum for 8 days using double-balloon enteroscopy [65], and Ramchandani *et al.* were able to remove a sewing needle that had partially penetrated the jejunal wall using single-balloon enteroscopy [66].

The exact endoscopic approach, technique, and equipment used will depend on the clinical scenario, including the nature and location of the ingested foreign material. Although experience matters, most endoscopists are capable of removing ingested foreign bodies from the gastrointestinal tract using flexible endoscopy equipment and commonly available accessories [67].

Patient preparation for endoscopy

Another issue to consider during ingested foreign body management is airway protection, particularly when endoscopy is indicated. In situations where endoscopic intervention using conscious sedation is appropriate and the ingested foreign material is amenable, use of an esophageal overtube can provide airway protection during foreign body extraction. In addition to standard clinical factors that should prompt the involvement of an anesthesiologist in providing sedation/anesthesia and airway support [68], there are several important issues to consider when preparing a patient for endoscopic removal of an ingested foreign body.

A complex endoscopic procedure to relieve a foreign body obstruction is likely to be more complicated and of longer duration as compared to a routine diagnostic endoscopy. As such, deeper levels of sedation may be required for a prolonged duration. In patients with a tenuous cardiopulmonary status (e.g. severe congestive heart failure, asthma, or emphysema), significant obstructive sleep apena, known history of laryngospasm, or risk of aspiration, general endotracheal anesthesia should be considered. General anesthesia should be used in most pediatric patients, particularly those with multiple ingested foreign bodies or difficult-to-remove objects, as most pediatric patients may not be able to understand or fully cooperate with instructions given during conscious sedation.

When considering or consenting patients for deep sedation or general anesthesia, it is important to convey the added benefits and to acknowledge the justifiable risks associated with procedures performed under these conditions. Although, the Institute of Medicine has approximated anesthesia-related mortality at 1 death per 200 000–300 000 cases, the medical literature supports a more realistic anesthesia-related mortality rate of 1 in 13 000 [69, 70].

Endoscopic equipment and accessories

Once the decision to proceed with endoscopic removal of ingested material has been made and issues regarding patient preparation have been addressed, the next step is to devise a strategy to efficiently and safely manage the clinical situation. A careful assessment of the available equipment, endoscopic accessories, and resources should be made. A diagnostic gastroscope may be sufficient to facilitate removal of an ingested sharp object or to cross a stricture, but a large-bolus food impaction may be better managed using a single- or double-channel therapeutic gastroscope, which will allow for better endoscopic suction. In some situations, the use of several different endoscopes may be required. As mentioned above, single-balloon enteroscopy, double-balloon enteroscopy, and overtube-assisted rotational enteroscopy are newer endoscopy platforms that can be used to remove dangerous foreign bodies from the jejunum and ileum. These deep enteroscopy platforms also enable the removal of ingested foreign bodies from patients with complicated surgically altered anatomy (such as a Roux-en-Y gastric bypass).

Several types of endoscopic accessories are available to facilitate safe and effective management of ingested foreign bodies. These include various grasping forceps, snares, wire baskets, retrieval nets, and retrieval balloons (Figure 37.7). Rubber or latex hoods are available that can be attached to the end of an endoscope in an inverted position to facilitate esophageal intubation [71]. Once the hood has been passed into the esophagus or stomach, it can be flipped into a forward-facing position by pulling back against the LES or UES. Such hoods allow for the safe capture and extraction of sharp and pointed objects through the UES and LES and out of the body (Figure 37.8). Prior to using a foreign body hood, it is important to determine if it is made of latex and if the patient has a latex allergy. The double-balloon enteroscope platform (Fujinon, Wayne, NJ, USA) also uses a latex balloon, and as such it should not be used in patients with latex sensitivity; in contrast, the single-balloon enteroscope

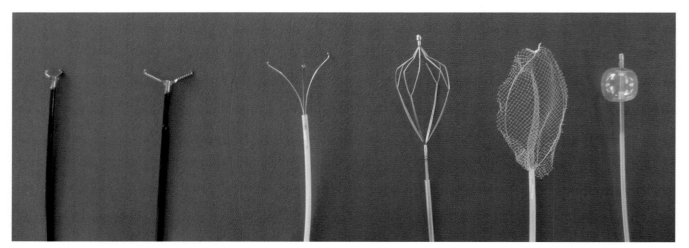

Figure 37.7 Examples of specialized endoscopic tools that facilitate foreign body extraction. From left to right: rat-tooth forceps, alligator-jaw forceps, tripod polyp retriever, wire basket, retrieval net, and biliary extraction balloon (inflated to 15 mm). Other standard devices that may also be used in foreign body removal include biopsy forceps and different sized and shaped polypectomy snares (not shown). The Roth retrieval net is manufactured by US Endoscopy, Mentor, OH, USA and the remaining devices by Olympus America, Center Valley, PA, USA.

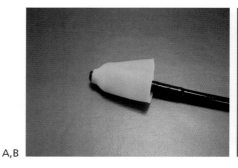 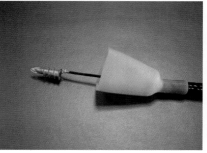 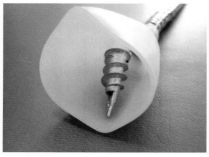

A,B   C

Figure 37.8 A soft foreign body hood can be used to retrieve sharp or pointed ingested foreign bodies. The hood is first affixed to the tip of the endoscope in the inverted or pulled-back position (A). Once the endoscope and hood have passed the upper or lower esophageal junctions, retraction of the scope against a sphincter deploys the hood. Once the object in question has been grasped with the pointed end trailing (B), it can then be brought back in to the hood (C) and then safely removed from the body by withdrawal of the endoscope.

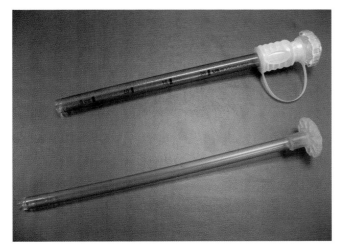

Figure 37.9 Example of an esophageal-length (25-cm long) two-tube–system overtube with an insufflation cap that prevents leakage of air during endoscopy (Guardus; US Endoscopy, Mentor, OH, USA).

platform (Olympus America, Center Valley, PA, USA) uses a silicone balloon and may be an alternative in patients who are latex sensitive. Esophageal and gastric overtubes are invaluable when the endoscope must be repeatedly inserted and removed from the body during management of impacted food or an ingested foreign body. In addition to protecting the airway during extraction of foreign material, overtubes also provide mucosal protection during extraction of sharp or pointed objects (Figure 37.9).

In addition to endoscopic accessories, an experienced assistant is an invaluable resource that can make the difference between success and failure when performing endoscopic foreign body and food bolus extraction. Furthermore, it is highly recommended that the endoscopist and assistant practice grasping and manipulating an object similar to the ingested foreign material outside of the body, prior to performing the procedure in the patient. Rehearsal using the tools anticipated to be of use in foreign body extraction can save time and reduce the risk of procedure-related complications.

Management strategies for various foreign bodies

In the following sections, we will describe the clinical features and recommended management strategies for different kinds of ingested foreign bodies.

Food bolus impaction
Food is the most common cause of esophageal impaction [72]. In the United States, the most commonly impacted foods are meat products [2, 73], including beef, chicken,

pork, and hot dogs [72]. More commonly in Asia or along costal areas, ingested fish bones that become lodged in the upper gastrointestinal tract are a clinical problem [37]. Fish bones and chicken bones, which also are on occasion inadvertently ingested, typically do not cause luminal blockage, rather they are prone to penetrate the mucosa of the hypopharynx or esophagus due to their pointed nature (see the following section on *sharp or pointed objects*).

Poor or absent dentition and/or improperly fitting dentures, which preclude efficient mastication, often contribute to food impaction. Food impaction can also occur in association with alcohol ingestion. Inebriated patients can swallow food without chewing sufficiently, from which the terms "steakhouse syndrome" [74] and "backyard barbecue syndrome" [1] have been coined. In cases of witnessed acute food impaction, if there are associated signs or symptoms of complete airway obstruction and asphyxiation, the Heimlich maneuver can be life saving. However, the Heimlich maneuver should not be performed unless there is definite evidence of airway compromise, as fractured ribs [75], esophageal rupture [76], hepatic rupture [77], and aortic dissection [78] have been reported.

Several non-endoscopic techniques have been used to either extract a food bolus or promote its passage into the stomach, although some of these practices are infrequently employed due to complications associated with their use. The best described pharmacologic agent administered in the setting of esophageal impaction is glucagon, which relaxes the smooth muscle of the LES; the upper third of the esophagus contains striated muscle and is not affected by glucagon. Glucagon is typically given in a dosage of 1–2 mg IV in adults and 0.02–0.03 mg/kg IV in children weighing less than 20 kg, with a maximum dose of 0.5 mg [8, 79]. Patients receiving glucagon in the setting of an esophageal impaction should be kept upright and given a small amount of water to ingest following the injection; patients at risk for aspiration should not be treated in this manner. A dose of glucagon may be repeated in 5–10 min if the first dose is ineffective. Most endoscopists who perform endoscopic retrograde cholangio-pancreatography (ERCP) are familiar with the use of glucagon, typically at doses ranging from 0.25 to 1 mg IV. However, when administered at a dose of 1 mg or greater, glucagon can cause nausea, vomiting, and hyperglycemia [80]. Glucagon is relatively contraindicated in patients with diabetes mellitus, and it is absolutely contraindicated in patients with insulinoma, pheochromocytoma, Zollinger–Ellison syndrome, or sensitivity to the drug.

When used to promote passage of an esophageal food impaction, glucagon has been shown to be variably effective in only 12–50% of cases [80], likely because it does not affect distal esophageal rings or strictures. In one multicenter, placebo-controlled, double-blind study that included 43 patients, a combination of glucagon and diazepam (n = 24) or placebo (n = 19) was administered to patients with an esophageal foreign body impaction [81]. These authors found no significant difference between the two study groups (rates of foreign body disimpaction were 38% and 32%, respectively). Most successful pharmacologic disimpactions actually occurred several hours after the medications were given, and the authors rejected their hypothesis that muscle spasm was an important cause of esophageal obstruction. Other agents such as nitroglycerin, calcium-channel blockers, atropine, and benzodiazepines have been used, but have not been shown to have any significant advantage over glucagon [8, 81].

Papain is a proteolytic enzyme that was used to digest esophageal meat impactions from the 1940s through the 1960s [82, 83]. However, the use of proteolytic enzymes to digest meat impactions has been eschewed since it became clear that papain use was associated with esophageal perforation and hemorrhagic pulmonary edema, and pneumonitis in cases of papain aspiration [84, 85]. Furthermore, other reports have questioned the effectiveness of papain in reducing the size of an impacted meat bolus and have suggested that it may worsen existing esophagitis [86].

Again, flexible endoscopy has become the treatment modality of choice when managing esophageal food impactions. Reported success rates using flexible endoscopy for relieving esophageal food impactions exceed 96% [59, 60]. The majority of patients who develop an esophageal food impaction have an underlying cause of luminal narrowing [2, 72, 73]. Most of these causes will be benign, such as a Schatzki's ring or peptic stricture, but an esophageal malignancy is also a possibility. Thus, unless an endoscope can be passed alongside the impacted food bolus into the distal esophagus, ruling out a stricture or obstructing lesion, one must avoid the temptation to blindly push an object through the gastroesophageal junction into the stomach [73]. In many cases, food impactions can be removed in one piece using a retrieval net, which also provides some protection against particles breaking off during extraction and causing airway compromise. In some instances, a large food bolus can be broken down into smaller pieces using a snare, grasping forceps, or a wire basket, after which the smaller particles can spontaneously pass or be gently pushed through into the stomach or be removed. Use of an esophageal-length overtube should be considered when it is necessary to sequentially remove multiple pieces of impacted food. In addition to providing airway protection, an overtube facilitates repeated intubation and retrieval episodes, and makes the entire procedure safer and better tolerated by the patient.

One novel technique for removing impacted meat uses a Stiegmann-Goff friction-fit adaptor (i.e. an endoscope cap) and an esophageal overtube to create a direct-vision suction device with which impacted material can be suctioned into the cap and removed from the body [72, 87, 88]. Although,

this method has been used successfully in small series, it has not gained widespread acceptance nor has it been proven to be safe and effective in large, prospective studies.

Sharp or pointed objects

Sharp and pointed objects account for one-third of all perforations caused by ingested foreign bodies, and if left untreated 15–35% of such objects can result in a gastrointestinal complication [1, 89]. Bones, toothpicks, and dental bridgework are the most common, inadvertently ingested sharp foreign objects. The common toothpick, which measures approximately 7 cm in length, and is sharp on both ends, has been reported to perforate and cause vascular fistulae [90], pericardial effusions [91], abdominal and liver abscesses [92], and pancreatitis [93]. Voluntary ingestion of more complex and varied foreign bodies, such as pens, razor blades, and metal wires, can be encountered in individuals with psychiatric illnesses or those who desire hospitalization as a secondary gain (Figure 37.10).

Although rigid endoscopy is utilized in some situations, flexible endoscopy is the diagnostic and therapeutic procedure of choice in managing ingested sharp or pointed objects. When retrieving ingested sharp or pointed foreign bodies, the axiom put forward by Chevalier Jackson, a pioneer in endoscopy, laryngoscopy, and foreign body removal, "advancing points puncture, trailing points do not" applies

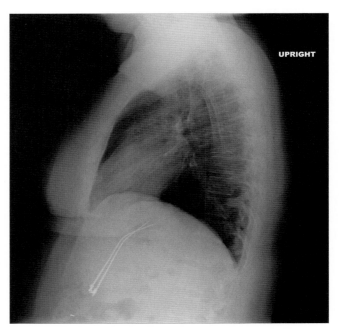

Figure 37.10 A pair of eyeglass arms were ingested by a prison inmate, presumably for purposes of secondary gain. The lateral radiograph showed the foreign bodies in the stomach. They were subsequently removed endoscopically using an esophageal overtube and rat-tooth forceps.

[94, 95]. Pointed objects should be removed in such a manner that the pointed end trails so as to minimize the risk of mucosal injury and perforation during extraction of the foreign body. A rubber foreign body hood or esophageal- or gastric-length overtube can also be used to protect the gastrointestinal tract during endoscopic removal of a sharp or pointed object. Sharp or pointed objects can usually be securely grasped with forceps (rat-tooth or alligator-jaw types) or a polypectomy snare.

Small, sharp objects lodged in the cervical esophagus may be especially difficult to visualize and remove. Zhang *et al.* described using a modified band-ligator cap to improve visualization in a small series of patients who had ingested fish bones. They reported 100% success and significantly shorter procedure times using this method [37]. Others have also used this technique to successfully remove ingested foreign bodies [96]. Similar caps are used for endoscopic mucosal resection and endoscopic submucosal dissection, and are commercially available for purchase.

Sharp objects beyond the reach of conventional endoscopy should be followed closely, typically with serial radiographs. Although most of these objects will spontaneously pass through the gastrointestinal tract, if an object does not progress; if the patient develops fever, abdominal pain, gastrointestinal bleeding, or symptoms of obstruction; or if there is evidence of perforation, then surgery is indicated.

Coins

Coins are a frequently ingested foreign body in children, with 3905 cases reported to poison control centers in 2004 [97]. Older patients rarely present with impacted dimes (18 mm in diameter), pennies (19 mm), or nickels (21 mm). However, quarters (24 mm) may become lodged at the level of the cricopharyngeus or in the esophagus, particularly in the pediatric population (Table 37.2).

Coins typically cause injury by pressure necrosis, but bleeding and perforation can occur. Newer pennies, minted after 1982, are composed primarily of zinc (97.6% zinc and 2.4% copper), as opposed to older pennies which are mostly copper (95% copper and 5% zinc). Zinc pennies are more corrosive than the older copper pennies, but zinc and copper are indistinguishable on radiographs. Furthermore, X-ray magnification can cause coins to appear larger than their actual size, making pennies and dimes difficult to distinguish. Therefore, coins lodged in the esophagus should be removed. An exception might be coins that have made it to the distal third of the esophagus, as most coins in this location will pass spontaneously—as such, a period of observation not exceeding 12 h is reasonable [3]. Objects 25 mm or smaller in size typically can pass through the pylorus. Thus, once a coin enters the stomach, with the exception of half dollars (30 mm) or silver dollars (38 mm), observation with a regular diet and conservative management is sufficient in most patients [1].

Table 37.2 Characteristics of ingested coins in a pediatric population from recently published studies.

	Waltzman *et al.* [98]	Arms *et al.* [101]*	Combined	
	Number	Number	Total	%
Type of coin				
Penny	26	229	255	37
Nickel	4	50	54	8
Dime	4	25	29	4
Quarter	15	180	195	29
Unknown	11	136	147	22
Total	**60**	**620**	**680**	**100**
Location in esophagus		Not specified		
Proximal	20		20	33
Middle	19		19	32
Distal	21		21	35
Total	**60**		**60**	**100**

*In this study, the number of coins in each category was extrapolated based on the percentages reported and the total number of patients included.

In a small prospective study by Waltzman *et al.* that included 60 pediatric patients, 25% of ingested coins passed spontaneously through the esophagus [98]. On multivariate analysis, adjusting for age, coins lodged in the distal half of the esophagus (OR 2.16; $P = .08$) and male gender (OR 3.30; $P = .08$) were predictors of spontaneous passage, which trended towards significance. In this study, neither size nor coin type was a predictor of spontaneous passage.

Coins lodged in the cervical esophagus may be amenable to removal by an experienced otolaryngologist using curved Magill forceps that are inserted through the mouth [99, 100]. Ingested coins in pediatric patients can also be effectively and relatively safely extracted using Foley balloon catheters passed blindly or under fluoroscopic guidance. A success rate of 88–90% and a rate of major complication of 1% has been reported [53, 54]. However, due to the risk of losing control of the coin at the level of the UES or posterior oropharynx, visual flexible endoscopic removal of ingested coins has largely supplanted Foley balloon catheter extraction in most centers.

Blind bouginage has been described as a treatment performed by emergency room physicians in children with confirmed coin ingestion. In a large retrospective series of 620 pediatric patients who had ingested coins, 372 underwent blind bouginage and 248 had flexible endoscopy for coin extraction [101]. Criteria used to select patients for bouginage included: (1) witnessed single coin ingestion; (2) ingestion less than 24 h before presentation; (3) coin position in the esophageal lumen confirmed by radiograph; and (4) no history of esophageal foreign body, esophageal surgery, strictures, or other esophageal disease. Bouginage was successful in 355 cases (94.6%) and in cases of failure, successful salvage endoscopy was performed. Flexible endoscopy was successful at alleviating the esophageal obstruction in all cases. There were no perforations sustained in either group. However, pushing ingested coins through the esophagus into the stomach by means of bouginage without the use of endoscopy, despite the reported success rates, is not a technique preferred by most emergency room physicians or gastroenterologists [102].

Although the above mentioned non-endoscopic techniques can effectively remove impacted coins from the esophagus, we recommend using flexible endoscopy, which allows for direct visualization during coin extraction and also offers superior control as compared to Foley catheter extraction or blind bouginage. A retrieval net is usually the best tool to use when removing ingested coins by flexible endoscopy. The thin edges or smooth hard surfaces present on most coins make them difficult to securely grasp using a wire basket, grasping forceps, or snare [60, 103].

Batteries

The National Capital Poison Center, affiliated with The George Washington University Medical Center, has an outstanding website and a 24-h hotline to which physicians and patients may be referred in cases of button-cell battery ingestion (http://www.poison.org/prevent/battery.asp, phone: 202-625-3333). Sixty-two percent of battery ingestions involve children under the age of 5 years, with a peak incidence in 1- and 2-year-olds [104]. Nearly half of ingested batteries are those intended for hearing aids [105], while 12% are from games or toys. There has been a nearly 70% decline (over an 8-year period) in the percentage of ingested batteries that come from games and toys, which reflects industry efforts to secure and "child proof" the battery compartments of these products [106]. In 8.5% of cases, multiple batteries are swallowed.

Button-cell batteries range in diameter from 6.8 mm to 23.0 mm, with the most popular standard sizes ranging from 7.9 mm to 11.6 mm. Most ingested batteries are smaller than 12–15 mm and have little potential to lodge in the esophagus [105, 106]. However, if a button-cell battery does lodge in the esophagus, it should be urgently removed as contact time of as little as 1 h can result in mucosal injury, and within 4 h full-thickness damage can occur [89]. Complications from unwitnessed button-cell battery ingestion in children have included aortoesophageal fistula and bilateral vocal cord paralysis [107]. Leakage and the generation of an external current are the major mechanisms of battery-induced tissue damage. Button-cells often contain potassium or sodium hydroxide electrolyte in concentrations of up to 45%. However, batteries do not have to leak to cause injury, since an external current can be established between the cathode and anode through adjacent tissue, causing hydrolysis of tissue fluids and generation of hydroxides. In 1996, federal legislation known as the "Mercury-Containing and Rechargeable Battery Management Act" (US Public law 104-142, http://www.epa.gov/epawaste/laws-regs/state/policy/p1104.pdf) was enacted by the 104th Congress. The purpose of this law was to phase out the use of mercury in batteries. Since its enactment, mercury or other heavy metal poisoning is no longer a concern when button-cell batteries are swallowed [106].

As previously mentioned, Foley balloon catheter extraction offers limited to no control of an ingested foreign object, such as a button-cell battery, in the cervical esophagus and posterior oropharynx. Foley catheters are of no value in removing button-cell batteries from the stomach or duodenum. Blind bouginage or pushing button-cell batteries into the stomach is not recommended as button-cell batteries can cause mucosal injury, full-thickness burns, and subsequent perforation. Therefore, flexible endoscopy is the procedure of choice to remove ingested button-cell batteries from the upper gastrointestinal tract. Faigel *et al.* reported their experience with endoscopic removal of various foreign bodies placed in the stomachs of live pigs. In their experiment, a button-disc battery could only be removed with a Roth net (United States Endoscopy Group Inc, Mentor, OH, USA) or Dormia basket (Olympus America, Center Valley, PA, USA), although the retrieval net was superior to the basket (100% vs 27% respective success; $P < .025$) [67].

Although button-cell batteries are easier to inadvertently ingest, suicidal, psychiatric, or incarcerated patients sometimes ingest larger alkaline batteries. Traditional AAA batteries (44 mm long and 10 mm wide) and AA batteries (50 mm long and 14 mm wide) that enter the stomach can pass through the pylorus by leading with their shorter axes, but this is not always the case given the length of their longer axes (Figure 37.11). As these larger batteries can take longer to pass the gastrointestinal tract, they should be removed endoscopically whenever possible.

Other foreign bodies

Other less commonly ingested foreign bodies include the ordinary toothbrush, aluminum can pull-tabs (pop-tops), and deliberately ingested narcotic packets as a means of illicit transport and drug trafficking. There are at least 31 cases of accidentally ingested toothbrushes in the medical literature [108]. Toothbrushes can become lodged in the pharynx, esophagus, or stomach, and have been reported to cause mucosal tears, gastritis, pressure necrosis, and perforation. In the published series, none of the ingested toothbrushes passed through to the stomach. Therefore, all ingested toothbrushes should be retrieved endoscopically and not observed [108].

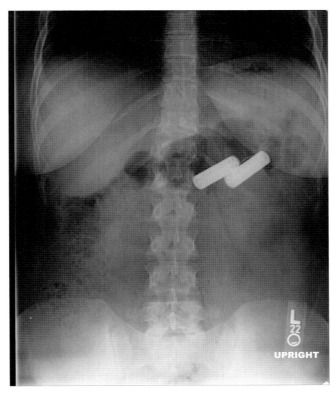

Figure 37.11 A pair of alkaline AA-batteries were ingested by a patient with a psychiatric illness. These batteries, which were retained in the stomach, were removed endoscopically to prevent caustic injury and obstruction.

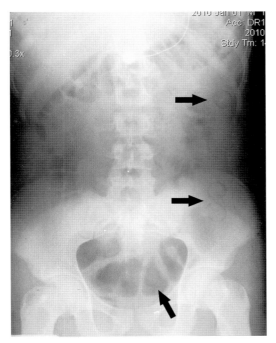

Figure 37.12 A man recently arrived from South America presented with symptoms of cocaine overdose. A radiograph revealed round radiolucencies (arrows) in the left colon representing condoms filled with cocaine, one of which had ruptured (reproduced courtesy of James M. Messmer MD and Hubert A. Shaffer Jr MD).

Pop-tops that are removed from aluminum beverage cans and subsequently ingested can be hazardous as they often can include pieces of attached, broken metal. As aluminum is not as dense or radio-opaque as other metals, these pop-tops can be difficult to identify on standard radiographs [109]. Rat-tooth forceps, retrieval nets, snares, and wire baskets can be used to remove pop-tops. However, if the pop-top cannot be firmly grasped using these devices, a long surgical ligature can be grasped using rat-tooth forceps and passed through the accessory channel of the endoscope into the esophagus or stomach. After the ligature has been guided through the opening in the center of the pop-top, the ligature is then grasped with the forceps, thereby securing the pop-top in a loop, after which it can be removed under endoscopic visualization.

Some patients ferry illicit drugs in their gastrointestinal tracts. These so-called "drug mules" or "body packers" swallow drugs in rubber or latex packets in an attempt to transport them across international borders without detection (Figure 37.12). Cocaine and heroin are the two most common internally smuggled substances. Body packers are typically encountered when they are brought in for medical attention by law enforcement officers with symptoms of drug intoxication or bowel obstruction. Fortunately, complications occur in fewer than 5% of hospitalized body packers [110]. However, intensive care unit-level monitoring is required to quickly recognize and treat acute drug intoxication if it occurs. Typically, a large number (20–50 packets) of drug packets will have been ingested, and they will be found throughout the small and large bowel. Endoscopy has little to no role in the management of body packers, as drug packets can rupture during attempted endoscopic removal and cause a drug overdose. Surgery is indicated in patients with acute drug intoxication or bowel obstruction [111]. A clear liquid diet with gentle use of polyethylene glycol (PEG) [112], mild laxatives, or observation without laxative administration [28] are recommended management strategies. These clinical approaches appear to have similar efficacies and complication rates. PEG can reduce cocaine toxicity by accelerating its removal from the gastrointestinal tract. Additionally, the relatively high pH of PEG can increase the conversion of cocaine to its inactive form, benzoylecgonine. Conversely, PEG may increase heroin toxicity by increasing its solubility [110].

Lastly, in the era of wireless video capsule endoscopy, it is important to note that capsule retention is a commonly observed complication, with an overall incidence of 1–2%; although reported rates vary widely from 0% to 21%

depending on the indication for the examination [113]. Wireless capsules can be retained at any level of the gastrointestinal tract, but fortunately in most cases the capsules eventually pass with no sequelae. However, symptomatic bowel obstruction requiring endoscopic or surgical removal of the impacted capsule can occur. Capsules lodged in the distal jejunum or ileum cannot be retrieved using standard endoscopy or push enteroscopy. Deep enteroscopy (using a single-balloon, double-balloon, or overtube-assisted rotational approach) offers the best chance to retrieve an impacted capsule in this situation.

Eosinophilic esophagitis

Eosinophilic esophagitis (EoE) is an increasingly recognized disorder that causes obstructive symptoms of the esophagus (see Chapter 36 for an in-depth review). Frequently, patients with EoE present with recurrent food impactions and solid food dysphagia [114]. The pathophysiology underlying EoE remains to be defined. In adults, EoE is more common in men (<50 years of age), who may have asthma, dysphagia, and present with food impactions [115]. Children present with a broader spectrum of symptoms, including frequent regurgitation, vomiting, abdominal pain, heartburn, odynophagia, chest pain, and food intolerance. Many EoE patients have a personal history of atopy, allergic rhinitis, or asthma [114]. Although this condition has mainly been described in Western countries, it is now being recognized and diagnosed in other areas of the world, including East Asia [116]. The prevalence of EoE in the United States appears to have increased in recent years [117, 118], and EoE has been reported in patients with severe GERD and also in patients with Schatzki's rings [119].

In patients who present with food impaction, but have an otherwise normal-appearing esophagus on endoscopy, EoE must be suspected. Although a normal esophagus can be seen in patients with EoE on upper endoscopy, other findings can include a ringed esophagus with or without strictures (Figure 37.13), a small-caliber esophagus (also visible on fluoroscopy; Figure 37.14), linear furrowing, erythema, edema, corrugation, white plaques (eosinophil microabscesses), granularity, and nodularity [114]. Although esophageal dilation can be effective and safely done in patients with EoE [120], treatment with ingested topical steroids and avoidance of any offending allergen are considered first-line therapies that can alleviate symptoms of dysphagia and prevent further food impaction [22]. In suspected cases of EoE, endoscopic biopsies should be taken from multiple levels in the esophagus to increase the sensitivity for diagnosing this disorder [121]. The defining histopathologic characteristic of EoE is an increased number of eosinophils (>15 eosinophils/HPF) [114].

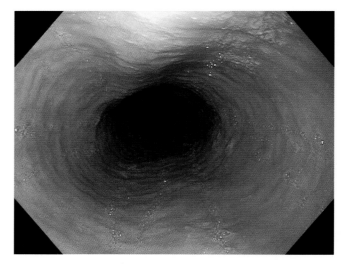

Figure 37.13 High-definition, white-light endoscopic image of a ringed-esophagus. Biopsies subsequently confirmed eosinophilic esophagitis, which was the cause of the patient's dysphagia and food impactions.

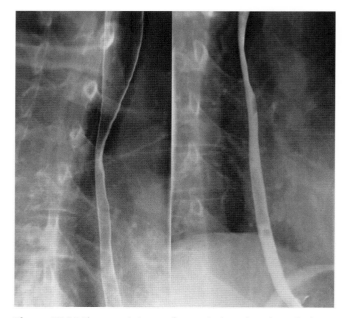

Figure 37.14 Fluoroscopic images from a single patient showed a long, smooth esophageal stricture due to long-standing, untreated, eosinophilic esophagitis. The patient reported having to chew carefully, requiring about 1.5 h in order to finish a normal meal, so as to minimize dysphagia and prevent food impaction.

Timing of esophageal dilation

After an esophageal food impaction has been relieved, often a Schatzki's ring or a peptic stricture will be found. If the impaction was transient (lasting only a few hours), and no underlying erythema, edema, or friability is found during endoscopy, then immediate dilation, preferably using a wire-guided bougie, can be performed [3]. However, if significant esophagitis or irritation is present after the food bolus has been removed, or if the impaction has been prolonged in duration, then it is advisable to place the patient on a proton pump inhibitor and to delay endoscopic dilation for 2–4 weeks. Patients should be counseled to eat slowly, chew their food well, and avoid particular foods that might cause another impaction during this waiting period. If no mechanical obstruction is seen after clearance of the food bolus, it is reasonable to obtain multiple cold biopsies in both the proximal and distal esophagus to evaluate for eosinophilic esophagitis. Pseudoachalasia should be suspected in patients with clinical features that are atypical for achalasia, and further evaluation with axial imaging [CT or magnetic resonance imaging (MRI)], endoscopic ultrasound, and specialized lab tests (anti-Hu antibodies) is warranted prior to considering pneumatic dilation or surgical myotomy [40].

Endoscopic complications

Aside from the baseline risks and complications associated with routine upper endoscopy [122], the overall complication rate of endoscopic treatment of an ingested foreign body or food impaction ranges from 0% to 1.8% [2, 16, 73, 123]. Mucosal injury can occur during endoscopic intervention to remove ingested foreign material, but the most common, serious complication associated with endoscopic extraction of foreign bodies is perforation. Other complications can include bleeding, aspiration, and cardiopulmonary issues related to sedation [1]. Although an overtube provides safety in terms of airway protection, its use also carries some risk. In patients who have high esophageal impactions associated with a stricture, or in patients who have previously undergone head and neck surgery or radiation therapy that can lead to stricture formation in the proximal esophagus [72], esophageal perforation due to overtube injury is a definite risk [88, 124]. Patients should be appropriately informed and counseled about the additional risks associated with endoscopic intervention in the setting of an ingested foreign body. However, as ingested foreign bodies and esophageal food impactions are considered medical emergencies, patients should also be informed that the potential benefits of endoscopic management far outweigh the inherent risks.

References

1. Pfau P. Ingested foreign objects and food bolus impactions. In: Ginsberg GG, Kochman ML, Norton ID, Gostout CJ, eds. *Clinical Gastrointestinal Endoscopy*. Philadelphia: Saunders-Elsevier, 2005, pp. 291–304.

2. Longstreth GF, Longstreth KJ, Yao JF. Esophageal food impaction: epidemiology and therapy. A retrospective, observational study. *Gastrointest Endosc* 2001;53:193–198.

3. Yeaton P, Peura DA. Foreign bodies. In: Castell DO, Richter JE, eds. *The Esophagus*, 3rd edn. Philadelphia: Lippincott Williams & Williams, 1999, pp. 335–348.

4. Nandi P, Ong GB. Foreign body in the oesophagus: review of 2394 cases. *Br J Surg* 1978;65:5–9.

5. Eisen GM, Baron TH, Dominitz JA, *et al.* Guideline for the management of ingested foreign bodies. *Gastrointest Endosc* 2002;55:802–806.

6. Clerf LH. Historical aspects of foreign bodies in the air and food passages. *South Med J* 1975;68:1449–1454.

7. Devanesan J, Pisani A, Sharma P, Kazarian KK, Mersheimer WL. Metallic foreign bodies in the stomach. *Arch Surg* 1977;112:664–665.

8. Benjamin SB, Noguera EC. Foreign bodies. In: Castell DO, Richer JE, eds. *The Esophagus*, 4th edn. Philadelphia: Lippincott Williams & Wilkins, 2003, pp. 340–353.

9. Perelman H. Toothpick perforations of the gastrointestinal tract. *J Abdom Surg* 1962;4:51–53.

10. Mok CK, Chiu CS, Cheung HH. Left subclavian arterioesophageal fistula induced by a foreign body. *Ann Thorac Surg* 1989;47:458–460.

11. Sloop RD, Thompson JC. Aorto-esophageal fistula: report of a case and review of literature. *Gastroenterology* 1967;53:768–777.

12. Janik JS, Bailey WC, Burrington JD. Occult coin perforation of the esophagus. *J Pediatr Surg* 1986;21:794–797.

13. Bozer AY, Saylam A, Ersoy U. Purulent pericarditis due to perforation of esophagus with foreign body. *J Thorac Cardiovasc Surg* 1974;67:590–592.

14. Welch TG, White TR, Lewis RP, Altieri PI, Vasko JS, Kilman JW. Esophagopericardial fistula presenting as cardiac tamponade. *Chest* 1972;62:728–731.

15. Brady PG. Esophageal foreign bodies. *Gastroenterol Clin North Am* 1991;20:691–701.

16. Webb WA. Management of foreign bodies of the upper gastrointestinal tract: update. *Gastrointest Endosc* 1995;41:39–51.

17. Koch H. Operative endoscopy. *Gastrointest Endosc* 1977;24:65–68.

18. Pellerin D, Fortier-Beaulieu M, Gueguen J. The fate of swallowed foreign bodies: experience of 1250 instances of subdiaphragmatic foreign bodies in children. *Prog Pediatr Radiol* 1969;2:286–302.

19. Webb WA. Management of foreign bodies of the upper gastrointestinal tract. *Gastroenterology* 1988;94:204–216.

20. Rothenberg ME. Biology and treatment of eosinophilic esophagitis. *Gastroenterology* 2009;137:1238–1249.

21. Liacouras CA, Spergel JM, Ruchelli E, *et al.* Eosinophilic esophagitis: a 10-year experience in 381 children. *Clin Gastroenterol Hepatol* 2005;3:1198–1206.

22. Furuta GT, Liacouras CA, Collins MH, *et al.* Eosinophilic esophagitis in children and adults: a systematic review and consensus recommendations for diagnosis and treatment. *Gastroenterology* 2007;133:1342–1363.

23. Desai TK, Stecevic V, Chang CH, Goldstein NS, Badizadegan K, Furuta GT. Association of eosinophilic inflammation with

esophageal food impaction in adults. *Gastrointest Endosc* 2005;61:795–801.

24. Wang AY, Kadkade R, Kahrilas PJ, Hirano I. Effectiveness of esophageal dilation for symptomatic cricopharyngeal bar. *Gastrointest Endosc* 2005;61:148–152.

25. Yamamoto S, Tsutsui S, Hayashi N. Esophageal intramural pseudodiverticulosis: A rare cause of esophageal stricture. *Clin Gastroenterol Hepatol* 2010;8:A28.

26. Teraishi F, Fujiwara T, Jikuhara A, *et al.* Esophageal intramural pseudodiverticulosis with esophageal strictures successfully treated with dilation therapy. *Ann Thorac Surg* 2006;82:1119–1121.

27. Bach KK, Postma GN, Koufman JA. Esophageal carcinoma discovered during evaluation of food impaction. *Ear Nose Throat J* 2002;81:620.

28. Brooks JW. Foreign bodies in the air and food passages. *Ann Surg* 1972;175:720–732.

29. McElhinney DB, Wernovsky G. Vascular ring, right aortic arch. *eMedicine* 2009; available at http://emedicine.medscape.com/article/899745-overview

30. Schunk JE, Corneli H, Bolte R. Pediatric coin ingestions. A prospective study of coin location and symptoms. *Am J Dis Child* 1989;143:546–548.

31. Herranz-Gonzalez J, Martinez-Vidal J, Garcia-Sarandeses A, Vazquez-Barro C. Esophageal foreign bodies in adults. *Otolaryngol Head Neck Surg* 1991;105:649–654.

32. Kimia A, Lee L, Shannon M, *et al.* Holiday ornament-related injuries in children. *Pediatr Emerg Care* 2009;25:819–822.

33. Schafer C, Graser A, Wagner A. Unusual cause for dysphagia: perforation of the proximal esophagus by a toothpick. *Endoscopy* 2008;40 (Suppl 2):E217–218.

34. Liu HJ, Liang CH, Huang B, Xie SF, Wang GY. Migration of a swallowed toothpick into the liver: the value of multiplanar CT. *Br J Radiol* 2009;82:e79–81.

35. Lacroix S, Ferland A, Gilbert P, Lemieux M, Bilodeau L, Poirier P. Cardiac hazard associated with eating habits. A case of infected intrapericardial foreign body due to an ingested toothpick. *Can J Cardiol* 2009;25:e263–264.

36. Dente M, Santi F, Solinas L, Bagarani M. Laparoscopic diagnosis and management of jejunal perforation resulting from accidental toothpick ingestion. *Am Surg* 2009;75:178–179.

37. Zhang S, Cui Y, Gong X, Gu F, Chen M, Zhong B. Endoscopic management of foreign bodies in the upper gastrointestinal tract in South China: A retrospective study of 561 cases. *Dig Dis Sci* 2010;55:1305–1312.

38. Ramadan MM, El-Desouky MEI-S. Images in clinical medicine. Esophageal foreign body. *N Engl J Med* 2009;361:e11.

39. Ginsberg GG. Management of ingested foreign objects and food bolus impactions. *Gastrointest Endosc* 1995;41:33–38.

40. Kahrilas PJ, Kishk SM, Helm JF, Dodds WJ, Harig JM, Hogan WJ. Comparison of pseudoachalasia and achalasia. *Am J Med* 1987;82:439–446.

41. Connolly AA, Birchall M, Walsh-Waring GP, Moore-Gillon V. Ingested foreign bodies: patient-guided localization is a useful clinical tool. *Clin Otolaryngol Allied Sci* 1992;17:520–524.

42. Yamamoto M, Mizuno H, Sugawara Y. A chopstick is removed after 60 years in the duodenum. *Gastrointest Endosc* 1985;31:51.

43. Adams DB. Endoscopic removal of entrapped coins from an intraluminal duodenal diverticulum 20 years after ingestion. *Gastrointest Endosc* 1986;32:415–416.

44. Kirberg AE. Long-standing esophageal foreign body. *Gastrointest Endosc* 1986;32:304–305.

45. Young CA, Menias CO, Bhalla S, Prasad SR. CT features of esophageal emergencies. *Radiographics* 2008;28:1541–1553.

46. Chang MY, Chang ML, Wu CT. Esophageal perforation caused by fish vertebra ingestion in a seven-month-old infant demanded surgical intervention: A case report. *World J Gastroenterol* 2006;12:7213–7215.

47. Marco De Lucas E, Sadaba P, Lastra Garcia-Baron P, *et al.* Value of helical computed tomography in the management of upper esophageal foreign bodies. *Acta Radiol* 2004;45:369–374.

48. Kobayashi M, Seto A, Nomura T, Yoshida T, Yamamoto M. [3D-CT highly useful in diagnosing foreign bodies in the paraesophageal orifice]. *Nippon Jibiinkoka Gakkai Kaiho* 2004;107:800–803.

49. James AE Jr, Montali RJ, Chaffee V, Strecker EP, Vessal K. Barium or gastrografin: which contrast media for diagnosis of esophageal tears? *Gastroenterology* 1975;68:1103–1113.

50. Goh GJ, Pilbrow WJ, Youngs GR. The use of gastrografin for esophageal perforation. *Gastroenterology* 1995;108:618.

51. Shaffer HA Jr, de Lange EE. Gastrointestinal foreign bodies and strictures: radiologic interventions. *Curr Prob Diag Radiol* 1994;23:205–249.

52. Kozarek RA, Sanowski RA. Esophageal food impaction: description of a new method for bolus removal. *Dig Dis Sci* 1980;25:100–103.

53. Schunk JE, Harrison AM, Corneli HM, Nixon GW. Fluoroscopic foley catheter removal of esophageal foreign bodies in children: experience with 415 episodes. *Pediatrics* 1994;94:709–714.

54. Little DC, Shah SR, St Peter SD, *et al.* Esophageal foreign bodies in the pediatric population: our first 500 cases. *J Pediatr Surg* 2006;41:914–918.

55. Adoga AA, Adoga AS, Nwaorgu OG. Experience with rigid esophagoscopy in Jos, north-central *Nigeria. Nigerian J Clin Pract* 2009;12:237–239.

56. Turkyilmaz A, Aydin Y, Yilmaz O, Aslan S, Eroglu A, Karaoglanoglu N. [Esophageal foreign bodies: analysis of 188 cases]. *Ulus Travma Acil Cerrahi Derg* 2009;15:222–227.

57. Berggreen PJ, Harrison E, Sanowski RA, Ingebo K, Noland B, Zierer S. Techniques and complications of esophageal foreign body extraction in children and adults. *Gastrointest Endosc* 1993;39:626–630.

58. Webb WA, McDaniel L, Jones L. Foreign bodies of the upper gastrointestinal tract: current management. *South Med J* 1984;77:1083–1086.

59. Katsinelos P, Kountouras J, Paroutoglou G, Zavos C, Mimidis K, Chatzimavroudis G. Endoscopic techniques and management of foreign body ingestion and food bolus impaction in the upper gastrointestinal tract: a retrospective analysis of 139 cases. *J Clin Gastroenterol* 2006;40:784–789.

60. Conway WC, Sugawa C, Ono H, Lucas CE. Upper GI foreign body: an adult urban emergency hospital experience. *Surg Endosc* 2007;21:455–460.

61. Yamamoto H, Sekine Y, Sato Y, *et al.* Total enteroscopy with a nonsurgical steerable double-balloon method. *Gastrointest Endosc* 2001;53:216–220.

62. Hartmann D, Eickhoff A, Tamm R, Riemann JF. Balloon-assisted enteroscopy using a single-balloon technique. *Endoscopy* 2007;39 (Suppl 1):E276.

63. Akerman PA, Agrawal D, Cantero D, Pangtay J. Spiral enteroscopy with the new DSB overtube: a novel technique for deep peroral small-bowel intubation. *Endoscopy* 2008;40:974–978.

64. Gerson LB. Outcomes associated with deep enteroscopy. *Gastrointest Endosc Clin North Am* 2009;19:481–496.

65. Neumann H, Fry LC, Rickes S, Jurczok C, Malfertheiner P, Monkemuller K. A 'double-balloon enteroscopy worth the money': endoscopic removal of a coin lodged in the small bowel. *Dig Dis (Basel)* 2008;26:388–389.

66. Ramchandani M, Reddy DN, Gupta R, *et al*. Diagnostic yield and therapeutic impact of single-balloon enteroscopy: series of 106 cases. *J Gastroenterol Hepatol* 2009;24:1631–1638.

67. Faigel DO, Stotland BR, Kochman ML, *et al*. Device choice and experience level in endoscopic foreign object retrieval: an in vivo study. *Gastrointest Endosc* 1997;45:490–492.

68. Lichtenstein DR, Jagannath S, Baron TH, *et al*. Sedation and anesthesia in GI endoscopy. *Gastrointest Endosc* 2008; 68:815–826.

69. Lagasse RS. Anesthesia safety: model or myth? A review of the published literature and analysis of current original data. *Anesthesiology* 2002;97:1609–1617.

70. Lagasse RS. Innocent prattle. *Anesthesiology* 2009;110: 698–699.

71. Bertoni G, Pacchione D, Conigliaro R, Sassatelli R, Pedrazzoli C, Bedogni G. Endoscopic protector hood for safe removal of sharp-pointed gastroesophageal foreign bodies. *Surg Endosc* 1992;6:255–258.

72. Mamel JJ, Weiss D, Pouagare M, Nord HJ. Endoscopic suction removal of food boluses from the upper gastrointestinal tract using Stiegmann-Goff friction-fit adaptor: an improved method for removal of food impactions. *Gastrointest Endosc* 1995;41:593–596.

73. Vizcarrondo FJ, Brady PG, Nord HJ. Foreign bodies of the upper gastrointestinal tract. *Gastrointest Endosc* 1983; 29:208–210.

74. Norton RA, King GD. "Steakhouse syndrome": the symptomatic lower esophageal ring. *Lahey Clinic Foundation Bull* 1963;13:55–59.

75. Drinka P. Broken ribs following CPR or the Heimlich maneuver. *J Am Med Dir Assoc* 2009;10:283–284.

76. Meredith MJ, Liebowitz R. Rupture of the esophagus caused by the Heimlich maneuver. *Ann Emerg Med* 1986;15:106–107.

77. Otero Palleiro MM, Barbagelata Lopez C, Fernandez Pretel MC, Salgado Fernandez J. Hepatic rupture after Heimlich maneuver. *Ann Emerg Med* 2007;49:825–826.

78. Desai SC, Chute DJ, Desai BC, Koloski ER. Traumatic dissection and rupture of the abdominal aorta as a complication of the Heimlich maneuver. *J Vasc Surg* 2008;48: 1325–1327.

79. Stack LB, Munter DW. Foreign bodies in the gastrointestinal tract. *Emerg Med Clin North Am* 1996;14:493–521.

80. Al-Haddad M, Ward EM, Scolapio JS, Ferguson DD, Raimondo M. Glucagon for the relief of esophageal food impaction does it really work? *Dig Dis Sci* 2006;51:1930–1933.

81. Tibbling L, Bjorkhoel A, Jansson E, Stenkvist M. Effect of spasmolytic drugs on esophageal foreign bodies. *Dysphagia* 1995;10:126–127.

82. Richardson JR. A new treatment for esophageal obstruction due to meat impaction. *Ann Otol Rhino Laryngol* 1945; 54:328–348.

83. Robinson AS. Meat impaction in the esophagus treated by enzymatic digestion. *JAMA* 1962;181:1142–1143.

84. Maini S, Rudralingam M, Zeitoun H, Osbourne JE. Aspiration pneumonitis following papain enzyme treatment for oesophageal meat impaction. *J Laryngol Otol* 2001;115:585–586.

85. Hall ML, Huseby JS. Hemorrhagic pulmonary edema associated with meat tenderizer treatment for esophageal meat impaction. *Chest* 1988;94:640–642.

86. Goldner F, Danley D. Enzymatic digestion of esophageal meat impaction. A study of Adolph's Meat Tenderizer. *Dig Dis Sci* 1985;30:456–459.

87. Saeed ZA, Michaletz PA, Feiner SD, Woods KL, Graham DY. A new endoscopic method for managing food impaction in the esophagus. *Endoscopy* 1990;22:226–228.

88. Berkelhammer C, Madhav G, Lyon S, Roberts J. "Pinch" injury during overtube placement in upper endoscopy. *Gastrointest Endosc* 1993;39:186–188.

89. Byrne WJ. Foreign bodies, bezoars, and caustic ingestion. *Gastrointest Endosc Clin North Am* 1994;4:99–119.

90. Blin O, Mestre D, Masson G, Serratrice G. Selective effects of low doses of apomorphine on spatiotemporal contrast sensitivity in healthy volunteers: a double-blind placebo-controlled study. *Br J Clin Pharmacol* 1991;32:551–556.

91. Liu YY, Tseng JH, Yeh CN, Fang JT, Lee HL, Jan YY. Correct diagnosis and successful treatment for pericardial effusion due to toothpick injury: a case report and literature review. *World J Gastroenterol* 2007;13:4278–4281.

92. Stoica M, Saftoiu A, Gheonea DI, Dumitrescu D, Surlin V. Pyogenic liver abscess caused by accidental ingestion of a wooden toothpick: role of preoperative imaging. *J Gastrointestin Liver Dis* 2007;16:221–222.

93. Kim KH, Woo EY, Rosato EF, Kochman ML. Pancreatic foreign body: Ingested toothpick as a cause of pancreatitis and hemorrhage. *Gastrointest Endosc* 2004;59:147–150.

94. Jackson C. New mechanical problems in the bronchoscopic extraction of foreign bodies from the lungs and eesophagus. *Ann Surg* 1922;75:1–30.

95. Jackson C, Jackson CL. *Diseases of the Air and Food Passages of Foreign Body Origin.* Philadelphia: WB Saunders, 1937.

96. Jeen YT, Chun HJ, Song CW, *et al*. Endoscopic removal of sharp foreign bodies impacted in the esophagus. *Endoscopy* 2001;33:518–522.

97. Watson WA, Litovitz TL, Rodgers GC Jr, *et al*. 2004 Annual report of the American Association of Poison Control Centers Toxic Exposure Surveillance System. *Am J Emerg Med* 2005;23:589–666.

98. Waltzman ML, Baskin M, Wypij D, Mooney D, Jones D, Fleisher G. A randomized clinical trial of the management of esophageal coins in children. *Pediatrics* 2005;116: 614–619.

99. Connors GP. A literature based comparison of the three methods of pediatric esophageal coin removal. *Pediatr Emerg Care* 1997;13:154–157.

100. Janik JE, Janik JS. Magill forceps extraction of upper esophageal coins. *J Pediatr Surg* 2003;38:227–229.

101. Arms JL, Mackenberg-Mohn MD, Bowen MV, *et al*. Safety and efficacy of a protocol using bougienage or endoscopy for the management of coins acutely lodged in the esophagus: a large case series. *Ann Emerg Med* 2008;51:367–372.

102. Dahshan AH, Kevin Donovan G. Bougienage versus endoscopy for esophageal coin removal in children. *J Clin Gastroenterol* 2007;41:454–456.

103. Raynor KM, Wu GY. 'Where the money is': a case report of the successful removal of a large number of coins by esophagogastroduodenoscopy utilizing a Roth net. *J Dig Dis* 2007;8:160–161.

104. Litovitz TL. Battery ingestions: product accessibility and clinical course. *Pediatrics* 1985;75:469–476.

105. Litovitz T, Schmitz BF. Ingestion of cylindrical and button batteries: an analysis of 2382 cases. *Pediatrics* 1992;89:747–757.

106. Swallowed a button Battery? Battery in the ear or nose? 2009. Available at http://www.poison.org/prevent/battery.asp

107. Hamilton JM, Schraff SA, Notrica DM. Severe injuries from coin cell battery ingestions: 2 case reports. *J Pediatr Surg* 2009;44:644–647.

108. Kirk AD, Bowers BA, Moylan JA, Meyers WC. Toothbrush swallowing. *Arch Surg* 1988;123:382–384.

109. Rogers LF, Igini JP. Beverage can pull-tabs. Inadvertent ingestion or aspiration. *JAMA* 1975;233:345–348.

110. Booker RJ, Smith JE, Rodger MP. Packers, pushers and stuffers–managing patients with concealed drugs in UK emergency departments: a clinical and medicolegal review. *Emerg Med J* 2009;26:316–320.

111. Yegane RA, Bashashati M, Hajinasrollah E, Heidari K, Salehi NA, Ahmadi M. Surgical approach to body packing. *Dis Colon Rectum* 2009;52:97–103.

112. Farmer JW, Chan SB. Whole body irrigation for contraband bodypackers. *J Clin Gastroenterol* 2003;37:147–150.

113. Karagiannis S, Faiss S, Mavrogiannis C. Capsule retention: a feared complication of wireless capsule endoscopy. *Scand J Gastroenterol* 2009;44:1158–1165.

114. Bohm M, Richter JE. Treatment of eosinophilic esophagitis: overview, current limitations, and future direction. *Am J Gastroenterol* 2008;103:2635–2644; quiz 2645.

115. Veerappan GR, Perry JL, Duncan TJ, *et al*. Prevalence of eosinophilic esophagitis in an adult population undergoing upper endoscopy: a prospective study. *Clin Gastroenterol Hepatol* 2009;7:420–426, 6 e1–2.

116. Lu HC, Lu CL, Chang FY. Eosinophilic esophagitis in an asymptomatic Chinese. *J Chin Med Assoc* 2008;71:362–364.

117. Kapel RC, Miller JK, Torres C, Aksoy S, Lash R, Katzka DA. Eosinophilic esophagitis: a prevalent disease in the United States that affects all age groups. *Gastroenterology* 2008; 134:1316–1321.

118. Gonsalves N. Eosinophilic esophagitis: history, nomenclature, and diagnostic guidelines. *Gastrointest Endosc Clin North Am* 2008;18:1–9; vii.

119. Rajagopalan J, Triadafilopoulos G. Ring(s)-related esophageal meat bolus impaction: biopsy first, dilate later. *Dis Esophagus* 2009;22:E14–16.

120. Schoepfer AM, Gonsalves N, Bussmann C, *et al*. Esophageal dilation in eosinophilic esophagitis: effectiveness, safety, and impact on the underlying Inflammation. *Am J Gastroenterol* 2010;105:1062–1070.

121. Gonsalves N, Policarpio-Nicolas M, Zhang Q, Rao MS, Hirano I. Histopathologic variability and endoscopic correlates in adults with eosinophilic esophagitis. *Gastrointest Endosc* 2006;64:313–319.

122. Eisen GM, Baron TH, Dominitz JA, *et al*. Complications of upper GI endoscopy. *Gastrointest Endosc* 2002;55:784–793.

123. Mosca S. Management and endoscopic techniques in cases of ingestion of foreign bodies. *Endoscopy* 2000;32:272–273.

124. Goldschmiedt M, Haber G, Kandel G, Kortan P, Marcon N. A safety maneuver for placing overtubes during endoscopic variceal ligation. *Gastrointest Endosc* 1992;38:399–400.

125. Nijhawan S, Shimpi L, Mathur A, Mathur V, Roop Rai R. Management of ingested foreign bodies in upper gastrointestinal tract: report on 170 patients. *Indian J Gastroenterol* 2003;22:46–48.

126. Khorshidi I, Maratchi LS, Ho S. Endoscopic management of food impaction in the upper gastrointestinal tract: A tertiary care center experience. *Gastrointest Endosc* 2007;65:AB330.

38 Pill-Induced Esophageal Injury

Patrick E. Young and James Walter Kikendall

National Naval Medical Center, Uniformed Services University of the Health Sciences, Division of Gastroenterology, Bethesda, MD, USA

Introduction

Most oral medications are administered as non-chewable tablets or capsules because these solid, compact pills are easily stored, transported, and consumed, and may be modified to regulate absorption. The tablets and capsules are designed to pass rapidly through the mouth and esophagus and to release their contents in the stomach or more distal regions of the gastrointestinal tract. On occasion, tablets and capsules may lodge in the esophagus and dissolve therein, releasing their undiluted contents directly onto the esophageal mucosa. If the concentrated medication thus released is sufficiently caustic, the esophageal wall may be injured, either directly or through interaction with refluxed gastric contents. This process is known as pill-induced esophageal injury [1]. This chapter reviews evidence from 1322 reported cases of pill-induced esophageal injury [1–330] caused by more than 100 different medications.

Clinical presentation and differential diagnosis

The abrupt onset of odynophagia in a patient taking potentially injurious pills is highly suggestive of pill-induced esophageal injury, the principal differential being infectious esophagitis [1]. The typical injured patient has no prior esophageal symptoms but experiences the sudden onset and progression over 1–4 days of retrosternal pain. The pain is almost always exacerbated by swallowing and may be perceived only with swallowing. The pain may remain mild or become so severe as to make swallowing impossible, compromising hydration and alimentation [4, 128, 255, 265]. Symptoms typically resolve in a few days to a few weeks.

Many patients relate that the tablet or capsule seemed to stick in the esophagus prior to the onset of symptoms.

Others admit that they have taken their pills with little or no water. Those patients who have been awakened from sleep by pain may relate that they took their pills immediately prior to going to bed. Many injured patients, however, have taken their pills entirely properly, and the absence of these predisposing features does not constitute evidence against the diagnosis of pill-induced esophageal injury.

Less typical symptoms may lead to diagnostic confusion. A burning quality to the pain may result in confusion with gastroesophageal reflux disease (GERD). Constant pain may suggest a myocardial infarction [15, 93, 173]. Slowly progressive painless dysphagia is uncommon with most medications, but is more commonly observed with injury due to alendronate, quinidine or potassium chloride pills. Slowly progressive dysphagia may suggest neoplasia. Hemorrhage occurs in fewer than 5% of reported cases, but pill-induced ulcers have indeed penetrated the left atrium and major vessels [59, 108, 169, 260]. Mediastinitis and free esophageal perforation have complicated injuries due to alendronate [83], ibuprofen [322], an Aspirin–caffeine compound pill [54], sustained-release ferrous sulfate [244], and sustained-release sodium valproate [284].

Diagnosis, pathology, and complications

When a patient states that a swallowed pill lodged in the chest prior to the onset of rapidly progressive retrosternal pain clearly exacerbated by swallowing, the diagnosis of pill-induced esophagitis is apparent. The evaluation of such a patient will properly be directed toward discovery of possible predisposing factors or complications and toward the planning of appropriate alternatives to the implicated oral medication.

While endoscopy may not be necessary for the patient with a typical, uncomplicated presentation and rapid recovery, endoscopy is indicated when symptoms are gradual

The Esophagus, Fifth Edition. Edited by Joel E. Richter, Donald O. Castell.

rather than acute in onset, atypical, or inordinately persistent, when the medication has not previously been associated with pill-induced esophageal injury, or when the relationship of symptoms to a previously reported potentially injurious pill is unclear. Endoscopy is also indicated in immunocompromised patients or in patients with hemorrhage.

Endoscopy is more sensitive than barium esophagography for subtle pill-induced esophageal lesions. With its biopsy capability, endoscopy is also more likely to provide a definitive alternative diagnosis, such as infectious esophagitis, cancer, or GERD. The only apparent advantages of esophagography over endoscopy are its lower initial cost and its higher sensitivity for extrinsic compression, which might lead to a recurrence of injury if undetected. The higher diagnostic yield of endoscopy make it the most cost-effective procedure if diagnostic testing is reserved for difficult cases as suggested above.

Endoscopy typically reveals one or more discrete ulcers with normal surrounding mucosa [1]. Discrete ulcers range from pinpoint to several centimeters in size. At times, diffuse inflammation is observed either without ulceration or surrounding the ulcer(s). Biopsies reveal acute inflammation without evidence for infection or neoplasia. Remnants of the offending pill may occasionally be identified [3, 34, 54, 115, 165, 207, 241].

Repetitive injury can lead to more extensive ulceration and nodularity suggesting neoplasia, as seen in a teenaged patient who persisted in taking doxycycline while recumbent every night for a full month after initially developing chest pain [323]. Especially when the injury is more chronic and cumulative, but at times with acute injury as well, exudates, edema, and nodularity may be so profuse as to suggest neoplasia, either at endoscopy or on barium swallow [1, 220, 234, 244, 266, 283]. Such inflammatory pseudotumors have been observed in patients injured by quinidine, especially the sustained-release form of quinidine [1, 220, 226, 283], sustained-release ferrous sulfate [244], and sustained-release naproxen [234]. Even such flamboyant inflammatory stenoses tend to resolve spontaneously if the offending pill is withdrawn. More ominously, large circumferential ulcers or repetitive injuries may lead to fibrotic strictures requiring dilatation or surgery.

Several cases of alendronate-induced esophageal injuries have demonstrated an unusual, thick, white pseudomembranous exudate [15, 221]. Biopsies in some of these cases have shown granulation tissue and birefringent, polarizable, crystalline material similar to a component of the alendronate tablet [15, 221]. The polarizable crystalline foreign material may be found in biopsies from alendronate-related injuries and may represent the filler rather than the active alendronate [308, 336].

Similarly, brown crystalline material in the mucosa or ulcer bed may suggest iron-induced injury and this can be confirmed with Perl's stain [298, 319, 325].

Any area of the esophagus may be injured [1]. The most common site of injury is the junction of the proximal and middle thirds of the esophagus where peristaltic amplitude is relatively low and where the esophagus may be compressed anteriorly by the aortic arch. Patients with left atrial enlargement are susceptible to injury at the site where the esophagus is compressed by the left atrium [48, 279, 287]. The most distal esophagus has uncommonly been reported as the site of injury, perhaps because of the difficulty in differentiating pill-induced injury from GERD in this location. Certainly, anatomic abnormalities may increase both the risk for pill-induced injury as well as the severity of the resulting complications. There have been several cases reports of massive upper gastrointestinal hemorrhage due to pill-induced injury to a Zenker's diverticulum [327, 328, 329, 330]. Often, these patients present with hemoptysis rather than hematemesis due to the anatomic positioning of the diverticulum near the tracheal orifice. Therefore, a high clinical suspicion is necessary in these cases.

Therapy and clinical course

The obvious first step in the treatment of pill-induced esophageal injury is withdrawal of the offending pill. Empiric antireflux therapy may be administered to prevent exacerbation of injury by refluxing acid. Swallowing a topical anesthetic will temporarily relieve severe pain. Most patients will become asymptomatic within a few days to a few weeks if the injury is not repeated [1]. Rarely, patients require parenteral hydration or parenteral alimentation. Complications of esophageal perforation, mediastinitis, hemorrhage, or fibrotic stricture require specific treatment.

Epidemiology and pathogenesis

Pill-induced esophageal injury was first reported in 1970 [129, 145, 207]. To date, 1322 cases have been reported or summarized in the medical literature. These cases represent only the tip of the iceberg. Cases are reported selectively, usually because of an unusual quality, such as a clustering of cases, a newly implicated pill, or a complication. The best estimate of the incidence of pill-induced esophageal injury is derived from 109 cases diagnosed in a region of Sweden during a 4-year period in the 1970s [44], an incidence of 4 cases per 100 000 population per year. The incidence of injury today is probably higher because of more frequent administration of medications. Still, pill-induced esophageal injury is an uncommon event considering the number of pills consumed each year.

Patients of all ages (3–98 years of age) have been injured (see Tables 38.1–4). Women have been injured in 67% of cases for which gender has been reported. More women

Table 38.1 Esophageal injury due to antibiotic, antiviral, and antiprotozoal pills.

Implicated pill	Cases	Gender		Age (years)			Number of complications			References
		M	F	Number for whom reported	Range	Mean	Hemorrhage	Stricture	Death	
Doxycycline	380	78	131	171	10–98	31	1	3	1	a
Tetracycline HCl	83	27	40	56	17–84	51	5	1	—	b
Unspecified tetracyclines	72	—	—	—	—	—	—	—	—	43, 198
Oxytetracycline	16	4	7	11	25–42	37	—	—	—	39, 43, 47, 71, 104, 133, 295
Demethylchlortetracycline	1	1	—	1	—	24	—	—	—	27
Minocycline	13	1	5	7	16–48	40	—	—	—	10, 126, 201, 253, 295
Florocycline	1	1	—	1	—	19	—	—	—	181
Metacycline	1	0	1	1	—	49	—	—	—	116
Methylenecycline	1	0	1	1	—	30	—	—	—	206
Pivmecillinam	32	2	30	32	—	35	—	—	—	184, 191
Penicillin	5	—	2	4	18–31	23	—	1	—	37, 40, 44,101, 259
Ampicillin	5	1	4	5	20–60	46	—	1	—	219, 228, 295
Pivampicillin	2	1	—	1	—	35	—	—	—	119, 228
Amoxicillin	3	2	—	2	39–70	51	—	—	—	51, 204, 270
Bacampicillin	1	1	—	1	—	28	—	—	—	299
Apocillin	2	—	—	—	—	—	—	—	—	71
Cloxacillin	1	—	—	—	—	—	—	—	—	201
Ampicillin/cloxacillin	2	2	0	2	21–24	22	—	—	—	285
Dicloxacillin + danzen	1	—	—	—	—	—	—	—	—	201
Trimethoprim-sulfamethoxazole	2	1	1	2	14–63	38	—	—	—	31, 243
Clindamycin	5	4	1	4	22–35	29	—	—	—	47, 93, 143, 235, 261
Lincomycin	1	—	1	1	—	28	—	—	—	242

(continued)

Table 38.1 (*continued*)

Implicated pill	Cases	Gender		Age (years)			Number of complications			References
		M	F	Number for whom reported	Range	Mean	Hemorrhage	Stricture	Death	
Spiramycine	1	1	0	1	—	70	—	—	—	211
Erythromycin	1	—	—	—	—	—	—	—	—	44
Clarithromycin	2	1	1	2	—	58	—	—	—	295
Telithromycin	1	1	0	1	—	43	—	—	—	305
Rifampicin	4	1	3	4	23–70	43	—	1	—	47, 250, 295
Sulfamethoxypyridazine	1	—	—	1	—	24	—	1	—	276
Cephotiam HCl	1	1	0	1	—	66	—	—	—	301
Cephalexin	1	0	1	1	—	15	—	—	—	79
Tinidazole	1	—	—	—	—	—	—	—	—	44
Metronidazole	1	0	1	1	—	25	—	—	—	178
Quinine sulfate	1	1	0	1	—	50	—	—	—	321
Grouped antibiotics[c]	4	3	1	2	33–77	55	1	—	—	196
Unidentified antibiotic	1	—	—	—	—	—	—	—	—	188
Nelfinavir	1	1	0	1	—	25	—	—	—	120
Zalcitibine	2	2	0	2	20–32	26	—	—	—	32, 122
Zidovudine	3	3	0	3	33–38	35	—	—	—	76
Totals	**656**	**141**	**231**	**324**	**10–98**	**36**	**7**	**8**	**1**	

[a]References for doxycycline: 1, 2, 7, 9, 14, 15, 18, 20, 24, 25, 28–30, 35, 36, 37, 43, 44, 47, 49, 50, 56–58, 62, 64, 66, 67, 81, 89–91, 94, 96, 97, 100, 107, 110, 116, 118, 123, 126, 128, 131–133, 135, 136, 141, 143, 144, 146, 147, 161, 171, 176, 177, 179, 185, 186, 188, 190, 192, 194, 196, 199, 201, 202, 205, 214, 216, 226, 235, 240, 248, 257, 263–265, 269, 272, 273, 275, 285, 303, 297, 300, 295, 304, 309, 311, 315, 320, 318, 323, 324.

[b]References for tetracycline: 1, 9, 25, 27, 29, 33, 36, 37, 41, 45, 57–59, 71, 72, 98, 126, 139–141, 154, 238, 239, 285, 309, 317.

[c]Erythromycin (two cases), josamycine (one case), clindamycin (one case).

Table 38.2 Esophageal injury due to Aspirin and other non-steroidal anti-inflammatory drug pills.

Implicated pill	Cases	Gender		Age (years)			Number of Complications			References
		M	F	Number for whom reported	Range	Mean	Hemorrhage	Stricture	Death	
Aspirin	38	21	10	19	16–89	51	14	5	2	1, 36, 37, 44, 122, 145, 225, 241, 280, 295, 326
Aspirin, caffeine	1	1	—	1	—	26	—	—	—	54
Aspirin, phenacetin, caffeine	1	1	—	1	—	54	1	—	—	281
Aspirin, anacin	1	0	1	1	—	41	1	—	—	258
Aspirin, ibuprofen	1	1	0	1	—	20	1	—	—	258
Doleron[a]	7	—	—	—	—	—	—	1	—	44
Decagesic[b]	1	1	—	1	Adolescent	—	—	—	—	73
Paraflex compound[c]	1	—	—	—	—	—	—	—	—	44
Naproxen										
Literature case reports	3	1	2	3	29–87	62	2	—	—	75, 234, 274
FDA reporting program	81	16	65	81	—	36	—	—	1	130
Indomethacin	15	4	1	5	28–82	62	2	1	—	8, 14, 23, 72, 73, 95
Ibuprofen	7	4	2	6	18–63	31	1	1	1	9, 50, 157, 188, 258, 322 (perf)
Piroxicam	5	4	1	5	20–79	33	—	1	—	69, 237
Meclofenamate sodium	2	0	2	2	36–47	41	—	—	—	187, 236
Mefenamic acid	2	2	0	2	35–63	49	1	1	—	63, 134
Tolmetin	2	2	0	2	11–27	19	—	—	—	60, 203
Diclofenac	3	0	3	3	20–74	39	—	—	—	121, 124, 300
Sulindac	1	1	0	1	—	36	—	—	—	158
Flurbiprofen	1	1	0	1	—	26	—	—	—	262
Ketoprofen	1	0	1	1	—	67	—	—	—	300
Phenylbutazone + prednisone	1	0	1	1	—	75	—	—	—	129
Grouped non-steroidal agents[d]	29	13	16	15	21–75	60	10	1	—	196, 295
Unspecified non-steroidals	8	—	—	—	—	—	—	—	—	198
Mesalamine	1	0	1	1	—	32	—	—	—	163
Acetominophen	2	—	1	1	—	55	—	—	—	71, 285
Acemetacin[e]	1	0	1	1	—	77	—	—	1	168
Percogesic[f]	1	0	1	1	—	31	—	—	—	197
Totals	**217**	**73**	**109**	**156**	**11–89**	**42**	**34**	**10**	**4**	

[a] Components of Doleron: Aspirin, dextropropoxyphene, phenothiazine carboxyl-10-hydrochloride, antipyrene, vinbarbital.
[b] Components of Decagesic: aspirin, dexamethasone, aluminum hydroxide gel.
[c] Components of Paraflex compound: aspirin, dextropropoxyphene, chlorzoxazone.
[d] Naproxen (14 cases), Oxyphenbutazone (three cases), indomethacin (nine cases), ibuprofen (three cases), diclofenac (one case).
[e] Patient also took verapamil, ferrous sulfate, and prednisone, but acemetacin was most closely related and likely causative.
[f] Components of Percogesic: acetaminophen, phenyltoloxamine citrate.

Table 38.3 Esophageal injury due to other pills available in the United States.

Implicated pill	Cases	Gender		Age (years)			Number of complications			References
		M	F	Number for whom reported	Range	Mean	Hemorrhage	Stricture	Death	
Potassium chloride (KCl)	45	14	23	35	14–77	64	6	19	6	[a]
Alendronate	142	11	128	127	23–90	67	4	28	1	[b]
Pamidronate	5	0	5	5	64–74	69	—	—	—	167
Etidronate	3	1	1	3	66–81	72	—	1	—	151, 172, 180
Ibandronate	1	0	1	1	—	67	—	—	—	314
Ferrous sulfate or succinate	28	6	12	18	62–94	80	4	6	1	3, 44, 147, 244, 298, 306, 319, 325
Quinidine	22	11	9	20	12–87	63	—	10	—	1, 34, 36, 38, 57, 183, 252, 266, 283, 295, 296
Quinidine + KCl	2	—	2	2	49–73	61	—	2	—	149, 222
Quinidine + other pills	3	—	3	3	69–77	73	—	2	—	72, 220
Mexiletine	4	1	2	3	72–77	74	—	—	—	6, 196, 209, 231
Captopril	1	0	1	1	—	84	1	—	—	13
Nifedipine	2	1	—	1	—	69	—	1	—	196, 249
Verapamil (+ zolpidem)	1	0	1	1	—	50	—	—	—	125
Bepridil	1	—	—	—	—	—	—	—	—	196
Unidentified antihypertensive	1	—	—	—	—	—	—	—	—	188
Theophylline/ aminophylline	7	2	1	3	28–31	30	—	—	—	80, 198, 245, 255
Corticosteroids	6	4	2	3	42–81	66	—	—	—	70, 196
Multivitamin + iron or minerals	3	2	—	3	3–62	29	—	—	—	37, 82, 212
Ascorbic acid	7	2	5	5	24–61	51	—	3	—	36, 142, 278, 295
13-cis-Retinoate	3	3	0	3	17–74	46	—	1	—	16, 85
Tryptophan	1	0	1	1	—	81	1	—	—	215
Valproic acid	1	1	0	1	—	49	—	—	—	284
Phenytoin sodium	1	1	0	1	—	36	—	1	—	36
Phenytoin + Phenobarbital	1	0	1	1	—	41	1	—	—	277
Warfarin	1	1	0	1	—	58	1	—	—	162
Copidogrel + warfarin	1	1	0	1	—	60	—	—	—	300
Lansoprazole	1	0	1	1	—	21	—	—	—	175
Thioridazine, slow-release	1	1	0	1	—	22	—	—	—	228
Clorazepate	1	0	1	1	—	25	—	—	—	182
Diazepam	1	0	1	1	—	45	—	—	—	109
Morphine sulfate, slow-release	1	—	—	—	—	—	1	—	—	114
Glyburide (glibenclamide)	2	—	1	1	—	82	—	—	—	119, 228
Estramustine phosphate	2	—	—	—	—	—	—	—	—	44
Eucalyptus-menthol	2	1	1	2	9–33	21	—	—	—	88, 246
Oral contraceptives	5	—	5	4	19–24	22	—	—	—	12, 51, 200, 310
Sildenafil	1	1	0	1	—	61	—	—	—	112
Tamsulosin required surgery	1	1	0	1	—	73	—	1	—	307
"Fat burner"	1	0	1	1	—	34	—	—	—	285
Totals	**312**	**66**	**209**	**257**	**3–94**	**64**	**19**	**75**	**8**	

[a]References for potassium chloride: 19, 21, 36, 38, 44, 48, 78, 108, 115, 153, 164, 165, 169, 188, 196, 198, 207, 213, 230, 233, 260, 264, 279, 295, 296, 316.

[b]References for alendronate: 4, 5, 42, 52, 65, 74, 83, 87, 99, 138, 141, 151, 152, 156, 159, 166, 174, 195, 217, 221, 223, 232, 251, 268, 271, 286, 295, 308, 312, 324.

Table 38.4 Esophageal injury due to pills not available in the United States.

Implicated pill	Cases	Gender		Age (years)			Number of complications			References
		M	F	Number for whom reported	Range	Mean	Hemorrhage	Stricture	Death	
Emepronium bromide	91	12	52	68	5–89	34	2	2	—	a
Alprenolol	12	—	3	3	32–73	59	—	7	—	44, 198, 254
Pinaverium bromide	14	4	7	11	17–48	33	—	—	—	17, 150, 196, 227, 256, 269
Thiazinium	5	1	3	4	21–53	30	—	—	—	196, 208
Naftidrofuryl	3	1	2	2	17–21	19	—	—	—	170, 173, 226
Pantogar[b]	1	0	1	1	—	21	—	—	—	146
Rhinasal[c]	3	2	—	1	—	27	—	—	—	11, 210, 224
Clomethiazol	1	1	0	1	—	55	—	—	—	228
Diltenate-tetra[d]	1	—	—	1	—	75	—	—	—	282
Traumanase-cyklin[e]	1	—	—	1	—	45	—	—	—	282
Acenocoumarol	1	—	—	—	—	—	—	—	—	196
Calcium dobesilate	1	—	—	1	—	45	—	—	—	86
Pantozyme	1	—	—	—	—	—	—	—	—	201
Minidril	1	—	—	—	—	—	—	—	—	51
Chlormadinone	1	0	1	1	—	50	—	—	—	61
Totals	**137**	**21**	**69**	**95**	**5–89**	**35**	**2**	**9**	**—**	

[a]References for emepronium bromide: 22, 26, 44, 46, 53, 55, 77, 84, 92, 102, 103, 105, 106, 111, 113, 116, 117, 119, 126, 127, 133, 135, 137, 146, 148, 155, 160, 189, 193, 218, 228, 229, 247, 267, 302.
[b]Components of Pantogar: thiamine HCl, calcium pantothenate, paraaminobenzoic acid, cystin, faex, keratin.
[c]Components of Rhinasal: thiazinium methylsulfate, acetaminophen, norephedrine chlorhydrate.
Components of Diltenate-tetra: tetracycline, theophylline, etafedrine, doxylamine succinate, phenylephrine, guaifenesin.
[e]Components of traumanase-cyklin: tetracycline, bromelaine.

than men have been injured by antibiotics, non-steroidal anti-inflammatory drugs (NSAIDs), alendronate (indicated for osteoporosis), and emepronium bromide (indicated for urinary frequency due to bladder irritability).

Most injured patients have normal esophageal structure and function. This is possible because pill transit through the esophagus is commonly interrupted even in normal subjects. When swallowed with water by upright subjects, gelatin capsules were retained in the esophagus longer than 5 min by 11 of 18 subjects [36]. Chasing pills with more water makes them more likely to pass rapidly to the stomach but does not guarantee transit [36]. Pills are even more likely to stick in the esophagus if taken without water or while supine, and these predisposing factors are frequently documented in literature case reports. Other factors favoring esophageal retention of pills include advanced patient age, decreased esophageal peristalsis, and extrinsic esophageal compression. Gelatin capsules are more likely to stick in the esophagus than tablets, and large pills are more likely to stick than small ones [288].

When a pill is retained in the esophagus, it may dissolve there and release its contents. If the contents are sufficiently caustic, injury will occur. The pathogenic mechanism for some pills, including the tetracyclines, ascorbic acid, and ferrous sulfate, may be production of an acid burn. Any of these pills dissolved in 10 ml of water produces a solution with a pH of 3.0 or less [36, 289]. Phenytoin sodium, 100 mg, dissolved in 10 mL of water produced a solution with a pH of 10.4, suggesting that it might produce an alkaline burn [36]. Other dissolved pills produce neutral solutions, so other mechanisms must be invoked. Postulated mechanisms include induction of GERD by anticholinergics and theophylline, production of local hyperosmolarity by potassium chloride [290], and intracellular poisoning after uptake of doxycycline [97], NSAIDs [291], and alprenolol [292, 293] directly from the esophageal lumen into the mucosa.

Several observations suggest that sustained-release medications may be more injurious to the esophagus than standard-release pills of the same medications. First, sustained-release preparations of potassium chloride, quinidine, ferrous sulfate, and alprenolol have caused most of the reported esophageal injuries and most of the reported complicated injuries due to these medications despite the widespread availability and use of standard-release preparations of the latter three medications. Isolated cases of complicated esophageal injury due to other sustained-release pills have also been reported: esophageal hemorrhage and pseudotumor due to slow-release naproxen [234], esophageal perforation due to sustained-release sodium valproate [284], and deep, circumferential esophageal ulceration and hemorrhage due to sustained-release morphine sulfate [114]. Finally, two small prospective clinical trials suggest that sustained-release pamidronate may be more injurious to the esophagus than the standard preparation of this drug [167]. Taken together, these observations demonstrate enhanced causticity for some sustained-release preparations.

Injuries due to specific pills

Antibiotics and antiviral pills

Antibiotics and antivirals have caused 656 of the 1322 reported cases of pill-induced esophageal injury (Table 38.1), nearly 50% of the esophageal injuries due to all medicinal pills combined. Doxycycline (most frequently the large-capsule form of this drug) and other tetracyclines have caused over 550 of these cases, but approximately 30 non-tetracycline antibiotics and antivirals have also been implicated. Predisposing factors other than improper pill-taking behavior have been rare. Almost all injured patients have presented with acute, severe retrosternal pain, and/or odynophagia. Mucosal injury is usually superficial, and symptoms almost always have resolved in a few days to a few weeks. Only 2.3% of reported cases have been complicated, seven by hemorrhage and eight by stricture.

Aspirin and other non-steroidal anti-inflammatory drugs

Table 38.2 documents 136 literature case reports of NSAID pill-induced esophageal injury and 81 cases compiled by the US Food and Drug Administration (FDA). Considering only the case reports, Aspirin and other NSAIDs have caused only 10% of the literature reports of pill-induced esophageal injury, but 34 of these NSAID-induced injuries have been complicated by hemorrhage. In contrast, only 28 esophageal injuries due to all other medications combined have been complicated by hemorrhage. NSAIDs are thus strikingly more likely than other pill classes to cause hemorrhage when they injure the esophagus.

Several of the NSAID-induced injuries have been devastating. A patient taking indomethacin suffered a fatal esophageal hemorrhage [8], and a patient whose injury was most likely due to acemetacin, a derivative of indomethacin, died of recurrent pulmonary infections due to a pill-induced

bronchoesophageal fistula [168]. Two patients died due to Aspirin pill-induced esophageal hemorrhage [295] and another required surgery [241]. A patient taking pills containing Aspirin and caffeine [54] and an 18-year-old male taking ibuprofen for a toothache [322] suffered esophageal perforations. Ten other patients injured by NSAIDs developed esophageal strictures.

Eighty-one of the cases of NSAID-related esophageal injury documented in Table 38.2 were due to over-the-counter naproxen sodium. These were not reported as literature case reports but were detected by the US FDA's Spontaneous Reporting System [130]. This system is a more sensitive surveillance system than review of literature case reports, especially for less serious injuries. Consequently, these 81 cases do not necessarily imply that naproxen is more likely than other NSAIDs to injure the esophagus. None of these 81 patients is known to have suffered a hemorrhage or stricture.

Bisphosphonates

Alendronate, pamidronate, etidronate, risedronate, and ibandronate are bisphosphonate inhibitors of bone resorption, and all but risedronate have been reported to cause pill-induced esophageal injury (Table 38.3). Since the initial marketing of alendronate in late 1995, 142 esophageal injuries due to this medication have been reported, 91 as case reports or case series, and 51 others with "serious" or "severe" adverse esophageal effects noted during the manufacturer's post-marketing survey [65]. Alendronate has been the most commonly reported cause of serious pill-induced esophageal injury in the past 15 years. Twenty-eight of the injured patients developed esophageal strictures. In one patient, an extensive stricture failed to respond to repetitive attempts at dilatation [232]. Another patient taking alendronate suffered fatal esophageal perforation [83]. Most patients injured by alendronate appear to have taken their pills improperly, either failing to remain upright after swallowing the pills or taking the pills with less than the 6 oz of water recommended by the manufacturer. Nonetheless, some patients appear to have been injured despite taking their pills entirely appropriately [4, 52, 65, 83, 156, 232].

Even though alendronate is a frequent offender compared to other medications, an individual patient taking alendronate properly is at only remote risk for serious esophageal injury. In 1998, only 65 patients were known to have been injured among more than 500 000 patients for whom prescriptions had been written [294].

Two controlled clinical trials provide the only documentation of esophageal injury due to oral pamidronate [167]. In these trials, four of 33 subjects taking timed-release pamidronate and one of 33 subjects taking standard pamidronate developed severe chest pain, dysphagia, and vomiting. Endoscopy revealed erosive and exudative distal esophagitis in each. No complications occurred.

Etidronate has been reported as causative in three cases of pill-induced esophageal injury [151, 172, 180], including one complicated by an esophageal stricture. Ibandronate, more recently introduced, has been the subject of a single case report of uncomplicated esophageal injury [314].

Much research has been conducted in both the *in vitro* and *in vivo* settings to better elucidate mitigating factors associated with bisphosphonate-associated esophageal injuries. Shakweh *et al.* performed experiments utilizing *ex vivo* pig esophagi and a texture analyzer to determine the maximal detachment force and adhesion work developed by both branded and several generic formulations of alendronate [331]. Significant differences were detected among the various formulations. Pills that contained hydroxypropylcellulose had a stronger adhesive force. Components such as carnuba wax tended to mitigate these forces. Experiments utilizing perfused canine esophagus have indicated that an acid environment appears to be necessary for injury to occur [332]. Perkins *et al.* have performed several *in vivo* experiments using radiolabeled tablets and scintigraphy to examine the esophageal transit properties of several bisphosphonates. In a study of 23 patients with documented osteoporosis, no association was found between esophageal transit time and the degree of kyphosis [333]. In a separate investigation in 20 healthy female volunteers, subjects were given different bisphosphonate preparations in both the erect and semi-supine (45 degrees) position [334]. As expected, the semi-supine position was significantly associated with delayed esophageal transit. The group had previously conducted a similar study comparing an oval, coated risedronate placebo to a round, uncoated placebo tablet of identical mass [335]. As expected, the uncoated tablets were substantially more likely to have delayed esophageal transit or esophageal stasis (defined as no movement for >20 s) than the coated tablets. The most interesting result of this study, however, was the effect that the volume of ingested water had on tablet adhesion. In those who drank only 30 mL of water, 17% had esophageal stasis versus 0% of those who drank 50 mL of water. Interestingly, none of the patients with esophageal stasis was aware of the tablet being lodged in their esophagus.

Potassium chloride, quinidine, ferrous sulfate or succinate, and alprenolol

Many of the 112 patients injured by potassium chloride, quinidine, ferrous sulfate or succinate, and alprenolol (a beta-blocker) (Tables 38.3 and 38.4) have presented with progressive dysphagia, often with little or no pain. Esophageal strictures have occurred in 46 (41%) of the patients injured by these four medications. This is nearly equal to the 56 strictures caused by all other medications combined.

At least 26 of the 45 patients injured by potassium chloride tablets (Table 38.3) have been predisposed to esophageal retention of pills by virtue of extrinsic esophageal compression or esophageal motor dysfunction. At least 22

had previously undergone cardiac surgery, which can result in entrapment of the esophagus between the aorta and vertebral column [279]. When the esophagus is fixed in position by adhesions and neighboring structures, it is especially susceptible to compression by an enlarged left atrium, predisposing these patients to pill retention and injury [279].

Potassium chloride-induced esophageal injuries have often been devastating. Nineteen patients have developed esophageal strictures, six have presented with hemorrhage, and six have died as a result of their injuries. Four patients suffered fatal esophageal hemorrhage, including one patient each with penetration of the aorta [169], the left atrium [260], and a bronchial collateral artery [108]. Another death was due to penetration of the mediastinum [230], and a patient with a potassium chloride-induced esophageal stricture died 1 week after surgical placement of a feeding jejunostomy [279]. All six deaths occurred in patients with cardiomegaly, and four of the six patients had previously undergone cardiac surgery.

Twenty-two cases of pill-induced esophageal injury in patients taking quinidine have been reported, and 10 of the 22 injured patients developed esophageal strictures. In contrast to the injuries due to potassium chloride, predisposing factors were identified in only two of these patients.

An unusual feature of quinidine-induced esophageal injury is the occasional presentation with flamboyant exudate that is so thick and tenacious as to suggest neoplasia on barium swallow [1, 220, 266, 283, 295]. This exudate may break up at endoscopy and reveal edematous, ulcerated underlying mucosa. Similar presentations have been documented in injuries due to sustained-release ferrous sulfate [244] and sustained-release naproxen [234]. Although these patients sometimes present with painless dysphagia suggesting a stricture or carcinoma, the lesions and symptoms may resolve without dilatation [296].

Prevention

Pills will not injure the esophagus directly unless they dissolve in the esophagus, so physicians, nurses, and pharmacists should instruct patients in a few simple and prudent steps to enhance esophageal transit of prescribed pills:

• Patients should drink at least 4 oz of fluid with any pill, twice this amount with pills that are especially likely to cause injury.

• Patients should remain upright for at least 10 min after taking most pills and for 30 min after taking pills likely to cause injury.

• Pills implicated as causing frequent or severe esophageal injury should be avoided in bedridden patients or patients with esophageal compression, stricture, or dysmotility.

These steps will greatly reduce the frequency of pill-induced esophageal injury but will not completely eliminate injury. A high index of suspicion is required to recognize pill-induced esophageal injury when it occurs, so that repetitive injury may be avoided by prompt withdrawal of the offending pill.

Disclaimer

The opinions and assertions contained herein are the personal views of the authors and are not to be construed as reflecting the views of the US Department of the Army or Department of Defense. This work was written by a government employee using government resources and is therefore not subject to copyright restrictions.

All previous writings by this author on this subject have similarly been written by a government employee using government resources.

"I certify that all individuals who qualify as authors have been listed; each has participated in the conception and design of this work, the analysis of data (when applicable), the writing of the document, and the approval of the submission of this version; that the document represents valid work; that if we used information derived from another source, we obtained all necessary approvals to use it and made appropriate acknowledgements in the document; and that each takes public responsibility for it. Nothing in the work implies any Federal/DOD/DON endorsement."

References

1. Kikendall JW, Friedman AC, Oyewole MA, Fleischer D, Johnson LF. Pill-induced esophageal injury: case reports and review of the medical literature. *Dig Dis Sci* 1983;28:174–182.
2. Aarons B, Bruns BJ. Oesophageal ulceration associated with ingestion of doxycycline. *NZ Med J* 1980;91:27.
3. Abbarah TR, Fredell JE, Ellenz GB. Ulceration by oral ferrous sulfate. *JAMA* 1976;236:2320.
4. Abdelmalek MF, Douglas DD. Alendronate-induced ulcerative esophagitis. *Am J Gastroenterol* 1996;91:1282–1283.
5. Abraham SC, Cruz-Correa M, Lee LA, Yardley JH, Wu T-T. Alendronate-associated esophageal injury: pathologic and endoscopic features. *Mod Pathol* 1999;12:1152–1157.
6. Adler JB, Goldberg RI. Mexiletine-induced pill esophagitis. *Am J Gastroenterol* 1990;85:629–630.
7. Adverse Drug Reactions Advisory Committee. Doxycycline-induced oesophageal ulceration. *Med J Aust* 1994;161:490.
8. Agdal N. Mediciniducerede esophagusskader. *Ugeskr Laeger* 1979;141:3019–3021.
9. Agha FP, Wilson JAP, Nostrand TT. Medication-induced esophagitis. *Gastrointest Radiol* 1986;11:7–11.
10. Algayres JP, Valmary J, Chabierski M, Daly JP, Rougier Y. Ulcère oesophagien après prise de minocycline. *Presse Med* 1989;18:541.
11. Allard C. Ulcére iatrogene de l'oesophage. *Gastroenterol Clin Biol* 1982;6:712.
12. Allmendinger G. Esophageal ulcer caused by the "pill." *Z Gastroenterol* 1985;23:531–533.
13. Al Mahdy H, Boswell GV. Captopril-induced oesophagitis. *Eur J Clin Pharmacol* 1988;34:95.
14. Alvares JF, Kulkarni SG, Bhatia SJ, Desai SA, Dhawan PS. Prospective evaluation of medication-induced esophageal injury and its relation to esophageal function. *Ind J Gastroenterol* 1999;18:115–117.
15. Amendola MA, Spera TD. Doxycycline-induced esophagitis. *JAMA* 1985;253:1009–1011.
16. Amichai B, Grunwald MH, Odes SH, Zirkin H. Acute esophagitis caused by isotretinoin. *Int J Dermatol* 1996;35:528–529.
17. Andre JM, Voiment YM, Marti RG. Ulcéres oesophagiens après prise de bromure de pinaverium. *Acta Endosc* 1980;10:289–291.
18. Anonymous. Esophageal injury in treatment with Doryx. *Lakartidningen* 1997;94:2665.
19. Ashour M, Salama FD, Morris A, Skinner J. Acute dysphagia induced by bendrofluazide-K. *Practitioner* 1984;228:524.
20. Barbier P, Dumont A, Dony A, Toussaint J, Thys O, Engelholm L. Ulcérations oesophagiennes induites par la doxycycline. *Acta Gastroenterol Belg* 1981;44:424–429.
21. Barbier P, Pringot J, Heimann R, Fiasse R, Jacobs E. Ulcérations digestives induites par le chlorure de potassium. *Acta Gastroenterol Belg* 1976;39:261–274.
22. Barrison IG, Trewby PN, Kane SP. Oesophageal ulceration due to emepronium bromide. *Endoscopy* 1980;12:197–199.
23. Bataille C, Soumagne D, Loly J, Brassinne A. Esophageal ulceration due to indomethacin. *Digestion* 1982;24:66–68.
24. Baumer VF, Kellner R, Neumaier U. Doxycyclin-induzierte ulzerose Osophagitis. *Fortschr Med* 1997;115:26–30.
25. Bell RL. Tetracycline induced esophagitis. *Alabama Med* 1986;55:47–50.
26. Bennett JR. Oesophageal ulceration due to emepronium bromide. *Lancet* 1977;1:810.
27. Berli DE, Salis GB, Chiocca JC. Lesion esofagica por drogas. *Acta Gastroent Latin Am* 1986;16:109–114.
28. Bezuidenhout DJJ. Iatrogene esofagitis. *S Afr Med J* 1980;57:1023.
29. Biller JA, Flores A, Buie T, Mazor S, Katz A. Tetracycline-induced esophagitis in adolescent patients. *J Pediatr* 1992;120:144–145.
30. Bissonnette B, Biron P. Ulcère oesophagien causé par la doxycycline. *Can Med Assoc J* 1984;131:1186–1188.
31. Bjarnason I, Bjornsson S. Oesophageal ulcers. *Acta Med Scand* 1981;209:431–432.
32. Blanco JR, Ibarra V, Oteo JA. Ulcera esofagica en paciente con sida. *Enferm Infect Microbiol Clin* 1997;15:269–270.
33. Bliss MR. Tablets and capsules that stick in the oesophagus. *J R Coll Gen Pract* 1984;34:301.
34. Bohane TD, Perrault J, Fowler RS. Oesophagitis and oesophageal obstruction from quinidine tablets in association with left atrial enlargement. *Aust Paediatr J* 1978;14:191–192.
35. Bokey L, Hugh TB. Oesophageal ulceration associated with doxycycline therapy. *Med J Aust* 1975;1:236–237.
36. Bonavina L, DeMeester TR, McChesney L, Schwizer W, Albertucci M, Bailey RT. Drug-induced esophageal strictures. *Ann Surg* 1987;206:173–183.

37. Bova JG, Dutton NE, Goldstein HM, Hoberman LJ. Medication-induced esophagitis: diagnosis by double-contrast esophagography. *AJR Am J Roentgenol* 1987;148:731–732.

38. Boyce HW Jr. Dysphagia after open heart surgery. *Hosp Pract* 1985;20:40–50.

39. Bretzke G. Tetrazyklin-ulkus der speiserohre. *Z Gesamte Inn Med* 1982;37:574–575.

40. Brochet E, Croisier G, Grimaldi A, Bosquet F. Stenose oesophagienne liée à la prise de phenoxylmethylpenicilline chez une diabetique insulin-dependante. *Presse Med* 1984;13:2392.

41. Burke EL. Acute oesophageal damage from one brand of tetracycline tablets. *Gastroenterology* 1975;68:1022.

42. Cameron RB. Esophagitis dissecans superficialis and alendronate: case report. *Gastrointest Endosc* 1997;46:562–563.

43. Carlborg B, Densert O, Lindqvist C. Tetracycline induced esophageal ulcers. A clinical and experimental study. *Laryngoscope* 1983;93:184–187.

44. Carlborg B, Kumlien A, Olsson H. Medikamentella esofagusstrikturer. *Lakartidningen* 1978;75:4609–4611.

45. Channer KS, Hollanders D. Tetracycline-induced oesophageal ulceration. *BMJ* 1981;282:1359–1360.

46. Chapman K. Emepronium bromide and the treatment of urge incontinence. *Med J Aust* 1978;1:103.

47. Chen CY, Wang LY, Liu HW, Jan CM, Chien CH. Esophageal ulcers caused by antibiotics. *J Formosan Med Assoc* 1982;81:618–625.

48. Chesshyre MH, Braimbridge MV. Dysphagia due to left atrial enlargement after mitral Starr valve replacement. *Br Heart J* 1971;33:799–802.

49. Cleau D. Ulcère oesophagien après prise de doxycycline. *Gastroenterol Clin Biol* 1982;6:510–511.

50. Coates AG, Nostrant TT, Wilson JAP, Elta GH, Agha FP. Esophagitis caused by nonsteroidal antiinflammatory medication: case reports and review of the literature on pill-induced esophageal injury. *South Med J* 1986;79:1094–1097.

51. Cocheton J-J, Bigot J-M, Penalba C. Les avatars du transit oesophagien des medicaments solides. *Concours Med* 1984;106:3895–3901.

52. Colina RA, Smith M, Kikendall JW, Wong RKH. A new, probably increasing cause of esophageal ulceration: alendronate. *Am J Gastroenterol* 1997;92:704–706.

53. Collins FJ, Matthews HR, Baker SE, Strakova JM. Drug-induced oesophageal injury. *BMJ* 1979;1:1673–1676.

54. Corsi PR, de Aguiar JR, de S Kronfly F, Saad R Jr, Rasslan S. Lesao esofagica provocada por ingestao de pilula. *Rev Assoc Med Brasil* 1995;41:360–364.

55. Cowan RE, Wright JT, Marsh F. Drug-induced oesophageal injury. *BMJ* 1979;2:132–133.

56. Craig JM, Giaffer MH, Talbot MD. Drug-induced oesophageal ulceration in a patient with acquired immunodeficiency syndrome. *Int J STD AIDS* 1996;7:370–371.

57. Creteur V, Laufer I, Kressel HY, *et al.* Drug-induced esophagitis detected by double-contrast radiography. *Radiology* 1983; 147:365–368.

58. Crowson TD, Head LH, Ferrante WA. Esophageal ulcers associated with tetracycline therapy. *JAMA* 1976;235:2747–2748.

59. Cummin ARC, Hangartner JRW. Oesophago-atrial fistual: a side effect of tetracycline? *J R Soc Med* 1990;83:745–746.

60. Cunningham JT. Induced esophageal ulceration. *Gastrointest Endosc* 1982;28:49–50.

61. Daghfous R, Hedi Loueslati M, El Aidli S, Srairi S, Lakhal M, Belkahia C. Atteinte inflammatoire du tractus digestif superieur probablement due à un progestatif de synthese. *Gastroenterol Clin Biol* 1995;19:853–854.

62. Daunt N, Brodribb TR, Dickey JD. Oesophageal ulceration due to doxycycline. *Br J Radiol* 1985;58:1209–1211.

63. de Caestecker JS, Heading RC. Iatrogenic oesophageal ulceration with massive haemorrhage and stricture formation. *Br J Clin Pract* 1988;42:212–214.

64. de Celis G, Sanchez J, Roig J, Gea E. Ulceracion esofagica unica por doxiciclina. *Med Clin (Barc)* 1998;110:118.

65. de Groen PC, Lubbe DF, Hirsch LJ, *et al.* Esophagitis associated with the use of alendronate. *N Engl J Med* 1996;335: 1016–1021.

66. Delpre G. Esophageal ulcers due to tetracycline. *Harefuah* 1981;101:281–282.

67. Delpre G, Kadish U. Esophageal ulceration due to enterocoated doxycycline therapy—further considerations. *Gastrointest Endosc* 1984;30:44.

68. del Valle Garcia Sanchez M, Gomez Camacho F, Poyato Gonzalez A, Vignote Alguacil M, Mino Fugarolas G. Ulcera esofagica por doxiciclina. *Gastroenterol Hepatol* 2001; 24:390–391.

69. Dertinger SH, Glossmann H, Reichsollner F, Drexel H, Feldkirch LKH. Ulcerative esophagitis and stricture due to long-term piroxicam therapy. *Gastroenterology* 1998;114:A101.

70. de Witte C, Dony A, Serste JP. Ulcere oesophagien iatrogene. *J Belge Radiol* 1972;55:655–656.

71. Djupesland G, Rolstad EA. Etsskader i oesophagus forarsaket av medikamenter. *Tidsskr Nor Laegeforen* 1978;98:696–697.

72. Doman DB, Ginsberg AL. The hazard of drug-induced esophagitis. *Hosp Pract* 1981;16:17–25.

73. *Drug Experience Report.* Spontaneous Reporting Program (1969–1980). Rockville, MD: Division of Drug Experience, U. S. Food and Drug Administration.

74. Duques P, Araujo RSA, de Amorim WPD. Ulceracao de anastomose esofago-enterica causada por alendronato. *Arq Gastroenterol* 2001;38:129–131.

75. Ecker GA, Karsh J. Naproxen induced ulcerative esophagitis. *J Rheumatol* 1992;19:646–647.

76. Edwards P, Turner J, Gold J, Cooper DA. Esophageal ulceration induced by zidovudine. *Ann Intern Med* 1990;112:65–66.

77. Eichenberger P, Blum AL. Drug-induced esophageal lesions. *Acta Endosc* 1980;10:273–283.

78. Eng J, Sabanathan S. Drug-induced esophagitis. *Am J Gastroenterol* 1991;86:1127–1133.

79. Engmann C, Kadish M, Truding RM. Picture of the month. *Arch Pediatr Adolesc Med* 2001;155:729–730.

80. Enzenauer RW, Bass JW, McDonnell JT. Esophageal ulceration associated with oral theophylline. *N Engl J Med* 1984;310:261.

81. Evenepoel C. Slokdarmzweren door gebruik van doxycycline. *Tijdschr Gastroenterol* 1977;20:293–296.

82. Ewert B, Ewert G, Glas JE, Thore M. Medikamentell hypofarynxskada. *Lakartidningen* 1979;76:739–740.

83. Famularo G, De Simone C. Fatal esophageal perforation with alendronate. *Am J Gastroenterol* 2001;96:3212–3213.

84. Fellows IW, Ogilvie AL, Atkinson M. Oesophageal stricture associated with emepronium bromide therapy. *Postgrad Med J* 1982;58:43–44.

85. Fennerty B, Sampliner R, Garewal H. Esophageal ulceration associated with 13-*cis*-retinoic acid therapy in patients with Barrett's esophagus. *Gastrointest Endosc* 1989;35:442–443.

86. Fernandez Rodriguez C, Moreira V, Boixeda D, Dominguez Rodriguez F, Garcia Plaza A. Ulcera esofagica por dobexilato calcico. *Gastroenterol Hepatol* 1986;9:102.

87. Ferrari Junior AP, Domingues SHS. Esophageal ulcer and alendronate. *Rev Paul Med* 1998;116:1882–1884.

88. Fiedorek SC, Casteel HB. Pediatric medication-induced focal esophagitis. *Clin Pediatr* 1988;27:455–456.

89. Florent C, Chagnon JP, Vivet P, Brun JG, Cattan D, Bernier JJ. Accidents oesophagiens associés à la prise orale de doxycycline. *Gastroenterol Clin Biol* 1980;4:888–892.

90. Foucaud P, Vincent MH, Scart G, Gaudelus J, Nathanson M, Perelman R. Premier cas chez l'enfant d'ulcère aigu oesophagien après pris de doxycycline. *Med Infantile* 1980;87:233–238.

91. Fraser GM, Odes HS, Krugliak P. Severe localised esophagitis due to doxycycline. *Endoscopy* 1987;19:86.

92. Freysteinsson H, Thorsson AV. Oesophageal ulcerations in two children taking emepronium bromide. *Acta Paediatr Scand* 1982;70:513–514.

93. Froese EH. Oesophagitis with clindamycin. *S Afr Med J* 1979;56:826.

94. Garcia Molinero MJ, Vidal Ruiz JV, Garcia Cabezudo J. Ulcera esofagica por doxiciclina. *Gastroenterol Hepatol* 1981;4:383.

95. Gardies A, Gevaudan J, Le Roux C, Cornet C, Warnet-Duboscq J, Viguie R. Ulcére iatrogene de l'oesophage. *Nouv Presse Med* 1978;7:1032.

96. Geschwind A. Oesophagitis and oesophageal ulceration following ingestion of doxycycline tablets. *Med J Aust* 1984;1:223.

97. Giger M, *et al.* Das tetracyclin-ulkus der speiserohre. *Dtsch Med Wochenschr* 1978;103:1038.

98. Ginaldi S. Drug-induced esophagitis. *Am Fam Physician* 1984;30:169–170.

99. Girelli C, Reguzzoni G, Rocca F. Esofagite da alendronato. *Recenti Prog Med* 1997;88:223–225.

100. Golindano C, Villalobos MM. Doxycycline esophageal ulcers: are they due to an irritant effect? *Gastrointest Endosc* 1985;31:408.

101. Gould PC, Bartolomeo RS, Sklarek HM. Esophageal ulceration associated with oral penicillin in Marfan's syndrome. *NY State J Med* 1985;85:199–200.

102. Guignard A, Savary M. L'oesophagite d'origine medicamenteuse. *Acta Endosc* 1980;10:263–272.

103. Habeshaw T, Bennett JR. Ulceration of mouth due to emepronium bromide. *Lancet* 1972;2:1422.

104. Haefeli W. Der fall aus der praxis. *Praxis* 1982;71:1396–1397.

105. Hale JE, Barnardo DE. Ulceration of mouth due to emepronium bromide. *Lancet* 1973;1:493.

106. Halter F, Scheurer U. Veratzung des distalen osophagus durch ein anticholinergikum. *Z Gastroenterol* 1978;16:699.

107. Hatheway GJ. Doxycycline-induced esophagitis. *Drug Intell Clin Pharmacy* 1982;16:879–880.

108. Henry JG, Shinner JJ, Martino JH, Cimino LE. Fatal esophageal and bronchial artery ulceration caused by solid potassium chloride. *Pediatr Cardiol* 1983;4:251–252.

109. Herrerias JM, Bonet M. Esofagitis por diacepam. *Med Clin (Barc)* 1984;83:690.

110. Herrerias JM, Bonet M, Jimenez M, Ariza A, Pellicer F. Oesophagite ulcérative et doxycycline. *Acta Endosc* 1984;14:141–143.

111. Higson RH. Oesophagitis as a side effect of emepronium. *BMJ* 1978;2:201.

112. Higuchi K, Ando K, Kim SR, *et al.* Sildenafil-induced esophageal ulcers. *Am J Gastroenterol* 2001;96:2516–2518.

113. Hillman LC, Scobie BA, Pomare EW, Austad WI. Acute oesophagitis due to emepronium bromide. *NZ Med J* 1981;94:4–6.

114. Hiraoka T, Okita M, Koganemaru S, Okada H, Sone Y. Hemorrhagic esophageal ulceration associated with slow-release morphine sulfate tablets. *Nippon Shokakibyo Gakkai Zasshi* 1991;88:1231.

115. Howie AD, Strachan RW. Slow release potassium chloride treatment. *BMJ* 1975;2:176.

116. Hugel HE, Schinko H, Bischof HP. Das medikamentos bedingte osophagusulkus. *Z Gastroenterol* 1982;20:599–603.

117. Hughes R. Drug-induced oesophageal injury. *BMJ* 1979;2:132.

118. Huizar JF, Podolsky I, Goldberg J. Ulceras esofagicas inducidas por doxiciclina. *Rev Gastroenterol Mex* 1998;63:101–105.

119. Hunert H, Ottenjann R. Drug-induced esophageal ulcers. *Gastrointest Endosc* 1979;25:41.

120. Hutter D, Akgun S, Ramamoorthy R, Dever LL. Medication bezoar and esophagitis in a patient with HIV infection receiving combination antiretroviral therapy. *Am J Med* 2000;108:684–685.

121. Imada T, Aoyama N, Amano T, Kolzumi H, Goto H. Esophageal ulceration associated with Voltaren therapy. *I To Cho* 1983;18:227–230.

122. Indorf A, Pegram PS. Esophageal ulceration related to Zalcitabine (ddC). *Ann Intern Med* 1992;117:133–134.

123. Isler M. Doxycycline-induced esophageal ulceration. *Mil Med* 2001;166:203, 222.

124. Isler M, Bahceci M. Cataflam-induced esophageal ulceration. *Am J Gastroenterol* 2001;96:1300–1301.

125. Jacques JP, Llau ME, Mercier JF, Vigreux P, Montastruc JL. Ulcération oesophagienne d'origine medicamenteuse. *Therapie* 1993;48:513.

126. Jeffery PC, Cullis SNR. Drug-induced oesophagitis. *S Afr Med J* 1983;64:1081.

127. Johnsen S, Koefoed-Nielsen B, Tos M. Emepron (Cetiprin) og aetsskader i mund og spiseror. *Ugeskr Laeger* 1982;144:1477–1479.

128. Jost PM. Drug-induced esophagitis. *JAMA* 1985;254:508.

129. Juncosa L. Ulcus peptico yatrogeno del esofago. *Rev Esp Enferm Apar Dig* 1970;30:457–458.

130. Kahn LH, Chen M, Eaton R. Over-the-counter naproxen sodium and esophageal injury. *Ann Intern Med* 1997;126:1006.

131. Kalar JG, Redwine JN, Persaud MV. Iatrogenic esophagitis. *Iowa Med* 1988;78:323–326.

132. Kato S, Kobayashi M, Sato H, Saito Y, Komatsu K, Harada Y. Doxycycline-induced hemorrhagic esophagitis: a pediatric case. *J Pediatr Gastroenterol Nutr* 1988;7:762–765.

133. Kato S, Komatsu K, Harada Y. Medication-induced esophagitis in children. *Gastroenterol Jpn* 1990;25:485–488.

134. Katsinelos P, Dimiropoulos S, Vasiliadis T, Fotiadis G, Xiarchos P, Eugenidis N. Oesophageal ulceration associated with ingestion of mefenamic acid capsules. *Eur J Gastroenterol Hepatol* 1999;11:1431–1432.

135. Kavin H. Oesophageal ulceration due to emepronium bromide. *Lancet* 1977;1:424–425.

136. Keegan AD. Drug-induced oesophageal ulceration. *Med J Austr* 1990;152:383.

137. Kenwright S, Norris ADC. Oesophageal ulceration due to emepronium bromide. *Lancet* 1977;1:548.

138. Kessenich CR. Differential diagnosis of chest pain: a case report. *Gastroenterol Nurs* 1999;22:10–12.

139. Khan SA. Esophageal ulceration related to oral ingestion of tetracycline capsules. *Gastrointest Endosc* 1983;29:163.

140. Khera DC, Herschman BR, Sosa F. Tetracycline-induced esophageal ulcers. *Postgrad Med* 1980;68:113, 115.

141. Kikendall JW. Pill esophagitis. In: Brandt LJ, ed. *Clinical Practice of Gastroenterology. Curr Med* 1999;91–96.

142. Kikendall JW, Schmidt M, Graeber GM, Burton NA, Fall SM, Johnson LF. Pill-induced esophageal ulceration and stricture following cardiac surgery. *Mil Med* 1986;151: 539–542.

143. Kimura K, Sakai H, Ido K, *et al.* Drug-induced esophageal ulcer. *Nippon Shokakibyo Gakkai Zasshi* 1978;75:64–70.

144. Klegar KL, Young TL. Pill-induced esophageal injury. *J Tenn Med Assoc* 1992;85:417–418.

145. Knauer CM, McLaughlin WT, Mark JBD. Esophago-esophageal fistula in a patient with achalasia. *Gastroenterology* 1970;58: 223–228.

146. Kobler E, Buhler H, Nuesch HJ, Deyhle P. Medikamentos induzierte osophagusulzera. *Dtsch Med Wochenschr* 1978;103: 1035–1037.

147. Kobler E, Nuesch HJ, Buhler H, Jenny S, Deyhle P. Medikamentos bedingte osophagusulzera. *Schweiz Med Wochenschr* 1979;109:1180–1182.

148. Kunert H. Medikamentos induzierte osophagusulzera. *Dtsch Med Wochenschr* 1978;103:1278.

149. Lambert JR, Newman A. Ulceration and stricture of the esophagus due to oral potassium chloride (slow release tablet) therapy. *Am J Gastroenterol* 1980;73:508–511.

150. Lamouliatte H, Plane D, Quinton A. Ulcére oesophagien après pris orale de bromure de pinaverium. *Gastroenterol Clin Biol* 1981;5:812–813.

151. Larsen K-O, Stray N, Engh V, Sandnes D. Oesophagus lesions associated with bisphosphonates. *Tidsskr Nor Laegeforen* 2000; 120:2397–2399.

152. Larzilliere I, Gargot D, Zleik T, Ramain JP. Oesophagite medicamenteuse: responsabilite de l'alendronate. *Gastroenterol Clin Biol* 1999;23:1098–1099.

153. Learmonth I, Weaver PC. Potassium stricture of the upper alimentary tract. *Lancet* 1976;1:251–252.

154. Lee MG, Hanchard B. Tetracycline-induced proximal oesophagitis. *West Ind Med J* 1990;39:124–127.

155. Leonard RCF, Adams PC, Parker S, Adams DM. Oesophageal injury associated with emepronium bromide (Ceteprin). *Br J Clin Pract* 1984;38:429–430.

156. Levine J, Nelson D. Esophageal stricture associated with alendronate therapy. *Am J Med* 1997;102:489–491.

157. Levine MS, Borislow SM, Rebesin SE, O'Brien C. Esophageal stricture caused by a Motrin tablet (Ibuporfen). *Abdom Imaging* 1994;19:6–7.

158. Levine MS, Rothstein RD, Laufer I. Giant esophageal ulcer due to Clinoril. *AJR Am J Roentgenol* 1991;156:955–956.

159. Lilley LL, Guanci R. Avoiding alendronate-related esophageal irritation. *Am J Nurs* 1997;97:12, 14.

160. Lind O. Medikamentindusert osofagitt. *Tidsskr Nor Laegeforen* 1978;98:742.

161. Llanos O, Guzman S, Duarte I. Doxycycline esophageal ulcer. *Gastrointest Endosc* 1985;31:407–408.

162. Loft DE, Stubington S, Clark C, Rees WDW. Oesophageal ulcer caused by warfarin. *Postgrad Med J* 1989;65:258–259.

163. Lopez-Cepero Andrada JM, Lopez Silva M, Salado Fuentes M, Benitez Roldan A. Ulcera esofagica por mesalazine. *Gastroenterol Hepatol* 2000;23:362.

164. Lowry N, Delaney P, O'Malley E. Oesophageal ulceration occurring secondary to slow release potassium tablets. *Irish J Med Sci* 1975;144:366.

165. Lubbe WF, Cadogan ES, Kannemeyer AHR. Oesophageal ulceration due to slow-release potassium in the presence of left atrial enlargement. *NZ Med J* 1979;90:377–379.

166. Luciani J, Pigatto V, Naves A, *et al.* [Esophagitis associated with use of alendronate in 5 postmenopausic patients]. *Acta Gastroenterol Latinoam* 2001;31:59–63.

167. Lufkin EG, Argueta R, Whitaker MD, *et al.* Pamidronate: an unrecognized problem in gastrointestinal tolerability. *Osteoporosis Int* 1994;4:320–322.

168. McAndrew NA, Greenway MW. Medication-induced oesophagial injury leading to broncho-oeophageal fistula. *Postgrad Med J* 1999;75:379–381.

169. McCall AJ. Slow-K ulceration of oesophagus with aneurysmal left atrium. *BMJ* 1975;3:230.

170. McCloy EC, Kane S. Drug-induced oesophageal ulceration. *BMJ* 1981;282:1703.

171. Macdonald L. Bulletin canadien sur les effets indesirables des medicaments. *CMAJ* 1998;158:945–946.

172. Macedo G, Azevedo F, Ribeiro T. Ulcerative esophagitis caused by etidronate. *Gastrointest Endosc* 2001;53:250–251.

173. McLean D. Drug-induced oesophageal ulceration. *BMJ* 1981;282:1975–1976.

174. Maconi G, Bianchi Porro G. Multiple ulcerative esophagitis caused by alendronate. *Am J Gastroenterol* 1995;90: 1889–1890.

175. Maekawa T, Ohji G, Inoue R, Shimoyama M, Shimada T, Misaki F. Pill-induced esophagitis caused by lansoprazole. *J Gastroenterol* 2001;36:790–791.

176. Maffioli C, Segal S, Diot J, Segal A. Oesophagite ulcéreuse a la doxycycline. *Acta Endosc* 1980;10:285–288.

177. Maffioli C, Segal S, Renard A, Diot J, Segal A. Ulcères oesophagiens à la doxycycline. *Nouv Presse Med* 1979;8:1264.

178. Marin Pineda R, Vila G. Ulcera esofagica inducida por metronidazol. Informe de un caso. *Rev Gastroenterol Mex* 1998;63: 106–107.

179. Markin RS, al-Turk M, Zetterman RK. Esophageal ulceration following doxycycline ingestion. *Postgrad Med* 1992;91:179–180.

180. Maroy B. Ulcere geant de l'oesophage probablement du a la prise d'etidronate. *Gastroenterol Clin Biol* 2001;25:917–918.

181. Maroy B. Ulcère oesophagien après prise de florocycline. *Gastroenterol Clin Biol* 1983;7:324.

182. Maroy B, Moullot P. Esophageal burn due to chlorazepate dipotassium (Tranxene^R). *Gastrointest Endosc* 1986;32:240.

183. Mason SJ, O'Meara TF. Drug-induced esophagitis. *J Clin Gastroenterol* 1981;3:115.

184. Matteo A, Eyssautier B, Rodor F, Gerolami A. Oesophagite ulcérée après prise de Selexid^R. *Gastroenterol Clin Biol* 1988;12:670–671.

185. Merino Angulo J, Perez de Diego I, Varas R, Casas JM. Dolor retrosternal y esofagitis inducida por doxiciclina. A proposito de dos observaciones. *Rev Clin Esp* 1986;179:431.

186. Meyboom RHB. Slokdarmbeschadiging door doxycycline en tetracycline. *Ned Tijdschr Geneeskd* 1977;121:1770.

187. Minocha A, Greenbaum DS. Pill-esophagitis caused by nonsteroidal antiinflammatory drugs. *Am J Gastroenterol* 1991;86:1086–1089.

188. Mohandas KM, Swaroop VS, Desai DC, *et al.* Medication induced esophageal injury. *Ind J Gastroenterol* 1991;10:20–22.

189. Morck HI, Nielsen VM, Kirkegaard P. Ulcus esophagei forarsaget af emeproniumbromid (Cetiprin). *Ugeskr Laeger* 1981;143: 623.

190. Morris TJ, Davis TP. Doxycycline-induced esophageal ulceration in the U. S. military service. *Mil Med* 2000;165:316–319.

191. Mortimer O, Wiholm BE. Oesophageal injury associated with pivmecillinam tablets. *Eur J Clin Pharmacol* 1989;37:605–607.

192. Muller, KD. Ulzerose osophagitis durch doxycyclin. *Z Arztl Fortbild (Jena)* 1990;84:659–660.

193. Murray K. Severe dysphagia from emepronium bromide associated with oesophageal diverticulum. *Br J Surg* 1982;69:439.

194. Mur Villacampa M, Guerrero Navarro L, Cabeza Lamban F. Ulcera esofagica por doxiciclina. *Rev Esp Enferm Apar Dig* 1989;76:67–69.

195. Naylor G, Davies MH. Oesophageal stricture associated with alendronic acid. *Lancet* 1996;348:1030–1031.

196. Netter P, Paille F, Trechot P, Bannwarth B, Royer RJ. Les complications oesophagiennes d'origine medicamenteuse. *Therapie* 1988;43:475–479.

197. Nwakama PE, Jenkins HJ Jr, Bailey RT Jr, Pelligrino J, DeMeester TR, Jones JB. Drug-induced esophageal injury: a case report *of Percogesic. Drug Intell Clin Pharmacy* 1989;23: 227–229.

198. Ollyo J-B, Fontolliet C, Monnier P, *et al.* L'oesophagite medicamenteuse et ses complications. *Schweiz Rundsch Med Prax* 1990;79:394–397.

199. O'Meara TF. A new endoscopic finding of tetracycline-induced esophageal ulcers. *Gastrointest Endosc* 1980;26:106–107.

200. Oren R, Fich A. Oral contraceptive-induced esophageal ulcer. Two cases and literature review. *Dig Dis Sci* 1991;36:1489–1490.

201. Ovartlarnporn B, Kulwichit W, Hiranniramol S. Medication-induced esophageal injury: report of 17 cases with endoscopic documentation. *Am J Gastroenterol* 1991;86:748–750.

202. Palmer KM, Selbst SM, Shaffer S, Proujansky R. Pediatric chest pain induced by tetracycline ingestion. *Pediatr Emerg Care* 1999;15:200–201.

203. Palop V, Juan-Martinez J, Andreu-Alapont E, Calvo-Penades I, Hernandez-Marco R. Tolmetin-induced esophageal ulceration. *Ann Pharmacother* 1997;31:929.

204. Palop V, Mir IM, Morales-Olivas FJ, Rubio E. Esofagitis relacionada con tabletas de amoxicilina de 750 mg. *Med Clin (Barc)* 1998;110:118–119.

205. Papazian A, Capron JP, Dupas JL. Doxycycline-induced esophageal ulcer. *Gastrointest Endosc* 1981;27:201.

206. Papazian A, Descombes P, Capron JP. Oesophagite ulcérée et mycotique après prise de Physiomycine^R. *Gastroenterol Clin Biol* 1984;8:389.

207. Pemberton J. Oesophageal obstruction and ulceration caused by oral potassium therapy. *Br Heart J* 1970;32:267–268.

208. Pen J, Van Meerbeeck J, Pelckmans P, Van Maercke Y. Thiazinium-induced oesophageal ulcerations. *Acta Clin Belg* 1986;41:278–283.

209. Penalba C. Ulcérations oesophagiennes induites par le chlorhydrate de mexiletine. *Ann Gastroenterol Hepatol (Paris)* 1986;22:267–268.

210. Penalba C, Eugene C. Oesophagite medicamenteuse due au Rhinasal. *Presse Med* 1983;12:1725–1726.

211. Perreard M, Klotz F. Oesophagite ulcérée après prise de spiramycine. *Ann Gastroenterol Hepatol (Paris)* 1989;25:313–314.

212. Perry PA, Dean BS, Krenelok EP. Drug induced esophageal injury. *Clin Toxicol* 1989;27:281–286.

213. Peters JL. Benign oesophageal stricture following oral potassium chloride therapy. *Br J Surg* 1976;63:698–699.

214. Petigny A, Moulinier B. Ulcères oesophagiens après prise de doxycycline. *Nouv Presse Med* 1979;8:439.

215. Piccione PR, Winkler WP, Baer J, Kotler DP. Pill-induced intramural esophageal hematoma. *JAMA* 1987;257:929.

216. Pinos T, Figueras C, Mas R. Doxycycline-induced esophagitis: treatment with liquid sucralphate. *Am J Gastroenterol* 1990;85:902.

217. Pizzani E, Valenzuela G. Esophagitis associated with alendronate sodium. *Va Med Q* 1997;124:181–182.

218. Puhakka HJ. Drug-induced corrosive injury of the oesophagus. *J Laryngol Otol* 1978;92:927–931.

219. Rambaud S, Elkharrat D, Gajdos P. Ulcération oesophagienne après prise d'ampicilline. *Ann Med Intern (Paris)* 1990;141: 275.

220. Ravich WJ, Kashima H, Donner MW. Drig-induced esophagitis simulating esophageal carcinoma. *Dysphagia* 1986;1:13–18.

221. Ribeiro A, DeVault KR, Wolfe JT III, Stark ME. Alendronate-associated esophagitis: endoscopic and pathologic features. *Gastrointest Endosc* 1998;47:525–528.

222. Riker J, Swanson M, Schweigert B. Esophageal ulceration caused by wax-matrix potassium chloride. *West J Med* 1978;128:542–543.

223. Rimmer DE, Rawls DE. Improper alendronate administration and a case of pill esophagitis. *Am J Gastroenterol* 1996;91:2648–2649.

224. Rives JJ, Olives JP, Ghisolfi J. Oesophagite aigue medicamenteuse. *Arch Fr Pediatr* 1985;42:33–34.

225. Rodino S, Sacca N, De Medici A, Giglio A. Multiple esophageal ulcerations caused by a granular formulation of aspirin. *Endoscopy* 1994;26:509–510.

226. Rodrigo Moreno M, Pleguezuelo Diaz J, Esteban Carretera J, Martinez Moreno J, Ruiz Cabello Jimenez M. Ulceraciones esofagicas de origen medicamentoso. Aportacion de dos casos y descripcion de un nuevo agente etiologico. *Gastroenterol Hepatol* 1985;8:311–315.

227. Rodriguez Agullo JL, Vidal Ruiz JV, Benita Leon V. Ulceras esofagicas causadas por una capsula de bromuro de pinaverium. *Gastroenterol Hepatol* 1983;6:362–365.

228. Rohner HG, Berges W, Wienbeck M. Clomethiazol tablets induce ulcers in the esophagus. *Z Gastroenterol* 1982;20:469–473.

229. Rose JDR, Tobin GB. Drug-induced oesophageal injury. *BMJ* 1980;1:110.

230. Rosenthal T, Adarj R, Militianu J, Deutsch V. Esophageal ulceration and oral potassium chloride ingestion. *Chest* 1974;65:463–465.

231. Rudolph R, Seggewiss H, Seckfort H. Oesophagus-ulcus durch Mexiletin. *Dtsch Med Wochenschr* 1983;108:1018–1020.

232. Ryan JM, Kelsey P, Ryan BM, Mueller PR. Alendronate-induced esophagitis: case report of a recently recognized form of severe esophagitis with esophageal stricture – radiographic features. *Radiology* 1998;206:389–391.

233. Ryan JR, McMahon FG, Akdamar K, Ertan A, Agrawal N. Mucosal irritant potential of a potassium-sparing diuretic and of wax-matrix potassium chloride. *Clin Pharmacol Ther* 1984;35:90–93.

234. Sacca N, Rodino S, De Medici A, De Siena M, Giglio A. NSAIDS-induced digestive hemorrhage and esophageal pseudotumor: a case report. *Endoscopy* 1995;27:632.

235. Sakai H, Seki H, Yoshida T, Ido K, Kimura K. Radiological study of drug-induced esophageal ulcer. *Rinsho Hoshasen* 1980;25:27–34.

236. Santalla Pecina F, Gomez Huelgas R, Sanchez Robles C. Sodium meclofenamate-induced esophageal ulcerations. *Am J Gastroenterol* 1991;86:786.

237. Santucci L, Patoia L, Fiorucci S, Farroni del Favero F, Morelli A. Oesophageal lesions during treatment with piroxicam. *BMJ* 1990;300:1018.

238. Scapa E, Shemesh E, Batt L. Fsophageal ulceration caused by tetracycline. *Harefuah* 1980;99:373–374.

239. Schmidt-Wilcke HA. Tetracyclin-ulkus der speiserohre. *Dtsch Med Wochenschr* 1978;103:2053.

240. Schneider R. Doxycycline esophageal ulcers. *Am J Dig Dis* 1977;22:805–807.

241. Schreiber JB, Covington JA. Aspirin-induced esophageal hemorrhage. *JAMA* 1988;259:1647.

242. Seaman WB. The case of the antibiotic dysphagia. *Hosp Pract* 1979;14:206, 208.

243. Seibert D, Al-Kawas F. Trimethoprim-sulfamethoxazole, hiccups, and esophageal ulcers. *Ann Intern Med* 1986;105:976.

244. Serck-Hanssen A, Stray N. Jerntablettinduserte oesophagu-slesjoner. *Tidsskr Nor Laegeforen* 1994;114:2129–2131.

245. Shaikh YM, Khan AH, Rao N, Rizvi IH, Hameed TA, Rana TA. Phyllocontin (theophylline) induced esophagitis. *J Pakistan Med Assoc* 1993;43:183.

246. Sharara AI. Lozenge-induced esophagitis. *Gastrointest Endosc* 2000;51:622–623.

247. Shepperd HWH. Iatrogenic reflux oesophagitis. *J Laryngol Otol* 1977;91:171–172.

248. Shiff AD. Doxycycline-induced esophageal ulcers in physicians. *JAMA* 1986;256:1893.

249. Simko V, Joseph D, Michael S. Increased risk in esophageal obstruction with slow-release medications. *J Assoc Acad Minority Physicians* 1997;8:38–42.

250. Smith SJ, Lee AJ, Maddix DS, Chow AW. Pill-induced esophagitis caused by oral rifampin. *Ann Pharmacother* 1999;33:27–31.

251. Sorrentino D, Trevisi A, Bernardis V, DeBiase F, Labombarda A, Bartoli E. Esophageal ulceration due to alendronate. *Endoscopy* 1996;28:529.

252. Stanely AJ, Eade OE, Hardwick D. Oesophageal ulceration secondary to potassium tablets. *Scot Med J* 1994;39:118–119.

253. Stillman AE, Martin RJ. Tetracycline-induced esophageal ulcerations. *Arch Dermatol* 1979;115:1005.

254. Stiris MG, Oyen D. Oesophagitis caused by oral ingestion of Aptin (alprenolol chloride) Durettes. *Eur J Radiol* 1982;2:38–40.

255. Stoller JL. Oesophageal ulceration and theophylline. *Lancet* 1985;2:328–329.

256. Stricker BHC. Slokdarmbeschadiging door pinaveriumbromide. *Ned Tijdschr Geneeskd* 1983;127:603–604.

257. Stricker BHC, van Overmeeren AB, Vegter AW. Doxycycline, tabletten of capsules? *Ned Tidschr Geneeskd* 1982;126:2200–2201.

258. Sugawa C, Takekuma Y, Lucas CE, Amamoto H. Bleeding esophageal ulcers caused by NSAIDs. *Surg Endosc* 1997;11:143–146.

259. Suissa A, Parason M, Lachter J, Eidelman S. Penicillin VK-induced esophageal ulcerations. *Am J Gastroenterol* 1987;82:482–483.

260. Sumithran E, Lim KH, Chiam HL. Atrio-oesophageal fistula complicating mitral valve disease. *BMJ* 1979;2:1552–1553.

261. Sutton DR, Gosnold JK. Oesophageal ulceration due to clindamycin. *BMJ* 1977;1:1598.

262. Takehana T, Imada T, Kubo A, Akaike M, *et al*. A case of drug-induced esophageal ulcer developed at the esophageal constriction due to the right aortic arch. *Nippon Kyobu Geka Gakkai Zasshi* 1992;40:1131–1134.

263. Tan HJ. Drug-induced oesophageal injury. *Hosp Med* 1998;59:938–939.

264. Tanaka S, Yamada A, Yoshida M, Hamano K, Endo M. Drug-induced esophageal ulcer—clinical report of 3 cases. *I To Cho* 1980;15:255–260.

265. Tankurt IE, Akbaylar H, Yenicerioglu Y, Simsek I, Gonen O. Severe, long-lasting symptoms from doxycycline-induced esophageal injury. *Endoscopy* 1995;27:626.

266. Teplick JG, Teplick SK, Ominsky SH, Haskin ME. Esophagitis caused by oral medication. *Radiology* 1980;134:23–25.

267. Tobias R, Cullis S, Kottler RE, Goodman H, Marks IN, Hatfield A. Emepronium bromide-induced oesophagitis. *S Afr Med J* 1982;61:368–370.

268. Toth E, Fork F-T, Lindelow K, Lindstrom E, Verbaan H, Veress B. Alendronate-induced oesophagitis; a rare, serious, but reversible side-effect. *Lakartidningen* 1998;95:3676–3680.

269. Tournier C, Lapuelle J, Gerardin A, Canard JM, Pillegand B, Claude R. Ulcères oesophagiens medicamenteux. *Rev Med Limoges* 1981;12:160.

270. Treille C. Ulcéres de l'oesophage secondaires à la prise d'amoxycilline (1 cas) et de mequitazine (1 cas). *Acta Endosc* 1985;15:41–49.

271. Tursi A, Cuoco L, Cammarota G, *et al*. Ulcerative oesophagitis due to alendronate. *Ital J Gastroenterol Hepatol* 1997;29:477–478.

272. Tzianetas I, Habal F, Keystone JS. Short report: severe hiccups secondary to doxycycline-induced esophagitis during treatment of malaria. *Am J Trop Med Hyg* 1996;54:203–204.

273. Ullah R, Golchin K, Hampton S, Primrose WJ. Oesophageal ulceration caused by doxycycline: an unusual complication. *J Laryngol Otol* 2000;114:467–468.

274. Vazquez Valdes E, Baptista MA, Barradas Guevara MC. Ulceras esofagicas producidas por medicamentos. Informe de un paciente. *Rev Gastroenterol Mex* 1987;52:119–121.

275. Viver JM, Bory F, Forne M, Garau J. Ulceraciones esofagicas medicamentosas a proposito de tres casos secundarios a ingestion de doxiciclina. *Ann Med Interna* 1986;3:600–602.

276. Voilque G. Oesophagite stenosante apparue au cours d'accidents digestifs graves par intolerance à la sulfamethoxypyridazine. *J Fr Otorhinolaryngol* 1973;22:923–925.

277. Walsh J, Kneafsey DV. Phenobarbitone induced oesophagitis. *Irish Med J* 1980;73:399.

278. Walta DC, Giddens JD, Johnson LF, Kelley JL, Waugh DF. Localized proximal esophagitis secondary to ascorbic acid ingestion and esophageal motor disorder. *Gastroenterology* 1976;70:766–769.

279. Whitney B, Croxon R. Dysphagia caused by cardiac enlargement. *Clin Radiol* 1972;23:147–152.

280. Wilcox CM, Schwartz DA, Clark WS. Esophageal ulceration in human immunodeficiency virus infection. *Ann Intern Med* 1995;122:143–149.

281. Williams JG. Drug-induced oesophageal injury. *BMJ* 1979;2:273.

282. Winckler K. Tetracycline ulcers of the oesophagus. Endoscopy, histology and roentgenology in two cases, and review of the literature. *Endoscopy* 1981;13:225–228.

283. Wong RKH, Kikendall JW, Dachman AH. Quinaglute-induced esophagitis mimicking an esophageal mass. *Ann Intern Med* 1986;105:62–63.

284. Yamaoka K, Takenawa H, Tajiri K, *et al.* A case of esophageal perforation due to a pill-induced ulcer successfully treated with conservative measures. *Am J Gastroenterol* 1996;91:1044–1045.

285. Yap I, Guan R, Kang JY, Tan CC, Gwee KA. Pill-induced esophageal injury. *Singapore Med J* 1993;34:257–258.

286. Yue Q-Y, Mortimer O. Alendronate – risk for esophageal stricture. *J Am Geriatr Soc* 1998;46:1581–1582.

287. Channer KS, Bell J, Virjee JP. Effect of left atrial size on the oesophageal transit of capsules. *Br Heart J* 1984;52:223–227.

288. Hey H, Jorgensen F, Sorensen K, Hasselbalch H, Wamberg T. Oesophageal transit of six commonly used tablets and capsules. *BMJ* 1982;285:1717–1719.

289. Carlborg B. Biverkningar vid accidentell losning av lakemedel i esofagus och bronker. *Lakartidningen* 1976;73:4201–4204.

290. Boley SJ, Allen AC, Schultz L, Schwartz S. Potassium-induced lesions of the small bowel. *JAMA* 1965;193:997–1000.

291. Semble EL, Wu WC, Castell DO. Nonsteroidal antiinflammatory drugs and esophageal injury. *Semin Arthritis Rheum* 1989;19:99.

292. Olovson SG, Bjorkman JA, Ek L, Havu N. The ulcerogenic effect on the esophagus of three B-adrenoceptor antagonists, investigated in a new porcine oesophagus test model. *Acta Pharmacol Toxicol (Copenh)* 1983;53:385–391.

293. Olovson SG, Havu N, Regardh CG, Sandberg A. Oesophageal ulcerations and plasma levels of different alprenolol salts: potential implications for the clinic. *Acta Pharmacol Toxicol (Copenh)* 1986;58:55–60.

294. Kikendall JW. Pill-induced esophageal injury. In: Castell DO, Richter JE, eds. *The Esophagus*, 3rd edn. Philadelphia: Lippincott Williams & Wilkins, 1999, pp. 527–537.

295. Abid S, Mumtaz K, Jafri W, *et al.* Pill-induced esophageal injury: Endoscopic features and clinical outcomes. *Endoscopy* 2005;37:740–744.

296. McCord GS, Clouse RE. Pill-induced esophageal strictures: Clinical features and risk factors for development. *Am J Med* 1990;88:512–518.

297. Akbayir N, Alkim C, Erdem L, Sakiz D, Mehmet S. A case report of doxycycline induced esophageal an gastric ulcer. *Turk J Gastroenterol* 2002;13:232–235.

298. Areia M, Gradiz R, Souto P, *et al.* Iron-induced esophageal ulceration. *Endoscopy* 2007;39:E326.

299. Bechade D, Desrame J, Raynaud J-J, Algayres J-P. Ulcere oesophagien secondaire a la prise de bacampicilline. *Presse Med* 2005;34:299–300.

300. Glumpak Z, Krznar J, Mihaldinec Z, Zlojtro M. Ostecenja jednjaka uzrokovana lijekovima. *Farmaceutski glasnik* 2009;65:291–296.

301. Adachi W, Watanabe H, Yazawa K, *et al.* A case of pill-induced esophagitis with mucosal dissection. *Diagn Therap Endosc* 1998;4:149–153.

302. Ahid S, Mounier G, Guy C, *et al.* Ulcere de l'oesophage secondaire a la prise de pinaverium. *Therapie* 2008;63:67–68.

303. Al-Mofarreh MA, Al Mofleh IA. Esophageal ulceration complicating doxycycline therapy. *World J Gastroenterol* 2003;9:609–611.

304. Banisaeed N, Truding RM, Chang C-H. Tetracycline-induced spongiotic esophagitis: a new endoscopic and histopathologic finding. *Gastrointest Endosc* 2003;58:292–294.

305. Buyukberber M, Demirci F, Savas MC, Kis C, Gulsen T, Koruk M. Pill esophagitis caused by telithromycin: A case report. *Turk J Gastroenterol* 2006;17:113–115.

306. Cerezo A, Costan G, Gonzalez A, *et al.* Esophagitis grave por la sobredosificacion de drageas de hierro. *Gastroenterol Hepatol* 2008;31:551–552.

307. D'Agostino L, Manguso F, Bennato R, Scaramuzzo A. A life-threatening case of stenosing pill hypopharynx-oesophagitis caused by a tamsulosin capsule. *Dig Liver Dis* 2004;36:632–634.

308. Fernandes PA, Pires MS, Gouvea AP. Esofagite ulcerativa associada ao uso de alendronato de sodio: achados histopatologicos e endoscopicos. *Arq Gastroenterol* 2002;39:173–176.

309. Gencosmanoglu R, Kurtkaya-Yapicier O, Tiftikci A, Avsar E, Tozun N, Oran ES. Mid-esophageal ulceration and candidiasis-associated distal esophagitis as two distinct clinical patterns of tetracycline or doxycycline-induced esophageal injury. *J Clin Gastroenterol* 2004;38:484–489.

310. Gulsen MT, Buyukberber NM, Karaca M, Kadayifci A. Cyproterone acetate and ethinylestradiol-induced pill oesophagitis: a case report. *Int J Clin Pract* 2005:59 (Suppl 147):79–81.

311. Grochenig HP, Tilg H, Vogetseder W. Clinical challenges and images in GI. *Gastroenterology* 2006:131:1365.

312. Hokama A, Ihama Y, Nakamoto M, Kinjo N, Kinjo F, Fujita J. Esophagitis dissecans superficialis associated with bisphosphonates. *Endoscopy* 2007;39:E91.

313. Kadayifci A, Gulsen MT, Koruk M, Savas MC. Doxycycline-induced pill esophagitis. *Dis Esophagus* 2004;17:168–171.

314. Lee C, Magee B. Oral bisphosphonates, concurrent thoracic radiotherapy and oesophagitis. *Clin Oncol* 2009;21:636–637.

315. Lutf AQ, Ghadban WK, Khan FY. Doxycycline-induced esophagitis. *Middle East J Emerg Med* 2006;6:36–38.

316. McCullough RW, Afzal ZA, Saifuddin T, Alba LM, Khan AH. Pill-induced esophagitis complicated by multiple esophageal septa. *Gastrointest Endosc* 2004;59:150–152.

317. Martinez Crespo JJ, Martinez de Guzman. Esofagitis medicamentosa: disfagia de etiologia poco frecuente. *Farm Hosp* 2005;29:71–72.

318. Misra SP, Dwivedi M. Pill-induced esophagitis. *Gastrointest Endosc* 2002;55:81.

319. Nandini CL, Lindop GB, Gillen D, Hendry A, Oien KA. Iron-induced oesophageal injury and pigmentation. *Histopathology* 2001;39:643–645.

320. Pociello Alminana N, Vilar Escrigas P, Luaces Cubells C. Esofagitis por doxiciclina. *Ann Pediatr (Barc)* 2005;62:171–173.

321. Sawadogo A, Ilboudo D. Les oesophagites medicamenteuses: la quinine aussi. *Gastroenterol Clin Biol* 2004;28:406–407.

322. Singh NP, Rizk JG. Oesophageal perforation following ingestion of over-the-counter ibuprofen capsules. *J Laryngol Otol* 2008;122:864–866.

323. Tahan V, Sayrak H, Bayar N, Erer B, Tahan G, Dane F. Doxycycline-induced ulceration mimicking esophageal cancer. *Cases J* 2008;1:144.

324. Valean S, Petrescu M, Catinean A, Chira R, Mircea PA. Pill esophagitis: Two case reports. *Romanian J Gastroenterol* 2005;14:159–163.

325. Zhang ST, Wong WM, Hu WHC, Trendell-Smith NJ, Wong BCY. Esophageal injury as a result of ingestion of iron tablets. *J Gastroenterol Hepatol* 2003;18:466–467.

326. Hirschowitz BI, Lanas A. Atypical and aggressive upper gastrointestinal ulceration associated with aspirin abuse. *J Clin Gastroenterol* 2002;34:523–528.

327. Kensing KP, White JG, Korompai F, Dyck WP. Massive bleeding From a Zenker's diverticulum: case report and review of the literature. *South Med J* 1994;87:1003–1004.

328. Hendren WG, Anderson T, Miller, JI. Massive bleeding in a Zenker's diverticulum. *South Med J* 1990;83:362.

329. Haas I, Gutman M, Paran H. Massive upper GI bleeding: a rare complication of Zenker's diverticulum. *J Postgrad Med* 2008;54: 209–210.

330. Ödemis B, Ataseven H, Basar Ö, Ertugrul I, Yüksel O, Tuhran N. Ulcer in the basis of Zenker's diverticulum mimicking esophageal malignancy. *J Nat Med Assoc* 2006;98:1177–1180.

331. Shakweh M, Bravo-Osuna I, Pinchel G. Comparative in vitro study of oesophageal adhesiveness of different commercial formulations containing alendronate. *Eur J Pharm Sci* 2007; 31:262–270.

332. Peter CP, Handt LK, Smith SM. Esophageal irritation due to alendronate sodium tablets: possible mechanisms. *Dig Dis Sci* 1998;43:1998–2002.

333. Perkins AC, Frier M, Blackshaw PE, *et al.* Esophageal transit of the weekly film-coated risendronate placebo tablet in subjects with kyphosis. *Int J Pharm* 2006;311:20–25.

334. Perkins AC, Blackshaw PE, Hay PD, *et al.* Esophageal transit and in vivo disintegration of branded risedronate sodium tablets and two generic formulations of alendronic acid tablets: a single-center, single-blind, six period crossover study in healthy female subjects. *J Clin Ther* 2008;30:834–844.

335. Perkins AC, Wilson CG, Frier M, *et al.* The use of scintigraphy to demonstrate the rapid esophageal transit of the oval film-coated placebo risedronate tablet compared to a round uncoated placebo tablet when administered with minimal volumes of water. *Int J Pharm* 2001;222:295–303.

336. Abraham SC, Cruz-Correa M, Lee LA, Yardley JH, Wu TT. Alendronate associated esophageal injury: pathologic and endoscopic features. *Mod Pathol* 1999;12:1152–1157.

39 Esophagitis in the Immunocompromised Host

C. Mel Wilcox

Department of Medicine, Division of Gastroenterology and Hepatology, University of Alabama at Birmingham, Birmingham, AL, USA

Introduction

Despite the great strides in immunosuppressive therapy, which now can more effectively target selective components of the immune system, use of antimicrobial prophylaxis for high-risk transplant patients, and the development of highly active antiretroviral therapy (HAART) for human immunodeficiency virus (HIV)-infected patients, esophageal infections remain important for the clinician. Infections of the esophagus are a relatively new problem. Before the 1960s, esophageal infections were uncommon and most often identified at autopsy [1]. The prevalence of these infections increased markedly from the 1970s through 1990s as organ transplantation grew and the acquired immunodeficiency syndrome (AIDS) exploded. Fortunately, the concurrent development and widespread adoption of endoscopy with biopsy defined the spectrum of causes, helped characterize these infections endoscopically and histologically, and became the gold standard for diagnosis.

More recently, there has been a reversal in the growing prevalence of esophageal infections. The incidence of esophagitis has been evolving in patients undergoing transplantation due to the selective administration of antimicrobial prophylaxis or pre-emptive therapy, particularly the use of strategies to prevent cytomegalovirus (CMV) disease [2, 3]. In the initial two decades of the AIDS epidemic in the United States, esophageal infections were one of the primary manifestations of the disease. However, since the availability of protease inhibitors in 1996, there has been a striking reduction overall in the incidence of opportunistic infections, including those involving the esophagus, at least in the developed world. Nevertheless, infections remain prevalent worldwide, linked to rampant AIDS in developing countries [4, 5]. Given the efficacy of therapies for virtually all esophageal infections, timely and accurate diagnosis is essential.

This chapter will focus on esophagitis in the immunocompromised host and review the epidemiology, pathology, presentation, diagnosis, and therapy for specific infections. Esophageal infections occurring in the normal host will be briefly discussed. Selected esophageal disorders associated with HIV infection and AIDS will also be reviewed.

Epidemiology

The epidemiology of esophageal infections continues to evolve. Much of the early data on the etiology and prevalence of esophageal infections were acquired from retrospective autopsy and radiographic series. Studies performed in the 1970s and 1980s ,which documented the incidence of esophageal infections following transplantation, are now largely outdated because of refinements in immunosuppressive therapy and overall management of the transplant patient. Similarly, the high incidence of esophageal infections, especially *Candida*, previously documented in patients with AIDS, is no longer the case today since the era of HAART in the developed world. In contrast, these infections are common in regions of the world without widespread exposure to HAART where infection mirrors what was seen here early in the AIDS epidemic [6, 7].

Esophageal infection is rare in an otherwise *normal person* in whom no permissive factor is present. In this setting, the most common symptomatic pathogen is herpes simplex virus (HSV) [8]. Although candidiasis has been observed in elderly patients without any obvious predisposing factors, almost uniformly, immunocompetent patients who develop esophageal infection have conditions that either weaken esophageal defense mechanisms and/or alter esophageal flora, such as disorders of esophageal emptying (achalasia, diverticula), use of corticosteroids or treatment with broad-spectrum antimicrobial agents.

The Esophagus, Fifth Edition. Edited by Joel E. Richter, Donald O. Castell.
© 2012 Blackwell Publishing Ltd. Published 2012 by Blackwell Publishing Ltd.

Esophageal infection following *solid organ transplantation* is usually due to *Candida* or herpes viruses (CMV, HSV) [9, 10]; coinfections have been described. The causes of esophageal infection following *bone marrow transplantation* are generally similar to those in other transplant patients [11]. As immunosuppressive therapy becomes even more targeted, it is likely that the prevalence of esophageal infection in all transplant patients will continue to decline.

Candida is the most common cause of esophageal infection associated with malnutrition, broad-spectrum antibiotics, and corticosteroids, both inhaled and ingested. Patients with *cancer* as well as *lymphoproliferative diseases* are well recognized to develop esophageal infections following chemotherapy, but *Candida* and viral esophagitis may also occur prior to such treatment.

Esophageal infections were common gastrointestinal complications of HIV infection, but as mentioned above, the efficacy of HAART has resulted in a striking reduction in the incidence of all opportunistic infections [4]. Before the development of these antiretroviral regimens and the widespread use of antifungal agents, prospective series of symptomatic patients found that *Candida* esophagitis was the most frequent cause of disease, seen in approximately 50% of patients [12–14]. Coinfections of *Candida* and viruses are common [15]. In contrast to other immunocompromised hosts, HSV esophagitis is less frequent than CMV esophagitis [16]. Patients with AIDS are also susceptible to a number of other unusual pathogens, which cause esophagitis, and these patients are commonly affected by the idiopathic esophageal ulcer (see below).

Predisposing factors

Esophageal infections are generally the result of humoral or cellular immune dysfunction or less commonly, arise from alterations in the normal esophageal flora. Numerous conditions are associated with immune dysfunction predisposing to infections, including diabetes mellitus, alcoholism, malnutrition, malignancies, and advanced age. In diabetes mellitus, hyperglycemia and ketoacidosis impair granulocyte function. Corticosteroids have many deleterious effects on the immune system which result in both lymphocyte and granulocyte dysfunction. Mucosal disruption of the oropharynx and esophagus commonly follows chemotherapy or radiation therapy, providing a portal of entry for pathogens. Depending on the specific type, transplantation predisposes to infection through both qualitative and quantitative effects on B and T cells due to immunosuppressive agents, chemotherapy, and neutropenia. A major risk factor for infection is episodes of rejection in recipients of solid organ transplant and graft-versus-host disease following allogeneic bone marrow transplantation, because these patients require additional potent immune suppression such as antithymo-cyte globulin. Broad-spectrum antibiotics, antacid therapy, prolonged intensive care unit (ICU) requirement or mechanical ventilation as well as surgical trauma further predispose to esophageal infections in the immunocompromised host.

Infection following solid organ transplantation has a relatively predictable time course [17]. Bacterial and fungal infections are most common during the initial months after transplantation, because it is during this period that granulocyte number and/or function are most compromised. Herpes simplex virus infection also tends to occur early after transplantation due to reactivation of disease, whereas CMV typically presents 2–6 months following transplantation at a time when neutropenia is common and T-cell function is most impaired. For HIV-infected patients, opportunistic infections reflect severe immunodeficiency (i.e. AIDS); esophageal infections typically become clinically manifest when the CD4 lymphocyte count falls below 200/mm^3, with most occurring below 100/mm^3 [18, 19]. A high HIV viral load is also a predisposing factor for opportunistic diseases [20].

General considerations

A number of factors guide the approach to the immunosuppressed patient with suspected esophageal infection. Given the breadth of potential causes of infection (Table 39.1), the differential diagnosis should be based on the cause, severity and timing of immunodeficiency, risk factors for infection, character of esophageal complaints, and findings on physical examination, particularly of the oropharynx. For HIV-infected patients, the absolute value of the CD4 lymphocyte count stratifies the risk for esophageal infection or other HIV-related process. Odynophagia is the most common presenting symptom of esophageal infection, and disorders resulting in esophageal ulceration almost uniformly cause odynophagia. Dysphagia may be observed with esophageal infections, especially *Candida* esophagitis, or may represent esophageal obstruction or dysmotility from some other cause. Bleeding may be the initial manifestation of esophageal ulceration, especially when there is an associated coagulopathy. Inspection of the oropharynx is essential when esophageal infection is suspected. Oropharyngeal candidiasis is commonly associated with esophageal candidiasis [21, 22]. However, the presence of oropharyngeal candidiasis does not prove *Candida* is the only cause of symptoms, nor does the absence of oropharyngeal candidiasis exclude *Candida* esophagitis. Coexistent oropharyngeal ulceration is common in patients with HSV esophagitis but is rarely observed in patients with CMV esophagitis [22, 23]. Patients with AIDS often have multiple coexisting esophageal disorders, which further complicate management [15].

Documentation of an infectious agent in tissue biopsies is the most specific means of diagnosis. Although barium

Table 39.1 Reported etiologies of esophageal infections.

Fungal	Viral	Bacterial	Mycobacterial	Parasitic
Candida sp.	CMV	Oral flora	TB	*Cryptosporidia*
Histoplasma	HSV	*Nocardia*	MAC	*Pneumocystis*
Blastomycosis	EBV	*Actinomyces*		*Leishmania*
Mucormycosis	HPV	*Bartonella*		*Trympanosoma*
Aspergillus	Varicella			

CMV, Cytomegalovirus; HSV, herpes simplex virus; EBV, Epstein–Barr virus; HPV, human papilloma virus; TB, tuberculosis; MAC, *Mycobacterium avium complex*.

radiography may suggest infectious esophagitis, rarely will these studies be definitive. Likewise, the clinical presentation may favor an infectious esophagitis, but the specific etiology can rarely be determined by history and physical examination alone.

At the time of endoscopy, the characteristics of the esophageal lesion(s) will provide diagnostic clues. The location, size, and appearance of all endoscopic abnormalities should be documented, because these features form the basis of the differential diagnosis and are useful for comparison on follow-up endoscopic examinations. The differential diagnosis of the lesion will dictate how the lesion(s) is sampled and what recommendations for diagnostic testing on the biopsy and/or cytologic specimens should be made. Based on the suspected cause clinically, endoscopically, and pathologically, additional stains for pathogens may be required, thereby necessitating close collaboration with the pathologist to accurately diagnose these infections. Since most esophageal infections can be diagnosed on tissue biopsy alone, multiple biopsies, which are safe to perform, should be obtained of endoscopic abnormalities to increase diagnostic yield. Esophageal brushings with cytologic evaluation may be diagnostically helpful in certain diseases such as those due to *Candida* and HSV. Viral culture of biopsy specimens may increase the diagnostic yield, although both false positives and false negatives occur. Overall multiple biopsies remain the best diagnostic method [24]. Serologic testing, such as assessment for CMV antigenemia, plays no significant role in the diagnosis of acute infectious esophagitis [25].

Fungal infections

Candida species

Epidemiology

Candida species are the most frequent esophageal pathogens. While *Candida albicans* is most common, other reported species include *C. dublenis, C. tropicalis, C. parapsilosis,* and *C. glabrata*. Overall, the rate of *C. albicans* infection is falling in the transplant setting, while that of non-*albicans* species is on the rise. Conditions predisposing to *Candida* esophagitis in the normal host include antibiotics, inhaled or ingested corticosteroids, antacid therapy or hypochlorhydric states, diabetes mellitus, alcoholism, malnutrition, old age, radiation therapy to the head, neck, and chest, and esophageal motility disturbances. Alterations in cellular immunity lead to candidal colonization and superficial infection, whereas humoral immunity (granulocytes) prevents invasive disease and dissemination. Chronic mucocutaneous candidiasis, a congenital immunodeficiency, is typically complicated by *Candida* esophagitis. As stated above, the use of immunosuppressive regimens (i.e. cyclosporine), which better target the immune system, combined with prophylactic antifungal therapy has reduced the incidence of candidal infections following solid organ and bone marrow transplantation. The incidence of *Candida* esophagitis in transplant patients administered prophylactic oral nystatin or azole therapy, typically fluconazole, is less than 5% [26]. For HIV-infected patients, the primary risk factor for esophageal candidiasis is the severity of immunodeficiency [13, 21, 27].

Pathology

The gross pathologic appearance of esophageal candidiasis ranges from a few white or yellow plaques on the mucosal surface to a dense, thick plaque coating the mucosa and encroaching on the esophageal lumen. Although occasionally misinterpreted as an "ulcer," this plaque material is composed of desquamated squamous epithelial cells, admixed with fungal organisms, inflammatory cells, and bacteria (Figure 39.1) [28]. True ulceration (granulation tissue) is rarely caused by *Candida* alone, and has been documented most commonly in immunosuppressed patients with profound granulocytopenia or when *Candida* is a coinfection with another cause of ulceration [15, 29].

Clinical manifestations

Although esophageal candidiasis may be an incidental finding in an asymptomatic patient, the usual clinical

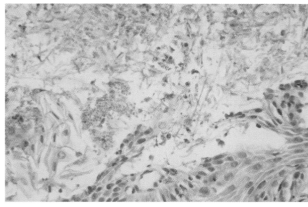

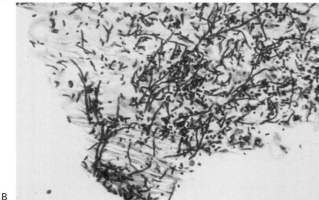

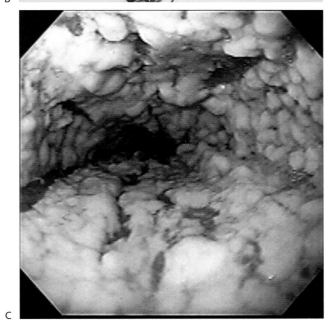

Figure 39.1 *Candida* esophagitis. (A) Diffuse plaque essentially coats the majority of the esophageal mucosa. No underlying ulcer is seen. (B) Biopsy of the mucosa and plaque shows that the plaque material is composed of desquamating epithelial cells admixed with bacteria and fungi. (C) Fungal stain shows numerous fungal pathogens.

Table 39.2. Presentations and complications of esophageal infections.

	Common	Uncommon
Candida spp	Dysphagia, odynophagia	Bleeding, chest pain
Other fungi	Dysphagia, odynophagia	Fistula
Viral	Odynophagia, chest pain	Fever, bleeding
Mycobacterial	Odynophagia, dysphagia, fever	Fistula
Bacterial	Odynophagia, fever	Dissemination
Parasitic	Odynophagia	

presentation is odynophagia with dysphagia [14, 21, 23] (Table 39.2). Symptoms are variable in severity, ranging from mild difficulty with swallowing to severe pain resulting in an inability to eat and secondary dehydration. When odynophagia is very severe, however, one must always consider causes other than *Candida* or coinfections, particularly in patients with AIDS.

Physical examination may be helpful in suggesting the diagnosis. Approximately two-thirds of patients with AIDS and esophageal candidiasis have oral candidiasis (thrush) [21, 22]. In other immunocompromised patients, oropharyngeal candidiasis is also commonly associated with esophageal candidiasis [23]. It should be recognized, however, that thrush may be absent if antifungal therapy, such as nystatin, is currently administered. In the oropharynx a diffuse erythema without plaque formation may be caused by *Candida*. Patients with chronic mucocutaneous candidiasis may have fungal involvement of various mucous membranes, hair, nails, and skin, and a history of adrenal or parathyroid dysfunction.

Complications

Complications from esophageal candidiasis are rare. Hemorrhage may occur when the disease is severe (erosion/ulcer) and there is an associated coagulopathy. Lumenal obstruction secondary to a mycetoma has also been described [30]. Fibrosis and stricture formation, and fistulization into the bronchial tree have been reported [31, 32], but these lesions probably represent *Candida* colonization of anatomic abnormalities caused by other underlying disorders or unrecognized coinfections.

Diagnosis

Esophageal candidiasis should be suspected in any patient at risk for esophageal infection, especially the immunocompromised patient, who complains of dysphagia or odynophagia. The presence of thrush further supports this diagnosis, but the absence of thrush does not exclude esophageal disease. Before endoscopy was developed, radiographic examination (barium esophagram) was the only diagnostic modality. The

Table 39.3 Pathologic findings of esophageal candidiasis infections

	Common	Uncommon
Candida	Plaques	Ulcer (rare)
Other fungi	Plaques, ulcer	Fistula
Viral	Ulcer	Mass lesions; nodules*
Mycobacteria		
TB	Ulcer, fistula	Mass lesions
MAC	Ulcer	
Bacteria	Ulcer, plaques	
Parasites	Plaque, ulcer	

*Human papilloma virus.
TB, *Mycobacterium tuberculosis;* MAC, *Mycobacterium avium* complex.

most characteristic radiographic feature of *Candida* esophagitis is the appearance of diffuse plaque-like lesions usually in a linear configuration. With disease progression, these plaques become confluent, causing a "shaggy" appearance of the esophagus, often described as ulcerations [33, 34]. Additional radiographic findings that have been reported include pseudomembranes, cobblestoning, polypoid nodules, fungus balls, strictures, esophagopulmonary fistulae, mucosal bridges, or large neoplastic-appearing esophageal ulcers and masses [29, 31–33]. A large, well-circumscribed ulceration should not be attributed to *Candida*. Importantly, a normal barium esophagram does not exclude mild esophageal candidiasis. In any patient, the presence of severe odynophagia limits the ability to drink barium, thereby hampering the potential utility of barium studies.

Endoscopic examination of the esophagus is the most sensitive and specific method of diagnosing esophageal candidiasis (Table 39.3) [35, 36]. The gross endoscopic appearance of *Candida* esophagitis is pathognomonic and may be graded according to published criteria (see Figure 39.1) [28]. During endoscopy, mucosal lesions can be brushed and submitted for cytologic evaluation or biopsied for histologic diagnosis [24]. When ulceration is identified endoscopically, multiple biopsies should be performed of the ulcer to exclude coexisting disorders [15]. The use of periodic acid-Schiff or Gomori methenamine silver stains help highlight the organisms. Cytologic examination of esophageal brushings is more sensitive than histologic examination of biopsy specimens in mild superficial candidiasis (i.e. grades 1 and 2) because organisms may be washed off tissue surfaces during processing of biopsy specimens [37]. As noted, the addition of esophageal brushings or cultures does not increase diagnostic yield over multiple biopsies alone [24]. A positive cytology but negative endoscopy and histology indicate colonization rather than infection. Skin testing and serologic tests for candidiasis are not useful for the diagnosis of *Candida* esophagitis.

In patients with AIDS and thrush, the presence of dysphagia and/or odynophagia usually indicates *Candida* esophagitis [14, 38]. Therefore, in the symptomatic patient with associated thrush, an empirical trial of systemic antifungal therapy should be instituted, reserving endoscopy for those patients who fail to respond. Further evaluation should be delayed for no longer than 1 week for patients with severe persistent symptoms since the response to antifungal therapy is rapid, with clinical improvement occurring in the majority of patients within days [14, 39]. If patients fail to improve with empirical antifungal therapy, endoscopy should be performed since disorders other than *Candida* are identified in most patients [14, 40]. This empirical strategy has not been critically studied in the transplant setting, yet clinical experience suggests it to be effective.

Treatment

A number of highly efficacious oral and intravenous medications are available for the treatment of *Candida* esophagitis (Table 39.4). In general, oral therapies should be initiated first, reserving intravenous treatment for refractory disease or when there are contraindications to orally administered medication. Although candidal species other than *C. albicans* cause esophagitis, speciation is neither widely employed nor necessary, as reliable culturing and sensitivity testing are lacking at most centers and the treatment is generally similar. For patients with mild disease, minimal immunocompromise, and/or readily reversible immunodeficiency, an abbreviated course of therapy with an oral azole should be given. Immunocompromised transplant patients and AIDS patients with *Candida* esophagitis are best treated with systemically active agents (azoles). In addition, patients with granulocytopenia are at significant risk for disseminated candidal infection, warranting the use of systemically acting agents. Drug interactions must always be kept in mind, particularly in transplant patients.

Orally administered systemically active agents which have efficacy for the treatment of *Candida* esophagitis include ketoconazole (Nizoral), fluconazole (Diflucan), and itraconazole (Sporanox). Posaconazole and voriconazole are the newest available agents, but they are used primarily for other situations. These agents, like other azoles, alter fungal cell membrane permeability by cytochrome P-450-dependent interference with ergosterol biosynthesis, resulting in fungal cell injury and death. The newer triazoles (itraconazole and fluconazole) have greater affinity then the imidazoles (miconazole and ketoconazole) for fungal P-450 enzymes. Although other agents such as clotrimazole and nystatin are effective for oral candidiasis and provide prophylaxis against esophageal involvement [41], they are significantly less effective than azoles as primary therapy for esophageal candidiasis. Ketoconazole therapy (200–400 mg/day) requires an acid milieu for optimal absorption, which limits its use in many patients [42]. Itraconazole absorption in the capsule

Table 39.4 Recommended treatment regimens for esophageal infections.

Pathogen	Drug	Dosage/route	Duration	Efficacy (%)
Candida	Ketoconazole	200–400 mg/day PO	7–14 days	<80
	Fluconazole	100 mg/day PO/IV	7–14 days	~80
	Itraconazole	200 mg/day PO	7–14 days	~80
	Amphotericin B	0.5 mg/kg/day PO/IV	7 days	>95
Histoplasma	Amphotericin B	IV		>90
	Ketoconazole			
Other fungi	Depends upon species			
CMV	Ganciclovir	5 mg/kg b.id IV	2–4 weeks	~75
	Foscarnet	90 mg/kg bid	2–4 weeks	~75
HSV	Acyclovir	400 mg 5x/day PO/IV	14 days	>90
	Valacyclovir	1 g tid PO	14 days	>90
	Famciclovir	500 mg tid PO	14 days	>90
	Foscarnet	90 mg/kg bid IV	14 days	>95
	Ganciclovir	5 mg/kg bid IV	14 days	>95
	Valganciclovir	900 mg bid PO	14 days	>90
Mycobacteria	Same as for pulmonary disease			
Bacteria	Based on infecting species			
Idiopathic ulcer	Prednisone	40 mg/day taper PO	4 weeks	>90
	Thalidomide	200–300 mg/day PO	4 weeks	>90

CMV, cytomegalovirus; HSV, herpes simplex virus.

formulation is also reduced by an increasing gastric pH [43]. Itraconazole is generally limited to those patients with mucosal *Candidiasis*, especially those who have experienced treatment failure with fluconazole.

Large randomized studies of patients with AIDS suggest that fluconazole (100 mg/day) has significantly greater efficacy than both ketoconazole (200 mg/day) and itraconazole for the treatment of *Candida* esophagitis [44, 45]. Unlike ketoconazole and itraconazole, fluconazole is highly water-soluble, is minimally protein bound or metabolized, and is excreted unchanged in the urine. The half-life of fluconazole is approximately 30 h if renal function is normal, and the presence of food or hypochlorhydria does not alter absorption. Fluconazole is available in oral and intravenous preparations, and both fluconazole and itraconazole are also available in equally effective oral solutions [46].

Adverse effects of ketoconazole, fluconazole, and itraconazole are primarily dose dependent and include nausea, hepatotoxicity, and inhibition of steroid production and cyclosporine metabolism. Due to the effects on hepatic microsomal enzymes, all three azoles inhibit the metabolism of cyclosporine, potentially resulting in an increase in cyclosporine blood levels; this effect is most pronounced with ketoconazole. In standard doses, however, fluconazole has no significant effect on cyclosporine metabolism. A number of other important drug interactions have been noted with these agents, although these tend to be more common with ketoconazole.

The other major family of antifungal agents is made up of the polyene antibiotics, represented by amphotericin and nystatin. These agents bind irreversibly to sterols in fungal cell membranes, thereby altering the permeability characteristics of the membrane and causing cell death. Nystatin is effective for treating thrush, but less so for esophageal disease. The efficacy, safety, and ease of administration of azoles have made nystatin a second-line agent. Although amphotericin B (Fungizone) is the most effective agent for systemic mycoses, its severe side effects in conjunction with the availability of azoles have limited its use for the treatment of esophageal candidiasis. When there is resistance to treatment with fluconazole or other azoles, low doses of intravenous amphotericin B (10–20 mg/day) are effective. Renal toxicity, which is usually reversible, is the most serious adverse effect of continued use of amphotericin B and can be troublesome in patients receiving cyclosporine. The liposomal form of amphotericin B has less toxicity, but the high cost has limited its use to patients with contraindications to amphotericin B, such as those at high risk for nephrotoxicity [47]. The total dose of amphotericin B for the treatment of esophageal candidiasis is approximately 100–200 mg. An oral suspension of amphotericin B is no longer available.

Flucytosine (Ancobon) is a fluorinated pyrimidine with a narrow spectrum of antifungal activity that acts by interfering with fungal translation of RNA. This oral agent, which is rarely used today, can be combined with amphotericin B or itraconazole [48], but it should not be used alone because fungi rapidly become resistant. Caspofungin, one of the new broad-spectrum antifungal agents of the echinocandid class, has been found to be as effective as amphotericin B for candidal esophagitis [49, 50]. These agents can only be given parenterally.

Prophylaxis

The prophylactic use of ketoconazole or nystatin for esophageal candidiasis in cancer and transplant patients has yielded mixed results. While the frequency of candidal infections is generally reduced, other mycoses still occur, and reductions in mortality have been difficult to establish. Prophylaxis is common in those undergoing liver transplantation because of a higher rate of candidal infection, but less so for other solid organ transplants [50, 51]. The use of azole prophylaxis in transplant patients may also be problematic in those receiving cyclosporine, mandating close monitoring of the blood level. Low doses of intravenous amphotericin B have been used successfully for prophylaxis in high-risk patients but are rarely needed today given the newer potent agents now available. While effective, primary prophylaxis against oropharyngeal and esophageal candidiasis is not currently recommended for patients with AIDS [52].

Drug resistance

Prior to HAART, because of widespread use, azole resistance was an important clinical problem, especially in AIDS patients. Both the cumulative dose of azole and severe immunodeficiency have been shown to be highly associated with the development of resistance and cross resistance [53, 54], and clinical resistance correlates with *in vitro* resistance. Prophylactic fluconazole has similarly been associated with resistance in transplant patients. When resistance occurs, increasing the dose of azole is often helpful. If higher doses fail, switching to another azole or use of an oral solution such as itraconazole [55] may be tried, but higher doses are often necessary because of cross-resistance. Intravenous amphotericin B is effective when high-dose (>400 mg/day fluconazole) therapy fails, achieving a satisfactory response rate. Resistance to amphotericin is rare. Efficacy and safety of the echinocandins has all but eliminated the need for amphotericin [50]. Posaconazole is another alternative [50]. Voriconazole or echinocandin may be required. With the availability of effective therapy for HIV infection, the current focus in these patients is on improving immune function with HAART as "therapy" for resistant candidal infections as well as prophylaxis for esophageal candidiasis [56].

Other fungi

Epidemiology

Esophageal involvement with other fungi is rare [57–65] and results from contiguously infected mediastinal lymph nodes, pulmonary parenchymal infection, primary esophageal disease, or widespread dissemination. Most instances of his-

toplasmosis and blastomycosis esophagitis represent secondary esophageal involvement from mediastinal lymph nodes rather than primary esophageal infection [57]. Although no particular geographic distribution within the United States has been reported for aspergillosis, blastomycosis, or mucormycosis, histoplasmosis is endemic in the midwestern states and Mississippi Valley. *Aspergillus*, principally a lung pathogen, has been reported to involve the esophagus in patients with leukemia and profound neutropenia [58, 59] after bone marrow or lung transplantation [66] and in AIDS [65]; contiguous pulmonary disease is usually present. Mucormycosis has been reported to involve the esophagus in a patient with AIDS [67], and only a few cases have been described in other immunocompromised patients [60].

Pathology, clinical manifestations, and complications

Other than the development of fistula, there are no unique pathologic features for these fungi (see Table 39.3). The principal clinical manifestation is usually odynophagia and/or dysphagia, and as such is non-specific. Pulmonary symptoms may predominate when there is fistula formation to the tracheobronchial tree or coexistent pulmonary involvement. With large lesions or fistulization, bleeding or perforation may occur [58]. Histoplasmosis and blastomycosis are more likely to cause focal lesions as a consequence of extension from mediastinal lymph nodes, but multiple lesions can occur during the course of dissemination [62]. Other sites of gastrointestinal involvement are common with disseminated histoplasmosis in immunocompromised patients, including those with AIDS [68].

Diagnosis

Histoplasmosis should be considered in endemic areas or in patients who have previously resided in these regions, especially if extraesophageal manifestations such as hilar adenopathy, calcified mediastinal lymph nodes, atelectasis of adjacent pulmonary tissue, or splenic calcification are present. Esophageal blastomycosis should be considered in patients with skin involvement and dysphagia; pulmonary disease may be present.

Recognition of these fungi depends on appropriate staining of endoscopic biopsy specimens with the identification of the characteristic fungal elements. Barium esophagram or endoscopy may show changes suggestive of *Candida*, malignancy [64], extrinsic compression due to lymph nodes usually in the region of the carina, or ulcer with or without fistula. Ulcerative lesions, which may be extensive, are common with all these fungi. Chest radiography may demonstrate acute or chronic pulmonary parenchymal changes, which frequently coexist in patients with esophageal histoplasmosis and aspergillosis. Endoscopy with biopsies and histologic examination (with cytologic brushings) may establish the diagnosis if the pathologist is able to differentiate the septate hyphae of *Aspergillus* species from the pseudohyphae of *Candida* species. Other fungi can be suggested by their appearance on staining of esophageal biopsies. Culture of biopsy material using fungal media can be diagnostic. Because *Histoplasma capsulatum* does not generally invade the esophageal mucosa and fibrosis is often marked, endoscopic brushings or biopsies are often non-diagnostic, thereby potentially requiring thoractomy or thoracscopy [57]. Serologic tests are not useful because of the high prevalence of positive results in endemic areas. A urine antigen test is sensitive and highly specific for disseminated histoplasmosis [69].

Treatment

While in the normal host pulmonary histoplasmosis may spontaneously resolve, therapy is required in those who are immunocompromised or have extrapulmonary disease. Itraconazole, voriconazole, and amphotericin B are effective against both histoplasmosis and blastomycosis [50]. Systemic aspergillosis should be treated with high-dose amphotericin B, although itraconazole has significant *in vitro* activity. Voriconazole or the echinocandins in combination with other agents may be a potential treatment. Surgery may be required for drainage of abscesses or excision of fistulae. Amphotericin should be administered with mucormycosis, and surgical debridement may be necessary.

Viral infections

With the implementation of *Candida* prophylaxis in selected patients undergoing transplantation and the widespread use of oral antifungal therapies in AIDS, viral esophagitis has assumed more etiologic importance in these immunosuppressed patients. Nevertheless, in the transplant setting, the incidence of clinically apparent viral esophageal disease, both HSV and CMV, has also been falling. One explanation for the decrease in herpetic esophagitis in the transplant patient is the frequent use of HSV prophylaxis. The fall in incidence of CMV disease is likely the result of use of CMV-seronegative organs and blood products for seronegative recipients, use of leukocyte-depleted platelets for patients following bone marrow transplantation, and the administration of pre-emptive ganciclovir or, more recently, valganciclovir for high-risk transplant patients [3]. Without antiviral prophylaxis, viral esophagitis is more common in bone marrow than solid organ transplant recipients because of the greater degree of immunosuppression required for these patients.

Herpes simplex virus

Epidemiology

HSV type 1 is one of three herpes viruses that affect the esophagus, the others being CMV and varicella zoster virus. HSV type 2 rarely involves the esophagus. After *Candida*

species, HSV is the next most frequent infectious agent that causes esophagitis. Although well recognized as an esophageal pathogen in otherwise healthy people [8], HSV esophagitis occurs most often in patients with some predisposing factor(s). Post transplant, HSV and CMV occur with equal frequency as causes of esophagitis [9, 66], whereas in patients with AIDS, HSV esophagitis is relatively uncommon and far less frequent than CMV. In a study of 100 HIV-infected patients with esophageal ulcer, HSV was only found in nine, in four of whom it was a copathogen with CMV [16].

Pathology

HSV infection is generally limited to squamous mucosa, where the earliest manifestation is a vesicle. As these vesicles enlarge and ulcerate, they coalesce to form larger superficial lesions, which are typically focal, leaving the intervening mucosa often normal [70]. Microscopic examination of the squamous epithelial cells at the ulcer edge reveals multinucleation, ground-glass nuclei, and eosinophilic Cowdry's type A inclusion bodies that may take up half of the nuclear volume (Figure 39.2). Over time, these inclusion bodies may be surrounded by haloes, become more basophilic, filling, enlarging, and deforming the nucleus [70].

Clinical manifestations and complications

HSV esophageal infection commonly presents with the sudden onset of severe odynophagia, heartburn or chest pain. Autopsy studies, however, suggest that esophageal symptoms may be absent [71]. Herpes labialis (i.e. cold sores) and oropharyngeal ulcers may coexist, antedate, or develop during the esophageal infection, whereas skin infection is rare [22, 23]. A number of systemic manifestations, including low-grade fever or symptoms of an upper respiratory infection, may precede the onset of esophageal symptoms. In untreated immunocompetent persons, spontaneous resolution of HSV esophageal infection occurs within 2 weeks of the onset of symptoms [8, 23, 72]. Complications are rare and include bleeding [8, 73], perforation [8, 74], tracheoesophageal fistula in association with other pathogens [75], or dissemination [71].

Diagnosis

Esophageal disease caused by HSV appears in barium radiographic studies as focal small ulceration(s) on a background of normal mucosa; vesicles are infrequently observed. These ulcers have been described as stellate or volcano-like in appearance, often with a thin halo of edema at the margin [72, 76]. There is less propensity to form the longitudinal or linear lesions that are typical for CMV infection [76]. Severe, diffuse herpetic esophagitis may result in a cobblestone or "shaggy" mucosal appearance resembling *Candida* esophagitis [77] (see Figure 39.2A). Although the radiographic appearance may be suggestive, definitive diagnosis of

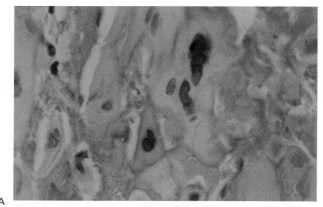

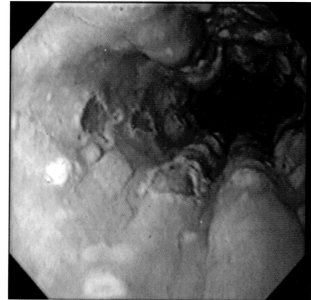

Figure 39.2 *Herpes simplex* virus esophagitis. (A) Multiple shallow ulcerations with normal intervening mucosa of the mid esophagus. (B) Characteristic multinucleated giant cells.

herpetic esophagitis requires endoscopic mucosal biopsies. The endoscopic characteristics of herpetic esophagitis reflect the pathologic changes (see Figure 39.2A), appearing as discrete, usually small (<1 cm), well-circumscribed shallow ulcers [78, 79], a diffuse erosive esophagitis, or rarely vesicles. Small, scattered lesions covered with exudate mimic esophageal candidiasis. Deep ulcers, as seen with CMV, are very rare. Cytologic brushings and endoscopic mucosal biopsies should be taken from the ulcer edge, as the viral cytopathic effect is best identified in epithelial cells rather than granulation tissue in the ulcer bed. Immunohistochemical staining on biopsy samples using specific monoclonal antibodies to HSV will help confirm the diagnosis when the viral cytopathic effect is difficult to appreciate. Viral culture of biopsy specimens helps establish a definitive diagnosis but takes several days for the results. As with other etiologies of

infectious esophagitis, serologic tests play no role in establishing the diagnosis.

Treatment

A number of uncontrolled trials and vast clinical experience in both immunocompetent and immunodeficient patients suggest the efficacy of acyclovir (Zovirax), a nucleoside analog, for the therapy of esophageal disease. In the largest study, which evaluated 34 patients with AIDS and HSV esophagitis, a clinical response was seen in essentially all treated patients [80]. More recently, valacyclovir, a prodrug of acyclovir, and famciclovir have been released. The advantage of these agents over acyclovir is that they can be administered three times per day at an equivalent cost. While large studies evaluating the use of these agents for esophagitis are lacking, trials for genital disease suggest equivalence to acyclovir [81]. Although spontaneous resolution of HSV esophagitis is common in the normal host, therapy is usually instituted regardless of immune status. When oral intake is hampered by severe odynophagia or when there is a question of drug absorption, intravenous administration is required. Side effects of these agents are few. Although rare, resistance should be suspected when there is clinical failure; in this setting, foscarnet (Table 39.4) is the drug of choice and will lead to clinical cure in most patients [82]. These agents are effective prophylaxis for HSV-antibody-positive patients undergoing transplantation [2]. Long-term secondary prophylaxis should be considered when immunodeficiency persists, because the relapse rate is high.

Cytomegalovirus

Epidemiology

Until the advent of transplantation, CMV disease was uncommon and it is extremely rare in normal individuals [83]. Currently, CMV is regarded as one of the most common opportunistic infections. Studies from developed countries have shown seropositivity rates of 50% or greater, and up to 90% seropositivity has been found in homosexual men, reflecting sexual transmission of the virus [84]. In transplant patients who receive no antiviral prophylaxis, CMV and HSV are equally common esophageal pathogens [2, 7, 66,]. As already noted, CMV is the most frequent cause of esophageal ulcer in patients with AIDS, comprising greater than 50% of esophageal ulcers in these patients [16].

Pathology

The histologic hallmark of CMV esophagitis is mucosal ulceration (see Table 39.3). Although variable, deep ulcers are very characteristic for disease in AIDS, whereas in other immunocompromised patients, lesions tend to remain more superficial. In contrast to HSV, the viral cytopathic effect of CMV is located in endothelial and mesenchymal cells in the granulation tissue of the ulcer base rather than squamous cells. Inclusions are large (cytomegalo) and often have an eosinophilic appearance that may be located either in the nucleus or cytoplasm. Because these inclusions can appear atypical, especially in patients with AIDS [85], immunohistochemical stains play a valuable role in selected patients for confirming the presence of CMV and often highlight more infected cells than are appreciated by routine hematoxylin and eosin staining. As with other esophageal infections, CMV may coexist with HSV or *Candida*, especially in patients with AIDS [15, 16]. The pathogenesis of CMV disease is not well understood. Mucosal ischemia has been hypothesized as an etiologic mechanism given the involvement of endothelial cells [86]. The high mucosal concentration of tumor necrosis factor- found in association with CMV esophagitis, which falls after ganciclovir treatment and ulcer healing, suggests an etiologic role for this proinflammatory cytokine [87].

Clinical manifestations and complications

Odynophagia is a cardinal symptom and is characteristically severe (see Table 39.2). Chest pain, weight loss, and fever may be reported. The onset of symptoms is often more subacute than the acute presentation of HSV. A prior or coexistent diagnosis of CMV infection in another organ (e.g. retinitis or colitis) is not infrequent. Although rare in transplant patients, retinitis may be observed in approximately 15% of AIDS patients at the time of diagnosis of gastrointestinal disease [88]. Complications include gastrointestinal bleeding (5% of patients) and rarely strictures, or fistulae to the tracheobronchial tree [89, 90].

Diagnosis

Like HSV, the radiologic appearance of CMV esophagitis is that of either focal or extensive ulceration, and will depend in large part on the epidemiologic setting. Barium esophagography of CMV esophagitis may reveal only thickening of mucosal folds, but more typically, well-circumscribed ulcers are present, which may be vertical, linear with central umbilication, solitary and deep, or occasionally diffuse and superficial [77, 91]. In patients with AIDS, these ulcers are often large and deep, exceeding 2 cm in size (Figure. 39.3). Rarely, the exuberant inflammatory response results in a lesion suggestive of a malignancy [92]. The endoscopic appearance of CMV esophagitis is similarly variable, ranging from multiple shallow ulcers, to solitary giant ulcers, to a diffuse superficial esophagitis (Figure 39.3) [93]. Given the high rate of prior exposure to CMV, serologic testing is not helpful. In addition, some immunosuppressed transplant patients fail to develop a brisk antibody response with acute infection. The absence of CMV DNA or antigenemia in the blood would, however, suggest an alternative diagnosis, but this test is neither sensitive nor specific [25].

Identification of viral cytopathic effect in mucosal biopsies is the best diagnostic method. Multiple biopsies (up to 10) may be required to establish the diagnosis in patients with AIDS and should be taken from the base of the ulcer [94].

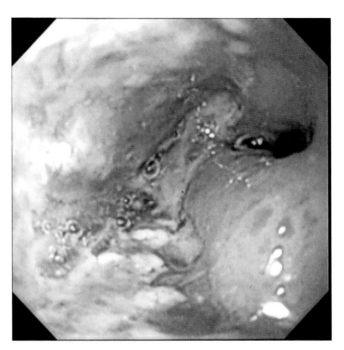

Figure 39.3 *Cytomegalovirus* esophagitis. Large, deep hemicircumferential ulceration in a patient with AIDS. These lesions may be indistinguishable from the idiopathic esophageal ulcer.

Viral culture of mucosal biopsies is less sensitive and specific than histology [24]. Use of shell vial techniques improves the turnaround time for the viral culture to 48 h. In contrast to *Candida* and HSV, cytologic specimens from esophageal lesions have very poor sensitivity for the diagnosis of CMV [24]. Since retinitis may coexist with gastrointestinal disease, a diagnosis of CMV gastrointestinal disease in any patient with AIDS warrants ophthalmologic examination [95].

Therapy

The therapies available for the treatment of CMV disease are generally efficacious but require intravenous administration and include ganciclovir, foscarnet, and cidofovir. A prospective open-label trial of ganciclovir therapy for CMV esophagitis in 35 AIDS patients documented clinical and endoscopic improvement in 77% of patients [88]. The time course of the clinical response to ganciclovir is variable; 1 week of therapy may be required before there is symptomatic improvement. The total treatment duration should be based on the clinical and endoscopic response, and a 2-4-week treatment course is usually adequate. If retinitis is absent and there has been a complete response, the patient may be followed closely without maintenance therapy, especially if immunodeficiency can be reversed with HAART. Because of low bioavailability (<10%), oral ganciclovir is not effective for the treatment of active infections, including those of the gastrointestinal tract [96]. Following acute CMV disease in transplantation patients, treatment should be given for 1–2 months until the immunosuppressive regimen is significantly reduced. Ganciclovir is well tolerated, with its major side effect being myelosuppression, which may be severe when other bone marrow suppressive drugs, such as azidothymidine, are coadministered. Clinical and virologic resistance has been recognized, usually in patients receiving prolonged therapy [97]. Combination therapy with foscarnet has been reported to treat refractory disease or when side effects are limiting, as lower doses of each agent may be utilized [98].

Foscarnet inhibits viral DNA polymerase and reverse transcriptase. A randomized trial comparing ganciclovir to foscarnet for AIDS patients with gastrointestinal CMV disease found clinical improvement in over 80% of patients, and there were no significant differences in efficacy between the two agents [99]. There is less information on the use of foscarnet in non-AIDS immunosuppressed patients. Foscarnet has been most frequently utilized when there is clinical resistance to ganciclovir or a major contradiction to ganciclovir use. The major side effect of foscarnet is reversible renal insufficiency [100]. This may be prevented by vigorous saline hydration prior to and during drug administration in combination with dose adjustments based on creatinine clearance. Electrolyte disturbances, which include hypocalcemia and hypophosphatemia, are also common during or shortly after infusion. Because of these side effects as well as higher cost, foscarnet remains second-line therapy.

Cidofovir is the newest systemic agent available for the therapy of CMV, but has only undergone evaluation for the treatment of retinitis in AIDS [101, 102]. Because of its long half-life, once-weekly administration is adequate, which makes it an ideal agent for selected patients. Like foscarnet, this drug is associated with renal insufficiency.

Valganciclovir is an oral agent for the treatment and prophylaxis of CMV infections [92]. In contrast to oral ganciclovir, this agent has excellent oral absorption, achieving therapeutic concentrations [103, 104]. While effective for retintitis, large studies for active gastrointestinal disease are lacking. Because of its low toxicity and oral bioavailability, it has become the agent of choice for prophylaxis in the transplant patient.

All drugs for herpes viruses only inhibit viral replication; thus, relapse is frequent when therapy is discontinued. The relapse rate for transplant patients also remains high until immunosuppressive therapy is reduced. In patients with AIDS, the relapse rate of CMV esophagitis is approximately 50%, similar to that for HSV [80, 88, 99]. With the advent of HAART, successful treatment of HIV-associated immunosuppression will serve to prevent relapse, thus negating the need for long-term antiviral therapy for CMV [105].

Prophylaxis

High-dose acyclovir has been used with some success for the prophylaxis of CMV infection in transplant patients, although intravenous ganciclovir has been shown to be superior [106]. Because of its cost, potential side effects, and intravenous route of administration, at most transplant centers intravenous prophylaxis is limited to high-risk patients, including CMV-seropositive patients, CMV-seronegative recipients who receive CMV-seropositive organs and/or blood products, and patients receiving potent immunosuppression for episodes of rejection [3]. With the availability of valganciclovir, most of these patients now receive this agent, negating the need for intravenous therapy [107]. While oral ganciclovir prophylaxis has been shown to decrease CMV disease in high-risk patients after liver transplantation [108], valganciclovir is now the drug of choice for such patients. Oral ganciclovir is effective prophylaxis for CMV retinitis in AIDS patients with a CD4 lymphocyte count of less than 200/mm^3, but is untested for either primary or secondary prophylaxis of gastrointestinal CMV disease [96]. Fortunately, despite long-term administration, resistance of CMV to ganciclovir and foscarnet is uncommon.

Other viruses

The frequency of esophageal involvement caused by varicella zoster virus during the course of chicken pox or herpes zoster infections is unknown but clinically uncommon [109, 110]. The esophagitis usually occurs when skin lesions are present, rather than antedating the cutaneous disease. Culture of mucosal biopsies is required to differentiate HSV from varicella zoster virus. The disease is self-limited in the immunocompetent patient. Papilloma virus may infect the esophagus in both normal and immunocompromised patients, and characteristically causes small polypoid lesions [111], which are usually asymptomatic, or symptomatic ulcers [112, 113]. Esophageal ulcers have been reported due to Epstein-Barr virus in patients with AIDS [114].

Mycobacterial infections

Epidemiology

Mycobacterial involvement of the esophagus is rare in both immunocompromised and immunocompetent patients with advanced pulmonary tuberculosis, even in countries with high prevalence rates. Previously, *Mycobacterium tuberculosis* (TB) involvement of the esophagus was considered a rare autopsy finding, found in fewer than 0.15% of necropsies [115]. In developing countries, the rate of TB is much higher, and extrapulmonary manifestations, including esophageal disease, are more common. The upsurge in reported cases of TB linked to the AIDS epidemic has increased the incidence of esophageal infection worldwide. *Mycobacterium avium* complex (MAC), a pathogen principally restricted to patients with AIDS, is primarily a small bowel pathogen with few reported cases of esophageal involvement [116–119].

Pathology

Most commonly, TB involves the mid esophagus at the level of the carina. Esophageal disease is caused by spread of infection from contiguous TB-infected mediastinal lymph nodes by way of a draining fistula or obstructed lymphatics, resulting in tracheoesophageal fistula. Rarely, TB involves the upper third of the esophagus by direct extension from tuberculous pharyngitis or laryngitis. Primary esophageal TB in the absence of extraesophageal disease is exceedingly rare [120, 121]. Granulomas are often present in ulcer tissue, with bacilli identifiable by mycobacterial staining. Unless multiple biopsies are taken, the diagnosis can be easily missed, especially if there is a significant fibrotic response.

Clinical manifestations and complications

The symptoms of esophageal TB depend on the degree and type of involvement. Systemic symptoms of fever and weight loss are common. Pulmonary complaints often predominate due to a fistula to the trachea, bronchus, or pleural space. Dysphagia may be prominent with the formation of long strictures or traction diverticula resulting from the fibrotic response or mediastinal fibrosis may be the cause of dysphagia [122]. Upper gastrointestinal hemorrhage from tuberculous esophageal ulcers [123] and tuberculous arterioesophageal fistulae [124] has been reported. Bleeding caused by extensive mucosal disease has been described in an AIDS patient with esophageal MAC [125].

Diagnosis

Esophageal TB should be suspected in patients with pulmonary or systemic TB who develop esophageal symptoms. Barium esophagram findings of ulceration and stricture are non-specific. A sinus tract or fistulous connection to the bronchial tree or mediastinum at the level of the hilum is highly suggestive of TB, but may be attributed to malignancy, which appears similarly, potentially delaying the diagnosis. An ulcerated tuberculous granulomatous mass may also mimic an esophageal neoplasm at endoscopy [121, 126]. When a fistula is present, sputum staining and culture can make the diagnosis of TB. Chest radiography is often abnormal and may suggest the diagnosis. Computed tomography of the chest usually demonstrates mediastinal lymphadenopathy, but again, carcinoma may appear similarly. Ulceration is usually present at the site of the fistula. Endoscopic biopsies from the edge of the lesions may reveal granulomas and/or acid-fast bacilli, and biopsy material should be cultured for further confirmation of the diagnosis and determination of sensitivities to antimycobacterial agents. Cytologic specimens may also be helpful.

Treatment

Even in the presence of immunodeficiency, a 9-month course of multidrug therapy (in the absence of drug resistance) will often cure esophageal TB and close fistulae. If fistulae do not close with medical therapy alone, surgical intervention will be required. Multidrug-resistant TB is becoming an increasingly complex problem; thus, knowing drug sensitivities to antituberculous therapy is essential to guide therapy.

The most effective agents for the treatment of MAC are clarithromycin and ethambutol [127]. Although a clinical and bacteriologic response is common, long-term therapy for MAC is required if immune function cannot be improved with highly active antiretroviral therapy.

Bacterial infections

Epidemiology

Bacterial esophagitis is a very rare cause of esophageal disease [128–131]. For the most part, this is a polymicrobial infection consisting of oral flora, particularly Gram-positive organisms, including *Streptococcus viridans,* staphylococci, and other bacilli. Bacterial esophagitis with these organisms occurs almost exclusively in patients with hematologic malignancies complicated by severe granulocytopenia [128], but occasionally following bone marrow transplantation [66], diabetic ketoacidosis [129], or steroid therapy. It is likely that these bacteria colonize and then invade mucosa damaged either from reflux disease, radiation therapy, or following chemotherapy, which leads to local infection; dissemination may occur when granulocyte function is poor and/or there is absolute granulocytopenia.

Other bacteria have been reported to involve the esophagus. *Brucella* presenting as a distal submucosal esophageal mass with dysphagia and fever has been noted in a normal host [132]. In patients with AIDS, *Bartonella hensellae,* the cause of cat scratch disease [133], actinomyces [134, 135], and *Nocardia* [136] have been described.

Pathology

The gross pathologic appearance of the esophagus in bacterial infection depends on the specific pathogen and ranges from diffuse, shallow ulcerations to ulcers associated with erythema, plaques, pseudomembranes, nodules, or hemorrhage [131]. Microscopic examination reveals pseudomembranes and bacterial invasion that may be superficial and limited to squamous epithelium or may be invasive and transmural with infiltration of blood vessels (i.e. phlegmonous esophagitis). Esophageal actinomycosis is characterized by ulceration and sinuses leading from abscess cavities, with sulfur granules and filamentous Gram-positive branching bacteria seen on tissue biopsies [65]. In the one reported case, *B. hensellae* esophagitis resulted in multiple nodules from a lobulated proliferation of capillary vessels lined by plump endothelial cells [133].

Clinical manifestations and complications

Bacterial esophagitis presents with odynophagia and dysphagia typical for any infectious esophagitis. Esophageal infection may serve as a focus for bacteremia and seeding of other organs [131]. Perforation has not been reported.

Diagnosis

The diagnosis of bacterial esophagitis should be considered in the clinical settings described above. Radiographic findings are non-specific, and endoscopic biopsy is required to establish this diagnosis. Additional stains, including Gram's stain, will be necessary to identify the etiologic bacteria. When suspected, bacterial cultures of biopsy material should be submitted. Positive blood cultures will also pinpoint the bacterial pathogen(s) and direct antimicrobial therapy.

Treatment

Since the infection may be polymicrobial, broad-spectrum antibiotics, which effectively treat both Gram-positive and Gram-negative oropharyngeal flora, are required. Treatment of other bacteria found in these patients is similar to infection in other locations.

Treponema pallidum

Although esophageal involvement by *Treponema pallidum* was well recognized many years ago, this disease is unheard of today in developed countries and is primarily of historical interest. The rarity of this esophageal infection has also not been altered by the AIDS epidemic. Tertiary syphilis of the esophagus may present as a submucosal gumma or diffuse inflammatory reaction with fibrosis, which often affects the upper third of the esophagus, and may be associated with mucosal ulcers and strictures [137, 138]. Given the rarity of esophageal syphilis, most patients with infectious esophagitis and positive serologic tests for syphilis will have another cause of esophagitis.

Protozoal infections

In developed countries, protozoal infections of the esophagus are very rare, having been reported almost exclusively in AIDS patients. In these patients, reported pathogens include *Pneumocystis carinii* [139], *Cryptosporidium parvum* [140], and *Leishmania donovani* [141]; coinfections were present in two of these cases [139, 140]. The clinical presentation is similar to other causes of infectious esophagitis. Ulceration(s) is the most common endoscopic finding and the diagnosis is established by appropriate histologic staining of mucosal biopsies. In normal hosts from endemic areas in South America, *Trypanosoma cruzi* may involve the myenteric plexus of the esophagus, resulting in Chagas' disease. This disease is indistinguishable clinically, radiographically, manometrically, and endoscopically from idiopathic achalasia. This diagnosis may be established by antibody testing.

Selected HIV-related esophageal disorders

In addition to the infections described above, there are other unique disorders causing esophageal disease in these patients.

Disorders associated with primary HIV infection

Although primary HIV infection is largely asymptomatic, in some patients, a mononucleosis-like illness occurs around the time of infection, consisting of fever, sore throat, and myalgias associated with a maculopapular rash [142]. Spontaneously resolving oropharyngeal and esophageal aphthous ulceration, candidal infection, or CMV esophagitis may also be observed with this seroconversion illness [143, 144]. During this primary infection, a brief period of immunodeficiency occurs and is likely the explanation for the development of opportunistic infections. Endoscopically, these aphthous esophageal ulcerations are multiple, small, and shallow [144]. In some of these patients, electron microscopic examination of biopsy specimens revealed enveloped virus-like particles with morphologic features compatible with retroviruses [144]. The diagnosis can be established at the time of presentation by the detection of HIV RNA in serum [142]. Serologic testing is unhelpful, as antibody positivity to HIV is delayed by 3–18 months after the illness.

Idiopathic esophageal ulcer

Epidemiology

Large, usually isolated esophageal ulcerations in which no specific etiology could be identified were recognized early in the AIDS epidemic. These ulcers, termed idiopathic esophageal ulcers (IEUs) or aphthous ulcers, are very common, comprising approximately 40% of esophageal ulcers in HIV-infected patients [16]. Like other esophageal infections in AIDS, IEUs are observed in patients with AIDS when the CD4 lymphocyte count is less than $100/mm^3$ [16]. These lesions appear to be unique to AIDS.

Pathology

IEUs are variable in size, may be quite large, and are uniformly well circumscribed [145, 145]. Ulcer tissue resembles that in cases of CMV and HSV esophagitis, except that viral cytopathic effect is absent. *Candida* coinfection is common [15]. The presence of a superficial candidal infection overlying a large, well-circumscribed lesion with histopathologic findings of granulation tissue but without viral cytopathic effect should still strongly suggest the diagnosis of IEU rather than *Candida* esophagitis. Since HIV has been observed in ulcer tissue by immunohistochemical staining, it has been suggested that HIV is the direct cause of these lesions. However, studies have found HIV histopathologically in esophageal biopsies from patients with *Candida,* CMV, and HSV esophagitis [147, 148]. HIV has been uniformly identified in inflammatory cells rather than in squamous epithelial cells, and the infected cells are few in number [147, 148]. In aggregate, these studies suggest that HIV does not cause IEU, at least based on a direct cytopathic mechanism.

Clinical manifestations and complications

The presentation of IEU is indistinguishable from other causes of esophageal ulcer. Coexistent oropharyngeal aphthous ulcers are infrequent [22], whereas thrush is common, especially if the patient has not received empirical antifungal therapy. Complications of IEU include bleeding and fistula to the stomach, but not to the tracheobronchial tree [145, 149], and esophageal strictures [90].

Diagnosis

The findings of IEU on barium esophagram are characteristically large, well circumscribed, and often deep ulcers [150, 151] (Figure 39.4). Because of the similarity to CMV esophagitis, a definitive diagnosis cannot be made on the radiographic appearance alone. As IEU is a diagnosis of exclusion, endoscopy with biopsy is required. Endoscopically, these ulcers are variable in size and appearance and larger ulcers are indistinguishable from CMV esophagitis (Figure 39.4) [93, 146]. Pill-induced esophagitis must be excluded by history since the pathologic findings of esophageal biopsies are similar. Likewise, distal esophageal ulcer may suggest gastroesophageal reflux disease (GERD), and the histopatho-

logic features cannot distinguish IEU from GERD. However, the clinical history is different, and the endoscopic appearance helps suggest reflux disease.

Treatment

These ulcers respond rapidly to either prednisone or thalidomide, with clinical and endoscopic cure seen in greater than 90% of cases [152, 153]. The prednisone regimen consists of 40 mg/day tapering 10 mg/ week for a 1-month treatment course. Intermittent azole therapy should be coadministered to reduce the likelihood of *Candida* complicating the use of high-dose corticosteroids. Steroid injection into the ulcers is effective, but requires repetitive endoscopy [145]. Thalidomide is given in a dose of 200 mg/day for 4 weeks. The main side effects are drowsiness, skin rash, and neurotoxicity. The horrific teratogenic effects are well recognized and limit its cautious use to male patients. The relapse rate for IEU is approximately 50%, and retreatment is usually successful. Long-term daily maintenance therapy may be required for the patient with frequent relapses. Like other opportunistic diseases in AIDS, improvement in immune function with HAART should prevent relapse.

References

1. Wong TW, Warner NE. Cytomegalic disease in adults. *Arch Pathol* 1962;74:403.
2. Momin F, Chandrasekaar PH. Antimicrobial prophylaxis in bone marrow transplantation. *Ann Intern Med* 1995;123:205–215.
3. Torres-Madriz G, Boucher HW. Perspectives in the treatment and prophylaxis of cytomegalovirus disease in solid-organ transplant recipients. *Clin Infect Dis* 2008;47:702–711.
4. Monkemuller KE, Call SA, Lazenby AJ, *et al.* Declining prevalence of opportunistic gastrointestinal disease in the era of combination antiretroviral therapy. *Am J Gastroenterol* 2000;95:457–462.
5. Braunstein SL, van de Wijgert JH, Nash D. HIV incidence in sub-Saharan Africa: a review of available data with implications for surveillance and prevention planning. *AIDS Rev* 2009;11:140–156.
6. Klotz SA, Nguyen HC, Pham TV, *et al.* Clinical features of HIV/AIDS patients presenting to an inner city clinic in Ho Chi Minh City, Vietnam. *Int J STD AIDS* 2007;18:482–485.
7. Chong VH, Lim CC. Human immunodeficiency virus and endoscopy: Experience of a general hospital in Singapore. *J Gastroenterol Hepatol* 2005;20:722–726.
8. Ramanathan J, Rammouni M, Baran J Jr, *et al.* Herpes simplex virus esophagitis in the immunocompetent host: an overview. *Am J Gastroenterol* 2000;95:2171–2176.
9. Alexander JA, Brouillette DE, Chien MC, *et al.* Infectious esophagitis following liver and renal transplantation. *Dig Dis Sci* 1988;33:1121–1126.
10. Bernabeu-Wittel M, Naranjo M, Cisneros JM, *et al.* Infections in renal transplant recipients receiving mycophenolate versus azathioprine –based immunosuppression. *Eur J Clin Microbiol Infect Dis* 2002;21:173–180.

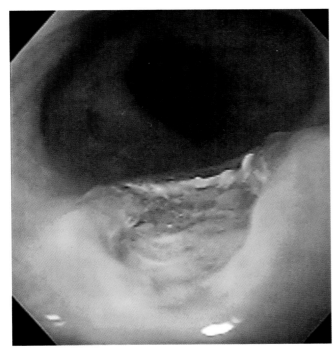

Figure 39.4 Idiopathic esophageal ulcer. Well circumscribed ulceration of the mid esophagus with a heaped up appearance

11. Vishny ML, Blades EW, Creger RJ, *et al*. Role of upper endoscopy in evaluation of upper gastrointestinal symptoms in patients undergoing bone marrow transplantation. *Cancer Invest* 1994;12:384–389.

12. Bonacini M, Young T, Laine L. The causes of esophageal symptoms in human immunodeficiency virus infection. *Arch Intern Med* 1991;151:1567–1572.

13. Connolly GM, Hawkins D, Harcourt-Webster JN, *et al*. Oesophageal symptoms, their causes, treatment, and prognosis in patients with the acquired immunodeficiency syndrome. *Gut* 1989;30:1033–1039.

14. Wilcox CM, Alexander LN, Clark WS, *et al*. Fluconazole compared with endoscopy for human immunodeficiency virus-infected patients with esophageal symptoms. *Gastroenterology* 1996;110:1803–1809.

15. Wilcox CM. Evaluation of a technique to evaluate the underlying mucosa in patients with AIDS and severe *Candida* esophagitis. *Gastrointest Endosc* 1995;42:360–363.

16. Wilcox CM, Schwartz DA, Clark WS. Esophageal ulceration in human immunodeficiency virus infection: causes, diagnosis, and management. *Ann Intern Med* 1995;123:143–149.

17. Rubin RR. Infections in the liver and renal transplant patient. In Rubin RH, Young LS, eds. *Clinical Approach to Infection in the Compromised Host*, 2nd edn. New York: Plenum Publishing, 1988, p. 561.

18. Bacellar H, Munoz A, Hoover DR, *et al*., for the Multicenter AIDS Cohort Study. Incidence of clinical AIDS conditions in a cohort of homosexual men with CD4+ cell counts <100/mm³. *J Infect Dis* 1994;170:1284–1287.

19. Wilcox CM, Saag MS. Gastrointestinal complications of HIV infection: changing priorities in the HAART era. *Gut* 2008;57:861–870.

20. Hammer SM, Eron JJ Jr, Reiss P, *et al*. Antiretroviral treatment of adult HIV infection: 2008 recommendations of the International AIDS Society–USA panel. *JAMA* 2008;300:555–570.

21. Lopez-Dulpa M, Mora Sanz P, Pintado Garcia V, *et al*. Clinical, endoscopic, immunologic, and therapeutic aspects of oropharyngeal and esophageal candidiasis in HIV-infected patients: a survey of 114 cases. *Am J Gastroenterol* 1992;87:1771–1774.

22. Wilcox CM, Straub RF, Clark WS. Prospective evaluation of oropharyngeal findings in human immunodeficiency virus-infected patients with esophageal ulceration. *Am J Gastroenterol* 1995;90:1938–1941.

23. Baehr PH, McDonald GB. Esophageal infections: risk factors, presentation, diagnosis, and treatment. *Gastroenterology* 1994; 106:509–532.

24. Wilcox CM, Rodgers W, Lazenby A. Prospective comparison of brush cytology, viral culture, and histology for the diagnosis of ulcerative esophagitis in AIDS. *Clin Gastroenterol Hepatol* 2004;2:564–567.

25. Jan E-Y, Park SY, Lee SJ, *et al*. Diagnostic performance of the cytomegalovirus (CMV) antigenemia assay in patients with CMV gastrointestinal disease. *Clin Infect Dis* 2009; 48:e121–124.

26. Frick T, Fryd DS, Goodale RL, *et al*. Incidence and treatment of *Candida* esophagitis in patients undergoing renal transplantation. Data from the Minnesota prospective randomized trial of cyclosporine versus antilymphocyte globulin-azathioprine. *Am J Surg* 1988;155:311–313.

27. Abgrall S, Charreau I, Joly V, *et al*. Risk factors for esophageal candidiasis in a large cohort of HIV-infected patients treated with nucleoside analogues. *Eur J Clin Microbiol Infect Dis* 2001;20:346–349.

28. Wilcox CM, Schwartz DA. Endoscopic-pathologic correlates of *Candida* esophagitis in acquired immunodeficiency syndrome. *Dig Dis Sci* 1996;41:1337–1345.

29. Eras P, Goldstein MJ, Sherlock P. *Candida* infection of the gastro-intestinal tract. *Medicine (Balt)* 1972;51:367–379.

30. Bhalodia MV, Vega KJ, DaCosta J, *et al*. Esophageal candidoma in a patient with acquired immunodeficiency syndrome. *J Assoc Acad Minor Phys* 1998;9:69–71.

31. Lewicki AM, Moore JP. Esophageal moniliasis: a review of common and less frequent characteristics. *AJR Am J Roentgenol* 1975;125:218–225.

32. Ott DJ, Gelfand DW. Esophageal stricture secondary to candidiasis. *Gastrointest Radiol* 1978;2:323–325.

33. Roberts L Jr, Gibbons R, Gibbons G, *et al*. Adult esophageal candidiasis: a radiographic spectrum. *Radiographics* 1987;7:289–307.

34. Glick SN. Barium studies in patients with Candida esophagitis: pseudoulcerations simulating viral esophagitis. *AJR Am J Roentgenol* 1994;163:349–352.

35. Bashir RM, Wilcox CM. Symptom-specific use of upper gastrointestinal endoscopy in human immunodeficiency virus-infected patients yields high dividends. *J Clin Gastroenterol* 1996;23:292–298.

36. Yang MT, Ko FT, Cheng NY, *et al*. Clinical experience of esophageal ulcers and esophagitis in AIDS patients. *Kaohsiung J Med Sci* 1996;12:624–629.

37. Kodsi BE, Wickremesinghe C, Kozinn PJ, *et al*. *Candida* esophagitis. A prospective study of 27 cases. *Gastroenterology* 1976;71:715–719.

38. Lai YP, Wu MS, Chen MY, *et al*. Timing and necessity of endoscopy in AIDS patients with dysphagia or odynophagia. *Hepatogastroenterology* 1998;45:186–189

39. Wilcox CM. Time course of clinical response to fluconazole for *Candida* oesophagitis in AIDS. *Aliment Pharmacol Ther* 1994;8:347–350.

40. Wilcox CM, Straub RF, Alexander LN, *et al*. Etiology of esophageal disease in human immunodeficiency virus-infected patients who fail antifungal therapy. *Am J Med* 1996;101:599–604.

41. Shepp DH, Klosterman A, Siegel MS. Comparative trial of ketoconazole and nystatin for prevention of fungal infection in neutropenic patients treated in a protective environment. *J Infect Dis* 1985;152:1257–1263.

42. Tavitian A, Raufman JP, Rosenthal LE. Ketaconazole-resistant *Candida* esophagitis in patients with acquired immunodeficiency syndrome. *Gastroenterology* 1986;90:443–445.

43. Lim SG, Sawyer AM, Hudson M, Sercombe J, Pounder RE. The absorption of fluconazole and itraconazole under conditions of low intragastric acidity. *Aliment Pharmacol Ther* 1993;7:317–321.

44. Laine L, Dretler RH, Contea CN, *et al*. Fluconazole compared to ketoconazole for the treatment of *Candida* esophagitis in AIDS. *Ann Intern Med* 1992;117:655–660.

45. Barbaro G, Barbarini G, Calderon W, *et al*. Fluconazole versus itraconazole for *Candida* esophagitis in acquired immunodeficiency syndrome. *Gastroenterology* 1996;111:1169–1177.

46. Wilcox CM, Darouiche RO, Laine L, *et al*. A randomized, double-blind comparison of itraconazole oral solution and fluconazole tablets in the treatment of esophageal candidiasis. *J Infect Dis* 1997;176:227–232.

47. Johnson PC, Wheat LJ, Cloud GA, *et al*. Safety and efficacy of liposomal amphotericin B compared with conventional amphotericin B for induction therapy of histoplasmosis in patients with AIDS. *Ann Intern Med* 2002;137:105–109

48. Barbaro G, Barbarini G, Di Lorenzo G. Fluconazole vs. itraconazole-flucytosine association in the treatment of esophageal candidiasis in AIDS patients. A double-blind, multicenter placebo-controlled study. The Candida Esophagitis Italian Study (CEMIS) Group. *Chest* 1996;110:1507–1514.

49. De Wet N, Llanos-Cuentas A, Suleiman J, *et al*. A randomized, double-blind, parallel-group, dose-response study of micafungin compared with fluconazole for the treatment of esophageal candidiasis in HIV-positive patients. *Clin Infect Dis* 2004;39:842–849.

50. Pappas PG, Kauffman CA, Andes D, *et al*. Clinical practice guidelines for the management of Candidasis: 2009 update by the Infectious Diseases Society of America. *Clin Infect Dis* 2009;48:503–535.

51. Salavert M. Prophylaxis, pre-emptive or empirical antifungal therapy: which is best in non-lung transplant recipients? *Int J Antimicrob Agents* 2008;32:S149–S153.

52. Kaplan JE, Benson C, Holmes KH, *et al*. Guidelines for prevention and treatment of opportunistic infections in HIV-infected adults and adolescents: recommendations from CDC, the National Institutes of Health, and the HIV Medicine Association of the Infectious Diseases Society of America. *MMWR Recomm Rep* 2009;58:1–207.

53. Fichtenbaum CJ, Koletar S, Yiannoutsos C, *et al*. Refractory mucosal candidiasis in advanced human immunodefiency virus infection. *Clin Infect Dis* 2000;30:749-56.

54. Mangi AA, Gaissert HA, Wright CD, *et al*. Benign bronchoesophageal fistula in the adult. *Ann Thorac Surg* 2002; 73:911–915.

55. Goldman M, Cloud GA, Smedema M, *et al*. Does long-term intraconazole prophylaxis result in in vitro azole resistance in mucosal Candida albicans isolates from persons with advanced human immunodeficiency virus infection? The National Institute of Allergy and Infectious Diseases Mycoses study group. *Antimicrob Agents Chemother* 2000; 44:1585–1587.

56. Cartledge JD, Midgley J, Gazzard BG. Itraconazole cyclodextrin solution: the role of *in vitro* susceptibility testing in predicting successful treatment of HIV-related fluconazole-resistant fluconazole-susceptible oral candidosis. *AIDS* 1997;11:163–168.

57. Marshall JB, Singh R, Demmy TL, *et al*. Mediastinal histoplasmosis presenting with esophageal involvement and dysphagia: case study. *Dysphagia* 1995;10:53–58.

58. Young RC, Bennett JE, Vogel CL, *et al*. Aspergillosis: the spectrum of the disease in 98 patients. *Medicine (Balt)* 1970;49:147–173.

59. Alioglu B, Avci Z, Canan O, *et al*. Invasive esophageal aspergillosis associated with acute myelogenous leukemia: successful therapy with combination caspofungin and liposomal amphotericin B. *Pediatr Hematol Oncol* 2007;24:63–68.

60. Neame P, Rayner D. Mucormycosis. *Arch Pathol* 1960;70:143.

61. Mezhir JJ, Mullane KM, Zarling J, *et al*. Successful nonoperative management of gastrointestinal mucormycosis: novel

therapy for invasive disease. *Surg Infect (Larchmt)* 2009; 10:447–451.

62. Forsmark CE, Wilcox CM, Darragh TM, *et al*. Disseminated histoplasmosis in AIDS: an unusual case of esophageal involvement and gastrointestinal bleeding. *Gastrointest Endosc* 1990; 36:604–605.

63. McKenzie R, Khakoo R. Blastomycosis of the esophagus presenting with gastrointestinal bleeding. *Gastroenterology* 1985;88:1271–1273.

64. Khandekar A, Moser D, Fidler WJ. Blastomycosis of the esophagus. *Ann Thorac Surg* 1980;30:76–79.

65. Spencer GM, Roach D, Skucas J. Actinomycosis of the esophagus in a patient with AIDS: findings on barium esophagograms. *AJR Am J Roentgenol* 1993;161:795–796.

66. McDonald GB, Sharma P, Hackman RC, *et al*. Esophageal infections in immunosuppressed patients after marrow transplantation. *Gastroenterology* 1985;88:1111–1117.

67. Washington K, Gottfried MR, Wilson MI. Gastrointestinal cyptococcosis. *Mod Pathol* 1991;4:707–711.

68. Baddley JW, Sankara IR, Rodriquez JM, *et al*. Histoplasmosis in HIV-infected patients in a southern regional medical center: poor prognosis in the era of highly active antiretroviral therapy. *Diagn Microbiol Infect Dis* 2008;62:151–156.

69. Scheel CM, Samayoa B, Herrera A, *et al*. Development and evaluation of an enzyme-linked immunosorbent assay to detect Histoplasma capsulatum antigenuria in immunocompromised patients. *Clin Vaccine Immunol* 2009;16:852–858.

70. Nash G, Ross JS. Herpetic esophagitis: a common cause of esophageal ulceration. *Hum Pathol* 1974;5:339–345.

71. Buss DH, Scharyj M. Herpes virus infection of the esophagus and other visceral organs in adults: incidence and clinical significance. *Am J Med* 1979;66:457–462.

72. Shortsleeve MJ, Levine MS. Herpes esophagitis in otherwise healthy patients: clinical and radiologic findings. *Radiology* 1992;182:859–861.

73. Byard RW, Champion MC, Orizaga M. Variability in the clinical presentation and endoscopic findings of herpetic esophagitis. *Endoscopy* 1987;19:153–155.

74. Cronstedt JL, Bouchama A, Hainau B, *et al*. Spontaneous esophageal perforation in herpes simplex esophagitis. *Am J Gastroenterol* 1992;87:124–127.

75. Obrecht WF, Richter JE, Olympio GA, *et al*. Tracheoesophageal fistula: a serious complication of infectious esophagitis. *Gastroenterology* 1984;83:1174–1179.

76. Levine MS, Loevner LA, Saul SH, *et al*. Herpes esophagitis: sensitivity of double-contrast esophagography. *AJR Am J Roentgenol* 1988;151:57–62.

77. Levine MS, Rubesin SE, Laufer I. Barium esophagography: a study for all seasons. *Clin Gastroenterol Hepatol* 2008; 6:11–25.

78. Agha FP, Horchang HL, Nostrant TT. Herpetic esophagitis: a diagnostic challenge in immunocompromised patients. *Am J Gastroenterol* 1986;81:246–253.

79. McBane RD, Gross JR Jr. Herpes esophagitis: clinical syndrome, endoscopic appearance, and diagnosis in 23 patients. *Gastrointest Endosc* 1991;37:600–603.

80. Genereau T, Lortholary O, Bouchaud O, *et al*. Herpes simplex esophagitis in patients with AIDS: report of 34 cases. *Clin Infect Dis* 1996;22:926–931.

81. Spruance SL, Tyring SK, DeGregorio B, *et al*. A large-scale, placebo-controlled, dose-ranging trial of peroral valaciclovir for episodic treatment of recurrent herpes genitalis. *Arch Intern Med* 1996;156:1729–1735.

82. Chatis PA, Miller CH, Schrager LE, *et al*. Successful treatment with foscarnet of an acyclovir-resistant mucocutaneous infection with herpes simplex virus in a patient with acquired immuno-deficiency syndrome. *N Engl J Med* 1989;320:297–300.

83. Altman C, Bedossa P, Dussaix E, *et al*. Cytomegalovirus infection of esophagus in immunocompetent adults. *Dig Dis Sci* 1995;40:606–608.

84. Shepp DH, Moses JE, Kaplan MH. Seroepidemiology of cytomegalovirus in patients with advanced HIV disease: influence on disease expression and survival. *J Acquir Immune Defic Syndr Hum Retroviruses* 1996;11:460–468.

85. Monkemuller KE, Bussian AH, Lazenby AJ, *et al*. Special histologic stains are rarely beneficial for the evaluation of HIV-related gastrointestinal infections. *Am J Clin Pathol* 2000;114:387–394.

86. Henson D. Cytomegalovirus inclusion bodies in the gastrointestinal tract. *Arch Pathol* 1972;93:477–482.

87. Wilcox CM, Harris PR, Redman TK, *et al*. High mucosal levels of tumor necrosis factor alpha messenger RNA in AIDS-associated cytomegalovirus-induced esophagitis. *Gastroenterology* 1998;114:77–82.

88. Wilcox CM, Straub RF, Schwartz DA. Cytomegalovirus esophagitis in AIDS: a prospective study of clinical response to ganciclovir therapy, relapse rate, and long-term outcome. *Am J Med* 1995;98:169–176.

89. Chalasani N, Parker KM, Wilcox CM. Bronchoesophageal fistula as a complication of cytomegalovirus esophagitis in AIDS. *Endoscopy* 1997;29:S28–S29.

90. Wilcox CM. Esophageal strictures complicating ulcerative esophagitis in patients with AIDS. *Am J Gastroenterol* 1999;94:339–343.

91. Balthazar EJ, Megibow AJ, Hulnick D, *et al*. Cytomegalovirus esophagitis in AIDS: radiographic features in 16 patients. *AJR Am J Roentgenol* 1987;149:919–923.

92. Laguna F, Garcia-Samaniego J, Alonso MJ, Alvarez I, Gonzalez-Lahoz JM. Pseudotumoral appearance of cytomegalovirus esophagitis and gastritis in AIDS patients. *Am J Gastroenterol* 1993;88:1108–1111..

93. Wilcox CM, Straub RA, Schwartz DA. Prospective endoscopic characterization of cytomegalovirus esophagitis in patients with AIDS. *Gastrointest Endosc* 1994;40:481–484.

94. Wilcox CM, Straub RF, Schwartz DA. A prospective evaluation of biopsy number for the diagnosis of viral esophagitis in patients with HIV infection and esophageal ulcer. *Gastrointest Endosc* 1996;44:587–593.

95. Yust I, Fox Z, Burke M, *et al*. Retinal and extraocular cytomegalovirus end-organ disease in HIV-infected patients in Europe: a EuroSIDA study, 1994–2001. *Eur J Clin Microbiol Infect Dis* 2004;23:550–559.

96. Biron KK. Antiviral drugs for cytomegalovirus diseases. *Antiviral Res* 2006;71:154–163.

97. Erice A, Chous S, Biron KK, *et al*. Progressive disease due to ganciclovir-resistant cytomegalovirus in immunocompromised patients. *N Engl J Med* 1989;320:289–293.

98. Dieterich DT, Poles MA, Lew EA, *et al*. Concurrent use of ganciclovir and foscarnet to treat cytomegalovirus infection in AIDS patients. *J Infect Dis* 1993;167:1184–1188.

99. Blanshard C, Benhamou Y, Dohin E, *et al*. Treatment of AIDS-associated gastrointestinal cytomegalovirus infection with foscarnet and ganciclovir: a randomized comparison. *J Infect Dis* 1995;172:622–628.

100. Jacobson MA. Review of the toxicities of foscarnet. *J Acquir Immune Defic Syndr* 1992;5:S11–S17.

101. Lalezari JP, Stagg RJ, Kuppermann BD, *et al*. Intravenous cidofovir for peripheral cytomegalovirus retinitis in patients with AIDS. *Ann Intern Med* 1997;126:257–263.

102. Studies of Ocular Complications of AIDS Research Group. Parenteral cidofovir for cytomegalovirus retinitis in patients with AIDS: The HPMPC peripheral cytomegalovirus retinitis trial. *Ann Intern Med* 1997;126:264–269.

103. Martin DF, Sierra-Madero J, Walmsley S, *et al*. A controlled trial of valganciclovir as induction therapy for cytomegalovirus retinitis. *N Engl J Med* 2002;11:1119–1126.

104. Czock D, Scholle C, Rasche FM, *et al*. Pharmacokinetics of valganciclovir and ganciclovir in renal impairment. *Clin Pharmacol Ther* 2002;72:142–150.

105. Kirk O, Reiss P, Uberti-Foppa U, *et al*. Safe interruption of maintenance therapy against previous infection with four common HIV-associated opportunistic pathogens during potent antiretroviral therapy. *Ann Intern Med* 2002;137:239–250.

106. Winston DJ, Wirin D, Shaked A, Busuttil RW. Randomised comparison of ganciclovir and high-dose acyclovir for long-term cytomegalovirus prophylaxis in liver-transplant recipients. *Lancet* 1995;346:69–74.

107. Kalil AC, Freifeld AG, Lyden ER, *et al*. Valganciclovir for cytomegalovirus prevention in solic organ transplant patients: an evidence-based reassessment of safety and efficacy. *PLoS One* 2009;4:e5512.

108. Gane E, Saliba F, Valdecasas GJC, *et al*. Randomised trial of efficacy and safety of oral ganciclovir in the prevention of cytomegalovirus disease in liver transplant recipients. *Lancet* 1997;350:1729–1733.

109. Kroneke MK, Cuadrado MR. Esophageal stricture following esophagitis in a patient with herpes zoster: case report. *Milit Med* 1984;149:479–481.

110. Gill RA, Gebhard RL, Dozenman RL, *et al*. Shingles esophagitis: endoscopic diagnosis in two patients. *Gastrointest Endosc* 1984;30:26–27.

111. Orlowska J, Jarosz D, Gugulski A, *et al*. Squamous cell papillomas of the esophagus: report of 20 cases and literature review. *Am J Gastroenterol* 1994;89:434–437.

112. Schechter M, Pannain VLN, de Oliveira AV. Papovavirus-associated esophageal ulceration in a patient with AIDS. *AIDS* 1991;5:238

113. Ouarto G, Sivero L, Somma P, *et al*. A case of infectious esophagitis caused by human papilloma virus. *Minerva Gastroenterol Dietol* 2008;54:317–321.

114. Kitchen VS, Helbert M, Francis ND, *et al*. Epstein-Barr virus associated oesophageal ulcers in AIDS. *Gut* 1990;31:1223–1225.

115. Lockard LB. Oesophageal tuberculosis. A critical review. *Laryngoscope* 1913;23:561

116. de Silva R, Stoopack PM, Raufman JP. Esophageal fistulas associated with mycobacterial infection in patients at risk for AIDS. *Radiology* 1990;175:449–453.

117. El-Serag HB, Johnston DE. *Mycobacterium avium* complex esophagitis. *Am J Gastroenterol* 1997;92:1561–1563.

118. Gray JR, Rabeneck L. Atypical mycobacterial infection of the gastrointestinal tract in AIDS patients. *Am J Gastroenterol* 1989;89:1521–1524.

119. Stoopack PM, de Silva R, Raufman JP. Inflammatory double-barrelled esophagus in two patients with AIDS. *Gastrointest Endosc* 1990;36:394–397.

120. Seivewright N, Feehally J, Wicks ACB. Primary tuberculosis of the esophagus. *Am J Gastroenterol* 1984;79:842–843.

121. Laajam MA. Primary tuberculosis of the esophagus: pseudo-tumoral presentation. *Am J Gastroenterol* 1984;79:839–841.

122. Ramakantan R, Shah R. Dysphagia due to mediastinal fibrosis in advanced pulmonary tuberculosis. *AJR Am J Roentgenol* 1990;154:61–63.

123. Porter JC, Friedland JS, Freedman AR. Tuberculosis bronch-oesophageal fistulae in patients infected with the human immunodeficiency virus: three case reports and review. *Clin Infect Dis* 1994;19:954–957.

124. Catinella FP, Kittle F. Tuberculous esophagitis with aortic aneurysm fistula. *Ann Thorac Surg* 1988;45:87–88.

125. Cappell MS, Gupta A. Gastrointestinal hemorrhage due to gastrointestinal *Mycobacterium avium intracellulare* of esopha-geal candidiasis in patients with the acquired immunodefi-ciency syndrome. *Am J Gastroenterol* 1992;87:224

126. Musoğlu A, Özütemiz, Tekin F, *et al*. Esophageal tuberculosis mimicking esophageal carcinoma. *Turk J Gastroenterol* 2005;16:105–107.

127. Shafran SD, Singer J, Zarowny DP, *et al*. A comparison of two regimens for the treatment of *Mycobacterium avium* complex bacteremia in AIDS: rifabutin, ethambutol, and clarithromycin versus rifampin, ethambutol, clofazimine, and ciprofloxacin. *N Engl J Med* 1996;335:377-383.

128. Gilver RL. Esophageal lesions in leukemia and lymphoma. *Dig Dis Sci* 1970;15:31

129. Ezzell JH, Bremer J, Adamec TA. Bacterial esophagitis: an often forgotten cause of odynophagia. *Am J Gastroenterol* 1990;85:296

130. Howlett SA. Acute streptococcal esophagitis. *Gastrointest Endosc* 1979;25:150–151.

131. Walsh TJ, Belitsos NJ, Hamilton SR. Bacterial esophagitis in immunocompromised patients. *Arch Intern Med* 1986; 146:1345–1348.

132. Laso FJ, Cordero M, Giarcia-Sanchez. Esophageal brucelosis: a new location of *Brucella* infection. *Clin Invest* 1994; 72:393–395.

133. Chang AD, Drachenberg CI, James SP. Bacillary angiomatosis associated with extensive esophageal polyposis: A new muco-cutaneous manifestation of acquired immunodeficiency disease (AIDS). *Am J Gastroenterol* 1996;91:2220–2223.

134. Poles MA, McMeeking AA, Scholes JV, *et al*. *Actinomyces* infec-tion of a cytomegalovirus esophageal ulcer in two patients with acquired immunodeficiency syndrome. *Am J Gastroenterol* 1994;89:1569–1572.

135. Ng FH, Wong SY, Chang CM, *et al*. Esophageal actinomycosis: a case report. *Endoscopy* 1997;29:133.

136. Kim J, Minamoto GY, Grieco MH. Nocardial infection as a complication of AIDS: report of six cases and review. *Rev Infect Dis* 1991;13:624–629.

137. Hudson TR, Head JR. Syphilis of the esophagus. *J Thoracic Surg* 1950;20:216.

138. Stone J, Friedberg SA. Obstructive syphilitic esophagitis. *JAMA* 1961;177:7116

139. Grimes MM, LaPook JD, Bar MH, *et al*. Disseminated *Pneumocystis carinii* infection in a patient with acquired immu-nodeficiency syndrome. *Hum Pathol* 1987;18:307–308.

140. Kazlow PG, Shah K, Benkov KJ, *et al*. Esophageal crypt-osporidiosis in a child with acquired immune deficiency syn-drome. *Gastroenterology* 1986;91:1301–1303.

141. Villanueva JL, Torre-Cisnero J, Jurado R, *et al*. *Leishmania* esophagitis in an AIDS patient: An unusual form of visceral leishmaniasis. *Am J Gastroenterol* 1994;89:273–275.

142. Schacker T, Collier AC, Hughes J, *et al*. Clinical and epidemio-logic features of primary HIV infection. *Ann Intern Med* 1996;125:257–264.

143. Kinloch-de-Los S, de Saussure P, Saurat JH, *et al*. Symptomatic primary infection due to human immunodeficiency virus type 1: review of 31 cases. *Clin Infect Dis* 1993;17:59–65.

144. Rabeneck L, Popovic M, Gartner S, *et al*. Acute HIV infection presenting with painful swallowing and esophageal ulcers. *JAMA* 1990;263:2318–2322..

145. Kotler DP, Reka S, Orenstein JM, *et al*. Chronic idiopathic esophageal ulceration in the acquired immunodeficiency syn-drome: characterization and treatment with steroids. *J Clin Gastroenterol* 1992;15:284–290.

146. Wilcox CM, Schwartz DA. Endoscopic characterization of idio-pathic esophageal ulceration associated with human immunode-ficiency virus infection. *J Clin Gastroenterol* 1993;16:251–256.

147. Smith PD, Eisner MS, Manischewitz JG, *et al*. Esophageal disease in AIDS is associated with pathologic processes rather than mucosal human immunodeficiency virus type 1. *J Infect Dis* 1993;167:547–552.

148. Wilcox CM, Zaki SR, Coffield LM, *et al*. Evaluation of idio-pathic esophageal ulcer for human immunodeficiency virus. *Mod Pathol* 1995;8:568–572.

149. Kimmel ME, Boylan JJ. Fistulous degeneration of a giant esophageal ulcer in a patient with acquired immunodeficiency syndrome. *Am J Gastroenterol* 1991;86:898–900.

150. Frager D, Kotler DP, Baer J. Idiopathic esophageal ulceration in the acquired immunodeficiency syndrome: radiologic reap-praisal in 10 patients. *Abdom Imaging* 1994;19:2–5.

151. Levine MS, Loercher G, Katzka DA, *et al*. Giant, human immu-nodeficiency virus-related ulcers in the esophagus. *Radiology* 1991;180:323–326.

152. Wilcox CM, Schwartz DA. Comparison of two corticosteroid regimens for the treatment of idiopathic esophageal ulcera-tions associated with HIV infection. *Am J Gastroenterol* 1994;89:2163–2167.

153. Alexander LN, Wilcox CM. A prospective trial of thalidomide for the treatment of HIV-associated idiopathic esophageal ulcers. *AIDS Res Hum Retroviruses* 1997;13:301–304.

40 Caustic Injuries of the Esophagus

Joseph R. Spiegel

Thomas Jefferson University, Philadelphia, PA, USA

Introduction

The Caustic Substances Labeling Act, passed in 1927, was perhaps the first consumer protection legislation. This law was enacted in large part due to the efforts of Chevalier Jackson, who recognized the hazards of caustic ingestion with the increasing prevalence of caustic substances [1]. Lye, used in soap making, was the original offending agent. In 1967, the introduction of liquid drain cleaners with their much higher alkaline concentrations greatly increased the risk of severe injuries secondary to ingestion. Some control of the problem was achieved as manufacturers reduced the concentration of caustic substances in their products in response to reports of injuries and the Poison Prevention Packaging Act and the Hazardous Substances Act of 1970. In some countries, lye has been outlawed, and the number of caustic ingestions has been reduced greatly, resulting in a trend toward a predominance of acid-induced injuries [2]. However, caustic substances remain ubiquitous and available in the United States and throughout most of the world.

Caustic ingestion can result in a range of injuries from a mild oral burn or sore throat to rapidly progressive life-threatening complications. After recovery from the initial injury, esophageal stricture may develop. Reducing the morbidity of these serious injuries depends on accurate early diagnosis, aggressive treatment of life-threatening complications, and attentive, long-term follow-up (Figure 40.1).

Incidence

Most caustic ingestions occur in children. The average age of an injured child is younger than 3 years, and this problem has been reported in neonates [3–5]. It is estimated that there are over 5000 accidental caustic ingestions each year in the United States [6]. There has been a decline in the incidence of caustic injuries in children in the United States, while an increasing incidence has been noted in developing countries such as Turkey and India [7]. In Denmark, the incidence of pediatric caustic ingestion has been measured at 34.6 per 100 000, with esophageal burns in 15.8/ per 100 000 [8]. Children are almost always the innocent victims of experimentation with substances found around the home. Even though traditional caustics, such as lye and drain cleaners, are now sold in child-protective containers, they are often transferred to cups or bottles. Other potential caustics, such as dishwasher detergent, denture cleanser, and small batteries, can be found easily by an adventurous toddler. In some cases, toxic ingestions can be part of a pattern of child abuse or neglect.

Caustic ingestions in adults are less common and are almost always associated with suicide attempts. In one study, 92% of 484 adults with caustic swallowing injuries treated in France were found to have attempted suicide [9]. In Denmark, incidence of caustic ingestion in adults has been measured at 1 per 100 000, with 61% of these representing suicide attempts. The remaining cases were mostly accidental ingestion by alcoholics [10]. In India, corrosive ingestion is a common mode of poisoning [11].

Pathophysiology

Alkali ingestion

The sequence of injury in lye burns of the esophagus was first described by Bosher *et al.* [12]: edema and congestion, principally of the submucosa; inflammation of the submucosa with thrombosis of its vessels; sloughing of the superficial layers; necrosis of the muscularis in varying degrees; organization and fibrosis of the deep layers; and delayed re-epithelialization. Superficial mucosal burns often heal without sequelae. Deeper burns into the muscularis can result in delayed healing with fibrosis. Usually, only

The Esophagus, Fifth Edition. Edited by Joel E. Richter, Donald O. Castell.
© 2012 Blackwell Publishing Ltd. Published 2012 by Blackwell Publishing Ltd.

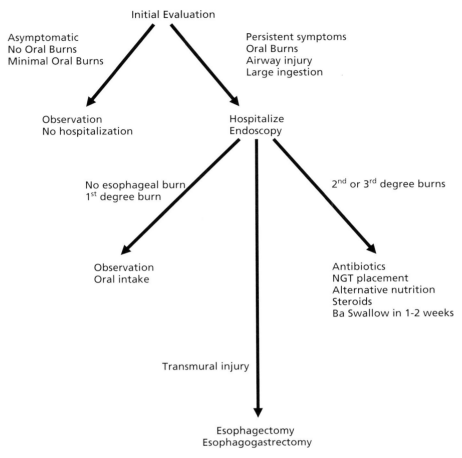

Figure 40.1 Algorithm for care of caustic ingestion. NGT, nasogastric tube.

circumferential burns cause strictures. For as long as 2 weeks, inflammation persists, necrotic tissue sloughs, granulation tissue forms, and new collagen is laid down. Between 3 and 4 weeks after the initial injury, the collagen begins to contract, and thus, the process of cicatrization begins [13]. When the liquefaction necrosis is transmural, esophageal perforation can result with its attendant high morbidity and mortality rates.

A clinical grading system for esophageal burns has been borrowed from the descriptions of thermal injuries of the skin. First-degree esophageal burns have superficial erythema and edema with only minimal tissue sloughing. Second-degree burns involve the muscularis with ulceration, necrosis, and usually some full-thickness mucosal slough. Third-degree burns are transmural with possible extension to extraesophageal structures [14].

The extent of injury is dependent on two factors: the concentration of the corrosive and the duration of exposure. Esophageal stricture has been induced experimentally with as little as a 0.5% NaOH solution (pH 13) and with an 8.8% ammonia solution (pH 12.5) [15]. However, most serious esophageal injuries result from ingestion of substances with

a pH of 14, and the closer the pH is to 14, the more likely the patient is to have an injury requiring treatment [16].

A list of common household products with their corrosive components and concentrations can be found in Table 40.1. Even after safety improvements made in the 1970s, all drain cleaners, oven cleaners, and detergents remain sufficiently concentrated to exert their toxic effects at a pH of 14 if swallowed in granular or solid form [17, 18]. Products with less concentrated alkali, such as Clinitests and denture cleaning tablets, can cause severe esophageal injury because their solid form allows them to lodge in the digestive tract and therefore prolong the duration of action [19]. Aluminum phosphide is a pesticide with increased use in the developing world because it is inexpensive and available in tablet form for easy storage. Its ingestion leads to lethal poisoning in most cases, but there is a high incidence of esophageal injuries in survivors. A recent report described 11 such survivors, 10 with esophageal strictures and one with a transesophageal fistula (TEF) [20]. The most common sites of these injuries are the three natural points of anatomic narrowing in the esophagus: cricopharyngeus, aortic arch, and cardia. Because foreign bodies can lodge at these sites,

Table 40.1 Common alkaline household corrosives (reproduced from Moore [6], with permission).

Type of corrosive	Product	Caustic ingredient
Bleaches	Clorox	Sodium hypochlorite (5.25%)
	Peroxide	Hydrogen peroxide (3%)
	Minute mildew remover	Calcium hypochlorite (48%)
	Tilex Instant mildew remover	Sodium hypochlorite (5%), sodium hydroxide (1%)
Detergents	Oxide laundry detergent	Sodium tripolyphosphate (25–49%)
	Electrasol dishwasher detergent	Sodium tripolyphosphate (20–40%)
	Calgonite dishwasher detergent	Sodium phosphates (<50%)
	Cascade dishwasher detergent	Phosphates (25–50%)
	Comet cleanser	Trisodium phosphate (14.5%)
	Provident powder	Sodium tripolyphosphate (<15%)
Alkalis	Drano (liquid)	Sodium hydroxide (9.5%)
	Drano Professional (liquid)	Sodium hydroxide (32.0%)
	Liquid Plumber	Sodium hydroxide (0.5–2%), sodium hypochlorite (5–10%)
	Dow oven cleaner (liquid)	Sodium hydroxide (4.0%)
	Crystal Drano (granular)	Sodium hydroxide (54.0%)
Thermal alkalis	Clinitest tablets	Sodium hydroxide (223 mg)
	Efferdent extra-strength tablets	Sodium hydroxide (0.5–1%)

Table 40.2 Common acidic household corrosives (reproduced from Moore [6], with permission).

Product	Caustic ingredient
Mister Plumber (liquid)	Sulfuric acid (99.5%)
SnoBol toilet cleaner (liquid)	Hydrochloric acid (15%)
Lysol toilet cleaner (liquid)	Hydrochloric acid (8.5%)
Cost Cutter toilet cleaner (liquid)	Hydrochloric acid (9.55%)
Saniflush toilet cleaner (granular)	Sodium bisulfate (75%)
Vanish toilet cleaner (granular)	Sodium bisulfate (75%)

battery ingestions have been found in children who wear hearing aids [23]. The injury in disk battery ingestion is secondary to both a caustic burn from leakage of alkali from inside the battery and a thermal burn from electrical discharge of the battery before it dissolves [24]. Because the battery lodges in the esophagus as a foreign body, its effects are concentrated and may lead to esophageal perforation or TEF [25, 26].

The liquid bleaches are much less concentrated, but they have also been shown to have the potential to cause esophageal injury in both experimental [27] and clinical settings [28]. It has long been thought that more viscous liquids, such as the liquid drain cleaners, are more dangerous because of their ability to coat the mucosal surface and thus have an increased duration of effect. However, this concept has recently been questioned in a study that found that relative viscosity of offending agents made no difference when their pH was also considered [15]. In recent years, hair relaxants have been involved commonly in caustic ingestions. Hair relaxants are mild alkalis, and although they can cause severe oral burns, they have never been implicated as a source of esophageal or more distal injury [29].

Acid ingestion

Esophageal injuries secondary to acid ingestion have been reported far less commonly than injuries due to alkaline products. The mechanism of injury differs, with a predominance of coagulation necrosis and the rapid formation of a protective eschar in tissues exposed to acid. This delays the progression of necrosis into the deeper tissues [30]. Additionally, most ingested acids have a rapid transit time in the esophagus, further limiting the opportunity for injury.

Table 40.2 lists the household products involved most often in acid ingestions. Sulfuric acid and hydrochloric acid are the most common offenders by far, but gastric injuries secondary to nitric and trichloroacetic acid, potassium and sodium hydroxide, sodium hypochloride, phenol, zinc chloride, mercurial salts, and formaldehyde have all been reported [31]. Even household vinegar has caused injury in young children [2].

substances other than traditional caustics can also lead to corrosive injury. A recent report reviewed nearly 100 pill-induced esophageal injuries [21]. Antibiotics were the most common offenders, but anti-inflammatories, potassium chloride, and quinidine led to a high incidence of secondary complications. There is an increased risk of pill-induced injuries in patients with left atrial enlargement, especially after cardiac surgery [21]. Similarly, there have been many reports of esophageal injury secondary to ingestion of small disk batteries [22]. These batteries are a problem in the pediatric population because they are small, shiny, and non-threatening in appearance. Over one-third of pediatric disk-

Acid injuries have long been thought to relatively spare the esophagus, although they can cause severe gastric injury [32, 33]. However, a study done in India, where acid ingestion is more common, revealed significant esophageal injury in as many as 85% of patients with gastric or duodenal injuries, and almost one-third of these patients went on to develop esophageal stricture [34]. Thus, patients with acid ingestion require the same rigorous assessment and follow-up as patients with caustic alkaline injuries.

Evaluation

History

Establishing an accurate history of the time of ingestion and the nature of the caustic substance is critical. Since these injuries are common in young children, this often involves sending a parent or guardian back to the home to retrieve a sample of the offending agent, ideally including the labeled bottle. An infant may demonstrate the same level of general distress initially whether a mild or severe corrosive was swallowed, so identifying the substance that was swallowed is often the single most important factor in determining the risk of severe injury. Victims of attempted suicide are often uncooperative historians, and family members or authorities who can investigate the scene of the incident must be interviewed.

Signs and symptoms

A wide variety of signs and symptoms are associated with caustic ingestion. Since the earliest investigations, there has been little correlation between the severity of presenting symptoms and the extent of the esophageal injury. As many as 10% of patients with significant esophageal injuries may have no early signs or symptoms [35, 36], while up to 70% of patients with oral and oropharyngeal burns will not have any significant distal lesion [37]. Recently, Riffat and Cheng reported that 12% of 50 children had no oral burns but were found to have esophageal burns on endoscopy [38]. Dogan *et al.* reported finding esophageal injury in 61% of 389 children without oral cavity burns undergoing endoscopy within 48 h of caustic ingestion; most were found to have first-degree burns [39]. However, reviews of pediatric patients alone have shown that there is little risk of subsequent problems in children who do not have symptoms and appear within hours following the ingestion [2, 40]. A review of 167 Italian children presenting after caustic ingestion showed a very low risk of third-degree lesions in patients without any early symptoms and the authors suggested that endoscopy is mandatory only for symptomatic patients [41].

Table 40.3 shows the mild-to-moderate signs and symptoms of caustic injuries categorized by the anatomic site affected. Oral and pharyngeal findings are established easily

Table 40.3 Mild-to-moderate signs and symptoms of caustic ingestion (reproduced from Moore [6], with permission).

Oral/pharyngeal	Laryngeal	Esophageal	Gastric
Pain	Hoarseness	Dysphagia	Abdominal
Odynophagia	Aphonia	Odynophagia	pain
Mucosal ulceration	Stridor	Chest pain	Vomiting
Drooling		Back pain	Hematemesis
Tongue edema			

Table 40.4 Severe signs and symptoms of caustic ingestion.

Airway obstruction	Aspiration	Perforation
Stridor	Cough	Pain
Agitation	Hypoxia	Tachycardia
Cyanosis	Fever	Fever
Hypoxia	Leukocytosis	Leukocytosis
		Shock

by observation and the use of a tongue depressor. Fiberoptic laryngoscopy provides a safe, easy method to complete the laryngeal and pharyngeal examination in almost any setting. Esophageal and gastric examinations must often be repeated to assess findings for signs of complications or long-term sequelae.

Life-threatening complications of airway obstruction, aspiration, or esophagogastric perforation can occur within seconds of the ingestion, or on a delayed basis as inflammation and necrosis progress. Table 40.4 lists the signs and symptoms of the most severe sequelae of caustic ingestions. Death is related to the amount and concentration of caustic substance ingested and has been noted uniformly in patients swallowing more than 6 mL of a concentrated substance, usually alkaline [43].

Endoscopy

Endoscopy is the single most valuable tool in the assessment of caustic trauma of the esophagus. The key is avoiding iatrogenic perforation of the weakened esophageal wall. Fear of endoscopic injury prompted some authors to suggest that endoscopy in patients suspected of having severe burns is contraindicated [34] or that, in children, it be restricted to patients with significant injuries 2 weeks after the ingestion [44]. A review of 115 children evaluated for caustic ingestion in Denmark has suggested that endoscopy is unnecessary in asymptomatic patients [45]. However, even earlier studies showed large numbers of patients who safely underwent diagnostic esophagoscopy for caustic injuries. Daly reported 105 consecutive patients [46] and Yarrington reported 70 consecutive patients [47], all having rigid esophagoscopy. More recently, Di Costanzo *et al.* reported 81 consecutive patients [48] and Rappert *et al.* reported 102 consecutive patients [49] who underwent evaluation for caustic injuries by flexible esophagoscopy, all without complication.

There are two important factors in performing safe esophagoscopy. First, the procedure should be used for diagnosis only. The procedure should be terminated before passing the scope beyond any area of severe or circumferential burn. Second, the endoscopy should be performed within 48 h of the ingestion, while the lumen wall retains its greatest strength. Some authors suggest a more aggressive approach with full esophagogastroscopy in all patients with severe injuries due to the risk of progressively more severe distal lesions that would otherwise be missed [50, 51]. The decision to proceed with endoscopy after encountering a severe circumferential burn must be made by an experienced endoscopist with full regard for the possible risks. With these caveats in mind, esophagoscopy is indicated if the history or any of the signs or symptoms raises the index of suspicion for a distal esophageal injury [52]. Adequate treatment of caustic ingestions in developing countries is often delayed, and a recent review of 40 children seen in Sierra Leone demonstrates the risk of late evaluation and treatment. The mortality rate was 58% for children seen with perforation after initial dilation at a referring hospital and 5.8% in patients undergoing dilation at the tertiary care hospital [53].

Either flexible or rigid instrumentation can be used. Flexible esophagoscopy can usually be accomplished under sedative anesthesia. A flexible, fiberoptic system is required to assess fully the cardia and stomach due to the anatomic narrowing and the need to "turn" the scope. However, it can be difficult to maintain visualization with the flexible scope in the presence of bleeding and necrotic tissue, so rigid instrumentation is sometimes necessary. An experienced endoscopist can often perform full rigid esophagoscopy with sedation alone, but general anesthesia with muscle relaxation is usually required. Endoscopic findings in the evaluation of acute caustic injuries are shown in Table 40.5.

Endoscopic findings are the best predictors of patient outcome. Fifty percent of patients with at least second-degree esophageal burns will go on to develop symptomatic stricture. Recently, a six-point grading system has been proposed to grade esophageal injury in caustic ingestion [54].

Radiology

A chest X-ray is probably the single most important radiographic study in the earliest stages of severe caustic injuries. Chest X-rays can reveal pulmonary infiltrates secondary to aspiration and signs of esophageal perforation (pneumothorax, pneumomediastinum, subcutaneous emphysema).

Contrast swallowing studies appear to be of little use in the early evaluation of caustic esophageal injuries. Findings of

Table 40.5 Endoscopic findings in esophageal burns.

First degree (superficial)	Non-ulcerative esophagitis Mild mucosal erythema and edema
Second degree (transmucosal)	Shallow to deep ulceration with possible extension to muscularis White exudate Severe erythema
Third degree (transmural)	Deep ulceration with possible perforation Dusky or blackened transmural tissue Little remaining mucosa Possible obliteration of lumen

atonic dilatation, intramural contrast dissection, and aperistalsis have been reported in severe injuries and have occasionally been precursors of perforation [55, 56]. However, even though the correlation of positive radiologic findings to endoscopic findings is reasonably high in some studies [57], other authors have found very high false-negative rates [58]. In the evaluation of acute injuries, contrast esophagograms are most useful to rule out and localize perforations. Initial examinations are performed with water-soluble contrast medium due to the risk of extravasation [59]. Once perforation is ruled out, studies with barium can proceed.

Contrast swallowing studies are much more important in the evaluation and treatment planning in the later stages of caustic esophageal injury. As patients with moderate-to-severe injuries are followed, smooth strictures can be noted radiologically as soon as 10 days to 2 weeks after ingestion. Other findings such as diverticulae and aperistaltic segments are not uncommon [52]. Contrast studies can demonstrate functional deficits, such as loss of muscle function or coordination, as well as demonstrate all areas of stricture without the risk of endoscopy [60].

New modalities are being studied to provide additional information about the depth of injury in the early stages. Technetium 99m-labeled sucralfate was used as an indicator of esophageal injury and was found to correlate with endoscopic findings in all cases [61]. Endosonography has also been used to assess depth of injury in the esophageal wall [62].

Treatment

Initial management

All patients who are thought to have suffered a serious caustic ingestion are hospitalized. Intravenous fluids are started, and if hypovolemia is present, central venous access is obtained. Intravenous antibiotics should be given prophylactically in any patient being treated for a presumed caustic ingestion.

Airway injury is not very common in adult caustic ingestions, but it is much more frequent in the pediatric population. Moulin *et al.* found significant laryngeal lesions in 14 of 33 children assessed after caustic ingestions, and seven children required intubation [63]. Obstruction may not be present initially but may develop over 24 h with progressive edema of the tongue and supraglottic larynx. If administered early, intravenous steroids can reduce upper airway swelling. If airway support is necessary, intubation is preferred when adequate visualization is possible. However, "blind" nasotracheal intubation should not be attempted because of the potential presence of necrotic tissue in the upper airway. Emergency tracheotomy is indicated in cases of rapidly progressive upper airway obstruction and when there has been a severe laryngeal burn.

After the patient has been stabilized, esophagoscopy should optimally take place within 24 h and should not be delayed beyond 48 h. Treatment is then determined based on the patient's general condition and the endoscopic findings. No treatment is necessary in patients with first-degree injuries. As soon as they are tolerating oral fluids, patients can be discharged from hospital. A follow-up barium swallow study is performed approximately 3 weeks after the injury. Further study is necessary only if symptoms develop or if the barium study identifies an abnormality. Strictures will rarely, if ever, occur in this group [33, 64].

In more extensive esophageal burns, the risk of severe complications and stricture is higher. Once the patient has been stabilized, there are many therapeutic options that can be considered.

Nutrition

Most clinicians agree that patients who can swallow should be allowed to take oral nutrition after they are stabilized.

Patients who are unable to swallow should receive total parenteral nutrition (TPN) or have a nasogastric (NG) tube placed under endoscopic guidance or undergo gastrostomy. If an NG tube is utilized, it should never be placed blindly due to the risk of perforation. It has been suggested that adequate nutrition alone is the most important factor in promoting healing of an esophageal burn [47].

Steroids

Steroids were originally advocated after they were found to be effective in preventing esophageal stricture in animal models with caustic injury [65–67]. Infectious complications of perforation and pneumonia were encountered, but were overcome by the addition of antibiotics [68, 69]. Subsequently, many clinical reports have supported the use of steroids to prevent the development of secondary esophageal stricture [35, 37, 52, 70, 71]. A review analyzing 13 prior studies (10 retrospective, three prospective) found evidence that steroids can prevent strictures in second- and third-degree burns [72]. Summarizing the findings of the studies that support

steroid use, the following clinical suggestions are noted: steroids are unnecessary in first-degree superficial burns; steroids are not beneficial and potentially dangerous in third-degree severe burns involving perforation or transmural necrosis; steroids should be given early and in high doses (e.g. prednisone 2 mg/kg/day or its equivalent); and steroids should always be given concomitantly with antibiotics. Finally, at least one study suggests that there may be increased effectiveness when steroids are used in conjunction with sucralfate and H_2 blockers [73].

Despite both the scientific logic and the clinical support for steroid use, other reports have questioned the effectiveness of this treatment. Ferguson *et al.* [74] and Kirsh *et al.* [75] found no difference in complication rates. Di Costanzo *et al.* avoided steroid use, advocating "therapeutic nihilism [48]." In this study, 94 patients were treated with supportive care alone, TPN in patients unable to swallow, and oral nutrition in the remaining patients. There were four deaths and five cases of stenosis, four of which required surgery. More recently, Anderson *et al.* reported a prospective study in which steroids were found to have no effect on stricture rates in patients with moderate and severe circumferential burns [76].

Thus, there is contradictory evidence regarding the efficacy of steroid use in caustic ingestions. However, if their use is limited to patients with endoscopically confirmed partial thickness injuries, they can be used safely in most cases and may help prevent late sequelae of the injury.

Stenting

The easiest and simplest stent is an NG tube. The endoscopically placed tube can be used to prevent stricture formation as well as to provide nutrition [77, 78]. A review of 48 children treated acutely for caustic ingestion showed excellent results for grade 2b and 3 lesions stented with an NG tube alone for 1 week [79]. In patients with deep partial thickness or transmural burns without perforation, a wider intraluminal stent can be considered. This practice was first described in animal models [80, 81] and has subsequently been used successfully in both children and adults [82–84]. Silicone-rubber or silastic is used. The stent can be placed endoscopically, but some surgeons routinely position the tube through a gastrostomy. Steroids and antibiotics have been utilized routinely, but a report by Berkovits *et al.* described excellent results using a custom-made, twin-tube silicone-rubber stent without steroids [85]. Stents can also be used in the treatment of refractory secondary strictures [86, 87]. Vandenplas *et al.* reported a 10-year-old child with esophageal stricture after corrosive ingestions who was successfully treated with a biodegradable stent [42].

Dilation

At one time, dilation was considered part of the early therapeutic regimen in caustic ingestions. This practice was abandoned due to the risk of perforation. However, early prophylactic dilation has been shown to reduce the severity of stricture formation in children [88]. Dilation is now utilized as the initial treatment for secondary esophageal strictures. The stenotic segments can often be managed with antegrade dilation. A rigid or mercury-weighted bougie system can be used with or without placement of a guidewire. More recently, both initial and secondary dilations can be accomplished with the balloon technique [89]. When stenotic segments are multiple, extensive, or involve the gastro-esophageal junction, retrograde dilation should be considered. The procedure was first popularized by Tucker [90] in the 1920s and involves having the patient swallow a string that is retrieved through a gastrostomy. Serial dilators are then passed over the string and pulled retrograde into the mouth. This method can now be performed as retrograde balloon dilation [91].

All dilations should be gentle with a goal of slow, progressive improvement. Perforation is a hazard with all manipulations of the stenotic lumen. Steroid and antibiotic treatment is not usually necessary in the secondary treatment of strictures. However, one report did describe an advantage with intralesional steroid injections in conjunction with dilations [92] and a recent double-blinded placebo controlled study showed benefit from intralesional steroid injections in peptic strictures [93]. A retrospective review of 117 patients who underwent balloon dilation for corrosive strictures showed 26% had no recurrence after a single procedure and an additional 20% improved after two to three dilations [94]. A review of 79 adults treated for corrosive esophageal strictures showed equivalent efficacy of bougie and balloon methods, and also that more dilations were necessary in acid-induced than alkali-induced strictures [95]. The complication rate in this series was only 0.56%. There are recent reports of the use of topical mitomycin-C at the time of dilation of caustic strictures, although the number of patients is not sufficient to determine efficacy [96, 97]. There remains a theoretical concern of carcinogenesis with mitomycin-C use, especially in the pediatric population. This will be very difficult to evaluate in the population of patients with caustic injuries who already have a very elevated lifetime risk for esophageal carcinoma.

The development of dysphagia after the initial injury may be due to more than the stricture alone. Dantas and Mamede reported disordered esophageal motility in almost all patients studied 1–53 years after their injury [98]. Other investigative studies, such as esophageal manometry, gastric emptying studies, and pH monitoring, should be considered in these patients.

Surgery

Surgical treatment is divided into emergency procedures to treat esophagogastric necrosis and perforation, and delayed reconstruction. Widespread necrosis with paraesophageal contamination secondary to a third-degree injury is life-threatening due to the rapid onset of mediastinitis, sepsis, tracheobronchial involvement, and shock. Patients with such severe injuries have routinely responded very poorly to conservative therapy, and thus an aggressive surgical philosophy has been adopted in many institutions [99–102]. Gastric necrosis with or without esophageal injury is seen in a high percentage of acid ingestions [103]. Often a laparotomy is indicated to diagnose the extent of the intraabdominal complications. These patients undergo emergency esophagogastrectomy and have reconstruction usually with a colon interposition graft on a delayed basis (at least 4–6 weeks later). Esophagectomy can be accomplished "bluntly," sparing the patient a thoracotomy [102, 104], but the esophagus can be left *in situ* if it is minimally burned [105], and it should not be resected when the trachea is involved. This aggressive approach has greatly reduced mortality and morbidity, and has also yielded acceptable swallowing rehabilitation [10, 74, 90]. A review of patients severely injured by caustic ingestion has shown excellent results utilizing early cervical esophagostomy and feeding jejunostomy, avoiding esophagectomy in most cases [106]. TEFs caused by disc battery ingestion can be considered for primary repair [107].

Reconstruction of the esophagus and pharynx is performed either as a planned second stage after an emergency resection or as an alternative to failed conservative treatment of a secondary stricture. If any swallowing can be preserved with periodic dilation, surgery should be avoided [108]. If esophageal replacement is necessary, the best results are obtained with vascularized grafts from the stomach or bowel. Colon interposition utilizes the right or transverse colon on a mesenteric pedicle. The bowel is passed through a retrosternal tunnel into the neck for esophagocolonic or pharyngocolonic anastomosis [109]. More recently, good functional results were obtained using colopharyngoplasty with a substernal approach in 58 adults requiring total esophageal reconstruction after corrosive ingestion [110]. When the stomach has not been damaged, it can be elongated, passed through the posterior mediastinum, and sutured to the pharynx for total esophageal replacement (a gastric "pull-up" procedure) [111]. This has been a useful reconstructive procedure in children as well as adults [112].

Microvascular free flaps and grafts have been adapted from use in head and neck cancer reconstruction of the pharynx and cervical esophagus. Free jejunal grafts have been utilized successfully in patients with caustic strictures [113]. More recently, use of thin-skin free flaps from the forearm and lateral thigh have provided improved outcomes in pharyngoesophageal reconstruction [114, 115]. Use of these flaps avoids the need for laparotomy. Refinements have allowed free jejunal grafts to be used for total esophageal reconstruction as well [116].

Conclusions

Caustic ingestion continues to be a complex clinical challenge. Even though most severe injuries are caused by lye or other solid alkalis, all caustic products have the potential to do harm. Acid ingestion must be evaluated with the same concern for serious complications. While safety measures have reduced the incidence of these injuries, they remain prevalent in developing countries.

Early diagnostic esophagoscopy is the crucial component of the initial evaluation. Contrast radiography is the mainstay of diagnosis in secondary strictures. The history of caustic ingestion is noteworthy as the risk of subsequent esophageal cancer is predicted to be 1000 times greater than that in the general population [117].

Superficial burns require no treatment and only limited follow-up. Partial thickness injuries are treated with nutritional support and close follow-up. Most clinicians also utilize steroids and antibiotics during the initial treatment interval. Long segments with circumferential burns can be successfully treated with intraluminal stents. Life-threatening perforations and severe, widespread necrosis are best treated by radical surgical resection and delayed reconstruction. Secondary strictures are treated with dilation or pharyngoesophageal reconstruction.

Although there have been important advances in the diagnosis and treatment of caustic injuries, much remains unknown. Even the use of steroids and antibiotics remains controversial. Studies of optimal management of caustic injuries are needed, and further refinements in clinical management should be anticipated.

References

1. Jackson C. Esophageal stenosis following the swallowing of caustic alkalis. *JAMA* 1921;77:22.
2. Nuutinen M, Uhari M, Karvali T, Kouvalainen K. Consequences of caustic ingestions in children. *Act Pediatric* 1994;83:1200–1205.
3. Casasnovas BA, Martinez E, Cives V. A retrospective analysis of ingestion of caustic substances by children. *Eur J Pediatr* 1997;156:410.
4. Kushimo T, Kane MM. Acid ingestion in a 2-day old baby. *W Aft J Med* 1997;16:121.
5. Turan C, Oscan U, Ozokutan BH, Ozdemir M, Okur H, Kuckaydin M. Corrosive injuries of the esophagus in newborns. *Pediatr Surg Int* 2000;16:483–484.
6. Moore WR. Caustic ingestions. *Clin Pediatr* 1986;25:192.
7. Arrival-Silva C, Elisha R, Wohlgelernter J, Elidan J, Gross M. Ingestion of caustic substances: a 15-year experience. *Laryngoscope* 2006;116:1422–1426.
8. Christesen HB. Epidemiology and prevention of caustic ingestion in children. *Acta Paediatr* 1994;83:212.
9. Sarfati E, Gossot D, Assens P, Celeries M. Management of caustic injuries in adults. *Br J Surg* 1987;74:146–148.
10. Christesen HB. Caustic ingestion in adults-epidemiology and prevention. *J Toxicol* 1994;32:557.
11. Zargar SA, Kochhar R, Nagi B, Mehta S, Mehta SK. Ingestion of strong corrosive alkalis: spectrum of injury to upper gastrointestinal tract and natural history. *Am J Gastroenterol* 1992;87:337.
12. Bosher LH, Burford TH, Ackerman L. The pathology of experimentally produced lye burns and strictures of the esophagus. *J Thorac Surg* 1951;21:483.
13. Waggoner LG. Diagnosis and management of chemical burns of the esophagus. *Laryngoscope* 1958;68:1790.
14. Holinger PH, Management of esophageal lesions caused by chemical burns. *Ann Otol Rhinol Laryngol* 1968;77:819.
15. Krey H. On treatment of corrosive lesions in the esophagus: experimental study. *Acta Otolaryngol Suppl* 1952;102:1.
16. Vancura EM, Clinton JE, Ruiz E, Krenzelok EP. Toxicity of alkaline solutions. *Ann Emerg Med* 1980;9:118–122.
17. Kynaston JA, Patrick MK, Shepherd RW, Raivadera PV, Cleghorn GI. The hazards of automatic-dishwasher detergent. *Med J Aust* 1989;151:5–7.
18. Vadarikan BA. Ingestion of dishwasher detergent by children. *Br J Clin Pediatr* 1996;44:35.
19. Burrington JD. Clinitest burns of the esophagus. *Ann Thorac Surg* 1975;20:400.
20. Darbari A, Tandon S, Chaudhary S, Bharadwaj M, Kumar A, Singh GP. Esophageal injuries due to aluminum phosphide tablet poisoning in India. *Asian Cardiovasc Thorac Ann* 2008;16:298–300.
21. Kikendall JW. Pill esophagitis. *J Clin Gastroenterol,* 1999;28:298–305.
22. Litovitz TL. Button battery ingestions: a review of 56 cases. *JAMA* 1983;249:2495.
23. Litovitz TL. Battery ingestions: product accessibility and clinical course. *Pediatrics* 1985;75:469.
24. Yasui T. Hazardous effects due to alkaline button battery ingestion: an experimental study. *Ann Emerg Med* 1986;15:901.
25. Weeks RS, Ravitch MM. The pathology of experimental injury to the cat esophagus by liquid chlorine bleach. *Laryngoscope* 1971;81:1532.
26. Mein JD. Caustic injury from household bleach too [letter]. *J Pediatr* 1986;108:328.
27. Weeks RS, Ravitch MM. The pathology of experimental injury to the cat esophagus by liquid chlorine bleach. *Laryngoscope* 1971;81:1532.
28. Mein JD. Caustic injury from household bleach too [letter]. *J Pediatr* 1986;108:328.
29. Cox AJ 3rd, Eisenbeis JF. Ingestion of caustic hair relaxer: is endoscopy necessary? *Laryngoscope* 1997;107:897.
30. Ashcraft KW, Padula RT. The effect of dilute corrosives on the stomach. *Pediatrics* 1974;53:226.
31. Gray HK, Holmes CL. Pyloric stenosis caused by ingestion of corrosive substances: report of a case. *Surg Clin North Am* 1948;28:1041.
32. Chodak GW Passaro E. Acid ingestion: need for gastric resection. *JAMA* 1978;239:225.
33. Penner GE. Acid ingestion: toxicology and treatment. *Ann Emerg Med* 1980;9:374.

34. Zargar SA, Kochhar R, Nagi B, Mehta S, Mehta SK. Ingestion of corrosive acids. *Gastroenterology* 1989;97:702–707.

35. Crain EF, Gershel JC, Mezey AP. Caustic ingestions: symptoms as predictors of esophageal injury. *Am J Dis Child* 1984;138:863.

36. Ferguson MK, Migliore M, Staszak VM, Little AG. Early evaluation and therapy for caustic esophageal injury. *Am J Surg* 1989;157:116–120.

37. Haller JA, Andrews G, White JJ, Tamer MA, Cleveland WW. Pathophysiology and management of acute corrosive burns of the esophagus: results of treatment in 285 children. *J Pediatr Surg* 1971;6:578–584.

38. Riffat F, Cheng A. Pediatric caustic ingestion: 50 consecutive cases and a review of the literature. *Dis Esophagus* 2009;22:89–94.

39. Dogan Y, Erkan T, Cokugras FC, Kutlu T. Caustic gastroesophageal lesions in childhood: an analysis of 473 cases. *Clin Pediatr* 2006;45:435–438.

40. Clausen JO, Nielsen TL, Fogh A. Admission of Danish hospitals after suspected ingestion of corrosives: a nationwide survey (1984–1988) comprising children aged 0–14 years. *Dan Med Bull* 1994;41:234.

41. Betalli P, Falchetti D, Giuliani S, *et al.* Caustic Ingestion Italian Study Group. Caustic ingestion in children: is endoscopy always indicated? The results of an Italian multicenter observational study. *Gastrointest Endosc* 2008;68:434–439.

42. Vandenplas Y, Hauser B, Devreker T, Urbain D, Renaert H, A biodegradable esophageal stent in the treatment of a corrosive esophageal stenosis in a child. *J Pediatr Gastroenterol Nutr* 2009;49:254–257.

43. Berthet B, Castellani P, Brioche MI, Assadourian R, Gauthier A. Early operation for severe corrosive injury of the upper gastrointestinal tract. *Eur J Surg* 1996;162:951–955.

44. Borja AR, Ransdell HT, Thomas TV, Johnson W. Lye injuries of the esophagus. *J Thorac Cardiovasc Surg* 1969; 57:533–538.

45. Christesen HB. Prediction of complications following unintentional caustic ingestion in children. Is endoscopy always necessary? *Acta Paediatr* 1995;84:1177.

46. Daly JF. Corrosive esophagitis. *Otolaryngol Clin North Am* 1968;1:119.

47. Yarrington C. Steroids, antibiotics and early esophagoscopy in caustic esophageal trauma. *NY State J Med* 1963;2960.

48. Di Costanzo J, Noirclerc M, Jouglard J, *et al.* New therapeutic approach to corrosive burns of the upper gastrointestinal tract. *Gut* 1980;21:370–375.

49. Rappert P, Preier L, Korab W, Nerbauer T. Diagnostic and therapeutic management of esophageal and gastric caustic burns in childhood. *Eur J Pediatr Surg* 1993;3:202.

50. Sellars SL, Spence RAJ. Chemical burns of the oesophagus. *J Laryngol Otol* 1987;101:1211.

51. Thompson J. Corrosive esophageal injuries I. A study of nine cases of concurrent accidental caustic ingestion. *Laryngoscope* 1987;97:1060.

52. Friedman EM, Lovejoy FH. The emergency management of caustic ingestions. *Emerg Med Clin North Am* 1984;2:77.

53. Contini S, Tesfaye M, Picone P, *et al.* Corrosive esophageal injuries in children. A shortlived experience in Sierra Leone. *Int J Pediatric Otolaryngol* 2007;71:1597–1604.

54. Cheng HT, Cheng CL, Lin CH, *et al.* Caustic ingestion in adults: the role of endoscopic classification in predicting outcome. *BMC Gastroenterol* 2008;8:31.

55. Chen YM, Ott DJ, Thompson JN, Gelfand DW. Progressive roentgenographic appearance of caustic esophagitis. *South Med J* 1988;81:724–728.

56. Franken EA. Caustic damage of the gastrointestinal tract: roentgen features. *AJR Am J Radiol* 1973;118:77.

57. Stannard MW. Corrosive esophagitis in children. *Am J Dis Child* 1978;132:596.

58. Mansson I. Diagnosis of acute corrosive lesions of the oesophagus. *J Laryngol Otol* 1978;92:499.

59. Martel WM. Radiologic features of esophagogastritis secondary to extremely caustic agents. *Radiology* 1972;103:31.

60. Ott DJ, Gelfand DW, Wu WC, Chen YM. Radiologic evaluation of dysphagia. *JAMA* 1986;256:2718.

61. Millar AJ, Numanoglu A, Mann M, Marven S, Rode H. Detection of caustic oesophageal injury with technetium 99m-labelled sucralfate. *J Pediatr Surg* 2001:36:262–265.

62. Bernhardt J, Ptok H, Wilhelm L, Ludwig K. Caustic acid burn of the upper gastrointestinal tract: first use of endosonography to evaluate the severity of the injury. *Surg Endosc* 2002;16:1004.

63. Moulin D, Bertrand JM, Buts JP, Nyakabasa M, Otte JB. Upper airway lesions in children after accidental ingestion of caustic substances. *Pediatrics* 1985;106:408.

64. Hawkins DB, Demeter MJ, Barnett TE. Caustic ingestion: controversies in management: a review of 214 cases. *Laryngoscope* 1980;90:98.

65. Floberg LE, Koch H. The effect of cortisone on the scarification in corrosive lesions of the esophagus. *Acta Otolaryngol* 1953;109 (Suppl):33.

66. Rosenberg N, Kunderman PJ, Vroman L, Moolten SE. Prevention of experimental lye strictures of the esophagus by cortisone. *Arch Surg* 1951;63:147.

67. Weisskopf A. Effects of cortisone on experimental lye burn of the esophagus. *Ann Otol Rhinol Laryngol* 1952;61:681.

68. Haller JA, Bachman K. The comparative effect of current therapy on experimental caustic burns of the esophagus. *Pediatrics* 1964;34:236.

69. Rosenberg N, Kunderman PJ, Vroman L, Moolten SE. Prevention of experimental lye strictures of the esophagus by cortisone II. Control of suppurative complications by penicillin. *Arch Surg* 1953;66:593.

70. Campbell GS, Burnett HF, Ransom JM, Williams GD. Treatment of corrosive burns of the esophagus. *Arch Surg* 1977;112:495.

71. Cleveland WW, Chandler JR, Lawson RB. Treatment of caustic burns of the esophagus. *JAMA* 1963;186:182.

72. Howell JM, Dalsey WC, Hartsell FW, Butzin CA. Steroids for the treatment of corrosive esophageal injury. *Am J Emerg Med* 1992;10:421.

73. Reddy AN, Budhraja M. Sucralfate therapy for lye-induced esophagitis. *Am J Gastroenterol* 1988;83:71.

74. Ferguson MK, Migliore M, Staszak VM, Little AG. Early evaluation and therapy for caustic esophageal injury. *Am J Surg* 1989;157:116.

75. Kirsh MM, Peterson A, Brown JW, Orringer MB, Ritter F, Sloan H. Treatment of caustic injuries of the esophagus: a ten-year experience. *Ann Surg* 1978;188:675.

76. Anderson KD, Rouse TM, Randolph JG. A controlled trial of corticosteroids in children with corrosive injury of the esophagus. *N Engl J Med* 1990;323:637.

77. Wijburg FA, Beukers MM, Heymans HS, Bartelsman JF, den Hartog Jager FC. Nasogastric intubation as sole treatment of caustic esophageal lesions. *Ann Otol Rhinol Laryngol* 1985;94:337.

78. Wijburg FA, Heymans HS, Urbanus NA. Caustic esophageal lesions in childhood: prevention of stricture formation. *J Pediatr Surg* 1989;24:171.

79. Gun F, Abbasoglu L, Celik A, Salman ET. Early and late term management in caustic ingestion in children: a 16 year experience. *Acta Chirurgica Belgica* 2007;107:49–52.

80. Fell SC, Denize A, Becker NH, Hurwitt ES. The effect of intraluminal splinting in the prevention of caustic stricture of the esophagus. *J Thorac Cardiovasc Surg* 1966;52:675.

81. Reyes HM, Lin CY, Schlunk FF, Replogle RL. Experimental treatment of corrosive esophageal burns. *J Pediatr Surg* 1974;9:317.

82. Coln D, Chang, JHT. Experience with esophageal stenting for caustic burns in children. *J Pediatr Surg* 1986;21:588.

83. Hill JL, Norberg HP, Smith MD, Young JA, Reyes HM. Clinical technique and success of the esophageal stent to prevent corrosive stenosis. *J Pediatr Surg* 1976;11:443.

84. Mills LJ, Estrera AS, Platt MR. Avoidance of esophageal stricture following severe caustic burns by the use of an intraluminal stent. *Ann Thorac Surg* 1979;28:60.

85. Berkovits RN, Bos CE, Wijburg FA, Holzki J. Caustic injury of the oesophagus. Sixteen years experience, and introduction of a new model oesophageal stent. *J Laryngol Otol* 1996;110:1041.

86. Atabek C, Surer I, Demirbag S, Caliskan B, Ozturk H, Cetinkursun S. Increasing tendency in caustic esophageal burns and long-term polytetrafluorethylene stenting in severe cases: 10 years experience. *J Pediatr Surg* 2007;42:636–640.

87. Vandenplas Y, Hauser B, Devreker T, Urbain D, Reynaert H. A biodegradable esophageal stent in the treatment of a corrosive esophageal stenosis in a child. *J Pediatr Gastoenterol Nutr* 2009;49:254–257.

88. Tiryaki T, Livanelioglu Z, Atayurt H. Early bougienage for relief of stricture formation following caustic esophageal burns. *Pediatr Surg Int* 2005;21;78–80.

89. Weintraub JL, Eubig J. Balloon catheter dilatation of benign esophageal strictures in children. *J Vasc Int Radiol* 2006;17:831–835.

90. Tucker G. Cicatricial stenosis of the esophagus. *Ann Otol Rhinol Laryngol* 1924;33:1180.

91. Oxford LE, Ducic Y. Retrograde dilation of complete cervical esophageal and hypopharyngeal strictures. *J Otolaryngol* 2006;35:327–331.

92. Holder TM, Ashcraft KW, Leape L. The treatment of patients with esophageal strictures by local steroid injections. *J Pediatr Surg* 1969;4:646.

93. Ramage JI Jr, Rumalla A, Baron TH, et al. A prospective, double-blinded, placebo-controlled trial of endoscopic steroid injection for recalcitrant esophageal peptic strictures. *Am J Gastroenterol* 2005;100:2419–2425.

94. Kim JH, Song HY, Kim HC, et al. Corrosive esophageal strictures: long-term effectiveness of balloon dilatation in 117 patients. *J Vasc Int Radiol* 2008;19:736–741.

95. Singhal S, Kar P. Management of acid- and alkali-induced esophageal strictures in 79 adults by endoscopic dilation: 8-years' experience in New Delhi. *Dysphagia* 2007;22:130–134.

96. Rosseneu S, Afzal N, Yerushalmi B, et al. Topical application of mitomycin-C in oesophageal strictures. *J Pediat Gastroenterol Nutr* 2007;44:336–341.

97. Heran MK, Baird R, Blair GK, Skarsgard ED. Topical mitomycin-C for recalcitrant esophageal strictures: a novel endoscopic/fluoroscopic technique for safe endoluminal delivery. *J Pediatr Surg* 2008; 43:815–818.

98. Dantas RO, Mamede RC. Esophageal motility in patients with esophageal caustic injury. *Am J Gastroenterol* 1996;91:2450.

99. Andreoni B, Farina ML, Biffi R, Crosta C. Esophageal perforation and caustic injury: emergency management of caustic ingestion. *Dis Esophagus* 1997;10:95.

100. Estrera A, Taylor W Mills LJ, Platt MR. Corrosive burns of the esophagus and stomach: a recommendation for an aggressive surgical approach. *Ann Thorac Surg* 1986;41:276.

101. Gossot D, Sarfati E, Celerier M. Early blunt esophagectomy in severe caustic burns of the upper digestive tract. *J Thorac Cardiovasc Surg* 1987;94:188.

102. Ray JF, Myers WO, Lawton BR, Lee FY, Wenzel FJ, Sautter RD. The natural history of liquid lye ingestion: rationale for an aggressive surgical approach. *Arch Surg* 1974;109:436.

103. Horvath OP, Olah T, Zentai G. Emergency esophagogastrectomy for treatment of hydrochloric acid injury. *Ann Thorac Surg* 1991;52:98.

104. Hwang TL, Shen-Chen SM, Chen ME Nonthoracotomy esophagectomy for corrosive esophagitis with gastric perforation. *Surg Gynecol Obstet* 1987;164:537.

105. Ribet ME. Esophagogastrectomy for acid injury [letter]. *Ann Thorac Surg* 1992;53:738.

106. Ribet M, Chambon JP, Pruvot FR. Oesophagectomy for severe corrosive injuries: is it always legitimate? *Eur J Cardiothorac Surg* 1990;4:347.

107. Okuyama H, Kubota A, Oue T, Kuroda S, Nara K, Takahashi T, Primary repair of tracheoesophageal fistula secondary to disc battery ingestion: a case report. *J Pediatr Surg* 2004;39:243–244.

108. Braghetto ACI. Surgical management of esophageal strictures. *Hepatogastroenterology* 1992;39:502.

109. Postlethwait RW, Sealy WC, Dillon ML, Young WG. Colon interposition for esophageal substitution. *Ann Thorac Surg* 1971;12: 89.

110. Chirica M, de Chaisemartin C, Goasguen N, et al. Colopharyngoplasty for the treatment of severe pharyngoesophageal caustic injuries. *Ann Surg* 2007;246:721–727.

111. Heimlich HJ. Esophagoplasty with reversed gastric tube. *Am J Surg* 1972;123:80.

112. Ein SH. Gastric tubes in children with caustic esophageal injury: a 32-year review. *J Pediatr Surg* 1998;33:1363–1365.

113. Wang TD, Sun YE, Chen Y. Free jejunal grafts for reconstruction of the pharynx and cervical esophagus. *Ann Otol Rhinol Laryngol* 1986;95:348.

114. Yang J, Tsai F, Chana J, Chuang S, Chang S, Huang W. Use of free thin anterolateral thigh flaps combined with cervicoplasty for reconstruction of postburn anterior cervical contractures. *Plastic Reconstr Surg* 2002;110:39–46.

115. Murray DJ, Novak CB, Neligan PC. Fasciocutaneous free flaps in pharyngolaryngo-oesophageal reconstruction: a critical review of the literature. *J Plast Reconstr Aesthet Surg* 2007;29:1148.

116. Chen H, Chana J, Chang C, Feng G, Ho-Asjoe M, Tang Y. A new method of subcutaneous placement of free jejunal flaps to reconstruct a diversionary conduit for swallowing in com-plicated pharyngoesophageal injury. *Plastic Reconstr Surg* 2003;112:1528–1533.

117. Kochhar R, Sethy P, Kochhar S, Nagi B, Gupta N. Corrosive induced carcinoma of esophagus: report of three patients and review of literature. *J Gastroenterol Hepatol* 2006;21:777–778.

41 Rupture and Perforation of the Esophagus

Harvey Licht and Robert S. Fisher

Temple University School of Medicine, Philadelphia, PA, USA

Introduction

Perforation of the esophagus is a catastrophic event associated with significant morbidity and mortality. There are multiple causes for esophageal perforation (Table 41.1 [1]). The most common cause is iatrogenic, i.e. secondary to instrumentation. The next most frequent etiology is vomiting, given the eponym Boerhaave's syndrome after the physician who first described this entity in 1723. Less common causes of esophageal perforation include trauma, operative injury, caustic injury, and ingestion of foreign bodies.

Several features of the esophagus make it especially susceptible to injury and perforation. First, it is a luminal organ lying within the negative pressure of the intrathoracic cavity. The esophagus may be exposed to abrupt elevations of transmural pressure during episodes of vomiting. This occurs when the esophagus becomes a common chamber with the stomach after relaxation of the lower esophageal sphincter (LES). The resulting pressure gradient between the lumen of the esophagus and the thoracic cavity can be very high, resulting in a tear through the wall of the esophagus. Postemetic perforation, i.e. Boerhaave's syndrome, leads to contamination of the mediastinum with oral and gastric contents. Second, the esophagus, unlike the other organs of the gastrointestinal tract, lacks a serosal layer. This reduces the strength of the wall and means it is less able to contain a perforation. Third, the esophagus and oropharynx are the first parts of the gastrointestinal tract to be exposed to noxious ingested materials that may damage the integrity of the esophageal wall.

Following transmural disruption of the esophagus, there is contamination of the mediastinum with oral secretions, ingested food and liquids, and gastric contents. Gastric acid and digestive enzymes cause a chemical inflammatory reaction within the mediastinum that can become infected and result in necrosis of surrounding tissue including the pleura.

This can lead to infection in the mediastinum or a communication with the pleural space, i.e. esophagopleural fistulae; with abscess formation or an empyema. Pleural effusion may also develop without a direct communication as a sympathetic response to a localized mediastinal inflammatory process. In addition to the serious intrathoracic infection, perforation frequently is associated with systemic infection and sepsis. Although there have been great strides in antibiotic therapy, surgical techniques, and perioperative care, the overall mortality rate for esophageal perforation, even with rapid diagnosis and treatment, is between 15% and 30%. It is dependent on the age and comorbid illnesses of the patient, in addition to the time between the perforation and its recognition and the initiation of treatment. Delayed diagnosis of greater than 24 h increases the likelihood of local and systemic infectious complications and may double the mortality rate to 50–60%.

Etiology: iatrogenic

The most common cause of esophageal perforation is iatrogenic, caused by instrumentation of the esophagus (Table 41.2 [2–16]). It is estimated that iatrogenic perforation associated with a medical procedure is the cause of almost 60% of cases of esophageal perforation. Esophageal intubation has become very frequent, and complications including perforation have increased with the number and types of interventions. Diagnostic endoscopy rarely causes perforation; however, the risk is increased if intubation of the esophagus is difficult. In this instance, the most common site of perforation is in the posterior cervical esophagus where the mucosa is not protected by a muscular layer. Anterior cervical osteophytes or a Zenker's diverticulum can increase the difficulty of passing the endoscope into the esophagus and increase the risk of iatrogenic injury to the cervical esophagus. It is more common for perforations to occur during

The Esophagus, Fifth Edition. Edited by Joel E. Richter, Donald O. Castell.
© 2012 Blackwell Publishing Ltd. Published 2012 by Blackwell Publishing Ltd.

Table 41.1 Causes of esophageal perforation [1].

Iatrogenic (instrumentation)	60%
Postemetic (Boerhaave's syndrome)	15%
Trauma	9%
Operative	2%
Caustic ingestion	<1%
Foreign body ingestion	12%
Infectious	<1%
Pill induced	<1%

Table 41.2 Incidence of iatrogenic esophageal perforation by procedure.

Procedure	Risk of perforation (%)
Endoscopy:	
Diagnostic	0.03 [2, 3]
Variceal sclerosis	1–6 [4, 5]
Variceal banding	0.7
Thermal coagulation	1–2 [6]
Endoscopic ultrasound	0.1 [7]
Esophageal cancer ablation	
Laser, photodynamic, bipolar coagulation	5 [8–10]
Esophageal stent placement	5–25 [11]
Esophageal manometry	Rare
Nasogastric intubation	Rare
Endotracheal intubation	Rare
Dilation:	0.4 [12, 13]
Maloney, Hurst, Savary–Gilliard	0.3 [14]
Through-the-scope (TTS)	2–6 [15, 16]
Pneumatic (for achalasia):	
Brown–McHardy	
Rigiflex	

interventions such as dilation of a stricture or ring or during pneumatic dilation for achalasia. Treatment using thermal energy, such as bipolar coagulation, laser or argon plasma coagulation for bleeding or tissue ablation for cancer can also be complicated by perforation. Variceal sclerosis or banding frequently causes esophageal ulceration. However, progression to perforation is typically only associated with sclerosis. This is due to a necroinflammatory response in the esophageal wall to the sclerosing agent. This may result in a delayed perforation several days to 1 week after variceal sclerosis.

Dilation of strictures

Type of dilator

Dilation of an esophageal stricture is the most frequent cause of perforation. Most, but not all, esophageal strictures are secondary to acid reflux. Dilation is performed to relieve dysphagia. Three types of dilators are available: mercury- or tungsten-filled bougies include Maloney dilators with a tapered end and blunt-ended Hurst dilators. Polyvinyl (Savary–Gilliard) dilators have a central core for passage over a guidewire. The third type of dilator is the "through the scope" (TTS) balloon dilator. The first two types of dilators apply both radial and longitudinal shearing forces on the stricture. In contrast, balloon dilators apply only radial forces. It is not proven that one type of dilator is more effective than another. However, it appears that the guidewire-directed Savary–Gilliard and TTS balloon dilators are safer, especially when treating a complex stricture. Strictures are classified as simple and complex [17]. A simple stricture is concentric, has a diameter larger than 12 mm, and allows passage of the gastroscope beyond the stricture. Complex strictures do not meet these criteria. Complex strictures have a greater risk of perforation when dilated with a Maloney bougie [18]. Risk of perforation is minimized if a guidewire is endoscopically or fluoroscopically passed through the stricture and placed into the stomach, over which a Savary dilator can be passed, or when a TTS balloon dilator is used (Table 41.2).

Technique of dilation

When dilating a fibrotic stricture, the technique is to gradually stretch the stricture rather than abruptly breaking the fibrotic bands. In order to minimize the risk of perforation, early guidelines [17] suggested that a session to dilate a stricture should be limited to the passage of three bougie dilators, each increasing in diameter by 1 mm (3F) after resistance to the passage of a dilator is met ("rule of threes"). However, experience has demonstrated that more aggressive dilation can be effectively and safely carried out with more than three dilators of increasing size at one session when using wire-guided Savary dilators or TTS balloon dilators. Vigorous dilation has been carried out with 2-mm increments until an adequate endpoint of 15 mm is reached [19]. At a diameter of 13–15 mm, most patients experience relief of dysphagia. Perforation complicating dilation of a stricture commonly occurs at the site of the stricture. The rate of perforation is not well established, but is probably less than 0.4% (1 in 250).

In addition to acid reflux causing benign strictures and peptic stenosis (Table 41.3), esophageal narrowing can also be caused by radiation, iatrogenic injection with sclerosing agents, caustic ingestion, and, rarely, infections. Rings and strictures are also found in patients with eosinophilic esophagitis. Other causes of esophageal narrowing include malignant strictures, which can be caused by a primary intrinsic esophageal cancer or by extrinsic compression of the esophagus secondary to malignant adenopathy or mediastinal mass. The risk of perforation complicating dilation of malignant strictures or corrosive strictures is increased compared to strictures of other etiology. Interestingly, radiation therapy does not appear to increase the risk of perforation when dilating a malignant stricture [20].

Table 41.3 Causes of esophageal stenosis.

Acid reflux:
   Stricture (irreversible)
   Peptic stenosis (reversible)
Caustic ingestion
Variceal sclerosis agents
Pill induced
Malignancy:
   Primary
   Extrinsic compression
Radiation therapy
Eosinophilic esophagitis
Rings or webs
Hypertensive lower esophageal sphincter:
   Achalasia
   Primary

Malignant strictures

Endoscopic tumor destruction and stent placement afford treatment for malignant strictures of the esophagus in patients who are not candidates for more conventional treatment, such as surgery, radiation therapy or chemotherapy, or in patients who have failed these treatments or who refuse to undergo these treatments. Similar use of ablative therapy, with and without endoscopic mucosal resection, has also been used for the treatment of early esophageal cancer [21]. Several techniques are available for tumor destruction of advanced cancers, which offer temporary palliation of dysphagia but carry risk of complications, including chest pain, mediastinitis, fever, and frank perforation. Tissue destruction can be achieved with endoscopic laser coagulation, photocoagulation, and bipolar coagulation.

After the lumen is opened to a sufficient diameter by tumor ablation or mechanical dilation, endoscopic placement of a stent can then offer more prolonged palliation of dysphagia. This technique is associated with rates of early perforation during ablative therapy and dilation of 5% and also can be complicated by late perforation secondary to migration of the stent. Late perforation occurs because of the pressure exerted by the expanding stent against the wall of the tumor. The rate of late perforation varies from 20% to 30% [22]. Self-expandable metal stents have replaced rigid stents, allowing placement of the stent into a narrower lumen. This reduces the early risk of perforation that was associated with dilation of the malignant stricture to a diameter large enough to accept the rigid stent. The self-expandable stent is deployed in a tightly coiled shape that bridges the cancer. This allows its placement into a narrower lumen. As it expands within the lumen, the lateral pressure against the tumor enlarges the lumen. Tumor growth into the stented lumen was a frequent cause of recurrent dysphagia, but occurs less often now that stents covered with silicone or plastic have replaced bare metal stents. Dysphagia now is more likely to occur from occlusion of the lumen at the stent orifice by an inflammatory reaction. Thus, perforation of the esophagus can occur during the tumor ablation or dilation that precedes stent placement or as a late complication a few weeks after placement of the expandable stent.

Endoscopic ablative therapy for benign disease

In addition to its palliative use to form a channel within the lumen of an advanced cancer, endoscopic ablative therapy can also be used to try to prevent or treat early cancer associated with Barrett's esophagus. Barrett's esophagus is defined by the presence of columnar epithelium with intestinal metaplasia replacing normal squamous mucosa. Observational studies suggest an annual rate of progression from metaplastic mucosa to adenocarcinoma of 0.5–1%. Usually there is a progression through stages of low-grade to high-grade dysplasia to cancer. Previously, the standard of care was to perform surveillance endoscopy and biopsy to screen for dysplasia, followed by esophagectomy if high-grade dysplasia or early cancer was found. Ablative therapy is now an alternative with the goal of cancer prevention through destruction of metaplastic tissue and replacement with normal squamous mucosa. Used in conjunction with ablative therapy, endoscopic mucosal resection to treat early cancer is an alternative to surgery in patients with intramucosal cancer. Studies are needed to determine if endoscopic ablation of metaplastic and dysplastic mucosa will lower the risk of progression to adenocarcinoma.

If a nodule is found in a field of Barrett's esophagus, there is great concern that this may represent a cancer. Endoscopic mucosal resection can be considered if computed tomography (CT) scan and endoscopic ultrasound demonstrate that the malignancy is limited to the mucosa. This technique provides a large, 2-cm sample of tissue for pathologic review and affords an endoscopic technique to remove early cancer that is limited to the mucosa. Endoscopic mucosal resection is performed with either a cap and internal snare or with a variceal ligation device or multiband ligator with an internal snare device. Saline is injected into the submucosa to raise the mucosa and separate the lesion from the muscular layer. The mucosal lesion is suctioned into the device, forming a pseudo-polyp which is then snared and removed. Hemorrhage and stricture formation are complications of this procedure. The risk of perforation varies from 0% to 9% and is dependent upon the ability to separate the mucosa from the muscular layer [23]. Ablative techniques are used in combination with mucosal resection to destroy the remaining Barrett's epithelium. Aggressive acid suppression is used to reduce reflux and allow re-epithelialization with squamous mucosa with the purpose to reduce future cancer risk that is associated with the metaplastic tissue.

Ablative techniques include those that direct thermal energy to tissue, such as laser, multipolar coagulation, and argon plasma coagulation. A recent review found all techniques are associated with a rare risk of perforation [24]. However, the first two techniques are not commonly used for ablative therapy because of the potential for deeper injury to the wall of the esophagus.

Energy can be applied for thermal tissue destruction using argon plasma coagulation through a stream of ionized argon gas directed endoscopically through a catheter at the diseased tissue. There is no direct tissue contact and depth of injury is limited to 1–3 mm, resulting in only a very small risk of perforation [25–27], Multipolar electrocoagulation applies electrical energy through a probe in direct contact with mucosa to cause tissue dessication. Thermal energy can also be applied using radiofrequency ablation, which transmits energy via an endoscopically placed balloon catheter with closely spaced electrodes. Two delivery systems are available that can either apply circumferential energy or treat a localized segment of the circumference of the involved esophagus. The energy applied is adjusted to produce thermal injury to a limited depth with preservation of the muscular layer, thereby minimizing the risk of perforation [28]. No perforations have been reported in a review of many large series [23] and only one perforation was attributed to radiofrequency ablation in another large review [29].

Photodynamic therapy is another ablative technique that leads to tissue destruction in a different manner [30]. A photosensitizing drug, such as porfirmir, is given intravenously and is absorbed by tissue throughout the body. Then, a light wave of specific wavelength is endoscopically directed, in the presence of oxygen, at the tissue to be ablated. This leads to formation of reactive oxygen species that cause local tissue destruction. There is apoptosis and death of the superficial mucosa, but the collagen layer is spared. Although it is associated with a high rate of stricture formation (20–30%), perforation is rare. Another complication that additionally limits the use of photodynamic therapy is generalized photosensitivity that may persist for 3 months, making it necessary for the patient to avoid exposure to direct sunlight during this time.

Cryotherapy is another endoscopic method used to cause tissue ablation [31, 32]. Extreme cold is applied by spraying liquid nitrogen through a catheter directed at the tissue to be destroyed. Initially, there is tissue destruction by the formation of extracellular crystals that lead to osmotic fluid shifts from within cells, thereby causing cell injury. Crystals can also form within cells, disrupting the cell membranes and leading to cell death. Extreme cooling also results in arterial vasoconstriction and ischemia, and then warming leads to vasodilation and increased vascular permeability. This sequence results in late tissue necrosis. There has been only limited experience with use for tumor destruction and Barrett's ablative therapy. A recent study of efficacy and safety for treatment of Barrett's esophagus noted a 3% stricture rate and no perforations [33].

Achalasia

Dilation of patients with achalasia represents a unique situation. Achalasia is a motor disorder of the esophagus with two features contributing to dysphagia. There is incomplete relaxation of the LES that results in mechanical obstruction to the passage of food into the stomach. Second, there is loss of peristaltic contractions of the body of the esophagus. This reduces the pressure gradient to advance the food bolus across the sphincter, resulting in functional obstruction (pump failure). Endoscopic treatment with pneumatic dilation is an attempt to replicate the surgical technique of myotomy of the LES to relieve the obstruction. In contrast to the incremental and gradual stretching of a benign stricture, the goal of pneumatic dilation in achalasia is to forcefully disrupt the muscle of the LES. Dilation is usually performed with a wire-guided balloon placed under fluoroscopic guidance and performed under fluoroscopic control. The perforation rate varies in the literature but the average rate is 3% to 4% [17]. Common practice is to perform a Gastrografin esophagram immediately after pneumatic dilation to evaluate for perforation. If a perforation is demonstrated and is localized and contained, it can be treated conservatively with nil by mouth, antibiotics, and parenteral nutrition. The patient must be carefully observed, with the help of a surgeon, for evidence of local spread of infection or clinical deterioration. Should either occur, surgery is necessary for drainage and repair of the perforation.

Eosinophilic esophagitis

Eosinophilic esophagitis also deserves special mention. This entity is being recognized with increasing frequency [34]. Symptoms of dysphagia or food impaction typically present in young males. Endoscopic findings of a feline ringed esophagus or longitudinal fissures in the esophagus increase suspicion for the disease and biopsy establishes the diagnosis. Many patients with eosinophilic esophagitis have motor disorders of the esophagus, but the relationship between the two is unknown. Case reports have described mucosal tears during diagnostic endoscopy. The apparent fragility of the mucosa has raised concern that there may be an increased risk of perforation with endoscopy or dilation. Case reports describe chest pain following dilation and suggest that a less aggressive course of dilation is advisable. Dilation is started with smaller dilators and a few and small incremental increases in size of the dilators are done at an individual session. The primary treatment of eosinophilic esophagitis is controversial. A recent retrospective review of a large number of dilations revealed no perforations and long-lasting relief of symptoms of dysphagia was achieved in over 80% of patients [35]. Prospective studies are needed to determine whether primary treatment with a medical regimen or dilation would be most beneficial for relief of symptoms and any benefit should be weighed against the risk of esophageal injury.

Etiology: not iatrogenic

Food impaction

Food impaction is an infrequent cause of esophageal perforation. A history of solid food dysphagia or food bolus impaction suggests an abnormality of the esophagus that may be structural. In addition to eosinophilic esophagitis, food impaction may occur because of narrowing of the esophagus by a stricture, ring or web. This is especially likely to occur in a setting in which food is not chewed well, as can occur in an edentulous person or in a patient with decreased attentiveness, such as an alcoholic. The risk of injury to the mucosa caused by pressure necrosis increases if the food impaction persists for longer than 24 h. This can result in perforation. Perforation can also occur during the endoscopic attempt to remove the food bolus. If the endoscope cannot pass beyond the food impaction, it is impossible to determine the course of the distal esophagus or whether there is an anatomic obstruction. Therefore, an attempt to push the food bolus blindly into the stomach is contraindicated because of the risk of scope trauma to the esophagus distal to the food bolus, which could result in perforation. Passing endoscopic instruments, such as nets or baskets, past the food impaction without direct visualization of the lumen must be done with caution for the same reason.

Foreign body ingestion

Ingestion of foreign bodies can also lead to perforation of the esophagus [36]. This may occur accidentally or purposefully by people desiring to injure themselves. People with psychiatric disease or diminished mental awareness, such as learning disability or alcoholism, are at increased risk for ingestion of foreign bodies. Edentulous people with dental appliances may also be at increased risk because they could swallow a loose appliance accidentally. The risk of injury and perforation is increased when there is ingestion of sharp objects, such as bones, paper clips, glass, needles, nails, and dental bridges. These must be removed emergently. Routine X-rays may not detect fish or chicken bones or some glass objects; therefore, there must be a heightened degree of suspicion in the appropriate clinical setting. When removal of a foreign body is performed with a flexible endoscope, an overtube or foreign body protector hood may be used to reduce risk of injury to the esophagus during extraction. Elective endotracheal intubation may also be done for airway protection. During extraction, the object should be grasped with the sharp point trailing to minimize injury to the esophagus. If the foreign body is in the cervical esophagus, extraction may be more safely and effectively accomplished with a rigid endoscope. Blunt objects, such as coins, are unlikely to cause esophageal injury with perforation. However, a special situation occurs when a disk or button battery is ingested. If the battery becomes impacted in the esophagus, this can lead to liquefaction necrosis resulting in perforation. To prevent this complication, batteries must be extracted urgently from the esophagus.

Medication injury

Injury to the esophagus can also occur from ingestion of prescribed or over-the-counter medications if these becomes lodged in the esophagus. This is more common in people who have a predisposing abnormality of the esophagus that can lead to stasis of pills, such as a motor disorder or a structural narrowing of the lumen. This may result in prolonged contact time of the medication with the mucosa and result in ulceration. This typically causes chest pain or odynophagia and usually resolves spontaneously. However, injury to the esophagus may be deep and result in stricture formation. Perforation is a rare complication documented in individual case reports. There are reports of many medications causing esophageal ulceration (see Chapter 38). The most frequently cited are antibiotics, such as tetracycline and doxycycline. Other medications have been reported to cause esophageal injury, including potassium supplements, quinidine, Aspirin and non-steroidal anti-inflammatory drugs, ferrous sulfate, ascorbic acid, and bisphosphonates, e.g. alendronate and risedronate. [37]. Case reports significantly under-represent the true incidence of pill-induced ulceration of the esophagus. Most patients are not evaluated if the typical history is obtained of developing chest pain after taking a pill without drinking enough fluid or after lying recumbent soon after taking the pill. A prior history of dysphagia is sometimes elicited that would suggest an underlying motor or structural disease of the esophagus.

As mentioned, despite the frequent occurrence of ulceration, perforation is extremely rare. A case was reported of an elderly woman at bed rest after a hip fracture who died from an empyema that complicated the postoperative course. Autopsy revealed an unexpected perforation of the esophagus as the cause of the chest infection. Iron deposits were found in the base of the perforated esophageal ulcer suggesting that oral iron pills were the cause of the perforation. [38]. Another case report described a perforation of an esophageal diverticulum in a patient taking alendronate. It is possible that there was stasis of the pill in the diverticulum leading to ulceration and perforation; however, this is presumptive and not proven [39].

Infectious esophagitis

Infectious esophagitis has a number of etiologies that may rarely lead to esophageal perforation. Only rare cases have been reported in which *Candida* esophagitis has led to severe necrosis and perforation. Affected patients were immunocompromised and presentations were atypical. One case report documented development of *Candida* empyema from an esophagopleural fistula as a complication of *Candida* esophagitis [40] and other cases presented with sepsis syndromes. There are also rare reports of esophageal perforation with herpes. One case report documented a patient with acquired immune deficiency syndrome (AIDS) presenting with a tracheoesophageal fistula. [41]. Although herpes esophagitis usually is found in immunocompromised patients, it infrequently can occur as a self-limited illness in immunocompetent people, and there has been a case report of herpes causing esophageal perforation in an immunocompetent person [42]. Perforation is rare because herpes infection usually causes discrete, small, superficial ulcers in the esophagus. In contrast, cytomegalovirus esophagitis usually causes large ulceration; however, surprisingly, perforation is rare. Cytomegalovirus virtually always occurs in immunocompromised patients

One review of patients with severe necrotizing infectious esophagitis documented an immunocompromised state in 84% of the patients [43]. Most had human immunodeficiency virus (HIV) disease, but others had leukemia or were on immunosuppressant drugs. Of the 25 patients in the series, 11 perforated, eight presented with esophageal fistulae to the trachea or bronchial tree, and six presented with necrosis. *Candida* and herpes accounted for the majority of infections and one patient had cytomegalovirus. Sepsis was the major cause of death in these patients. Unlike the treatment of other causes of perforation in which the esophagus can be repaired with surgical closure, all patients with complications of infectious necrotizing esophagitis required esophagectomy. The overall mortality rate was 48% while the mortality rate in those who did not undergo surgery was 90%.

Caustic ingestion

Caustic ingestion may also cause esophageal injury [44, 45]. The ingestion of alkaline agents is more likely to cause injury to the esophagus than the stomach. The reverse is true for acidic agents. The oropharynx and hypopharynx are also frequently affected by alkaline agents; although injury to these sites from ingestion of liquid alkaline agents may be less severe than injury to the esophagus due to decreased exposure time secondary to rapid swallowing. However, when there is ingestion of alkaline crystals or solids, they can adhere to the oropharyngeal mucosa and cause focal injury and pain that prevents people from swallowing the agent, thereby minimizing esophageal exposure and subsequent injury. Thus, one cannot predict involvement or severity of esophageal injury from the degree of injury affecting the oropharynx. Alkaline ingestion causes liquefactive necrosis of tissue. This leads to cell death, thrombosis of vessels, and edema. The severity of the injury frequently occurs rapidly and is related to the duration of contact with the tissue, the amount of substance ingested, and the pH of

the substance. Other characteristics of the material, such as the concentration of the agent and its ability to penetrate tissue also factor into the severity of the tissue injury.

The severity of the injury and risk of complications are related to the depth of the injury. Endoscopy within the first 24 h following ingestion offers the ability to assess the severity of injury and provides insight into the prognosis. Findings of erythema and edema are indicative of a first-degree burn, which has an excellent prognosis without treatment. A second-degree burn causes ulceration and exudates, and a third-degree burn is defined by transmural involvement with necrosis that may appear as blackened tissue. One series found a perforation rate of 30% with second- or third-degree burns [46]. An additional 20% of those with third-degree burns required emergency esophagectomy. The majority of the other patients with this degree of injury developed strictures. Another series suggested temporary placement of an esophageal stent as an alternative to emergency esophagectomy in those with severe caustic injury [47].

Common alkaline substances that are ingested include drain cleaning products, ammonia-containing cleaners, and some detergents. Household bleach usually does not cause serious injury unless large amounts are ingested because it is a weak base. Injury caused by strong alkaline agents leads to mucosal injury that occurs within seconds and continues for several hours, but sloughing of mucosa typically occurs later within the first week after ingestion. Collagen deposition does not begin until the second week so the strength of the wall of the esophagus is decreased during the first 2–3 weeks after which the risk of perforation decreases. Stricture formation can progress over the next several months.

Acidic caustic ingestion injures the stomach more frequently than the esophagus and can lead to coagulative necrosis which causes dessication of tissue. The major determinant of the severity of the injury and the risk of perforation is the pH of the material. Chemicals that are strong acids with a pH below 3 or alkaline agents with a pH above 12 cause the greatest damage and are associated with the greatest risk of necrosis and perforation. Acidic ingestion can result in the formation of an eschar, which may limit initial exposure of the underlying tissue to the caustic agent. However, in cases with deep injury, a delayed perforation may occur when the eschar detaches after 3–4 days. Common acidic agents that are ingested include toilet bowl cleaning products and car battery fluid.

Trauma

Trauma may also result in esophageal perforation. Penetrating trauma is most easily suspected in the setting of a gun shot or knife stabbing to the chest or neck or from injury related to shattered glass. Penetrating trauma that causes esophageal injury and perforation must not be overlooked when evaluating an acutely ill patient who may also have injury to other vital organs. Perforation of the esophagus is much less likely to occur after blunt trauma. Blunt trauma causing esophageal injury rarely occurs as a complication of rapid speed auto accidents or falls from high elevations [48]. In this setting, injury is usually at the cervical or upper thoracic esophagus and diagnosis is often delayed because of other life-threatening injury. Suspicion for esophageal perforation is usually low and findings such as pneumothorax and pneumomediastinum are often attributed to other injuries that are sustained, such as rib fracture and lung injury, resulting in delayed diagnosis of esophageal perforation. Esophageal perforation may not be diagnosed until sepsis or chest abscess or empyema develops. Diagnosis can be difficult to establish and in the setting of penetrating trauma, gastroscopy has been proposed as the test most likely to definitively demonstrate the esophageal injury [49].

Esophageal perforation is also an infrequent complication of surgery and has been reported after fundoplication for acid reflux and cardiomyotomy for achalasia. In rare cases, it has been reported after other chest surgical procedures, such as aneurysm repair, pneumonectomy, and vagotomy. Rarely, esophageal perforation has been observed after anterior cervical spine surgery and even after intraesophageal echocardiographic monitoring during cardiac surgery. In the latter case, perforation may occur because of prolonged pressure on the esophagus by the ultrasound probe.

Postemetic "spontaneous" rupture

Spontaneous rupture is the second most common cause of esophageal perforation. This may occur after any process associated with a rapid rise in intra-abdominal pressure, such as forceful vomiting or retching. This leads to a sudden increased pressure within the esophagus transmitted from the abdomen across the open LES. If the upper esophageal sphincter does not relax, a closed common chamber is formed, causing the intraluminal esophagus to be exposed to the high intra-abdominal pressure. This causes a high pressure differential across the esophageal wall that may result in rupture. This was initially described in 1723 by Hermann Boerhaave, physician to the admiral of the Dutch navy who developed severe pain after an episode of prolonged vomiting caused by excessive consumption of food and alcohol. He became progressively ill and died. Postmortem exam demonstrated perforation of the esophagus and soilage of the chest. The most common site of postemetic perforation is the left lateral wall of the distal esophagus because of the relative weakness of the wall in this region. This presents as pain in the left chest or left upper abdomen that is quickly followed by shock and sepsis. There also may be pulmonary symptoms with shortness of breath.

Presentation of clinical symptoms

Symptoms and signs of esophageal perforation vary depending on the site of perforation. As noted, spontaneous esophageal rupture caused by vomiting usually occurs at the distal left wall of the esophagus and causes profound and immediate pain in the left chest or upper abdomen. Contamination of the mediastinum occurs immediately and the patient is usually in acute distress with shock and sepsis when seen in the emergency room. Perforation complicating iatrogenic dilation usually occurs at or just proximal to the obstruction being dilated and may present as left- or right-sided chest pain. In a similar fashion, perforation of the cervical esophagus will present with neck pain. The triad of pain, fever, and mediastinal or subcutaneous air is classic, but is not always present with esophageal perforation. Pain is typically acute in onset with spontaneous rupture; although it is sometimes delayed with iatrogenic perforation. Fever usually develops following pain, but may be delayed for hours or longer after perforation and corresponds to the onset of sepsis, mediastinitis, empyema or abscess formation. On physical examination the finding of a pleural effusion can represent a sympathetic effusion or an infected pleural space. Crepitus on palpation of the neck or chest or a crunching sound with systole on cardiac auscultation (Hamman's sign) are uncommon, but suggest the presence of mediastinal air. Any unexpected symptom, such as pain, fever or pulmonary complaints, following a procedure involving the esophagus should raise the concern for esophageal perforation.

Evaluation for perforation

Investigation for the suspicion of esophageal perforation should include radiologic evaluation. An upright X-ray of the chest can be diagnostic when it reveals subcutaneous emphysema or pneumomediastinum (Figure 41.1) or pneumohydrothorax. Although non-specific, other findings that could suggest esophageal perforation include pleural effusion or pulmonary infiltrate. Thoracentesis supports the diagnosis of perforation if the pH of the fluid is less than 2, if food particles are found, or if the pleural fluid amylase is significantly elevated. The latter occurs from salivary amylase leaking through the perforation. These findings would indicate the presence of an esophagopleural fistula. The chest X-ray can be normal soon after perforation. Air in the mediastinum and effusions may take several hours to manifest. Contrast studies are performed if there is a suspicion of perforation. Water-soluble Gastrografin is used instead of barium if there is concern for leakage into the mediastinum because of the inflammatory response caused by barium [50]. However, if Gastrografin does not document a suspected perforation, then barium is used because its better coating of the esophageal wall results in a greater likelihood of documenting the tear (Figure 41.2). CT scan of the chest or neck is more sensitive than a regular chest X-ray or contrast esophagram for demonstrating extraluminal air

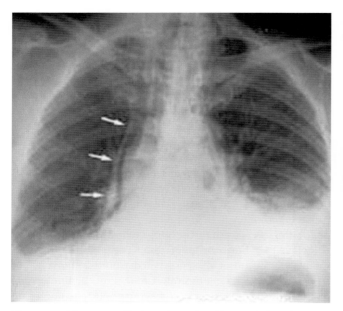

Figure 41.1 Pneumomediastinum (reproduced by permission of Elsevier).

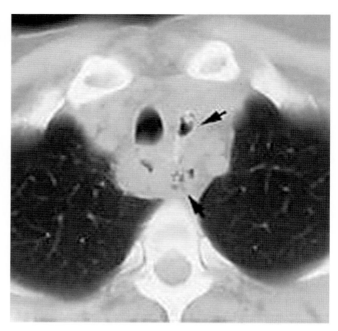

Figure 41.3 CT scan revealing pneumomediastinum secondary to esophageal perforation (reproduced by permission of Elsevier).

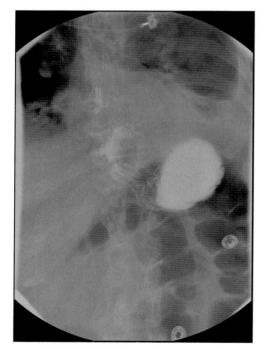

Figure 41.2 Contrast extravasation.

[51, 52]. In addition, it might demonstrate extravasation through the perforation, fistulization, and evidence of abscess in the chest or neck (Figure 41.3).

Early diagnosis is critical to decreasing the morbidity and mortality associated with esophageal perforation. Mediastinal

contamination with gastric and oral contents frequently leads to widespread infection of the mediastinum that in turn may lead to abscess and sepsis, which carry a high mortality. The absence of a serosal layer of the esophageal wall in addition to the loose tissue planes of the mediastinum result in spread of infection throughout the mediastinum. In contrast, perforation of the cervical esophagus is more likely to remain a localized infection because of the compartmentalization in the neck and the attachment of the esophagus to the prevertebral fascia.

Management of perforation

The management of esophageal perforation most frequently requires surgery [53]. Drainage of infection is necessary, and repair of the perforation is desirable and should be done if possible. However, when closure of a perforation is performed in an infected field, this may result in wound dehiscence at the repaired site. Therefore, in patients with intra-abdominal or thoracic perforation with severe infection and soilage of the surgical field, esophageal diversion with future repair or esophagectomy are considered instead of primary closure. The decision by a knowledgeable and experienced surgeon determines which surgery is appropriate for the patient. Morbidity and mortality increase dramatically with delay in diagnosis. The mortality after rapid diagnosis of an iatrogenic perforation is approximately 20%

but increases to greater than 35% after spontaneous or postemetic perforation. This may be attributable to contamination of the mediastinum and pleural space by food and gastric contents in the postemetic perforation as compared to soilage from an empty stomach in the patient who has not eaten in preparation for a procedure. When diagnosis is delayed for longer than 1 day the mortality is increased almost two-fold.

If CT scan or X-ray contrast studies demonstrate a small and well-contained perforation with a small amount of extravasation and the patient is stable and not septic, medical management can be initiated with careful observation [54–56]. This would include a regimen of esophageal rest with nil by mouth, broad-spectrum antibiotics, and parenteral nutrition. If the patient demonstrates clinical deterioration or failure to improve or if there is radiologic evidence of spread of the infection or abscess formation, then surgery becomes imperative. If there is an adequate clinical response, the patient can be followed with contrast studies. When closure of the tear is demonstrated with no extravasation of contrast on follow-up X-ray study, clear liquids by mouth can be started. Sometimes there may be an extended period of time over which extravasation into a contiguous and contained cavity persists, but if contrast flows back into the esophagus freely and the patient is clinically responding to treatment, clear liquids can be started in this situation also. Medical management of esophageal tears may be successful and small tears may seal without surgical intervention in up to 75% of cases within 1–2 weeks, although it may take longer. Tears in the cervical esophagus also may be successfully treated with medical management unless the infection is not contained or an abscess develops.

In the unique situation when there is rapid recognition of a perforation complicating pneumatic dilation of achalasia, if there is no significant soilage, the tear is closed and a definitive surgical procedure done with myotomy of the wall opposite the site of perforation, accompanied by a partial fundoplication. It is always important to relieve a distal obstruction during surgical closure of a perforation to reduce the risk of postoperative leakage at the closure site.

Conclusions

Esophageal perforation continues to present challenges in diagnosis and treatment. Morbidity and mortality are reduced by rapid recognition of this complication and urgent treatment that should be coordinated between the gastroenterologist, radiologist, and surgeon. Early involvement from the time of initial consideration of the diagnosis of perforation with a multidisciplinary approach between these specialists aids in diagnostic and therapeutic decision-making, which should help to improve patient outcome. The level of suspicion must remain high if any unexpected symptoms develop after a procedure involving the esophagus or in the settings discussed above.

References

1. Brinster C, Singhal S, Lee L, *et al.* Evolving options in the management of esophageal perforation. *Ann Thorac Surg* 2004; 77:1475–1483.
2. Dawson J, Cockel R. Oesophageal perforation at fiberoptic gastroscopy. *BMJ* 1981;283:583.
3. Katz D. Morbidity and mortality in standard and flexible gastrointestinal endoscopy. *Gastrointest Endosc* 1967;14:134.
4. Clouse T, Takriti M, Gordon WH, Just-Viera JO. Surgical repair of esophageal perforation in cirrhotic patients with varices. *Chest* 1994;105:1896.
5. Lee J, Lieberman D. Complications related to endoscopic hemostasis techniques. *Gastrointest Endosc Clin North Am* 1996;6:305.
6. Fleischer D. Therapy for gastrointestinal bleeding. In: Geenen J, Fleischer D, Waye J, eds. *Techniques in Therapeutic Endoscopy*, 2nd edn. New York: Gower Medical Publishing, 1992, p. 25.
7. ASGE Technical Assessment Committee. *Status Evaluation: Endoscopic Ultrasound.* Chicago: American Society for Gastrointestinal Endoscopy, 1991.
8. Ell C, Riemann J, Lux G, *et al.* Palliative laser treatment of malignant stenoses in the upper gastrointestinal tract. *Endoscopy* 1986;18 (Suppl 1):21.
9. Lightdale C, *et al.* A multi-center phase III trial of photodynamic therapy versus Nd YAG laser in the treatment of malignant dysphagia. *Gastrointest Endosc* 1993;39:283A.
10. Johnston J, Fleischer D, Pertrini J, *et al.* Palliative bipolar electrocoagulation of obstructing esophageal cancer. *Gastrointest Endosc* 1987;33:349.
11. Tytgat G, den Hartos Jager F, Bartelman J. Endoscopic prosthesis for advanced esophageal cancer. *Endoscopy* 1986;18 (Suppl 3):32.
12. Cox J, Bennett J. Benign esophageal strictures. In: Bennett J, Hunt R, eds. *Therapeutic Endoscopy and Radiology of the Gut*, 2nd edn. Baltimore; Williams & Wilkins, 1990, p. 11.
13. Silvis S, Nebel O, Rogers G, Sugawa C, Mandelstam P. Endoscopic complications: results of the 1974 American Society for Gastrointestinal Endoscopy survey. *JAMA* 1976;235:928.
14. Kozarek R. Hydrostatic balloon dilatation of gastrointestinal stenoses; a national survey. *Gastrointest Endosc* 1986;23:15.
15. White R, Morris D. Diagnosis and management of esophageal perforations. *Am Surg* 1992;58:112.
16. Nair L, Reynolds JC, Parkman HP, *et al.* Complications during pneumatic dilatation for achalasia or diffuse esophageal spasm: analysis of risk factors, early clinical characteristics, and outcome. *Dig Dis Sci* 1993;38:1893.
17. American Society of Gastrointestinal Endoscopy Guideline—Esophageal dilation. *Gastrointest Endosc* 2006;63:755–760.
18. Hernandez LJ, Jacobson JW, Harris MS. Comparison among the perforation rates of Maloney, balloon and Savary dilation of esophageal strictures. *Gastrointest Endosc* 2000;51:460–462.
19. Kozarek RA, Patterson DJ, Ball TJ, *et al.* Esophageal dilation can be done safely using selective fluoroscopy and single dilating sessions. *J Clin Gastroenterol* 1995;20:184–188.

20. American Society of Gastrointestinal Endoscopy Guideline—Complications of upper GI endoscopy. *Gastrointest Endosc* 2002;55:784–793.

21. Das A, Singh V, Fleischer D, *et al*. A comparison of endoscopic treatment and surgery in early esophageal cancer: an analysis of surveillance epidemiology and end results data. *Am J Gastroenterol* 2008;103:1340–1345.

22. Schembre D. Recent advances in the use of stents for esophageal disease. *Gastrointest Endosc Clin North Am* 2010;20:103–121.

23. Wolfsen H. Endoluminal therapy for Barrett's Esophagus. *Gastrointest Endosc Clin North Am* 2007;17:59–82.

24. Wani S, Sayara H, Sharma P. Endoscopic eradication of Barrett's esophagus. *Gastrointest Endosc* 2010;71:147–166.

25. Dulai G, Jensen D, Cortina G, *et al*. Randomized trial of argon plasma coagulation vs. multipolar electrocoagulation for ablation of Barrett's esophagus. *Gastrointest Endosc* 2005;61:232–240.

26. Yeh R, Triadafilopoulos G. Endoscopic therapy for Barrett's esophagus. *Gastrointest Endosc Clin North Am* 2005;15:377–397.

27. Sampliner R. Endoscopic ablative therapy for Barrett's esophagus: current status. *Gastrointest Endosc* 2004;59:66–69.

28. vanVilsteren F. Endoscopic therapy using radiofrequency ablation for esophageal dysplasia and cancer in Barrett's esophagus. *Gastrointest Endosc Clin North Am* 2010;20:55–74.

29. Rees JRE, Lao-Siriex P, Wong A, Fitzgerald RC. Treatment for Barrett's esophagus. *Cochrane Database Syst Rev* 2010;(1):CD004060.

30. Gross S, Wolfsen H. The role of photodynamic therapy in the esophagus. *Gastrointest Endosc Clin N Am* 2010;20:35–53.

31. Helsey K, Greenwald B. Cryotherapy in the management of esophageal dysplasia and malignancy. *Gastrointest Endosc Clin North Am* 2010;20:75–87.

32. Dumot J, Vargo J, Falk G, *et al*. An open-label, prospective trial of cryospray ablation for Barrett's esophagus high grade dysplasia and early esophageal cancer in high risk patients. *Gastrointest Endosc* 2009;70:635–644.

33. Shaheen N, Greenwald B, Peery A, *et al*. Safety and efficacy of endoscopic spray cryotherapy for Barrett's esophagus with high grade dysplasia. *Gastrointest Endosc* 2010;71:680–685.

34. Atkins D, Kramer R, Capocelli K, *et al*. Eosinophilic esophagitis: the newest esophageal inflammatory disease. *Nat Rev Gastroenterol Hepatol* 2009;6:267–278.

35. Dellon E, Gibbs W, Rubinas T, *et al*. Esophageal dilation in eosinophilic esophagitis: safety and predictors of complications. *Gastrointest Endosc* 2010;71:706–712.

36. American Society of Gastrointestinal Endoscopy Guideline for the management of ingested foreign bodies. *Gastrointest Endosc* 2002;55:802–806.

37. Kikendall JW. Pill induced esophageal injury. *Gastroenterol Clin North Am* 1991;20:835–846.

38. Patel J, Sahota O, Kaye P. Fatal esophageal perforation caused by oral iron. *Scand J Gastroenterol* letter to the editor 2/17/2010 on line.

39. Famulano G, DeSimone C. Fatal esophageal perforation with alendronate. *Am J Gastroenterol* 2001;96:3212–3213.

40. Al-Shawwa B, D'Andrea L, Quintero D. Candida esophageal perforation and esophagopleural fistula: a case report. *J Med Case Rep* 2008;2:209–211.

41. Cirillo N, Lyon D, Schuller A. Tracheoesophageal fistula complicating herpes esophagitis in AIDS. *Am J Gastroenterol* 2008;88:587–589.

42. Cronstedt J, Bouchama A, Hainau B. Spontaneous esophageal perforation in herpes simplex esophagitis. *Am J Gastroenterol* 2008;87:124–127.

43. Gaissart H, Roper C, Patterson G, *et al*. Infectious Necrotizing Esophagitis: outcome after medical and surgical interventions. *Ann Thorac Surg* 2003;75:342–347.

44. Ramasany K, Gumaste V. Corrosive ingestion in adults. *J Clin Gastroenterol* 2003;37:119–124.

45. Salzman M, O'Malley R. Update on the evaluation and management of caustic ingestion. *Emerg Med Clin North Am* 2007;25:459–476.

46. Kirsh M, Peterson A, Brown J, *et al*. Treatment of caustic injuries of the esophagus: a ten year experience. *Ann Surg* 1978;188:675–678.

47. Zwischenberger J, Savage C, Bidani A. Surgical aspects of esophageal disease: perforation and caustic injury. *Am J Respir Crit Care Med* 2002;165:1037–1040.

48. Beal S, Pottmeyer E, Spisso J. Esophageal perforation following external blunt trauma. *J Trauma* 1998;28:1425–1432.

49. Horwitz B, Krevsky B, Buckman Jr R, *et al*. Endoscopic evaluation of penetrating esophageal injuries. *Am J Gastroenterol* 1993;88:1249–1253.

50. Richter J, Castell D. Balloon dilatation for the treatment of achalasia. In: Bennett J, Hunt R, eds. *Therapeutic Endoscopy and Radiology of the Gut*, 2nd edn. Baltimore: Williams & Wilkins, 1990, p. 82.

51. Bladergroen M, Lowe J, Posthelwaite R. Diagnosis and recommended management of esophageal perforation and rupture. *Ann Thorac Surg* 1986;42:235.

52. Kim-Deobald J, Kozarek R. Esophageal perforation: an 8-year review of a multispecialty clinic's experience. *Am J Gastroenterol* 1992;87:1112.

53. Brinster C, Singhal S, Lee L, *et al*. Evolving options in the management of esophageal perforation. *Ann Thorac Surg* 2004;77:1475–1483.

54. Cameron J, Kieffer R, Hendrix T, *et al*. Selective nonoperative management of contained intrathoracic esophageal disruptions. *Ann Thorac Surg* 1979;27:404–408.

55. Shaffer H, Valenzuela G, Mittal R. Esophageal perforation. A reassessment of the criteria for choosing medical or surgical therapy. *Arch Intern Med* 1992;152:757.

56. Altorjay A, Kiss J, Voros A, *et al*. Non-operative management of esophageal perforations. Is it justified? *Ann Surg* 1997;225:415.

42 Cutaneous Diseases and the Esophagus

Pamela A. Morganroth,[1,2] **Victoria P. Werth**[1,2] **and David A. Katzka**[3]

[1]Philadelphia VA Medical Center, Philadelphia, PA, USA
[2]Department of Dermatology, University of Pennsylvania School of Medicine, Philadelphia, PA, USA
[3]Department of Gastroenterology, University of Pennsylvania School of Medicine, Philadelphia, PA, USA

Introduction

As the skin and the esophagus are both lined by stratified squamous epithelium, it is not surprising that many diseases have pathologic manifestations in both organs. Most diseases affecting both the skin and the esophagus fall into the following categories: connective tissue diseases, bullous diseases, infectious diseases, and malignancy or malignancy-associated diseases. There are also several miscellaneous acquired diseases and inherited syndromes that do not fit into the above categories but are still worthy of mention. This chapter summarizes the main cutaneous findings and the range of esophageal pathology that can be seen in diseases with involvement of both the skin and the esophagus. It is important for both dermatologists and gastroenterologists to be aware of the multidisciplinary characteristics of these diseases to enable early diagnosis, appropriate referrals, and improved patient care. Table 42.1 lists the classic skin findings of the diseases discussed in this chapter.

Connective tissue diseases

Scleroderma

Scleroderma (systemic sclerosis) is a connective tissue disease that affects the skin as well as many internal organs, including the esophagus, lungs, heart, and kidney. The pathogenesis of scleroderma involves vasculopathy, activation of the immune system, and excessive fibrosis [1]. Scleroderma is divided into two categories, which are named to reflect the degree of skin involvement. In limited cutaneous scleroderma, cutaneous fibrosis is limited predominantly to the face, hands, and arms (distal to the elbows) [2]. Raynaud's phenomenon develops long before symptoms of fibrosis, and approximately 70% of patients have anticentromere antibodies [3]. Limited cutaneous scleroderma was

formerly entitled CREST (calcinosis cutis, Raynaud's syndrome, esophageal dysmotility, sclerodactyly, and telangiectasia) syndrome, but this acronym has fallen out of favor. Diffuse cutaneous scleroderma is a rapidly progressive disease characterized by more widespread skin fibrosis and increased internal organ involvement. Onset of Raynaud's phenomenon is typically concurrent with onset of symptomatic skin fibrosis [4]. Patients with severe disease of the internal organs and skin tend to develop the severe disease within the first 3 years after scleroderma onset and have a high mortality rate [5]. Those who do not develop severe organ involvement in the first few years have a reduced chance of developing such disease in subsequent years and have a much higher survival rate [5]. Approximately 30% of patients with diffuse cutaneous scleroderma have antibodies to topoisomerase I (Scl 70) [3].

The hallmark cutaneous manifestation of scleroderma is thick, hardened skin that feels tight due to decreased elasticity, but edema and erythema may be present in early lesions. Cutaneous involvement typically begins in the fingers (sclerodactyly; Figure 42.1), hands, and face (microstomy, beak-like nose, facial stiffening), but patients with diffuse cutaneous sclerosis have extension of skin disease to the proximal limbs and trunk [2, 4]. Other characteristic skin findings include: calcinosis cutis (firm nodules, typically located over joints), dilation and drop out of nailfold capillaries, digital ulcers (due to local ischemia and vascular insufficiency), salt-and-pepper pigmentation (areas of skin hyper- and hypo-pigmentation), and telangiectasias [4]. Telangiectasias are commonly found on the face, hands, trunk, and lips, but may rarely also be seen on the esophagus, stomach, small intestines, colon, and larynx [6, 7].

Esophageal dysmotility occurs in approximately 60–80% of both limited cutaneous and diffuse cutaneous scleroderma patients [3]. Patients with esophageal dysmotility may complain of dysphagia, but many patients with less severe esophageal dysfunction are asymptomatic [8].

The Esophagus, Fifth Edition. Edited by Joel E. Richter, Donald O. Castell.
© 2012 Blackwell Publishing Ltd. Published 2012 by Blackwell Publishing Ltd.

Table 42.1 Classic skin findings of diseases with cutaneous and esophageal involvement.

Disease	Category	Classic skin findings
Scleroderma	Connective tissue disease	Thick and hardened skin on the hands and face, microstomy, sclerodactyly
Dermatomyositis	Connective tissue disease	Gottron's papules, heliotrope rash
Mixed connective tissue disease	Connective tissue disease	Skin findings of lupus erythematosus, dermatomyositis, or scleroderma
Systemic lupus erythematosus	Connective tissue disease	Malar erythema, oral ulcers
Pemphigus vulgaris	Bullous	Flaccid blisters or erosions on skin, erosions on oral mucosa
Paraneoplastic pemphigus	Bullous	Painful erosions and crusting on oral mucosa and lips
Mucous membrane pemphigoid	Bullous	Painful oral cavity erosions, conjunctivitis
Epidermolysis bullosa acquisita	Bullous	Trauma-induced bullae and erosions (typically acral)
Dystrophic epidermolysis bullosa	Bullous	Trauma-induced bullae and erosions (acral or generalized)
Stevens–Johnson syndrome and toxic epidermal necrolysis	Bullous	Erosions and crusting on oral mucosa and lips, full-thickness skin detachment, macular or atypical target lesions on skin
Herpes simplex virus	Infectious	Vesicles or erosions on an erythematous base
Candidiasis	Infectious	White patches on tongue and oral mucosa; erythematous, hyperkeratotic plaques on skin
Melanoma	Malignancy	Changing macular brown lesion with variegate pigmentation and asymmetric borders
Cutaneous T-cell lymphoma	Malignancy	Slow progression (years) from patches to plaques to tumors; initial lesions on buttocks and other sun-shielded areas
Kaposi's sarcoma	Malignancy	Red or violaceous papular lesions concentrated on lower extremities, head, and neck
Acanthosis nigricans	Malignancy associated	Symmetrical, hyperpigmented, velvety plaques on intertriginous areas and the neck
Plummer–Vinson syndrome (Paterson–Brown–Kelly syndrome, sideropenic dysphagia)	Malignancy associated	Angular cheilitis, atrophic glossitis, koilonychia
Bazex syndrome (acrokeratosis paraneoplastica)	Malignancy associated	Erythematous or violaceous hyperkeratotic lesions which begin in acral areas
Palmoplantar keratoderma, tylosis, Howel–Evans syndrome	Malignancy associated	Hyperkeratosis of palms and soles
Cowden syndrome (multiple hamartoma syndrome)	Malignancy associated	Oral fibromas, facial trichilemmomas, acral and palmoplantar keratoses
Dyskeratosis congenita (Zinsser–Engman–Cole syndrome)	Malignancy associated	Reticular hyperpigmentation of skin, oral leukoplakia, nail dystrophy
Lichen planus	Miscellaneous acquired	Pruritic, violaceous, polygonal plaques on flexor surfaces of skin
Behcet's disease	Miscellaneous acquired	Recurrent oral ulcers, recurrent genital ulcers, papulopustular skin lesions, erythema nodosum
Nephrogenic systemic fibrosis	Miscellaneous acquired	Symmetric fibrotic plaques on extremities and trunk
Ehlers–Danlos syndrome	Miscellaneous syndrome	Soft, velvety, hyperextensible skin; cigarette-paper scars; thin skin with visible underlying vessels; bruises
Hereditary hemorrhagic telangiectasia (Osler–Weber–Rendu syndrome)	Miscellaneous syndrome	Telangiectasias on skin and oral mucosa
Focal dermal hypoplasia (Goltz syndrome, Goltz–Gorlin syndrome)	Miscellaneous syndrome	Linear atrophic lesions following the lines of Blashko, papillomas at junctions between skin and mucosa

Scleroderma affects the lower two-thirds of the esophagus, resulting in decreased or absent peristalsis and relaxation of the lower esophageal sphincter. This puts scleroderma patients at high risk for gastroesophageal reflex disease (GERD) and the sequelae of chronic acid reflux, such as esophagitis, stricture formation, Barrett's esophagus, and esophageal adenocarcinoma [8–13]. Scleroderma patients with esophageal dysmotility may also develop *Candida* esophagitis (due to esophageal stasis, acid suppression, or immunosuppressive medications) and pill-induced esophagitis (if taking drugs with the potential to irritate the esophageal mucosa, such as doxycycline, tetracyclines,

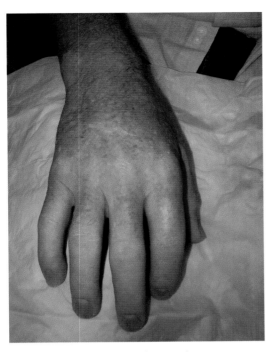

Figure 42.1 Sclerodactyly in a scleroderma patient.

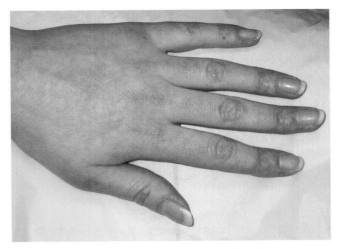

Figure 42.2 Gottron's papules in a dermatomyositis patient.

non-steroidal anti-inflammatory drugs, bisphosphonates, and potassium chloride) [14–16]. Behavioral modifications and medical therapy (mainly with high-dose proton pump inhibitors) are the primary treatments for GERD in scleroderma patients [17, 18]. Surgical interventions may be useful in patients with severe refractory GERD, but fundoplication is generally less successful in scleroderma patients than in those with idiopathic GERD [17, 19]. Roux-en-Y gastric bypass may be a more effective surgical option than fundoplication for scleroderma patients with refractory GERD [19].

Dermatomyositis

Dermatomyositis is defined by a set of hallmark cutaneous manifestations, including Gottron's papules and the heliotrope rash. The extent of muscle disease in dermatomyositis is highly variable and ranges from no evidence of muscle involvement to profound weakness requiring hospitalization. Striated muscles in various organs and organ systems may be involved, including respiratory muscles (chest wall and diaphragm), esophagus (upper one-third), and heart (myocarditis) [20–23]. Patients with muscle weakness (generally proximal and symmetric) and objective evidence of skeletal muscle disease are classified as classic dermatomyositis, whereas those with no clinically significant muscle disease are termed clinically amyopathic dermatomyositis. Objective measures of muscle disease include muscle enzymes (creatine kinase and aldolase), magnetic resonance

imaging, electromyography, and muscle biopsy. Both classic and clinically amyopathic dermatomyositis may be associated with interstitial lung disease and with underlying malignancy, and patients should be screened for these diseases.

Gottron's papules, erythematous papules that frequently occur over the metacarpal and interphalangeal joints (Figure 42.2), but may also be found overlying the elbows or knees, are the classic dermatologic finding. Macular erythema over the joints is called Gottron's sign and is less specific for dermatomyositis [24]. Photosensitive erythema, involving the V-neck area (V-sign), upper back (shawl sign), and/or face is also common. Other skin changes may include the heliotrope rash (violaceous erythema of the eyelids), periorbital edema, periungual telangiectasias and/or erythema, cuticular dystrophy, and hyperkeratosis on the palms or lateral fingers (mechanic's hands).

Dysphagia is estimated to occur in approximately 10–50% of dermatomyositis and polymyositis patients [25–28]. Although dermatomyositis characteristically causes disease of striated muscles, patients may have dysfunction of both the striated muscles of the oropharynx and upper esophagus, as well as the smooth muscles of the distal esophagus. Typical pathologic findings include a prolonged pharyngeal phase of swallowing and severe electromyographic abnormalities of the cricopharyngeal sphincter muscle during swallowing [25]. In addition, distal esophageal dysmotility similar to that seen in scleroderma has been demonstrated in dermatomyositis and polymyositis patients (without scleroderma overlap) via manometry and fluoroscopy [29]. Dysphagia has occasionally been reported as the presenting symptom of dermatomyositis [30], although this appears to occur more commonly in inclusion body myositis [22]. High-dose systemic steroids are the mainstay of treatment for symptomatic muscle disease (including esophageal disease) in dermatomyositis, but after therapy is initiated the dysphagia can take a longer time to improve than other muscle symptoms. Although it does not directly treat the myositis, speech therapy may be a helpful addition to the management plan. Dysphagia in dermatomyositis patients may also rarely be secondary to esophageal cancer [31].

Mixed connective tissue disease

Although there is debate within the literature as to whether mixed connective tissue disease is a specific clinical entity, the term is still frequently used in the clinical setting [32]. Mixed connective tissue disease is an overlap syndrome that combines features of scleroderma, dermatomyositis, and systemic lupus erythematosus (SLE). By definition, patients have high titers of antibodies to U1-ribonucleoprotein (RNP) [32–34]. The most common manifestations are arthritis or arthralgias, Raynaud's phenomenon, esophageal symptoms, decreased diffusing capacity for carbon monoxide, hand edema, and myositis [32]. Skin findings typical of lupus erythematosus, dermatomyositis, and scleroderma can also be seen. Esophageal manifestations resemble those seen in scleroderma; patients have decreased or absent peristalsis of the lower esophagus and frequently complain of dysphagia and heartburn [35].

Systemic lupus erythematosus

Esophageal involvement in SLE is not as prominent as in scleroderma, dermatomyositis, or mixed connective tissue disease [36]. Dysphagia occurs in fewer than 15% of SLE patients and may have a variety of etiologies, including decreased salivation from secondary Sjögren syndrome and reduced esophageal peristalsis [36–38]. Other considerations in patients with SLE and esophageal symptoms include GERD, esophageal ulcers, esophageal infection, and medication-induced esophagitis [37, 39–41]. The erythematous malar "butterfly" rash is the classic skin finding associated with SLE, but SLE patients may also have a wide variety of other cutaneous lesions.

Bullous diseases

Pemphigus vulgaris

Pemphigus vulgaris is an acquired antibody-mediated autoimmune bullous disease which is typically diagnosed in the fourth to sixth decades of life [42]. Autoantibodies are directed against desmogleins 1 and 3, desmosomal transmembrane proteins found on stratified squamous epithelial cells. Patients with mucocutaneous pemphigus vulgaris typically have antibodies against desmogleins 1 and 3, whereas patients with mucosal-predominant pemphigus vulgaris have antibodies targeting desmoglein 1 but not desmoglein 3 [43]. Pemphigus vulgaris results in suprabasilar epidermal cleavage, which has a characteristic histologic appearance on

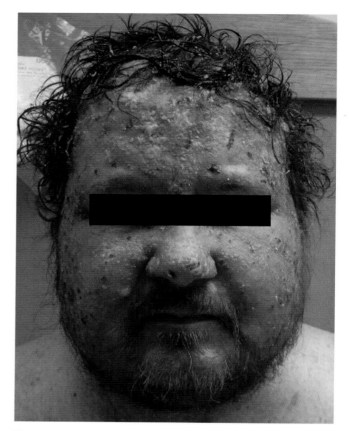

Figure 42.3 Pemphigus vulgaris patient with lesions predominantly on the head.

biopsy. Direct and indirect immunofluorescence show intercellular immunoreactants distributed along the border of keratinocytes in the epidermis, which helps to confirm the diagnosis [44].

Clinically, pemphigus vulgaris patients present with flaccid blisters that easily rupture to form superficial erosions. Pemphigus vulgaris patients may display the Nikolsky sign (induction of blisters when normal-appearing skin is rubbed). Lesions are most common (and tend to occur earliest) on the oral mucosa, but also frequently occur on the skin [42]. The head, upper chest, and back are typical areas for cutaneous blisters (Figure 42.3). In addition, any other stratified squamous epithelium may be involved, including the nasal, pharyngeal, laryngeal, anogenital, conjunctival, and esophageal mucosa [45–49]. A recent investigation of 26 pemphigus vulgaris patients (23 with oral involvement) experiencing acute pemphigus flares found upper gastrointestinal symptoms (dysphagia, odynophagia, or retrosternal burning) in 81% and biopsy-proven esophageal pemphigus lesions in 46% [47]. There was also a high incidence of non-pemphigus gastrointestinal disease associated with hyperacidity, including gastritis in 42%, esophagitis in 8%, and peptic ulcer disease in 4%. Patients (both with and without a prior diagnosis of pemphigus vulgaris) may rarely have pemphigus vulgaris isolated to the esophagus [50]. Like lesions on the skin, esophageal lesions may be flaccid blisters or erosions, but they may also appear as red longitudinal lines along the entire esophagus [51]. Very rarely, esophagitis dissecans superficialis (vomiting a cast of the esophageal mucosal membrane) has been reported in association with pemphigus vulgaris [52].

Endoscopic evaluation of pemphigus vulgaris patients with esophageal symptoms may help direct treatment, and endoscopy and biopsies are essential for the definitive diagnosis of pemphigus vulgaris. However, such procedures may induce an esophageal Nikolsky sign, resulting in aggravation of esophageal blistering [53]. The risk of complications in pemphigus vulgaris patients is increased not only by the fragile esophageal mucosa, but also by the need for multiple and deep biopsies (specimens should include the entire esophageal mucosa and basement membrane). Although endoscopy and biopsy are safe when performed by experienced physicians [54], these procedures should be done carefully. When performing an endoscopy on a pemphigus vulgaris patient, it is helpful to wait 30–60 s between biopsies to observe for hemorrhage and profound sloughing before continuing with the procedure. Like cutaneous and oral pemphigus, esophageal pemphigus is generally treated with corticosteroids (moderate to high dose) [55]. Combination therapy with steroid-sparing immunosuppressants may also be helpful.

Paraneoplastic pemphigus

Paraneoplastic pemphigus is an autoimmune bullous disorder that has been reported most frequently in association with neoplasms of lymphoreticular origin, including non-Hodgkin's lymphoma, chronic lymphocytic leukemia, Castleman's disease, thymoma, and Waldenstrom's macroglobulinemia [56]. Clinically, patients present with painful, often extensive oral mucosal bullae and erosions. The erosions may extend into the oropharynx, hypopharynx, nasopharynx, and esophagus, resulting in dysphagia and throat pain [57]. Pulmonary involvement may also occur, sometimes resulting in fatal respiratory failure [58]. Patients may develop a wide variety of cutaneous lesions that can be difficult to distinguish clinically from other bullous diseases [56, 57]. Histopathologic examination of cutaneous lesions (showing dyskeratosis and vacuolar interface dermatitis in addition to pemphigus vulgaris-like suprabasilar epidermal acantholysis) and indirect and direct immunofluorescence testing (showing deposition of immunoreactants in the epidermal intercellular spaces and/or at the basement membrane) are helpful in establishing the diagnosis [56]. Patient sera contain antibodies against numerous proteins in the plakin family, including desmoplakin, bullous pemphigoid antigen I, envoplakin and periplakin, and desmogleins 1 and 3 [59].

Mucous membrane pemphigoid

Mucous membrane pemphigoid (cicatricial pemphigoid) is an acquired subepidermal bullous disorder that typically begins in adulthood. In mucous membrane pemphigoid, the bullae primarily localize to the mucous membranes, whereas in bullous pemphigoid, the lesions mainly affect the skin. The most frequent sites of bullae in mucous membrane pemphigoid are (in descending order): mouth, eyes, pharynx, nose, larynx, genitalia, skin, anus, and esophagus [60]. Compatible clinical and immunohistopathologic findings are required for the diagnosis. Histopathology demonstrates subepithelial blisters, and direct immunofluorescence shows linear deposits of immunoreactants (IgG, IgA, and/or C3) in the basement membrane zone [61]. Indirect immunofluorescence on sodium chloride-split skin has variable findings. At least 10 basement membrane zone antigens have been identified, including bullous pemphigoid antigens 1 and 2 [61].

Biopsy procedures for suspected mucous membrane pemphigoid are the same as those for other autoimmune bullous diseases. The biopsy specimen that is sent for direct immunofluorescence should be obtained from perilesional uninvolved skin or mucosa and is typically stored in a special non-formalin medium (e.g. Michel's medium) to preserve tissue-bound immunoreactants. Alternatively, some prefer storing biopsies in saline, providing the laboratory will receive the biopsies within 24 h [62]. For esophageal biopsies, the endoscopist must remember to place biopsies that are to be sent for direct immunofluorescence into saline (rather than formalin) at the time of the procedure and before sending the biopsies to pathology.

Mucous membrane pemphigoid lesions often heal with scarring, which can lead to blindness and laryngeal or esophageal stenosis [60]. Esophageal involvement occurs in fewer than 15% of patients and can present as many as 10 years after disease onset [63]. Esophageal manifestations may also be the isolated presentation of mucous membrane pemphigoid [64]. Imaging of the esophagus typically shows erosions, strictures, or webs, and patients complain of dysphagia and odynophagia [63, 65]. Bullae may also be seen, particularly after dilatation or other esophageal trauma. Although topical steroids and dapsone are recommended as the first-line treatment of oral and cutaneous disease, treatment of severe orocutaneous disease and disease involving other organs (including the esophagus) generally requires both systemic corticosteroids and steroid-sparing immunosuppressants [63, 66]. Mycophenolate mofetil is often helpful for mucous membrane pemphigoid patients [67], but those with severe scarring may require treatment with cyclophosphamide. There are also case reports documenting successful use of tumor necrosis factor-alpha inhibitors [68] and rituximab [69] in refractory patients. Endoscopic dilatation is an option for severe esophageal disease, but this must be done carefully to avoid mucosal injury [63, 70]. Colonic interposition has also been used for refractory esophageal disease [71].

Epidermolysis bullosa acquisita

Epidermolysis bullosa acquisita (EBA) is an acquired subepidermal bullous disorder associated with antibodies to type VII collagen, which is a component of anchoring fibrils in the basement membrane of stratified squamous epithelium. Patients typically present in the fourth to fifth decades of life with tense bullae on trauma-prone skin surfaces that heal with scarring and milia [72, 73]. Immunofluorescence is required for diagnosis because the clinical presentation and histopathology are non-specific. Direct immunofluorescence demonstrates linear deposition of IgG at the basement membrane zone, and indirect immunofluorescence on sodium chloride-split skin shows antibody deposition on the dermal side of the split. Patients with EBA may rarely develop esophageal webs or strictures and associated dysphagia, which can be responsive to dilatation [73–75].

Dystrophic epidermolysis bullosa

Dystrophic epidermolysis bullosa (EB) is an inherited bullous disease that results from mutations in *COL7A1*, the gene encoding type VII collagen (the EBA antigen) [76]. Like EBA, dystrophic EB is characterized by antibodies to type VII collagen and results in tense subepidermal bullae that heal with scarring and milia [73]. The bullae are generally acral (on the extremities) in EBA, whereas dystrophic EB patients may have acral or generalized bullae [73]. Dystrophic EB presents at birth or during childhood and is inherited as an autosomal dominant or recessive trait, whereas EBA is an acquired disorder that tends to present in adults.

Dysphagia and esophageal strictures are much more common in dystrophic EB than in EBA. In the recessively inherited forms of dystrophic EB, approximately 70–95% of patients develop esophageal stenosis or strictures by age 50 years [77]. Strictures are commonly encountered in pediatric practices and are seen in children with recessive dystrophic EB as young as 1 year of age [77]. In contrast, fewer than 10% of patients with dominant dystrophic EB develop strictures by age 50 years, and stricture onset is typically in adulthood [77].

The childhood onset of strictures and dysphagia in recessive dystrophic EB is particularly problematic as it can result in malnutrition, growth impairment, and failure to thrive. Treatment of esophageal strictures in children with dystrophic EB is challenging because instrumentation of the esophagus may induce the formation of bullae. However, fluoroscopically-assisted balloon dilatation is safe and effective when performed by experienced physicians and is considered to be the first-line treatment [78]. When dilatations fail, children may require gastrostomy tubes to avoid severe malnutrition [79]. A non-endoscopic percutaneous image-guided approach to gastrostomy tube insertion may help minimize trauma to the skin and pharyngoesophageal mucosa in these patients [80]. Successful esophagectomy with colonic interposition has been reported in some patients with severe, refractory esophageal disease [81]. Pathology of the oral cavity, including blisters, progressive microstomia, ankyloglossia, and dental caries (secondary to difficult dental access), also contributes to feeding difficulties [79].

Stevens–Johnson syndrome and toxic epidermal necrolysis

Stevens–Johnson syndrome (SJS) and toxic epidermal necrolysis (TEN) are systemic reactions classically characterized by fever, full-thickness epidermal detachment, and blistering of the mucous membranes (Figure 42.4). Discrete macular or atypical target lesions may also be present on the skin. When epidermal detachment involves less than 10% of the body surface area, the term SJS is used, whereas TEN describes patients with greater than 30% body surface area involvement [82, 83]. Intermediate percentages of body surface involvement are called SJS/TEN overlap syndrome.

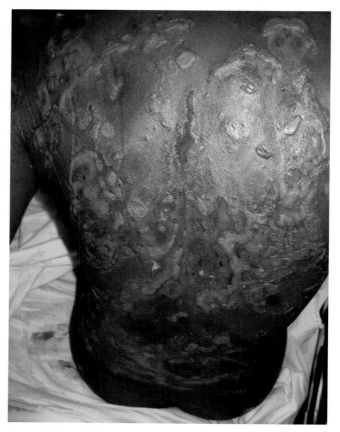

Figure 42.4 Full thickness epidermal detachment involving a large surface area in a patient with toxic epidermal necrolysis (reproduced courtesy of William James MD, University of Pennsylvania, Department of Dermatology).

The mortality rates of TEN and SJS are approximately 30–50% and 1–3%, respectively [84]. Medications are the most frequent cause of TEN and SJS. Commonly used drugs that are associated with a high risk of SJS or TEN include nevirapine, lamotrigine, carbamazepine, phenytoin, phenobarbital, anti-infective sulfonamides, sulfasalazine, allopurinol, and oxicam non-steroidal anti-inflammatory drugs [85]. Mucous membrane involvement is present in nearly all SJS and TEN patients and can affect the conjunctiva, oral cavity, pharynx, nasal cavity, genitalia, and esophagus [86]. Esophageal disease may range from minor erosions to frank necrosis [87]. Many TEN patients have severe oropharyngeal or esophageal mucosal involvement that results in dysphagia and odynophagia and prevents adequate oral intake [86]. When a patient is unable to maintain oral intake, enteral feeding should be considered. The key principles for management of TEN and SJS are to stop any potential causative medications and deliver supportive care. Options for adjunctive treatment include systemic corticosteroids and intravenous immunoglobulin, but there is no consensus regarding the effectiveness of these treatments [88, 89]. Esophageal stricture has been reported as a rare sequela in survivors of TEN [90].

Infectious diseases

Herpes simplex virus

Herpes simplex virus (HSV) presents on the skin as painful clustered vesicles or erosions on an erythematous base (Figure 42.5). Orolabial lesions are more frequently caused by HSV-1 and genital lesions by HSV-2, but both viruses can cause lesions anywhere on the body [91]. Symptomatic reactivation is typically less severe than primary infection. HSV esophagitis, which is usually caused by HSV-1 [92], is a well-recognized disease in immunocompromised patients, and the esophagus is the most frequently involved internal organ in disseminated HSV [93]. Transplant recipients are particularly susceptible to HSV and cytomegalovirus (CMV) esophagitis [94, 95], whereas *Candida* species and CMV are more common sources of esophagitis than HSV in human immunodeficiency virus (HIV) patients with low CD4 counts [96]. HSV esophagitis has also been reported in immunocompetent children and adults [97, 98].

Common symptoms of HSV esophagitis include fever, odynophagia, chest pain, and dysphagia [92, 97, 98]. Endoscopy and radiology characteristically demonstrate multiple ulcers and friable mucosa, predominantly involving the distal esophagus [92, 97]. Case reports document severe pathology, including esophageal perforation and tracheoesophageal fistulae [99–101]. Concurrent orolabial HSV may occur more frequently in immunocompromised than immunocompetent HSV esophagitis patients [97, 102]. Virus isolation from esophageal tissue and histopathologic

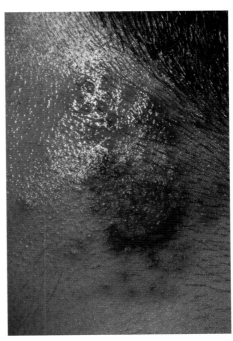

Figure 42.5 Cutaneous infection with herpes simplex virus presenting as grouped vesicles on an erythematous base (reproduced courtesy of William James MD, University of Pennsylvania, Department of Dermatology).

examination aid in the diagnosis of HSV esophagitis [97]. Depending on the severity of the esophageal disease and the underlying health of the patient, treatment options may include intravenous or oral acyclovir and/or symptomatic treatment [92, 97].

Candidiasis

Candidiasis, which is most frequently caused by *Candida albicans* [103], manifests on the skin as erythematous hyperkeratotic plaques. Infection localized to the oropharyngeal mucosa results in white patches. Oropharyngeal candidiasis (Figure 42.6) is a common infection that may be seen in a variety of patients, including infants and the elderly, denture-wearing patients, patients with xerostomia (secondary to Sjögren's syndrome, radiation therapy, or chemotherapy), immunodeficient patients, and patients treated with glucocorticoids or systemic antibiotics [103]. In contrast, esophageal candidiasis is more common in HIV patients and others with impaired cellular immunity (hematologic malignancies, transplant patients) [104]. Esophageal candidiasis is also occasionally seen in immunocompetent patients with marked esophageal stasis, such as those with advanced-stage achalasia [105] or scleroderma with esophageal involvement [106] (Figure 42.7). Immunocompetent patients using inhaled steroids are also at risk for esophageal candidiasis, especially if they swallow the steroids for treatment of eosinophilic esophagitis [107]. Candidal infections of the

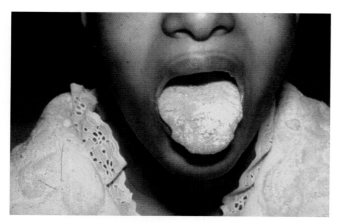

Figure 42.6 White plaques on the tongue of a patient with oral candidiasis (reproduced courtesy of William James MD, University of Pennsylvania, Department of Dermatology).

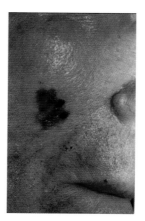

Figure 42.8 Melanoma with variegate pigmentation, asymmetric borders, and a large diameter.

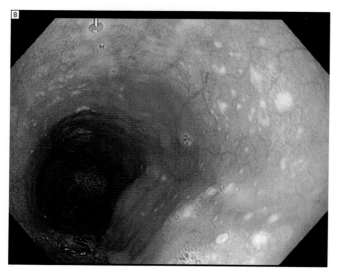

Figure 42.7 White adherent exudates in the distal esophagus of a scleroderma patient with esophageal candidiasis.

high prevalence of esophageal candidiasis in HIV patients, some recommend treating HIV-infected patients with esophagitis symptoms empirically with antifungals, reserving endoscopy for those with refractory symptoms [110].

Malignancies and malignancy-associated diseases

Malignancies

Cutaneous melanoma is classically a macular brown lesion with variegate pigmentation and asymmetric borders (Figure 42.8). A large diameter (>6 mm), symptoms (itching, tenderness), bleeding, and changing color, shape, and size are also worrisome features of pigmented lesions that may indicate melanoma [111]. Cutaneous melanoma may occasionally metastasize to the esophagus, resulting in dysphagia [112, 113]. Primary esophageal melanoma, an extremely rare malignancy, can be difficult to distinguish from metastatic melanoma, both clinically and histopathologically [113]. Although the prognosis is poor with both diseases, metastatic melanoma of the esophagus has a worse prognosis than primary esophageal melanoma [112, 113]. Distinguishing between the two diseases is important as this information may alter treatment decisions.

The most common type of cutaneous T-cell lymphoma is mycosis fungoides, a lymphoma that is characterized by malignant clonal T cells with an affinity for the epidermis [114]. Mycosis fungoides lesions classically begin as chronic erythematous patches on sun-shielded areas (Figure 42.9). Over the course of years, the patches progress to plaques, then tumors. The lesions may be difficult to distinguish from benign dermatoses, such as atopic dermatitis and psoriasis [114]. The medical literature documents few cases of symptomatic esophageal involvement in mycosis fungoides [115]. Dysphagia in mycosis fungoides patients may indicate

esophagus tend to be less invasive when they complicate achalasia, scleroderma, and eosinophilic esophagitis in immunocompetent patients than when they occur in patients with impaired cellular immunity.

Esophageal candidiasis characteristically presents as odynophagia, dysphagia, and/or chest pain. Endoscopy demonstrates scattered or coalescent yellow–white mucosal plaques [108]. Mild oropharyngeal candidiasis may be treated with topical clotrimazole or nystatin, whereas oral fluconazole is needed for moderate and severe oropharyngeal candidiasis and esophageal infections [109]. Intravenous fluconazole, an echinocandin, or amphotericin B deoxycholate are appropriate options for esophageal candidiasis patients who cannot tolerate oral therapy [109]. Given the

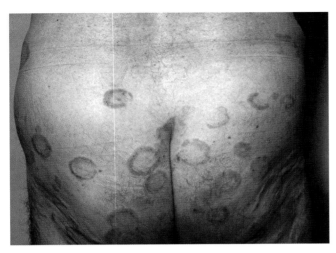

Figure 42.9 Mycosis fungoides patient with erythematous lesions in sun-shielded areas (reproduced courtesy of Alain Rook MD, University of Pennsylvania, Department of Dermatology).

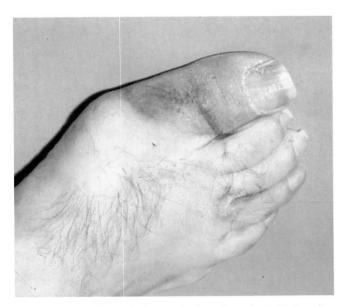

Figure 42.10 Violaceous lesions on the foot of a patient with Kaposi's sarcoma.

malignant lesions of the oropharynx, pharynx, and/or larynx, as these structures appear to be more frequently involved than the esophagus [115].

Kaposi's sarcoma (KS) is a vascular spindle cell malignancy caused by human herpesvirus 8 and seen at a greatly increased prevalence in HIV-infected patients and transplant recipients [116]. Patients with cutaneous KS typically present with red or violaceous papular lesions concentrated on the lower extremities, head, and neck (Figure 42.10). Gastrointestinal KS is a common form of visceral KS and

may occur with or without concurrent cutaneous KS lesions [117, 118]. The small bowel is the most frequently involved site in the gastrointestinal tract, but lesions may also occur in the stomach, esophagus, and colon [118, 119]. Endoscopy classically shows small (<5 mm), red maculopapular lesions [117, 119]. Although gastrointestinal KS is often asymptomatic, patients may experience gastrointestinal bleeding, resulting in chronic anemia or gross hemorrhage [119, 120].

Acanthosis nigricans

Acanthosis nigricans characteristically presents as symmetrical, hyperpigmented, velvety plaques on intertriginous areas and the neck (Figure 42.11). Papillomatous lesions may also develop in the oral cavity and have rarely been reported on the esophageal mucosa [121, 122]. Acanthosis nigricans is typically seen in association with obesity and insulin resistance, but some cases are associated with gastric carcinoma or a variety of other malignancies [123, 124]. Oral and esophageal involvement in acanthosis nigricans are more frequently associated with internal malignancy than is isolated cutaneous acanthosis nigricans [121, 122].

Malignancy-associated syndromes

Plummer–Vinson syndrome (Paterson–Brown–Kelly syndrome, sideropenic dysphagia) is a syndrome of unknown pathogenesis characterized by the triad of cervical dysphagia, esophageal webs, and chronic iron-deficiency anemia [125]. Orocutaneous features are related to iron deficiency and include angular cheilitis, atrophic glossitis, and koilonychia. Patients are at an increased risk for upper gastrointestinal tract carcinomas, including squamous cell carcinoma of the esophagus [126, 127]. The syndrome is most commonly seen in white women in the fourth to seventh decades of life but may also occur in children [125]. Figure 42.12 shows a ring-like esophageal stricture in a patient with Plummer–Vinson syndrome.

Bazex syndrome (acrokeratosis paraneoplastica) is a paraneoplastic dermatosis that presents with erythematous or violaceous hyperkeratotic lesions beginning on acral areas [128]. The ears, nose, hands (including the nails), and feet are the most frequent locations of skin disease, but lesions may also occur on the trunk as the disease progresses [128, 129]. Skin symptoms often precede the diagnosis of the malignancy and usually progress and regress in parallel with the malignancy [128, 129]. Most malignancies are squamous cell carcinomas of the upper gastrointestinal tract (including the esophagus) or the respiratory tract [128, 129]. The syndrome is typically seen in men over the age of 40 years [130].

The palmoplantar keratodermas are a large group of dermatoses characterized by hyperkeratosis of the palms and soles (Figure 42.13). Numerous hereditary and acquired palmoplantar keratodermas have been described [131, 132]. Tylosis is a rare autosomal dominant hereditary

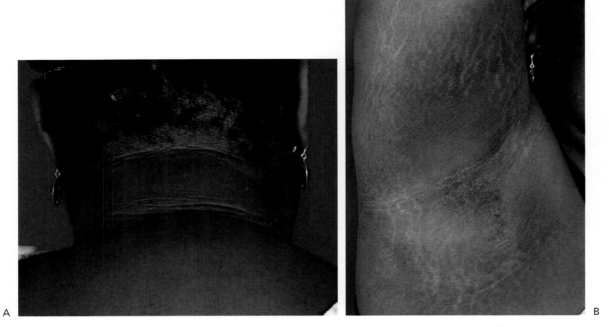

Figure 42.11 Hyperpigmented velvety plaques on the (A) neck and (B) axilla of an acanthosis nigrans patient (reproduced courtesy of the Department of Dermatology Photographic Collection, University of Pennsylvania).

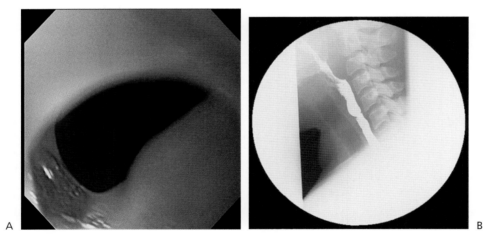

Figure 42.12 Esophageal web in a patient with Plummer–Vinson syndrome. (A) endoscopy and (B) radiography.

palmoplantar keratoderma that has a strong association with squamous cell esophageal carcinoma. Linkage analysis studies have mapped the disease locus (termed the tylosis esophageal cancer gene) to chromosome 17q23 [133]. Studies of families with tylosis estimate that at least 90% of patients with tylosis die of esophageal cancer by the age of 70 years [134]. Esophageal cancer in association with tylosis is called Howel–Evans syndrome [135]. Acquired palmoplantar keratoderma has many causes but may rarely be a paraneoplastic phenomenon and has been reported in association with malignancies of multiple organs, including the esophagus [132].

Cowden syndrome (multiple hamartoma syndrome) is an autosomal dominant disease that is frequently associated with a mutation in the tumor suppressor gene *PTEN* on chromosome 10q22–23 [136]. Clinically, the disease presents with multiple hamartomas involving several organ systems and an increased risk of breast and thyroid cancer [136]. At least 90% of patients have mucocutaneous lesions, including facial trichilemmomas (papular hamartomas of the hair-follicle infundibulum), oral mucosal papillomatosis, acral keratoses (smooth or verrucous growths on the dorsal hands and feet), and palmoplantar keratoses (punctate keratotic lesions on the palms and soles) [136]. Gastrointestinal

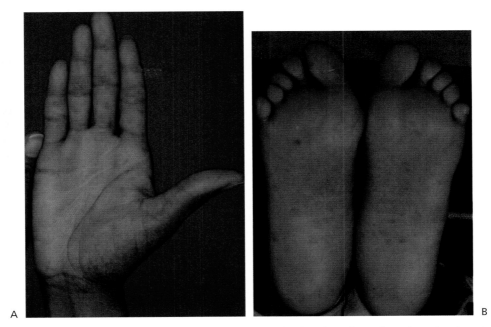

Figure 42.13 Diffuse hyperkeratosis of the (A) palms and (B) soles of a patient with palmoplantar keratoderma (reproduced courtesy of the Department of Dermatology Photographic Collection, University of Pennsylvania).

polyps (primarily hamartomatous) are seen in approximately 40–80% of patients [136]. Polyps are most common in the colon but may also be found in the stomach, small intestine, and esophagus [137]. Although the gastrointestinal hamartomatous polyps are typically benign, malignant transformation to invasive adenocarcinoma has been reported [138]. Esophageal glycogenic acanthosis is another characteristic finding in Cowden syndrome, and some authors suggest that the finding of extensive esophageal glycogenic acanthosis in addition to benign gastrointestinal polyposis should be considered pathognomonic for Cowden syndrome [139].

Dyskeratosis congenita (Zinsser–Engman–Cole syndrome) is an inherited syndrome associated with mutations in the telomerase complex genes [140]. X-linked recessive, autosomal dominant, and autosomal recessive forms have been described [140]. The classic clinical triad of dyskeratosis congenita is reticular hyperpigmentation of the skin, oral leukoplakia, and nail dystrophy [141]. Each of these mucocutaneous features is seen in approximately 80–90% of dyskeratosis congenita patients [140]. Dyskeratosis congenita is associated with esophageal pathology, including strictures (congenital and acquired), webs, and diverticula [140, 142–144]. Esophageal strictures occur in approximately 15% of patients [140]. Other important features of dyskeratosis congenita are bone marrow failure (over 80% of patients) and malignancy (approximately 10% of patients) [140, 145]. The most common malignancy is squamous cell carcinoma of the head and neck, but a variety of other

cancers may be seen, including squamous cell carcinoma of the esophagus [145].

Miscellaneous acquired diseases

Lichen planus

Lichen planus is a mucocutaneous disease of unknown etiology that has an association with hepatitis C virus infection in some cases [146, 147]. Patients generally present in the fourth to seventh decades of life [148]. Individual patients may have disease limited to either the skin or the mucous membranes or may have combined mucocutaneous disease [148]. The skin lesions are pruritic, violaceous, polygonal papules or plaques (Figure 42.14) that classically occur on the flexor surfaces of the extremities, but can also be found in other areas, including the scalp, vulva, and penis. Close examination of skin lesions often reveals Wikham's striae (white lace-like lines on the lesion surface). Mucous membrane lesions may consist of isolated Wikham's striae, plaques, atrophic areas, or erosions. These lesions classically occur on the buccal mucosa and the tongue, but the mucous membrane disease may also involve other areas of the oral cavity and the esophagus, conjunctiva, nose, larynx, stomach, bladder, and anus [148]. Figure 42.15 shows a classic picture of lichen planus of the palate.

Esophageal lichen planus may occur in up to 25–50% of patients with lichen planus, but most patients are asymptomatic or have only minor symptoms [149, 150]. However,

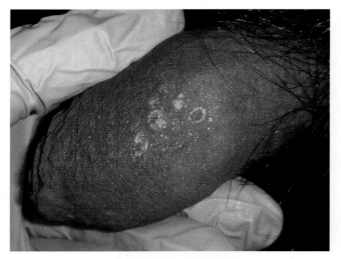

Figure 42.14 Shiny, violaceous, polygonal papules and plaques on a patient with lichen planus (reproduced courtesy of Kenneth Katz MD).

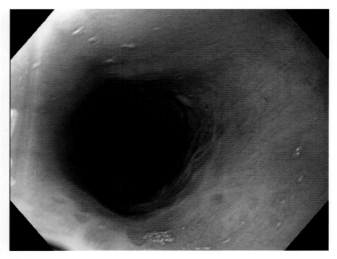

Figure 42.16 Eoesophageal endoscopy in a patient with lichen planus shows a proximal stricture and a white lacy pattern on the mucosa.

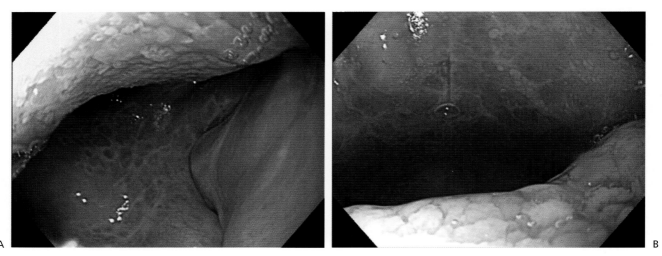

A   B

Figure 42.15 White lacy pattern of lichen planus of the palate. (A) Tongue is on top. (B) Tongue is on bottom.

patients with severe esophageal lichen planus often develop strictures and may present with dysphagia, odynophagia, and weight loss [151]. Strictures are typically proximal but may be variable in length, sometimes involving most of the esophageal body. Although the vast majority of published cases of esophageal lichen planus occur in patients with pre-existing oral, cutaneous, and/or vaginal lichen planus, patients may also present with esophageal lichen planus in the absence of extraesophageal disease [151, 152].

Histopathologic examination of esophageal lichen planus shows a characteristic lymphohistiocytic interface inflammatory infiltrate and apoptotic basal keratinocytes (similar to the pattern seen in cutaneous lichen planus) [149]. In con-

trast, endoscopic findings of lichen planus can be subtle and non-specific, and include peeling mucosa, hyperemic focal abnormalities, and submucosal plaques or papules [149, 151]. Figure 42.16 shows endoscopic findings from a patient with esophageal lichen planus. Histopathology consistent with lichen planus may also been seen in samples taken from grossly normal-appearing esophageal mucosa [149]. High-dose systemic steroids are often successful in treating esophageal lichen planus, but relapse is common when steroids are tapered [151]. Dilatation and intralesional steroids can alleviate the symptoms associated with strictures, but these symptoms frequently recur in less than a year, necessitating repeat dilatations [153]. Oral fluticasone has also been tried, but the experience is anecdotal. Case reports of squamous cell carcinoma in esophageal lichen planus patients indicate that the esophageal lesions may have malignant potential [154, 155].

Behçet's disease

Behçet's disease is a unique vasculitis because it can involve arteries and veins of all sizes [156]. Diagnosis of Behçet's disease requires recurrent oral ulcers plus two or more of the following: recurrent genital ulcers, typical eye lesions (including anterior or posterior uveitis and retinal vasculitis), typical skin lesions, and a positive pathergy test [157]. Disease may also occur in the joints, nervous system, kidneys, heart, lungs, and gastrointestinal tract. The most common cutaneous manifestations seen in the United States are papulopustular lesions and erythema nodosum, but patients may also have pseudofolliculitis, acneiform nodules, and ulcerative lesions that may resemble pyoderma gangrenosum [158]. The prevalence of gastrointestinal ulcers, which usually occur in the ileocecum and colon, varies by country from 0% to 60%, with the lowest frequency reported in Israel, the highest in Japan, and an intermediate frequency in the United States [159]. Esophageal ulcers are uncommon, occurring in fewer than 15% of patients [159, 160]. The ulcers are typically located in the middle third of the esophagus and are often associated with ulcers in the stomach, ileum, or colon [159]. Rare esophageal lesions that have been reported in Behçet's disease include strictures, varices (associated with venous thrombosis), and fistulae connecting with the trachea [161–163].

Nephrogenic systemic fibrosis

Nephrogenic systemic fibrosis (originally called nephrogenic fibrosing dermopathy) is a disease of systemic fibrosis that occurs in patients with chronic renal insufficiency who receive gadolinium contrast (commonly used for magnetic resonance imaging and magnetic resonance angiography). The disease was first identified in 1997 and, as of 2009, over 300 cases were documented in the International Nephrogenic Systemic Fibrosis Registry at Yale University [164, 165]. Cutaneous lesions are generally symmetric fibrotic papules or plaques, which may be erythematous [166]. Coalescing plaques result in diffuse thickening and hardening of the skin. Lesions typically occur on the extremities and trunk. In contrast to scleroderma, lesions tend to spare the face and only occasionally cause edema of the hands [166]. Skin fibrosis can limit joint mobility, resulting in contractures and rapid debilitation. The skin lesions may also be associated with pain and pruritus [167, 168]. Systemic fibrosis has been documented in a variety of organs, including skeletal muscles and their fascia, the heart and pericardium, lungs and pleura, diaphragm, and skeletal muscle of the proximal esophagus [167–170].

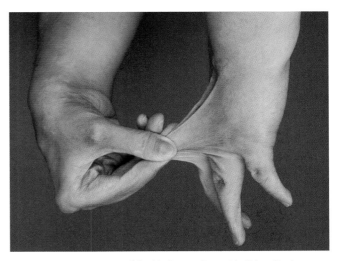

Figure 42.17 Hyperextensible skin in a patient with Ehlers–Danlos syndrome (reproduced courtesy of William James MD, University of Pennsylvania, Department of Dermatology).

Miscellaneous inherited syndromes

Ehlers–Danlos syndrome (EDS) refers to a group of inherited connective tissue diseases resulting from a genetic defect in collagen. Different types of EDS have varied clinical features, but common manifestations are hypermobile joints, hyperextensible skin (Figure 42.17), easy bruising, and poor wound healing [171]. Characteristic cutaneous features include cigarette-paper scars (Figure 42.18), soft skin with a velvety texture, and thin skin with visible underlying vessels [171, 172]. Hiatal hernias are common, and case reports document other structural esophageal defects, such as giant epiphrenic diverticula and megaesophagus [173–175]. Spontaneous esophageal rupture may also be seen [176, 177].

Hereditary hemorrhagic telangiectasia (Osler–Weber–Rendu syndrome) is an autosomal dominant disease that results in telangiectasias, arteriovenous malformations, and bleeding. Telangiectasias may involve the skin, oral and nasal mucosa, gastrointestinal tract, and conjunctiva [178]. Larger arteriovenous malformations can also occur in the gastrointestinal tract as well as in the lungs, central nervous system, and liver [178]. Telangiectasias on the skin and buccal mucosa are largely a cosmetic problem, but telangiectasias on the nasal mucosa and in the gastrointestinal tract can result in severe chronic anemia or acute life-threatening hemorrhage [179–181]. Telangiectasias are more common in the stomach, duodenum, and jejunum than in the esophagus [182].

Focal dermal hypoplasia (Goltz syndrome or Goltz–Gorlin syndrome) is an X-linked dominant syndrome characterized by mesoectodermal developmental abnormalities. The disorder is associated with over 20 different pathogenic

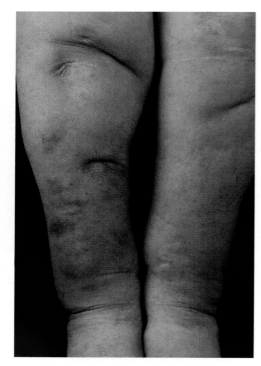

Figure 42.18 Abnormal scarring and bruises on the legs of a patient with Ehlers–Danlos syndrome (reproduced courtesy of William James MD, University of Pennsylvania, Department of Dermatology).

mutations in the *PORCN* gene on the X chromosome [183]. Focal dermal hypoplasia is frequently lethal in males (*in utero*), although there are case reports of the disease in live male patients [184]. Females present with disease of variable severity due to different patterns of X chromosome inactivation [185]. Focal dermal hypoplasia has manifestations in many organs, including the skin and esophagus. The hallmark cutaneous findings are linear atrophic lesions following the lines of Blashko and papillomatous lesions (often perineal, perivulvar, and perianal) [186, 187]. Papillomas in the esophagus may be numerous and can be associated with strictures and dysphagia [188]. Hiatal laxity with marked gastroesophageal reflux has also been reported [189].

References

1. Sakkas LI. New developments in the pathogenesis of systemic sclerosis. *Autoimmunity* 2005;38:113–116.
2. Walker JG, Pope J, Baron M, *et al.* The development of systemic sclerosis classification criteria. *Clin Rheumatol* 2007;26:1401–1409.
3. Gabrielli A, Avvedimento EV, Krieg T. Scleroderma. *N Engl J Med* 2009;360:1989–2003.
4. Krieg T, Takehara K. Skin disease: a cardinal feature of systemic sclerosis. *Rheumatology (Oxf)* 2009;48 (Suppl 3):iii 14–18.
5. Steen VD, Medsger TA Jr. Severe organ involvement in systemic sclerosis with diffuse scleroderma. *Arthritis Rheum* 2000;43:2437–2444.
6. Ueda M, Abe Y, Fujiwara H, *et al.* Prominent telangiectasia associated with marked bleeding in CREST syndrome. *J Dermatol* 1993;20:180–184.
7. Khanlou H, Malhotra A, Friedenberg F, Rothstein K. Jejunal telangiectasias as a cause of massive bleeding in a patient with scleroderma. *Rev Rheum Engl Ed* 1999;66:119–121.
8. Kaye SA, Siraj QH, Agnew J, Hilson A, Black CM. Detection of early asymptomatic esophageal dysfunction in systemic sclerosis using a new scintigraphic grading method. *J Rheumatol* 1996;23:297–301.
9. Halpert RD, Laufer I, Thompson JJ, Feczko PJ. Adenocarcinoma of the esophagus in patients with scleroderma. *AJR Am J Roentgenol* 1983;140:927–930.
10. Wipff J, Allanore Y, Soussi F, *et al.* Prevalence of Barrett's esophagus in systemic sclerosis. *Arthritis Rheum* 2005; 52:2882–2888.
11. Zamost BJ, Hirschberg J, Ippoliti AF, Furst DE, Clements PJ, Weinstein WM. Esophagitis in scleroderma. Prevalence and risk factors. *Gastroenterology* 1987;92:421–428.
12. Katzka DA, Reynolds JC, Saul SH, *et al.* Barrett's metaplasia and adenocarcinoma of the esophagus in scleroderma. *Am J Med* 1987;82:46–52.
13. Recht MP, Levine MS, Katzka DA, Reynolds JC, Saul SH. Barrett's esophagus in scleroderma: increased prevalence and radiographic findings. *Gastrointest Radiol* 1988;13:1–5.
14. Hendel L, Svejgaard E, Walsoe I, Kieffer M, Stenderup A. Esophageal candidosis in progressive systemic sclerosis: occurrence, significance, and treatment with fluconazole. *Scand J Gastroenterol* 1988;23:1182–1186.
15. Winstead NS, Bulat R. Pill esophagitis. *Curr Treat Options Gastroenterol* 2004;7:71–76.
16. Ebert EC. Esophageal disease in scleroderma. *J Clin Gastroenterol* 2006;40:769–775.
17. Ntoumazios SK, Voulgari PV, Potsis K, Koutis E, Tsifetaki N, Assimakopoulos DA. Esophageal involvement in scleroderma: gastroesophageal reflux, the common problem. *Semin Arthritis Rheum* 2006;36:173–181.
18. Forbes A, Marie I. Gastrointestinal complications: the most frequent internal complications of systemic sclerosis. *Rheumatology (Oxf)* 2009;48 (Suppl 3):iii 36–39.
19. Kent MS, Luketich JD, Irshad K, *et al.* Comparison of surgical approaches to recalcitrant gastroesophageal reflux disease in the patient with scleroderma. *Ann Thorac Surg* 2007;84: 1710–1715; discussion 1715–1716.
20. Haupt HM, Hutchins GM. The heart and cardiac conduction system in polymyositis-dermatomyositis: a clinicopathologic study of 16 autopsied patients. *Am J Cardiol* 1982;50:998–1006.
21. Dickey BF, Myers AR. Pulmonary disease in polymyositis/dermatomyositis. *Semin Arthritis Rheum* 1984;14:60–76.
22. Oh TH, Brumfield KA, Hoskin TL, Stolp KA, Murray JA, Bassford JR. Dysphagia in inflammatory myopathy: clinical characteristics, treatment strategies, and outcome in 62 patients. *Mayo Clin Proc* 2007;82:441–447.
23. Teixeira A, Cherin P, Demoule A, *et al.* Diaphragmatic dysfunction in patients with idiopathic inflammatory myopathies. *Neuromusc Disord* 2005;15:32–39.

24. Dugan EM, Huber AM, Miller FW, Rider LG, International Myositis Assessment and Clinical Studies Group. Photoessay of the cutaneous manifestations of the idiopathic inflammatory myopathies. *Dermatol Online J* 2009;15:1.

25. Ertekin C, Secil Y, Yuceyar N, Aydogdu I. Oropharyngeal dysphagia in polymyositis/dermatomyositis. *Clin Neurol Neurosurg* 2004;107:32–37.

26. Bohan A, Peter JB, Bowman RL, Pearson CM. Computer-assisted analysis of 153 patients with polymyositis and dermatomyositis. *Medicine (Balt)* 1977;56:255–286.

27. Cunningham JD Jr, Lowry LD. Head and neck manifestations of dermatomyositis-polymyositis. *Otolaryngol Head Neck Surg* 1985;93:673–677.

28. Sonies BC. Evaluation and treatment of speech and swallowing disorders associated with myopathies. *Curr Opin Rheumatol* 1997;9:486–495.

29. Jacob H, Berkowitz D, McDonald E, Bernstein LH, Beneventano T. The esophageal motility disorder of polymyositis. A prospective study. *Arch Intern Med* 1983;143:2262–2264.

30. Scola RH, Werneck LC, Prevedello DM, Toderke EL, Iwamoto FM. Diagnosis of dermatomyositis and polymyositis: a study of 102 cases. *Arq Neuropsiquiatr* 2000;58:789–799.

31. Iftikhar I, Abdelmannan D, Daw HA. Dermatomyositis and esophageal cancer. *South Med J* 2006;99:777–779.

32. Venables PJ. Mixed connective tissue disease. *Lupus* 2006; 15:132–137.

33. Sharp GC, Irvin WS, Tan EM, Gould RG, Holman HR. Mixed connective tissue disease—an apparently distinct rheumatic disease syndrome associated with a specific antibody to an extractable nuclear antigen (ENA). *Am J Med* 1972;52:148–159.

34. Sharp GC, Irvin WS, May CM, *et al.* Association of antibodies to ribonucleoprotein and Sm antigens with mixed connective-tissue disease, systematic lupus erythematosus and other rheumatic diseases. *N Engl J Med* 1976;295:1149–1154.

35. Marshall JB, Kretschmar JM, Gerhardt DC, *et al.* Gastrointestinal manifestations of mixed connective tissue disease. *Gastroenterology* 1990;98:1232–1238.

36. Lapadula G, Muolo P, Semeraro F, *et al.* Esophageal motility disorders in the rheumatic diseases: a review of 150 patients. *Clin Exp Rheumatol* 1994;12:515–521.

37. Sultan SM, Ioannou Y, Isenberg DA. A review of gastrointestinal manifestations of systemic lupus erythematosus. *Rheumatology (Oxf)* 1999;38:917–932.

38. Rhodus NL, Colby S, Moller K, Bereuter J. Quantitative assessment of dysphagia in patients with primary and secondary Sjogren's syndrome. *Oral Surg Oral Med Oral Pathol Oral Radiol Endod* 1995;79:305–310.

39. Jimenez-Alonso J, Estev D, Vera C, Sabio JM, Grupo Lupus Virgen de las Nieves. Dysphagia in patients with systemic lupus erythematosus. *Lupus* 2003;12:493.

40. Colina RE, Smith M, Kikendall JW, Wong RK. A new probable increasing cause of esophageal ulceration: alendronate. *Am J Gastroenterol* 1997;92:704–706.

41. Hokama A, Ihama Y, Nakamoto M, Kinjo N, Kinjo F, Fujita J. Esophagitis dissecans superficialis associated with bisphosphonates. *Endoscopy* 2007;39 (Suppl 1):E91.

42. Bystryn JC, Rudolph JL. Pemphigus. *Lancet* 2005;366:61–73.

43. Amagai M, Tsunoda K, Zillikens D, Nagai T, Nishikawa T. The clinical phenotype of pemphigus is defined by the anti-desmoglein autoantibody profile. *J Am Acad Dermatol* 1999; 40:167–170.

44. Mihai S, Sitaru C. Immunopathology and molecular diagnosis of autoimmune bullous diseases. *J Cell Mol Med* 2007;11:462–481.

45. Daoud YJ, Cervantes R, Foster CS, Ahmed AR. Ocular pemphigus. *J Am Acad Dermatol* 2005;53:585–590.

46. Espana A, Fernandez S, del Olmo J, *et al.* Ear, nose and throat manifestations in pemphigus vulgaris. *Br J Dermatol* 2007; 156:733–737.

47. Calka O, Akdeniz N, Tuncer I, Metin A, Cesur RS. Oesophageal involvement during attacks in pemphigus vulgaris patients. *Clin Exp Dermatol* 2006;31:515–519.

48. Malik M, El Tal AE, Ahmed AR. Anal involvement in pemphigus vulgaris. *Dis Colon Rectum* 2006;49:500–506.

49. Malik M, Ahmed AR. Involvement of the female genital tract in pemphigus vulgaris. *Obstet Gynecol* 2005;106:1005–1012.

50. Faias S, Lage P, Sachse F, *et al.* Pemphigus vulgaris with exclusive involvement of the esophagus: case report and review. *Gastrointest Endosc* 2004;60:312–315.

51. Mignogna MD, Lo Muzio L, Galloro G, Satriano RA, Ruocco V, Bucci E. Oral pemphigus: clinical significance of esophageal involvement: report of eight cases. *Oral Surg Oral Med Oral Pathol Oral Radiol Endod* 1997;84:179–184.

52. Cesar WG, Barrios MM, Maruta CW, Aoki V, Santi GG. Oesophagitis dissecans superficialis: an acute, benign phenomenon associated with pemphigus vulgaris. *Clin Exp Dermatol* 2009;34:e614–616.

53. Revuz J. Oesophageal involvement in pemphigus vulgaris. *Lancet* 2000;355:656.

54. Galloro G, Mignogna M, de Werra C, *et al.* The role of upper endoscopy in identifying oesophageal involvement in patients with oral pemphigus vulgaris. *Dig Liver Dis* 2005;37:195–199.

55. Jessop S, Khumalo NP. Pemphigus: a treatment update. *Am J Clin Dermatol* 2008;9:147–154.

56. Sehgal VN, Srivastava G. Paraneoplastic pemphigus/paraneoplastic autoimmune multiorgan syndrome. *Int J Dermatol* 2009;48:162–169.

57. Sklavounou A, Laskaris G. Paraneoplastic pemphigus: a review. *Oral Oncol* 1998;34:437–440.

58. Nousari HC, Deterding R, Wojtczack H, *et al.* The mechanism of respiratory failure in paraneoplastic pemphigus. *N Engl J Med* 19996;340:1406–1410.

59. Zhu X, Zhang B. Paraneoplastic pemphigus. *J Dermatol* 2007;34:503–511.

60. Hardy KM, Perry HO, Pingree GC, Kirby TJ Jr. Benign mucous membrane pemphigoid. *Arch Dermatol* 1971;104:467–475.

61. Chan LS, Ahmed AR, Anhalt GJ, *et al.* The first international consensus on mucous membrane pemphigoid: definition, diagnostic criteria, pathogenic factors, medical treatment, and prognostic indicators. *Arch Dermatol* 2002;138:370–379.

62. Vodegel RM, de Jong MC, Meijer HJ, Weytingh MB, Pas HH, Jonkman MF. Enhanced diagnostic immunofluorescence using biopsies transported in saline. *BMC Dermatol* 2004;4:10.

63. Syn WK, Ahmed MM. Esophageal involvement in cicatricial pemphigoid: a rare cause of dysphagia. *Dis Esophagus* 2004;17:180–182.

64. Sallout H, Anhalt GJ, Al-Kawas FH. Mucous membrane pemphigoid presenting with isolated esophageal involvement: a case report. *Gastrointest Endosc* 2000;52:429–433.

65. Tang SJ. Electronic clinical challenges and images in GI. Esophageal involvement in mucous membrane pemphigoid. *Gastroenterology* 2009;136:e6–7.

66. Chan LS, Ahmed AR, Anhalt GJ, et al. The first international consensus on mucous membrane pemphigoid: definition, diagnostic criteria, pathogenic factors, medical treatment, and prognostic indicators. *Arch Dermatol* 2002;138:370–379.

67. Megahed M, Schmiedeberg S, Becker J, Ruzicka T. Treatment of cicatricial pemphigoid with mycophenolate mofetil as a steroid-sparing agent. *J Am Acad Dermatol* 2001;45:256–259.

68. Canizares MJ, Smith DI, Conners MS, Maverick KJ, Heffernan MP. Successful treatment of mucous membrane pemphigoid with etanercept in 3 patients. *Arch Dermatol* 2006; 142:1457–1461.

69. Taverna JA, Lerner A, Bhawan J, Demierre MF. Successful adjuvant treatment of recalcitrant mucous membrane pemphigoid with anti-CD20 antibody rituximab. *J Drugs Dermatol* 2007;6:731–732.

70. Warren LJ, Wojnarowska F, Wilkinson JD. Oesophageal involvement in cicatricial pemphigoid. *Aust J Dermatol* 1997; 38:148–151.

71. Popovici Z, Deac M, Rotaru M, Vestemeanu P, Vargatu V. Stenosis of the esophagus in cicatricial pemphigoid resolved by colon interposition: report of a case. *Surg Today* 1997; 27:234–237.

72. Lehman JS, Camilleri MJ, Gibson LE. Epidermolysis bullosa acquisita: concise review and practical considerations. *Int J Dermatol* 2009;48:227–235; quiz 235–236.

73. Shipman AR, Agero AL, Cook I, et al. Epidermolysis bullosa acquisita requiring multiple oesophageal dilatations. *Clin Exp Dermatol* 2008;33:787–789.

74. Stewart MI, Woodley DT, Briggaman RA. Epidermolysis bullosa acquisita and associated symptomatic esophageal webs. *Arch Dermatol* 1991;127:373–377.

75. Weinman D, Stewart MI, Woodley DT, Garcia G. Epidermolysis bullosa acquisita (EBA) and esophageal webs: a new association. *Am J Gastroenterol* 1991;86:1518–1522.

76. Dang N, Murrell DF. Mutation analysis and characterization of COL7A1 mutations in dystrophic epidermolysis bullosa. *Exp Dermatol* 2008;17:553–568.

77. Fine JD, Johnson LB, Weiner M, Suchindran C. Gastrointestinal complications of inherited epidermolysis bullosa: cumulative experience of the National Epidermolysis Bullosa Registry. *J Pediatr Gastroenterol Nutr* 2008;46:147–158.

78. Azizkhan RG, Stehr W, Cohen AP, et al. Esophageal strictures in children with recessive dystrophic epidermolysis bullosa: an 11-year experience with fluoroscopically guided balloon dilatation. *J Pediatr Surg* 2006;41:55–60.

79. Azizkhan RG, Denyer JE, Mellerio JE, et al. Surgical management of epidermolysis bullosa: Proceedings of the IInd International Symposium on Epidermolysis Bullosa, Santiago, Chile, 2005. *Int J Dermatol* 2007;46:801–808.

80. Stehr W, Farrell MK, Lucky AW, Johnson ND, Racadio JM, Azizkhan RG. Non-endoscopic percutaneous gastrostomy placement in children with recessive dystrophic epidermolysis bullosa. *Pediatr Surg Int* 2008;24:349–354.

81. Demirogullari B, Sonmez K, Turkyilmaz Z, et al. Colon interposition for esophageal stenosis in a patient with epidermolysis bullosa. *J Pediatr Surg* 2001;36:1861–1863.

82. Letko E, Papaliodis DN, Papaliodis GN, Daoud YJ, Ahmed AR, Foster CS. Stevens-Johnson syndrome and toxic epidermal necrolysis: a review of the literature. *Ann Allergy Asthma Immunol* 2005;94:419–436; quiz 436–438, 456.

83. Bastuji-Garin S, Rzany B, Stern RS, Shear NH, Naldi L, Roujeau JC. Clinical classification of cases of toxic epidermal necrolysis, Stevens-Johnson syndrome, and erythema multiforme. *Arch Dermatol* 1993;129:92–96.

84. Abood GJ, Nickoloff BJ, Gamelli RL. Treatment strategies in toxic epidermal necrolysis syndrome: where are we at? *J Burn Care Res* 2008;29:269–276.

85. Mockenhaupt M, Viboud C, Dunant A, et al. Stevens-Johnson syndrome and toxic epidermal necrolysis: assessment of medication risks with emphasis on recently marketed drugs. The EuroSCAR-study. *J Invest Dermatol* 2008;128:35–44.

86. Clayton NA, Kennedy PJ. Management of dysphagia in toxic epidermal necrolysis (TEN) and Stevens-Johnson syndrome (SJS). *Dysphagia* 2007;22:187–192.

87. Mahe A, Keita S, Blanc L, Bobin P. Esophageal necrosis in the Stevens-Johnson syndrome. *J Am Acad Dermatol* 1993;29:103–104.

88. Schneck J, Fagot JP, Sekula P, Sassolas B, Roujeau JC, Mockenhaupt M. Effects of treatments on the mortality of Stevens-Johnson syndrome and toxic epidermal necrolysis: A retrospective study on patients included in the prospective EuroSCAR Study. *J Am Acad Dermatol* 2008;58:33–40.

89. Pehr K. The EuroSCAR study: cannot agree with the conclusions. *J Am Acad Dermatol* 2008;59:898–899; author reply 899–900.

90. Herman TE, Kushner DC, Cleveland RH. Esophageal stricture secondary to drug-induced toxic epidermal necrolysis. *Pediatr Radiol* 1984;14:439–440.

91. Fleming DT, McQuillan GM, Johnson RE, et al. Herpes simplex virus type 2 in the United States, 1976 to 1994. *N Engl J Med* 1997;337:1105–1111.

92. Genereau T, Lortholary O, Bouchaud O, et al. Herpes simplex esophagitis in patients with AIDS: report of 34 cases. The Cooperative Study Group on Herpetic Esophagitis in HIV Infection. *Clin Infect Dis* 1996;22:926–931.

93. Buss DH, Scharyj M. Herpesvirus infection of the esophagus and other visceral organs in adults. Incidence and clinical significance. *Am J Med* 1979;66:457–462.

94. McDonald GB, Sharma P, Hackman RC, Meyers JD, Thomas ED. Esophageal infections in immunosuppressed patients after marrow transplantation. *Gastroenterology* 1985;88:1111–1117.

95. Mosimann F, Cuenoud PF, Steinhauslin F, Wauters JP. Herpes simplex esophagitis after renal transplantation. *Transpl Int* 1994;7:79–82.

96. Bonacini M, Young T, Laine L. The causes of esophageal symptoms in human immunodeficiency virus infection. A prospective study of 110 patients. *Arch Intern Med* 1991;151:1567–1572.

97. Ramanathan J, Rammouni M, Baran J Jr, Khatib R. Herpes simplex virus esophagitis in the immunocompetent host: an overview. *Am J Gastroenterol* 2000;95:2171–2176.

98. Rodrigues F, Brandao N, Duque V, Ribeiro C, Antonio AM. Herpes simplex virus esophagitis in immunocompetent children. *J Pediatr Gastroenterol Nutr* 2004;39:560–563.

99. Dieckhaus KD, Hill DR. Boerhaave's syndrome due to herpes simplex virus type 1 esophagitis in a patient with AIDS. *Clin Infect Dis* 1998;26:1244–1245.

100. Cirillo NW, Lyon DT, Schuller AM. Tracheoesophageal fistula complicating herpes esophagitis in AIDS. *Am J Gastroenterol* 1993;88:587–589.

101. Cronstedt JL, Bouchama A, Hainau B, *et al.* Spontaneous esophageal perforation in herpes simplex esophagitis. *Am J Gastroenterol* 1992;87:124–127.

102. Connolly GM, Hawkins D, Harcourt-Webster JN, Parsons PA, Husain OA, Gazzard BG. Oesophageal symptoms, their causes, treatment, and prognosis in patients with the acquired immunodeficiency syndrome. *Gut* 1989;30:1033–1039.

103. Epstein JB, Polsky B. Oropharyngeal candidiasis: a review of its clinical spectrum and current therapies. *Clin Ther* 1998;20:40–57.

104. Vazquez JA. Invasive oesophageal candidiasis: current and developing treatment options. *Drugs* 2003;63:971–989.

105. Ganatra JV, Bostwick HE, Medow MS, Beneck D, Berezin S. Candida esophagitis in a child with achalasia. *J Pediatr Gastroenterol Nutr* 1996;22:330–333.

106. Hendel L, Svejgaard E, Walsoe I, Kieffer M, Stenderup A. Esophageal candidosis in progressive systemic sclerosis: occurrence, significance, and treatment with fluconazole. *Scand J Gastroenterol* 1988;23:1182–1186.

107. Schaefer ET, Fitzgerald JF, Molleston JP, *et al.* Comparison of oral prednisone and topical fluticasone in the treatment of eosinophilic esophagitis: a randomized trial in children. *Clin Gastroenterol Hepatol* 2008;6:165–173.

108. Wilcox CM, Schwartz DA. Endoscopic-pathologic correlates of Candida esophagitis in acquired immunodeficiency syndrome. *Dig Dis Sci* 1996;41:1337–1345.

109. Pappas PG, Kauffman CA, Andes D, *et al.* Clinical practice guidelines for the management of candidiasis: 2009 update by the Infectious Diseases Society of America. *Clin Infect Dis* 2009;48:503–535.

110. Wilcox CM, Alexander LN, Clark WS, Thompson SE, 3rd. Fluconazole compared with endoscopy for human immunodeficiency virus-infected patients with esophageal symptoms. *Gastroenterology* 1996;110:1803–1809.

111. Abbasi NR, Shaw HM, Rigel DS, *et al.* Early diagnosis of cutaneous melanoma: revisiting the ABCD criteria. *JAMA* 2004;292:2771–2776.

112. Schneider A, Martini N, Burt ME. Malignant melanoma metastatic to the esophagus. *Ann Thorac Surg* 1993;55:516–517.

113. Sanchez AA, Wu TT, Prieto VG, Rashid A, Hamilton SR, Wang H. Comparison of primary and metastatic malignant melanoma of the esophagus: clinicopathologic review of 10 cases. *Arch Pathol Lab Med* 2008;132:1623–1629.

114. Hwang ST, Janik JE, Jaffe ES, Wilson WH. Mycosis fungoides and Sezary syndrome. *Lancet* 2008;371:945–957.

115. Redleaf MI, Moran WJ, Gruber B. Mycosis fungoides involving the cervical esophagus. *Arch Otolaryngol Head Neck Surg* 1993;119:690–693.

116. Serraino D, Angeletti C, Carrieri MP, *et al.* Kaposi's sarcoma in transplant and HIV-infected patients: an epidemiologic study in Italy and France. *Transplantation* 2005;80:1699–1704.

117. Barrison IG, Foster S, Harris JW, Pinching AJ, Walker JG. Upper gastrointestinal Kaposi's sarcoma in patients positive for HIV antibody without cutaneous disease. *Br Med J (Clin Res Ed)* 1988;296:92–93.

118. Reed WB, Kamath M, Weiss L. Kaposi sarcoma, with emphasis on the internal manifestations. *Arch Dermatol* 1974;110:115–118.

119. Lin CH, Hsu CW, Chiang YJ, Ng KF, Chiu CT. Esophageal and gastric Kaposi's sarcomas presenting as upper gastrointestinal bleeding. *Chang Gung Med J* 2002;25:329–333.

120. Calzona A, Naso P, Puliatti C, Veroux PF, Leone F, Russo A. Massive gastrointestinal hemorrhage in a renal transplant recipient due to visceral Kaposi's sarcoma. *Endoscopy* 2002;34:179.

121. Cairo F, Rubino I, Rotundo R, Prato GP, Ficarra G. Oral *Acanthosis nigricans* as a marker of internal malignancy. A case report. *J Periodontol* 2001;72:1271–1275.

122. Kozlowski LM, Nigra TP. Esophageal acanthosis nigricans in association with adenocarcinoma from an unknown primary site. *J Am Acad Dermatol* 1992;26:348–351.

123. Higgins SP, Freemark M, Prose NS. Acanthosis nigricans: a practical approach to evaluation and management. *Dermatol Online J* 2008;14:2.

124. Rigel DS, Jacobs MI. Malignant acanthosis nigricans: a review. *J Dermatol Surg Oncol* 1980;6:923–927.

125. Atmatzidis K, Papaziogas B, Pavlidis T, Mirelis C, Papaziogas T. Plummer–Vinson syndrome. *Dis Esophagus* 2003;16:154–157.

126. Chisholm M. The association between webs, iron and post-cricoid carcinoma. *Postgrad Med J* 1974;50:215–219.

127. Messmann H. Squamous cell cancer of the oesophagus. *Best Pract Res Clin Gastroenterol* 2001;15:249–265.

128. Bolognia JL, Brewer YP, Cooper DL. Bazex syndrome (acrokeratosis paraneoplastica). An analytic review. *Medicine (Balt)* 1991;70:269–280.

129. Louvel G, Vauleon E, Boucher E, Raoul JL. Acrokeratosis paraneoplastica (Bazex' syndrome) associated with metastatic squamous cell esophageal carcinoma. *J Clin Oncol* 2008;26:5128–5129.

130. Poligone B, Christensen SR, Lazova R, Heald PW. Bazex syndrome (acrokeratosis paraneoplastica). *Lancet* 2007;369:530.

131. Itin PH, Fistarol SK. Palmoplantar keratodermas. *Clin Dermatol* 2005;23:15–22.

132. Patel S, Zirwas M, English JC 3rd. Acquired palmoplantar keratoderma. *Am J Clin Dermatol* 2007;8:1–11.

133. Kelsell DP, Risk JM, Leigh IM, *et al.* Close mapping of the focal non-epidermolytic palmoplantar keratoderma (PPK) locus associated with oesophageal cancer (TOC). *Hum Mol Genet* 1996;5:857–860.

134. Ellis A, Field JK, Field EA, *et al.* Tylosis associated with carcinoma of the oesophagus and oral leukoplakia in a large Liverpool family—a review of six generations. *Eur J Cancer B Oral Oncol* 1994;30B:102–112.

135. Howel-Evans W, McConnell RB, Clarke CA, Sheppard PM. Carcinoma of the oesophagus with keratosis palmaris et plantaris (tylosis): a study of two families. *Q J Med* 1958;27:413–429.

136. Pilarski R. Cowden syndrome: a critical review of the clinical literature. *J Genet Couns* 2009;18:13–27.

137. Salem OS, Steck WD. Cowden's disease (multiple hamartoma and neoplasia syndrome). A case report and review of the English literature. *J Am Acad Dermatol* 1983;8:686–696.

138. Bosserhoff AK, Grussendorf-Conen EI, Rubben A, *et al.* Multiple colon carcinomas in a patient with Cowden syndrome. *Int J Mol Med* 2006;18:643–647.

139. Kay PS, Soetikno RM, Mindelzun R, Young HS. Diffuse esophageal glycogenic acanthosis: an endoscopic marker of Cowden's disease. *Am J Gastroenterol* 1997;92:1038–1040.

140. Kirwan M, Dokal I. Dyskeratosis congenita: a genetic disorder of many faces. *Clin Genet* 2008;73:103–112.

141. Vulliamy T, Dokal I. Dyskeratosis congenita. *Semin Hematol* 2006;43:157–166.

142. Berezin S, Schwarz SM, Slim MS, Beneck D, Brudnicki AR, Medow MS. Gastrointestinal problems in a child with dyskeratosis congenita. *Am J Gastroenterol* 1996;91:1271–1272.

143. Sirinavin C, Trowbridge AA. Dyskeratosis congenita: clinical features and genetic aspects. Report of a family and review of the literature. *J Med Genet* 1975;12:339–354.

144. de Roux-Serratrice C, Serratrice J, Escoffier JM, Granel B, Disdier P, Weiller PJ. Esophageal web in Zinsser-Engman-Cole-Fanconi disease. *Gastrointest Endosc* 2000;52:561–562.

145. Alter BP, Giri N, Savage SA, Rosenberg PS. Cancer in dyskeratosis congenita. *Blood* 2009;113:6549–6557.

146. Chuang TY, Stitle L, Brashear R, Lewis C. Hepatitis C virus and lichen planus: A case-control study of 340 patients. *J Am Acad Dermatol* 1999;41:787–789.

147. Carrozzo M, Pellicano R. Lichen planus and hepatitis C virus infection: an updated critical review. *Minerva Gastroenterol Dietol* 2008;54:65–74.

148. Scully C, el-Kom M. Lichen planus: review and update on pathogenesis. *J Oral Pathol* 1985;14:431–458.

149. Quispel R, van Boxel OS, Schipper ME, *et al.* High prevalence of esophageal involvement in lichen planus: a study using magnification chromoendoscopy. *Endoscopy* 2009;41:187–193.

150. Dickens CM, Heseltine D, Walton S, Bennett JR. The oesophagus in lichen planus: an endoscopic study. *BMJ* 1990;300:84.

151. Westbrook R, Riley S. Esophageal lichen planus: case report and literature review. *Dysphagia* 2008;23:331–334.

152. Harewood GC, Murray JA, Cameron AJ. Esophageal lichen planus: the Mayo Clinic experience. *Dis Esophagus* 1999;12:309–311.

153. Wedgeworth EK, Vlavianos P, Groves CJ, Neill S, Westaby D. Management of symptomatic esophageal involvement with lichen planus. *J Clin Gastroenterol* 2009;43:915–919.

154. Chryssostalis A, Gaudric M, Terris B, Coriat R, Prat F, Chaussade S. Esophageal lichen planus: a series of eight cases including a patient with esophageal verrucous carcinoma. A case series. *Endoscopy* 2008;40:764–768.

155. Schwartz MP, Sigurdsson V, Vreuls W, Lubbert PH, Smout AJ. Two siblings with lichen planus and squamous cell carcinoma of the oesophagus. *Eur J Gastroenterol Hepatol* 2006;18:1111–1115.

156. Calamia KT, Schirmer M, Melikoglu M. Major vessel involvement in Behcet disease. *Curr Opin Rheumatol* 2005;17:1–8.

157. Criteria for diagnosis of Behcet's disease. International Study Group for Behcet's Disease. *Lancet* 1990;335:1078–1080.

158. Balabanova M, Calamia KT, Perniciaro C, O'Duffy JD. A study of the cutaneous manifestations of Behcet's disease in patients from the United States. *J Am Acad Dermatol* 1999;41:540–545.

159. Bayraktar Y, Ozaslan E, Van Thiel DH. Gastrointestinal manifestations of Behcet's disease. *J Clin Gastroenterol* 2000;30:144–154.

160. Yi SW, Cheon JH, Kim JH, *et al.* The prevalence and clinical characteristics of esophageal involvement in patients with Behcet's disease: a single center experience in Korea. *J Korean Med Sci* 2009;24:52–56.

161. Asaoka M, Sakai Y, Kimura J, Ichihara T, Seki A, Ishii M. A case of tracheoesophageal fistula in Behcet's disease repaired with pericardial patch and gastric roll. *Nippon Kyobu Geka Gakkai Zasshi* 1990;38:1549–1553.

162. Orikasa H, Ejiri Y, Suzuki S, *et al.* A case of Behcet's disease with occlusion of both caval veins and "downhill" esophageal varices. *J Gastroenterol* 1994;29:506–510.

163. Bottomley WW, Dakkak M, Walton S, Bennett JR. Esophageal involvement in Behcet's disease. Is endoscopy necessary? *Dig Dis Sci* 1992;37:594–597.

164. The International Center for Nephrogenic Fibrosing Dermopathy Research. Available at: http://www.icnfdr.org/ [accessed September 8 2009].

165. Cowper SE, Robin HS, Steinberg SM, Su LD, Gupta S, LeBoit PE. Scleromyxoedema-like cutaneous diseases in renal-dialysis patients. *Lancet* 2000;356:1000–1001.

166. Firoz BF, Hunzeker CM, Soldano AC, Franks AG Jr. Nephrogenic fibrosing dermopathy. *Dermatol Online J* 2008; 14:11.

167. Ting WW, Stone MS, Madison KC, Kurtz K. Nephrogenic fibrosing dermopathy with systemic involvement. *Arch Dermatol* 2003;139:903–906.

168. Jimenez SA, Artlett CM, Sandorfi N, *et al.* Dialysis-associated systemic fibrosis (nephrogenic fibrosing dermopathy): study of inflammatory cells and transforming growth factor beta1 expression in affected skin. *Arthritis Rheum* 2004; 50:2660–2666.

169. Kucher C, Steere J, Elenitsas R, Siegel DL, Xu X. Nephrogenic fibrosing dermopathy/nephrogenic systemic fibrosis with diaphragmatic involvement in a patient with respiratory failure. *J Am Acad Dermatol* 2006;54 (2 Suppl):S31–34.

170. Daram SR, Cortese CM, Bastani B. Nephrogenic fibrosing dermopathy/nephrogenic systemic fibrosis: report of a new case with literature review. *Am J Kidney Dis* 2005; 46:754–759.

171. Callewaert B, Malfait F, Loeys B, De Paepe A. Ehlers-Danlos syndromes and Marfan syndrome. *Best Pract Res Clin Rheumatol* 2008;22:165–189.

172. Sidhu-Malik NK, Wenstrup RJ. The Ehlers-Danlos syndromes and Marfan syndrome: inherited diseases of connective tissue with overlapping clinical features. *Semin Dermatol* 1995; 14:40–46.

173. van der Peet DL, Klinkenberg-Knol EC, Berends FJ, Cuesta MA. Epiphrenic diverticula: minimal invasive approach and repair in five patients. *Dis Esophagus* 2001;14:60–62.

174. Toyohara T, Kaneko T, Araki H, Takahashi K, Nakamura T. Giant epiphrenic diverticulum in a boy with Ehlers-Danlos syndrome. *Pediatr Radiol* 1989;19:437.

175. Solomon JA, Abrams L, Lichtenstein GR. GI manifestations of Ehlers-Danlos syndrome. *Am J Gastroenterol* 1996;91:2282–2288.

176. Reis ED, Martinet OD, Mosimann F. Spontaneous rupture of the oesophagus in an adolescent with type IV Ehlers-Danlos syndrome. Ehlers-Danlos and spontaneous oesophageal rupture. *Eur J Surg* 1998;164:313–316.

177. Habein HC. Ehlers-Danlos syndrome with spontaneous rupture of the esophagus. Report of first case. *Rocky Mt Med J* 1977;74:78–80.

178. Shovlin CL, Letarte M. Hereditary haemorrhagic telangiectasia and pulmonary arteriovenous malformations: issues in clinical management and review of pathogenic mechanisms. *Thorax* 1999;54:714–729.

179. Lesnik GT, Ross DA, Henderson KJ, Joe JK, Leder SB, White RI Jr. Septectomy and septal dermoplasty for the treatment of

severe transfusion-dependent epistaxis in patients with hereditary hemorrhagic telangiectasia and septal perforation. *Am J Rhinol* 2007;21:312–315.

180. Kjeldsen AD, Kjeldsen J. Gastrointestinal bleeding in patients with hereditary hemorrhagic telangiectasia. *Am J Gastroenterol* 2000;95:415–418.

181. Gallitelli M, Pasculli G, Fiore T, Carella A, Sabba C. Emergencies in hereditary haemorrhagic telangiectasia. *Q J Med* 2006; 99:15–22.

182. Proctor DD, Henderson KJ, Dziura JD, Longacre AV, White RI Jr. Enteroscopic evaluation of the gastrointestinal tract in symptomatic patients with hereditary hemorrhagic telangiectasia. *J Clin Gastroenterol* 2005;39:115–119.

183. Clements SE, Mellerio JE, Holden ST, McCauley J, McGrath JA. PORCN gene mutations and the protean nature of focal dermal hypoplasia. *Br J Dermatol* 2009;160:1103–1109.

184. Miteva L. Focal dermal hypoplasia syndrome in a male. *Acta Derm Venereol* 2001;81:218–219.

185. Clements SE, Mellerio JE, Holden ST, McCauley J, McGrath JA. PORCN gene mutations and the protean nature of focal dermal hypoplasia. *Br J Dermatol* 2009;160:1103–1109.

186. Goltz RW. Focal dermal hypoplasia syndrome. An update. *Arch Dermatol* 1992;128:1108–1111.

187. Sacoor MF, Motswaledi MH. Three cases of focal dermal hypoplasia (Goltz syndrome). *Clin Exp Dermatol* 2005;30:35–37.

188. Brinson RR, Schuman BM, Mills LR, Thigpen S, Freedman S. Multiple squamous papillomas of the esophagus associated with Goltz syndrome. *Am J Gastroenterol* 1987;82:1177–1179.

189. Boothroyd AE, Hall CM. The radiological features of Goltz syndrome: focal dermal hypoplasia. A report of two cases. *Skeletal Radiol* 1988;17:505–508.

43 Esophageal Disease in Older Patients

Kenneth R. DeVault and Sami R. Achem
Department of Medicine, Mayo Clinic, Jacksonville, FL, USA

Introduction

The aging population has become a major social, economic, and political issue. Whereas only 13% of the population was aged 65 years or older in 1990, it is estimated that 21% of the population will be aged 65 years or older by 2030. Currently, older individuals account for one-third of total healthcare expenditures in the United States, and each year persons aged older than 75 years make six times as many office visits to an internist as do young adults. In 2004, the per capita healthcare expense of patients over age 85 years was over US$25 000 per year in comparison to just over US$5000 per year for those aged 45–54 years [1]. The old are more likely than the young to have multiple chronic and often terminal illnesses. They are also more likely to be on multiple medications, which may have unwanted side effects and drug–drug interactions.

Esophageal diseases are common in all age groups, including the old [2]. In a survey in the Netherlands, 16% of a cohort of residents aged older than 87 years described symptoms of swallowing dysfunction [3]. Some esophageal diseases are unique to the older patients, including Zenker's diverticulum, cervical osteophytes, and dysphagia aortica. Other disorders may pose special diagnostic considerations in the old [4]. For example, in the older patient with achalasia there is a higher possibility of secondary achalasia due to a distal esophageal malignancy than in a young patient presenting with achalasia. In some cases, diagnosis may be made more complex because of atypical presentations or coexisting illnesses. Chest pain due to chronic gastroesophageal reflux disease (GERD) may be more difficult to diagnose because of associated coronary artery disease or lack of heartburn in older patients. In addition, there is a clear association between GERD and cardiovascular disease (myocardial infarction, angina, and stroke), likely due to these disorders existing in the same demographic group rather than one disorder

causing the other [5]. Esophageal physiology is adversely affected by many chronic diseases and it appears that, at least for diabetes, the longer the duration of the disease, the more likely it is that there will be changes [6]. Finally, there is a greater potential for older patients to develop complications of long-standing GERD. For example, the frequencies of Barrett's esophagus and adenocarcinoma of the esophagus increase with the duration of chronic GERD.

The diagnosis of esophageal disorders in older patients is complicated by changes brought about by "normal" aging. The concept of presbyesophagus was proposed to explain age-related decreases in esophageal peristaltic pressures, abnormal contractions in the esophageal body, and incomplete lower esophageal sphincter (LES) relaxation and dilation of the esophagus on barium examination in patients aged older than 90 years [7]. With the advent of esophageal manometry, this concept was challenged and the majority of older patients with abnormal peristalsis are now classified into one of the described motility disorders (achalasia, diffuse esophageal spasm, etc.), although a large number are labeled as "non-specific" disorders or more recently as a disorder of ineffective peristalsis [8]. The fate of esophageal peristalsis with aging in both the normal population and in those with symptoms has been extensively debated. Although many have discarded the concept of presbyesophagus, there are certainly changes in the esophagus with aging. These changes are manifest both in the physiology of the esophagus and in the presenting symptoms in older patients, which are often atypical to those seen in younger patients. Up to 10% of patients aged older than 50 years have dysphagia, although they often do not report these symptoms to their healthcare provider [9]. Another study found at least some swallowing difficulty in 15% of subjects aged older than 85 years [3]. In the older patient with esophageal disease, diagnosis is more likely to be delayed compared to younger patients because symptoms are often attributed to underlying cardiac and pulmonary

The Esophagus, Fifth Edition. Edited by Joel E. Richter, Donald O. Castell.
© 2012 Blackwell Publishing Ltd. Published 2012 by Blackwell Publishing Ltd.

disorders. Moreover, older patients are more likely than younger ones to experience complications resulting from aspiration and malnutrition, which often accompany inadequately treated esophageal diseases [10].

In this chapter, we review changes in pharyngoesophageal function with aging and the unique aspects of esophageal diseases, including clinical presentation, diagnosis, and management, in older individuals.

Changes in esophageal physiology with aging

Motility

Upper esophageal sphincter/pharynx

Dysfunction of the proximal aspects of swallowing—upper esophageal sphincter (UES) and pharynx—has been described with both normal aging and with disease in older subjects. Reduction in lean muscle mass throughout the body occurs with age; therefore, the skeletal muscles involved in the oral and pharyngeal phase of swallowing may be affected by aging. In one autopsy study, an age-associated decrease in the number of type 1 (slow-acting) muscle fibers of the pharyngeal constrictor was found [11]. The strength of the tongue and the ability to propel a bolus to the back of the mouth also decreases with aging [12].

These age-related changes may result in functional changes during the oropharyngeal phase of swallowing. Using videofluoroscopy, Ekberg and Feinberg found swallowing to be normal, as defined in young persons, in only 16% of 56 older persons without dysphagia [13]. In another study of 100 asymptomatic individuals aged older than 65 years, 22 had pharyngeal muscle weakness and abnormal cricopharyngeal relaxation on barium swallow, with pooling of barium in the valleculae and piriform sinuses. Some subjects also demonstrated tracheal aspiration of barium [14]. Aging has been reported to affect the coordination of swallowing in some [15], but not other studies [16].

UES function is affected by aging. Using a solid-state intraluminal transducer system, Fulp *et al.* found that compared to persons aged younger than 60 years, healthy persons aged older than 60 years have a lower resting UES pressure and delayed UES relaxation after swallowing (Figure 43.1) [17]. On the other hand, Wilson *et al.* found only marginally lower resting UES pressures, but higher pharyngeal contraction pressures and a reduction in the duration of upper esophageal contractions in older subjects compared to younger ones [18]. We studied the function of the pharynx and UES in a group of asymptomatic patients aged older than 75 years in comparison to a younger control population aged 20–35 years [19]. Both resting UES pressure and the ability of the UES to relax were decreased in the older "normal" population. These findings suggest that resistance

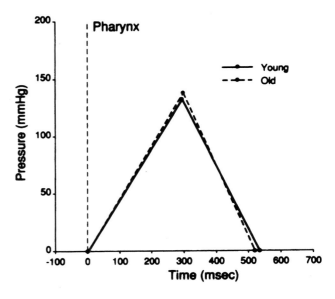

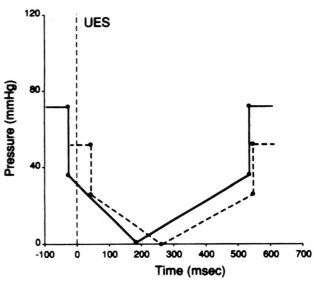

Figure 43.1 A simplified representation of pharyngeal and upper esophageal sphincter (UES) coordination based on computer analysis for pressure dynamics for wet swallows. There is a trend toward delayed UES relaxation in the normal elderly (reproduced from Fulp *et al.* [17], with permission).

to flow across the UES is increased because of decreased compliance with age. Indeed, the duration of oropharyngeal swallowing, as measured by videofluoroscopy, is significantly longer in older than in younger persons [16, 20]. The sensory threshold for initiating a swallow has also been reported to increase with age [21, 22]. Modern imaging techniques suggest that older patients require more central (cortical) input to initiate and maintain a swallow, which may be due to less effective subcortical and peripheral processes [23]. These changes have the net effect of the bolus staying in the oropharyngeal area longer, during which time laryngeal penetration or even aspiration may occur. Some authors have suggested that the reported changes in UES function with age reflect an increased frequency of concurrent illnesses in the old, rather than age-related physiologic changes *per se* [24, 25]. It would seem that the above data support age-related changes in both health and disease.

Esophageal body

Although the effects of aging on the esophageal body remain unclear, some data from pathology studies are available. In the human esophagus, the number of myenteric neurons decreases with aging [26]. This could result in dysmotility related to a relative deinnervation, producing disorders similar to idiopathic achalasia and diffuse spasm. In fact, the pathologic changes seen in the esophagus with aging are very similar to the changes seen in patients with the more specific spastic esophageal motility disorders [27]. Loss of esophageal innervation also most likely underlies the loss of balloon distention-induced secondary peristalsis in older healthy subjects [28]. Secondary peristalsis is dependent on the sensory and motor function of the esophagus, either one of which could be affected with aging. In a study by Hollis and Castell, edrophonium chloride did not increase pressures as readily in older compared to younger patients. They suggested that this indicated weakening in muscle, but not neurologic function [29].

There has long been controversy as to whether "normal" aging itself leads to disordered esophageal function. In 1964, Soergel *et al.* found frequent non-propulsive, tertiary contractions, delayed esophageal emptying, esophageal dilation, decreased LES relaxation, and an intrathoracic location of the LES (indicative of a hiatal hernia) in 15 nonagenarians studied with intraluminal manometry and barium radiography [7]. They concluded that these abnormalities represented "presbyesophagus" and resembled diffuse esophageal spasm. In contrast, in 1974, Hollis and Castell were unable to detect an increase in abnormal esophageal motility in a group of men aged 70–87 years when compared to a control group of young adults aged 19–27 years [29]. However, in a subgroup of 80-year-old men, an age-related reduction in the amplitude of esophageal contractions was noted, implying that the neural system was intact, but that there was weakening of the smooth muscle [30].

In 1987, Richter *et al.*, using more advanced manometric techniques, found an increase in distal esophageal amplitude and duration with age until age 50 years, after which values decreased [31]. In this study, age had no effect on peristaltic velocity, basal LES pressure, or the frequency of double- and triple-peaked waveforms. In another study, manometric findings and diagnoses were compared between a group of patients aged older than 75 years and another group younger than 50 years [32]. The older patients were more likely to be evaluated for dysphagia and less likely to be evaluated

for chest pain. The LES was no different in the two groups, but the older patients were more likely to have ineffective peristalsis. Furthermore, in patients referred for esophageal motility and pH testing, the only subgroup with frequent peristaltic failure was the older patients who had the highest percentage acid exposure [33].

Aperistalsis not otherwise explained by an underlying disease such as achalasia or scleroderma is more common in older persons with dysphagia than in their younger counterparts [34] (Figure 43.2). If presbyesophagus truly exists, these patients with aperistalsis may represent its most advanced manifestation. On the other hand, it is often difficult to truly declare that patients without peristalsis do not actually have achalasia with a different onset or even different pathogenesis, since it has been long suggested that there is a second peak of achalasia in the later years. The differentiation of achalasia from other forms of aperistalsis (including "presbyesophagus") is often difficult and requires a careful comparison of the patient's history as well as manometry, radiologic and endoscopic studies. The prevalence of secondary achalasia related to malignancy seems to increase with age, emphasizing the need for a careful endoscopy and, on occasion, other selected tests such as a computed tomography (CT) scans and endoscopic ultrasound.

The clinical significance of age-related esophageal manometric changes described above is unclear. An increased frequency of radiographic and scintigraphic transit abnormalities in older patients (e.g. "tertiary contractions") has not been shown to correlate with esophageal symptoms [35]. The amount of gastric acid refluxed, as measured by an ambulatory pH system, was shown in one study to increase with age [36]. However, another study found no difference in the frequency of spontaneous reflux between a group of normal volunteers with a mean age of 49 years and a group with a mean age of 22 years [37]. Moreover, Richter *et al.* found no independent effect of age on ambulatory esophageal pH parameters, although older men experienced a significantly greater number of reflux episodes longer than 5 min than did women and younger men [38]. The effect of age on GERD will be extensively discussed in a following section. Age-associated changes of the esophageal mucosa have not been studied critically, but the perception of pain on esophageal distention or infusion of acid has been reported to decline with age [39, 40].

Thus, on the basis of the studies available, it appears that in normal healthy individuals, the physiologic function of the esophagus is preserved with increasing age, with the possible exception of the very old (>80 years), in whom the amplitude of esophageal contractions is decreased. In addition, there are some newer data that suggest an association of GERD with the peristaltic dysfunction that does occur. Finally, there is evidence to suggest that the perception of pain on distention of the esophagus or infusion of acid declines with age, which will be discussed below.

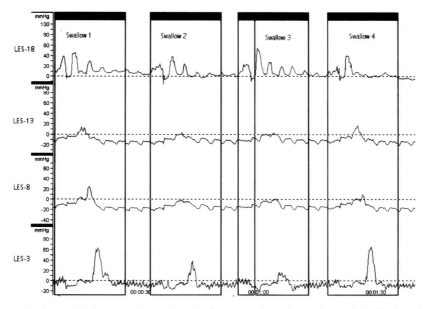

Figure 43.2 Weak, non-transmitted peristalsis from an older patient. The four channels are (top to bottom) 18, 13, 8, and 3 cm from the upper border of the lower esophageal sphincter. A weak peristaltic sequence is seen in the first and fourth swallow, whereas minimal to no activity is seen following the second and third swallows.

Lower esophageal sphincter

In 1977, Khan *et al.* found an increased frequency of abnormal LES responses to deglutition, including a reduced amplitude of the after contraction, compared to results in a group of healthy persons aged younger than 40 years [41]. The older persons also showed reduced amplitude of peristaltic contractions in the upper and lower esophagus, reduced peristaltic velocity, and an increased frequency of simultaneous contractions. Basal LES pressures were similar between the two groups, as has been the case in other manometric studies in healthy older patients. We confirmed this in our study that suggested a fall in LES pressure with increasing amounts of acid exposure independent of age [33]. The length of the LES in addition to the pressure seems to be preserved with aging. Paradoxically, hiatal hernias (both routine and paraesophageal) seem to increase in prevalence with age [42]. We discuss specific issues related to the LES and GERD in a following section, but the majority of the available evidence suggests minimal to no changes in LES pressure with aging. Transient LES relaxations have not been adequately studied in an older population.

Sensory function

Aging has been noted to attenuate visual and gustatory sensation in healthy control subjects [43, 44]. A recent study found that pulses of air initiated the swallowing reflux in younger, but did not in older subjects [45]. It is possible that this sensory impairment could underlie some of the abnormalities seen in the oropharyngeal phase of swallowing studies in both older normals and patients.

Secondary peristalsis tends to fail with aging, which could be due to a loss of the sensory function of the esophagus. Changes in esophageal sensation with aging were demonstrated in a study by Lasch *et al.* [39]. In this study, there was a clear distinction between the volume of balloon distention required to produce pain in a group of older patients compared to younger controls. In fact, in the 17 patients aged older than 65 years, 10 experienced no pain in at least one of the two trials performed, even when the balloon was filled with 30 mL of air. No younger subject was able to tolerate this degree of distention. Weusten *et al.* noted similar findings in a study where there were age-related alterations in cerebral potentials evoked by esophageal balloon distention [46]. The technique of impedance planimetry has been preliminarily reported to document reduced visceral pain perception from both the proximal and mid esophagus of a group of normal older subjects [47]. When older patients undergo a modified Bernstein test of acid sensitivity, they have a longer lag time to symptoms and experience less intense symptoms than younger patients [48]. This decreased esophageal acid sensitivity has also been noted in patients with Barrett's esophagus, and a study suggested that these changes might be related to aging and not just to the Barrett's esophagus [40].

It is reasonable to assume that many of the esophageal motility changes seen with aging are related to nerve dysfunction. While some of these changes are probably intramural, others are most certainly related to degeneration in central innervation. Failure of transmission of afferent, sensory information is most assuredly part of this equation.

One can also assume that impaired sensory perception may lead to a delay in clinical presentation and the presentation at a more advanced or complicated stage of esophageal disease in the older patient.

Gastroesophageal reflux disease in older patients

GERD is common, with the prevalence of its major symptom—heartburn—ranging from 10% to 48% in large population-based studies [49]. The estimated lifetime prevalence of GERD in the US population is 25–30% [50]. There is controversy as to whether GERD is more common in the old than the young. A Gallup survey found that 22% of respondents aged older than 50 years used antacids and other antidyspeptic medications two or more times weekly compared to only 9% of those aged younger than 50 years [51]. In a Finnish survey of 487 older subjects aged older than 65 years, the frequency of daily symptoms suggestive of GERD was 8% in men and 15% in women, and 54% of men and 66% of women reported symptoms at least once per month [52]. In a survey from the United States, heartburn at least once a week was reported by 22% of persons aged older than 65 years [53]. On the other hand, among 476 predominantly male veterans who underwent upper endoscopy to evaluate upper gastrointestinal symptoms, the frequency and severity of esophagitis were similar in those aged older than 65 years and those under age 65 years [54]. Moreover, in a random sample of 2200 residents aged 25–74 years of Olmsted County, Minnesota, the overall prevalence of heartburn or acid regurgitation at least weekly was 20 per 100, and no significant increase in prevalence occurred with age. In fact, the prevalence of heartburn, but not acid regurgitation, declined with age, which supports the previously discussed concepts of impaired sensory function [55]. There may also be some differences in the cause of "atypical" GERD symptoms in older patients. For example, when nearly 3000 patients were studied, GERD [in addition to angiotensin-converting enzyme (ACE) inhibitor therapy] was more commonly found to be the cause of cough in older patients [56]. In general older patients with GERD are less likely to have typical symptoms and are more likely to have symptoms such as anorexia, weight loss, anemia, vomiting, and dysphagia [57]. Whether or not they have GERD, many older patients are treated with acid-suppressing medication. In a review of 98 admissions to a long-term care center, over 60% of patients were on acid blockers [the vast majority on proton pump inhibitors (PPIs)] [58].

Could changes in physiology with aging result in the paradox of more severe reflux disease with less severe symptoms? The risk of complications due to GERD seems to be higher in older patients. For example, Collen *et al.* found erosive esophagitis in 81% of GERD patients aged older than

60 years compared to 47% in those aged younger than 60 years. Barrett's esophagus was also more common in older patients (25% vs 15%) [59]. A recent case–control study from the Veterans Administration found more erosions, ulcers, and strictures in older patients, particularly older, white males [60]. In addition, in persons aged older than 80 years, esophagitis seems to account for a higher-than-expected proportion of patients with gastrointestinal bleeding [61]. These older GERD patients are treated with both medical and surgical therapy, and in a study from Scotland, patients in their 70s were actually 10 times more likely to undergo antireflux surgery than patients in their 50s [62].

Changes in gastroesophageal reflux disease-related physiology with aging

The change in esophageal physiology in disease and in normal older patients was discussed earlier. Many of the purported age-related changes in the esophageal body, LES, and anatomy (hiatal hernia) predispose to GERD. Transient LES relaxations are the single most common cause of reflux, yet the frequency of transient LES relaxations in older patients has not been evaluated. An age-dependent fall in salivary bicarbonate production has been reported, which may increase esophageal acid exposure due to a delay in acid clearance [63]. The integrity of esophageal mucosal resistance and the status of gastric emptying or duodenogastric reflux in older patients have also not been well evaluated.

The effect of aging on the LES has been examined in a series of 95 normal control subjects where age did not seem to adversely affect LES pressure [31]. A hypotensive LES was suggested to be an uncommon finding in GERD, especially in those with mild or moderate GERD [64], while other studies have suggested an inverse correlation between the severity of esophageal damage from GERD and LES pressures [65]. These studies did not focus specifically on the effect of age on the LES, while we recently demonstrated that LES pressure remains similar regardless of age even when patients were segregated by percentage of acid exposure. The lowest LES pressures occurred in those subjects with the most prolonged acid exposure independent of age. An additional study showed an increased esophageal acid exposure with age and that these changes in acid exposure were associated with a decrease in both abdominal LES length and a weakening in esophageal motility [66].

An increased proportion of abnormal peristalsis and delayed esophageal acid clearance has been reported in older patients [67]. It is possible that the variable changes in motility seen in older patients are more related to long-term esophageal acid exposure than to the effects of aging on esophageal smooth muscle. We have found that failed peristalsis occurs more commonly in the group of older patients with the most severe degree of acid exposure [33]. These observations suggest that the increased prevalence of GERD complications may be due to impaired esophageal motility and hence delayed clearance. Additionally, older patients may fail to perceive esophageal reflux episodes due to a defective visceral sensory mechanism. Sustained and prolonged acid exposure experienced over time coupled with blunted sensory perception may be the most plausible explanations for the severity of GERD recognized in patients aged over 65 years. This has not been documented in all studies, but was seen by Zhu *et al.* when they observed that among patients with symptoms of GERD who underwent prolonged ambulatory esophageal pH monitoring, the mean percentage time that the pH was below 4 was 32.5% among 24 older patients with a mean age of 69 years, compared to 12.9% among 147 younger patients with a mean age of 45 years [68].

GERD in the elderly certainly could be influenced by coexisting diseases that affect the esophagus, including diabetes, Parkinson's disease, Alzheimer's disease, amyotrophic lateral sclerosis, and others. One factor likely to be important in the elderly is the use of medications known to decrease LES pressure and thereby increase GER. Drugs such as theophylline, nitrates, calcium antagonists, benzodiazepines, anticholinergics, antidepressants, lidocaine, and prostaglandins are more likely to be administered to the elderly than to the young and may therefore contribute to GERD [69]. An increase in body weight with age may also predispose to GERD [70], which is important since our older population is now more likely to be obese than in the past.

In conclusion, it is clear that esophageal peristaltic dysfunction is common in older patients with more severe GERD, while the fall in LES pressure seen with increased acid exposure does not seem to be age dependent. This impairment in esophageal function may result in a prolongation of acid exposure and potentially could increase older patients' risk for complications of GERD, including ulcers, strictures, and Barrett's esophagus. Additional studies are needed to determine how these physiologic abnormalities translate into differences in clinical outcome in older patients with GERD. It will also be important to determine whether these motility abnormalities are caused by acid reflux or are the cause of the reflux. This may be an unanswerable question, but perhaps a little of each is true. In some patients, reflux may impair motility, which subsequently worsens reflux and sets up a spiraling feedback loop that eventually results in both complications of GERD and impaired peristalsis. These events seem to be more common in older patients.

Role of *Helicobacter pylori* infection and other gastric factors

The acid-peptic injury produced at the esophageal mucosa secondary to chronic GERD is predominantly related to the acid content of the stomach and the resulting activation of pepsinogen. Although gastric acid secretion does not decrease because of aging *per se* [71], gastric acid secretion may decline in older persons with long-standing *Helicobacter pylori*

infection in whom atrophic gastritis develops. Conversely, eradication of *H. pylori* has been reported to provoke reflux esophagitis, possibly by eliminating gastric ammonia, which is produced by *H. pylori* and may serve to neutralize acid in the esophagus [72]. Thus, in the majority of older persons who are infected with *H. pylori*, refluxed material is less acidic than in the young, an observation that may explain in part a lower frequency of heartburn in older patients with GERD compared to young patients and the under recognition of GERD in older people. Curing *H. pylori* infection may actually provoke reflux esophagitis in some patients [73]. Since the prevalence of *H. pylori* seems to be decreasing in the Western world, one might hypothesize that more patients will retain their ability to secrete acid into old age. It is probable that this decrease in *H. pylori* prevalence has more to do with improved public health and increased use of antibiotics than it does with specific attempts at eradication. This increased acid secretion may result in a group of older patients with failing esophageal motility, who now have more acid gastric content and are at a greater risk for GERD and its complications.

Mold and Rankin observed a surprisingly high frequency of distal esophageal alkalinity (>30%) among older patients undergoing ambulatory esophageal pH testing; such persons had a lower frequency of heartburn, but a higher frequency of pulmonary symptoms compared to those with acid reflux [74]. A role for duodenogastroesophageal reflux in more severe grades of reflux esophagitis has been suggested [75].

Obesity and aging

The population in Western counties (particularly the United States) and in many developing countries is becoming obese at an alarming rate. This includes the older age groups as well. For example, in people aged 65–74 years, the overweight status has increased from 57% to 73% and obesity from 18% to 36% comparing 1976–1980 to 1990–2002 [76]. Obesity is an independent risk factor for both GERD symptoms and erosive esophagitis [77]. Increased body mass index (BMI) is associated with complicated GERD, including Barrett's esophagus [78] and esophageal adenocarcinoma [79]. It therefore appears that at least some of the increase in GERD associated with aging may well be related to the concomitant increase in obesity.

Differences in presentation

Compared to younger patients, older patients with GERD are less likely to report heartburn, possibly because of a decline in esophageal sensitivity with age, as previously discussed. On the other hand, dysphagia, chest pain, respiratory symptoms, and vomiting are common [80, 81], and in persons aged older than 80 years, esophagitis may account for a greater percentage of cases of upper gastrointestinal bleeding than in younger persons [61]. Because the severity of symptoms often does not correlate with the degree of esophagitis, diagnostic endoscopy should be considered in all older patients with a new onset of symptoms suggestive of GERD. It may be particularly challenging for the clinician to differentiate chest pain of cardiac origin from that of esophageal origin [82, 83]. Pulmonary and otolaryngologic manifestations of GERD in the elderly, as in the young, include asthma, bronchitis, aspiration pneumonia, pulmonary fibrosis, hiccups, and laryngitis [84]. In a study of 195 older patients with a mean age of 74 years, Raiha *et al.* found that among those with esophagitis on endoscopy, heartburn was absent in 50% and the presence of heartburn did not correlate with the degree of reflux on ambulatory pH study [81]. On the other hand, respiratory symptoms and dysphagia were common, and vomiting occurred in 25%. On surveying 487 subjects aged 65 years or older, these same investigators also found that typical symptoms of GERD were often associated with abdominal symptoms, chest pain, or respiratory symptoms [52]. Restrictive ventilatory defects [85] and lung parenchymal scars and pleural thickening [86] in particular were more common in older patients with increased acid exposure on 24-h esophageal pH studies than in those without abnormal results.

Special considerations related to Barrett's esophagus in older patients

Because GERD is a chronic persistent disorder, it seems likely that the frequency of associated complications increases with increasing duration of disease and thus with age. In 1969, Brunnen *et al.* reported that in Northern Scotland over an 11-year period (1951–1962), the incidence of patients referred for surgery for severe esophagitis was 18 per 100 000 in persons aged 60–69 years compared to only 1.7 per 100 000 in those aged 40–49 years [62]. Despite milder heartburn, older patients may be more likely to have severe esophagitis, strictures, and Barrett's esophagus [68, 87]. The incidence of Barrett's esophagus rises with age. Moreover, older patients with Barrett's esophagus are less symptomatic than younger patients with Barrett's esophagus [40]. On the other hand, older patients with GERD seem to need a greater degree of acid suppression to control symptoms and heal esophagitis than younger patients [59, 88].

Once Barrett's esophagus is diagnosed in older patients, they usually are entered into a surveillance program. Many authors have advocated an end to Barrett's esophagus surveillance at some point as the patient ages. This was because of the unacceptable outcome of esophagectomy in older patients with high-grade dysplasia or cancer. The advent of less-invasive, albeit still experimental, approaches to dysplastic Barrett's esophagus and early-stage adenocarcinoma, such as photodynamic therapy, catheter-based ablation, and localized mucosal resection, has resulted in older patients continuing with surveillance into advanced age. It is important to discuss the goals of Barrett's esophagus surveillance with all patients. If the patient does not agree to endoscopic or surgical treatment for high-grade dysplasia or cancer, continued surveillance is unreasonable.

Differences in Treatment of Older Patients

Therapy of GERD is similar in the elderly and young. However, care must be taken in prescribing drugs to older patients with GERD, because certain medications are more likely to result in adverse effects in older patients. In addition, there is a greater frequency of adverse drug interactions in older patients, because they are more likely to be taking a variety of drugs for multiple medical conditions.

Lifestyle and patient-directed therapy

Changes in lifestyle can be effective in controlling episodes of heartburn and dyspepsia in the elderly as in the young. In fact, emphasis on lifestyle therapy may be particularly appropriate in older patients, in whom additional drug therapy may be undesirable and difficult to afford. The patient should be instructed to eat three meals per day, with the evening meal taken at least 3 h before bedtime, in order to avoid recumbency with a full stomach. Older patients may be more able to comply with these changes due to a more flexible lifestyle. Napping after lunch is common in older patients and may be refluxogenic, especially if lunch is the largest meal of the day. Obese patients should be advised to lose weight. For patients with nocturnal symptoms, the head of the bed should be elevated by at least 6 inches by placing blocks or other elevators under the legs of the bed. Elevation of the head of the bed may be effective in decreasing nocturnal esophageal acid exposure, as assessed by overnight pH monitoring [89]. Alternatively, placing a foam rubber wedge (10 inches high) on top of the mattress and under the patient's head may be as effective as elevating the entire head of the bed [90] and this may be more convenient for some older patients.

Dietary recommendations include a decrease in the total fat content of the diet, because fat lowers esophageal sphincter pressure and thereby increases gastric acid reflux. Agents that may irritate the esophagus such as citrus juices, tomato products, coffee, and probably alcohol should be restricted. Smoking decreases LES pressure and should be discouraged. As noted earlier, medications that may decrease LES pressure should be avoided if possible. Dietary changes in older patients may be effective, but care should be taken in prescribing an overly restrictive diet. Older patients may already be avoiding some foods due to advice on other medical conditions, may have decreased appetite and gustatory sensation, and may be living alone with little desire to prepare meals. Physician advice on diet can on occasion result in unwanted weight loss and contribute to malnutrition in an older patient who is zealous in following recommendations. In many patients the best approach is to help them discover foods and behaviors that trigger their symptoms and then encourage them to avoid those triggers.

The intermittent use of antacids, alginic acid, or over-the-counter H_2-receptor antagonists (H_2RAs) is also appropriate. Antacids must be used with caution because of an increased risk of toxicity in older individuals, including salt overload, constipation, diarrhea, hypercalcemia, and interference with the absorption of other drugs. H_2RAs (especially generic over-the-counter formulations) may provide low-cost therapy for older patients with mild reflux symptoms. Over-the-counter and generic formulations of several PPIs have been approved in the United States and offer an alternative for some older reflux patients.

Medical therapy

Acid suppression is the mainstay of GERD therapy in all age groups. Available agents include H_2RAs (cimetidine, nizatidine, famotidine, ranitidine) and PPIs (esomeprazole, lansoprazole, omeprazole, pantoprazole, rabeprazole, dexlansoprazole). The PPIs provide the greatest degree of acid suppression and are effective for the majority of patients, regardless of age, while H_2RAs are effective in patients with milder disease.

PPIs may be particularly useful in older patients with GERD, who seem to require a greater degree of acid suppression than younger patients to heal esophagitis [53, 79, 91]. Analysis of controlled trials has suggested that, as in younger patients, therapy with PPIs is more effective than that with H_2RAs in older patients with esophagitis [92, 93]. On the other hand, a study comparing pantoprazole to nizatidine or placebo found that the PPI was superior in healing regardless of age and there were no age-related differences within each treatment arm [94]. Rabeprazole and pantoprazole have also been demonstrated to be highly effective in the therapy of GERD [95, 96]. Comparisons of clinical efficacy among agents are limited, although there have been several physiologic studies suggesting small benefits of one agent over another. A large study randomized patients with esophagitis to receive either omeprazole 20 mg or lansoprazole 30 mg daily. There were no significant differences between the outcomes of the two groups, with identical healing at 8 weeks [97]. Similarly, approximately 200 patients with esophagitis were randomized to either omeprazole 20 mg or rabeprazole 20 mg and had identical healing at both 4 and 8 weeks [93]. Finally, another trial of around 200 patients with esophagitis found no difference between omeprazole 20 mg daily and pantoprazole 40 mg daily [98]. Esomeprazole (the s-isomer of omeprazole) has been purified and found to have superior activity to racemic omeprazole in physiology and gastric pH studies. In a large trial, this agent (esomeprazole 40 mg) was found to be clinically superior (in terms of symptoms and esophagitis) to omeprazole 20 mg, with an 8-week healing rate of 94% for esomeprazole and 87% for omeprazole ($P < .05$) [99]. This difference was particularly impressive in patients with more severe grades of esophagitis. Agents with longer durations of action

may be attractive when treating older patients who often need more aggressive acid control, e.g. a new formulation of dual release, dexlansoprazole has been developed and suggested to have a longer duration of action. Another advantage of this agent is that it can be taken independent of meals [100]. An immediate-release formulation of omeprazole combined with an antacid has also been introduced and may have better absorption and also does not need to be taken with a meal [101]. There is a substantial sodium load associated with this product, which needs to be considered in older patients with hypertension.

When using PPIs, particularly in older patients, several issues need to be considered. Plasma clearance of PPIs decreases with age, but no reduction in the dose of PPIs is necessary in older patients, even those with impaired renal or hepatic function [102]. Omeprazole and lansoprazole are metabolized by hepatic cytochrome P450 and may affect the metabolism of other drugs, but the effects have been shown to be clinically insignificant with the exception of one reported issue [103, 104]. That issue involves the interaction between PPIs and clopidogrel, which are more likely to be prescribed together in older patients. Clopidogrel is a prodrug that is metabolized to its active form by the same cytochromes that metabolize most PPIs, and caution is advised when considering giving these medications together since in some patients cotherapy may decrease the efficacy of clopidogrel and lead to adverse vascular events [105]. Long-term use of a PPI may lead to a reduction in protein-bound vitamin B_{12} absorption [106], but is unlikely to cause clinical B_{12} deficiency. Significant fat or carbohydrate malabsorption due to bacterial overgrowth is unlikely with these agents [107]. The effect of PPI therapy on calcium absorption and subsequent bone density has become a topic of concern, especially among older patients, given a 2006 report suggesting an association between PPI therapy and hip fractures [108]. Other possible, but infrequent, associations that should be remembered include an increased risk of community-acquired pneumonia and *Clostridium difficile* infection [109]. Another rare complication of PPI therapy is interstitial nephritis. This does seem to be more common in older patients with a mean age in one series of 78 years [110].

While PPIs have become the treatment of choice for GERD, some patients may be managed on standard doses of H_2RAs. For example, in maintenance trials, PPIs are usually superior to H_2RAs, but up to 50% of patients can be successfully stepped down from PPI therapy. Patients with severe or refractory GERD or with complications of gastroesophageal disease may require higher doses of H_2RAs to promote relief of symptoms and heal esophagitis [111], and in fact are usually better served with PPI therapy. In the older patients, caution is required in using higher doses of H_2RAs. Mental status changes have been described in older patients, particularly those with renal and liver dysfunction, with both cimetidine and ranitidine [112]. Cimetidine in particular may affect the metabolism of drugs by the hepatic cytochrome P450 system, including warfarin sodium (Coumadin), theophylline, and benzodiazepines. Famotidine and nizatidine appear to be associated with low rates of side effects [111], but in patients with renal insufficiency, the doses of all H$_2$RAs may need to be reduced [113].

The routine use of promotility agents for the treatment of GERD should be discouraged. Metoclopramide, a dopamine antagonist that increases LES pressure and improves gastric emptying [114], must be used with caution in older patients because of side effects in up to one-third of patients, including muscle tremors, spasms, agitation, anxiety, insomnia, drowsiness, and even frank confusion or tardive dyskinesia [115]. This has led regulatory agencies in the United States to place a "black box" warning on metoclopramide. Domperidone is a similar agent, but with little to no central nervous system (CNS) interactions, although it has not been proven to be very effective in GERD and is not available in the United States. Cisapride can cause cardiac arrhythmias and has been removed from the market in the United States. Bethanecol, which increases resting LES pressure, is rarely used and is associated with various side effects, including urinary frequency, abdominal pain, blurred vision, and worsening glaucoma, all of which are more likely in an older patient.

Surgery

Surgery can be performed successfully in selected older patients who are reasonable operative risks, but should be avoided in patients with concomitant medical problems that make such surgery hazardous. A recent study found laparoscopic antireflux surgery to be safe and effective in both young and older patients with well-documented GERD [116]. When a group of surgical patients over age 70 years was compared to a group under age 60 years, pre- and postoperative reflux symptom scores and postoperative dysphagia were lower in the older patients, but all other outcomes and complications were similar between the two groups [117]. An additional series also reported similar outcomes with the only significant findings being more atypical symptoms and more impaired preoperative motility in the older patients [118]. Large, paraesophageal hernias are an additional surgical problem in the older patient with GERD, although most suggest that these only be repaired when they are symptomatic or producing complications. Laparoscopic repair of these hernias is technically challenging and also associated with higher complication and recurrence rates, but it can be successful even in very old patients [119]. Regardless of the type of hernia (standard hiatal, paraesophageal, or mixed), older patients are at risk for weak peristalsis and for postoperative dysphagia. We continue to use the preoperative esophageal motility study to guide surgery, particularly in older patients.

Dysphagia

Dysphagia may be caused by many of the diseases that can afflict the young as well as others unique to the elderly. Eating disorders in older patients may result not only from pharyngoesophageal disease, but also from disturbances not associated with the gastrointestinal tract, including cognitive or psychiatric problems, physical disability of the upper limbs, deterioration of the muscles of mastication, sensory discrimination in the oral cavity, dental disease, medications, cervical spine disease (osteophytes), and osteoporosis affecting the mandible [120, 121].

Prevalence and importance

Dysphagia is a frequent symptom in the geriatric population. As the population ages, it was projected that in 2010, 16.5 million people will require treatment of dysphagia [122]. Estimates of the prevalence of dysphagia in the elderly are variable and depend on the population sampled. In studies from Europe, dysphagia occurs in 8–10% of persons aged older than 50 years, yet most do not consult a physician regarding this problem [9, 123]. In a survey in the US Midwest, Talley *et al.* estimated the prevalence at 6.9% [124]. The prevalence of dysphagia is even higher in selected populations, such as patients residing in homes for the aged. Siebens *et al.* reported that 30–40% of older nursing home residents have dysphagia [125]. Difficulties at mealtime were observed in up to 87% of 349 residents in a home for the aged [126]. Oropharyngeal dysphagia in particular may occur in up to 50% of nursing home residents. One study reported that even in older patients without dysphagia, videofluoroscopy shows abnormalities in up to 63% [13]. Irreversible eating and swallowing disturbances are associated with a poor prognosis, regardless of the cause. In a study of 240 residents in a skilled nursing facility, persons who could eat without help had a significantly lower mortality rate at 6 months compared to those requiring assistance in eating [125–128]. Determination of the cause of a patient's inability to maintain adequate nutrition may therefore be of vital prognostic importance.

As in the young, dysphagia in the elderly can be divided into two categories: abnormalities affecting the neuromuscular mechanisms controlling movements of the tongue, pharynx, and UES (oropharyngeal dysphagia), and disorders affecting the esophagus itself (esophageal dysphagia).

Oropharyngeal dysphagia

Oropharyngeal dysphagia (OPD) refers to the inability to initiate the act of swallowing, so that food cannot be transferred from the mouth to the upper esophagus. Patients with OPD generally complain of food sticking in the throat, difficulty initiating a swallow, nasal regurgitation, and coughing during swallowing. Because of associated muscle

Table 43.1 Causes of oropharyngeal dysphagia in older patients.

Central nervous system disease
Stroke
Parkinson's disease
Multiple sclerosis
Wilson's disease
Brainstem tumors
Alzheimer's disease

Other neurologic and muscular disease
Peripheral neuropathy
Poliomyelitis and post-polio syndrome
Paraneoplastic syndromes
Myasthenia gravis
Muscular dystrophy
Polymyositis and dermatomyositis
Amyotropic lateral sclerosis
Inclusion body myositis
Hyper- and hypo-thyroidism
Hypercalcemia
Drugs (botulinum toxin, procainamide, cytotoxics, phenotiazine,
    benzodiazepine, etc.)

Local lesions
Radiation therapy
Oropharyngeal tumors
Abscess
Esophageal webs
Thyromegaly
Cervical osteophytes
Upper esophageal sphincter (UES) dysfunction
Zenker's diverticulum
Isolated cricopharyngeal (UES) dysfunction

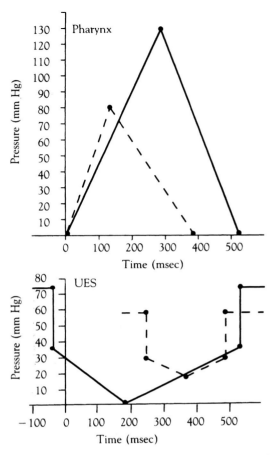

Figure 43.3 Schematic representation of pressures and timings obtained during computed manometry of the pharynx and upper esophageal sphincter in a normal person (solid lines) and in a patient following a stroke (broken lines) (reproduced from Castell [2],).

weaknesses, they may also have dysarthria or nasal speech. In fact, OPD is usually one of several manifestations of a local, neurologic, or muscular disease (Table 43.1).

Central nervous system diseases

OPD can be caused by any disorder that affects the swallowing center in the brainstem or the nerves that modulate the swallowing process, including the fifth, seventh, ninth, 10th, and 12th cranial nerves.

Stroke

Strokes are a common source of neurogenic dysphagia. At least 400 000–500 000 people in the United States are affected each year with a stroke at an estimated cost of more than US$50 billion dollars in direct and indirect costs, and approximately half of them die [127]. The incidence of stroke rises with age and two-thirds of all strokes occur in people aged over 65 years. It is estimated that up to one-half of stroke survivors experience OPD [128–130]. Patients with major strokes often manifest dysphagia as part of their neurologic deficit [131] (Figure 43.3). In a study involving 128 patients with acute first-ever stroke, clinical and videofluor-

oscopic evidence of a swallowing disorder was noted in 51% [132]. Notably, videofluoroscopic evaluations have shown that a large proportion of these patients develop silent aspiration [133]. Stroke-related swallowing difficulties lead to an increased rate of complications such as aspiration pneumonia, dehydration, malnutrition [134], and depression. Dysphagia is associated with pulmonary infections in 32% of stroke victims [132] and carries a high mortality rate at 90 days [135, 136].

Strokes interrupt the normal neurophysiology of swallowing by affecting the transmission of impulses through the corticobulbar pathways, which extend from the inferior frontal region of the cortex to the lower brainstem nuclei. Although the corticobulbar pathways are bilateral, unilateral strokes can induce swallowing difficulties. In cortical strokes, lingual and pharyngeal paresis may be unilateral, thus allowing for a compensatory strategy of turning the head to the paretic side so as to exclude the weakened musculature from the path of the food bolus [131]. Right cortical strokes affect the pharyngeal phase of swallowing, resulting in pooling of secretions and possible aspiration. Left cortical strokes impair the oral phase of swallowing, resulting in pseudobulbar palsy due to disruption of the upper motor neuron. Symptoms include swallowing apraxia and impaired coordination of the oral mastication muscles. In anterior cortical strokes, the motor cortex controlling tongue movement may be affected and thereby results in poor oral control of a food bolus. Dysphagia is more likely with larger cortical strokes than with smaller ones [137]. Other symptoms associated with stroke include dysarthria, ataxia, vertigo, ipsilateral facial numbness, and contralateral body paresthesias. Dysphagia may occur in pseudobulbar palsy or in the Wallenberg syndrome, a lesion in the distribution of the posterior inferior cerebellar artery. Brainstem strokes may affect the swallowing center beneath the nucleus of the solitary tract, which coordinates pharyngeal swallowing, or the nucleus ambiguus, which controls the muscles used in swallowing [24]. Rarely, dysphagia has been observed as the sole manifestation of bilateral strokes [138] or an otherwise occult brainstem stroke [139]. Lacunar strokes are small infarcts resulting from occlusion of penetrating arterioles into the brain and brainstem. These mini-strokes are associated with aging, diabetes, and hypertension, and may produce dysphagia as their sole manifestation. The diagnosis is based primarily on physical findings related to the deficits supplied by an artery. Magnetic resonance imaging (MRI) is frequently used to evaluate the stroke victim but may not be sensitive enough to detect small infarctions [140].There are little data regarding the effect of stroke on the tubular esophagus. The evaluation of esophageal peristalsis by manometry can be challenging in stroke victims, since they often have enough oropharyngeal dysfunction to make initiation of swallows difficult. Repetitive swallowing often results in loss of peristalsis due to deglutive inhibition.

An important concern in patients with stroke is the potential risk of aspiration, which occurs in 33–66% of patients with brainstem stroke [141]. The ability of the patient to maintain protective airway reflexes is essential to prevent aspiration. Multiple approaches have been proposed to identify patients who are at risk for aspiration given the high mortality of this complication. Patients frequently undergo a videofluoroscopic assessment of their potential risk of aspiration. Although there are no controlled clinical trials validating this approach, it is intuitive to speculate that the likelihood of aspiration pneumonia may be predicted by findings on videofluoroscopy. Recent studies suggest that patients suffering with a more severe stroke and those with lesions of the insular and frontal region on brain imaging are more likely to develop prolonged dysphagia and require a feeding tube [142]. The longitudinal course of post-stroke dysphagia remains insufficiently understood. Aspiration persisted at 1 year in 12% of anterior territory lesions versus 58% of posterior territory lesions. Oropharyngeal reflex abolition, pala-

toglossal seal alteration, and pharyngeal delay time at baseline were also risk factors for aspiration [143]. A fiberoptic endoscopic dysphagia severity scale for acute stroke patients may help identify prognostic risk factors as well [144]. Hyoid–larynx approximation is an essential part of the swallowing process, and is related to airway protection. In a recent study, ultrasound evaluation of hyoid–larynx approximation was significantly reduced in stroke patients with dysphagia when compared to controls [145]. Thus, use of these techniques may allow better classification of risk factors for the prevention of aspiration in stroke victims.

Parkinson's disease

Parkinson's disease (PD) is a disorder resulting from gradual degeneration of dopaminergic neurons in the CNS that are thought to be replaced by cholinergic neurons, leading to disorganized control of the central swallowing center [146]. This disorder increases with age demonstrating an incidence of 12 per 100 000 for ages 55–64 years; 108 per 100 000 for ages 65–74; and 257 per 100 000 for ages 75–84 years [147]. Dysphagia develops in approximately 50% of patients and may be due to damage to both the central and enteric nervous systems [148, 149]. The median survival time from onset of dysphagia to death in PD and neurodegenerative disorders (Lewi body) ranges from 15 to 24 months [150].

In patients with PD, OPD may result from tremor of the tongue or hesitancy in swallowing; dysfunction of the pharyngeal phase of swallowing is also likely [151, 152]. Self-report of "no difficulty" with swallowing is not a reliable marker for lack of swallowing dysfunction. In a study of 137 untreated patients with PD who were asked to drink 150 mL of water as quickly as possible, 23% could not completely drink the full 150 mL of water and 84% had functional impairment of swallowing (unable to drink at the speed of published standards). There was a poor correlation between dysphagia reporting and the water swallowing test [153]. PD patients with depression and anxiety may have a higher prevalence of dysphagia than those without those traits [154]. Drooling, tremor, and speech disturbances have been reported to correlate with swallowing difficulties in some patients [155].

Abnormalities may be detected on videofluoroscopy even in the absence of symptoms [156]. These patients not only experience dysfunction of the oral, pharyngeal, and esophageal phases of swallowing, but also have great difficulty in feeding themselves. Using a dynamic videofluoroscopic swallowing function study of 71 patients with PD, a variety of abnormalities have been reported [157]. The most common abnormalities observed during the pharyngeal phase included impaired motility, vallecular and pyriform sinus stasis, supraglotic and glottic aspiration, and deficient epiglotic positioning and range of motion. Esophageal abnormalities included delayed transport, stasis, bolus redirection, and tertiary contractions. Using electromyography and esophageal scintigraphy, 18 patients with PD and 22 healthy control subjects were investigated. This study demonstrated delayed triggering of the swallowing reflex, and prolongation of laryngeal movement and of the esophageal phase of swallowing in PD patients [158]. Bassotti *et al.* reported esophageal manometric abnormalities in 61% (n = 18) of patients with PD, including repetitive contractions, simultaneous contractions, reduced LES pressure, and high amplitude contractions [159]. However, only 33% of patients had both symptoms and manometric abnormalities. Other manometric studies have also shown diminished pharyngeal contraction pressures, pharyngosphincteric incoordination, or synchronous pressure waves, and failure of UES relaxation in up to 25% of cases [160, 161]. Treatment of dysphagia in PD is challenging and two critical reviews have suggested that no specific treatment has been found to be clearly superior and the treatment of choice [162, 163]. Promising results have been described during acute studies involving 14 patients with PD who underwent subthalamic nuclei deep brain stimulation. This treatment induced a significant improvement in pharyngeal motor activity, but not in oral phase or hyoid bone activity [164]. Small open trials also have shown that after swallowing training exercises, dysphagia may improve in patients with PD [165]. A large randomized clinical trial assigned 515 patients with PD or dementia who had documented aspiration of liquids on a video swallow study to drink all liquids in a chin-down posture (n = 259) or to use thickened nectar (n = 133) or honey-thick (n = 123) diets. The main outcome was development of pneumonia by chest X-ray or three respiratory indicators [166]. At 3-month follow-up no significant differences were observed among treatment modalities. An uncontrolled report of four patients with PD showed that percutaneous injection of botulinum A of both cricopharyngeal muscles guided with electromyography resulted in dysphagia improvement, albeit temporarily [167]. Cricophayngeal myotomy has been shown to be effective in small series but it cannot be recommended at this time without more objective data [168]. Clearly, more research is needed in this area. Until then, patients with PD are treated with therapeutic principles similar to those applied to patients with stroke.

Multiple sclerosis

Multiple sclerosis (MS) is the most common inflammatory demyelinating disease of the CNS. It affects between 25 000 and 350,000 people in the United States and about 2.5 million people worldwide [169]. It is a major cause of disability in both the young and elderly [170]. In a study of 143 consecutive patients with MS, 34% reported dysphagia. This percentage rises to 65% in the severely affected patient with brainstem involvement [171, 172].

The disorder typically affects the young; two-thirds are patients between the ages of 20 and 40 years, but in a dis-

tinctive proportion it can develop in later adult life (50s and 60s). Women have a two to three times higher incidence compared to men. The factors more closely correlating with the prevalence of dysphagia in MS are bulbar involvement and severity of the illness [173]. Noseworthy *et al.* compared patients with the onset of MS after 50 years (n = 79) versus those with onset before age 50 years (n = 527). Older patients had a faster progression of disability when compared to the younger cohort [174].

A study of hospitalized patients with MS found documentable swallowing disturbances during a quantitative water test in up to 43%. However, almost half of these patients did not actually report swallowing difficulties [175]. The diagnosis of MS rests on clinical grounds and has recently been revised by an international panel of MS experts in order to include the contribution of MRI and to involve progressive forms of the disease. Details are beyond of the scope of this review but the reader is referred to these sources for more information [176, 177].

Similar to other neurologic conditions, identifying patients at risk for aspiration is a concern [178]. Clinical features associated with aspiration include: dysphonia/aphonia, harsh phonation, breathy phonation, wet phonation, wet spontaneous cough, abnormal palatal gag on either or both sides, some or no swallowing of secretions, abnormal or absent laryngeal elevation, and reclining or lying posture [179]. A recent study validated a 10-item dysphagia questionnaire that may be a useful tool to identify patients at risk for aspiration [180].

Other neuromuscular disorders

OPD may also result from disorders affecting the peripheral nervous system or muscles involving the tongue, pharynx, or UES. In older patients, such disorders include peripheral neuropathy caused by diabetes mellitus, muscular dystrophies, polymyositis and dermatomyositis, hypothyroidism, and hyperthyroidism. In some cases, dysphagia may be the presenting or sole manifestation of the disorder. Depending on the degree of pharyngeal muscular involvement, polymyositis and dermatomyositis may result in weakness of the muscles controlling pharyngeal function and may lead to nasal regurgitation or aspiration, with abnormal pharyngeal transfer demonstrated on barium swallow [181]. These abnormalities may reverse with treatment of the muscular inflammation. Occasionally, abnormal motility of the distal esophagus is also observed [182]. An inflammatory myopathy isolated to the pharynx has also been described [183].

Inclusion body myositis (IBM) is an inflammatory myopathy of unknown cause and distinguishable from other myopathic disorders by its characteristic histologic feature: filamentous inclusions that may be intracytoplasmic or intranuclear. IBM is considered now as the most common acquired muscle disease in subjects over the age of 50 years [184]. Epidemiologic data suggest that 7.9 million new cases of IBM occur in the United States with a prevalence rate of 70.6 million [185]. Clinical features include male preponderance and onset in the 60s or 70s. There is weakness of the distal musculature, which may manifest as falling (due to involvement of the quadriceps), and the involvement of finger flexors presents as difficulty with certain tasks such as turning keys, tying knots, and holding golf clubs. Other features include absence of connective tissue disease, a mixed pattern of myopathic/neurogenic process on electromyography, resistance to steroids, and a protracted course [186]. Dysphagia has been reported in up to 60% of cases [187]. Videofluoroscopy and motility studies usually disclose weak pharyngeal motility. Although several therapeutic attempts have been made, thus far none has resulted in significant benefit.

In the elderly with OPD, it is particularly important to consider hyper- or hypo-thyroidism, since the clinical presentation may otherwise be occult. Thyrotoxicosis can manifest with dysphagia and the clinician should remain alert to this possibility since it is a treatable and reversible condition [188]. Post-polio muscular atrophy results from dysfunction of the residual motor neurons that were unaffected by the original viral infection. Up to 20% of patients who experienced acute paralytic polio are now suffering from residual dysphagia [189].

Myasthenia gravis

Myasthenia gravis (MG) is a disease of the neuromuscular junction affecting the motor endplate. MG is relatively rare with a reported annual incidence of 3–4 million and a prevalence of about 4 per 100 000, although a report suggested a higher prevalence of 9–10 million [190]. There appears to be a higher prevalence in the United States at 20 per 100 000 [191], likely reflecting increased recognition. Although the disease is commonly seen in young women, recent data suggest that the elderly are also affected with the incidence becoming higher in men after age 50 years [192].

The disease is characterized by global fluctuating muscle fatigue that increases with effort. Typical clinical features can vary according to the muscle system involved: ocular (ptosis, diplopia), bulbar (dysarthria, dysphagia, nasal speech or regurgitation, jaw claudication), facial (eyelid closure issues, facial movements) or limb (proximal muscles, arms greater than legs).

Estimates of the prevalence of dysphagia are missing but some reports claim that up to 28% of patients may experience dysphagia at the onset of MG [190]. Unexplained dysphagia can be the first presenting symptom prior to the recognition of other clinical features of this illness. Bulbar muscle weakness causes dysphagia and dysarthria labeled as "flaccid dysarthria" (hypernasality, imprecise articulation, and continuous breathiness with progression and an increase in severity with prolonged speaking). Some cases may not improve even with aggressive treatment [193]. Atrophy of

the tongue with paresis and eventually atrophy of other muscles of the palate and uvula have been described [194].

Videofluoroscopic evaluation may reveal decreased pharyngeal motility, laryngeal penetration, and silent aspiration [193]. Associated motility disturbances include decreased amplitude and duration of the peristaltic sequence and low cricopharyngeal sphincter pressures with normal coordination [195]. Myasthenia-like symptoms might be induced by certain medications (procainamide, amynoglicosides, or penicillamine).

The diagnosis is confirmed by detecting anti-acetylcholine receptor (AChR) antibodies, which are present in 85% of patients and are highly specific [196]. In patients who are seronegative for AChR, and in particular those with predominant bulbar or respiratory muscle involvement, anti–muscle-specific tyrosine kinase (anti-MuSK) antibodies may be present. The edrophonium (Tensilon) stimulation has a diagnostic sensitivity of 72–95% in patients with generalized disease [197]. In this bedside test, the intravenous administration of edrophonium induces resolution of eyelid ptosis or improvement of a paretic extraocular eye muscle. Single-fiber electromyographic (EMG) recording is the most sensitive diagnostic test (95–99%) [198]. Patients with thymoma may present with MG and a mediastinal scan looking for this unusual tumor should be considered in patients with MG.

Treatment includes cholinesterase inhibitors (pyridostigmine). In patients requiring rapid improvement, the use of plasma exchange and intravenous immunoglobulin are effective. Immunosuppressive therapy using a variety of agents, such as steroids, azathioprine, mycophenolate mofetil, cyclosporine, tacrolimus, cyclophosphamide and rituximab, has been reported in small studies [199].

Amyotrophic lateral sclerosis

Amyotrophic lateral sclerosis (ALS), commonly called Lou Gehrig's disease, is a devastating condition and the most common degenerative motor neuron disorder in adults. It is estimated that 30 000 Americans currently have the disease with an annual incidence of 1–2 per 100 000 [200]. The etiology remains unknown, although much research continues to focus on the potential role of glutamate, neurotoxins, and neurotrophic factors. The disease can begin at any time during adulthood but is most commonly diagnosed in middle age and affects more men than women.

ALS is characterized by loss of motor neurons in the cortex, brainstem, and spinal cord, manifested by upper and lower motor neuron signs and symptoms affecting bulbar, limb, and respiratory muscles. It usually presents with problems in dexterity or gait resulting from muscle weakness. The bulbar phase is signaled by the appearance of dysarthria and dysphagia. OPD is characteristically progressive and severe, resulting in frequent aspiration, which usually indicates a preterminal phase of the disease [201]. Studies have reported dysarthria in 93%, dysphagia in 86%, and tongue fasciculations in 64% of patients with ALS who have bulbar symptoms [202].

The patient eventually becomes paralyzed, and approximately 50% of patients die within 3 years after the onset of symptoms, usually due to respiratory failure [200]. Two mechanisms have been described as sources of OPD: delay in triggering the swallowing reflex for the voluntarily initiated swallow, and hyperreflexia and hypertension of the UES [203]. Much of the treatment is directed at controlling symptoms of muscle weakness. Management of the dysphagia is usually a multidisciplinary task. Swallowing therapy can help to ensure oral alimentation for as long as possible and also helps prevent aspiration. Drooling can be a difficult problem. Some patients may be managed with anticholinergic agents such as scopolamine transdermal patches [204]. Nutritional deficiency induced by OPD frequently requires supplemental gastrostomy feeding [205]. The need for placement of a gastrostomy is a poor prognostic sign, in that median survival after gastrostomy placement, at least in one study, was confined to 185 days [206]. In patients with ALS, a marked reduced forced vital capacity (FVC) predicts high mortality (within 30 days) for patients undergoing gastrostomy [207]. A study in the Netherlands found that provided the FEV was 1 L or more and P_{CO_2} 45 mmHg or less, the success rate of gastrostomy placement and feeding in a group of patients with ALS was 89% [208].

Upper esophageal sphincter dysfunction

The high-pressure zone of the UES results from contraction of the cricopharyngeus muscle and the adjacent hypopharyngeal musculature [209]. Cricopharyngeal dysfunction is incompletely understood but may contribute to the development of OPD. As noted above, aging itself has been associated with a decrease in UES tone, although this does not appear to directly result in dysphagia [17]. The term cricopharyngeal achalasia is often used inappropriately to describe putative cricopharyngeal dysfunction when the cricopharyngeal muscle is actually able to relax. The true abnormality is often an inability of the muscle to function in synchrony with other components of the swallowing mechanism or weakness of the pharyngeal muscles, resulting in inability to initiate the opening of the cricopharyngeus muscle [2]. Patients are suspected of having this disorder when they have dysphagia associated with a prominent indentation of the UES area on barium testing and no other additional abnormalities to explain the dysphagia. This radiologic finding is often seen in both symptomatic and asymptomatic individuals. A small recent study of UES histopathology in patients suspected to suffer from cricopharyngeal achalasia found a combination of neuropathic and myopathic features [210]. More studies are needed to understand the etiopathology of this disorder. Other abnormalities in the UES that may result in OPD in the elderly

include truly abnormal UES relaxation, a spectrum of disorders that includes oculopharyngeal muscular dystrophy (true cricopharyngeal achalasia) [211] and premature closure of the UES, or delayed relaxation of the sphincter, as in familial dysautonomia. It has been suggested that dysphagia patients with a manometrically abnormal UES may respond to dilation of this area [212].

Local structural lesions

Various lesions may lead to OPD as a result of obstruction. In older patients, especially if they have been tobacco users, consideration must always be given to the possibility of head and neck tumors. Other obstructing lesions include inflammatory processes, such as an abscess, congenital web, prior surgical resection, an enlarged thyroid gland, and cervical hypertrophic osteoarthropathy. Although cervical osteoarthritis is frequent in the elderly, dysphagia secondary to compression of the esophagus by hypertrophic spurs of the anterior portion of cervical vertebrae is unusual. In a series of 116 patients evaluated for cervical osteophytes, only seven reported dysphagia [213]. The disease is most prevalent in men after age 50 years and the typical clinical presentation includes difficulty swallowing solid foods, but on occasion, they may also have odynophagia, a foreign body sensation or globus, cough, hoarseness, and an urge to clear the throat. Compression by the osteophytes is most common at the C5–C7 levels, with 41% of reported cases occurring at that level [214]. Barium swallow with lateral views suggests the diagnosis, and since osteophytes are so common, dysphagia should not be blamed on the condition unless a solid bolus is documented to be delayed or stopped at the level of the osteophyte. Endoscopy should be performed to exclude an obstructing neoplasm, although the lesions may increase the difficulty of endoscopic intubation. This can be a particular problem with larger diameter and side-viewing instruments. Many patients respond to dietary modification and reassurance. For those with persistent symptoms, surgical excision of the osteophytes may be considered.

Diffuse idiopathic skeletal hyperostosis (DISH or Forestier disease), is characterized by new bone formation and affects 10% of the population [215]. It is both more common and severe in men and its prevalence increases with age. The process begins with ossification of the anterior longitudinal ligament followed by cartilaginous metaplasia and ossification of the posterior longitudinal ligament. Spinal rigidity of a variable degree is the most common clinical presenting feature. Protrusion of hyperostotic formations may cause esophageal compression and lead to dysphagia [216]. The diagnosis rests on plain radiographs of the spine showing a flowing ossification along the anterolateral aspect of at least four contiguous vertebrae in the absence of degenerative or inflammatory changes. Medical management includes anti-inflammatory medications, muscle relaxants, and reassurance, with surgical intervention only for those with unrelenting symptoms [217]. A recent study provided long-term clinical follow up of a limited number of patients (n = 5) who underwent surgical resection of osteophytes. All improved after surgery and at a median follow-up period of 53 months none had recurrent dysphagia [218]. Other common conditions such as ankylosing spondylitis and cervical spondylosis may also cause pronounced anterior osteophyte formation of the cervical vertebrae and consequent dysphagia.

Finally, thyroid cancer can present with dysphagia. The incidence typically peaks in the sixth to seventh decades of life. Neck imaging such as CT and MRI are useful in defining the extent of the disease [219].

Zenker's diverticulum

A Zenker's diverticulum (ZD) is an outpouching in the posterior pharyngeal wall immediately above the UES (Killian's triangle), and is found almost exclusively in persons aged over 50 years. The disorder is more common in males than females [220]. A community study from the UK estimates an annual incidence of 2 per 100 000/year [221]. However, the true incidence may be difficult to evaluate since many patients with small pouches may not seek medical attention [222]. The pathogenesis of ZD is thought to relate to decreased compliance of the cricopharyngeus muscle, which results in increased resistance to the passage of a bolus [223, 224]. Intermittent dysphagia is often the earliest symptom, but when the diverticulum becomes large enough to retain food, patients may develop more classic symptoms of cough, fullness and gurgling in the neck, post-prandial regurgitation, and aspiration. A ZD may become large enough to produce a visible mass, which may gurgle on palpation (Boyce's sign) or to obstruct the esophagus by compression, thereby contributing to esophageal dysphagia. A sudden increase in the severity of symptoms, particularly progressive dysphagia or aphagia, pain, or hemoptysis may suggest the development of malignancy (squamous carcinoma) [225].

Treatment is indicated for all symptomatic patients with or without associated complications. The treatment of choice is surgical and the approach may be external or endoscopic. External surgical treatment of ZD is effective in 80–100% of patients. The preferred approach involves the resection of the pouch (diverticulectomy) plus cricopharyngeal myotomy through a left cervicotomy. Endoscopic procedures involve division of the common muscular septum that separates the esophagus and the pouch. This approach is equivalent to performing an internal cricopharyngeal myotomy and creating a single lumen. Although the pouch has not been removed, it no longer fills and food passes into the esophagus, resulting in symptomatic improvement [226]. The endoscopic approach provides similar efficacy and less morbidity and potential mortality than open surgical approaches. Originally, rigid endoscopes were used but now flexible instruments are preferred with good results reported in over

80% of patients [227]. Recurrence rates are 5–15% and complications occurred in 3–5%, including perforation into the mediastinal space [228]. More recently, endoscopic stapling devices that seal the edges of the incision and, in particular, the end of the dissection line at the bottom of the diverticulum have emerged as more popular treatment methods [229], but there are little comparative data with other procedures and scant information on long-term outcome studies. An Italian study compared transoral stapling (n = 181) to an open approach (n = 116) (stapled diverticulectomy and cricopharyngeal myotomy) [230]. Overall, 92% of patients undergoing the endosurgical approach and 94% of those undergoing the open approach were symptom free or were significantly improved after a median follow-up of 27 and 48 months, respectively. At a minimum follow-up of 5 and 10 years, most patients were asymptomatic after both procedures, except for those individuals undergoing an endosurgical procedure for a small diverticulum (<3 cm). Endoscopic therapies offer advantages over external surgical techniques: short procedure and anesthesia time, short hospital stay (1–2 days) with resumed oral intake within 24 h and a lower complication rate. They can also be used for patients with a recurrent diverticulum following a surgical approach. However, in some situations, such as an elderly, medically unfit patient with minimal symptoms, clinical observation might be the best therapeutic option. Recent reports have noted lodging of endoscopic capsules in a ZD pouch [231]. Patients known to have ZD should be considered for endoscopic insertion of capsule endoscopy.

Diagnostic approach to oropharyngeal dysphagia

In evaluating the patient with OPD, a careful history and physical examination may provide clues to the diagnosis. For example, evidence of a systemic neurologic disorder should be sought. Careful examination of the head and neck for a neoplasm is also important. The diagnosis of ZD may be suggested by a typical history. The major diagnostic study in the evaluation of OPD is a barium X-ray of the pharynx and UES with videofluoroscopy (also referred as the modified barium swallow). Rapid-sequence pictures must be obtained because bolus transfer from the mouth to the upper esophagus requires only approximately 1 s [232, 233]. Use of thick barium or a solid bolus is particularly helpful in assessing the ability of the patient to transfer food from the mouth to the esophagus [234]. The main difference between videofluoroscopy and the standard barium swallow is that the former is specifically aimed at analyzing functional impairment of the swallowing mechanism. Such an evaluation permits the detection of: (1) dysfunction or inability to initiate the pharyngeal swallow; (2) aspiration; (3) nasal regurgitation; (4) obstruction (mechanical or functional) to the normal barium flow, and (5) residual bolus in the pharynx after swallowing. The development of improved computerized manometric techniques has simplified diagnostic testing, particularly in the evaluation of abnormalities of pharyngeal and UES coordination [17, 234]. Identification of an elevated pharyngeal bolus pressure or failure of UES relaxation have been suggested as important manometric findings to guide the decision for cricopharyngeal myotomy or UES dilation [235]. However, manometric evaluation of UES dysfunction is limited due to catheter motion during swallowing, necessitating the use of simultaneous radiography (manofluorography) to determine the location of the sensors [236]. The recent introduction of high-resolution manometry offers a new approach to the evaluation of dynamics of the UES and its disorders. Future studies using this technique may contribute to a better understanding of these challenging patients [237].

EMG recording of the cricopharyngeal muscle is a promising technique that might provide additional helpful information in the evaluation of patients with OPD. Larger studies are needed to determine the exact role of this test in patients with OPD [238]. Evaluation of the cause of unexplained neurogenic dysphagia should include consultation by a neurologist, MRI of the brain, blood tests (routine studies and muscle enzymes, thyroid screening, vitamin B_{12}, and selected antibodies, EMG and nerve conduction studies, and, in certain cases, muscle biopsy or cerebrospinal fluid examination) [128]. Consideration of the risk of aspiration pneumonia should also be part of the evaluation strategy in patients with OPD. A videofluoroscopic swallow and other clinical techniques (see Stroke section above) should be used to identify patients at risk for this complication.

Treatment

Treatment of OPD depends on the underlying cause. OPD associated with systemic illnesses, such as parkinsonism, myasthenia gravis, polymyositis, and thyroid dysfunction, often improves with treatment of the underlying disorder. Neoplasms require resection and, in some cases, chemotherapy or radiotherapy. Unfortunately, treatment itself may also result in dysphagia, because of the removal or loss of function of structures critical to normal swallowing. Dysphagia following a stroke may respond to techniques aimed at rehabilitation of the physical components of swallowing [239]. Manipulation of the diet and proper positioning of the head may facilitate swallowing in these patients. There is less risk for aspiration with thickened liquids (honey-like consistency). In some cases, radiographic assessment of swallowing with various types of food (liquids, semi-solids, and solids) in different head positions may permit recommendations that lead to improved swallowing. Consultation with a speech pathologist trained in swallowing therapy is helpful. There is some encouraging evidence showing that many patients will recover some swallowing function with this approach [127]. To date, pharmacologic therapy for the management of neurogenic dysphagia has

received scant attention with the exception of PD. A small pilot study (n = 17; double-blind, placebo-controlled) reported that nifedipine 30 mg orally resulted in improvement in swallowing in eight patients (five medication, three placebo) at the end of 4 weeks [240]. The exact mechanism of action resulting in improved swallow in these patients remains speculative. For those with permanently impaired swallowing, a feeding gastrostomy or jejunostomy may be the only option.

In patients with neurologic disorders, including stroke and degenerative conditions, who present with pharyngeal dysphagia due to discoordination of the pharynx and UES, myotomy may also be considered, particularly in those with inadequate and incomplete sphincter relaxation and "adequate" tongue/pharyngeal propulsion and laryngeal/hyoid elevation. Studies in small groups of patients with pharyngeal dysphagia have revealed good-to-excellent results with cricopharyngeal myotomy in patients with strokes, motor neuron disease, head trauma, poliomyelitis, and neoplastic or post-surgical nerve injury [241–243]. Obstruction to thick or solid barium at the UES or hypopharyngeal bar of 50% or greater of the lumen throughout the swallow would indicate a defective opening UES. Additionally, the "adequacy" of tongue/pharyngeal and laryngeal/thyroid peristalsis should be established during this study. Cineradiographic studies have shown that myotomy produces improvement in the motor function of the entire pharyngoesophageal segment, not just the UES [244]. Injection of botulinum toxin may provide an alternative approach to cricopharyngeal dysfunction, but its exact role in therapy remains to be defined [245]. In one trial, in 10 patients with well-defined UES dysfunction (incomplete or delayed opening primarily), OPD was improved but not resolved [246]. Passing a large-diameter dilator (18–20 mm) may improve dysphagia, particularly in patients in whom manometric studies show high UES pressure or impaired relaxation [212].

Esophageal dysphagia

Esophageal dysphagia is characterized by difficulty in the transport of ingested material down the esophagus and can result from a variety of neuromuscular (motility) disorders or mechanically obstructing lesions. A careful history usually allows the physician to place a patient into one of these two main categories of esophageal dysphagia. In approaching the patient with esophageal dysphagia, the three most important questions to answer are: (1) Is swallowing liquids or solids associated with dysphagia? (2) Is the dysphagia intermittent or progressive? (3) Is there associated heartburn? The presence of additional associated symptoms, including chest pain, and nocturnal symptomatology and/or weight loss may also provide helpful clues to the diagnosis (see Chapter 1) [247].

The major neuromuscular (motility) disorders to be considered in older patients include achalasia, distal esophageal

Table 43.2 Esophageal causes of dysphagia in older patients.

Motility disorders
Achalasia
Spastic disorders
Scleroderma
Gastroesophageal reflux disease (GERD)-related dysmotility
Diabetic dysmotility
Non-specific aperistalsis or weak esophagus

Structural lesions
GERD-related strictures
Lower esophageal ring
Carcinoma
Esophageal webs
Medication injury
Neoplasms
Dysphagia aortica
Adenopathy
Mid and distal esophageal diverticula

spasm and related disorders, and scleroderma. As noted above, in some elderly patients with dysphagia, the principal manometric finding is aperistalsis not associated with a classic primary motility disorder [34]. The major mechanical causes of esophageal dysphagia in the elderly include esophageal carcinoma, peptic strictures, rings or webs, vascular lesions, and medication-induced esophageal injury (Table 43.2). In general, motility disorders are characterized by dysphagia for both solids and liquids, whereas mechanical obstructing lesions initially cause dysphagia for solids only.

Achalasia

Achalasia is an esophageal disorder of undetermined etiology with an estimated annual incidence of 0.3–1 per 100 000, depending on the country where the disease is studied [248]. It is characterized by slowly progressive dysphagia for solids and liquids followed by gradual weight loss (see Chapter 13). The onset of achalasia is usually between ages 20 and 40 years, but the incidence of the disease increases with age with a second peak occurring in the elderly [249].

The clinical and manometric presentation of achalasia in the elderly is similar to that observed in younger counterparts. However, Clouse *et al.* found in a small study (n = 13) of older patients with idiopathic achalasia (mean age 79 ± 2 years) that fewer complained of chest pain (27% vs 53%), and the pain was less severe. In addition the LES residual pressure was significantly lower [249]. In a large retrospective study in older patients, achalasia was associated with a significant increase in risk for pulmonary complications, malnutrition, and gastroesophageal cancer [250]. In the older patient with long-standing achalasia, extreme dilatation and tortuosity of the esophagus as seen on barium X-ray may result in the so-called sigmoid esophagus.

In an older patient with achalasia, it is important to perform an upper endoscopy (including a retroflexed view of the gastroesophageal junction), with biopsy of any suspicious area to exclude the possibility of secondary achalasia caused by a cancer that may produce clinical, radiographic, and manometric abnormalities similar to these associated with idiopathic achalasia [251]. Tumors most likely to be associated with secondary achalasia are proximal gastric cancers and distal esophageal cancers. Occasionally, pancreatic cancer, lung cancer, breast cancer, mesothelioma, hepatocellular carcinoma, sarcoma, and lymphoma can present in this manner [252–254]. Secondary achalasia should be suspected in a patient with the clinical triad of age over 50 years, dysphagia of less than 1 year's duration, and weight loss of more than 15 lb [247]. However, this triad is not specific and can also be associated with idiopathic achalasia. Moreover, squamous cell carcinoma may complicate long-standing achalasia [255]. Endoscopic ultrasonography may be particularly sensitive in detecting small neoplasms before they are visible at endoscopy [256], but the role of routine endoscopic ultrasound to exclude malignancy in achalasia has not been established.

As in the young patient with achalasia, treatment of the older patient can be medical or surgical, and the choice depends on the preference and expertise of the treating physicians, the overall health of the patient, and the patient's preference after being properly apprised of the techniques, risks, and expected outcomes. The principal options are pneumatic dilatation, surgical myotomy, and injection of botulinum toxin. One report has suggested that pneumatic dilatation may be particularly suitable for older patients in whom improvement in dysphagia is often sustained after pneumatic dilatation and the need for surgical myotomy is infrequent [257]. In fact, patients younger than 40 years had a significantly poorer response to pneumatic dilatation (2-year remission rate of 67%) than did patients older than 40 years (2-year remission rate of 29%) [258]. More prolonged relief in older patients may be related to a weaker tissue resistance with aging, which allows for easier disruption of the smooth muscle fibers. On the other hand, an esophageal perforation after pneumatic dilation may be particularly devastating in an older patient with a risk of considerable morbidity and potential mortality. Myotomy of the abnormal sphincter (Heller procedure) has also been followed by a good outcome in carefully selected older patients, although surgery is generally associated with a higher frequency of side effects, including GER, compared to pneumatic dilatation [259]. In 1991, Shimi *et al.* described the first case of achalasia treated by a minimally invasive approach [260]. In 1992, Pellegrini *et al.* published the first series in the English literature including 17 cases treated via a thoracoscopic approach [261]. Minimally invasive surgery via the abdominal laparoscopic approach provides effective short-term improvement in achalasia that compares favorably with the open surgical approach [262]. The abdominal approach allows for an easy to perform antireflux procedure and offers several other technical advantages over the thoracoscopic approach [263]. Therefore, laparoscopic myotomy has emerged as a preferred technique for the surgical management of achalasia. A recent study noted a three-fold increase in Heller myotomies in the USA from 1993 to 2005 with an improved shorter hospital stay in higher volume centers [264]. A European study of 26 patients with advanced age showed that Heller myotomy with a Toupe funduplicaton was effective and safe even in older patients (mean age 69.7 years) [265]. Patient selection remains influenced by the ability of the older patient to tolerate general anesthesia (although the same can be said of pneumatic dilation with its inherent risk of perforation, which usually requires a thoracotomy).

With increasing age, potential complications such as squamous carcinoma or even Barrett esophagus and adenocarcinoma (following surgical disruption of the LES barrier) can occur. In fact, 8.5% of a series of 331 patients treated by esophageal balloon dilation developed Barrett's esophagus; one had high-grade dysplasia and three adenocarcinoma [266].

In the older patient with other serious medical problems in whom both pneumatic dilatation and surgery are high risk (American Society of Anesthesiology class ≥ III) or those with challenging anatomic risk factors, such as a tortuous megaesophagus or epiphrenic diverticulum), injection of botulinum toxin into the LES may provide symptomatic relief, at least temporarily [267, 268]. Unfortunately, treatment frequently has to be repeated due to symptom recurrence, resulting in increasing costs. Although botulinum toxin is devoid from major side effects [269], recent troubling reports described a death in a patient suffering from a fatal heart block following therapy with this agent and urinary retention in another case [270, 271].

Self-expanding stents may offer temporary relief in older patients unable to undergo surgery but in need to improve quality of life [272]. An uncontrolled, prospective study of 75 patients with achalasia in China used a specially designed 30-mm self-expanding metal stent, and found a 96% clinical remission at 1-year follow-up and sustained remission at 5 and 10 years in 100% and 83% of patients, respectively [273]. Stent migration, a common problem with stents in benign strictures, occurred only in 5.3% of the cases and no patient developed a perforation or obstruction. If this study can be confirmed, a specially designed stent may be useful and perhaps safer than pneumatic dilation.

Medical therapy with smooth muscle-relaxing agents, such as isosorbide dinitrate or nifedipine given sublingually before meals, has not proven effective [274]. Sildenafil (Viagara) has recently emerged as a drug that may have a potential application for the treatment of achalasia. In a preliminary study of 14 patients with achalasia, sildenafil

caused a significant decrease in LES pressure lasting for less than 1 h. No data were provided regarding the effects on clinical parameters [275]. Further studies are needed to determine the clinical efficacy and safety of this agent in patients with achalasia. For the rare patient with refractory dysphagia to repeated attempts at balloon dilation and/or surgical myotomy and botulinum toxin injection, experienced surgeons at tertiary centers have resorted, as a last option, to esophagectomy through a transhiatal approach using the stomach as esophageal substitute [276]. This is a major operation of last resort that must be reserved for the medically fit patient; gastrostomy feeding may be a better alternative for the older patient, particularly if they have considerable comorbidities.

Distal esophageal spasm and related disorders

Esophageal motility testing in patients with chest pain and/or dysphagia commonly reveals a spectrum of abnormal patterns whose cause, pathophysiology, and importance remain to be determined. In an effort to provide a critical frame of reference that may serve as a tool for clinicians and investigators alike, Spechler and Castell have proposed a new classification of esophageal motility abnormalities applicable to all ages (see Chapter 8) [277]. A recent Australian audit of 452 esophageal motility studies found that older patients (132 patients were >65 years) tended to have more spastic motor disorders (P < .06) than younger counterparts [278]. Diffuse esophageal spasm is a term used for over 100 years to describe patients with intermittent dysphagia for both solids and liquids, often in association with chest pain. Esophageal manometry shows normal peristalsis interrupted by simultaneous (non-peristaltic) contractions. Data in 53 patients found that the abnormality is confined to the distal esophagus and is not seen in the proximal areas; thus, the authors recommended the term "distal esophageal spasm" (DES) rather than "diffuse" spasm to describe this entity [279]. There are no data on the impact of age, gender, or race on the prevalence of DES. The etiology of DES has not been established. Rao *et al.*, using esophageal impedance planimetry and balloon distention studies, found that disturbed esophageal sensory processing is more likely to correlate with symptoms than abnormal esophageal motility [280]. These findings support the theory that esophageal dysmotility may represent a marker associated with a patient's symptoms rather than the cause. Others argue that the abnormal esophageal motility originates in deeper layers of the muscularis that are not amenable to detection by conventional manometry but can be observed during esophageal intraluminal sonography [281]. The structural basis for these abnormal esophageal motility patterns has been difficult to study since most affected subjects do not require surgery and the benign nature of the disease does not result in death and subsequent autopsy. Whether some of these patients represent an early spectrum of achalasia is unclear. Disorders of the autonomic nervous system have also been noted in some patients [282]. Increased frequency of psychiatric diagnoses has been reported in patients with spastic esophageal disorders [283]. To date, no single explanation has provided a satisfactory basis for these patients' abnormal motility, although many of the changes noted could be explained by a loss of innervation or loss of muscle function, which may be particularly important in the older patient with a motility disorder.

The aim of treatment of DES is to correct peristaltic dysfunction and improve symptoms. Agents such as nitrates, calcium antagonists (nifedipine or diltiazem), sedatives, and anticholinergic compounds may be helpful; however, there is poor correlation between improvement in motility changes and clinical response. These agents should be used carefully in older patients who may be taking other drugs that could predispose them to orthostatic changes and put them at risk of falling. We, as well as others, have reported the frequent coexistence of GERD in patients with spastic dysmotility, underscoring the importance of an initial therapeutic antireflux trial in this population [284, 285]. Occasionally, esophageal dilatation provides relief, and in severe, refractory cases, esophageal myotomy may be considered [286]. Many patients improve after being reassured that their chest pain is esophageal, not cardiac, in origin.

Nitric oxide (NO) is a major inhibitory neurotransmitter in the gastrointestinal tract. *In vivo* studies in humans have shown that by removing NO or inhibiting its production with N-monomethyl-L-arginine, the simultaneous contractions characteristic of DES can be induced [287, 288]. Therefore, pharmacologic agents that result in augmentation of NO may improve the clinical and manometric patterns of patients with hypercontractile responses. In a small study of six healthy volunteers and 11 patients with a variety of spastic motility disorders, sildenafil (Viagra) significantly reduced LES pressure vector volume and distal esophageal amplitude in healthy controls. Manometric improvement was also observed in nine of the 11 patients with hypercontractile esophageal motility; however, only four of these reported symptomatic improvement and two of these four discontinued drug therapy due to side effects [289]. Larger, placebo-controlled trials are needed to determine whether this compound or other related agents may be of benefit to patients with spastic esophageal disorders. Contraindications for use of this agent may be more common in older patients and include use of nitrates, cardiovascular disease, bleeding disorders, and active peptic ulcer disease. Miller *et al.* completed an open-label trial of botulinum toxin in 29 patients with spastic motility disorders other than achalasia [290]. They found that 72% of the patients experienced symptomatic improvement. No information was provided regarding the effects of botulinum toxin on esophageal manometry. The mean duration of response was 6.2 months and six of the nine responders required a third dose to sustain remis-

sion. Placebo-controlled trials are needed to confirm the results of this study, although the risk of botulinum toxin therapy is low enough that offering it to patients with spastic dysmotility of the esophagus seems reasonable [291]. Surgical treatment of DES is used as a last resort for those patients refractory to medical therapy. This approach is tempered by the fact we understand neither the cause of this disorder nor the long-term course of these patients [292]. A comprehensive review of published literature of surgical series showed that there are no clinical controlled trials, and that outcomes for success are variable [293]. For those highly selected patients, when referred to surgery, a myotomy and partial fundoplication is the preferred surgical approach.

Scleroderma

Scleroderma (systemic sclerosis) is a multisystem disease affecting women three to four times more commonly than men, with symptoms occurring in their 20s to 40s. It is a relatively rare disease with 10 new cases per 1 million adults per year [294]. Recent medical advances and improvements in therapy now allow these patients to reach middle age or beyond. Esophageal involvement occurs in more than 80% of patients with scleroderma and correlates with the presence of Raynaud's phenomenon (see Chapter 18) [295, 296]. Those with a positive anticentromere antibody have more pronounced esophageal involvement when compared to those who are positive for other markers commonly observed in scleroderma, such as anti-Sc170 antibodies or antinuclear antibodies [297]. Patients with scleroderma often experience slowly progressive dysphagia for both solids and liquids, as in achalasia. However, in scleroderma, unlike achalasia, heartburn is a prominent symptom and up to 40% of patients with GERD due to scleroderma develop a peptic esophageal stricture and many develop Barrett's esophagus [298]. Manometric findings in scleroderma include decreased LES pressure and feeble peristalsis in the lower esophagus with preserved peristalsis in the upper esophagus. Videoradiology and manometry can demonstrate abnormalities in up to 80%, but up to a third of these patients may be asymptomatic, underscoring the lack of relationship between tests and symptoms [299]. Any patient with aperistalsis of the distal esophagus and a weak LES should be examined for signs of systemic scleroderma, and selected patients should have antibody testing to exclude the disease. This is particularly important in older patients where these motility changes may be inaccurately ascribed to presbyesophagus. Recent studies using 24-h impedance–pH monitoring off-PPI therapy have shown a more severe acid and non-acid reflux and more proximal extent of the refluxate in patients with scleroderma and interstitial lung disease [300].

The treatment of esophageal involvement in scleroderma includes measures to treat severe GERD, primarily using high doses of PPIs. Surgery has been avoided since fundoplication has the potential for worsening dysphagia in the setting of poor esophageal peristalsis. Other options, such as biliary diversion and esophagectomy, have been described, but carry a high morbidity, especially in the elderly. Given the rarity of the disease and the even more infrequent referral of patients for surgery, most surgical series consist of few patients and uncontrolled studies, which makes it difficult to draw objective conclusions [301, 302].

Esophageal cancer

In any older patient with new-onset dysphagia, cancer should be the primary initial diagnostic consideration. In esophageal cancer, dysphagia is usually progressive, initially for solids and then for liquids, and is associated with weight loss. In patients with squamous cell carcinoma of the esophagus, there is often a history of tobacco and alcohol use. The principal risk factor for adenocarcinoma is Barrett's esophagus in long-standing GERD, and over the past two decades, the incidence of adenocarcinoma of the esophagus (as well as of the gastric cardia) has risen faster than that of most other cancers [303]. In addition to aging and longer duration of disease, additional risk factors have been identified and include gender, race, obesity, reflux symptoms, smoking, and diet. Factors that may protect against the development of adenocarcinoma include infection with *H. pylori*, a diet rich in fruits and vegetables, and consumption of aspirin and non-steroidal anti-inflammatory drugs (NSAIDs0 [304].

The diagnosis of esophageal cancer may be suggested from a barium X-ray study, but confirmation with tissue diagnosis requires endoscopy with biopsy, which is safe and well tolerated in the elderly [305]. The treatment of choice for esophageal cancer is surgical resection (with or without preoperative chemotherapy and radiation, depending on the stage of the cancer), which can be performed successfully in selected older patients with no or few coexisting medical problems [306–309]. Studies in the 1980s showed a higher surgical mortality for patients aged over 80 years when compared to younger counterparts [310]. More contemporary, albeit small series, suggest that age alone should not be used as a selection criteria not to undergo esophageal resection [311]. Unfortunately, many older patients are poor operative risks, and the disease is often unresectable at the time of diagnosis. CT scanning and endoscopic ultrasonography should be used to determine stage and potential for resection. Endoscopic ultrasonography with biopsy of any suspicious lymph nodes may be even more important in the older patient, since accurate staging may avoid unnecessary surgery in these patients with greater risk of operative morbidity and mortality. Laser ablation and photodynamic therapy also have shown promise in the treatment of Barrett's esophagus, with or without dysplasia or early cancer [312–314]. In patients who are poor operative risks or who have unresectable disease, palliation with radio-

therapy, chemotherapy, or both may be considered. For relief of dysphagia, bougienage or laser photocoagulation of obstructing esophageal lesions, photodynamic therapy, or endoscopic insertion of an expandable mesh stent or silastic prosthesis are options (see Chapter 34). In general, the prognosis of esophageal cancer is poor, with a 5-year survival rate of less than 5%. The prognosis is much better when cancer is detected early as part of endoscopic surveillance in Barrett's esophagus.

Peptic stricture

Peptic strictures are estimated to occur in 7–23% of patients with untreated reflux disease, especially older men [315]. Patients with peptic strictures usually present with progressive dysphagia for solids in the setting of a long history of heartburn and other symptoms of GERD. Patients with strictures are usually older than patients with GERD but no stricture, presumably because strictures form over a long period of time [316]. Peptic strictures can be demonstrated by barium radiography, but endoscopy is mandatory to exclude carcinoma. The strictures are typically smooth, tapered, and of varying lengths. If they are located above the distal esophagus, Barrett's esophagus may be found.

Most patients with a peptic stricture can be managed with intermittent dilatation using standard Maloney or Savary dilators in combination with aggressive long-term antireflux therapy. Recurrence of esophageal stricture necessitating repeated dilation treatment is more likely in those patients reporting a history of weight loss, and less likely in those reporting heartburn at initial presentation [317]. Data indicate that following dilation of peptic esophageal strictures, treatment with a PPI significantly decreases the need for esophageal dilation and maybe more cost-effective [318, 319]. If the stricture does not respond to conservative therapy, intralesional endoscopic steroid injection may be a useful adjunctive therapy to esophageal dilation [320]. A number of studies have shown the benefits of laparoscopic antireflux surgery in patients with refractory peptic strictures. For instance, Klingler *et al.* noted a significant decrease in the need for esophageal dilation after surgery when compared to preoperative intervention [321]. For patients with recalcitrant strictures not responding to medical therapy, preliminary reports suggest that self-expandable stents may offer a potential rescue approach [322]. However, complications such as chest pain, bleeding, esophageal perforation, worsening GERD, and stent migration have been described.

Rings or webs

Rings or webs usually present with intermittent dysphagia for solids. Most symptomatic rings present after age 50 years, and there is no difference in the prevalence of rings based on gender. Rings are seen in 6–18% of routine barium examinations, while symptomatic rings occur in about 0.5%

of examinations [323]. The first episode of dysphagia frequently occurs while the patient is eating steak or bread, so the disorder has been termed the "steakhouse syndrome." Often the bolus can be forced down by drinking liquids, but occasionally it must be regurgitated, after which the meal can usually be finished without difficulty. Barium swallow with a solid bolus makes the best diagnosis, and endoscopy is indicated to facilitate dilation and if there is any question about the diagnosis.

The most common type of ring is a Schatzki's ring, which is composed of invaginated mucosa located at the gastro-esophageal mucosal junction [324]. The cause of a lower esophageal ring remains a subject of debate. Theories range from a congenital lesion to pill-induced esophageal inflammation. There is conflicting information about the association of these rings with GERD [325, 326]. Experience from 41 patients identified GERD in 68% [327]. On barium swallow, rings are seen approximately 3–4 cm above the diaphragm. They produce symptoms when the lumen is narrowed to less than 12 or 13 mm. Treatment usually consists of dilatation of the esophagus with a large-caliber bougie. If symptoms occur infrequently, careful chewing of food may suffice. In patients who do not respond to standard bougienage, electrocautery incision and even neodynium–yttrium–aluminium–garnet (Nd:YAG) have been reported to provide successful outcome in small number of cases (see Chapter 15). A small study from Greece showed that in patients randomized to esophageal dilation and PPI therapy versus dilation and no PPI therapy there was a higher relapse in those not receiving acid inhibition [328]. Hiatal hernias predispose to Schatzki's ring and are more common with age. Other factors that may increase the incidence of symptomatic rings in older patients include oropharyngeal and dental difficulties, which decrease mastication and weaken peristaltic pressures.

Eosinophilic esophagitis (EoE) is a disorder characterized by an increased eosinophilic infiltration of the esophageal mucosa coupled with esophageal symptoms, typically recurrent dysphagia and history of food impaction [329]. Endoscopic findings include multiple concentric rings, vertical furrows, and white specs [330].This disease was recognized first in the pediatric literature but it is now well known to affect adults also [331]. Although the disease typically has a tendency to affect younger male adults, a number of reports have also identified older patients with EoE. This disorder is discussed in detail in Chapter 36.

Vascular compression

The term dysphagia aortica was first used by Pape [332] in 1932 to describe difficulty in swallowing caused by external compression from a tortuous or aneurysmal aorta (Figure 43.4). Dysphagia aortica is a disorder of the elderly hypertensive patient who is more often female [333]. Radiographic findings include a prominent indentation of aortic arch on

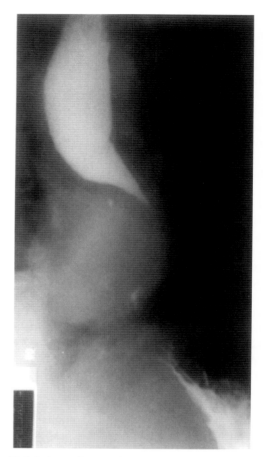

Figure 43.4 Barium radiograph from a 72-year-old patient with dysphagia aortica from a thoracic aortic aneurysm. Compression of the barium-filled distal esophagus produces a pseudoachalasia appearance.

a plain chest radiograph. On barium swallow, features include a partial esophageal obstruction at the aortic arch area, pulsatile movement of barium synchronous with aortic pulsation, and a flattened contour of the left margin of the esophagus [334]. Endoscopic findings include stenosis, band-like pulsatile extrinsic compression, or kinking of the esophagus [335]. Esophageal manometry may reveal a localized high-pressure barrier with superimposed oscillations synchronous with aortic pulsation confined to one transducer [336]. This manometric finding is interesting, but lacks specificity. Mittal *et al.* [336] and Nguyen *et al.* [337] reported similar patterns in healthy controls and in dysphagia lusoria (compression of the esophagus by an aberrant subclavian vessel). Surprisingly, CT has not been found as helpful in the evaluation of dysphagia aortica, but the incorporation of CT angiography may improve diagnostic yield; vascular MRI may prove to be a more useful diagnostic technique. Treatment is usually conservative, such as dietary modifications, and occasionally for those unable to swallow the insertion of a feeding tube. Esophageal dilation would seem contraindicated for theoretical fear of injury to the aorta, but it has been used in some cases. Surgery has also been performed on a number of cases but is rarely the treatment of choice due to the advanced age of these patients and coexisting comorbities [338].

Occasionally, the esophagus may be compressed by a markedly enlarged left atrium [339]. Rarely, exsanguinating hemorrhage may result from penetration of an esophageal ulcer into an adjacent major blood vessel [340]. Several cases have been identified of aortaoesophageal fistulas. This is a rare and lethal complication caused by fistulization of an expanding atherosclerotic thoracic aortic aneurysm into the esophagus, or less commonly, by a reflux-associated ulcer into the aorta [341]. Aortosophageal fistulas can be also caused by a penetrating carcinoma of the esophagus after esophageal surgery, following radiation to the mediastinum, tuberculosis of the mediastinum, mycotic aneurysm, pseudoaneurysm, foreign bodies, and after repair of a thoracic aortic aneurysm. All of these disorders disproportionately affect older individuals.

Medication-induced esophageal injury

Medication-induced esophageal injuries occur when caustic medicinal preparations dissolve in the esophagus rather than passing into the stomach as intended. Injury of this type has been termed pill esophagitis or pill-induced esophageal injury. This is a common disorder with nearly 1000 documented cases reported in the world's literature and an estimated 10 000 cases per year occurring in the United States [342]. Elderly patients are at particular risk of medication-induced esophageal injury for several reasons: They take more medications than younger patients, are more likely to have anatomic or motility disorders or the esophagus, spend more time in a recumbent position, and may have reduced salivary production and/or impaired esophageal motility. A retrospective study addressing the frequency of medication-induced injury in patients over 65 years with dysphagia, odynophagia or chest pain found that of 250 patients, 68 (27%) had suffered from this condition [343]. Women appear to suffer from pill-induced injury at twice the rate of men, which is possibly related to the more common use of agents to treat osteoporosis (alendronate) and bladder disturbances (emepronium bromide) in women, although the precise reason has not been critically appraised. Patients with scleroderma, esophageal motility disorders, cardiomegaly (atrial compression of the esophagus), decreased salivary production, and neurologic diseases may also be more predisposed to pill esophagitis.

Acute esophageal injury may result from ingestion of a variety of medications (see Chapter 38). Several observations indicate that sustained-release preparations may be more injurious than standard preparations of the same medications [344]. Large pills or those with sticky surfaces are most likely to induce injury [345]. Other factors that predispose to drug-induced esophageal injury include the patient's position at the time the drug is ingested and the volume of fluid ingested with the drug. It has been well established that the likelihood of passage of a pill through the esophagus is reduced when the medication is ingested by a patient in a recumbent position and with less than 15 mL of water [346]. It is thus particularly ill advised to administer medications at bedtime with small sips of water, as is common practice. The majority of patients with medication-induced esophageal lesions do not have underlying esophageal abnormalities. The site of injury probably relates primarily to anatomic factors, as injury occurs most frequently in the mid esophagus at the level of the aortic arch or distally in the area adjacent to the left atrium or above the LES.

The most commonly reported cause of pill esophagitis is alendronate (ALN). There are nearly 100 documented cases, of which nine were complicated with the development of a stricture and three with hemorrhage [347]. Most patients are able to tolerate this medication, as demonstrated by a multicenter, double-blind, placebo-controlled trial of postmenopausal women with osteoporosis, which found no more upper gastrointestinal issues in patients taking ALN compared to those taking placebo [348]. Concomitant use of ALN and Aspirin may increase the risk of esophageal injury. Lesions vary from an erythematous patch to an ulcer or stricture. Most strictures tend to occur in the proximal esophagus [349]. Occasional deaths from hemorrhage and perforation have been reported in patients with potassium chloride-induced esophagitis [350]. However, most medication-induced esophageal lesions heal with discontinuation of the causative agent and short-term therapy with antacids. Occasionally, more aggressive antireflux therapy is required and, in rare instances, resulting strictures must be dilated [351]. Strictures are most likely to occur with esophageal injury from potassium chloride and quinidine preparations (47% of patients exposed to these agents), and older age has been shown to be a significant risk factor for the development of such strictures.

NSAIDs, which are very commonly used by older patients, account for about 8% of reported cases of pill esophagitis. Recent experience suggests that as many as 20% of patients on NSAID therapy have coexisting esophagitis [352]. Whether this is the result of a direct effect of the medications on the esophagus or underlying chronic GERD remains to be determined. In one report [353], evidence of recent Aspirin or NSAID use was found in 62% of patients with endoscopically verified esophagitis, compared to 26% of control subjects. Patients with a hiatal hernia taking NSAIDs appear to be at particular risk of developing esophageal ulcers [354]. NSAIDs have been frequently associated with the development of esophageal strictures [355, 356]. Concomitant therapy with PPIs is protective against gastric injury caused by NSAID use, but the effect of this combination on esophageal disease has not been studied.

Miscellaneous conditions

Spontaneous intramural hematoma of the esophagus is a rare condition usually affecting middle-aged and older women, and presents with acute substernal or epigastric pain and dysphagia or hematemesis. The pathogenesis is uncertain and symptoms usually resolve with conservative therapy [357]. In other cases, endoscopy or a forced Valsalva maneuver has also been identified as precipitating events [358, 359]. The endoscopic appearance may resemble an esophageal neoplasm.

Acute esophageal necrosis (AEN) is another rare disorder that tends to occur more commonly in older individuals. Of 25 recognized cases in the literature, only three occurred in subjects aged under 50 years (in two additional cases age was not reported) [360]. AEN was first described in 1990 at endoscopy, although two post-mortem cases had previously been reported [361, 362]. The etiology is unknown, although spontaneous rupture of the thoracic aorta, hypercoagulable state, Stevens–Johnson syndrome, and gastric outlet obstruction are noted associations. Ischemic esophageal infarction due to shock has been described in the elderly [363]. For patients undergoing endoscopy, the appearance of the esophageal mucosa is that of a black, necrotic-appearing esophagus with a pink transition zone at the gastroesophageal junction. Biopsies confirm mucosa and submucosa necrosis.

Spontaneous hemorrhage into a parathyroid adenoma has also been reported to cause acute dysphagia [364]. Intramural esophageal pseudodiverticulosis is another disease associated with dysphagia in persons aged over 60 years. The disorder is characterized by multiple small circumferential invaginations of the esophageal wall, either diffusely or focally, presumably as a result of dilatation of the secretory ducts of the submucosal glands [365]. In addition to pseudodiverticulosis, stenoses or areas of reduced distensibility are found, usually in the upper esophagus. The etiology is unknown, but many affected patients have associated *Candida albicans* colonization of the esophageal mucosa. Another entity, termed chronic esophagitis dessicans and characterized by chronic dysphagia, shedding of the esophageal mucosa, and localized esophageal strictures, has been described in five older patients with a mean age of 66 years [366].

Conclusions

In general, the classic symptoms of dysphagia, heartburn, and chest pain are the presenting manifestations of esophageal disorders in the elderly, as in the young. Several unique conditions may occur in the elderly, including ZD and vascular compression of the esophagus. Certain disorders increase in frequency with age, such as OPD due to neurologic disorders. Treatment approaches are similar in older and younger patients, but the potential for adverse drug effects and drug interactions is greater in the elderly than in the young. Endoscopy and surgery can also be used to treat esophageal disease, although procedure-related complications may be more devastating in older patients. GERD may present differently and be more difficult to treat in the older patient.

The special psychosocial, economic, and humanistic aspects of caring for the aged are just as important as the medical ones. Factors that may have an impact on illness in an older person include the losses and disability associated with aging; feelings of isolation; a reticence to discuss certain embarrassing problems; and the variety of settings for healthcare, including nursing homes, home care communities, geriatric units, geropsychiatric units, rehabilitation units, and hospices. The multiplicity of medical problems that often lead to contradictory and mutually exclusive management options and the frequency of multiple-drug use and adverse drug reactions may pose great challenges to treatment of an older patient. In addition, many older patients have a limited income and may not be able to afford expensive medications. Clearly, just as children are not "little adults," the elderly are not "big adults," and the delivery of care to older patients requires special expertise and sensitivity.

References

1. www.cms.hhs.gov/NationalHealthExpendData
2. Castell DO. Esophageal disorders in the elderly. *Gastroenterol Clin North Am* 1990;19:235–254.
3. Bloem BR, Lagaay AM, van Beek W, *et al*. Prevalence of subjective dysphagia in community residents aged over 87. *BMJ* 1990;300:721–722.
4. Tack J, Vantrappen G. The aging oesophagus. *Gut* 1997; 41:422–424.
5. Jansson C, Nordenstedt H, Wallander MA, *et al*. Severe symptoms of gastro-oesophageal reflux disease are associated with cardiovascular disease, but not diabetes: a population-based study. *Aliment Pharmacol Ther* 2008;27:58–65.
6. Kinekawa F, Kubo F, Matsuda K, *et al*. Esophageal function worsens with long duration of diabetes. *J Gastroenterol* 2008; 43:338–344.
7. Soergel KH, Zboralske FF, Amberg JRl. Presbyesophagus: Esophageal motility in nonagenarians. *J Clin Invest* 1964;43:1472–1479.
8. Leite LP, Johnston BT, Barrett J, *et al*. Ineffective esophageal motility (IEM): the primary finding in patients with nonspecific esophageal motility disorder. *Dig Dis Sci* 1997; 42:1859–1865.
9. Lindgren S, Janzon L. Prevalence of swallowing complaints and clinical findings among 50–79-year-old men and women in an urban population. *Dysphagia* 1991;6:187–192.
10. Gorman RC, Morris JB, Kaiser LR. Esophageal disease in the elderly patient. *Surg Clin North Am* 1994;74:93–112.

11. Leese G, Hopwood D. Muscle fibre typing in the human pharyngeal constrictors and oesophagus: the effect of ageing. *Acta Anat* 1986;127:77–80.

12. Youmans SR, Youmans GL, Stierwalt JAG. Differences in tongue strength across age and gender: is there a diminished strength reserve? *Dysphagia* 2009;24:57–65.

13. Ekberg O, Feinberg MJ. Altered swallowing function in elderly patients without dysphagia: radiologic findings in 56 cases. *AJR Am J Roentgenol* 1991;156:1181–1184.

14. Piaget F, Fouillet J. Le pharynx et l'oesophage seniles: etude clinique radiologique et radiocinematographique. *J Med Lyon* 1959;40:951.

15. Nilsson H, Ekberg O, Olsson R, et al. Quantitative aspects of swallowing in an elderly nondysphagic population. *Dysphagia* 1996;11:180–184.

16. Shaw DW, Cook IJ, Gabb M, et al. Influence of normal aging on oral-pharyngeal and upper esophageal sphincter function during swallowing. *Am J Physiol* 1995;268:G389–396.

17. Fulp SR, Dalton CB, Castell JA, et al. Aging-related alterations in human upper esophageal sphincter function. *Am J Gastroenterol* 1990;85:1569–1572.

18. Wilson JA, Pryde A, Macintyre CC, et al. The effects of age, sex, and smoking on normal pharyngoesophageal motility. *Am J Gastroenterol* 1990;85:686–691.

19. DeVault KR, Kingler PJ, Bammer T, et al. Manofluorographic evaluation of swallowing and pharyngeal function in the young and aged. *Gastroenterology* 1998;116:A985.

20. Robbins J, Hamilton JW, Lof GL, et al. Oropharyngeal swallowing in normal adults of different ages. *Gastroenterology* 1992;103:823–829.

21. Aviv JE, Martin JH, Jones ME, et al. Age-related changes in pharyngeal and supraglottic sensation. *Ann Otol Rhinol Laryngol* 1994;103:749–752.

22. Shaker R, Ren J, Zamir Z, et al. Effect of aging, position, and temperature on the threshold volume triggering pharyngeal swallows. *Gastroenterology* 1994;107:396–402.

23. Humbert IA, Fitzgeral ME, McLaren DG, et al. Neurophysiology of swallowing: effects of age and bolus type. *Neuroimage* 2009;44:982–991

24. Ergun GA, Kahrilas PJ. Oropharyngeal dysphagia in the elderly. *Pract Gastroenterol* 1993;17:9.

25. Feinberg MJ, Ekberg O, Segall L, et al. Deglutition in elderly patients with dementia: findings of videofluorographic evaluation and impact on staging and management. *Radiology* 1992;183:811–814.

26. Eckhardt VF, LeCompte PM. Esphageal ganglia and smooth muscle in the elderly. *Am J Dig Dis* 1978;23:443.

27. Adams CW, Brain RH, Trounce JR. Ganglion cells in achalasia of the cardia. *Virchows Arch A Pathol Anat Histol* 1976;372:75–79.

28. Ren J, Shaker R, Kusano M, et al. Effect of aging on the secondary esophageal peristalsis: presbyesophagus revisited. *Am J Physiol* 1995;268:G772–779.

29. Hollis JB, Castell DO. Esophageal function in elderly man. A new look at "presbyesophagus". *Ann Intern Med* 1974;80:371–374.

30. Goekas MD, Conteas CN, Majumdar AP. The aging gastrointestinal tract, liver, and pancreas. *Clin Geriatr Med* 1985;1:177.

31. Richter JE, Wu WC, Johns DN, et al. Esophageal manometry in 95 healthy adult volunteers. Variability of pressures with age and frequency of "abnormal" contractions. *Dig Dis Sci* 1987;32:583–592.

32. Ribeiro AC, Klingler PJ, Hinder RA, et al. Esophageal manometry: a comparison of findings in younger and older patients. *Am J Gastroenterol* 1998;93:706–710.

33. Achem AC, Achem SR, Stark ME, et al. Failure of esophageal peristalsis in older patients: association with esophageal acid exposure. *Am J Gastroenterol* 2003;98:35–39.

34. Meshkinpour H, Haghighat P, Dutton C. Clinical spectrum of esophageal aperistalsis in the elderly. *Am J Gastroenterol* 1994;89:1480–1483.

35. Grishaw EK, Ott DJ, Frederick MG, et al. Functional abnormalities of the esophagus: a prospective analysis of radiographic findings relative to age and symptoms. *AJR Am J Roentgenol* 1996;167:719–723.

36. Smout AJ, Breedijk M, van der Zouw C, et al. Physiological gastroesophageal reflux and esophageal motor activity studied with a new system for 24-hour recording and automated analysis. *Dig Dis Sci* 1989;34:372–378.

37. Spence RA, Collins BJ, Parks TG, et al. Does age influence normal gastro-oesophageal reflux? *Gut* 1985;26:799–801.

38. Richter JE, Bradley LA, DeMeester TR, et al. Normal 24-hr ambulatory esophageal pH values. Influence of study center, pH electrode, age, and gender. *Dig Dis Sci* 1992;37:849–856.

39. Lasch H, Castell DO, Castell JA. Evidence for diminished visceral pain with aging: studies using graded intraesophageal balloon distension. *Am J Physiol* 1997;272:G1–3.

40. Grade A, Pulliam G, Johnson C, et al. Reduced chemoreceptor sensitivity in patients with Barrett's esophagus may be related to age and not to the presence of Barrett's epithelium. *Am J Gastroenterol* 1997;92:2040–2043.

41. Khan TA, Shragge BW, Crispin JS, et al. Esophageal motility in the elderly. *Am J Dig Dis* 1977;22:1049–1054.

42. Stilson WL, Sanders I, Gardiner GA, et al. Hiatal hernia and gastroesophageal reflux. A clinicoradiological analysis of more than 1,000 cases. *Radiology* 1969;93:1323–1327.

43. Gray LS, Heron G, Cassidy D, et al. Comparison of age-related changes in short-wavelength-sensitive cone thresholds between normals and patients with primary open-angle glaucoma. *Optom Vis Sci* 1995;72:205–209.

44. de Graaf C, Polet P, van Staveren WA. Sensory perception and pleasantness of food flavors in elderly subjects. *J Gerontol* 1994;49:93–99.

45 Theurer JA, Czachorowski KA, Martin LP, Martin RE. Effects of oropharyngeal air-pulse stimulation on swallowing in healthy older adults. *Dysphagia* 2009;24:302–313.

46. Weusten BL, Lam HG, Akkermans LM, et al. Influence of age on cerebral potentials evoked by oesophageal balloon distension in humans. *Eur J Clin Invest* 1994;24:627–631.

47. Patel R, Rao S. Biochemical and sensory parameters of the human oesophagus vary with age. *Am J Gastroenterol* 1995;90:1567 (abst).

48. Fass R, Pulliam G, Johnson C, et al. Symptom severity and oesophageal chemosensitivity to acid in older and young patients with gastro-oesophageal reflux. *Age Ageing* 2000;29:125–130.

49. Heading RC. Prevalence of upper gastrointestinal symptoms in the general population: a systematic review. *Scand J Gastroenterol* 1999;231 (Suppl):3–8.

50. Scott M, Gelhot AR. Gastroesophageal reflux disease: diagnosis and management. *Am Fam Physician* 1999;59:1161–1169, 1199.

51. Gallup Organization. *A Gallup Survey on Heartburn Across America*. Princeton, NJ: Gallup Organization, 1988.

52. Raiha IJ, Impivaara O, Seppala M, *et al*. Prevalence and characteristics of symptomatic gastroesophageal reflux disease in the elderly. *J Am Geriatr Soc* 1992;40:1209–1211.

53. Talley NJ, O'Keefe EA, Zinsmeister AR, *et al*. Prevalence of gastrointestinal symptoms in the elderly: a population-based study. *Gastroenterology* 1992;102:895–901.

54. Triadafilopoulos G, Sharma R. Features of symptomatic gastroesophageal reflux disease in elderly patients. *Am J Gastroenterol* 1997;92:2007–2011.

55. Locke GR 3rd, Talley NJ, Fett SL, *et al*. Prevalence and clinical spectrum of gastroesophageal reflux: a population-based study in Olmsted County, Minnesota. *Gastroenterology* 1997; 112:1448–1456.

56. Wei W, Yu L, Lu, H, *et al*. Comparisons of cause distribution between elderly and non-elderly patients with cough. *Respiration* 2009;77:259–264.

57. Pilotto A, Franceschi M, Leandro G, *et al*. Clinical features of reflux esophagitis in older people: a study of 840 consecutive patients. *J Am Geriatrics Soc* 2006;54:1537–1542.

58. Glew CM, Rentler RJ. Use of proton pump inhibitors and other acid suppressive medications in newly admitted nursing facility patients. *J Am Med Direct Assoc* 2008;8:607–609.

59. Collen MJ, Abdulian JD, Chen YK. Gastroesophageal reflux disease in the elderly: more severe disease that requires aggressive therapy. *Am J Gastroenterol* 1995;90:1053–1057.

60. El-Serag HB, Sonnenberg A. Associations between different forms of gastro-oesophageal reflux disease. *Gut* 1997;41:594–599.

61. Zimmerman J, Shohat V, Tsvang E, *et al*. Esophagitis is a major cause of upper gastrointestinal hemorrhage in the elderly. *Scand J Gastroenterol* 1997;32:906–909.

62. Brunnen PL, Karmody AM, Needham CD. Severe peptic oesophagitis. *Gut* 1969;10:831–837.

63. Sonnenberg A, Steinkamp U, Weise A, *et al*. Salivary secretion in reflux esophagitis. *Gastroenterology* 1982;83:889–895.

64. Dent J, Holloway RH, Toouli J, *et al*. Mechanisms of lower oesophageal sphincter incompetence in patients with symptomatic gastrooesophageal reflux. *Gut* 1988;29:1020–1028.

65. Iascone C, DeMeester TR, Little AG, *et al*. Barrett's esophagus. Functional assessment, proposed pathogenesis, and surgical therapy. *Arch Surg* 1983;118:543–549.

66. Lee J, Anggiansha A, Anggiansah R, *et al*. Effects of age on the gastroesophageal junction, esophageal motility, and reflux disease. *Clin Gastroenterol Hepatol* 2007;5:1392–1398.

67. Ferriolli E, Oliveira RB, Matsuda NM, *et al*. Aging, esophageal motility, and gastroesophageal reflux. *J Am Geriatr Soc* 1998;46:1534–1537.

68. Zhu H, Pace F, Sangaletti O, *et al*. Features of symptomatic gastroesophageal reflux in elderly patients. *Scand J Gastroenterol* 1993;28:235–238.

69. Richter JE, Castell DO. Gastroesophageal reflex. Pathogenesis, diagnosis, and therapy. *Ann Intern Med* 1982;97:93–103.

70. Wajed SA, Streets CG, Bremner CG, *et al*. Elevated body mass disrupts the barrier to gastroesophageal reflux. *Arch Surg* 2001;136:1014–1019.

71. Hurwitz A, Brady DA, Schaal SE, *et al*. Gastric acidity in older adults. *JAMA* 1997;278:659–662.

72. Vakil NB. Review article: gastro-oesophageal reflux disease and *Helicobacter pylori* infection. *Aliment Pharmacol Ther* 2002;16 (Suppl 1):47–51.

73. Labenz J, Blum AL, Bayerdorffer E, *et al*. Curing *Helicobacter pylori* infection in patients with duodenal ulcer may provoke reflux esophagitis. *Gastroenterology* 1997;112:1442–1447.

74. Mold JW Rankin RA. Symptomatic gastroesophageal reflux in the elderly. *J Am Geriatr Soc* 1987;35:649–659.

75. Champion G, Richter JE, Vaezi ME, *et al*. Duodenogastroesophageal reflux: relationship to pH and importance in Barrett's esophagus. *Gastroenterology* 1994;107:747–754.

76. Older Americans 2004: Key Indicators of Well-Being. http://www.agingstats.gov/agingstatsdotnet/Main_Site/Data/Data_2008.aspx

77. El-Serag, HB, Graham DY, Satia JA, Rabenek L. Obesity is an independent risk factor for GERD symptoms and erosive esophagitis. *Am J Gastroenterol* 2005;100:1243–1250.

78. Cook MB, Greenwood DC, Hardie IJ, *et al*. A systemic review and meta-analysis of increasing adiposity on Barrett's esophagus. *Am J Gastroenterol* 2008;103:292–300.

79. Anderson LA, Watson RG, Murphy SJ, *et al*. Risk factors for Barrett's oesophagus and oesophageal adenocarcinoma: Results from the FINBAR study. *World J Gastroenterol* 2007; 13:1585–1594.

80. Nano M, Ferrara L, Camandona M. Sliding hiatal hernia in the elderly: a clinical entity. *J Am Geriatr Soc* 1981;29:463–464.

81. Raiha I, Hietanen E, Sourander L. Symptoms of gastrooesophageal reflux disease in elderly people. *Age Ageing* 1991;20:365–370.

82. Browning TH. Diagnosis of chest pain of esophageal origin. A guideline of the Patient Care Committee of the American Gastroenterological Association. *Dig Dis Sci* 1990;35:289–293.

83. Richter JE, Bradley LA, Castell DO. Esophageal chest pain: current controversies in pathogenesis, diagnosis, and therapy. *Ann Intern Med* 1989;110:66–78.

84. Deschner WK, Benjamin SB. Extraesophageal manifestations of gastroesophageal reflux disease. *Am J Gastroenterol* 1989;84:1–5.

85. Raiha IJ, Ivaska K, Sourander LB. Pulmonary function in gastro-oesophageal reflux disease of elderly people. *Age Ageing* 1992;21:368–373.

86. Raiha I, Manner R, Hietanen E, *et al*. Radiographic pulmonary changes of gastro-oesophageal reflux disease in elderly patients. *Age Ageing* 1992;21:250–255.

87. Richter JE. Gastroesophageal reflux disease in the elderly. *Geriatr Med Today* 1989;8:27.

88. James OF, Parry-Billings KS. Comparison of omeprazole and histamine H$_2$-receptor antagonists in the treatment of elderly and young patients with reflux oesophagitis. *Age Ageing* 1994;23:121–126.

89. Johnson LF, DeMeester TR. Evaluation of elevation of the head of the bed, bethanechol, and antacid form tablets on gastroesophageal reflux. *Dig Dis Sci* 1981;26:673–680.

90. Hamilton JW, Boisen RJ, Yamamoto DT, *et al*. Sleeping on a wedge diminishes exposure of the esophagus to refluxed acid. *Dig Dis Sci* 1988;33:518–522.

91. Garnett WR, Garabedian-Ruffalo SM. Identification, diagnosis, and treatment of acid-related diseases in the elderly: implications for long-term care. *Pharmacotherapy* 1997;17:938–958.

92. Hetzel DJ, Dent J, Reed WD, *et al*. Healing and relapse of severe peptic esophagitis after treatment with omeprazole. *Gastroenterology* 1988;95:903–912.

93. Skoutakis VA, Joe RH, Hara DS. Comparative role of omeprazole in the treatment of gastroesophageal reflux disease. *Ann Pharmacother* 1995;29:1252–1262.

94. DeVault KR, Morgenstern DM, Lynn RB, Metz DC. Effect of pantoprazole in older patients with erosive esophagitis. *Dis Esophagus* 2007;20:411–415.

95. Cloud ML, Enas N, Humphries TJ, *et al*. Rabeprazole in treatment of acid peptic diseases: results of three placebo-controlled dose-response clinical trials in duodenal ulcer, gastric ulcer, and gastroesophageal reflux disease (GERD). The Rabeprazole Study Group. *Dig Dis Sci* 1998;43:993–1000.

96. Dettmer A, Vogt R, Sielaff F, *et al*. Pantoprazole 20 mg is effective for relief of symptoms and healing of lesions in mild reflux oesophagitis. *Aliment Pharmacol Ther* 1998;12:865–872.

97. Castell DO, Richter JE, Robinson M, *et al*. Efficacy and safety of lansoprazole in the treatment of erosive reflux esophagitis. The Lansoprazole Group. *Am J Gastroenterol* 1996;91:1749–1757.

98. Dekkers CP, Beker JA, Thjodleifsson B, *et al*. Double-blind comparison of rabeprazole 20 mg vs. omeprazole 20 mg in the treatment of erosive or ulcerative gastro-oesophageal reflux disease. The European Rabeprazole Study Group. *Aliment Pharmacol Ther* 1999;13:49–57.

99. Richter JE, Kahrilas PJ, Johanson J, *et al*. Efficacy and safety of esomeprazole compared with omeprazole in GERD patients with erosive esophagitis: a randomized controlled trial. *Am J Gastroenterol* 2001;96:656–665.

100. Lee RD, Vakily M, Mulford D, Wu J, Atkinson SN. Clinical trial: the effect and timing of food on the pharmacokinetics and pharmacology of dexlansoprazole MR, a novel dual delayed release formulation of a proton pump inhibitor-evidence for dosing flexibility. *Aliment Pharmacol Ther* 2009;29:824–833.

101. Katz PO, Koch FK, Ballard ED, *et al*. Comparison of the effects of immeridate-relase omeprazole oral suspension, delayed-release lansoprazole capsules and delayed-release esomeprazole capsules on nocturnal gastric acidity after bedtime. *Aliment Pharmacol Ther* 2007;25:197–205.

102. McTavish D, Buckley MM, Heel RC. Omeprazole. An updated review of its pharmacology and therapeutic use in acid-related disorders. *Drugs* 1991;42:138–170.

103. Andersson T. Pharmacokinetics, metabolism and interactions of acid pump inhibitors. Focus on omeprazole, lansoprazole and pantoprazole. *Clin Pharmacokinet* 1996;31:9–28.

104. Petersen KU. Review article: omeprazole and the cytochrome P450 system. *Aliment Pharmacol Ther* 1995;9:1–9.

105. Laine L, Hennekens C. Proton pump inhibitor and clopidogrel interaction: fact or fiction? *Am J Gastroenterol* 2010;105:34–41.

106. Saltzman JR, Kemp JA, Golner BB, *et al*. Effect of hypochlorhydria due to omeprazole treatment or atrophic gastritis on protein-bound vitamin B12 absorption. *J Am Coll Nutr* 1994;13:584–591.

107. Saltzman JR, Kowdley KV, Pedrosa MC, *et al*. Bacterial overgrowth without clinical malabsorption in elderly hypochlorhydric subjects. *Gastroenterology* 1994;106:615–623.

108. Yang YX, Lewis JD, Epstein S, Metz DC. Long-term proton pump inhibitor therapy and risk of hip fracture. *JAMA* 2006;296:2947–2953.

109. DeVault KR, Talley NJ. Insights into the future of gastric acid suppression. *Nat Rev Gastroenterol Hepatol* 2009;6:524–532.

110. Sierra F, Suarez M, Rey M, Vela MF. Systematic review: Proton pump inhibitor-associated acute interstial nephritis. *Aliment Pharmacol Ther* 2007;26:545–553.

111. Colin-Jones DG. Histamine-2-receptor antagonists in gastrooesophageal reflux. *Gut* 1989;30:1305–1308.

112. Lipsy RJ, Fennerty B, Fagan TC. Clinical review of histamine2 receptor antagonists. *Arch Intern Med* 1990;150:745–751.

113. Hatlebakk JG, Berstad A. Pharmacokinetic optimisation in the treatment of gastro-oesophageal reflux disease. *Clin Pharmacokinet* 1996;31:386–406.

114. Lieberman DA, Keeffe EB. Treatment of severe reflux esophagitis with cimetidine and metoclopramide. *Ann Intern Med* 1986;104:21–26.

115. Verlinden M. Review article: a role for gastrointestinal prokinetic agents in the treatment of reflux oesophagitis? *Aliment Pharmacol Ther* 1989;3:113–131.

116. Richardson WS, Hunter JG, Waring JP. Laparoscopic antireflux surgery. *Semin Gastrointest Dis* 1997;8:100–110.

117. Cowgill SM, Arnaoutakis D, Villadolid D, *et al*. Results after laparoscopic fundoplication: does age matter? *Am Surg* 2006;72:448–483.

118. Pizza F, Rossetti G, Limongelli P, *et al*. Influence of age on outcome of total laparoscopic fundoplication for gastroesophageal reflux disease. *World J Gastroenterol* 2007;13:740–747.

119. Gupta A, Change D, Steele KE, *et al*. Looking beyond age and co-morbidities as predictors of outcome in paraesophageal hernia repair. *J Gastrointest Surg* 2008;12:2119–2124..

120. Gutmann E. Muscle. In: Finch CE, Hayflick L, eds. *Handbook of the Biology of Aging*. New York: Van Nostrand Reinhold, 1977, p. 709.

121. Steele CM, Greenwood C, Ens I, *et al*. Mealtime difficulties in a home for the aged: not just dysphagia. *Dysphagia* 1997; 12:43–51.

122. Robbins J, Langmore S, Hind JA, Erlichman M. Dysphagia research in the 21st century and beyond: proceedings of the Dysphagia Experts Meeting, August 21. *J Rehab* 2002; 39:543–548

123. Tibbling L, Gustafsson B. Dysphagia and its consequences in the elderly. *Dysphagia* 1991;6:200–202.

124. Talley NJ, Weaver AL, Zinsmeister AR, *et al*. Onset and disappearance of gastrointestinal symptoms and functional gastrointestinal disorders. *Am J Epidemiol* 1992;136:165–177.

125. Siebens H, Trupe E, Siebens A, *et al*. Correlates and consequences of eating dependency in institutionalized elderly. *J Am Geriatr Soc* 1986;34:192–198.

126. Trupe EH, *et al*. Prevalence of feeding and swallowing disorders in a nursing home. *Arch Phys Med Rehab* 1984;65:651.

127. American Heart Association. *1992 Heart and Stroke Facts*. Dallas, American Heart Association, 1991.

128. Buchholz DW. Dysphagia associated with neurological disorders. *Acta Otorhinolaryngol Belg* 1994;48:143–155.

129. Horner J, Massey EW, Riski JE, *et al*. Aspiration following stroke: clinical correlates and outcome. *Neurology* 1988;38:1359–1362.

130. Palmer JB, DuChane AS. Rehabilitation of swallowing disorders due to strokes. *Phys Med Rehab Clin North Am* 1991;2:259.

131. Gordon C, Hewer RL, Wade DT. Dysphagia in acute stroke. *Br Med J (Clin Res Ed)* 1987;295:411–414.

132. Mann G, Hankey GJ, Cameron D. Swallowing disorders following acute stroke: prevalence and diagnostic accuracy. *Cerebrovasc Dis* 2000;10:380–386.

133. Daniels SK, Brailey K, Priestly DH, *et al*. Aspiration in patients with acute stroke. *Arch Phys Med Rehab* 1998;79:14–19.

134. Foley NC, Martin RE, Salter KL, Teasell RW. A review of the relationship between dysphagia and malnutrition following stroke. *J Rehab Med* 2009;41:707–713.

135. Sharma JC, Fletcher S, Vassallo M, *et al*. What influences outcome of stroke-pyrexia or dysphagia? *Int J Clin Pract* 2001;55:17–20.

136. Smithard DG, O'Neill PA, Parks C, *et al*. Complications and outcome after acute stroke. Does dysphagia matter? *Stroke* 1996;27:1200–1204.

137. Alberts MJ, Horner J, Gray L, *et al*. Aspiration after stroke: lesion analysis by brain MRI. *Dysphagia* 1992;7:170–173.

138. Celifarco A, Gerard G, Faegenburg D, *et al*. Dysphagia as the sole manifestation of bilateral strokes. *Am J Gastroenterol* 1990;85:610–613.

139. Buchholz DW. Neurogenic dysphagia: what is the cause when the cause is not obvious? *Dysphagia* 1994;9:245–255.

140. Buchholz DW. Clinically probable brainstem stroke presenting primarily as dysphagia and nonvisualized by MRI. *Dysphagia* 1993;8:235–238.

141. Gordon C,Hewer RL,Wade DT. Dysphagia in acute stroke. *Br Med J* 1987;295:411.

142. Steinhagen V, Grossmann A, Benecke R, Walter U. Swallowing disturbance pattern relates to brain lesion location in acute stroke patients. *Stroke* 2009;40:1903–1906.

143. Terre R, Mearin F. Resolution of tracheal aspiration after the acute phase of stroke-related oropharyngeal Dysphagia. *Am J Gastroenterol* 2009;104:923–932.

144. Warnecke T, Ritter MA, Kroger B, *et al*. Fiberoptic endoscopic dysphagia severity scale predicts outcome after acute stroke. *Cerebrovasc Dis* 2009;28:283–289.

145. Huang YL, Hsieh SF, Chang YC, Chen HC, Wang TG. Ultrasonographic evaluation of hyoid-larynx approximation in dysphagic stroke patients. *Ultrasound Med Biol* 2009;35:1103–1118.

146. Bramble MG, Cunliffe J, Dellipiani AW. Evidence for a change in neurotransmitter affecting oesophageal motility in Parkinson's disease. *J Neurol Neurosurg Psychiatry* 1978;41:709–712.

147. van de Vijver DA, Roos RA, Jansen PA, *et al*. Estimation of incidence and prevalence of Parkinson's disease in the elderly using pharmacy records. *Pharmacoepidemiol Drug Saf* 2001;10:549–554.

148. Edwards LL, Quigley EM, Pfeiffer RF. Gastrointestinal dysfunction in Parkinson's disease: frequency and pathophysiology. *Neurology* 1992;42:726–732.

149. Pfeiffer RE Gastrointestinal dysfunction in Parkinson's disease. *Clin Neurosci* 1998;5:136–146.

150. Muller J, Wenning GK, Verny M, *et al*. Progression of dysarthria and dysphagia in postmortem-confirmed parkinsonian disorders. *Arch Neurol* 2001;58:259.

151. Logemann JA, Blonsky ER, Boshes B. Dysphagia in Parkinsonism [Editorial]. *JAMA* 1975;231:69–70.

152. Silbiger ML, Pikielney R, Donner MW. Neuromuscular disorders affecting the pharynx. Cineradiographic analysis. *Invest Radiol* 1967;2:442–448.

153. Miller N, Allcock L, Hildreth AJ, *et al*. Swallowing problems in Parkinson disease: frequency and clinical correlates. *J Neurol Neurosurg Psychiatry* 2009;80:1047–1049.

154. Manor Y, Balas M, Giladi N, *et al*. Anxiety, depression and swallowing disorders in patients with Parkinson's disease. *Parkinsonism Relat Disord* 2009;15:453–456.

155. Nobrega AC, Rodrigues B, Torres AC, Scarpel RD, Neves CA, Melo A. Is drooling secondary to a swallowing disorder in patients with Parkinson's disease? *Parkinsonism Relat Disord* 2008;14:243–245.

156. Bird MR, Woodward MC, Gibson EM, *et al*. Asymptomatic swallowing disorders in elderly patients with Parkinson's disease: a description of findings on clinical examination and videofluoroscopy in sixteen patients. *Age Ageing* 1994;23:251–254.

157. Leopold NA, Kagel MC. Pharyngo-esophageal dysphagia in Parkinson's disease. *Dysphagia* 1997;12:11–20.

158. Potulska A, Friedman A, Krolicki L, Spychala A. Swallowing disorders in Parkinson's disease. *Parkinsonism Relat Disord* 2003;9:349–353.

159. Bassotti G, Germani U, Pagliaricci S, *et al*. Esophageal manometric abnormalities in Parkinson's disease. *Dysphagia* 1998;13:28–31.

160. Ali GN, Wallace KL, Schwartz R, *et al*. Mechanisms of oralpharyngeal dysphagia in patients wit Parkinson's disease. *Gastroenterology* 1996;110:383.

161. Hurwitz AL, Nelson JA, Haddad JK. Oropharyngeal dysphagia: manometric and cine-esophagographic findings. *Am J Dig Dis* 1975;20:313.

162. Baijens LW, Speyer R. Effects of therapy for dysphagia in Parkinson's disease: systematic review. *Dysphagia* 2009; 24:91–102.

163. Deane KH, Whurr R, Clarke CE, Playford ED, Ben-Shlomo Y. Non-pharmacological therapies for dysphagia in Parkinson's disease. *Cochrane Database Syst Rev* 2001;(1):CD002816.

164. Ciucci MR, Barkmeier-Kraemer JM, Sherman SJ. Subthalamic nucleus deep brain stimulation improves deglutition in Parkinson's disease. *Mov Disord* 2008;23:676–683.

165. Nagaya M. Kachi T. Yamada T. Effect of swallowing training on swallowing disorders in Parkinson's disease. *Scand J Rehab Med* 200;32:11–15.

166. Robbins J, Gensler G, Hind J, *et al*. Comparison of 2 interventions for liquid aspiration on pneumonia incidence: a randomized trial. *Ann Intern Med* 2008;148:509–518.

167. Restivo DA. Palmeri A. Marchese-Ragona R. Botulinum toxin for cricopharyngeal dysfunction in Parkinson's disease. *N Engl J Med* 2002;346:1174–1175.

168. Cook IJ. Oropharyngeal dysphagia. *Gastroenterol Clin North Am* 2009;38:411–431.

169. Anderson DW, Ellenberg JH, Leventhal CM, *et al*. Revised estimate of the prevalence of multiple sclerosis in the United States. *Ann Neurol* 1992;31:333–336.

170. Rodriguez M, Siva A, Ward J, *et al*. Impairment, disability, and handicap in multiple sclerosis: a population-based study in Olmsted County, Minnesota. *Neurology* 1994;44:28–33.

171. Calcagno P, Ruoppolo G, Grasso MG, *et al*. Dysphagia in multiple sclerosis—prevalence and prognostic factors. *Acta Neurol Scand* 2002;105:40–43.

172. Crayton HJ, Rossman HS Managing the symptoms of multiple slcerosis: a multimodal approach. *Clin Ther* 2006;28:445–460.

173. Calcagno P, Ruoppolo G, Grasso MG, *et al*. Dysphagia in multiple sclerosis-prevalence and prognostic factors. *Acta Neurol Scand* 2002;105:40–43.

174. Noseworthy J, Paty D, Wonnacott T, Feasby, T, Ebers G. Multiple sclerosis after age 50. *Neurology* 1983;33:1537–1544.

175. Thomas FJ, Wiles CM. Dysphagia and nutritional status in multiple sclerosis. *J Neurol* 1999;246:677–682.

176. McDonald WI, Compston A, Edan G, *et al*. Recommended diagnostic criteria for multiple sclerosis: guidelines from the International Panel on the diagnosis of multiple sclerosis. *Ann Neurol* 2001;50:121–127.

177. Lövblad KO, Anzalone N, Dörfler A, *et al*. MR imaging in multiple sclerosis: Review and recommendations for current practice. *Am J Neuroradiol* 2010;31:983–989.

178. Tassorelli C, Bergamaschi R, Buscone S, *et al*. Dysphagia in multiple sclerosis: from pathogenesis to diagnosis. *Neurol Sci* 2008;Suppl 4:S360–363.

179. Linden P, Kuhlemeier KV, Patterson C. The probability of correctly predicting subglottic penetration from clinical observations. *Dysphagia* 1993;8:170–179.

180. Bergamaschi R, Rezzani C, Minguzzi S, *et al*. Validation of the DYMUS questionnaire for the assessment of dysphagia in multiple sclerosis. *Funct Neurol* 2009;24:159–162.

181. Grunebaum M, Salinger H. Radiologic findings in polymyositis-dermatomyositis involving the pharynx and upper oesophagus. *Clin Radiol* 1971;22:97–100.

182. Jacob H, Berkowitz D, McDonald E, *et al*. The esophageal motility disorder of polymyositis. A prospective study. *Arch Intern Med* 1983;143:2262–4.

183. Shapiro J, Martin S, DeGirolami U, *et al*. Inflammatory myopathy causing pharyngeal dysphagia: a new entity. *Ann Otol Rhinol Laryngol* 1996;105:331–335.

184. Machado P, Miller A, Holton J, Hanna M. Sporadic inclusion body myositis: an unsolved mystery. *Acta Rheumatol Port* 2009;34:161–182.

185. Wilson FC, Ytterberg SR, St Sauver JL, Reed AM. Epidemiology of sporadic inclusion body myositis and polymyositis in Olmsted County, Minnesota. *J Rheumatol* 2008;35:445–447.

186. Darrow DH, Hoffman HT, Barnes GJ, *et al*. Management of dysphagia in inclusion body myositis. *Arch Otolaryngol Head Neck Surg* 1992;118:313–317.

187. Badrising UA, Maat-Schieman ML, van Houwelingen JC, *et al*. Inclusion body myositis. Clinical features and clinical course of the disease in 64 patients. *J Neurol* 2005;252:1448–1454.

188. Chiu WY, Yang CC, Huang IC, Huang TS. Dysphagia as a manifestation of thyrotoxicosis: report of three cases and literature review. *Dysphagia* 2004;19:120–124.

189. Dalakas MC, Elder G, Hallett M, *et al*. A long-term follow-up study of patients with post-poliomyelitis neuromuscular symptoms. *N Engl J Med* 1986;314:959–963.

190. Schon F, Drayson M, Thompson RA. Myasthenia gravis and elderly people. *Age Ageing* 1996;25:56–58.

191. Phillips LH 2nd. The epidemiology of myasthenia gravis. *Ann N Y Acad Sci* 2003;998:407–412.

192. Gilhus NE. Autoimmune myasthenia gravis. *Expert Rev Neurother* 2009;9:351–358.

193. Kluin KJ, Bromberg MB, Feldman EL, *et al*. Dysphagia in elderly men with myasthenia gravis. *J Neurol Sci* 1996;138:49–52.

194. De Assis JL, Marchiori PE, Scaff M. Atrophy of the tongue with persistent articulation disorder in myasthenia gravis: report of 10 patients. *Auris Nasus Larynx* 1994;21:215–218.

195. Huang MH, King KL, Chien KY. Esophageal manometric studies in patients with myasthenia gravis. *J Thorac Cardiovasc Surg* 1988;95:281–285.

196. Meriggioli MN. Myasthenia gravis with anti-acetylcholine receptor antibodies. *Front Neurol Neurosci* 2009;26:94–108.

197. Pascuzzi RM. The edrophonium test. *Semin Neurol* 2003; 23:83–88.

198. Sanders DB, Howard JF, Johns TR. Single fi ber electromyography in myasthenia gravis. *Neurology* 1979;29:68–76.

199. Meriggioli MN, Sanders DB. Autoimmune myasthenia gravis: emerging clinical and biological heterogeneity. *Lancet Neurol* 2009;8:475–490.

200. Walling AD. Amyotrophic lateral sclerosis: Lou Gehrig's disease. *Am Fam Physician* 1999;59:1489–1496.

201. Robbins J. Swallowing in ALS and motor neuron disorders. *Neurol Clin* 1987;5:213–229.

202. Chen A, Garrett CG. Otolaryngologic presentations of amyotrophic lateral sclerosis. *Otolaryngol Head Neck Surg* 2005; 132:500–504.

203. Ertekin C, Aydogdu I, Yuceyar N, *et al*. Pathophysiological mechanisms of oropharyngeal dysphagia in amyotrophic lateral sclerosis. *Brain* 2000;123:125–140.

204. Kühnlein P, Gdynia HJ, Sperfeld AD, *et al*. Diagnosis and treatment of bulbar symptoms in amyotrophic lateral sclerosis. *Nat Clin Pract Neurol* 2008;4:366–374.

205. Borasio GD, Voltz R, Miller RG. Palliative care in amyotrophic lateral sclerosis. *Neurol Clin* 2001;19:829–847.

206. Chio A, Finocchiaro E, Meineri P, *et al*. Safety and factors related to survival after percutaneous endoscopic gastrostomy in ALS. ALS Percutaneous Endoscopic Gastrostomy Study Group. *Neurology* 1999;53:1123–1125.

207. Kasarskis EJ, Scarlata D, Hill R, *et al*. A retrospective study of percutaneous endoscopic gastrostomy in ALS patients during the BDNF and CNTF trials. *J Neurol Sci* 1999;169:118–125.

208. Mathus-Vliegen LM, Louwerse LS, Merkus MP, *et al*. Percutaneous endoscopic gastrostomy in patients with amyotrophic lateral sclerosis and impaired pulmonary function. *Gastrointest Endosc* 1994;40:463–469.

209. Gerhardt DC, Shuck TJ, Bordeaux RA, *et al*. Human upper esophageal sphincter. Response to volume, osmotic, and acid stimuli. *Gastroenterology* 1978;75:268–274.

210. Merati AL, Tseng J, Blumin JH, *et al*. Comparative neuromuscular histopathology of cricopharyngeal achalasia patients with and without previous botulinum toxin treatment. *Ann Otol Rhinol Laryngol* 2007;116:375–380.

211. Fradet G, Pouliot D, Robichaud R, *et al*. Upper esophageal sphincter myotomy in oculopharyngeal muscular dystrophy: long-term clinical results. *Neuromusc Disord* 1997;7 (Suppl 1):S90–S95.

212. Hatlebakk JG, Castell JA, Spiegel J, *et al*. Dialtion therapy for dysphagia in patients with upper esophageal sphincter dysfunction: manometric and symptomatic response. *Dis Esophagus* 1998;11:254–259.

213. Saffouri MH, Ward PH. Surgical correction of dysphagia due to cervical osteophytes. *Ann Otol Rhinol Laryngol* 1974; 83:65–70.

214. Ladenheim SE, Marlowe FI. Dysphagia secondary to cervical osteophytes. *Am J Otolaryngol* 1999;20:184–189.

215. Lulkuneii I, Lleinonen OP, Knekl P, Maalela I. The epidemiology of hyperostosis of the spine together with its symptoms and related mortality in a general population. *Scand J Rheumatol* 1975;4:23–27.

216. Ebo D, Goethals L, Bracke P, *et al*. Dysphagia in a patient with giant osteophytes: case presentation and review of the literature. *Clin Rheumatol* 2000;19:70–72.

217. Oppenlander ME, Orringer DA, La Marca F, *et al*. Dysphagia due to anterior cervical hyperosteophytosis. *Surg Neurol* 2009;72:266–270.

218. Urrutia J, Bono CM. Long-term results of surgical treatment of dysphagia secondary to cervical diffuse idiopathic skeletal hyperostosis. *Spine J* 2009;9:e13–17.

219. Chiacchio S, Lorenzoni A, Boni G, *et al*. Anaplastic thyroid cancer: prevalence, diagnosis and treatment. *Minerva Endocrinol* 2008;33:341–357.

220. Maran AG, Wilson JA, Al Muhanna AH. Pharyngeal diverticula. *Clin Otolaryngol* 1986;11:219–225.

221. Laing MR, Murthy P, Ah-See KW, *et al*. Surgery for pharyngeal pouch: audit of management with short- and long-term follow-up. *J R Coll Surg Edinb* 1995;40:315–318.

222. Siddiq MA, Sood S, Strachan D. Pharyngeal pouch (Zenker's diverticulum). *Postgrad Med J* 2001;77:506–511.

223. Cook IJ, Blumbergs P, Cash K, *et al*. Structural abnormalities of the cricopharyngeus muscle in patients with pharyngeal (Zenker's) diverticulum. *J Gastroenterol Hepatol* 1992; 7:556–562.

224. Cook IJ, Gabb M, Panagopoulos V, *et al*. Pharyngeal (Zenker's) diverticulum is a disorder of upper esophageal sphincter opening. *Gastroenterology* 1992;103:1229–1235.

225. Bradley PJ, Kochaar A, Quraishi MS. Pharyngeal pouch carcinoma: real or imaginary risks? *Ann Otol Rhinol Laryngol* 1999;108:1027–1032.

226. Ishioka S, Felix VN, Sakai P, *et al*. Manometric study of the upper esophageal sphincter before and after endoscopic management of Zenker's diverticulum. *Hepatogastroenterology* 1995;42:628–632.

227. Visosky AM, Parke RB, Donovan DT. Endoscopic management of Zenker's diverticulum: factors predictive of success or failure. *Ann Otol Rhinol Laryngol* 2008;117:531–537.

228. Sakai P.Endoscopic treatment of Zenker's diverticulum. *Gastrointest Endosc* 2007;65:1054–1055.

229. Feussner H. Endoscopic therapy for Zenker diverticulum—the good and the bad. *Endoscopy* 2007;39:154–155.

230. Bonavina L, Bona D, Abraham M, Saino G, Abate E. Long-term results of endosurgical and open surgical approach for Zenker diverticulum. *World J Gastroenterol* 2007; 13:2586–2589.

231. Ford RM, Affronti J, Cohen R, *et al*. Zenker's diverticulum: a contraindication for wireless capsule endoscopy? *J Clin Gastroenterol* 2005;39:257.

232. Dodds WJ, Logemann JA, Stewart ET. Radiologic assessment of abnormal oral and pharyngeal phases of swallowing. *AJR Am J Roentgenol* 1990;154:965–974.

233. Dodds WJ, Stewart ET, Logemann JA. Physiology and radiology of the normal oral and pharyngeal phases of swallowing. *AJR Am J Roentgenol* 1990;154:953–963.

234. Castell JA, Castell DO. Upper esophageal sphincter and pharyngeal function and oropharyngeal (transfer) dysphagia. *Gastroenterol Clin North Am* 1996;25:35–50.

235. Cook IJ. Oropharyngeal dysphagia. *Gastroenterol Clin North Am* 2009;38:411–431.

236. McConnel FM. Analysis of pressure generation and bolus transit during pharyngeal swallowing. *Laryngoscope* 1988;98:71–78.

237. Pandolfino JE, Kahrilas PJ. New technologies in gastrointestinal clinic and research: impedance and high-resolution manometry. *World J Gastroenterol* 2009;15:131–138.

238. Jaradeh SS, Shaker R, Toohill RB. Electromyographic recording of the cricopharyngeus muscle in humans. *Am J Med* 2000;108 (Suppl 4a):40S–42S.

239. Elmstahl S, Bulow M, Ekberg O, *et al*. Treatment of dysphagia improves nutritional conditions in stroke patients. *Dysphagia* 1999;14:61–66.

240. Perez I, Smithard DG, Davies H, *et al*. Pharmacological treatment of dysphagia in stroke. *Dysphagia* 1998;13:12–16.

241. Bonavina L, Khan NA, DeMeester TR. Pharyngoesophageal dysfunctions. The role of cricopharyngeal myotomy. *Arch Surg* 1985;120:541–549.

242. David VC. Relief of dysphagia in motor neurone disease with cricopharyngeal myotomy. *Ann R Coll Surg Engl* 1985; 67:229–231.

243. Ellis FH Jr, Crozier RE. Cervical esophageal dysphagia: indications for and results of cricopharyngeal myotomy. *Ann Surg* 1981;194:279–289.

244. Ekberg O, Lindgren S. Effect of cricopharyngeal myotomy on pharyngoesophageal function: pre- and postoperative cineradiographic findings. *Gastrointest Radiol* 1987;12:1–6.

245. Schneider I, Thumfart WF, Pototschnig C, *et al*. Treatment of dysfunction of the cricopharyngeal muscle with botulinum A toxin: introduction of a new, noninvasive method. *Ann Otol Rhinol Laryngol* 1994;103:31–35.

246. Alberty J, Oelerich M, Ludwig K, et al. Efficacy of botulinum toxin A for treatment of upper esophageal sphincter dysfunction. *Laryngoscope* 2000;110:1151–1156.

247. Cattau EL Jr, Castell DO. Symptoms of esophageal dysfunction. *Adv Intern Med* 1982;27:151–181.

248. Mayberry JE Epidemiology and demographics of achalasia. *Gastrointest Endosc Clin North Am* 2001;11:235–248.

249. Clouse RE, Abramson BK, Todorczuk JR. Achalasia in the elderly. Effects of aging on clinical presentation and outcome. *Dig Dis Sci* 1991;36:225–228.

250. Sonnenberg A, Massey BT McCarty DJ, *et al*. Epidemiology of hospitalization for achalasia in the United States. *Dig Dis Sci* 1993;38:233–244.

251. Tucker HJ, Snape WJ Jr, Cohen S. Achalasia secondary to carcinoma: manometric and clinical features. *Ann Intern Med* 1978;89:315–318.

252. Herrera JL. Case report: esophageal metastasis from breast carcinoma presenting as achalasia. *Am J Med Sci* 1992;303:321–323.

253. Kahrilas PJ, Kishk SM, Helm JF, *et al*. Comparison of pseudoachalasia and achalasia. *Am J Med* 1987;82:439–446.

254. Subramanyam K. Achalasia secondary to malignant mesothelioma of the pleura. *J Clin Gastroenterol* 1990;12:183–187.

255. Meijssen MA, Tilanus HW, van Blankenstein M, *et al*. Achalasia complicated by oesophageal squamous cell carcinoma: a prospective study in 195 patients. *Gut* 1992;33:155–158.

256. Dancygier H, Classen M. Endoscopic ultrasonography in esophageal diseases. *Gastrointest Endosc* 1989;35:220–225.

257. Robertson CS, Fellows IW Mayberry JF, *et al*. Choice of therapy for achalasia in relation to age. *Digestion* 1988;40:244–250.

258. Eckardt VF, Aignherr C, Bernhard G. Predictors of outcome in patients with achalasia treated by pneumatic dilation. *Gastroenterology* 1992;103:1732–1738.

259. Csendes A, Velasco N, Braghetto I, *et al*. A prospective randomized study comparing forceful dilatation and esophagomyotomy in patients with achalasia of the esophagus. *Gastroenterology* 1981;80:789–795.

260. Shimi S, Nathanson LK, Cuschieri A. Laparoscopic cardiomyotomy for achalasia. *J R Coll Surg Edinb* 1991;36:152–154.

261. Pellegrini C, Wetter LA, Patti M, *et al*. Thoracoscopic esophagomyotomy. Initial experience with a new approach for the treatment of achalasia. *Ann Surg* 1992;216:291–299.

262. Sharp KW, Khaitan L, Scholz S, *et al*. 100 consecutive minimally invasive Heller myotomies: lessons learned. *Ann Surg* 2002;235:631–639.

263. Berreca M, Oelschlager BK, Pellegrini CA. Minimally invasive surgery for the treatment of achalsia. *Endoscopia* 2002; 14:59–66.

264. Wang YR, Dempsey DT, Friedenberg FK, Richter JE. Trends of Heller myotomy hospitalizations for achalasia in the United States, 1993–2005: effect of surgery volume on perioperative outcomes. *Am J Gastroenterol* 2008;103:2454–2564.

265. Kala Z, Weber P, Marek F, *et al*. Achalasia—which method of treatment to choose for senior patients? *Gerontol Geriatr* 2009;42:408–411.

266. Leeuwenburgh I, Haringsma J, Van Dekken H, *et al*. Long-term risk of oesophagitis, Barrett's oesophagus and oesophageal cancer in achalasia patients. *Scand J Gastroenterol* 2006;243 (Suppl):7–10.

267. Gordon JM, Eaker EY. Prospective study of esophageal botulinum toxin injection in high-risk achalasia patients. *Am J Gastroenterol* 1997;92:1812–1817.

268. Pasricha PJ, Rai R, Ravich WJ, *et al*. Botulinum toxin for achalasia: long-term outcome and predictors of response. *Gastroenterology* 1996;110:1410–1415.

269. Schiano TD, Parkman HP, Miller LS, *et al*. Use of botulinum toxin in the treatment of achalasia. *Dig Dis* 1998;16:14–22.

270. Malnick SD, Metchnik L, Somin M, *et al*. Fatal heart block following treatment with botulinum toxin for achalasia. *Am J Gastroenterol* 2000;95:3333–3334.

271. Khurana V Nehme O, Khurana R, *et al*. Urinary retention secondary to detrusor muscle hypofunction after botulinum toxin injection for achalasia. *Am J Gastroenterol* 2001; 96:3211–3212.

272. Díaz Roca AB, Sampascual SB, Calderón AJ, *et al*. Self-expanding metal stents for endoscopic treatment of esophageal achalasia unresponsive to conventional treatments. *Gastrointest Endosc* 2009;69:980.

273. Zhao JG, Dong LY, Sheng CY, *et al*. Long-term safety and outcome of a temporary self-expanding metallic stent for achalasia: a prospective study with a 13-year single-center experience. *Eur Radiol* 2009;19:1973–1980.

274. Ghosh S, Heading RC, Palmer KR. Achalasia of the oesophagus in elderly patients responds poorly to conservative therapy. *Age Ageing* 1994;23:280–282.

275. Bortolotti M, Mari C, Lopilato C, *et al*. Effects of sildenafil on esophageal motility of patients with idiopathic achalasia. *Gastroenterology* 2000;118:253–257.

276. Devaney EJ, Lannettoni MD, Orringer MB, *et al*. Esophagectomy for achalasia: patient selection and clinical experience. *Ann Thorac Surg* 2001;72:854–858.

277. Spechler SJ, Castell DO. Classification of oesophageal motility abnormalities. *Gut* 2001;49:145–151.

278. Andrews JM, Heddle R, Hebbard GS, *et al*. Age and gender affect likely manometric diagnosis: Audit of a tertiary referral hospital clinical esophageal manometry service. *J Gastroenterol Hepatol* 2009;24:125–128.

279. Sperandio M, Tutuian R, Gideon RM, *et al*. Diffuse esophageal spasm: not diffuse but distal esophageal spasm (DES). *Dig Dis Sci* 2003;48:1380–1384.

280. Rao SS, Hayek B, Summers RW. Functional chest pain of esophageal origin: hyperalgesia or motor dysfunction. *Am J Gastroenterol* 2001;96:2584–2589.

281. Balaban DH, Yamamoto Y, Liu J, *et al*. Sustained esophageal contraction: a marker of esophageal chest pain identified by intraluminal ultrasonography. *Gastroenterology* 1999; 116:29–37.

282. Pirtniecks A, Smith LF, Thorpe JA. Autonomic dysfunction in nonspecific disorders of oesophageal motility. *Eur J Cardiothorac Surg* 2000;17:101–105.

283. DeVault KR, Achem SR, Stark ME, *et al*. Nutcracker esophagus: a statistical aberrancy associated with psychopathology? *Am J Gastroenterol* 2002;97:S33.

284. Achem SR, Kolts BE, MacMath T, *et al*. Effects of omeprazole versus placebo in treatment of noncardiac chest pain and gastroesophageal reflux. *Dig Dis Sci* 1997;42:2138–2145.

285. Borjesson M, Pilhall M, Rolny P, *et al*. Gastroesophageal acid reflux in patients with nutcracker esophagus. *Scand J Gastroenterol* 2001;36:916–920.

286. Champion JK, Delisle N, Hunt T. Laparoscopic esophagomyotomy with posterior partial fundoplication for primary esophageal motility disorders. *Surg Endosc* 2000;14:746–749.

287. Murray JA, Ledlow A, Launspach J, *et al*. The effects of recombinant human hemoglobin on esophageal motor functions in humans. *Gastroenterology* 1995;109:1241–1248.

288. Konturek JW, Thor P, Lukaszyk A, *et al*. Endogenous nitric oxide in the control of esophageal motility in humans. *J Physiol Pharmacol* 1997;48:201–209.

289. Eherer AJ, Schwetz I, Hammer HF, *et al*. Effect of sildenafil on oesophageal motor function in healthy subjects and patients with oesophageal motor disorders. *Gut* 2002;50:758–764.

290. Miller LS, Pullela SV, Parkman HP, *et al*. Treatment of chest pain in patients with noncardiac, nonreflux, nonachalasia spastic esophageal motor disorders using botulinum toxin injection into the gastroesophageal. *Am J Gastroenterol* 2002;97:1640–1646.

291. Achem SR. Noncardiac chest pain-treatment approaches. *Gastroenterol Clin North Am* 2008;37:859–878.

292. Almansa C, Achem SR. Diffuse esophageal spasm (DES). Practical concepts of diagnosis and treatment. *Rev Gastroenterol Mex* 2007;72:136–145.

293. Almansa C, Hinder RA, Smith CD, Achem SR. A comprehensive appraisal of the surgical treatment of diffuse esophageal spasm. *J Gastrointest Surg* 2008;12:1133–1145.

294. Le Roy EC, Black C, Fleischemajer R, *et al.* Scleroderma (systemic sclerosis): classification, subsets, and pathogenesis. *J Rheumatol* 1988;15:202–205.

295. Zamost BJ, Hirschberg J, Ippoliti AF, *et al.* Esophagitis in scleroderma. Prevalence and risk factors. *Gastroenterology* 1987;92:421–428.

296. Ebert EC. Esophageal disease in scleroderma. *J Clin Gastroenterol* 2006;40:769–775.

297. Gonzalez R, Storr M, Bloching H, *et al.* Autoantibody profile in progressive systemic sclerosis as markers for esophageal involvement. *J Clin Gastroenterol* 2001;32:123–127.

298. Katzka DA, Reynolds JC, Saul SH, *et al.* Barrett's metaplasia and adenocarcinoma of the esophagus in scleroderma. *Am J Med* 1987;82:46–52.

299. Ipsen P, Egekvist H, Aksglaede K, *et al.* Oesophageal manometry and video-radiology in patients with systemic sclerosis: a retrospective study of its clinical value. *Acta Derm Venereol* 2000;80:130–133.

300. Savarino E, Bazzica M, Zentilin P, *et al.* Gastroesophageal reflux and pulmonary fibrosis in scleroderma: a study using pH-impedance monitoring. *Am J Respir Crit Care Med* 2009;179:408–413.

301. Poirer T, Taillefer R, Topart P, *et al.* Antireflux operations in patients with scleroderma, *Ann Thorac Surg* 1994;58:66–72.

302. Kent MS, Luketich JD, Irshad K, *et al.* Comparison of surgical approaches to recalcitrant gastroesophageal reflux disease in the patient with scleroderma. *Ann Thorac Surg* 2007;84:1710–1715.

303. Kelsen D. Multimodality therapy for adenocarcinoma of the esophagus. *Gastroenterol Clin North Am* 1997;26:635–645.

304. Falk GW. Risk factors for esophageal cancer development. *Surg Oncol Clin North Am* 2009;18:469–485.

305. Bannister P, Stanners AJ, Mountford RA. Dysphagia in the elderly: what does it mean to the endoscopist? *J R Soc Med* 1990;83:552–553.

306. Adam DJ, Craig SR, Sang CT, *et al.* Esophagectomy for carcinoma in the octogenarian. *Ann Thorac Surg* 1996;61:190–194.

307. Jougon JB, Ballester M, Duffy J, *et al.* Esophagectomy for cancer in the patient aged 70 years and older. *Ann Thorac Surg* 1997;63:1423–1427.

308. Muehrcke DD, Kaplan DK, Donnelly RJ. Oesophagogastrectomy in patients over 70. *Thorax* 1989;44:141–145.

309. Thomas P, Doddoli C, Neville P, *et al.* Esophageal cancer resection in the elderly. *Eur J Cardiothorac Surg* 1996;10:941–946.

310. Wong J. Management of carcinoma of oesophagus: art or science? *J R Coll Surg Edinb* 1981;26:138–149.

311. Kuwano H, Morita M, Baba K, *et al.* Surgical treatment of esophageal carcinoma in patients eighty years of age and older. *J Surg Oncol* 1993;52:36–39.

312. Ertan A, Zimmerman M, Younes M. Esophageal adenocarcinoma associated with Barrett's esophagus: long- term management with laser ablation. *Am J Gastroenterol* 1995;90:2201–2203.

313. Overholt BF, Panjehpour M. Barrett's esophagus: photodynamic therapy for ablation of dysplasia, reduction of specialized mucosa, and treatment of superficial esophageal cancer. *Gastrointest Endosc* 1995;42:64–70.

314. Salo JA, Salminen JT, Kiviluoto TA, *et al.* Treatment of Barrett's esophagus by endoscopic laser ablation and antireflux surgery. *Ann Surg* 1998;227:40–44.

315. Richter JE. Gastroesophageal reflux disease in the older patient: presentation, treatment, and complications. *Am J Gastroenterol* 2000;95:368–373.

316. Marks RD, Richter JE. Peptic strictures of the esophagus. *Am J Gastroenterol* 1993;88:1160–1173.

317. Agnew SR, Pandya SP, Reynolds RP, *et al.* Predictors for frequent esophageal dilations of benign peptic strictures. *Dig Dis Sci* 1996;41:931–936.

318. Barbezat GO, Schlup M, Lubcke R. Omeprazole therapy decreases the need for dilatation of peptic oesophageal strictures. *Aliment Pharmacol Ther* 1999;13:1041–1045.

319. Marks RD, Richter JE, Rizzo J, *et al.* Omeprazole versus H_2-receptor antagonists in treating patients with peptic stricture and esophagitis. *Gastroenterology* 1994;106:907–915.

320. Zein NN, Greseth JM, Perrault J. Endoscopic intralesional steroid injections in the management of refractory esophageal strictures. *Gastrointest Endosc* 1995;41:596–598.

321. Klingler PJ, Hinder RA, Cina RA, *et al.* Laparoscopic antireflux surgery for the treatment of esophageal strictures refractory to medical therapy. *Am J Gastroenterol* 1999;94:632–636.

322. Dua KS, Vleggaar FP, Santharam R, *et al.* Removable self-expanding plastic esophageal stent as a continuous, non-permanent dilator in treating refractory benign esophageal strictures: a prospective two-center study. *Am J Gastroenterol* 2008;103:2988–2994.

323. DeVault KR. Lower esophageal (Schatzki's) ring: pathogenesis, diagnosis and therapy. *Dig Dis* 1996;14:323–329.

324. Schatzki R. The lower esophageal ring. *AJR Am J Roentgenol* 1963;90:805.

325. Marshall JB, Kretschmar JM, Diaz-Arias AA. Gastroesophageal reflux as a pathogenic factor in the development of symptomatic lower esophageal rings. *Arch Intern Med* 1990;150:1669–1672.

326. Ott DJ, Ledbetter MS, Chen MY, *et al.* Correlation of lower esophageal mucosal ring and 24-h pH monitoring of the esophagus. *Am J Gastroenterol* 1996;91:61–64.

327. Jalil S, Castell DO. Schatzki's ring: a benign cause of dysphagia in adults. *J Clin Gastroenterol* 2002;35:295–298.

328. Sgouros SN. Vlachogiannakos J. Karamanolis G, *et al.* Long-term acid suppressive therapy may prevent the relapse of lower esophageal (Schatzki's) rings: a prospective, randomized, placebo-controlled study. *Am J Gastroenterol* 2005;100:1929–1934.

329. Garrean C, Hirano I. Eosinophilic esophagitis: pathophysiology and optimal management. *Curr Gastroenterol Rep* 2009;11:175–181.

330. Fox VL. Eosinophilic esophagitis: endoscopic findings. *Gastrointest Endosc Clin North Am* 2008;18:45–57.

331. Gonsalves N, Kahrilas PJ. Eosinophilic oesophagitis in adults. *Neurogastroenterol Motil* 2009;21:1017–1026.

332. Pape R. Uber einen abnormen verlauf ("tiefe Rechtslage") der mesa aortitischen aorta descendes. *Fortschr Roetgenstr* 1932;46:257–269.

333. Sundaram U, Traube M. Radiologic and manometric study of the gastroesophageal junction in dysphagia aortica. *J Clin Gastroenterol* 1995;21:275–277.

334. Birnholz JC, Ferrucci JT, Wyman SM. Roentgen features of dysphagia aortica. *Radiology* 1974;111:93–96.

335. Hanna A, Derrick JR. Dysphagia caused by tortuosity of the thoracic aorta. *J Thorac Cardiovasc Surg* 1969;57:134–137.

336. Mittal RK, Siskind BN, Hongo M, et al. Dysphagia aortica. Clinical, radiological, and manometric findings. *Dig Dis Sci* 1986;31:379–384.

337. Nguyen P, Gideon RM, Castell DO. Dysphagia lusoria in the adult: associated esophageal manometric findings and diagnostic use of scanning techniques. *Am J Gastroenterol* 1994;89:620–623.

338. Hilli ES, Mueli NA, Keller AS. Dysphagia aortica. *Ann Intern Med* 2005;142:230–231.

339. Kress S, Martin WR, Benz C, et al. Dysphagia secondary to left atrial dilatation. *Z Gastroenterol* 1997;35:1007–1011.

340. Mo KM, Craig GM, Clark JV, et al. Sudden death from perforation of a benign oesophageal ulcer into a major blood vessel. *Postgrad Med J* 1988;64:687–689.

341. Luketich JD, Sommers KE, Griffith BP, et al. Successful management of secondary aortoesophageal fistula. *Ann Thorac Surg* 1996;62:1852–1854.

342. Kikendall JW. Pill esophagitis. *J Clin Gastroenterol* 1999;28:298–305.

343. Akhtar AJ. Oral medication-induced esophageal injury in elderly patients. *Am J Med Sci* 2003;326:133–135.

344. Hiraoka T, Okita M, Koganemaru S, et al. [Hemorrhagic esophageal ulceration associated with slow-release morphine sulfate tablets]. *Nippon Shokakibyo Gakkai Zasshi* 1991;88:1231–1234.

345. Hey H, Jorgensen F, Sorensen K, et al. Oesophageal transit of six commonly used tablets and capsules. *Br Med J (Clin Res Ed)* 1982;285:1717–1719.

346. Perkins AC. Blackshaw PE. Hay PD, et al. Esophageal transit and in vivo disintegration of branded risedronate sodium tablets and two generic formulations of alendronic acid tablets: a single-center, single-blind, six-period crossover study in healthy female subjects. *Clin Ther* 2008;30:834–844.

347. de Groen PC, Lubbe DF, Hirsch LJ, et al. Esophagitis associated with the use of alendronate. *N Engl J Med* 1996;335:1016–1021.

348. Adachi JD, Faraawi RY, O'Mahony MF, et al. Upper gastrointestinal tolerability of alendronate sodium monohydrate 10 mg once daily in postmenopausal women: a 12-week, randomized, double-blind, placebo-controlled, exploratory study. *Clin Ther* 2009;31:1747–1753.

349. McCord GS, Clouse RE. Pill-induced esophageal strictures: clinical features and risk factors for development. *Am J Med* 1990;88:512–518.

350. Bott S, Prakash C, McCallum RW. Medication-induced esophageal injury: survey of the literature. *Am J Gastroenterol* 1987;82:758–763.

351. Bonavina L, DeMeester TR, McChesney L, et al. Drug-induced esophageal strictures. *Ann Surg* 1987;206:173–183.

352. Semble EL, Wu WC, Castell DO. Nonsteroidal antiinflammatory drugs and esophageal injury. *Semin Arthritis Rheum* 1989;19:99–109.

353. Lanas A, Hirschowitz BI. Significant role of aspirin use in patients with esophagitis. *J Clin Gastroenterol* 1991;13:622–627.

354. Shallcross TM, Wyatt JI, Rathbone BJ, et al. Non-steroidal antiinflammatory drugs, hiatus hernia, and *Helicobacter pylori*, in patients with oesophageal ulceration. *Br J Rheumatol* 1990;29:288–290.

355. Heller SR, Fellows IW, Ogilvie AL, et al. Non-steroidal antiinflammatory drugs and benign oesophageal stricture. *Br Med J (Clin Res Ed)* 1982;285:167–168.

356. Wilkins WE, Ridley MG, Pozniak AL. Benign stricture of the oesophagus: role of nonsteroidal anti- inflammatory drugs. *Gut* 1984;25:478–480.

357. Ackert JJ, Sherman A, Lustbader IJ, et al. Spontaneous intramural hematoma of the esophagus. *Am J Gastroenterol* 1989;84:1325–1328.

358. McIntyre AS, Ayres R, Atherton J, et al. Dissecting intramural haematoma of the oesophagus. *Q J Med* 1998;91:701–705.

359. Thomson A, Fleischer DE, Epstein B. Submucosal hemorrhage of the esophagus associated with endoscopy in a patient with cervical osteophytes. *J Clin Gastroenterol* 1998;27:267–268.

360. Lacy BE, Toor A, Bensen SP, et al. Acute esophageal necrosis: report of two cases and a review of the literature. *Gastrointest Endosc* 1999;49:527–532.

361. Goldenberg SP, Wain SL, Marignani P. Acute necrotizing esophagitis. *Gastroenterology* 1990;98:493–496.

362. Lee KR, Stark E, Shaw FE. Esophageal infarction complicating spontaneous rupture of the thoracic aorta. *JAMA* 1977;237:1233–1234.

363. Haviv YS, Reinus C, Zimmerman J. "Black esophagus": a rare complication of shock. *Am J Gastroenterol* 1996;91:2432–2434.

364. Korkis AM, Miskovitz PE. Acute pharyngoesophageal dysphagia secondary to spontaneous hemorrhage of a parathyroid adenoma. *Dysphagia* 1993;8:7–10.

365. Medeiros LJ, Doos WG, Balogh K. Esophageal intramural pseudodiverticulosis: a report of two cases with analysis of similar, less extensive changes in "normal" autopsy esophagi. *Hum Pathol* 1988;19:928–931.

366. Ponsot P, Molas G, Scoazec JY, et al. Chronic esophagitis dissecans: an unrecognized clinicopathologic entity? *Gastrointest Endosc* 1997;45:38–45.

Index

4125

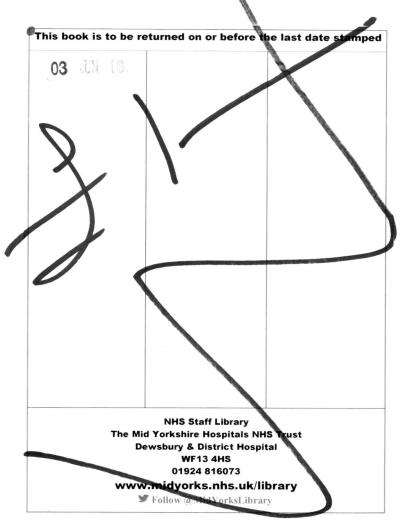

This book is to be returned on or before the last date stamped

03 JUN 16.